# Marks'
# Essentials of Medical Biochemistry
## A Clinical Approach
### Second Edition

D1294384

# Marks'
# Essentials
# of Medical
# Biochemistry
## A Clinical Approach
### Second Edition

**Michael Lieberman, PhD**
Distinguished Teaching Professor
Department of Molecular Genetics, Biochemistry, and Microbiology
University of Cincinnati College of Medicine
Cincinnati, Ohio

**Alisa Peet, MD**
Associate Professor of Clinical Medicine
Director, Medicine Clerkship
Department of Internal Medicine
Temple University School of Medicine
Philadelphia, Pennsylvania

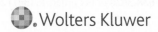. Wolters Kluwer

Philadelphia · Baltimore · New York · London
Buenos Aires · Hong Kong · Sydney · Tokyo

*Publisher:* Michael Tully
*Acquisitions Editor:* Tari Broderick
*Product Manager:* Stacey Sebring
*Marketing Manager:* Joy Fisher-Williams
*Production Editor:* Bridgett Dougherty
*Designer:* Steve Druding
*Manufacturing Coordinator:* Margie Orzech
*Compositor:* Absolute Service, Inc.

2nd Edition
Copyright © 2015, 2007 Lippincott Williams & Wilkins, a Wolters Kluwer business.

351 West Camden Street
Baltimore, MD 21201

Two Commerce Square
2001 Market Street
Philadelphia, PA 19103

Printed in China

9  8  7  6  5  4  3  2  1

**Library of Congress Cataloging-in-Publication Data**

Lieberman, Michael, 1950- , author.
  [Marks' essential medical biochemistry]
  Marks' essentials of medical biochemistry : a clinical approach / Michael Lieberman, Alisa Peet. — Second edition.
    p. ; cm.
  Essentials of medical biochemistry
  Includes indexes.
  Preceded by: Marks' essential medical biochemistry / Michael Lieberman, Allan Marks, Colleen Smith. c2007.
  Based on: Marks' basic medical biochemistry / Michael Lieberman, Allan Marks, Alisa Peet. 4th ed. c2013.
  ISBN 978-1-4511-9006-9
  I. Peet, Alisa, author. II. Lieberman, Michael, 1950- Marks' basic medical biochemistry. Based on (work): III. Title. IV. Title: Essentials of medical biochemistry.
  [DNLM: 1. Biochemical Phenomena. 2. Clinical Medicine. 3. Metabolism. QU 34]
  QP514.2
  612'.015—dc23
                                                                                                      2014026258

## DISCLAIMER

Care has been taken to confirm the accuracy of the information present and to describe generally accepted practices. However, the authors, editors, and publisher are not responsible for errors or omissions or for any consequences from application of the information in this book and make no warranty, expressed or implied, with respect to the currency, completeness, or accuracy of the contents of the publication. Application of this information in a particular situation remains the professional responsibility of the practitioner; the clinical treatments described and recommended may not be considered absolute and universal recommendations.

The authors, editors, and publisher have exerted every effort to ensure that drug selection and dosage set forth in this text are in accordance with the current recommendations and practice at the time of publication. However, in view of ongoing research, changes in government regulations, and the constant flow of information relating to drug therapy and drug reactions, the reader is urged to check the package insert for each drug for any change in indications and dosage and for added warnings and precautions. This is particularly important when the recommended agent is a new or infrequently employed drug.

Some drugs and medical devices presented in this publication have Food and Drug Administration (FDA) clearance for limited use in restricted research settings. It is the responsibility of the health care provider to ascertain the FDA status of each drug or device planned for use in their clinical practice.

To purchase additional copies of this book, call our customer service department at **(800) 638-3030** or fax orders to **(301) 223-2320**. International customers should call **(301) 223-2300**.

Visit Lippincott Williams & Wilkins on the Internet: http://www.lww.com. Lippincott Williams & Wilkins customer service representatives are available from 8:30 am to 6:00 pm, EST.

# Preface

*Marks' Essential Medical Biochemistry, Second Edition* is based on the fourth edition of *Marks' Medical Biochemistry: A Clinical Approach.* It has been streamlined to focus primarily on only the most essential biochemical concepts important to medical students. If further detail is needed, the larger "parent" book can be consulted.

Medical biochemistry has often been the least appreciated course taken by medical students during their 4 years of training. Many students fail to understand how the biochemistry they are learning will be applicable to their clinical years. Too often, in order to make it through the course, students fall into the trap of rote memorization instead of understanding the key biochemical concepts. This is unfortunate, as medical biochemistry provides a molecular basis and scaffold on which all future courses in medical school are built. Biochemistry provides the foundation on which disease can be understood at the molecular level. Biochemistry provides the tools on which new drug treatments and therapies are based. It is very difficult to understand today's practice of medicine without comprehending the basic principles of biochemistry.

As the student proceeds through the text, two important objectives will be emphasized: an understanding of protein structure and function and an understanding of the metabolic basis of disease. In order to accomplish this, the student will learn how large molecules are synthesized and used (DNA, RNA, and proteins), and how energy is generated, stored, and retrieved (metabolism). Once these basic concepts are understood, it will be straightforward to understand how alterations in the basic processes can lead to a disease state.

Inherited disease is caused by alterations in a person's DNA, which leads to a variant protein being synthesized. The metabolic pathway which depends on the activity of that protein is then altered, which leads to the disease state. Understanding the consequences of a block in a metabolic pathway (or in signaling or regulating a pathway) will enable the student to better understand the signs and symptoms of a specific disease. Type I diabetes, for example, is caused by a lack of synthesized insulin, but how do the myriad of symptoms which accompany this type of diabetes come about? Understanding how insulin affects, and regulates, normal metabolic pathways will enable the student to figure out its effects and not just memorize them from a list.

This text presents patient cases to the students as the biochemistry is being discussed. This strengthens the link between biochemistry and medicine and allows the student to learn about this interaction as the biochemistry is presented. As more biochemistry is learned, patients reappear and more complicated symptoms and treatments are discussed. In this manner, the medical side of biochemistry is reinforced as the book progresses.

It has been 8 years since the first edition of the essentials text was published, and in preparing the second edition of the text, the authors focused on updating the patient cases to reflect current care guidelines as well as updating the basic science chapters where required. This is particularly evident for Chapter 14, which describes recombinant DNA technology and how such technology can be used for diagnosis of disease. One chapter (Chapter 15) was also added to the text on the molecular biology of cancer, and while building upon Chapter 14 also reflects some recent trends in cancer therapeutics.

*Michael Lieberman, PhD*
*Alisa Peet, MD*

## HOW TO USE THIS BOOK

Icons identify the various components of the book: the patients who are presented at the start of each chapter; the clinical notes, questions, and answers that appear in the margins; and the clinical comments that are found at the end of each chapter.

Each chapter starts with an outline and key points that summarize the information so that students can recognize the key words and concepts they are expected to learn. The next component of each chapter is the "Waiting Room," containing patients with complaints and a description of the events that lead them to seek medical help.

 Indicates a female patient

 Indicates a male patient

 Indicates a patient who is a baby or young child

As each chapter unfolds, icons identify information related to the material presented in the text:

 Indicates a clinical note usually related to the patients in the "Waiting Room" for that chapter. These notes explain signs or symptoms of a patient or give some other clinical information relevant to the text.

 Indicates a book note, which elaborates on some aspect of the basic biochemistry presented in the text. These notes provide tidbits, pearls, or just reemphasize a major point of the text.

 Refers the reader to extra material that can be found online on thePoint.

Questions and answers also appear in the margin and should help to keep students thinking as they read the text:

 Indicates a question

 Indicates the answer to the question. The answer to a question is always located on the next page. If two questions appear on one page, the answers are given in order on the next page.

Each chapter ends with "Clinical Comments" and "Review Questions":

 Indicates clinical comments that give additional clinical information, often describing the treatment plan and the outcome.

 Indicates chapter review questions. These questions highlight and reinforce the take-home messages in each chapter.

Disease tables are also listed at the end of each chapter, serving as a summary of the diseases discussed in each chapter.

A companion website on thePoint contains animations, depicting key biochemical concepts; interactive question bank with more than 350 questions and complete rationales; full patient summaries for each patient discussed in the text; a comprehensive list of disorders covered in the text with relevant web links; suggested readings for each chapter for students interested in exploring a topic in more depth; and supplemental chapter content.

# Acknowledgments

The authors would like to thank all of the reviewers who worked hard to inspect the chapters and who made excellent suggestions for revisions. Matt Chansky, the illustrator and animator, has done a great job in taking the author's stick figures and creating easy to understand diagrams and amazing animations. Stacey Sebring, the product development editor, displayed immense patience with the authors as they worked with updating the first edition of the text while still keeping the page count to a manageable size. Her assistance was invaluable.

Any errors in the text are the authors' responsibility, and Dr. Lieberman would appreciate being informed of such errors (lieberma@ucmail.uc.edu). And finally, Dr. Lieberman would like to thank the past 30 years of first year medical students at the University of Cincinnati College of Medicine who have put up with my various attempts at teaching biochemistry while always keeping in the back of my mind "how is this relevant to medicine?" The comments these students have made have greatly influenced the manner in which I teach this material and how this material is presented in this text.

# Table of Contents

# 1    An Overview of Fuel Metabolism

## CHAPTER OUTLINE

## KEY POINTS

- Fuel is provided in the form of carbohydrates, fats, and proteins in our diet.
- Energy is obtained from the fuel by oxidizing it to $CO_2$ and $H_2O$.
- Unused fuel can be stored as triacylglycerol (fat) or glycogen (carbohydrate) within the body.
- Weight loss or gain is a balance between the energy required each day to drive the basic functions of our body and our physical activity versus the amount of fuel consumed.
- Two endocrine hormones, insulin and glucagon, primarily regulate fuel storage and retrieval.

continued

- The predominant carbohydrate in the blood is glucose. Blood glucose levels regulate the release of insulin and glucagon from the pancreas.
- During fasting, when blood glucose levels drop, glucagon is released from the pancreas. Glucagon signals the liver to utilize its stored carbohydrate to release glucose into the circulation, primarily for use by the brain.
- After fasting for 3 days, the liver releases ketone bodies (derived from fat) as an alternative fuel supply for the brain.
- The resting metabolic rate (RMR) is a measure of the energy required to maintain life (this is also known as the basal metabolic rate [BMR]).
- The body mass index (BMI) is a rough measure of determining an ideal weight for an individual and whether a person is underweight or overweight.
- In addition to nutrients, the diet provides vitamins and essential fatty acids and amino acids.

## THE WAITING ROOM

**Ivan A.** is a 56-year-old accountant who has been obese for many years. He exhibits a pattern of central obesity, called an "apple shape," which is caused by excess adipose tissue deposited in the abdominal area. His major recreational activities are watching TV while drinking scotch and soda and doing occasional gardening. At a company picnic, he became very "winded" while playing softball and decided it was time for a general physical examination. At the examination, he weighed 264 lb at 5 feet 10 inches tall. His blood pressure was elevated, 155 mm Hg systolic and 95 mm Hg diastolic (hypertension is defined as >140 mm Hg systolic and >90 mm Hg diastolic). For a male of these proportions, a BMI of 18.5 to 24.9 would correspond to a weight between 129 and 173 lb. Mr. A. is currently almost 100 lb overweight, and his BMI of 37.9 is in the range defined as obesity.

**Ann R.** is a 23-year-old buyer for a woman's clothing store. Despite the fact that she is 5 feet 7 inches tall and weighs 99 lb, she is convinced she is overweight. About 2 months ago, she started a daily exercise program that consists of 1 hour of jogging every morning and 1 hour of walking every evening. She also decided to consult a physician about a weight reduction diet. If patients are above (like Ivan A.) or below (like Ann R.) their ideal weight, the physician, often in consultation with a registered dietician, prescribes a diet designed to bring the weight into the ideal range.

**Otto S.** is a 25-year-old medical student who was very athletic during high school and college and is now out of shape. Since he started medical school, he has been gaining weight. He is 5 feet 10 inches tall, and began medical school weighing 154 lb. By the time he finished his last examination in his first year, he weighed 187 lb. He has decided to consult a physician at the student health service before the problem gets worse, as he would like to reduce his weight of 187 lb (BMI of 27) to his previous level of 154 lb (BMI of 22, the middle of the healthy range).

## I. GENERAL INTRODUCTION

This chapter of the book contains an **_overview_** of basic metabolism (the generation and storage of energy and biosynthetic intermediates from the foods that we eat), which allows patients to be presented at a simplistic level and to whet the student's appetite for the biochemistry to come. Its goal is to enable the student to taste and preview what biochemistry is all about. It is not designed to be all inclusive, as all of these topics will be discussed in greater detail in Sections 4 through 6 of the text. The next section of the text (Section 2) begins with the basics of biochemistry and the relationship of basic chemistry to processes which occur in all living cells.

## II. DIETARY FUELS

The major fuels we obtain from our diet are **carbohydrates**, **proteins**, and **fats**. When these fuels are oxidized to $CO_2$ and $H_2O$ in our cells (the process of **catabolism**), energy is released by the transfer of electrons to $O_2$. The energy from this oxidation process generates heat and **adenosine triphosphate (ATP)** (Fig. 1.1). Carbon dioxide travels in the blood to the lungs where it is expired, and water is excreted in urine, sweat, and other secretions. Although the heat that is generated by fuel oxidation is used to maintain body temperature, the main purpose of fuel oxidation is to generate ATP. ATP provides the energy that drives most of the energy-consuming processes in the cell, including biosynthetic reactions (**anabolism**), muscle contraction, and active transport across membranes. As these processes utilize energy, ATP is converted back to adenosine diphosphate (ADP) and inorganic phosphate ($P_i$). The generation and utilization of ATP is referred to as the **ATP-ADP cycle**.

The oxidation of fuels to generate ATP is called **respiration** (Fig. 1.2). Prior to oxidation, carbohydrates are converted principally to glucose, fat to fatty acids, and protein to amino acids. The pathways for oxidizing glucose, fatty acids, and amino acids have many features in common. They first oxidize the fuels to **acetyl CoA**, a precursor of the **tricarboxylic acid (TCA) cycle**. The TCA cycle is a series of reactions that completes the oxidation of fuels to $CO_2$ (see Chapter 17). Electrons lost from the fuels during oxidative reactions are transferred to $O_2$ by a series of proteins in the electron transport chain (see Chapter 18). The energy of electron transfer is used to convert ADP and $P_i$ to ATP by a process known as **oxidative phosphorylation**.

In discussions of metabolism and nutrition, energy is often expressed in units of **calories**. A calorie in this context (a nutritional calorie) is equivalent to 1 **kilocalorie (kcal)** in energy terms. Thus, a 1-calorie soft drink actually has 1 kcal of energy. Energy is also expressed in **joules**. One kilocalorie equals 4.18 kilojoules (kJ). Physicians tend to use units of calories, in part because that is what their patients use and understand.

### A. Carbohydrates

The major carbohydrates in the human diet are starch, sucrose, lactose, fructose, and glucose. The polysaccharide **starch** is the storage form of carbohydrates in plants. **Sucrose** (table sugar) and **lactose** (milk sugar) are disaccharides, and **fructose** and **glucose** are monosaccharides. Digestion converts the larger carbohydrates to monosaccharides, which can be absorbed into the bloodstream. Glucose, a monosaccharide, is the predominant sugar in human blood (Fig. 1.3).

Oxidation of carbohydrates to $CO_2$ and $H_2O$ in the body produces approximately 4 kcal/g. In other words, every gram of carbohydrate we eat yields approximately 4 kcal of energy. Note that carbohydrate molecules contain a significant amount of oxygen and are already partially oxidized before they enter our bodies (see Fig. 1.3).

### B. Proteins

Proteins are composed of **amino acids** that are joined to form linear chains (Fig. 1.4). In addition to carbon, hydrogen, and oxygen, proteins contain about 16% nitrogen by weight. The digestive process breaks down proteins to their constituent amino acids, which enter the blood. The complete oxidation of proteins to $CO_2$, $H_2O$, and $NH_4^+$ in the body yields approximately 4 kcal/g.

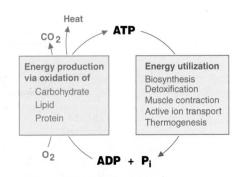

**FIG. 1.1.** The ATP–ADP cycle. The energy-generating pathways are shown in *red*; the energy-utilizing pathways in *blue*.

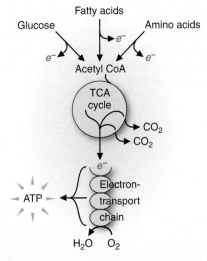

**FIG. 1.2.** Generation of ATP from fuel components during respiration. Glucose, fatty acids, and amino acids are oxidized to acetyl CoA, a substrate for the TCA cycle. In the TCA cycle, they are completely oxidized to $CO_2$. As fuels are oxidized, electrons ($e^-$) are transferred to $O_2$ by the electron transport chain, and the energy is used to generate ATP.

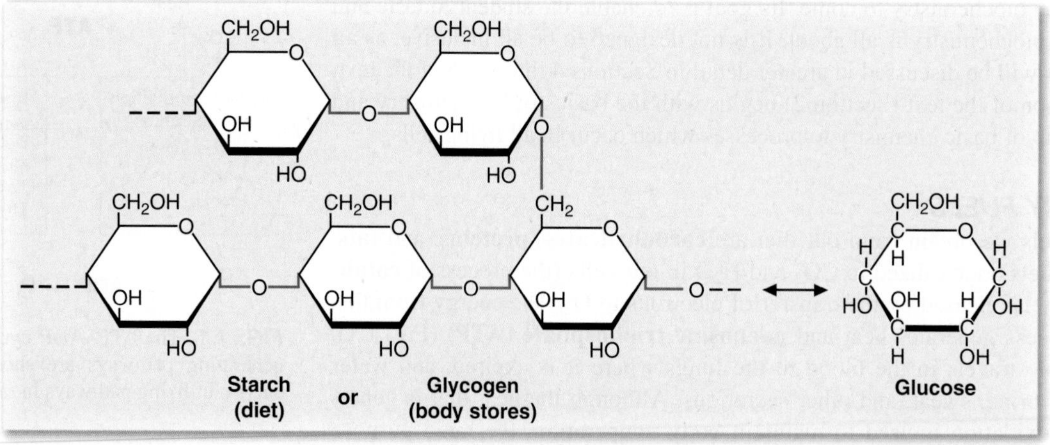

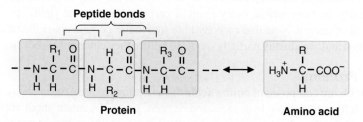

**FIG. 1.3.** Structure of starch and glycogen. Starch, our major dietary carbohydrate, and glycogen, the body's storage form of glucose, have similar structures. They are polysaccharides (many sugar units) composed of glucose, which is a monosaccharide (one sugar unit). Dietary disaccharides are composed of two sugar units.

### C. Fats

**Fats** are lipids composed of **triacylglycerols** (also called **triglycerides**). A triacylglycerol molecule contains three **fatty acids** esterified to one **glycerol** moiety (Fig. 1.5).

Fats contain much less oxygen than is contained in carbohydrates or proteins. Therefore, fats are more reduced and yield more energy when oxidized. The complete oxidation of triacylglycerols to $CO_2$ and $H_2O$ in the body releases approximately 9 kcal/g, more than twice the energy yield from an equivalent amount of carbohydrate or protein.

### D. Alcohol

**Alcohol** (**ethanol**, in the context of the diet) has considerable caloric content. Ethanol ($CH_3CH_2OH$) is oxidized to $CO_2$ and $H_2O$ in the body and yields about 7 kcal/g; that is, more than carbohydrate but less than fat.

### III. BODY FUEL STORES

Humans carry supplies of fuel within their bodies (Table 1.1). These fuel stores are light in weight, large in quantity, and readily converted into oxidizable substances. Most of us are familiar with **fat**, our major fuel store, which is located in **adipose tissue**. Although fat is distributed throughout our body, it tends to increase in quantity in our hips and thighs and in our abdomen as we advance into middle age. In addition to our fat stores, we also have important, although much smaller, stores of carbohydrate in the form of **glycogen** located mainly in our liver and muscles (see Fig. 1.3). Body protein, particularly the protein of our large muscle masses, also serves to a small extent as a fuel store, and we draw on it for energy when we fast.

**Q:** An analysis of **Ann R.**'s diet showed she ate 100 g of carbohydrate, 20 g of protein, and 15 g of fat each day, whereas **Ivan A.** ate 585 g of carbohydrates, 150 g of protein, and 95 g of fat each day. In addition, he drank 45 g of alcohol daily. Approximately how many calories did Ann and Ivan consume per day?

**FIG. 1.4.** General structure of proteins and amino acids. Each amino acid in this figure is indicated by a different color. Different amino acids have different side chains. For example, $R_1$ might be $-CH_3$; $R_2$, $-CH_2OH$; $R_3$, $-CH_2-COO^-$. In a protein, the amino acids are linked by peptide bonds. *R*, side chain.

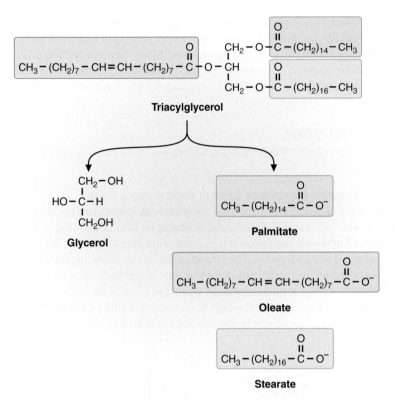

**Ann R.** consumed 400 kcal as carbohydrate ($4 \times 100$), 80 kcal as protein ($4 \times 20$), and 135 kcal as fat ($15 \times 9$), for a total of 615 calories per day. **Ivan A.**, on the other hand, consumed 4,110 calories per day $[(585 \times 4) + (150 \times 4) + (95 \times 9) + (45 \times 7)]$.

**FIG. 1.5.** Structure of a triacylglycerol. Palmitate and stearate are saturated fatty acids (i.e., they have no double bonds). Oleate is monounsaturated (one double bond). Polyunsaturated fatty acids have more than one double bond.

## A. Glycogen

Our stores of glycogen in liver, muscle, and other cells are relatively small in quantity but are nevertheless important. Liver glycogen is used to maintain blood glucose levels between meals. Thus, the size of this glycogen store fluctuates during the day; an average 70-kg man might have 200 g or more of liver glycogen after a meal but only 80 g after an overnight fast. Muscle glycogen supplies energy for muscle contraction during exercise. At rest, the 70-kg man has about 150 g of muscle glycogen. Almost all cells, including neurons, maintain a small emergency supply of glucose as glycogen.

## B. Protein

Protein serves many important roles in the body, and it is, therefore, not solely a fuel store like fat and glycogen. Muscle protein is essential for **body movement**. Other proteins serve as **enzymes** (catalysts of biochemical reactions) or as **structural components** of cells and tissues. Only a limited amount of body protein can be degraded, about 6 kg in the average 70-kg man, before our body functions are compromised.

## C. Fat

Our major fuel store is adipose triacylglycerol (triglyceride), a lipid more commonly known as fat. The average 70-kg man has about 15 kg of stored triacylglycerol, which accounts for about 85% of his total stored calories (see Table 1.1).

**Table 1.1   Fuel Composition of the Average 70-kg Man after an Overnight Fast**

| Fuel | Amount (kg) | Percent of Total Stored Calories |
|---|---|---|
| Glycogen | | |
| Muscle | 0.15 | 0.4 |
| Liver | 0.08 | 0.2 |
| Protein | 6.0 | 14.4 |
| Triglyceride | 15 | 85 |

Two characteristics make adipose triacylglycerol a very efficient fuel store: the fact that triacylglycerol contains more calories per gram than carbohydrate or protein (9 kcal/g vs. 4 kcal/g) and the fact that adipose tissue does not contain much water. Adipose tissue contains only about 15% water, compared to tissues like muscle that contains about 80%. Thus, the 70-kg man with 15 kg of stored triacylglycerol has only about 18 kg of adipose tissue.

## IV. THE FED STATE

The period during which digestion and absorption of nutrients occurs is considered the fed state.

### A. Changes in Hormone Levels following a Meal

After a typical high-carbohydrate meal, the **pancreas** is stimulated to release the hormone **insulin**, and release of the hormone **glucagon** is inhibited (Fig. 1.6, *circle 4*). **Endocrine hormones** are released from endocrine glands, such as the pancreas, in response to a specific stimulus. They travel in the blood, carrying messages between tissues concerning the overall physiological state of the body. At their target tissues, they adjust the rate of various metabolic pathways to meet the changing conditions. The endocrine hormone insulin, which is secreted from the pancreas in response to a high-carbohydrate meal, carries the message that dietary glucose is available and

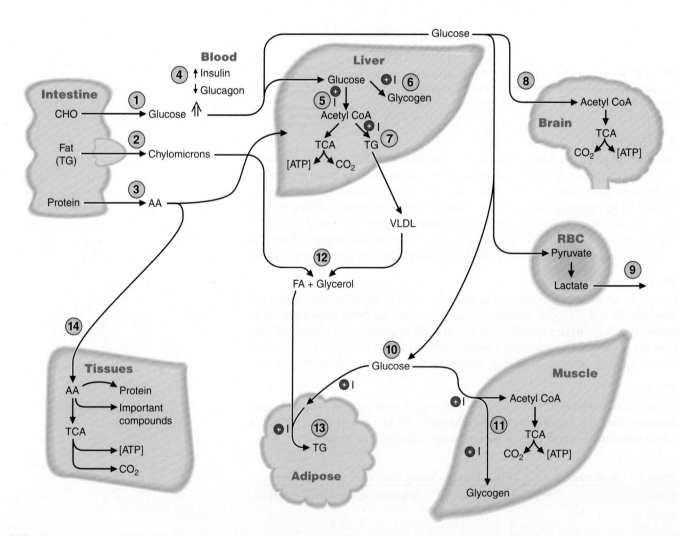

**FIG. 1.6.** The fed state. The circled numbers indicate the approximate order in which the processes occur. *TG*, triacylglycerols; *FA*, fatty acid; *AA*, amino acid; *RBC*, red blood cell; *VLDL*, very low density lipoprotein; *I*, insulin; ⊕, stimulated by.

can be transported into cells, utilized, and stored. The release of another hormone, glucagon, is suppressed by glucose and insulin. Glucagon carries the message that glucose must be generated from endogenous fuel stores. The subsequent changes in circulating hormone levels cause changes in the body's metabolic patterns, involving a number of different tissues and metabolic pathways.

## B.  Absorption, Digestion, and Fate of Nutrients

After a meal is consumed, foods are **digested** (broken down into simpler components) by a series of **enzymes** in the mouth, stomach, and small intestine. Enzymes are proteins that **catalyze** biochemical reactions; that is, they increase the speed at which reactions occur. Digestive enzymes convert the dietary components into smaller, more manageable, subunits. The products of digestion eventually are absorbed into the blood. The fate of dietary carbohydrates, proteins, and fats is summarized in Table 1.2 and Figure 1.7.

## 1.  FATE OF GLUCOSE

### a.  Conversion to Glycogen, Triacylglycerols, and CO₂ in the Liver

Because glucose leaves the intestine via the hepatic portal vein (a blood vessel which carries blood from the intestine to the liver), the liver is the first tissue it passes through. The liver extracts a portion of this glucose from the blood. Some of the glucose that enters **hepatocytes** (liver cells) is oxidized in ATP-generating pathways to meet the immediate energy needs of these cells, and the remainder is converted to glycogen and triacylglycerols or used for biosynthetic reactions. In the liver, insulin promotes the uptake of glucose by increasing its use as a fuel and its storage as glycogen and triacylglycerols (see Fig. 1.6, *circles 5–7*).

As glucose is being oxidized to $CO_2$, it is first oxidized to pyruvate in the pathway of **glycolysis** (discussed in more detail in Chapter 19), a series of reactions common to the metabolism of many carbohydrates. Pyruvate is then oxidized to acetyl CoA. The acetyl group enters the TCA cycle, where it is completely oxidized to $CO_2$. Energy from the oxidative reactions is used to generate ATP (see Fig. 1.2).

Liver glycogen stores reach a maximum of about 200 to 300 g after a high-carbohydrate meal, whereas the body's fat stores are relatively limitless. As the glycogen stores begin to fill, the liver also begins converting some of the excess glucose it receives to triacylglycerols. Both the glycerol and the fatty acid moieties of the triacylglycerols can be synthesized from glucose. The fatty acids are also obtained preformed from the blood (these are the dietary fatty acids). The liver does not store triacylglycerol, however, but packages it along with proteins, **phospholipids**, and

 The laboratory studies ordered at the time of his second office visit show that **Ivan A.** has hyperglycemia, an elevation of blood glucose above normal values. At the time of this visit, his blood glucose level determined after an overnight fast was 162 mg/dL. Because this blood glucose measurement was significantly above normal, the fasting blood glucose levels were tested the next day, with a result of 170 mg/dL. A diagnosis of type 2 diabetes mellitus, due to two significantly elevated readings of Ivan's fasting blood glucose levels, was made. In this disease, liver, muscle, and adipose tissue are relatively resistant to the action of insulin in promoting glucose uptake into cells and storage as glycogen and triacylglycerols. Therefore, more glucose remains in his blood. This is in contrast to individuals with type 1 diabetes mellitus who cannot produce any insulin in response to increases in blood glucose levels.

**Table 1.2  Digestion of Dietary Nutrients**

| Dietary Form | Enzymes Required and Source of Enzymes* | End Products |
|---|---|---|
| Starch | α-Amylase (found in saliva and secreted from pancreas for use in the intestine) | Glucose |
| Sucrose (table sugar) | Sucrase (intestinal brush-border enzyme) | Glucose and fructose |
| Lactose (found in milk) | Lactase (intestinal brush-border enzyme) | Glucose and galactose |
| Proteins | Proteases (e.g., pepsin and trypsin; found in the stomach, secreted from the pancreas for use in the intestine, and some native to the intestine) | Amino acids |
| Fats (including triacylglycerol and cholesterol) | Lipases (secreted from the pancreas for use in the intestine) | Chylomicrons (a protein-lipid particle which allows the transport of the dietary lipid, which is insoluble, throughout the bloodstream) |

*The action of enzymes is described in more detail in Chapter 6.

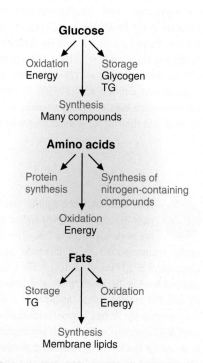

**FIG. 1.7.** Major fates of fuels in the fed state. *TG,* triacylglycerol.

Fuel metabolism is often discussed as though the body consisted only of brain, skeletal and cardiac muscle, liver, adipose tissue, red blood cells, kidney, and intestinal epithelial cells ("the gut"). These are the dominant tissues in terms of overall fuel economy, and they are the tissues we will describe most often. Of course, all tissues require fuels for energy, and many have very specific fuel requirements.

Unfortunately, **Ivan A.**'s efforts to lose weight had failed dismally. In fact, he now weighed 270 lb, an increase of 6 lb since his first visit 2 months ago. Ivan reported that the recent death of his 45-year-old brother from a heart attack had made him realize that he must pay more attention to his health. Because Mr. A.'s brother had a history of hypercholesterolemia and because Mr. A.'s serum total cholesterol had been significantly elevated (296 mg/dL) at his first visit, his blood lipid profile was determined, his blood glucose level was measured, and a number of other tests were ordered. The blood lipid profile is a test that measures the content of the various triacylglycerol- and cholesterol-containing particles in the blood. His blood pressure was 162 mm Hg systolic and 98 mm Hg diastolic or 162/98 mm Hg (normal = 120/80 mm Hg or less; with prehypertension = 120–139/80–89; with hypertension defined as >140/90). His waist circumference was 48 inches (healthy values for men, less than 40; for women, less than 35).

**Ivan A.**'s total cholesterol level is now 315 mg/dL, slightly higher than his previous level of 296. (The currently recommended level for total serum cholesterol is 200 mg/dL or less.). His triacylglycerol level is 250 mg/dL (normal is between 60 and 160 mg/dL). These lipid levels clearly indicate that Mr. A. has a hyperlipidemia (high level of lipoproteins in the blood) and therefore is at risk for the future development of atherosclerosis and its consequences, such as heart attacks and strokes.

**cholesterol** into the lipoprotein complexes known as **very low density lipoproteins (VLDL)**, which are secreted into the bloodstream. Some of the fatty acids from the VLDL are taken up by tissues for their immediate energy needs, but most are stored in adipose tissue as triacylglycerol.

### b.  Glucose Metabolism in Other Tissues

The glucose from the intestine that is not metabolized by the liver travels in the blood to peripheral tissues (most other tissues), where it can be oxidized for energy. Glucose is the one fuel that can be utilized by all tissues. In the following paragraphs, we examine how glucose is used in the brain, red blood cells, muscle, and adipose tissue

The brain and other neural tissues are dependent on glucose for their energy needs. They generally oxidize glucose via glycolysis and the TCA cycle completely to $CO_2$ and $H_2O$, generating ATP (see Fig. 1.6, *circle 8*). Except under conditions of starvation, glucose is their only major fuel. Glucose is also a major precursor of **neurotransmitters**, the chemicals that convey electrical impulses (as ion gradients) between neurons. If our blood glucose drops much below normal levels, we become dizzy and light-headed. If blood glucose continues to drop, we become comatose and ultimately die. Under normal, nonstarving conditions, the brain and the rest of the nervous system require about 150 g of glucose each day.

Red blood cells use glucose as their only fuel source because they lack **mitochondria**. Fatty acid oxidation, amino acid oxidation, the TCA cycle, the electron transport chain, and oxidative phosphorylation occur principally in mitochondria. Glucose, in contrast, generates ATP from **anaerobic glycolysis** (glycolysis in the absence of oxygen) in the **cytosol**, and thus, red blood cells obtain all their energy by this process. In anaerobic glycolysis, the pyruvate formed from glucose is converted to **lactate** and then released into the blood (see Fig. 1.6, *circle 9*).

Without glucose, red blood cells could not survive. Red blood cells carry $O_2$ from the lungs to the tissues. Without red blood cells, most of the tissues of the body would suffer from a lack of energy because they require $O_2$ in order to completely convert their fuels to $CO_2$ and $H_2O$.

Exercising skeletal muscles can use glucose from the blood or from their own glycogen stores, converting glucose to lactate via glycolysis or oxidizing it completely to $CO_2$ and $H_2O$. Muscle also uses other fuels from the blood, such as fatty acids (Fig. 1.8). After a meal, glucose is used by muscle to replenish the glycogen stores that were depleted during exercise. Glucose is transported into muscle cells and converted to glycogen by processes that are stimulated by insulin.

Insulin stimulates the transport of glucose into adipose cells as well as into muscle cells. Adipocytes oxidize glucose for energy, and they also use glucose as the source of the **glycerol** moiety of the triacylglycerols they store (see Fig. 1.6, *circle 10*).

### 2.  LIPOPROTEINS

Two types of **lipoproteins, chylomicrons** and **VLDL**, are produced in the fed state. The major function of these lipoproteins is to provide a blood transport system for triacylglycerols, which are insoluble in water. However, these lipoproteins also contain the lipid cholesterol, which is also somewhat insoluble in water. The triacylglycerols of chylomicrons are formed in intestinal epithelial cells from the products of digestion of dietary triacylglycerols. The triacylglycerols of VLDL are synthesized in the liver.

When these lipoproteins pass through blood vessels in adipose tissue, their triacylglycerols are degraded to fatty acids and glycerol (see Fig. 1.6, *circle 12*). The fatty acids enter the adipose cells and combine with a glycerol moiety that is produced from blood glucose. The resulting triacylglycerols are stored as large fat droplets in the adipose cells. The remnants of the chylomicrons are cleared from the blood by the liver. The remnants of the VLDL can be cleared by the liver, or they can form **low density lipoprotein (LDL)**, which is cleared by the liver or by peripheral cells.

Most of us have not even begun to reach the limits of our capacity to store triacylglycerols in adipose tissue. The ability of humans to store fat appears to be limited only by the amount of tissue we can carry without overloading the heart.

## 3. AMINO ACIDS

The amino acids derived from dietary proteins travel from the intestine to the liver in the hepatic portal vein (see Fig. 1.6, *circle 3*). The liver uses amino acids for the synthesis of serum proteins, as well as its own proteins, and for the biosynthesis of nitrogen-containing compounds that need amino acid precursors, such as the nonessential amino acids, **heme**, hormones, neurotransmitters, and **purine** and **pyrimidine bases** (which are required for the synthesis of the nucleic acids RNA and DNA). Many amino acids will enter the peripheral circulation, where they can be used by other tissues for protein synthesis and various biosynthetic pathways or oxidized for energy (see Fig. 1.6, *circle 14*). Proteins undergo **turnover**; they are constantly being synthesized and degraded. The amino acids released by protein breakdown enter the same pool of free amino acids in the blood as the amino acids from the diet. This free amino acid pool in the blood can be utilized by all cells to provide the right ratio of amino acids for protein synthesis or for biosynthesis of other compounds. In general, each individual biosynthetic pathway using an amino acid precursor is found in only a few tissues in the body.

## V.  THE FASTING STATE

Blood glucose levels peak about an hour after eating (the postprandial state) and then decrease as tissues oxidize glucose or convert it to storage forms of fuel. By 2 hours after a meal, the level returns to the fasting range (between 80 and 100 mg/dL). This decrease in blood glucose causes the pancreas to decrease its secretion of insulin, and the serum insulin level falls. The liver responds to this hormonal signal by starting to degrade its glycogen stores (**glycogenolysis**) and release glucose into the blood.

If we eat another meal within a few hours, we return to the fed state. However, if we continue to fast for a 12-hour period, we enter the basal state (also known as the postabsorptive state). A person is generally considered to be in the basal state after an overnight fast, when no food has been eaten since dinner the previous evening. By this time, the serum insulin level is low and glucagon is rising. Figure 1.9 illustrates the main features of the basal state.

## A.  Metabolic Changes During a Brief Fast

In the initial stages of fasting, stored fuels are used for energy (see Fig. 1.9). Fatty acids, which are released from adipose tissue by the process of **lipolysis** (the splitting of triglycerides to produce glycerol and fatty acids), serve as the body's major fuel during fasting (see Fig. 1.9, *circle 5*). The liver oxidizes most of its fatty acids only partially, converting them to ketone bodies, which are released into the blood. Thus, during the initial stages of fasting, blood levels of fatty acids and ketone bodies begin to increase. Muscle uses fatty acids, ketone bodies, and (when exercising and while supplies last) glucose from muscle glycogen. Many other tissues use either fatty acids or ketone bodies. However, red blood cells, the brain, and other neural tissues use mainly glucose.

## 1.  BLOOD GLUCOSE AND THE ROLE OF THE LIVER DURING FASTING

Because the liver maintains blood glucose levels during fasting, its role in survival is critical. Most neurons lack enzymes required for oxidation of fatty acids but can use ketone bodies to a limited extent. Red blood cells can utilize only glucose as a fuel. Therefore, it is imperative that blood glucose not decrease too rapidly nor fall too low.

Initially, liver glycogen stores are degraded to supply glucose to the blood, but these stores are limited. Although liver glycogen levels may increase to 200 to 300 g after a meal, only about 80 g remain after an overnight fast. When blood glucose

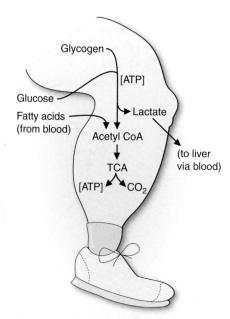

**FIG. 1.8.** Oxidation of fuels in exercising skeletal muscle. Exercising muscle uses more energy than resting muscle, and therefore, fuel utilization is increased to supply more ATP.

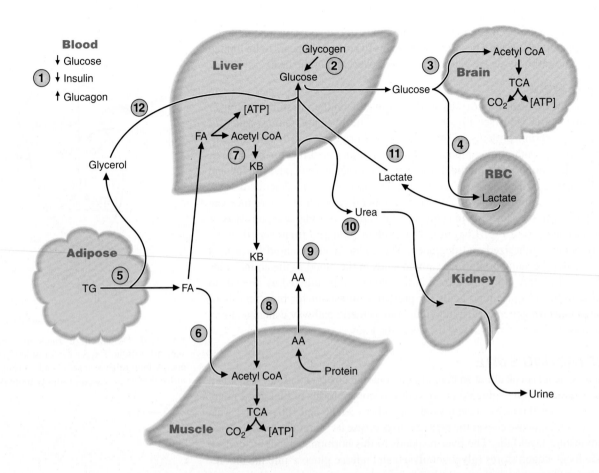

***FIG. 1.9.*** Basal state. This state occurs after an overnight (12-hour) fast. The circled numbers serve as a guide indicating the approximate order in which the processes begin to occur. *KB*, ketone bodies; *TG*, triacylglycerols; *FA*, fatty acid; *AA*, amino acid; *RBC*, red blood cell.

levels drop, the liver replenishes blood glucose via **gluconeogenesis**. In gluconeogenesis, lactate, glycerol, and amino acids are used as carbon sources to synthesize glucose. As fasting continues, gluconeogenesis progressively adds to the glucose produced by **glycogenolysis** in the liver.

Because our muscle mass is so large, most of the amino acid is supplied from degradation of muscle protein. The amino acids, lactate, and glycerol travel in the blood to the liver, where they are converted to glucose by gluconeogenesis. Because the nitrogen of the amino acids can form ammonia, which is toxic to the body, the liver converts this nitrogen to urea. Urea has two amino groups for just one carbon ($NH_2$-CO-$NH_2$). It is a very soluble, nontoxic compound that can be readily excreted by the kidneys and is thus an efficient means for disposing of excess ammonia. As fasting progresses, gluconeogenesis becomes increasingly more important as a source of blood glucose. After about a day of fasting, liver glycogen stores are depleted and gluconeogenesis is the only source of blood glucose.

## 2.  ROLE OF ADIPOSE TISSUE DURING FASTING

Adipose triacylglycerols are the major source of energy during fasting. They supply fatty acids, which are quantitatively the major fuel for the human body. Fatty acids are not only oxidized directly by various tissues of the body, they are also partially oxidized in the liver to four-carbon products called **ketone bodies**. Ketone bodies are subsequently oxidized as a fuel by other tissues.

It is important to realize that most fatty acids cannot provide carbon for gluconeogenesis. Thus, of the vast store of food energy in adipose tissue triacylglycerols, only the small glycerol portion travels to the liver to enter the gluconeogenic pathway.

Fatty acids serve as a fuel for muscle, kidney, and most other tissues. They are oxidized to acetyl CoA and subsequently to $CO_2$ and $H_2O$ in the TCA cycle, producing energy in the form of ATP. In addition to the ATP required to maintain cellular integrity, muscle uses ATP for contraction, and the kidney uses it for urinary transport processes.

Most of the fatty acids that enter the liver are converted to ketone bodies rather than being completely oxidized to $CO_2$. The process of conversion of fatty acids to acetyl CoA produces a considerable amount of energy (ATP), which drives the reactions of the liver under these conditions. The acetyl CoA is converted to the ketone bodies **acetoacetate** and **β-hydroxybutyrate**, which are released into the blood (see Figure 2.4 to view their structures). A third ketone body, acetone, is produced by nonenzymatic decarboxylation of acetoacetate. However, acetone is expired in the breath and not metabolized to a significant extent in the body.

The liver lacks an enzyme required for ketone body oxidation. However, ketone bodies can be further oxidized by most other cells with mitochondria, such as muscle and kidney. In these tissues, acetoacetate and β-hydroxybutyrate are converted to acetyl CoA and then oxidized in the TCA cycle, with subsequent generation of ATP.

## B. Metabolic Changes during a Prolonged Fast

If the pattern of fuel utilization that occurs during a brief fast were to persist for an extended period, the body's protein would be quite rapidly consumed to the point where critical functions would be compromised. Fortunately, metabolic changes occur during prolonged fasting that conserve (spare) muscle protein by causing muscle protein turnover to decrease. Figure 1.10 shows the main features of metabolism during prolonged fasting (starvation).

 **Ann R.** was receiving psychological counseling for anorexia nervosa but with little success. She saw her gynecologist because she had not had a menstrual period for 5 months. She also complained of becoming easily fatigued. The physician recognized that Ann's body weight of 85 lb was now less than 65% of her ideal weight. (Her BMI was now 13.7.) Immediate hospitalization was recommended. The admission diagnosis was severe malnutrition secondary to anorexia nervosa. Clinical findings included decreased body core temperature, blood pressure, and pulse (adaptive responses to malnutrition). Her physician ordered measurements of blood glucose and ketone body levels and made a spot check for ketone bodies in the urine as well as ordering tests to assess the functioning of her heart and kidneys.

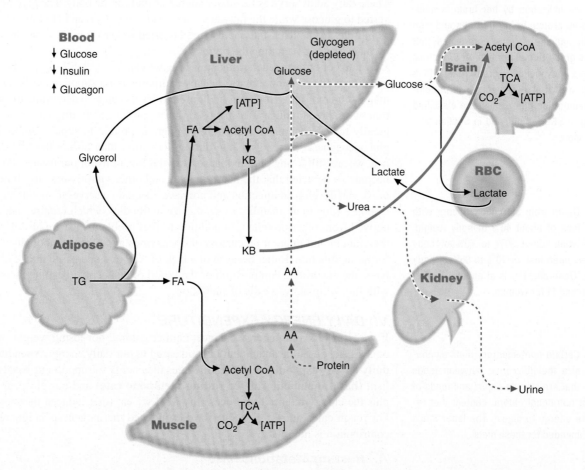

**FIG. 1.10.** Starved state. *Broken blue lines* indicate processes that have decreased, and the *heavy red solid line* indicates a process that has increased relative to the fasting state. *KB*, ketone bodies; *TG*, triacylglycerols; *FA*, fatty acid; *AA*, amino acid; *RBC*, red blood cell.

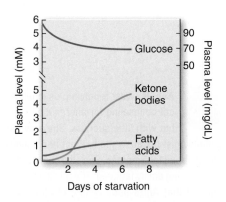

**FIG. 1.11.** Changes in the concentration of fuels in the blood during prolonged fasting.

🩺 **Ann R.**'s admission laboratory studies revealed a blood glucose level of 65 mg/dL (normal fasting blood glucose = 80 to100 mg/dL). Her serum ketone body concentration was 4,200 μM (normal = ~70 μM). The Ketostix urine test was moderately positive, indicating that ketone bodies were present in the urine. In her starved state, ketone body utilization by her brain is helping conserve protein in her muscles and vital organs. In addition, it was determined that Ms. R. has grade III malnutrition. At 67 inches, she needs a body weight of greater than 118 lb to achieve a BMI of 18.5. Degrees of protein-energy malnutrition (marasmus) are classified according to BMI, as outlined in Section VI.C of this chapter.

🩺 Death from starvation occurs with loss of about 40% of body weight, when about 30% to 50% of body protein has been lost, or 70% to 95% of body fat stores. Generally, this is at about a BMI of 13 for men and 11 for women.

🩺 Certain contemporary diets emphasize the difference between foods that are easy to digest and foods of equivalent nutritional caloric content that require more energy to digest. The latter foods are recommended for these diets.

## 1. ROLE OF LIVER DURING PROLONGED FASTING

After 3 to 5 days of fasting, when the body enters the starved state, muscle decreases its use of ketone bodies and depends mainly on fatty acids for its fuel. The liver, however, continues to convert fatty acids to ketone bodies. The result is that the concentration of ketone bodies in the blood rises (Fig. 1.11). The brain begins to take up these ketone bodies from the blood and to oxidize them for energy. Therefore, the brain needs less glucose than it did after an overnight fast.

Because the stores of glycogen in the liver are depleted by about 30 hours of fasting, gluconeogenesis is the only process by which the liver can supply glucose to the blood if fasting continues. The amino acid pool, produced by the breakdown of protein, continues to serve as a major source of carbon for gluconeogenesis. A fraction of this amino acid pool is also being utilized for biosynthetic functions (e.g., synthesis of heme and neurotransmitters) and new protein synthesis, processes that must continue during fasting. However, as a result of the decreased rate of gluconeogenesis during prolonged fasting due to ketone body utilization, protein is spared; less protein is degraded to supply amino acids for gluconeogenesis.

While converting amino acid carbon to glucose in gluconeogenesis, the liver also converts the nitrogen of these amino acids to urea. Consequently, because glucose production decreases during prolonged fasting compared to early fasting, urea production also decreases.

## 2. ROLE OF ADIPOSE TISSUE DURING PROLONGED FASTING

During prolonged fasting (no food intake), adipose tissue continues to break down its triacylglycerol stores, providing fatty acids and glycerol to the blood (lipolysis). These fatty acids serve as the major source of fuel for the body. The glycerol is converted to glucose while the fatty acids are oxidized to $CO_2$ and $H_2O$ by tissues such as muscle. In the liver, fatty acids are converted to ketone bodies that are oxidized by many tissues, including the brain.

A number of factors determine how long we can fast and still survive. The amount of adipose tissue is one factor, because adipose tissue supplies the body with its major source of fuel. However, body protein levels can also determine the length of time we can fast. Glucose is still used during prolonged fasting (starvation) but in greatly reduced amounts. Although we degrade protein to supply amino acids for gluconeogenesis at a slower rate during starvation than during the first days of a fast, we are still losing protein that serves vital functions for our tissues. Protein can become so depleted that the heart, kidney, and other vital tissues stop functioning, or we can develop an infection and not have adequate reserves to mount an immune response (due to an inability to synthesize antibodies, which requires amino acids derived from other proteins). In addition to fuel problems, we are also deprived of the vitamin and mineral precursors of coenzymes and other compounds necessary for tissue function. Either because of a lack of ATP or a decreased intake of electrolytes, the electrolyte composition of the blood or cells could become incompatible with life. Ultimately, we die of starvation.

## VI. DAILY ENERGY EXPENDITURE

If we want to stay in energy balance, neither gaining nor losing weight, we must, on average, consume an amount of food equal to our daily energy expenditure. The **daily energy expenditure (DEE)** includes the energy to support our basal metabolism (**basal metabolic rate** or **resting metabolic rate**) and our physical activity, plus the energy required to process the food we eat (diet-induced thermogenesis). For rough calculations, the value for diet-induced thermogenesis is ignored, as its contribution is minimal.

### A. Resting Metabolic Rate

The **resting metabolic rate (RMR)** is a measure of the energy required to maintain life: the functioning of the lungs, kidneys, and brain; the pumping of the heart;

**Table 1.3  Factors Affecting Basal Metabolic Rate Expressed as Calories Required per Kilogram Body Weight**

Gender (males higher than females)
Body temperature (increased with fever)
Environmental temperature (increased in cold)
Thyroid status (increased in hyperthyroidism)
Pregnancy and lactation (increased)
Age (decreases with age)

the maintenance of ionic gradients across membranes; the reactions of biochemical pathways; and so forth. Another term used to describe basal metabolism is the **basal metabolic rate** (**BMR**). It is also sometimes called the **resting energy expenditure** (**REE**). The RMR and BMR differ very little in value.

The BMR, which is usually expressed in kilocalories per day, is affected by a number of factors. It is proportional to the amount of metabolically active tissue (including the major organs) and to the lean (or fat free) body mass. Other factors which affect the BMR are outlined in Table 1.3. Additionally, there are large variations in BMR from one adult to another, determined by genetic factors.

A rough estimate of the BMR for the resting individual may be obtained by assuming it is 24 kcal/day/kg body weight and multiplying by the body weight. An easy way to remember this is 1 kcal/kg/hour. This estimate works best for young individuals who are near their ideal weight. More accurate methods for calculating the BMR use empirically derived equations for different gender and age groups (see Table A1.1 @ ), but even these calculations do not take into account variation among individuals.

## B.  Physical Activity

In addition to the RMR, the energy required for **physical activity** contributes to the DEE. The difference in physical activity between a student and a lumberjack is enormous, and a student who is relatively sedentary during the week may be much more active during the weekend.

A rough estimate of the energy required per day for physical activity can be made by using a value of 30% of the RMR (per day) for a very sedentary person (such as a medical student who does little but study) and a value of 60% to 70% of the RMR (per day) for a person who engages in about 2 hours of moderate exercise a day. A value of 100% or more of the RMR is used for a person who does several hours of heavy exercise a day.

The total DEE is usually calculated as the sum of the RMR (in kcal/day) plus the energy required for the amount of time spent in each of the various types of physical activity. For example, a very sedentary medical student would have a DEE equal to the RMR plus 30% of the RMR (or 1.3 × RMR) and an active person's daily expenditure could be two times the RMR.

## C.  Healthy Body Weight

Ideally, we should strive to maintain a weight consistent with good health. Overweight people are frequently defined as more than 20% above their ideal weight. But what is the ideal weight? The **body mass index** (**BMI**), calculated as **weight/height$^2$ (kg/m$^2$)**, or weight (pounds × 704)/height$^2$ (inches squared), is currently the preferred method for determining whether a person's weight is in the healthy range. It is based on two simple measurements, height without shoes and weight with minimal clothing. Patients can be shown their BMI in a nomogram and need not use calculations (see Fig. A1.1 @ ).

In general, adults with BMI values below 18.5 are considered underweight. Those with BMIs between 18.5 and 24.9 are considered to be in the healthy weight range, between 25 and 29.9 are in the overweight or preobese range, and above 30 are in the obese range. Degrees of **protein-energy malnutrition** (**marasmus**) are classified

A person whose weight consists primarily of lean muscle mass (such as body builders) is not obese but may be classified as such by their BMI.

Are **Ivan A.** and **Ann R.** in a healthy weight range? Calculate their respective BMIs.

**Ivan A.**'s weight is classified as obese. His BMI is 264 lb × 704/(70 in)$^2$ = 37.9.
**Ann R.** is underweight. Her BMI is 99 lb × 704/(67 in)$^2$ = 15.5.

according to BMI. A BMI of 17.0 to 18.4 is degree I; values of 16.0 to 16.9 is degree II; and any value less than 16.0 is degree III, the most severe.

### D. Weight Gain and Loss

To maintain our body weight, we must stay in **caloric balance**. We are in caloric balance if the kilocalories in the food we eat equal our DEE. If we eat less food than we require for our DEE, our body fuel stores supply the additional calories and we lose weight. On the other hand, if we eat more food than we require for our energy needs, the excess fuel is stored (mainly in our adipose tissue) and we gain weight.

When we draw upon our adipose tissue to meet our energy needs, we lose approximately 1 lb whenever we expend about 3,500 calories more than we consume. In other words, if we eat 500 calories less than we expend per day, we will lose about 1 lb/week. Because the average food intake is only about 2,000 to 3,000 calories/day, eating one-third to one-half the normal amount will cause a person to lose weight rather slowly. Fad diets that promise a loss of weight much more rapid than this have no scientific merit. In fact, the rapid initial weight loss the fad dieter typically experiences is due largely to loss of body water. This loss of water occurs in part because muscle tissue protein and liver glycogen are degraded rapidly to supply energy during the early phase of the diet. When muscle tissue (which is about 80% water) and glycogen (about 70% water) are broken down, this water is excreted from the body.

### VII. DIETARY REQUIREMENTS, NUTRITION, AND GUIDELINES

In addition to supplying us with fuel and with general-purpose building blocks for biosynthesis, our diet also provides us with specific nutrients that we need to remain healthy. We must have a regular supply of **vitamins** and **minerals** and of the **essential fatty acids** and **essential amino acids**. "Essential" means that they are essential in the diet; the body cannot synthesize these compounds from other molecules and must therefore obtain them from the diet. Nutrients that the body requires in the diet only under certain conditions are called "conditionally essential."

The **Recommended Dietary Allowance (RDA)** and the **Adequate Intake (AI)** provide quantitative estimates of nutrient requirements. The RDA for a nutrient is the average daily dietary intake level necessary to meet the requirement of nearly all (97% to 98%) healthy individuals in a particular gender and life stage group. Life stage group is a certain age range or physiological status (i.e., pregnancy or lactation). The RDA is intended to serve as a goal for intake by individuals. The AI is a recommended intake value that is used when there is not enough data available to establish an RDA.

### A. Carbohydrates

No specific carbohydrates have been identified as dietary requirements. Carbohydrates can be synthesized from amino acids, and we can convert one type of carbohydrate to another. However, health problems are associated with the complete elimination of carbohydrate from the diet, partly because a low-carbohydrate diet must contain higher amounts of fat to provide us with the energy we need. High-fat diets are associated with obesity, atherosclerosis, and other health problems.

### B. Essential Fatty Acids

Although most lipids required for cell structure, fuel storage, or hormone synthesis can be synthesized from carbohydrates or proteins, we need a minimal level of certain dietary lipids for optimal health. These lipids, known as **essential fatty acids**, are required in our diet because we cannot synthesize fatty acids with these particular arrangements of double bonds. The essential fatty acids **α-linoleic** and **α-linolenic acid** are supplied by **dietary plant oils**, and they can be used to produce **eicosapentaenoic acid (EPA)** and **docosahexaenoic acid (DHA)**, which are also supplied in **fish oils**. These latter compounds are the precursors of the **eicosanoids**

Malnutrition, the absence of an adequate intake of nutrients, occurs in the United States principally among children of families with incomes below the poverty level, the elderly, individuals whose diet is influenced by alcohol and drug usage, and those who make poor food choices. Over 15 million children in the United States live in families with incomes below the poverty level. Of these, about 10% have clinical malnutrition, most often anemia from a lack of adequate iron intake. A larger percentage have mild protein and energy malnutrition and exhibit growth retardation, sometimes as a result of parental neglect. Childhood malnutrition may also lead to learning failure and chronic illness later in life. A weight-for-age measurement is one of the best indicators of childhood malnourishment because it is easy to measure, and weight is one of the first parameters to change during malnutrition.

The term "kwashiorkor" refers to a disease originally seen in African children with a protein deficiency. It is characterized by marked hypoalbuminemia, anemia, edema, pot belly, loss of hair, and other signs of tissue injury. This is due to the inability of the liver to synthesize new proteins as a result of the deficiency of essential amino acids. The term "marasmus" is used for prolonged protein-calorie malnutrition, particularly in young children.

(a set of hormone-like molecules that are secreted by cells in small quantities and have numerous important effects on neighboring cells). The eicosanoids include the **prostaglandins**, **thromboxanes**, **leukotrienes**, and other related compounds.

## C. Protein

The RDA for protein is about 0.8 g of high-quality protein per kilogram of ideal body weight, or about 60 g/day for men and 50 g/day for women. **High-quality protein** contains all the essential amino acids in adequate amounts. Proteins of animal origin (milk, egg, and meat proteins) are of high quality. The proteins in plant foods are generally of lower quality, which means they are low in one or more of the essential amino acids. Vegetarians may obtain adequate amounts of the essential amino acids by eating mixtures of vegetables that complement each other in terms of their amino acid composition.

### 1. ESSENTIAL AMINO ACIDS

Different amino acids are used in the body as precursors for the synthesis of proteins and other nitrogen-containing compounds. Of the 20 amino acids commonly required in the body for synthesis of protein and other compounds, nine amino acids are essential in the diet of an adult human because they cannot be synthesized in the body. These are **lysine**, **isoleucine**, **leucine**, **threonine**, **valine**, **tryptophan**, **phenylalanine**, **methionine**, and **histidine**.

Certain amino acids are conditionally essential, that is, required in the diet only under certain conditions. Children and pregnant women have a high rate of protein synthesis to support growth and require some arginine in the diet, although it can be synthesized in the body. Histidine is essential in the diet of the adult in very small quantities because adults efficiently recycle histidine. The increased requirement of children and pregnant women for histidine is, therefore, much larger than their increased requirement of other essential amino acids. Tyrosine and cysteine are considered conditionally essential. Tyrosine is synthesized from phenylalanine, and it is required in the diet if phenylalanine intake is inadequate or if an individual is congenitally deficient in an enzyme required to convert phenylalanine to tyrosine (the congenital disease phenylketonuria). Cysteine is synthesized using sulfur from methionine, and it may also be required in the diet under certain conditions.

### 2. NITROGEN BALANCE

The proteins in the body undergo constant turnover; that is, they are constantly being degraded to amino acids and resynthesized. When a protein is degraded, its amino acids are released into the pool of free amino acids in the body. The amino acids from dietary proteins also enter this pool. Free amino acids can have one of three fates: They are used to make proteins, they serve as precursors for synthesis of essential nitrogen-containing compounds (e.g., heme, DNA, RNA), or they are oxidized as fuel to yield energy. When amino acids are oxidized, their nitrogen atoms are excreted in the urine, principally in the form of urea. The urine also contains smaller amounts of other nitrogenous excretory products (uric acid, creatinine, and $NH_4^+$) derived from the degradation of amino acids and compounds synthesized from amino acids. Some nitrogen is also lost in sweat, feces, and cells that slough off.

**Nitrogen balance** is the difference between the amount of nitrogen taken into the body each day (mainly in the form of dietary protein) and the amount of nitrogen in compounds lost. If more nitrogen is ingested than excreted, a person is said to be in positive nitrogen balance. Positive nitrogen balance occurs in growing individuals (e.g., children, adolescents, and pregnant women) who are synthesizing more protein than they are breaking down. On the other hand, if less nitrogen is ingested than excreted, a person is said to be in negative nitrogen balance. A negative nitrogen balance develops in a person who is eating either too little protein or protein that is deficient in one or more of the essential amino acids. Amino acids are continuously being mobilized from body proteins. If the diet is lacking an essential amino acid or if the intake of protein is too low, new protein cannot be synthesized and the unused amino acids will be degraded, with the nitrogen appearing in the urine. If a negative nitrogen balance persists for too long, bodily function will be impaired by the net loss of critical proteins. In contrast, healthy adults are in nitrogen balance (neither positive nor negative), and the amount of nitrogen consumed in the diet equals its loss in urine, sweat, feces, and other excretions.

## D. Vitamins

Vitamins are a diverse group of organic molecules required in very small quantities in the diet for health, growth, and survival (Latin *vita*, life). The absence of a vitamin from the diet or an inadequate intake results in characteristic deficiency signs and ultimately death. Table A1.2 @ lists the signs or symptoms of deficiency for each vitamin, its RDA or AI for young adults, and common food sources. The amount of each vitamin required in the diet is small (in the microgram or milligram range) compared to essential amino acid requirements (in the gram range). The vitamins are often divided into two classes: **water-soluble vitamins** and **fat-soluble vitamins** (**A**, **D**, **E**, and **K**). This classification has little relationship to their function but is related to the absorption and transport of fat-soluble vitamins with lipids.

Most vitamins are utilized for the synthesis of **coenzymes**, complex organic molecules that assist enzymes in catalyzing biochemical reactions, and the deficiency symptoms reflect an inability of cells to carry out certain reactions. However, some vitamins also act as hormones. We will consider the roles played by individual vitamins as we progress through the subsequent chapters of this text.

Vitamins, by definition, cannot be synthesized in the body or are synthesized from a very specific dietary precursor in insufficient amounts. For example, we can synthesize the vitamin niacin from the essential amino acid tryptophan but not in sufficient quantities to meet our needs. It is, therefore, still classified as a vitamin.

Excessive intake of many vitamins, both fat soluble and water soluble, may cause deleterious effects. For example, high doses of vitamin A, a fat-soluble vitamin, can cause desquamation of the skin and birth defects. High doses of vitamin C cause diarrhea and gastrointestinal disturbances. One of the Dietary Reference Intakes is the **Tolerable Upper Intake Level (UL)**, which is the highest level of daily nutrient intake that is likely to pose no risk of adverse effects to almost all individuals in the general population. As intake increases above the UL, the risk of adverse effects increases. Table A1.2 @ includes the UL for vitamins known to pose a risk at high levels. Intake above the UL occurs most often with dietary or pharmacologic supplements of single vitamins and not from foods.

## E. Minerals

Many **minerals** are required in the diet. They are generally divided into the classification of **electrolytes** (inorganic ions that are dissolved in the fluid compartments of the body), minerals (required in relatively large quantities), **trace minerals** (required in smaller quantities), and **ultratrace** minerals. Table A1.3 @ lists the minerals which fall into each group.

**Sodium** ($Na^+$), **potassium** ($K^+$), and **chloride** ($Cl^-$) are the major **electrolytes** (ions) in the body. They establish ion gradients across membranes, maintain water balance, and neutralize positive and negative charges on proteins and other molecules.

**Calcium** and **phosphorus** serve as structural components of bones and teeth and are thus required in relatively large quantities. Calcium ($Ca^{2+}$) plays many other roles in the body; for example, it is involved in hormone action and blood clotting. Phosphorus is required for the formation of ATP and of phosphorylated intermediates in metabolism. Magnesium activates many enzymes and also forms a complex with ATP. **Iron** is a particularly important mineral because it functions as a component of hemoglobin (the oxygen-carrying protein in the blood) and is part of many enzymes. Other minerals, such as **zinc** and **molybdenum**, are required in very small quantities (trace or ultratrace amounts).

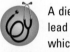 A dietary deficiency of calcium can lead to osteoporosis, a disease in which bones are insufficiently mineralized and consequently are fragile and easily fractured. Osteoporosis is a particularly common problem among elderly women. Deficiency of phosphorus results in bone loss along with weakness, anorexia, malaise, and pain. Iron deficiencies lead to anemia, a decrease in the concentration of hemoglobin in the blood.

Sulfur is ingested principally in the amino acids cysteine and methionine. It is found in connective tissue, particularly in cartilage and skin. It has important functions in metabolism, which we will describe when we consider the action of **Coenzyme A** (**CoA**), a compound used to activate carboxylic acids. Sulfur is excreted in the urine as sulfate.

Minerals, like vitamins, have adverse effects if ingested in excessive amounts. Problems associated with dietary excesses or deficiencies of minerals will be described in subsequent chapters in conjunction with their normal metabolic functions.

### F. Water

Water constitutes one-half to four-fifths of the weight of the human body. The intake of water required per day depends on the balance between the amount produced by body metabolism and the amount lost through the skin, through expired air, and in the urine and feces.

### G. Dietary Guidelines

Dietary guidelines or goals are recommendations for food choices that can reduce the risk of developing chronic or degenerative diseases while maintaining an adequate intake of nutrients. Many studies have shown an association between diet and exercise and decreased risk of certain diseases including hypertension, atherosclerosis, stroke, diabetes, certain types of cancer, and osteoarthritis. Thus, the American Heart Association and the American Cancer Society, as well as several other groups, have developed dietary and exercise recommendations to decrease the risk of these diseases. The *Dietary Guidelines for Americans* (2010), prepared under the joint authority of the U.S. Department of Agriculture (USDA) and the U.S. Department of Health and Human Services, merges many of these recommendations (see http://www.healthierus.gov/nutrition.html @ ). Issues of special concern for physicians who advise patients are included in the Appendix, Section A1.

### H. Xenobiotics

In addition to nutrients, our diet also contains a large number of chemicals called **xenobiotics** that have no nutritional value, are of no use in the body, and can be harmful if consumed in excessive amounts. These compounds occur naturally in foods, can enter the food chain as contaminants, or can be deliberately introduced as food additives.

Dietary guidelines of the American Cancer Society and the American Institute for Cancer Research make recommendations relevant to the ingestion of xenobiotic compounds, particularly carcinogens. The dietary advice that we eat a variety of food helps to protect us against the ingestion of a toxic level of any one xenobiotic compound (such as pesticides). It is also suggested that we reduce consumption of salt-cured, smoked, and charred foods, which contain chemicals that can contribute to the development of cancer (such as nitrites and benzopyrene). Other guidelines encourage ingestion of fruits and vegetables that contain protective chemicals called **antioxidants**.

## CLINICAL COMMENTS

A summary of the diseases discussed in this chapter is presented in Table 1.4.

**Ivan A.** Ivan was advised that his obesity represents a risk factor for future heart attacks and strokes. He was told that his body has to maintain a larger volume of circulating blood to service his extra fat tissue. This expanded blood volume not only contributes to his elevated blood pressure (itself a risk factor for vascular disease) but also puts an increased workload on his heart. This increased load will cause his heart muscle to thicken and eventually to fail.

**Table 1.4   Diseases and Disorders Discussed in Chapter 1**

| Disorder or Condition | Genetic or Environmental | Comments |
|---|---|---|
| Obesity | Both | Long-term effects of obesity affect the cardiovascular system and may lead to metabolic syndrome. |
| Anorexia | Environmental | Self-induced reduction of food intake, distorted body image, considered at least in part a psychiatric disorder |
| Kwashiorkor | Environmental | Protein and mineral deficiency yet normal amount of calories in the diet. Leads to marked hypo-albuminemia, anemia, edema, pot belly, loss of hair, and other indications of tissue injury. |
| Marasmus | Environmental | Prolonged calorie and protein malnutrition |
| Osteoporosis/osteomalacia | Environmental | Calcium-deficient diet leading to insufficient mineralization of the bones, which produces fragile and easily broken bones. |
| Type 2 diabetes mellitus | Both | Impaired response by tissues to insulin, resulting in hyperglycemia. |
| Hypercholesterolemia | Both | Elevated cholesterol due to mutation within a specific protein or excessive cholesterol intake. |
| Hyperlipidemia | Both | High levels of blood lipids may be due to mutations in specific proteins or ingestion of high-fat diets. |
| Malnutrition | Both | Reduced nutrient uptake may be due to genetic mutation in specific proteins or dietary habit. May lead to increased ketone body production and reduced liver protein synthesis. |

*Note.* Diseases which may have a genetic component are indicated as genetic; disorders due to environmental factors (with or without genetic influences) are indicated as environmental.

Cholesterol is obtained from the diet and synthesized in most cells of the body. It is a component of cell membranes and the precursor of steroid hormones and of the bile salts used for fat absorption. High concentrations of cholesterol in the blood, particularly the cholesterol in lipoprotein particles called low density lipoproteins (LDL), contribute to the formation of atherosclerotic plaques. These plaques (fatty deposits within arterial walls) are associated with heart attacks and strokes. A high content of saturated fat in the diet tends to increase circulatory levels of LDL cholesterol and contributes to the development of atherosclerosis.

Mr. A.'s increasing adipose mass has also contributed to his development of type 2 diabetes mellitus characterized by hyperglycemia (high blood glucose levels). The mechanism behind this breakdown in his ability to maintain normal levels of blood glucose is, at least in part, a resistance by his triacylglycerol-rich adipose cells to the action of insulin.

In addition to type 2 diabetes mellitus, Mr. A. has a hyperlipidemia (high blood lipid level—elevated cholesterol and triacylglycerol), another risk factor for cardiovascular disease. A genetic basis for Mr. A.'s disorder is inferred from a positive family history of hypercholesterolemia and premature coronary artery disease in a brother.

At this point, the first therapeutic steps should be nonpharmacologic. Mr. A.'s obesity should be treated with caloric restriction and a carefully monitored program of exercise. A reduction of dietary fat and sodium would be advised in an effort to correct his hyperlipidemia and his hypertension, respectively. He should also monitor his carbohydrate intake because of his type 2 diabetes. The body can make fatty acids from a caloric excess of carbohydrate and proteins. These fatty acids, together with the fatty acids of chylomicrons (derived from dietary fat), are deposited in adipose tissue as triacylglycerols. Thus, Ivan's increased adipose tissue is coming from his intake of all fuels in excess of his caloric need.

It was also noted that **Ivan**'s waist circumference indicates he has the android pattern of obesity (apple shape). Fat stores are distributed in the body in two different patterns: android and gynecoid. After puberty, men tend to store fat in and on their abdomens and upper body (an android pattern) while women tend to store fat around their breasts, hips, and thighs (a gynecoid pattern). Thus, the typical overweight male tends to have more of an apple shape than the typical overweight female who is more pear shaped. Abdominal fat carries a greater risk for hypertension, cardiovascular disease, hyperinsulinemia, diabetes mellitus, gallbladder disease, stroke, and cancer of the breast and endometrium. It also carries a greater risk of overall mortality. Because more men than women have the android distribution, they are more at risk for most of these conditions. Likewise, women who deposit their excess fat in a more android manner have a greater risk than women whose fat distribution is more gynecoid.

**Ann R.** Ann R. has anorexia nervosa, a chronic disabling disease in which poorly understood psychological and biological factors lead to disturbances in the patient's body image. These patients typically pursue thinness in spite of the presence of severe emaciation and a "skeletal appearance."

They generally have an intense fear of being overweight and deny the seriousness of their low body weight.

Amenorrhea (lack of menses) usually develops during anorexia nervosa and other conditions when a woman's body fat content falls to about 22% of her total body weight. The immediate cause of amenorrhea is a reduced production of the gonadotropic protein hormones (luteinizing hormone and follicle-stimulating hormone) by the anterior pituitary; the connection between this hormonal change and body fat content is not yet understood.

Ms. R. is suffering from the consequences of prolonged and severe protein and caloric restriction. Fatty acids, released from adipose tissue by lipolysis, are being converted to ketone bodies in the liver, and the level of ketone bodies in the blood is extremely elevated (4,200 μM vs. normal of 70 μM). The fact that her kidneys are excreting ketone bodies is reflected in the moderately positive urine test for ketone bodies noted on admission.

Although Ms. R.'s blood glucose is below the normal fasting range (65 mg/dL vs. normal of 80 mg/dL), she is experiencing only a moderate degree of hypoglycemia (low blood glucose) despite her severe, near starvation diet. Her blood glucose level reflects the ability of the brain to utilize ketone bodies as a fuel when they are elevated in the blood, thereby decreasing the amount of glucose that must be synthesized from amino acids provided by protein degradation.

Ms. R.'s BMI shows that she is close to death through starvation. She was, therefore, hospitalized and placed on enteral nutrition (nutrients provided through tube feeding). The general therapeutic plan of nutritional restitution and identification and treatment of those emotional factors leading to the patient's anorectic behavior was continued. As a consequence of her treatment, she was able to eat small amounts of food while hospitalized.

 **Otto S.**  Mr. S. sought help in reducing his weight of 187 lb (BMI of 27) to his previous level of 154 lb (BMI of 22, in the middle of the healthy range). Otto is 5 feet 10 inches tall, and he calculated that his maximum healthy weight was 173 lb. He planned on becoming a family physician and knew that he would be better able to counsel patients in healthy behaviors involving diet and exercise if he practiced them himself. With this information and assurances from the physician that he was otherwise in good health, Otto embarked on a weight loss program. One of his strategies involved recording all the food he ate and the proportions. To analyze his diet for calories, saturated fat, and nutrients, he used the MyPlate web site (www.choosemyplate.gov) available online from the USDA Food and Nutrition Information Center.

 When a patient develops a metabolic problem, it is difficult to examine cells to determine the cause. In order to obtain tissue for metabolic studies, biopsies must be performed. These procedures can be difficult, dangerous, or even impossible, depending on the tissue. Cost is an additional problem. However, both blood and urine can readily be obtained from patients, and measurements of substances in the blood and urine can help in diagnosing a patient's problem. Concentrations of substances that are higher or lower than normal indicate which tissues are malfunctioning. For example, if high levels of ketone bodies are found in the blood or urine, the patient's metabolic pattern is that of the starved state. If the high levels of ketone bodies are coupled with elevated levels of blood glucose, the problem is most likely a deficiency of insulin; that is, the patient probably has type 1 diabetes mellitus (these patients are usually young). Without insulin, fuels are mobilized from tissues rather than being stored.

These relatively easy and inexpensive tests on blood and urine can be used to determine which tissues need to be studied more extensively to diagnose and treat the patient's problem. A solid understanding of fuel metabolism helps in the interpretation of these simple tests.

## REVIEW QUESTIONS-CHAPTER 1

1. Which one of the following occurs to fuels in the process of respiration?
    A. They are stored as triacylglycerols.
    B. They release energy principally as heat.
    C. They combine with $CO_2$ and $H_2O$.
    D. They are oxidized to generate ATP.
    E. They combine with other dietary components in anabolic pathways.

2. The resting metabolic rate (RMR) is best described by which one of the following?
    A. It is equivalent to the caloric requirement of our major organs and resting muscle.
    B. It is generally higher per kilogram body weight in women than in men.
    C. It is generally lower per kilogram body weight in children than adults.
    D. It is decreased in a cold environment.
    E. It is approximately equivalent to the daily energy expenditure

3. Which one of the following will occur after digestion of a high-carbohydrate meal?

   A. Glucagon is released from the pancreas.
   B. Insulin stimulates the transport of glucose into the brain.
   C. Skeletal muscles convert glucose to fatty acids.
   D. Red cells oxidize glucose to $CO_2$.
   E. Adipose tissue and skeletal muscle will use glucose as their major fuel.

4. Which one of the following is most likely to occur 24 to 30 hours after a fast is initiated?

   A. Muscle glycogenolysis provides glucose to the blood.
   B. Gluconeogenesis in the liver will become the major source of blood glucose.
   C. Muscle converts amino acids to blood glucose.
   D. Fatty acids released from adipose tissue provide carbon for synthesis of glucose.
   E. Ketone bodies provide carbon for gluconeogenesis.

5. Jim Smith, an overweight medical student, discovered he could not exercise enough during his summer clerkship rotations to lose 2 to 3 lb/week. He decided to lose weight by eating only 300 kcal/day of a dietary supplement that provided half the calories as carbohydrate and half as protein. In addition, he consumed a multivitamin supplement. Which one of the following is most likely to occur during the first 7 days on this diet?

   A. His protein intake will have met the RDA for protein.
   B. His carbohydrate intake will have met the fuel needs of his brain.
   C. He will remain in nitrogen balance.
   D. He will have developed severe hypoglycemia.
   E. Both his adipose mass and his muscle mass will be decreased.

# 2 Water, Acids, Bases, and Buffers

## CHAPTER OUTLINE

**I. WATER**
- A. Fluid compartments in the body
- B. Hydrogen bonds in water
- C. Electrolytes
- D. Osmolality and water movement

**II. ACIDS AND BASES**
- A. The pH of water
- B. Strong and weak acids

**III. BUFFERS**

**IV. METABOLIC ACIDS AND BUFFERS**
- A. The bicarbonate buffer system
- B. Bicarbonate and hemoglobin in the red blood cell
- C. Intracellular pH
- D. Urinary hydrogen, ammonium, and phosphate ions
- E. Hydrochloric acid

## KEY POINTS

- Approximately 60% of our body is water.
- Water is distributed between intracellular and extracellular (interstitial fluids, blood, lymph) compartments.
- Because water is a dipolar molecule with an uneven distribution of electrons between the hydrogen and oxygen atoms, it forms hydrogen bonds with other polar molecules and acts as a solvent.
- Many of the compounds produced in the body and dissolved in water contain chemical groups that act as acids or bases, releasing or accepting hydrogen ions.
- The hydrogen ion content and the amount of body water are controlled to maintain homeostasis, a constant environment for the cells.
- The pH of a solution is the negative log of its hydrogen ion concentration.
- Acids release hydrogen ions; bases accept hydrogen ions.
- Strong acids dissociate completely in water, whereas only a small percentage of the total molecules of a weak acid dissociate.
- The dissociation constant of a weak acid is designated as $K_a$.
- The Henderson-Hasselbalch equation defines the relationship between the pH of a solution, the $K_a$ of an acid, and the extent of the acid dissociation.
- A buffer, a mixture of an undissociated acid and its conjugate base, resists changes in pH when either $H^+$ or $OH^-$ is added.
- Buffers work best within a range of 1 pH unit either above or below the $pK_a$ of the buffer, where the $pK_a$ is the negative log of the $K_a$.
- Normal metabolism generates metabolic acids (lactate, ketone bodies), inorganic acids (sulfuric acid, hydrochloric acid), and carbon dioxide.
- Carbon dioxide reacts with water to form carbonic acid.
- Physiological buffers include bicarbonate, phosphate, and the protein hemoglobin.

# THE WAITING ROOM

**Di A.** has ketoacidosis. When the amount of insulin she injects is inadequate, she remains in a condition similar to a fasting state even though she ingests food (see Chapter 1). Her liver continues to metabolize fatty acids to the ketone bodies acetoacetic acid and β-hydroxybutyric acid. These compounds are weak acids that dissociate to produce anions (acetoacetate and β-hydroxybutyrate, respectively) and hydrogen ions, thereby lowering her blood and cellular pH below the normal range.

**Dianne (Di) A.** is a 26-year-old woman who was diagnosed with type 1 diabetes mellitus at the age of 12 years. She has an absolute insulin deficiency resulting from autoimmune destruction of the β-cells of her pancreas. As a result, she depends on daily injections of insulin to prevent severe elevations of glucose and ketone bodies in her blood. When **Di A.** could not be aroused from an afternoon nap, her roommate called an ambulance, and Di was brought to the emergency department of the hospital in a coma. Her roommate reported that Di had been feeling nauseated and drowsy and had been vomiting for 24 hours. Di is clinically dehydrated and her blood pressure is low. Her respirations are deep and rapid, and her pulse rate is rapid. Her breath has the "fruity" odor of acetone.

Blood samples are drawn for measurement of her arterial blood pH, arterial partial pressure of carbon dioxide ($PaCO_2$), serum glucose, and serum bicarbonate ($HCO_3^-$). In addition, serum and urine are tested for the presence of ketone bodies, and Di is treated with intravenous normal saline and insulin. The lab reports that her blood pH is 7.08 (reference range 7.36 to 7.44) and that ketone bodies are present in both blood and urine. Her blood glucose level is 648 mg/dL (reference range = 80 to 110 mg/dL after an overnight fast and no higher than 200 mg/dL in a casual glucose sample taken without regard to the time of a last meal).

**Dennis V.**, age 3 years, was brought to the emergency department by his grandfather, **Percy V.** While Dennis was visiting his grandfather, he climbed up on a chair and took a half-full 500-tablet bottle of 325-mg aspirin (acetylsalicylic acid) tablets from the kitchen counter. Mr. V. discovered Dennis with a mouthful of aspirin, which he removed, but he could not tell how many tablets Dennis had already swallowed. Although Dennis was acting bright and alert, Mr. V. rushed Dennis to the hospital.

## I.  WATER

Water is the solvent of life. It bathes our cells, dissolves and transports compounds in the blood, provides a medium for movement of molecules into and throughout cellular compartments, separates charged molecules, dissipates heat, and participates in chemical reactions. Most compounds in the body, including proteins, must interact with an aqueous medium in order to function. In spite of the variation in the amount of water we ingest each day and produce from metabolism, our body maintains a nearly constant amount of water that is about 50% to 60% of our body weight (Fig. 2.1).

### A.  Fluid Compartments in the Body

Total body water is about 50% to 60% of body weight in adults and about 75% of body weight in children. Because fat has relatively little water associated with it, obese people tend to have a lower percentage of body water than thin people, females tend to have a lower percentage than males, and older people have a lower percentage than younger people.

Approximately 60% of the total body water is intracellular and 40% extracellular. The extracellular water includes the fluid in plasma (blood after the cells have been removed) and interstitial water (the fluid in the tissue spaces, lying between cells). Transcellular water is a small, specialized portion of extracellular water that includes gastrointestinal secretions, urine, sweat, and fluid that has leaked through capillary walls due to such processes as increased hydrostatic pressure or inflammation.

**A. Total body water**

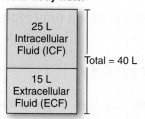

**B. Extracellular fluid**

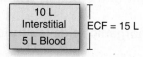

*FIG. 2.1.* **A,B.** Fluid compartments in the body based on an average 70-kg male.

## B. Hydrogen Bonds in Water

The dipolar nature of the water ($H_2O$) molecule allows it to form hydrogen bonds, a property that is responsible for the role of water as a solvent. In $H_2O$, the oxygen atom has two unshared electrons that form an electron-dense cloud around it. This cloud lies above and below the plane formed by the water molecule (Fig. 2.2). In the covalent bond formed between the hydrogen and oxygen atoms, the shared electrons are attracted toward the oxygen atom, which gives the oxygen atom a partial negative charge and the hydrogen atom a partial positive charge. As a result, the oxygen side of the molecule is much more electronegative than the hydrogen side, creating a dipolar molecule.

Both the hydrogen and oxygen atoms of the water molecule form hydrogen bonds and participate in hydration shells. A hydrogen bond is a weak noncovalent interaction between the hydrogen of one molecule and the more electronegative atom of an acceptor molecule. The oxygen of water can form hydrogen bonds with two other water molecules, so that each water molecule is hydrogen-bonded to about four close neighboring water molecules in a fluid three-dimensional lattice (see Fig. 2.2).

Polar organic molecules and inorganic salts can readily dissolve in water because water also forms hydrogen bonds and electrostatic interactions with these molecules. Organic molecules containing a high proportion of electronegative atoms (generally oxygen or nitrogen) are soluble in water because these atoms participate in hydrogen bonding with water molecules (Fig. 2.3). Chloride ($Cl^-$), bicarbonate ($HCO_3^-$), and other anions are surrounded by a hydration shell of water molecules arranged with their hydrogen atoms closest to the anion. In a similar fashion, the oxygen atom of water molecules interacts with inorganic cations like $Na^+$ and $K^+$ to surround them with a hydration shell.

Although hydrogen bonds are strong enough to dissolve polar molecules in water and to separate charges, they are weak enough to allow movement of water and solutes. The strength of the hydrogen bond between two water molecules is only around 4 kcal/mole, about one-twentieth of the strength of the covalent O—H bond in the water molecule. Thus, the extensive water lattice is dynamic and has many strained bonds that are continuously breaking and reforming. As a result, hydrogen bonds between water molecules and polar solutes continuously dissociate and reform, thereby permitting solutes to move through water and water to pass through channels in cellular membranes.

## C. Electrolytes

Both extracellular fluid (ECF) and intracellular fluid (ICF) contain **electrolytes**, a general term applied to bicarbonate and inorganic anions and cations. The electrolytes are unevenly distributed between compartments; $Na^+$ and $Cl^-$ are the major electrolytes in the ECF (plasma and interstitial fluid), and $K^+$ and phosphates such as $HPO_4^{-2}$ are the major electrolytes in cells (Table 2.1). This distribution is maintained principally by energy-requiring transporters which pump $Na^+$ out of cells in exchange for $K^+$ (see Chapter 8).

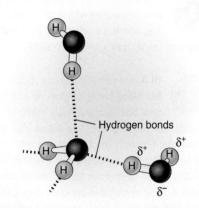

*FIG. 2.2.* Hydrogen bonds between water molecules. The oxygen atoms are shown in *black*.

The structure of water also allows it to resist temperature change. Its heat of fusion is high, so it takes a large drop in temperature to convert liquid water to the solid state, ice. The thermal conductivity of water is also high, thereby facilitating heat dissipation from high energy-using areas like the brain into the blood and the total body water pool. Its heat capacity and heat of vaporization are remarkably high, so that as liquid water is converted to a gas and evaporates from the skin, we feel a cooling effect. Water responds to the input of heat by decreasing the extent of hydrogen bonding and to cooling by increasing the bonding between water molecules.

**Table 2.1    Distribution of Ions in Body Fluids**

|  | ECF* mmol/L | ICF |
|---|---|---|
| Cations |  |  |
| Na$^+$ | 145 | 12 |
| K$^+$ | 4 | 150 |
| Anions |  |  |
| Cl$^-$ | 105 | 5 |
| HCO$_3^-$ | 25 | 12 |
| Inorganic Phosphate | 2 | 100 |

*The content of inorganic ions is very similar in plasma and interstitial fluid, the two components of the extracellular fluid. ECF, extracellular fluid; ICF, intracellular fluid.

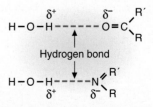

*FIG. 2.3.* Hydrogen bonds between water and polar molecules. *R* denotes additional atoms.

In the emergency department, **Di A.** was rehydrated with intravenous saline, which is a solution of 0.9% NaCl. Why was saline used instead of water?

**Di A.** has osmotic diuresis. Because her blood levels of glucose and ketone bodies are so high, these compounds are passing from the blood into the glomerular filtrate in the kidneys and then into the urine. As a consequence of the high osmolality of the glomerular filtrate, much more water is being excreted in the urine than usual. Thus, Di has polyuria (increased urine volume). As a result of water lost from the blood into the urine, water passes from inside cells into the interstitial space surrounding those cells and then moves into the blood, resulting in an intracellular dehydration. The dehydrated cells in the brain are unable to carry out their normal functions. The result is that Di is in a coma.

## D.  Osmolality and Water Movement

Water is distributed between the different fluid compartments according to the concentration of solutes, or osmolality, of each compartment. The **osmolality** of a fluid is proportionate to the total concentration of all dissolved molecules including ions, organic metabolites, and proteins (usually expressed as milliosmoles per kilogram of water). The semipermeable cellular membrane that separates the extracellular and intracellular compartments contains a number of ion channels through which water, but not other molecules, can freely move. Likewise, water can freely move through the capillaries separating the interstitial fluid and the plasma. As a result, water will move from a compartment with a low concentration of solutes (lower osmolality) to one with a higher concentration to achieve an equal osmolality on both sides of the membrane. The force it would take to keep water from moving across the membrane under these conditions is called the **osmotic pressure**.

As water is lost from one fluid compartment, it is replaced with water from another to maintain a nearly constant osmolality. The blood contains a high content of dissolved negatively charged proteins and the electrolytes needed to balance these charges. As water is passed from the blood into the urine to balance the excretion of ions, the blood volume is replenished with water from interstitial fluid. When the osmolality of the blood and interstitial fluid is too high, water moves out of the cells. The loss of cellular water can also occur in hyperglycemia (high blood glucose levels), because the high concentration of glucose increases the osmolality of the blood.

## II.  ACIDS AND BASES

**Acids** are compounds that donate a hydrogen ion ($H^+$) to a solution, and **bases** are compounds (like the $OH^-$ ion) that accept hydrogen ions. Water itself dissociates to a slight extent, generating hydrogen ions ($H^+$), which are also called protons, and hydroxide ions ($OH^-$). An acid can also be defined as a substance that accepts a pair of electrons to form a covalent bond, whereas bases are substances which can donate a pair of electrons to form a covalent bond.

### A.  The pH of Water

The extent of dissociation by water molecules into $H^+$ and $OH^-$ is very slight, and the hydrogen ion concentration of pure water is only 0.0000001 M, or $10^{-7}$ mol/L. The concentration of hydrogen ions in a solution is usually denoted by the term **pH**, which is the negative $\log_{10}$ of the hydrogen ion concentration expressed in moles per liter (Equation 2.1). Therefore, the pH of pure water is 7.

#### Equation 2.1. Definition of pH

$$pH = -\log [H^+]$$

The dissociation constant for water, $K_d$, expresses the relationship between the hydrogen ion concentration [$H^+$], the hydroxide ion concentration [$OH^-$], and the concentration of water [$H_2O$] at equilibrium (Equation 2.2). Because water dissociates to such a small extent, [$H_2O$] is essentially constant at 55.5 mol/L. Multiplication of the $K_d$ for water (about $1.8 \times 10^{-16}$ mol/L) by 55.5 mol/L gives a value of about $10^{-14}$ $(mol/L)^2$, which is called the ion product of water ($K_w$) (Equation 2.3) . Because $K_w$, the product of [$H^+$] and [$OH^-$], is always constant, a decrease of [$H^+$] must be accompanied by a proportionate increase of [$OH^-$].

A pH of 7 is termed neutral because [$H^+$] and [$OH^-$] are equal. Acidic solutions have a greater hydrogen ion concentration and a lower hydroxide ion concentration than pure water (pH <7.0), and basic solutions have a lower hydrogen ion concentration and a greater hydroxide ion concentration (pH >7.0).

#### Equation 2.2. Dissociation of water

$$K_d = \frac{[H^+][OH^-]}{[H_2O]}$$

#### Equation 2.3. The ion product of water

$$K_w = [H^+][OH^-] = 1 \times 10^{-14}$$

### B.  Strong and Weak Acids

During metabolism, the body produces a number of acids that increase the hydrogen ion concentration of the blood or other body fluids and tend to lower the pH (for examples, see Table A2.1 @ ). These metabolically important acids can be classified

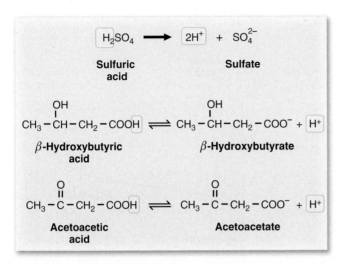

**FIG. 2.4.** Dissociation of acids. Sulfuric acid is a strong acid that dissociates into $H^+$ ions and sulfate. The ketone bodies acetoacetic acid and β-hydroxybutyric acid are weak acids that partially dissociate into $H^+$ and their conjugate bases.

 A 0.9% NaCl solution is 0.9 g NaCl/100 mL, equivalent to 9 g/L. NaCl has a molecular weight of 58 g/mole, so the concentration of NaCl in isotonic saline is 0.155 M, or 155 mM. If all of the NaCl were dissociated into $Na^+$ and $Cl^-$ ions, the osmolality would be 310 mOsm/kg of water. Because NaCl is not completely dissociated and some of the hydration shells surround undissociated NaCl molecules, the osmolality of isotonic saline is about 290 mOsm/kg of water. The osmolality of plasma, interstitial fluids, and intracellular fluids is also about 290 mOsm/kg of water, so that no large shifts of water or swelling occur when isotonic saline is given intravenously.

as weak acids or strong acids by their degree of dissociation into a hydrogen ion and a base (the anion component). Inorganic acids such as sulfuric acid ($H_2SO_4$) and hydrochloric acid (HCl) are strong acids that dissociate completely in solution (Fig. 2.4). Organic acids containing carboxylic acid groups (e.g., the ketone bodies acetoacetic acid and β-hydroxybutyric acid) are weak acids that dissociate in water only to a limited extent. In general, a weak acid (HA), called the **conjugate acid**, dissociates into a hydrogen ion and an anionic component ($A^-$), called the **conjugate base**. The name of an undissociated acid usually ends in "-ic acid" (e.g., acetoacetic acid) and the name of the dissociated anionic component ends in "-ate" (e.g., acetoacetate).

The tendency of the acid (HA) to dissociate and donate a hydrogen ion to solution is denoted by its $K_a$, the equilibrium constant for dissociation of a weak acid (Equation 2.4). The higher the $K_a$, the greater the tendency to dissociate a proton, therefore the stronger the acid.

In the **Henderson-Hasselbalch equation**, the formula for the dissociation constant of a weak acid is converted to a convenient logarithmic equation (Equation 2.5). The term $pK_a$ represents the negative log of $K_a$. If the $pK_a$ for a weak acid is known, this equation can be used to calculate the ratio of the unprotonated to the protonated form at any pH. From this equation, you can see that a weak acid will be 50% dissociated at a pH equal to its $pK_a$.

Most metabolic carboxylic acids have a $pK_a$ between 2 and 5, depending on the other groups on the molecule. The $pK_a$ reflects the strength of an acid. Acids with a $pK_a$ of 2 are stronger acids than those with a $pK_a$ of 5 because, at any pH, a greater proportion is dissociated.

*Equation 2.4. The $K_{acid}$*

For the reaction

$$HA \leftrightarrow A^- + H^+$$

$$K_a = \frac{[H^+][A^-]}{HA}$$

*Equation 2.5.*
*The Henderson-Hasselbalch equation*

$$pH = pK_a + \log\frac{[A^-]}{[HA]}$$

## III. BUFFERS

**Buffers** consist of a weak acid and its conjugate base. They cause a solution to resist changes in pH when hydrogen ions or hydroxide ions are added. In Figure 2.5, the pH of a solution of the weak acid acetic acid is graphed as a function of the amount of $OH^-$ that has been added. The $OH^-$ is expressed as equivalents of total acetic acid present in the dissociated and undissociated forms. At the midpoint of this curve, 0.5 equivalent of $OH^-$ has been added and one-half of the conjugate acid has dissociated, so that $[A^-]$ equals [HA] (the $pK_a$ has been obtained). As you add more $OH^-$ ions and move to the right on the curve, more of the conjugate acid (HA) molecules dissociate to generate $H^+$ ions, which combine with the added $OH^-$ ions

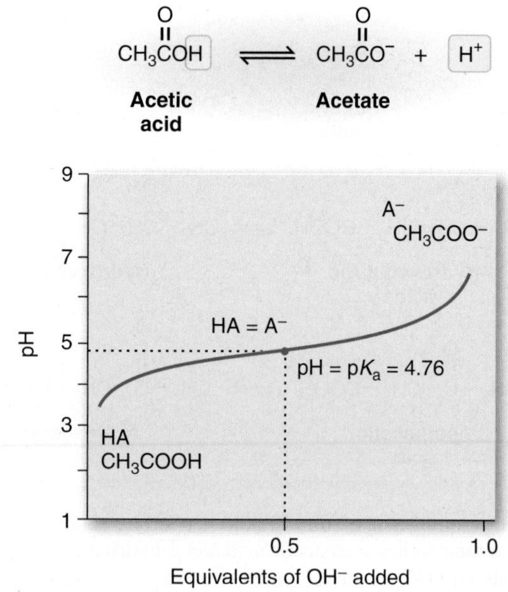

$$CH_3\overset{\overset{\displaystyle O}{\|}}{C}OH \rightleftharpoons CH_3\overset{\overset{\displaystyle O}{\|}}{C}O^- + \boxed{H^+}$$

**Acetic**       **Acetate**
**acid**

**FIG. 2.5.** Titration curve for acetic acid.

**Dennis V.** has ingested an unknown number of acetylsalicylic acid (aspirin) tablets. Acetylsalicylic acid is rapidly converted to salicylic acid in the body. The initial effect of aspirin is to induce an alkalosis caused by an effect on the hypothalamus that increases the rate of breathing and the expiration of $CO_2$. As the $CO_2$ levels drop, $HCO_3^-$ combines with a proton to form $H_2CO_3$, which is converted to $CO_2$ and $H_2O$. The decrease in proton concentration leads to the initial alkalosis. This is followed by a complex metabolic acidosis (a lowering of fluid pH) caused partly by the dissociation of salicylic acid (salicylic acid $\leftrightarrow$ salicylate$^-$ + $H^+$, $pK_a$ about 3.5). Salicylate also interferes with mitochondrial ATP production (acting as an uncoupler, see Chapter 18), resulting in increased generation of $CO_2$ and accumulation of lactate (due to stimulation of glycolysis, see Chapter 19) and other organic acids in the blood. Subsequently, salicylate may impair renal function, resulting in the accumulation of strong acids of metabolic origin, such as sulfuric acid and phosphoric acid. Usually, children who ingest toxic amounts of aspirin are acidotic by the time they arrive in the emergency department.

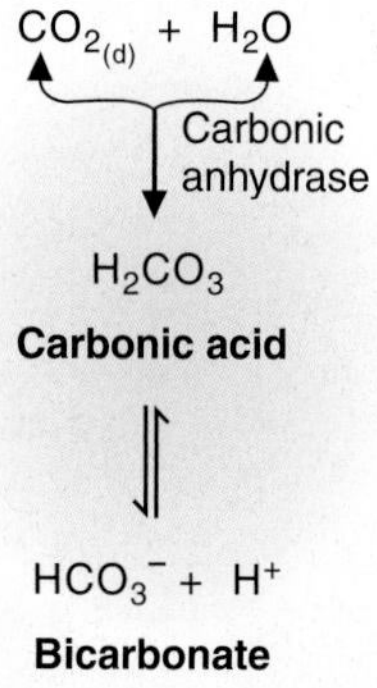

**FIG. 2.6.** The bicarbonate buffer system. $CO_{2(d)}$ refers to carbon dioxide dissolved in water and not in the gaseous state.

to form water. Consequently, there is little increase in pH. If you add hydrogen ions to the buffer at its $pK_a$ (moving to the left of the midpoint in Fig. 2.5), conjugate base molecules ($A^-$) combine with the added hydrogen ions to form HA, and there is almost no fall of pH.

As can be seen from Figure 2.5, a buffer can only compensate for an influx or removal of hydrogen ions within about 1 pH unit of its $pK_a$. As the pH of a buffered solution changes from the $pK_a$ to one pH unit below the $pK_a$, the ratio of $[A^-]$ to HA changes from 1:1 to 1:10. If more hydrogen ions were added, the pH would fall rapidly because there is relatively little conjugate base remaining. Likewise, at one pH unit above the $pK_a$ of a buffer, relatively little undissociated acid remains. More concentrated buffers are more effective simply because they contain a greater total number of buffer molecules per unit volume that can dissociate or recombine with hydrogen ions.

## IV. METABOLIC ACIDS AND BUFFERS

An average rate of metabolic activity produces about 22,000 mEq of acid per day. If all of this acid were dissolved at one time in unbuffered body fluids, their pH would be less than 1. However, the pH of the blood is normally maintained between 7.36 and 7.44 and intracellular pH around 7.1 (between 6.9 and 7.4). The widest range of extracellular pH over which the metabolic functions of the liver, the beating of the heart, and conduction of neural impulses can be maintained is 6.8 to 7.8. Thus, until the acid produced from metabolism can be excreted as $CO_2$ in expired air and as ions in the urine, it needs to be buffered in the body fluids. The major buffer systems in the body are the bicarbonate–carbonic acid buffer system, which operates principally in ECF; the hemoglobin buffer system in red blood cells; the phosphate buffer system in all types of cells; and the protein buffer system of cells and plasma.

## A. The Bicarbonate Buffer System

The major source of metabolic acid in the body is the gas $CO_2$, produced principally from fuel oxidation in the tricarboxylic acid (TCA) cycle. Under normal metabolic conditions, the body generates over 13 moles of $CO_2$ per day (about 0.5 to 1 kg). $CO_2$ dissolves in water and reacts with water to produce carbonic acid, $H_2CO_3$, a reaction accelerated by the enzyme carbonic anhydrase (Fig. 2.6). Carbonic acid is a weak acid that partially dissociates into $H^+$ and bicarbonate anion, $HCO_3^-$.

Carbonic acid is both the major acid produced by the body and its own buffer. The $pK_a$ of carbonic acid itself is only 3.8, so at the blood pH of 7.4, it is almost completely dissociated and theoretically unable to buffer and generate bicarbonate. However, carbonic acid can be replenished from $CO_2$ in body fluids and air because the concentration of dissolved $CO_2$ in body fluids is about 500 times greater than that of carbonic acid. As the concentration of base is increased in body fluids and $H^+$ is removed, $H_2CO_3$ dissociates into hydrogen and bicarbonate ions, forcing dissolved $CO_2$ to react with $H_2O$ to replenish the $H_2CO_3$ (see Fig. 2.6). Dissolved $CO_2$ is in equilibrium with the $CO_2$ in air in the alveoli of the lungs, and thus the availability of $CO_2$ can be increased or decreased by an adjustment in the rate of breathing and the amount of $CO_2$ expired. The $pK_a$ for the bicarbonate buffer system in the body thus combines $K_h$ (the hydration constant for the reaction of water and $CO_2$ to form $H_2CO_3$) with the chemical $pK_a$ to obtain the value of 6.1 used in the Henderson-Hasselbalch equation (Equation 2.6). In the clinical setting, the dissolved $CO_2$ is expressed as a fraction of the partial pressure of $CO_2$ in arterial blood, $PaCO_2$.

The respiratory center within the hypothalamus that controls the rate of breathing is sensitive to changes in pH. As the pH falls, individuals breathe more rapidly and expire more $CO_2$. As the pH rises, they breathe more shallowly. Thus, the rate of breathing contributes to regulation of pH through its effects on the dissolved $CO_2$ content of the blood.

## B. Bicarbonate and Hemoglobin in the Red Blood Cell

The bicarbonate buffer system and hemoglobin in red blood cells cooperate in buffering the blood and transporting $CO_2$ to the lungs. Most of the $CO_2$ produced from tissue metabolism in the TCA cycle diffuses into the interstitial fluid, then into the blood plasma, and then into red blood cells (Fig. 2.7, *circle 1*). Although there is no carbonic anhydrase in blood plasma or interstitial fluid, the red blood cells contain high amounts of this enzyme, and $CO_2$ is rapidly converted to carbonic acid ($H_2CO_3$) within these cells (*circle 2*). As the carbonic acid dissociates (*circle 3*), the $H^+$ released is also buffered by combination with certain amino acid side chains in hemoglobin (Hb, *circle 4*). The bicarbonate anion is transported out of the red blood cell into the blood in exchange for chloride anion, and thus bicarbonate is relatively high in the plasma (*circle 5*) (see Table 2.1).

As the red blood cell approaches the lungs, the direction of the equilibrium reverses. $CO_2$ is released from the red blood cell, causing more carbonic acid to dissociate into $CO_2$ and water and more hydrogen ions to combine with bicarbonate. Hemoglobin loses some of its hydrogen ions, a feature that allows it to bind oxygen more readily (see Chapter 5). Thus, the bicarbonate buffer system is intimately linked to the delivery of oxygen to tissues.

Bicarbonate and carbonic acid, which diffuse through the capillary wall from the blood into interstitial fluid, provide a major buffer for both plasma and interstitial fluid. However, blood differs from interstitial fluid in that the blood contains a high content of extracellular proteins, such as albumin, which contribute to its buffering capacity through amino acid side chains that are able to accept and release protons. The protein content of interstitial fluid is too low to serve as an effective buffer.

## C. Intracellular pH

Phosphate anions and proteins are the major buffers involved in maintaining a constant pH of ICF. The inorganic phosphate anion $H_2PO_4^-$ dissociates to generate $H^+$ and the conjugate base, $HPO_4^{-2}$, with a $pK_a$ of 7.2 (see Fig. 2.7, *circle 6*). Thus, phosphate anions play a major role as an intracellular buffer in the red blood cell and in other types of cells, where their concentration is much higher than in blood and interstitial fluid (See Table 2.1, extracellular fluid). Organic phosphate anions, such as glucose-6-phosphate and adenosine triphosphate (ATP), also act as buffers. ICF contains a high content of proteins that contain histidine and other amino acids that can accept protons in a fashion similar to hemoglobin (see Fig. 2.7, *circle 7*).

The $pK_a$ for dissociation of bicarbonate anion ($HCO_3^-$) into $H^+$ and carbonate ($CO_3^{-2}$) is 9.8, so that only trace amounts of carbonate exist in body fluids.

***Equation 2.6. The Henderson-Hasselbalch equation for the bicarbonate buffer system***

$$pH = pK_a + \log\frac{[HCO_3^-]}{[H_2CO_3]}$$

The $pK_a = 3.5$, so

$$pH = 3.5 + \log\frac{[HCO_3^-]}{[H_2CO_3]}$$

$[H_2CO_3]$ is best estimated as $[CO_2]_d/400$, where $[CO_2]_d$ is the concentration of dissolved $CO_2$, so substituting this value for $[H_2CO_3]$ we get

$$pH = 3.5 + \log 400 + \log\frac{[HCO_3^-]}{[CO_2]_d}$$

or

$$pH = 6.1 + \log\frac{[HCO_3^-]}{[CO_2]_d}$$

Because only 3% of the gaseous $CO_2$ is dissolved, $[CO_2]_d = 0.03\ PaCO_2$, so

$$pH = 6.1 + \log\frac{[HCO_3^-]}{0.03\ PaCO_2}$$

The $HCO_3^-$ is expressed as milliequivalents per milliliter (mEq/mL) and $PaCO_2$ as millimeters of mercury (mm Hg).

The partial pressure of $CO_2$ ($PaCO_2$) in **Di A.'s** arterial blood was 28 mm Hg (reference range = 37 to 43), and her serum bicarbonate level was 8 mEq/L (reference range = 24 to 28). Elevated levels of ketone bodies had produced a ketoacidosis, and **Di A.** was exhaling increased amounts of $CO_2$ by breathing deeply and frequently (Kussmaul breathing) to compensate. Why does this occur? Ketone bodies are weak acids that partially dissociate, increasing $H^+$ levels in the blood and the interstitial fluid surrounding the metabolic respiratory center in the hypothalamus that controls the rate of breathing. A drop in pH elicits an increase in the rate of breathing. Bicarbonate combines with protons, producing $H_2CO_3$, thereby lowering bicarbonate levels. The $H_2CO_3$ is converted to $CO_2$ and $H_2O$, which increases the $CO_2$ concentration which is exhaled. This increase in the $CO_2$ concentration leads to an increase in the respiratory rate, causing a fall in the partial pressure of arterial $CO_2$ ($PaCO_2$). As shown by Di's low arterial blood pH of 7.08, the Kussmaul breathing was unable to fully compensate for the high rate of acidic ketone body production.

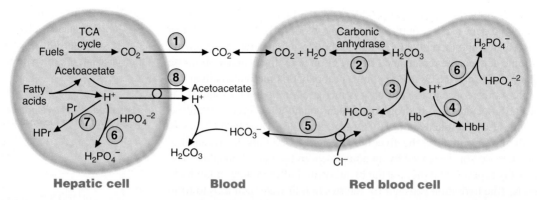

**FIG. 2.7.** Buffering systems of the body. $CO_2$ produced from cellular metabolism is converted to bicarbonate and $H^+$ in the red blood cells. Within the red blood cells, the $H^+$ is buffered by hemoglobin (Hb) and phosphate ($HPO_4^{-2}$) (*circles 4 and 6*). The bicarbonate is transported into the blood to buffer $H^+$ generated by the production of other metabolic acids, like the ketone body acetoacetic acid (*circle 5*). Other proteins (Pr) also serve as intracellular buffers. (Numbers refer to the text discussion.)

The transport of hydrogen ions out of the cell is also important for maintenance of a constant intracellular pH. Metabolism produces a number of other acids in addition to $CO_2$. For example, the metabolic acids acetoacetic acid and β-hydroxybutyric acid are produced from fatty acid oxidation to ketone bodies in the liver, and lactic acid is produced by glycolysis in muscle and other tissues. The $pK_a$ for most metabolic carboxylic acids is below 5, so these acids are completely dissociated at the pH of blood and cellular fluid. Metabolic anions are transported out of the cell together with $H^+$ (see Fig. 2.7, *circle 8*). If the cell becomes too acidic, more $H^+$ is transported out in exchange for $Na^+$ ions by a different transporter. If the cell becomes too alkaline, more bicarbonate is transported out in exchange for $Cl^-$ ions.

### D. Urinary Hydrogen, Ammonium, and Phosphate Ions

The nonvolatile acid (acid which cannot be converted to a gaseous form) that is produced from body metabolism is excreted in the urine. Most nonvolatile acid hydrogen ions are excreted as undissociated acid that generally buffers the urinary pH between 5.5 and 7.0. A pH of 5.0 is the minimum urinary pH. The acid secretion includes inorganic acids like phosphate and ammonium ions, as well as uric acid, dicarboxylic acids, and tricarboxylic acids like citric acid. One of the major sources of nonvolatile acid in the body is sulfuric acid ($H_2SO_4$). Sulfuric acid is generated from the sulfate-containing compounds ingested in foods and from metabolism of the sulfur-containing amino acids cysteine and methionine. It is a strong acid that is dissociated into $H^+$ and sulfate anion ($SO_4^{-2}$) in the blood and urine (see Fig. 2.4). Urinary excretion of $H_2PO_4^-$ helps to remove acid. To maintain metabolic homeostasis, we must excrete the same amount of phosphate in the urine that we ingest with food as phosphate anions or organic phosphates like phospholipids. Whether the phosphate is present in the urine as $H_2PO_4^-$ or $HPO_4^{-2}$ depends on the urinary pH and the pH of blood.

Ammonium ions are major contributors to buffering urinary pH but not blood pH. Ammonia ($NH_3$) is a base that combines with protons to produce ammonium ($NH_4^+$) ions ($NH_3 + H^+ \leftrightarrow NH_4^+$), a reaction that occurs with a $pK_a$ of 9.25. Ammonia is produced from amino acid catabolism or absorbed through the intestine and kept at very low concentrations in the blood because it is toxic to neural tissues.

### E. Hydrochloric Acid

HCl, also called gastric acid, is secreted by parietal cells of the stomach into the stomach lumen, where the strong acidity denatures ingested proteins so they can be degraded by digestive enzymes. When the stomach contents are released into the lumen of the small intestine, gastric acid is neutralized by bicarbonate secreted from pancreatic cells and by cells in the intestinal lining.

## CLINICAL COMMENTS

Diseases discussed in this chapter are summarized in Table 2.2.

**Dianne A.** Di A. has type 1 diabetes mellitus (formerly called juvenile or insulin-dependent diabetes mellitus, IDDM). Because the β-cells of her pancreas have a very limited ability to synthesize and secrete insulin, she maintains her blood insulin level by giving herself two daily subcutaneous (under the skin) injections of insulin. If her blood insulin levels fall too low, free fatty acids leave her adipocytes (fat cells) and are converted by the liver to the ketone bodies acetoacetic acid and β-hydroxybutyric acid. As these acids accumulate in the blood, a metabolic acidosis known as diabetic ketoacidosis (DKA) develops. Until insulin is administered to reverse this trend, several compensatory mechanisms operate to minimize the extent of the acidosis. One of these mechanisms is a stimulation of the respiratory center in the hypothalamus induced by the acidosis, which leads to deeper and more frequent respiration (Kussmaul breathing). $CO_2$ is expired more rapidly than normal, and the lowered blood pH rises toward normal. The results of the laboratory studies performed on **Di A.** in the emergency department were consistent with a moderately severe DKA. Her arterial blood pH and serum bicarbonate were low and ketone bodies were present in her blood and urine (normally, ketone bodies are not present in the urine). In addition, her serum glucose level was 648 mg/dL (reference range = 80 to 110 mg/dL fasting and no higher than 200 mg/dL in a random glucose sample). Her hyperglycemia, which induces osmotic diuresis, contributed to her dehydration and the hyperosmolality of her body fluids.

Treatment was initiated with intravenous saline solutions to replace fluids lost with the osmotic diuresis and hyperventilation. The osmotic diuresis resulted from increased urinary water volume required to dilute the large amounts of glucose and ketone bodies excreted in the urine. Hyperventilation increased the water of respiration lost with expired air. A loading dose of regular insulin was given as an intravenous bolus followed by an insulin drip, giving her continuous insulin intravenously. The patient's metabolic response to the treatment was monitored closely.

**Dennis V.** Dennis is alert in the emergency department. While awaiting the report of his initial serum salicylate level, his stomach was lavaged and several white tablets were found in the stomach aspirate. He was examined repeatedly and showed none of the early symptoms of salicylate toxicity, such as respiratory stimulation, upper abdominal distress, nausea, or headache.

His serum salicylate level was reported as 92 μg/mL (usual level in an adult on a therapeutic dosage of 4 to 5 g/day is 120 to 350 μg/mL, and a level of 800 μg/mL is considered potentially lethal). He was admitted for overnight observation and continued to do well. A serum salicylate level the following morning was 24 μg/mL. He was discharged later that day.

Diabetes mellitus is diagnosed by the concentration of plasma glucose (plasma is blood from which the red blood cells have been removed by centrifugation). Because plasma glucose normally increases after a meal, the normal reference ranges and the diagnostic level are defined relative to the time of consumption of food or to consumption of a specified amount of glucose during an oral glucose tolerance test. After an overnight fast, a fasting plasma glucose level below 100 mg/dL is considered normal; a level above 126 mg/dL defines diabetes mellitus. Fasting plasma glucose values greater or equal to 100 and less than 126 mg/dL define an intermediate condition termed impaired fasting glucose or prediabetes. Normal random plasma glucose levels (random is defined as any time of day without regard to the time since a last meal) should not be above 200 mg/dL. Normal subjects generally do not increase their blood sugar above 140 mg/dL, even after a meal. Thus, a 2-hour postprandial (after a meal or after an oral glucose load) plasma glucose level between 140 and 199 mg/dL defines a condition known as impaired glucose tolerance or prediabetes, whereas a level above 200 mg/dL defines overt diabetes mellitus. Diabetes mellitus is also diagnosed by measuring the hemoglobin $A_{1c}$ (HbA$_{1c}$) values, which is a measure of glycosylated hemoglobin in the red blood cells. This is a nonenzymatic reaction that is dependent on glucose concentration; so as the glucose concentration increases, the levels of HbA$_{1c}$ increase. Normal levels of HbA$_{1c}$ are 4% to 6% of total hemoglobin, and a value of greater than 6.5% HbA$_{1c}$ defines diabetes mellitus.

**Table 2.2   Diseases Associated with Chapter 2**

| Disorder or Condition | Genetic or Environmental | Comments |
| --- | --- | --- |
| Type 1 diabetes | Environmental | Lack of insulin production leads to type 1 diabetes. One consequence of untreated type 1 diabetes is ketoacidosis (elevated levels of ketone bodies in the blood). |
| Salicylate overdose | Environmental | Complex effects on respiratory center and basic metabolism, causing alterations in acid/base management, amongst other effects. Leads to impaired renal function |

## REVIEW QUESTIONS-CHAPTER 2

1. A decrease of blood pH from 7.5 to 6.5 would be accompanied by which one of the following changes in ion concentration?

    A. A 10-fold increase in hydrogen ion concentration
    B. A 10-fold increase in hydroxyl ion concentration
    C. An increase in hydrogen ion concentration by a factor of 7.5/6.5
    D. A decrease in hydrogen ion concentration by a factor of 7.5/6.5
    E. A shift in concentration of buffer anions, with no change in hydrogen ion concentration

2. Which one of the following best describes a universal property of buffers?

    A. Buffers work best at one pH unit lower than the $pK_a$.
    B. Buffers work equally well at all concentrations.
    C. Buffers work best at the pH at which they are 50% dissociated.
    D. Buffers are usually composed of a mixture of strong acids and strong bases.
    E. Buffers work best at the pH at which they are completely dissociated.

3. A patient with enteropathy (intestinal disease) produced large amounts of ammonia ($NH_3$) from bacterial overgrowth in the intestine. The ammonia was absorbed through the intestine into the portal vein and entered the circulation. Which of the following is a likely consequence of his ammonia absorption?

    A. A decrease of blood pH
    B. A decreased concentration of bicarbonate in the blood
    C. Kussmaul breathing
    D. Increased expiration of $CO_2$
    E. Conversion of ammonia to ammonium ion in the blood

4. Which one of the following physiological or pathological conditions is most likely to result in alkalosis, provided that the body could not fully compensate?

    A. Production of lactic acid by muscles during exercise
    B. Repeated vomiting of stomach contents, including hydrochloric acid (HCl)
    C. Production of ketone bodies by a patient with diabetes mellitus
    D. Diarrhea with loss of the bicarbonate anions secreted into the intestine
    E. An infection resulting in a fever and hypercatabolism

5. Effective buffering of blood is best described by which one of the following?

    A. It maintains blood pH in the normal range of 7.43 to 6.43.
    B. It is required because normal metabolism produces strong bases.
    C. It utilizes principally the phosphate buffering system.
    D. It requires a high concentration of carbonic anhydrase in serum (blood after cells have been removed).
    E. It utilizes the amino acid side chains of serum proteins.

# 3 Structures of the Major Compounds of the Body

## CHAPTER OUTLINE

## KEY POINTS

- Carbohydrates, commonly known as sugars, can be classified by a number of criteria:
  - Type of carbonyl group (aldo or keto sugars)
  - Number of carbons (pentoses [five carbons], hexoses [six carbons])
  - Positions of hydroxyl groups on asymmetric carbon atoms (D or L configuration, stereoisomers, epimers)
  - Substituents (amino sugars)
  - Number of monosaccharides joined through glycosidic bonds (disaccharides, oligosaccharides, polysaccharides)
- Lipids are structurally diverse compounds that are not very soluble in water (i.e., they are hydrophobic).
  - The major lipids are fatty acids.
  - Triacylglycerol (triglycerides) consist of three fatty acids esterified to the carbohydrate glycerol.
  - Phosphoacylglycerols (phosphoglycerides or phospholipids) are similar to triacylglycerol but contain a phosphate in place of a fatty acid.

continued

■ Sphingolipids are built upon sphingosine.
■ Cholesterol is a component of membranes and a precursor for molecules which contain the steroid nucleus, such as bile salts and steroid hormones.
■ Nitrogen is found in a variety of compounds in addition to amino sugars.
  ■ Amino acids and heterocyclic rings contain nitrogens, which carry a positive charge at neutral pH.
  ■ Amino acids contain a carboxyl group, an amino group, and a side chain attached to a central carbon.
  ■ Proteins consist of a linear chain of amino acids.
  ■ Purines, pyrimidines, and pyridines have heterocyclic nitrogen-containing ring structures.
  ■ Nucleosides consist of a heterocyclic ring attached to a sugar.
  ■ A nucleoside plus phosphate is a nucleotide.
■ Glycoproteins and proteoglycans have sugars attached to protein components.

# THE WAITING ROOM

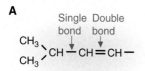

**Di A.** had a metabolic acidosis resulting from an increased hepatic production of ketone bodies. Her response to therapy was followed with screening tests for ketone bodies in her urine that employed a paper strip containing nitroprusside, a compound that reacts with keto groups. Her blood glucose was measured with an enzymatic assay that is specific for the sugar D-glucose and will not react with other sugars.

**Di A.** recovered from her bout of diabetic ketoacidosis and was discharged from the hospital (see Chapter 2). She has returned for a follow-up visit as an outpatient. She reports that she has been compliant with her recommended diet and that she faithfully gives herself insulin by subcutaneous injection usually four times daily. She self-monitors her blood glucose levels at least four times a day and reports the results to her physician.

**Lotta T.** is a 54-year-old woman who came to the physician's office complaining of a severe throbbing pain in the right great toe that began 8 hours earlier. The toe has suffered no trauma but appears red and swollen. It is warmer than the surrounding tissue and is exquisitely tender to even light pressure. Ms. T. is unable to voluntarily flex or extend the joints of the digit and passive motion of the joints causes great pain.

## I. FUNCTIONAL GROUPS ON BIOLOGICAL COMPOUNDS

### A. Biological Compounds

The organic molecules of the body consist principally of carbon, hydrogen, oxygen, nitrogen, sulfur, and phosphorus joined by covalent bonds. The key element is carbon, which forms four covalent bonds with other atoms. Carbon atoms are joined through double or single bonds to form the carbon backbone for structures of varying size and complexity (Fig. 3.1). Groups containing one, two, three, four, and five carbons plus hydrogen are referred to as methyl, ethyl, propionyl, butyl, and pentanyl groups, respectively. If the carbon chain is branched, the prefix "iso-" is used. If the compound contains a double bond, "-ene" is sometimes incorporated into the name. Carbon structures that are straight or branched with single or double bonds, but do not contain a ring, are called **aliphatic**.

Carbon-containing rings are found in a number of biological compounds. One of the most common is the six-member carbon-containing benzene ring, sometimes called a phenyl group (see Fig. 3.1). This ring has three double bonds, but the electrons are shared equally by all six carbons and delocalized in planes above and below the ring. Compounds containing the benzene ring or a similar ring structure with benzene-like properties are called **aromatic**.

### B. Functional Groups

Biochemical molecules are defined both by their carbon skeleton and by structures called **functional groups** that usually involve bonds between carbon and

**A**

**Aliphatic isopentenyl group**

**B**

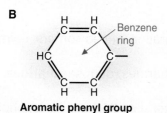

**Aromatic phenyl group**

*FIG. 3.1.* Examples of aliphatic and aromatic compounds. **A.** An **isoprene** group, which is an aliphatic group. The "iso-" prefix denotes branching and the "-ene" denotes a double bond. **B.** A benzene ring (or phenyl group), which is an aromatic group.

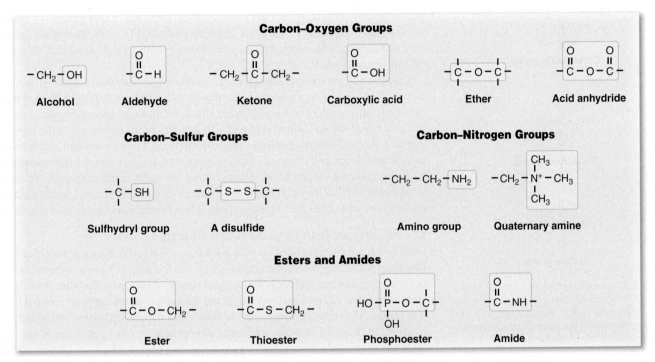

*FIG. 3.2.* Major types of functional groups found in biochemical compounds of the human body.

oxygen, carbon and nitrogen, carbon and sulfur, and carbon and phosphate groups (Fig. 3.2). In carbon-carbon and carbon-hydrogen bonds, the electrons are shared equally between atoms, and the bonds are nonpolar and relatively unreactive. In carbon-oxygen and carbon-nitrogen bonds, the electrons are shared unequally and the bonds are polar and more reactive. Thus, the properties of the functional groups usually determine the types of reactions that occur and the physiological role of the molecule.

Functional group names are often incorporated into the common name of a compound. For example, a ket**one** might have a name that ends in "-one" like acet**one**, and the name of a compound that contains a hydroxyl (alcoh**ol** or OH group) might end in "-ol" (e.g., ethan**ol**). The acyl group is the portion of the molecule that provides the carbonyl (—C═O) group in an **ester** or amide linkage. It is denoted in a name by a "-yl" ending. For example, the fat stores of the body are tri**acyl**glycer**ols**. Three acyl (fatty acid) groups are esterified to glycer**ol**, a compound containing three alcohol groups. In the remainder of this chapter, we will bold the portions of names of compounds that refer to a class of compounds or a structural feature.

## 1.  OXIDIZED AND REDUCED GROUPS

The carbon-carbon and carbon-oxygen groups are described as "oxidized" or "reduced" according to the number of electrons around the carbon atom. **Oxidation** is the loss of electrons and results in the loss of hydrogen atoms together with one or two electrons or the gain of an oxygen atom or hydroxyl group. **Reduction** is the gain of electrons and results in the gain of hydrogen atoms or loss of an oxygen atom. Thus, the carbon becomes progressively more oxidized (and less reduced) as we go from an alcohol to an aldehyde or a ketone to a carboxyl group (see Fig. 3.2). Carbon-carbon double bonds are more oxidized (and less reduced) than carbon-carbon single bonds.

## 2.  GROUPS THAT CARRY A CHARGE

Acidic groups contain a proton that can dissociate, usually leaving the remainder of the molecule as an **anion** with a negative charge (see Chapter 2). In biomolecules,

**Q:** The ketone bodies synthesized in the liver are β-hydroxybutyrate and acetoacetate. A third ketone body, acetone, is formed by the nonenzymatic decarboxylation of acetoacetate.

$$CH_3 - \overset{\overset{\displaystyle OH}{|}}{C}H - CH_2 - COO^-$$

**β-Hydroxybutyrate**

$$CH_3 - \overset{\overset{\displaystyle O}{\|}}{C} - CH_2 - COO^-$$

**Acetoacetate**

$$CH_3 - \overset{\overset{\displaystyle O}{\|}}{C} - CH_3$$

**Acetone**

Acetone is volatile and accounts for the fruity and alcohol-like odor in the breath of patients like **Dianne A.** when they have ketoacidosis. What functional groups are present in each of these ketone bodies?

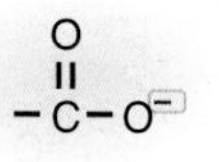

$$\begin{array}{c} O \\ \| \\ -C-O^{\ominus} \end{array}$$

**Carboxylate group**

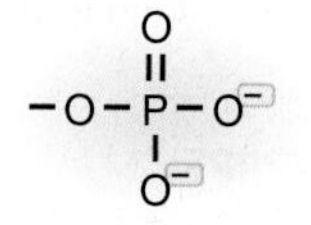

$$\begin{array}{c} O \\ \| \\ -O-P-O^{\ominus} \\ | \\ O^{\ominus} \end{array}$$

**Phosphate group**

$$\begin{array}{c} O \\ \| \\ -O-S-O^{\ominus} \\ \| \\ O \end{array}$$

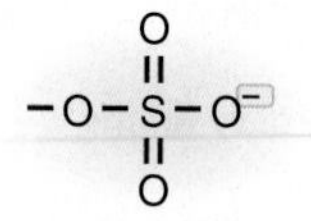

**Sulfate group**

**FIG. 3.3.** Examples of anions formed by dissociation of acidic groups. At physiological pH, carboxylic acids, phosphoric acid, and sulfuric acid are dissociated into hydrogen ions and negatively charged anions.

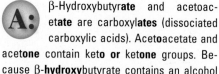

**A:** β-Hydroxybutyr**ate** and acetoac-**etate** are carboxylates (dissociated carboxylic acids). Acetoacetate and acet**one** contain ket**o** or ket**one** groups. Because β-**hydroxy**butyrate contains an alcohol (**hydroxyl**) group and not a keto group, the general name of ketone bodies for these compounds is really a misnomer.

Dopamine structure:

HO—⟨ring⟩—$CH_2$—$CH_2$—$\overset{+}{N}H_3$

with OH on ring

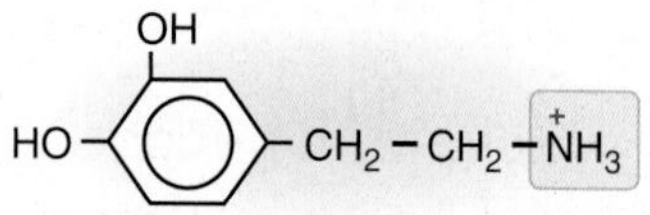

**Dopamine** (a primary amine)

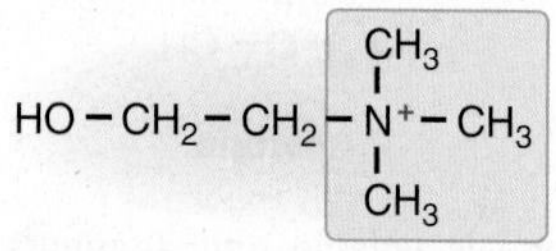

Choline structure:

$$HO-CH_2-CH_2-\overset{\overset{\displaystyle CH_3}{|}}{\underset{\underset{\displaystyle CH_3}{|}}{N^+}}-CH_3$$

**Choline** (a quaternary amine)

**FIG. 3.4.** Examples of amines. At physiological pH, many amines carry positive charges.

the major anionic substituents are carboxyl**ate** groups, phosph**ate** groups, or sulf**ate** groups (the "-ate" suffix denotes a negative charge) (Fig. 3.3). Phosphate groups attached to metabolites are often abbreviated as P with a circle around it, or just as "P", as in glucose 6-**P**.

Compounds containing nitrogen are usually basic and can acquire a positive charge (Fig. 3.4). Nitrogen has five electrons in its valence shell. If only three of these electrons form covalent bonds with other atoms, the nitrogen has no charge. If the remaining two electrons form a bond with a hydrogen ion or a carbon atom, the nitrogen carries a positive charge. **Amines** consist of nitrogen attached through single bonds to hydrogen atoms and to one or more carbon atoms. Primary amines, like dop**amine**, have one carbon-nitrogen bond. These amines are weak acids with a $pK_a$ of about 9, so that at pH 7.4, they carry a positive charge. Secondary, tertiary, and quaternary amines have two, three, and four nitrogen-carbon bonds, respectively (see Fig. 3.4).

## C. Polarity of Bonds and Partial Charges

Polar bonds are covalent bonds in which the electron cloud is denser around one atom (the atom with the greater electronegativity) than the other. Oxygen is more electronegative than carbon, and a carbon-oxygen bond is therefore polar, with the oxygen atom carrying a partial negative charge and the carbon atom carrying a partial positive charge. In nonpolar carbon-carbon bonds and carbon-hydrogen bonds, the two electrons in the covalent bond are shared almost equally. Nitrogen, when it has only three covalent bonds, also carries a partial negative charge relative to carbon and the carbon-nitrogen bond is polarized. Sulfur can carry a slight partial negative charge.

### 1. SOLUBILITY

Water is a dipolar molecule in which the oxygen atom carries a partial negative charge and the hydrogen atoms carry partial positive charges (see Chapter 2). In order for molecules to be soluble in water, they must contain charged or polar groups that can associate with the partial positive and negative charges of water. Thus, the solubility of organic molecules in water is determined by both the proportion of polar to nonpolar groups attached to the carbon–hydrogen skeleton and to their relative positions in the molecule. Polar groups or molecules are called **hydrophilic** (water loving) and nonpolar groups or molecules are **hydrophobic** (water fearing). Sugars such as glucose-6-phosphate, for example, contain so many polar groups (many hydroxyl and one phosphate) that they are very hydrophilic and almost infinitely water soluble. The water molecules interacting with a polar or ionic compound form a hydration shell around the compound.

Compounds that have large nonpolar regions are relatively water insoluble. They tend to cluster together in an aqueous environment and form weak associations through van der Waals interactions and hydrophobic interactions. Hydrophobic compounds are essentially pushed together (the hydrophobic effect) as the water molecules maximize the number of energetically favorable hydrogen bonds they can form with each other in the water lattice. Thus, lipids will form droplets or separate layers in an aqueous environment (e.g., vegetable oils in a salad dressing).

### 2. REACTIVITY

Another consequence of bond polarity is that atoms which carry a partial (or full) negative charge will be attracted to atoms which carry a partial (or full) positive charge and vice versa. These partial or full charges dictate the course of biochemical reactions.

The partial positive charge on the carboxyl carbon attracts more negatively charged groups and accounts for many of the reactions of carboxylic acids. An ester is formed when a carboxylic acid and an alcohol combine, splitting out water (Fig. 3.5). Similarly, a thioester is formed when an acid combines with a sulfhydryl group and an amide is formed when an acid combines with an amine. Similar reactions result in the formation of a phosphoester from phosphoric acid and an alcohol and in the formation of an anhydride from two acids.

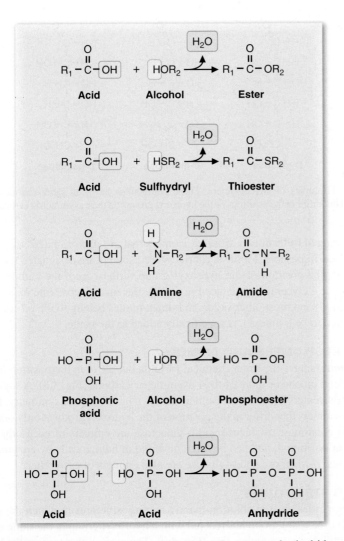

FIG. 3.5. Formation of esters, thioesters, amides, phosphoesters, and anhydrides.

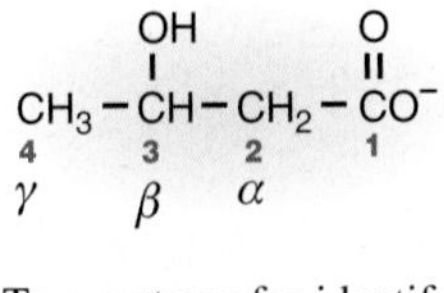

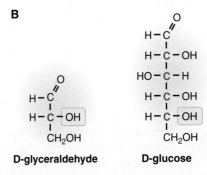

*FIG. 3.6.* Two systems for identifying the carbon atoms in a compound. This compound is called 3-hydroxybutyrate or β-hydroxybutyrate.

## D. Nomenclature

Biochemists use two systems for the identification of the carbons in a chain. In the first system, the carbons in a compound are numbered, starting with the carbon in the most oxidized group (e.g., the carboxyl group). In the second system, the carbons are given Greek letters, starting with the carbon next to the most oxidized group. Hence, the compound shown in Figure 3.6 is known as 3-hydroxybutyrate or β-hydroxybutyrate.

## II. CARBOHYDRATES

### A. Monosaccharides

Simple **monosaccharides** consist of a linear chain of three or more carbon atoms, one of which forms a carbonyl group via a double bond with oxygen. The other carbons of an unmodified monosaccharide contain hydroxyl groups, which results in the general formula for an unmodified sugar of $C_nH_{2n}O_n$. The suffix "-ose" is used for the names of sugars. If the carbonyl group is an aldehyde, the sugar is an aldose; if the carbonyl group is a ketone, the sugar is a ketose. Monosaccharides are also classified according to their number of carbons: Sugars containing three, four, five, six, and seven carbons are called trioses, tetroses, pentoses, hexoses, and heptoses, respectively.

### 1. D- AND L-SUGARS

A carbon atom that contains four different chemical groups forms an asymmetric (or chiral) center (Fig. 3.7A). The groups attached to the asymmetric carbon atom

*FIG. 3.7.* **A.** D- and L-Glyceraldehyde. The carbon in the center contains four different substituent groups arranged around it in a tetrahedron. A different arrangement creates an isomer that is a nonsuperimposable mirror image. If you rotate the mirror image structure so that groups 1 and 2 align, group 3 will be in the position of group 4, and group 4 will be in position 3. **B.** D-Glyceraldehyde and D-glucose. These sugars have the same configuration at the asymmetric carbon atom farthest from the carbonyl group. Both belong to the D series. Asymmetric carbons are shown in *red.*

$$
\begin{array}{ccc}
\text{H}-\overset{\displaystyle O}{\overset{\|}{\text{C}}} & \text{H}-\overset{\displaystyle O}{\overset{\|}{\text{C}}} & \text{H}-\overset{\displaystyle O}{\overset{\|}{\text{C}}} \\
\text{H}-\text{C}-\text{OH} & \text{HO}-\text{C}-\text{H} & \text{H}-\text{C}-\text{OH} \\
\text{HO}-\text{C}-\text{H} & \text{HO}-\text{C}-\text{H} & \text{HO}-\text{C}-\text{H} \\
\text{H}-\text{C}-\text{OH} & \text{H}-\text{C}-\text{OH} & \text{HO}-\text{C}-\text{H} \\
\text{H}-\text{C}-\text{OH} & \text{H}-\text{C}-\text{OH} & \text{H}-\text{C}-\text{OH} \\
\text{CH}_2\text{OH} & \text{CH}_2\text{OH} & \text{CH}_2\text{OH} \\
\textbf{D-glucose} & \textbf{D-mannose} & \textbf{D-galactose}
\end{array}
$$

*FIG. 3.8.* Examples of stereoisomers. These compounds have the same chemical formula ($C_6H_{12}O_6$) but differ in the positions of the hydroxyl groups on their asymmetric carbons (in *red*).

The stereospecificity of D-glucose is still frequently denoted in medicine by the use of its old name, dextrose. A solution used for intravenous infusions in patients is a 5% (5 g/100 mL) solution of dextrose.

**Q:** Are D-mannose and D-galactose stereoisomers? Are they epimers of each other? (see Fig.3.8)

Proteoglycans contain many long unbranched polysaccharide chains attached to a core protein. The polysaccharide chains, called glycosaminoglycans, are composed of repeating disaccharide units containing oxidized acid sugars (such as glucuronic acid), sulfated sugars, and *N*-acetylated amino sugars. The large number of negative charges causes the glycosaminoglycan chains to radiate out from the protein so that the overall structure resembles a bottlebrush. The proteoglycans are essential parts of the extracellular matrix, the aqueous humor of the eye, secretions of mucus-producing cells, and cartilage.

can be arranged to form two different isomers that are mirror images of each other and not superimposable. Monosaccharide stereoisomers are designated D or L based on whether the position of the hydroxyl group furthest from the carbonyl carbon matches D or L glyceraldehyde (see Fig. 3.7B). Because glucose (the major sugar in human blood) and most other sugars in human tissues belong to the D series, sugars are assumed to be D unless L is specifically added to the name.

### 2. STEREOISOMERS AND EPIMERS

**Stereoisomers** have the same chemical formula but differ in the position of the hydroxyl group on one or more of their asymmetric carbons (Fig. 3.8). A sugar with **n** asymmetric centers has $2^n$ stereoisomers unless it has a plane of symmetry. **Epimers** are stereoisomers that differ in the position of the hydroxyl group at only one of their asymmetric carbons. D-Glucose and D-galactose are epimers of each other, differing only at position 4, and can be interconverted in human cells by enzymes called **epimerases**. D-Mannose and D-glucose are also epimers of each other.

### 3. RING STRUCTURES

Monosaccharides exist in solution mainly as ring structures in which the carbonyl (aldehyde or ketone) group has reacted with a hydroxyl group in the same molecule to form a five- or six-member ring (Fig. 3.9). The oxygen that was on the hydroxyl group is now part of the ring, and the original carbonyl carbon, which now contains an —OH group, has become the anomeric carbon atom. A hydroxyl group on the anomeric carbon drawn down below the ring is in the α-position; drawn up above the ring, it is in the β-position. In the actual three-dimensional structure, the ring is not planar but usually takes a "chair" conformation in which the hydroxyl groups are located at a maximal distance from each other.

In solution, the hydroxyl group on the anomeric carbon spontaneously (nonenzymatically) changes from the α- to the β-position through a process called **mutarotation**. When the ring opens, the straight chain aldehyde or ketone is formed. When the ring closes, the hydroxyl group may be either in the α- or the β-position. This process occurs more rapidly in the presence of cellular enzymes called **mutarotases**. However, if the anomeric carbon forms a bond with another molecule, that bond is fixed in the α or β-position, and the sugar cannot mutarotate. Enzymes are specific for α or β-bonds between sugars and other molecules and react with only one type.

### 4. SUBSTITUTED SUGARS

Sugars frequently contain phosphate groups, amino groups, sulfate groups, or *N*-acetyl groups. Most of the free monosaccharides within cells are phosphorylated at their terminal carbons, which prevents their transport out of the cell. Amino sugars, such as galacto**samine** and glucos**amine**, contain an amino group instead of a hydroxyl group on one of the carbon atoms, usually carbon 2. Frequently, this amino group has been acetylated to form an *N*-acetylated sugar. In complex molecules

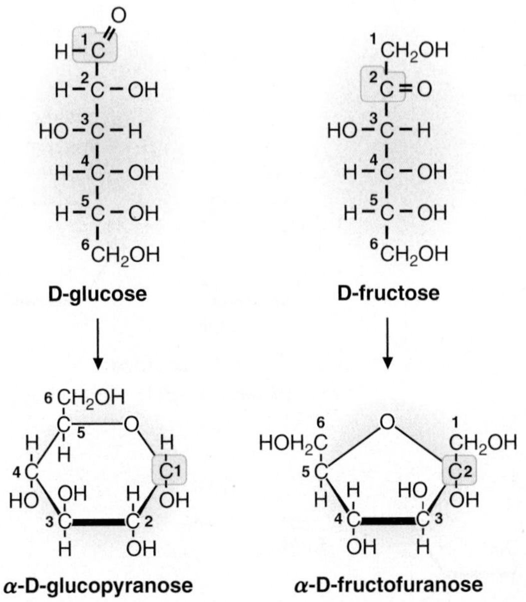

**D-glucose**

**D-fructose**

**α-D-glucopyranose**

**α-D-fructofuranose**

*FIG. 3.9.* Pyranose and furanose rings formed from glucose and fructose. The anomeric carbons are highlighted (carbon 1 of glucose and carbon 2 of fructose).

termed proteoglycans, many of the *N*-acetylated sugars also contain negatively charged sulfate groups attached to a hydroxyl group on the sugar.

## 5.  OXIDIZED AND REDUCED SUGARS

Sugars can be oxidized at the aldehyde carbon to form an acid. Technically, the compound is no longer a sugar, and the ending on its name is changed from "-ose" to "-onic acid" or "-onate" (e.g., glu**onic** acid, Fig. 3.10). If the carbon containing the terminal hydroxyl group is oxidized, the sugar is called a uronic acid (e.g., glu**curonic** acid).

If the aldehyde of a sugar is reduced, all the carbon atoms contain alcohol (hydroxyl) groups and the sugar is a poly**ol** (e.g., sorbit**ol**) (see Fig. 3.10). If one of the hydroxyl groups of a sugar is reduced so that the carbon contains only hydrogen, the sugar is a deoxysugar, such as the **deoxy**ribose in DNA.

## B. Glycosides

### 1.  N- AND O-GLYCOSIDIC BONDS

The hydroxyl group on the anomeric carbon of a monosaccharide can react with an —OH or —NH group of another compound to form a glyc**osidic** bond. The linkage may be either α or β, depending on the position of the atom attached to the anomeric carbon of the sugar. *N*-glycosidic bonds are found in nucle**osides** and nucle**otides**. For example, in the adenosine moiety of adenosine triphosphate (ATP), the nitrogenous base adenine is linked to the sugar ribose through a β-*N*-glycosidic bond (Fig. 3.11). In contrast, *O*-glycosidic bonds, such as those found in lactose, join sugars to each other or attach sugars to the hydroxyl group of an amino acid on a protein.

### 2.  DISACCHARIDES, OLIGOSACCHARIDES, AND POLYSACCHARIDES

A **disaccharide** contains two monosaccharides joined by an *O*-glycosidic bond. Lactose, which is the sugar in milk, consists of galactose and glucose linked through a β(1→4) bond formed between the β —OH group of the anomeric carbon of galactose and the hydroxyl group on carbon 4 of glucose (see Fig. 3.11). **Oligosaccharides** contain 3 to about 12 monosaccharides linked together. They are often found attached through *N*- or *O*-glycosidic bonds to proteins to form **glyco**proteins

 They are stereoisomers but not epimers of each other. They have the same chemical formula but differ in the position of two hydroxyl groups.

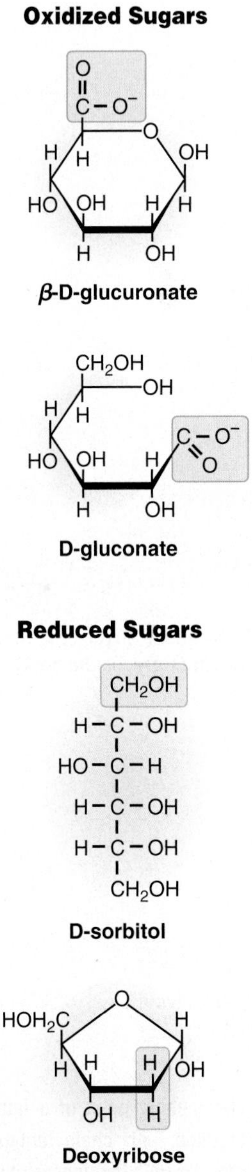

**Oxidized Sugars**

**β-D-glucuronate**

**D-gluconate**

**Reduced Sugars**

**D-sorbitol**

**Deoxyribose**

*FIG. 3.10.* Oxidized and reduced sugars. The affected group is shown in the colored box. Gluconic acid (D-gluconate) is formed by oxidation of the glucose aldehyde carbon. Glucuronic acid is formed by oxidation of the glucose terminal —OH group. Sorbitol, a sugar alcohol, is formed by reduction of the glucose aldehyde group. Deoxyribose is formed by reduction of ribose.

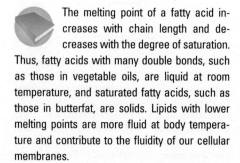

*FIG. 3.11.* *N*- and *O*-glycosidic bonds. ATP contains a β-, *N*-glycosidic bond. Lactose contains an *O*-glycosidic β(1→4) bond. Starch contains α-1,4 and α-1,6 *O*-glycosidic bonds. The glycosidic bonds are shown in *red*.

(see Chapter 4). **Polysaccharides** contain tens to thousands of monosaccharides joined by glycosidic bonds to form linear chains or branched structures. Amylopectin (a form of starch) and glycogen (the storage form of glucose in human cells) are branched polymers of glucosyl residues linked through α(1→4) and α(1→6) bonds.

## III.  LIPIDS

### A.  Fatty Acids

**Fatty acids** are usually straight aliphatic chains with a methyl group at one end (called the ω-carbon) and a carboxyl group at the other end (Fig. 3.12). Most fatty acids in the human have an even number of carbon atoms, usually between 16 and 20. **Saturated fatty acids** have single bonds between the carbons in the chain, and **unsaturated fatty acids** contain one or more double bonds. The most common saturated fatty acids present in the cell are palmitic acid (C16) and stearic acid (C18). Although these two fatty acids are generally called by their common names, shorter fatty acids are often called by the Latin word for the number of carbons, such as octanoic acid (8 carbons) and decanoic acid (10 carbons).

**Monounsaturated fatty acids** contain one double bond, and **polyunsaturated fatty acids** contain two or more double bonds (see Fig. 3.12). The position of a double bond is designated by the number of the carbon in the double bond that is closest to the carboxyl group. For example, oleic acid, which contains 18 carbons

The melting point of a fatty acid increases with chain length and decreases with the degree of saturation. Thus, fatty acids with many double bonds, such as those in vegetable oils, are liquid at room temperature, and saturated fatty acids, such as those in butterfat, are solids. Lipids with lower melting points are more fluid at body temperature and contribute to the fluidity of our cellular membranes.

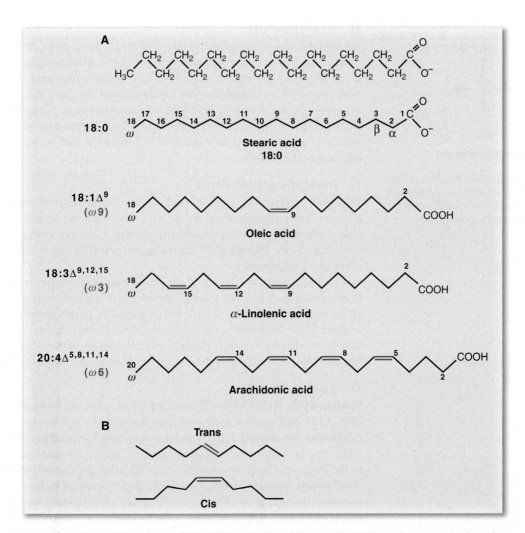

**FIG. 3.12. A.** Saturated fatty acids and unsaturated fatty acids. In stearic acid, the saturated fatty acid at the top of the figure, all the atoms are shown. A more common way of depicting the same structure is shown beneath the top structure. The carbons are either numbered starting with the carboxyl group or given Greek letters starting with the carbon next to the carboxyl group. The methyl (or ω) carbon at the end of the chain is always called the ω-carbon regardless of the chain length. The symbol 18:0 refers to the number of carbon atoms (18) and the number of double bonds (0). In the unsaturated fatty acids shown, not all of the carbons are numbered, but note that the double bonds are *cis* and spaced at three-carbon intervals. Both ω3 and ω6 fatty acids are required in the diet, as humans cannot synthesize these molecules. **B.** *Cis* and *trans* double bonds in fatty acid side chains. Note that the *cis* double bond causes the chain to bend.

and a double bond between positions 9 and 10, is designated 18:1, $\Delta^9$. The number 18 denotes the number of carbon atoms, 1 (one) denotes the number of double bonds, and $\Delta^9$ denotes the position of the double bond between the 9th and 10th carbon atoms. Oleic acid can also be designated 18:1(9), without the $\Delta$. Fatty acids are also classified by the distance of the double bond closest to the ω end (the methyl group at the end farthest from the carboxyl group). Thus, oleic acid is an ω9 fatty acid and linolenic acid is an ω3 fatty acid. Arachidonic acid, a polyunsaturated fatty acid with 20 carbons and 4 double bonds, is an ω6 fatty acid that is completely described as 20:4, $\Delta^{5,8,11,14}$.

The double bonds in most naturally occurring fatty acids are in the *cis* configuration. The designation *cis* means that the hydrogens are on the same side of the double bond and the acyl chains on the other side. In *trans* fatty acids, the acyl chains are on opposite sides of the double bond. Trans **fatty acids** are produced by the chemical hydrogenation of polyunsaturated fatty acids in vegetable oils and are not a natural food product.

*Trans* fatty acid consumption has been linked in some studies to an increased risk of heart disease. These findings, however, have been challenged by the food industry. The FDA now mandates the labeling of foods with trans fatty acid content, and the use of trans fatty acids in commercial food preparation has been banned in certain localities in the United States.

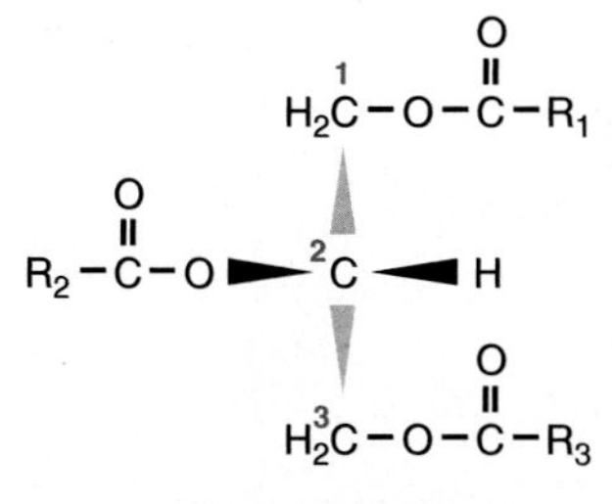

**Triacyl-*sn*-glycerol**

*FIG. 3.13.* A triacylglycerol. Note that carbons 1 and 3 of the glycerol moiety are not identical. The broad end of each *arrowhead* is closer to the reader than the narrow, pointed end.

## B.  Acylglycerols

An **acyl**glycer**ol** is composed of glycerol with one or more fatty acids (the **acyl** group) attached through ester linkages (Fig. 3.13). Monoacylglycerols, diacylglycerols, and triacylglycerols contain one, two, or three fatty acids esterified to glycerol, respectively. Tri**acyl**glycer**ols** rarely contain the same fatty acid at all three positions and are therefore called mixed triacylglycerols. Unsaturated fatty acids, when present, are most often esterified to carbon 2. In the three-dimensional configuration of glycerol, carbons 1 and 3 are not identical, and enzymes are specific for one or the other carbon.

## C.  Phosphoacyglycerols

**Phospho**acylglycerols contain fatty acids esterified to positions 1 and 2 of glycerol and a phosphate (alone or with a substituent) attached to carbon 3. If only a phosphate group is attached to carbon 3, the compound is **phospha**tidic acid (Fig. 3.14). Phosphatidic acid is a precursor for the synthesis of the other phosphoacylglycerols.

Phosphatidylchol**ine** is one of the major phosphoacylglycerols found in membranes (see Fig. 3.14). The am**ine** is positively charged at neutral pH and the phosphate negatively charged. Thus, the molecule is **amphipathic**, meaning that it contains large polar and nonpolar regions. Phosphatidylcholine is also called lecithin. Removal of a fatty acyl group from a phosphoacylglycerol leads to a *lyso*lipid. For example, removing the fatty acyl group from lecithin forms lysolecithin.

## D.  Sphingolipids

**Sphingolipids** do not have a glycerol backbone; they are formed from sphingosine (Fig. 3.15). Sphingos**ine** is derived from ser**ine** and a specific fatty acid, palmitate. Cer**amides** are **amides** formed from sphingosine by attaching a fatty acid to the amino group. Various sphingolipids are then formed by attaching different groups to the hydroxyl group on ceramide. As reflected in the names for cerebr**osides** and gangli**osides**, these sphingolipids contain sugars attached to the hydroxyl group of ceramide through glycosidic bonds. They are glycolipids (more specifically, glycosphingolipids). Sphingomyelin, which contains a phosphorylcholine group attached to ceramide, is a component of cell membranes and the myelin sheath around neurons.

## E.  Steroids

**Steroids** contain a four-ring structure called the steroid nucleus (Fig. 3.16). In human cells, cholesterol is the steroid precursor from which all of the steroid hormones are synthesized by modifications to the ring or C20 side chain. Although cholesterol is not very water soluble, it is converted to amphipathic water-soluble bile salts like cholic acid. Bile salts line the surfaces of lipid droplets called micelles in the lumen of the intestine, where they keep the droplets emulsified in the aqueous environment.

Cholesterol is one of the compounds synthesized in the human from branched five-carbon units with one double bond called an isoprenyl unit (see Fig. 3.1A).

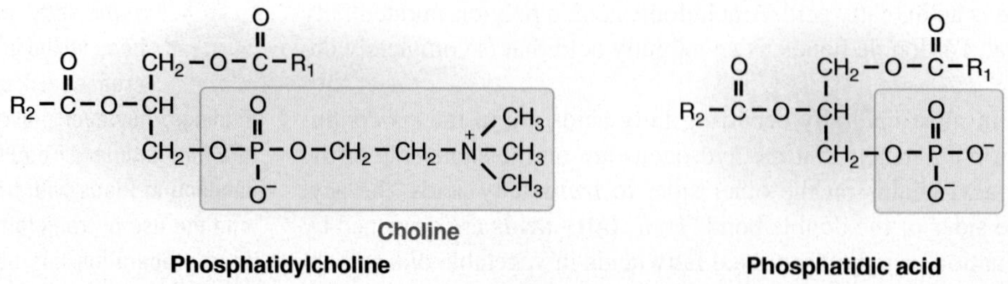

**Phosphatidylcholine**

**Phosphatidic acid**

*FIG. 3.14.* Phosphoacylglycerols. Phospholipids found in membranes, such as phosphatidylcholine, have a polar group attached to the phosphate.

Isoprenyl units are combined in long chains to form other structures, such as the side chains of coenzyme Q in humans and vitamin A in plants.

## IV. NITROGEN-CONTAINING COMPOUNDS

Nitrogen, as described in Section I.B.2, is an electronegative atom with three unshared electrons in its outer valence shell. At neutral pH, the nitrogen in amino groups is usually bonded to four other atoms and carries a positive charge. However, the presence of a nitrogen atom in an organic compound will increase its solubility in water, whether the nitrogen is charged or uncharged.

### A. Amino Acids

**Amino acids** are compounds that contain an amino group and a carboxylic acid group. In proteins, the amino acids are always L-α-amino acids (the amino group is attached to the α carbon in the L-configuration) (Fig. 3.17). These same amino acids also serve as precursors of nitrogen-containing compounds in the body, such as phosphatidylcholine (see Fig. 3.14) and are the basis of most human amino acid metabolism. However, our metabolic reactions occasionally produce an amino acid that has a β or γ amino group, such as the neurotransmitter γ-aminobutyric acid (see Fig. 3.17). However, only α-amino acids are incorporated into proteins.

### B. Nitrogen-Containing Ring Structures

#### 1. PURINES, PYRIMIDINES, AND PYRIDINES

Nitrogen is also a component of ring structures referred to as heterocyclic rings or nitrogenous bases. The three most common types of nitrogen containing rings in the body are pur**ines** (e.g., aden**ine**), pyrimid**ines** (e.g., thym**ine**), and pyrid**ines** (e.g., the vitamins nicot**ine**ic acid, also called niacin, and pyridox**ine**, also called vitamin B₆) (Fig. 3.18). The suffix "**-ine**" denotes the presence of nitrogen (am**ine**) in the ring. The pyrimidine uracil is an exception to this general type of nomenclature. The utility of these nitrogen-containing ring structures lies in the ability of the nitrogen to form hydrogen bonds and to accept and donate electrons while still part of the ring. In contrast, the unsubstituted aromatic benzene ring in which electrons are distributed equally among all six carbons (see Fig. 3.1) is nonpolar, hydrophobic, and relatively unreactive.

#### 2. NUCLEOSIDES AND NUCLEOTIDES

Nitrogenous bases form nucleosides and nucleotides. A **nucleoside** consists of a nitrogenous base joined to a sugar, usually ribose or deoxyribose, through an *N*-glycosidic bond (see Fig. 3.11). If phosphate groups are attached to the sugar, the compound becomes a **nucleotide**. In the name of the nucleotide ATP, the addition of the ribose is indicated by the name change from adenine to aden**osine** (for the gly**cosidic** bond). Monophosphate, diphosphate, or triphosphate are added to the name

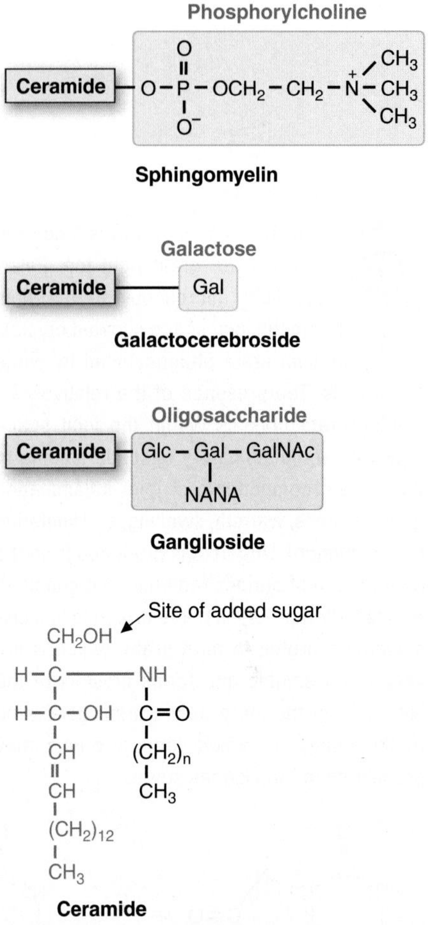

**FIG. 3.15.** Sphingolipids, derivatives of ceramide. The structure of ceramide is shown at the bottom of the figure. The portion of ceramide shown in *red* is sphingosine. The —NH and —OH were contributed by serine. Different groups are added to the hydroxyl group of ceramide to form sphingomyelin, galactocerebrosides, and gangliosides. *NANA*, N-acetylneuraminic acid, also called sialic acid; *Glc*, glucose; *Gal*, galactose; *GalNAc*, N-acetylgalactosamine.

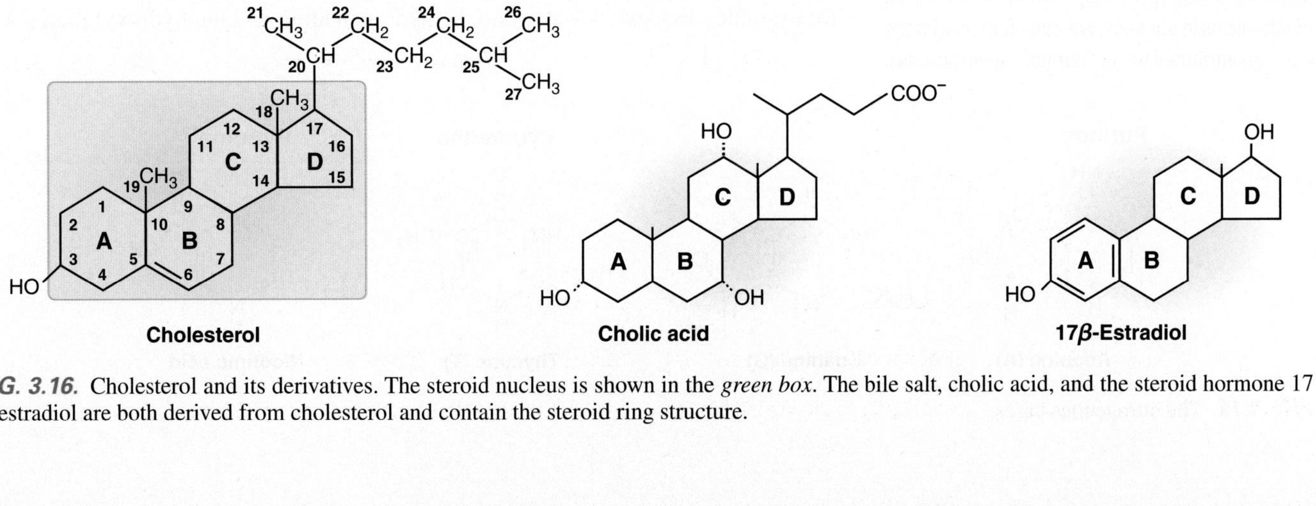

**FIG. 3.16.** Cholesterol and its derivatives. The steroid nucleus is shown in the *green box*. The bile salt, cholic acid, and the steroid hormone 17 β-estradiol are both derived from cholesterol and contain the steroid ring structure.

L-alanine D-alanine γ-Aminobutyrate

*FIG. 3.17.* The structure of the α-amino acid alanine (both the D- and L-configuration) and the γ-amino acid γ-aminobutyrate.

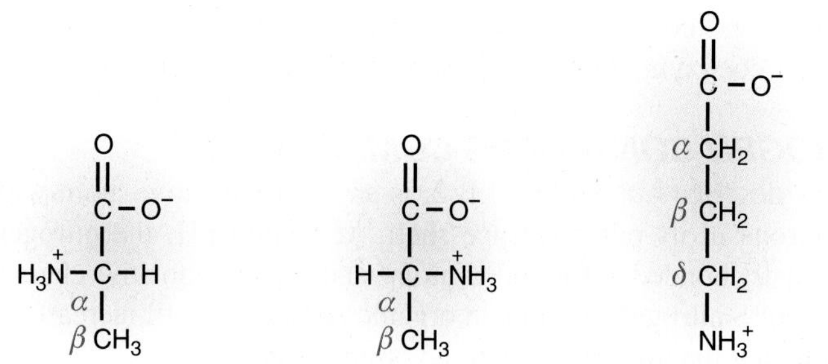

**Lotta T.** has gouty arthritis (podagra) involving her great right toe. Polarized light microscopy of the fluid aspirated from the joint space showed crystals of monosodium urate phagocytosed by white blood cells. The presence of the relatively insoluble urate crystals within the joint space activates an inflammatory cascade leading to the classic components of joint inflammation (pain, redness, warmth, swelling, and limitation of joint motion). Uric acid is produced from the degradation of purines (adenine and guanine). At a blood pH of 7.4, all of the uric acid has dissociated a proton to form urate, which is not very water soluble and forms crystals of the $Na^+$ salt. In the more acidic urine generated by the kidney, the acidic form, uric acid, may precipitate to form kidney stones.

to indicate the presence of one, two, or three phosphate groups in the nucleotide. The structures of the nucleotides that serve as precursors of DNA and RNA are discussed in more detail in Chapter 9.

### 3. TAUTOMERS

In many of the nitrogen-containing rings, the hydrogen can shift to produce a **tautomer**, a compound in which the hydrogen and double bonds have changed position (i.e., —N=C—OH → —NH—C=O ). Tautomers are considered the same compound, and the structure may be represented either way. Generally, one tautomeric form is more reactive than the other. For example, in the two tautomeric forms of uric acid, a proton can dissociate from the enol form to produce urate.

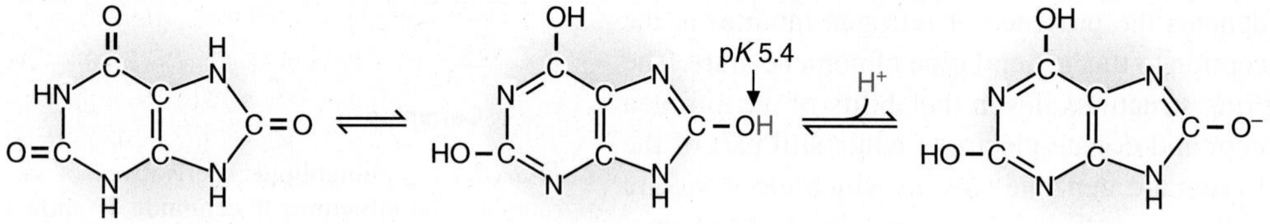

**Uric acid** (keto form) **Uric acid** (enol form) **Urate**

Free radicals are not just esoteric reactants; they are the agents of cell death and destruction. They are involved in all chronic disease states (e.g., coronary artery disease, diabetes mellitus, arthritis, and emphysema) as well as acute injury (e.g., radiation, strokes, myocardial infarction, and spinal cord injury). Through free radical defense mechanisms in our cells, we can often restrict the damage attributed to the "normal" aging process.

## *V. FREE RADICALS*

**Radicals** are compounds which have a single electron, usually in an outer orbital. Free radicals are radicals that exist independently in solution or in a lipid environment. Although many enzymes generate radicals as intermediates in reactions, these are not usually released into the cell to become free radicals.

Many of the compounds in the body are capable of being converted to free radicals by natural events that remove one of their electrons or by radiation. Radiation, for example, dissociates water into the hydrogen atom and the hydroxyl radical:

$$H_2O \leftrightarrow H\bullet + OH\bullet$$

**Purines** **Pyrimidine** **Pyridine**

**Adenine (A)** **Guanine (G)** **Thymine (T)** **Nicotinic acid**

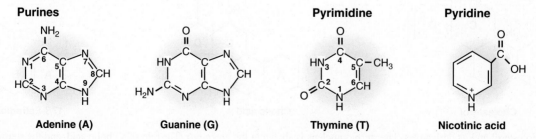

*FIG. 3.18.* The nitrogenous bases.

In contrast, water normally dissociates into a proton and the negatively charged hydroxyl ion. The hydroxyl radical forms organic radicals by taking one electron (as H•) from a compound like an unsaturated membrane lipid, which then has a single unpaired electron and is a new radical.

Compounds that are radicals may be written with or without the radical showing. For example, nitrogen dioxide, a potent reactive toxic radical present in smog and cigarette smoke, may be designated in medical and lay literature as $NO_2$ rather than $NO_2$•. Superoxide, a radical produced in the cell that is the source of much destruction, is correctly written as the superoxide anion, $O_2^-$. However, to emphasize its free radical nature, the same compound is sometimes written as $O_2^-$•. If a compound is designated as a radical in the medical literature, you can be certain that it is a reactive radical and that its radical nature is important for the pathophysiology under discussion. (Reactive oxygen- and nitrogen-containing free radicals are discussed in more detail in Chapter 18).

## VI. ENVIRONMENTAL TOXINS

As a result of human endeavor, toxic compounds containing chlorinated benzene rings have been widely distributed in the environment. These have serious implications for human health, and are described in Section A2, Environmental Toxins, in the online resources associated with the text @.

## CLINICAL COMMENTS

Diseases discussed in Chapter 3 are summarized in Table 3.1.

**Dianne A. (Di A.)** The severity of clinical signs and symptoms in patients with diabetic ketoacidosis (DKA), such as **Di A.** is directly correlated with the concentration of ketone bodies in the blood. Direct quantitative methods for measuring acetoacetate and β-hydroxybutyrate are not routinely available. As a result, clinicians usually rely on semiquantitative reagent strips (Ketostix) or tablets (Acetest) to estimate the level of acetoacetate in the blood and the urine. The nitroprusside on the strips and in the tablets reacts with acetoacetate and to a lesser degree with acetone (both of which have ketone groups) but does not react with β-hydroxybutyrate (which does not have a ketone group). β-Hydroxybutyrate is the predominant ketone body present in the blood of a patient in DKA, and its concentration could decline at a disproportionately rapid rate compared to acetoacetate and acetone. Therefore, tests employing the nitroprusside reaction to monitor the success of therapy in such a patient may be misleading. As a result, clinicians will follow the "anion gap" in the blood, which in DKA represents the increase in ketone bodies.

In contrast to the difficulty of ketone body measurements, diabetic patients can self-monitor blood glucose levels at home, thereby markedly decreasing the time

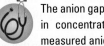 The anion gap refers to the difference in concentration between routinely measured anions (chloride and bicarbonate) and cations (sodium and potassium) in the blood. Because these cations are in most cases in greater concentration than the measured anions, the difference in value is known as the anion gap. The normal value for the anion gap is 12 ($\pm$4). If the anion gap is greater than normal, it is indicative of unknown anions being present in excess, and in the case of type 1 diabetics, most often reflects the production of ketone bodies.

**Table 3.1    Diseases Discussed in Chapter 3**

| Disorder of Condition | Genetic or Environmental | Comments |
| --- | --- | --- |
| Gout | Both | May be due to mutations in specific proteins or dietary habits. Leads to a buildup of uric acid in the blood and precipitation of the uric acid in the joints and/or kidney (producing kidney stones). |
| Type 1 diabetes | Both | Appropriate management of type 1 diabetes requires insulin injections and frequent monitoring of blood glucose levels throughout the day. Without such careful monitoring, ketone bodies may be produced inappropriately. |

and expense of the many blood glucose determinations they need. Capillary blood obtained from a finger prick is placed on the pad of a plastic strip. The strip has been impregnated with an enzyme (usually the bacterial enzyme glucose oxidase) that specifically converts the glucose in the blood to a compound (hydrogen peroxide, $H_2O_2$) that reacts with a dye to produce a color. The intensity of the color, which is directly proportionate to the concentration of glucose in the patient's blood, is read on an instrument called a blood glucose monitor.

 **Lotta T.** Ms. T. has acute gouty arthritis (podagra) involving her right great toe. Initially, Lotta was treated with colchicine (aceto-trimethyl-colchinic acid) for the acute attack of gout affecting her great toe. After taking two doses of colchicine, the throbbing pain in her toe had abated significantly. The redness and swelling also seemed to have lessened slightly. Colchicine will reduce the effects of the inflammatory response to the urate crystals. Several weeks later Lotta was started on allopurinol (150 mg, twice daily), which inhibits the enzyme that produces uric acid. Within several days of starting allopurinol therapy, Lotta's uric acid levels began to decrease.

## REVIEW QUESTIONS-CHAPTER 3

1. Which one of the following is a universal characteristic of water-soluble organic compounds?

    A. They are composed of carbon and hydrogen atoms.
    B. They contain polar groups that can hydrogen bond with water.
    C. They must contain a group that has a full negative charge.
    D. They must contain a group that has a full positive charge.
    E. They contain aromatic groups.

2. A patient was admitted to the hospital emergency room in a coma. Laboratory tests found high levels of the following compound in her blood.

    $$CH_2OH—CH_2—CH_2—COO^-$$

    On the basis of its structure (and your knowledge of the nomenclature of functional groups), you identify the compound as which one of the following?

    A. Methanol (wood alcohol)
    B. Ethanol (alcohol)
    C. Ethylene glycol (antifreeze)
    D. β-hydroxybutyrate (a ketone body)
    E. γ-hydroxybutyrate (the "date rape" drug)

3. A patient was diagnosed with a deficiency of the lysosomal enzyme α-glycosidase. The name of the deficient enzyme suggests it hydrolyzes a glycosidic bond, which is a bond formed via which one of the following?

    A. Between the anomeric carbon of a sugar and an O-H (or N) of another molecule

    B. Through multiple hydrogen bonds between two sugar molecules
    C. Between two anomeric carbons in polysaccharides
    D. Internally between the anomeric carbon of a monosaccharide and its own fifth carbon hydroxyl group.
    E. Between the carbon containing the aldo or keto group and the α-carbon

4. A patient was diagnosed with a hypertriglyceridemia. This condition is named for the high blood levels of lipids composed of which one of the following?

    A. A glycerol lipid containing a phosphorylcholine group
    B. A sphingolipid containing three fatty acyl groups
    C. Three glycerol moieties attached to a fatty acid
    D. Three fatty acyl groups attached to a glycerol backbone
    E. Three glyceraldehyde moieties attached to a fatty acid

5. A patient was diagnosed with one of the sphingolipidoses, which are congenital diseases involving the inability to degrade sphingolipids. All sphingolipids have in common which one of the following?

    A. Phosphorylcholine
    B. Ceramide
    C. A glycerol backbone
    D. *N*-acetylneuraminic acid (NANA)
    E. A steroid ring structure to which sphingosine is attached

# 4 Amino Acids and Proteins

## CHAPTER OUTLINE

I. **GENERAL STRUCTURE OF THE AMINO ACIDS**

II. **CLASSIFICATION OF AMINO ACID SIDE CHAINS**
   A. Nonpolar, aliphatic amino acids
   B. Aromatic amino acids
   C. Aliphatic, polar, uncharged amino acids
   D. Sulfur-containing amino acids
   E. The acidic and basic amino acids

III. **VARIATIONS IN PRIMARY STRUCTURE**
   A. Polymorphism in protein structure
   B. Tissue and developmental variations in protein structure
      1. Developmental variation
      2. Tissue-specific isoforms

   C. Species variations in the primary structure of insulin

IV. **MODIFIED AMINO ACIDS**
   A. Glycosylation
   B. Fatty acylation or prenylation
   C. Regulatory modifications
   D. Other amino acid posttranslational modifications
   E. Selenocysteine

## KEY POINTS

- A protein's unique characteristics including its three-dimensional folded structure are dictated by its linear sequence of amino acids, termed its **primary structure**.
- The primary structures of all of the diverse human proteins are synthesized from 20 amino acids arranged in a linear sequence determined by the genetic code.
- Each three base (nucleotide) sequence within the coding region of a gene (the genetic code) specifies which amino acid should be present in a protein. The genetic code is discussed further in Chapter 12.
- All amino acids contain a central $\alpha$-carbon, joined to a carboxylic acid group, an amino group, a hydrogen, and a side chain, which varies between the 20 different amino acids.
- At physiological pH, the amino acids are zwitterions; the amino group is positively charged, and the carboxylate is negatively charged.
- In proteins, amino acids are joined into linear polymers called polypeptide chains via peptide bonds, which are formed between the carboxylic acid of one amino acid and the amino group of the next amino acid.
- Amino acid side chains can be classified either by polarity (charged, nonpolar hydrophobic, or uncharged polar) or structural features (aliphatic, cyclic, or aromatic).
- Depending on their side chain characteristics, certain amino acids cluster together to exclude water (hydrophobic effect), whereas others participate in hydrogen bonding. Cysteine can form disulfide bonds, whereas charged amino acids can form ionic bonds.

continued

■ Amino acids in proteins can be modified by phosphorylation, carboxylation, or other reactions after the protein is synthesized (posttranslational modifications).

■ Alterations in the genetic code may lead to mutations in the protein's primary structure, which can affect the protein's function.

■ Proteins with the same function but different primary structure (isoforms and isozymes) can exist in different tissues or during different phases of development.

## THE WAITING ROOM

**Will S.** is a 17-year-old boy who presented to the hospital emergency department with severe pain in his lower back, abdomen, and legs, which began after a 2-day history of nausea and vomiting caused by gastroenteritis. He was diagnosed as having sickle cell disease at age 3 years and has been admitted to the hospital on numerous occasions for similar vaso-occlusive sickle cell crises. Sickle cell anemia is caused by a mutation of DNA that changes just one amino acid in the hemoglobin β chains from a glutamic acid to a valine. Hemoglobin is the protein present in red blood cells that reversibly binds oxygen and transports it to the tissues. The adult hemoglobin consists of four polypeptide chains, two α chains and two β chains.

On admission, the patient's hemoglobin level in peripheral venous blood was 7.8 g/dL (reference range, 12 to 16 g/dL). The hematocrit or packed cell volume (the percentage of the total volume of blood made up by red blood cells) was 23.4% (reference range, 41% to 53%). His serum total bilirubin level (a pigment derived from hemoglobin degradation) was 2.3 mg/dL (reference range, 0.2 to 1.0 mg/dL). A radiograph of his abdomen showed radiopaque stones in his gallbladder. With chronic hemolysis (red blood cell destruction), the amount of heme degraded to bilirubin is increased. These stones are the result of the chronic excretion of excessive amounts of bilirubin from the liver into the bile leading to bilirubinate crystal deposition in the gallbladder lumen.

**Di A.,** who has type 1 diabetes mellitus, was giving herself subcutaneous injections of Iletin II NPH beef insulin several times daily after her disease was first diagnosed (see Chapters 2 and 3). Subsequently, her physician switched her to Humulin (synthetic human insulin). At this visit, her physician changed her insulin therapy and has written a prescription for Humalog mix 75/25, a mixture of Humalog in protamine suspension (75%) and unbound Humalog insulin (25%).

**Anne J.** is a 54-year-old woman who is 68 inches tall and weighs 198 lb. She has a history of high blood pressure and elevated serum cholesterol levels. Following a heated argument with a neighbor, **Mrs. J.** experienced a "tight pressure-like band of pain" across her chest, associated with shortness of breath, sweating, and a sense of light-headedness.

After 5 hours of intermittent chest pain, she went to the hospital emergency department, where her electrocardiogram showed changes consistent with an acute infarction of the anterior wall of her heart. She was admitted to the cardiac care unit. Blood was sent to the laboratory for various tests, including the total creatine kinase (CK) level, the MB ("muscle-brain") fraction of CK in the blood, and cardiac troponin T (Tn-T) levels.

The term *angina* describes a crushing or compressive pain. The term *angina pectoris* is used when this pain is located in the center of the chest or pectoral region, often radiating to the neck or arms. The most common mechanism for the latter symptom is a decreased supply of oxygen to the heart muscle caused by atherosclerotic coronary artery disease, which results in obstruction of the vessels that supply arterial blood to cardiac muscle.

## I. GENERAL STRUCTURE OF THE AMINO ACIDS

Twenty different amino acids are commonly found in proteins. They are all α-amino acids, amino acids in which the amino group is attached to the α-carbon (the carbon atom next to the carboxylate group) (Fig 4.1A). The α-carbon has two additional substituents, a hydrogen atom and an additional chemical group called a **side chain** (−R). The side chain is different for each amino acid.

At a physiological pH of 7.4, the amino group on these amino acids carries a positive charge, and the carboxylic acid group is negatively charged (see Fig. 4.1B). The $pK_a$ of the primary carboxylic acid groups for all of the amino acids is around 2 (1.8 to 2.4). At pH values much lower than the $pK_a$ (higher hydrogen ion concentrations), all of the carboxylic acid groups are protonated. At the $pK_a$, 50% of the molecules are dissociated into carboxylate anions and protons, and at a pH of 7.4, over 99% of the molecules are dissociated (see Chapter 2). The $pK_a$ for all of the α-amino groups is around 9.5 (8.8 to 11.0), so that at the lower pH of 7.4, most of the amino groups are fully protonated and carry a positive charge. The form of an amino acid that has both a positive and a negative charge is called a **zwitterion**. Because these charged chemical groups can form hydrogen bonds with water molecules, all of these amino acids are water soluble at physiological pH.

In all of the amino acids but glycine (where the side chain is a hydrogen), the α-carbon is an asymmetric carbon atom that has four different substituents and can exist in either the D or L configuration (see Fig. 3.7). The amino acids in mammalian proteins are all L-amino acids, and these same amino acids serve as precursors of nitrogen-containing compounds synthesized in the body. Thus, human amino acid metabolism is centered on L-amino acids. The amino acid glycine is neither D nor L because the α-carbon atom contains two hydrogen atoms and is not an asymmetric carbon.

The chemical properties of the amino acids give each protein its unique characteristics. Proteins are composed of one or more linear **polypeptide chains** and may contain hundreds of amino acids. The sequence of amino acids, termed the **primary structure**, is determined by the genetic code for the protein. In the polypeptide chains, amino acids are joined through **peptide bonds** between the carboxylic acid of one amino acid and the amino group of the adjacent amino acid (Fig. 4.2). Thus, the amino group, the α-carbon, and the carboxyl groups form the peptide backbone, and the side chains of the amino acids extend outward from this backbone. The side chains interact with the peptide backbone of other regions of the chain or with the side chains of other amino acids in the protein to form hydrophobic regions, electrostatic bonds, hydrogen bonds, or disulfide bonds. These interactions dictate the folding pattern of the molecule. The three-dimensional folding of the protein forms distinct regions called **binding sites** that are lined with amino acid side chains that interact specifically with another molecule termed a *ligand* (such as heme in hemoglobin). Thus, the chemical properties of the side chains determine how the protein folds, how it binds specific ligands, and how it interacts with its environment (such as the aqueous media of the cytoplasm). Each chain will have a **carboxy terminal** and an **amino terminal**. The amino terminal is the first amino acid in the chain, which contains a free amino group. The carboxy terminal is the last amino acid in the chain, which contains a free carboxylate group.

## II. CLASSIFICATION OF AMINO ACID SIDE CHAINS

In Figure 4.3, the 20 amino acids used for protein synthesis are grouped into different classifications according to the polarity and structural features of the side chains. These groupings can be helpful in describing common functional roles or metabolic pathways of the amino acids. However, some amino acid side chains fit into a number of different classifications and are therefore grouped differently in different textbooks. Two of the characteristics of the side chain that are useful for classification are its $pK_a$ and its **hydropathic** index, which are indicated in Table A4.1, found in the online supplement @. The hydropathic index is a scale used to denote

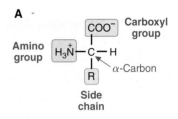

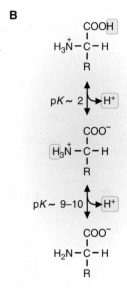

*FIG. 4.1.* Amino acid structure. **A.** General structure of the amino acids found in proteins. The carbon contains four substituents; an amino group, a carboxyl group, a hydrogen atom, and a side chain (R). Both the amino and carboxyl groups carry a charge at physiological pH. **B.** Dissociation of the α-carboxyl and α-amino groups of amino acids. At physiological pH (~7), a form in which both the α-carboxyl and α-amino groups are charged predominates. Some amino acids also have ionizable groups on their side chains.

*FIG. 4.2.* Peptide bonds. Amino acids in a polypeptide chain are joined through peptide bonds between the carboxyl group of one amino acid and the amino group of the next amino acid in the sequence.

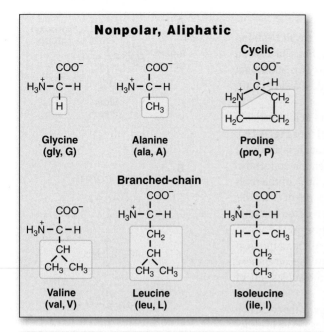

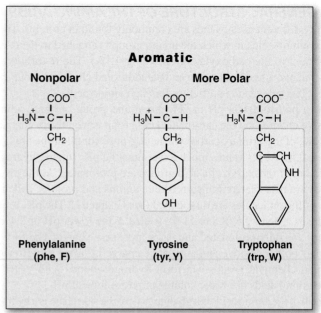

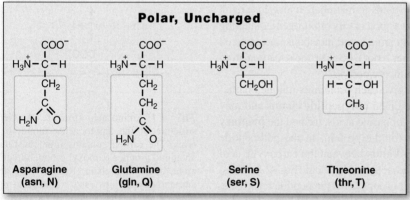

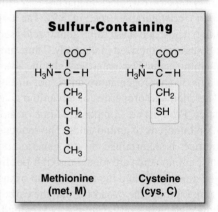

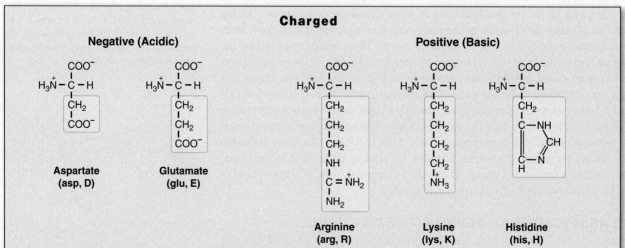

**FIG. 4.3.** The side chains of the amino acids. The side chains are highlighted. The amino acids are grouped by the polarity and structural features of their side chains. These groupings are not absolute, however. Tyrosine and tryptophan, often listed with the nonpolar amino acids, are more polar than other aromatic amino acids because of their phenolic and indole rings, respectively. The single- and three-letter codes are also indicated for each amino acid.

the hydrophobicity of the side chain; the more positive the hydropathic index, the greater the tendency to cluster with other nonpolar molecules and exclude water in the hydrophobic effect. These hydrophobic side chains tend to occur in membranes or in the center of a folded protein, where water is excluded. The more negative the hydropathic index of an amino acid, the more hydrophilic is its side chain.

The names of the different amino acids have been given three-letter and one-letter abbreviations (see Fig. 4.3). The three-letter abbreviations use the first two letters in the name plus the third letter of the name or the letter of a characteristic sound, such as "trp" for tryptophan. The one-letter abbreviations use the first letter of the name of the most frequent amino acid in proteins (such as an "A" for alanine). If the first letter has already been assigned, the letter of a characteristic sound is used (such as an "R" for arginine). Single-letter abbreviations are usually used to denote the amino acids in a polypeptide sequence.

## A. Nonpolar, Aliphatic Amino Acids

Glycine is the simplest amino acid and really does not fit well into any classification because its side chain is only a hydrogen atom. Because the side chain of glycine is so small compared to that of other amino acids, it causes the least amount of steric hindrance in a protein (i.e., it does not significantly impinge on the space occupied by other atoms or chemical groups). Therefore, glycine is often found in bends or in the tightly-packed chains of fibrous proteins.

Alanine and the branched chain amino acids (valine, leucine, and isoleucine) have bulky, nonpolar, **aliphatic** (open-chain hydrocarbon) side chains and exhibit a high degree of hydrophobicity. Electrons are shared equally between the carbon and hydrogen atoms in these side chains, so that they cannot hydrogen bond with water, and therefore, the side chains do not interact with water. Within proteins, these amino acid side chains will cluster together to form hydrophobic cores. Their association is also promoted by van der Waals forces between the positively charged nucleus of one atom and the electron cloud of another. This force is effective over short distances when many atoms pack closely together.

The role of proline in amino acid structure differs from those of the nonpolar amino acids. The amino acid proline contains a ring involving its α-carbon and its α-amino group, which are part of the peptide backbone. It is an imino acid. This rigid ring causes a kink in the peptide backbone that prevents it from forming its usual configuration, and it will restrict the conformation of the protein at that point.

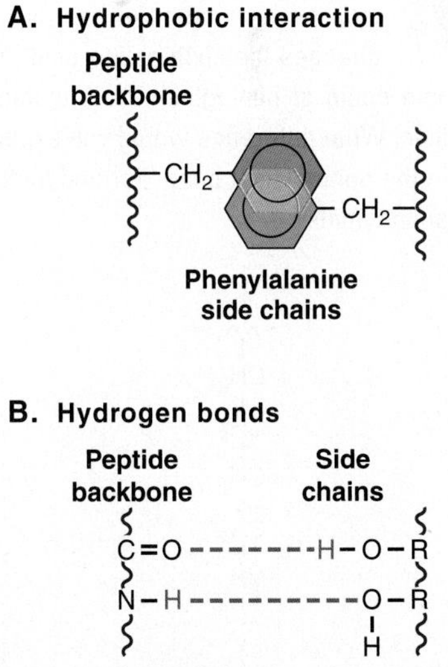

## B. Aromatic Amino Acids

The **aromatic** amino acids have been grouped together because they all contain ring structures with similar properties, but their polarity differs a great deal. The aromatic ring is a six-member carbon-hydrogen ring with three conjugated double bonds (the benzene ring or phenyl group). These hydrogen atoms do not participate in hydrogen bonding. The substituents on this ring determine whether the amino acid side chain engages in polar or hydrophobic interactions. In the amino acid phenylalanine, the ring contains no substituents, and the electrons are shared equally between the carbons in the ring, resulting in a very nonpolar hydrophobic structure in which the rings can stack on each other (Fig. 4.4A). In tyrosine, a hydroxyl group on the phenyl ring engages in hydrogen bonds, and the side chain is therefore more polar and more hydrophilic. The more complex ring structure in tryptophan is an indole ring with a nitrogen that can engage in hydrogen bonds. Tryptophan is therefore also more polar than phenylalanine.

## C. Aliphatic, Polar, Uncharged Amino Acids

Amino acids with side chains that contain an amide group (asparagine and glutamine) or a hydroxyl group (serine and threonine) can be classified as aliphatic, polar, uncharged amino acids. Asparagine and glutamine are amides of the amino acids aspartate and glutamate. The hydroxyl groups and the amide groups in the side

**FIG. 4.4.** Hydrophobic and hydrogen bonds. **A.** Strong hydrophobic interactions occur with the stacking of aromatic groups in phenylalanine side chains. **B.** Examples of hydrogen bonds in which a hydrogen atom is shared by a nitrogen in the peptide backbone and an oxygen atom in an amino acid side chain or between an oxygen in the peptide backbone and an oxygen in an amino acid side chain.

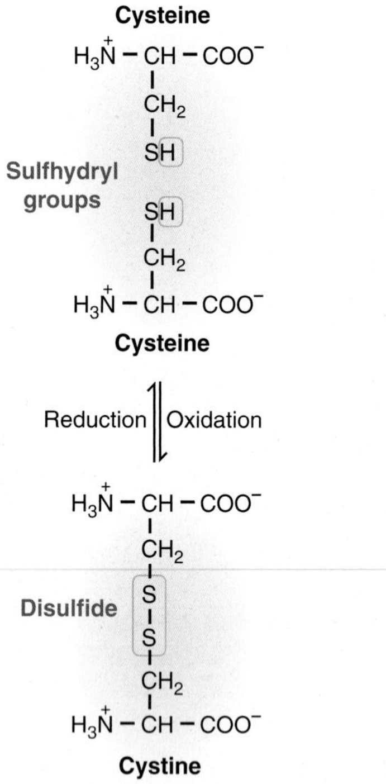

**Cysteine**

$$H_3\overset{+}{N} - CH - COO^-$$

$$CH_2$$

$$SH$$

Sulfhydryl groups

$$SH$$

$$CH_2$$

$$H_3\overset{+}{N} - CH - COO^-$$

**Cysteine**

Reduction ⇅ Oxidation

$$H_3\overset{+}{N} - CH - COO^-$$

$$CH_2$$

$$S$$

Disulfide

$$S$$

$$CH_2$$

$$H_3\overset{+}{N} - CH - COO^-$$

**Cystine**

*FIG. 4.5.* A disulfide bond. Covalent disulfide bonds may be formed between two molecules of cysteine or between two cysteine residues in a protein. The disulfide compound is called cystine. The hydrogens of the cysteine sulfhydryl groups are removed during oxidation.

**Q:** **Will S.** has sickle cell anemia caused by a point mutation in his DNA that changes the sixth amino acid in the β-globin chain of hemoglobin from glutamate to valine. What difference would you expect to find in the noncovalent bonds formed by these two amino acids?

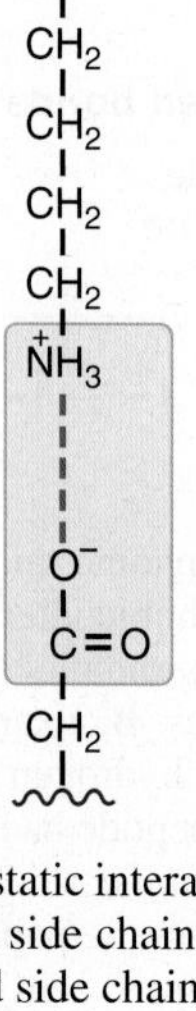

$$CH_2$$

$$CH_2$$

$$CH_2$$

$$CH_2$$

$$\overset{+}{N}H_3$$

$$O^-$$

$$C = O$$

$$CH_2$$

*FIG. 4.6.* Electrostatic interaction between the positively charged side chain of lysine and the negatively charged side chain of aspartate.

chains allow these amino acids to form hydrogen bonds with water, with each other and the peptide backbone, or with other polar compounds in the binding sites of the proteins (see Fig. 4.4B). As a consequence of their hydrophilicity, these amino acids are frequently found on the surface of water-soluble globular proteins.

## D. Sulfur-containing Amino Acids

Both cysteine and methionine contain sulfur. The side chain of cysteine contains a sulfhydryl group that has a $pK_a$ of about 8.4 for dissociation of its hydrogen, so cysteine is predominantly undissociated and uncharged at the physiological pH of 7.4. The free cysteine molecule in solution can form a covalent disulfide bond with another cysteine molecule through spontaneous (nonenzymatic) oxidation of their sulfhydryl groups. The resultant amino acid, cystine, is present in blood and tissues, and is not very water-soluble. In proteins, the formation of a cystine disulfide bond between two appropriately positioned cysteine sulfhydryl groups often plays an important role in holding two polypeptide chains or two different regions of a chain together (Fig. 4.5). Methionine, although it contains a sulfur group, is a nonpolar amino acid with a large bulky side chain that is hydrophobic. It does not contain a sulfhydryl group, and cannot form disulfide bonds. Its important and central role in metabolism is related to its ability to transfer the methyl group attached to the sulfur atom to other compounds.

## E. The Acidic and Basic Amino Acids

The amino acids aspartate and glutamate have carboxylic acid groups that carry a negative charge at physiological pH (see Fig. 4.3). The basic amino acids histidine, lysine, and arginine have side chains containing nitrogen that can be protonated and positively charged at physiological and lower pH values.

The positive charges on the basic amino acids enables them to form ionic bonds (electrostatic bonds) with negatively charged groups, such as the side chains of acidic amino acids or the phosphate groups of coenzymes (Fig. 4.6). The acidic and basic amino acid side chains also participate in hydrogen bonding and the formation of salt bridges (such as the binding of an inorganic ion like $Na^+$ between two partially or fully negatively charged groups).

The charge on these amino acids at physiological pH is a function of their $pK_a$s for dissociation of protons from the α-carboxylic acid groups, the α-amino groups, and the side chains. The titration curve of histidine illustrates the changes in amino acid structure that occur as the pH of the solution is changed from less than 1 to 14 by the addition of hydroxide ions (Fig. 4.7). At low pH, all groups carry protons, amino groups have a positive charge, and carboxylic acid groups have zero charge. As the pH is increased by the addition of alkali ($OH^-$), the proton dissociates from the carboxylic acid group, and its charge changes from zero to negative, with a $pK_a$ of about 2, the pH at which 50% of the protons have dissociated.

The histidine side chain is an imidazole ring with a $pK_a$ of about 6 that changes from a predominantly protonated positively charged ring to an uncharged ring at this pH. The amino group on the α-carbon titrates at a much higher pH (between 9 and 10), and the charge changes from positive to zero as the pH rises. The pH at which the net charge on the molecules in solution is zero is called the **isoelectric point** (pI).

**Electrophoresis,** a technique used to separate proteins on the basis of charge, has been extremely useful in medicine to identify proteins with different amino acid composition. The net charge on a protein at a certain pH is a summation of all of the positive and negative charges on all of the ionizable amino acid side chains plus the N-terminal amino and C-terminal carboxyl groups. Theoretically, the net charge of a protein at any pH could be determined from its amino acid composition by calculating the concentration of positively and negatively charged groups from the Henderson-Hasselbalch equation (see Chapter 2). However, hydrogen bonds and ionic bonds between amino acid side chains in the protein make this calculation unrealistic.

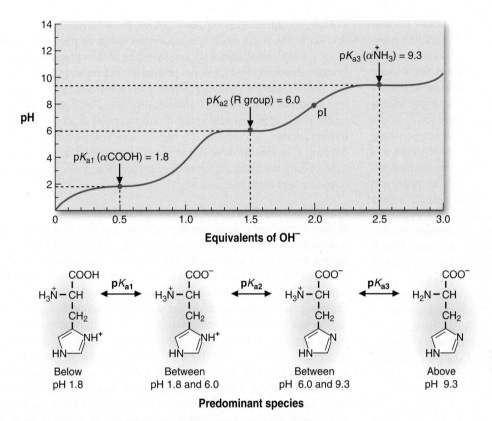

**FIG. 4.7.** Titration curve of histidine. The ionic species that predominates in each region is shown below the graph. pI is the isoelectric point (the pH at which there is no net charge on the molecule).

At this pH, the molecules will not migrate in an electric field toward either a positive pole (cathode) or a negative pole (anode) because the number of negative charges on each molecule is equal to the number of positive charges.

Amino acid side chains change from uncharged to negatively charged or from positively charged to uncharged as they release protons. The acidic amino acids lose a proton from their carboxylic acid side chains at a pH of about 4 and are thus negatively charged at pH 7.4. Cysteine and tyrosine lose protons at their $pK_a$ (~8.4 and 10.5, respectively), so their side chains are uncharged at physiological pH. Histidine, lysine, and arginine side chains change from positively charged to neutral at their $pK_a$. The side chains of the two basic amino acids arginine and lysine have $pK_a$ values above 10, so that the positively charged form always predominates at physiological pH. The side chain of histidine ($pK_a$ ~6.0) dissociates near physiological pH, so only a portion of the histidine side chains carry a positive charge (see Fig. 4.7).

In proteins, only the amino acid side chains and the amino group at the amino terminal and carboxyl group at the carboxyl terminal have dissociable protons. All of the other carboxylic acid and amino groups on the α-carbons are joined in peptide bonds that have no dissociable protons. The amino acid side chains might have a very different $pK_a$ than those of the free amino acids if they are involved in hydrogen or ionic bonds with other amino acid side chains. The $pK_a$ of the imidazole group of histidine, for example, is often shifted to a higher value (between 6 and 7) so that it adds and releases a proton in the physiological pH range.

## III. VARIATIONS IN PRIMARY STRUCTURE

Although almost every amino acid in the primary structure of a protein contributes to its conformation (three-dimensional structure), the primary structure of a protein

 Glutamate carries a negative charge on its side chain at physiological pH and, thus, can engage in ionic bonds or hydrogen bonds with water or other side chains. Valine is a hydrophobic amino acid and, therefore, tends to interact with other hydrophobic side chains to exclude water. (The effect of this substitution on hemoglobin structure is described in more detail in Chapter 7.)

For the most part, human chromosomes occur as homologous pairs, with each member of a pair containing the same genetic information. One member of the pair is inherited from the mother and one from the father. Genes are arranged linearly along each chromosome. A genetic locus is a specific position or location on a chromosome. Alleles are alternative versions of a gene at a given locus. For each locus (site), we have two alleles of each gene, one from our mother and one from our father. If both alleles of a gene are identical, the individual is homozygous for this gene; if the alleles are different, the individual is heterozygous for this gene. **Will S.** has two identical alleles for the sickle variant of the β-globin gene that results in substitution of a valine for a glutamate residue at the sixth position of the β-globin chain. He is therefore homozygous for the sickle cell allele and has sickle cell anemia. Individuals with one normal gene and one sickle cell allele are heterozygous. They are carriers of the disease and have sickle cell trait.

can vary to some degree between species. Even within the human species, the amino acid sequence of a normal functional protein can vary somewhat among individuals, tissues of the same individual, and the stage of development. These variations in the primary structure of a functional protein are tolerated if they are confined to noncritical regions (called variant regions), if they are conservative substitutions (replace one amino acid with one of similar structure), or if they confer an advantage. If many different amino acid residues are tolerated at a position, the region is called **hypervariable**. In contrast, the regions that form binding sites or are critical for forming a functional three-dimensional structure are usually invariant regions that have exactly the same amino acid sequence from individual to individual, tissue to tissue, or species to species.

## A. Polymorphism in Protein Structure

Within the human population, the primary structure of a protein may vary slightly among individuals. The variations generally arise from mutations in DNA that are passed to the next generation. The mutations can result from the substitution of one base for another in the DNA sequence of nucleotides (a point mutation), from deletion or insertions of bases into DNA, or from larger changes (see Chapter 12). For many alleles, the variation has a distinct phenotypic consequence that contributes to our individual characteristics, produces an obvious dysfunction (a congenital or genetically inherited disease), or increases susceptibility to certain diseases. A defective protein may differ from the most common allele by as little as a single amino acid that is a nonconservative substitution (replacement of one amino acid with another of a different polarity or very different size) in an invariant region. Such mutations might affect the ability of the protein to carry out its function, catalyze a particular reaction, reach the appropriate site in a cell, or be degraded. For other proteins, the variations appear to have no significance.

Variants of an allele that occur with a significant frequency in the population are referred to as **polymorphisms**. Thus far in studies of the human genome, almost one-third of the genetic loci appear to be polymorphic. When a particular variation of an allele, or polymorphism, increases in the general population to a frequency of more than 1%, it is considered stable. The sickle cell allele is an example of a point mutation that is stable in the human population. Its persistence is probably due to selective pressure for the heterozygous mutant phenotype, which confers some protection against malaria.

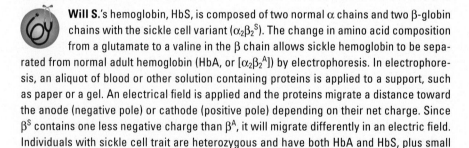

**Will S.**'s hemoglobin, HbS, is composed of two normal α chains and two β-globin chains with the sickle cell variant ($\alpha_2\beta_2^S$). The change in amino acid composition from a glutamate to a valine in the β chain allows sickle hemoglobin to be separated from normal adult hemoglobin (HbA, or [$\alpha_2\beta_2^A$]) by electrophoresis. In electrophoresis, an aliquot of blood or other solution containing proteins is applied to a support, such as paper or a gel. An electrical field is applied and the proteins migrate a distance toward the anode (negative pole) or cathode (positive pole) depending on their net charge. Since $\beta^S$ contains one less negative charge than $\beta^A$, it will migrate differently in an electric field. Individuals with sickle cell trait are heterozygous and have both HbA and HbS, plus small amounts of fetal hemoglobin, HbF ($\alpha_2\gamma_2$).

In heterozygous individuals with sickle cell trait, the sickle cell allele provides some protection against malaria. In **Will S.** and other homozygous individuals with sickle cell anemia, however, the red blood cells sickle more frequently than in heterozygotes, especially under conditions of low oxygen tension (see Chapter 5). The result is a vaso-occlusive crisis in which the sickled cells clog capillaries and prevent oxygen from reaching cells (ischemia), thereby causing pain. The enhanced destruction of the sickled cells by the spleen results in anemia. Consequently, the sickle cell allele is of little advantage to homozygous individuals.

## B. Tissue and Developmental Variations in Protein Structure

Within the same individual, different **isoforms** or **isozymes** of a protein may be synthesized during different stages of fetal and embryonic development, may be present in different tissues, or may reside in different intracellular locations. Isoforms of a protein all have the same function. If they are isozymes (isoforms of enzymes), they catalyze the same reactions. However, isoforms have somewhat different properties and amino acid structure.

### 1. DEVELOPMENTAL VARIATION

Hemoglobin isoforms provide an example of variation during development. Hemoglobin is expressed as the fetal isozyme HbF during the last trimester of pregnancy until after birth, when it is replaced with HbA. HbF is composed of two hemoglobin α and two hemoglobin γ polypeptide chains, in contrast to the adult hemoglobin, hemoglobin A, which is two α and two β chains. During the embryonic stages of development, chains with a different amino acid composition, the embryonic ε and ζ chains are produced. The fetal and embryonic forms of hemoglobin have a much higher affinity for $O_2$ than the adult forms and thus confer an advantage at the low $O_2$ tensions to which the fetus is exposed. At different stages of development, the globin genes specific for that stage are expressed and translated.

### 2. TISSUE-SPECIFIC ISOFORMS

Proteins that differ somewhat in primary structure and properties from tissue to tissue, but retain essentially the same function, are called **tissue-specific isoforms** or **isozymes**. The enzyme creatine kinase (CK) is an example of a protein that exists as tissue-specific isozymes, each composed of two subunits with 60% to 72% sequence homology (similarity between sequences). Of the two CKs that bind to the muscle sarcomere, the M form is produced in skeletal muscle and the B polypeptide chains are produced in the brain. The protein is composed of two subunits, and skeletal muscle therefore produces an MM creatine kinase and the brain produces a BB form. The heart produces both types of chains and therefore forms a heterodimer, MB, as well as the homodimers. Two more CK isozymes are found in mitochondria, a heart mitochondrial CK and the "universal" isoform found in other tissues. In general, most proteins that are present in both the mitochondria and cytosol will be present as different isoforms. The advantage conferred upon different tissues by having their own isoform of CK is unknown. However, tissue-specific isozymes such as MB creatine kinase are useful in diagnosing sites of tissue injury and cell death.

## C. Species Variations in the Primary Structure of Insulin

Species variations in primary structure are also important in medicine, as illustrated by the comparison of human, beef, and pork insulin. **Insulin** is one of the hormones that are highly conserved between species, with very few amino acid substitutions and none in the regions that affect activity. Insulin is a polypeptide hormone of 51 amino acids that is composed of two polypeptide chains (Fig. 4.8). It is synthesized as a single polypeptide chain, but is cleaved in three places prior to secretion to form the C peptide and the active insulin molecule containing the A and B chains. The folding of the A and B chains into the correct three-dimensional structure is promoted by the presence of one intrachain and two interchain disulfide bonds formed by cysteine residues. The invariant residues consist of the cysteine residues engaged in disulfide bonds and the residues that form the surface of the insulin molecule that binds to the insulin receptor. The amino acid substitutions in bovine and porcine insulin (shown in red in Fig. 4.8) are not in amino acids that affect its activity. Consequently, bovine and pork insulin were used for many years for the treatment of diabetes mellitus. However, even with only a few different amino acids, some patients developed an adverse immune response to these forms of insulin.

 A myocardial infarction (heart attack) is caused by an atheromatous obstruction and/or a severe spasm in a coronary artery that prevents the flow of blood to an area of heart muscle distal to the obstruction. Thus, heart cells in this region suffer from a lack of oxygen and blood-borne fuel. Because the cells cannot generate ATP, the membranes become damaged, and enzymes leak from the cells into the blood.

Creatine kinase (CK or CPK) is one of these enzymes. The protein is composed of two subunits, which may be either of the muscle (M) or the brain (B) type. The MB form, containing one M and one B subunit, is found primarily in cardiac muscle. It can be separated electrophoretically from other CK isozymes, and the amount in the blood used to determine if a myocardial infarction has occurred. On admission to the hospital, **Anne J.**'s total CK was 182 units/L (reference range, 38 to 174 units/L). Her MB fraction was 6.8% (reference range 5% or less of the total CK). Although these values are only slightly elevated, they are typical of the phase immediately following a myocardial infarction. Additional information was provided by measuring cardiac troponin T (Tn-T) levels in the blood.

 Although bovine (beef) insulin is identical to human insulin in those amino acid residues essential for activity, the amino acid residues that are in the variable regions can act as antigens and stimulate the formation of antibodies against bovine insulin. Consequently, recombinant DNA techniques have been used for the synthesis of human insulins, such as Humulin (intermediate-acting), or Humalog (rapid-acting), also known as lispro. (See Chapter 14 for information on recombinant DNA technology.) Although **Di A.** had not yet experienced an allergic response to her beef insulin, the cost of Humulin is now sufficiently low that most patients are being changed from beef insulin to the synthetic forms of human insulin.

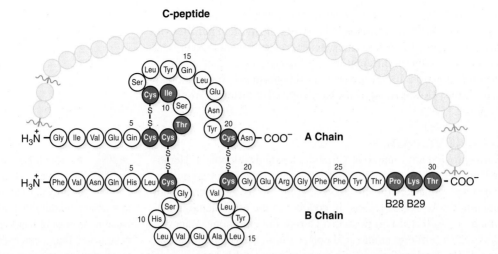

**FIG. 4.8.** The primary structure of human insulin. The substituted amino acids in bovine (beef) and porcine (pork) insulin are shown in *red*. Threonine 30 at the carboxy terminal of the B chain is replaced by alanine in both beef and pork insulin. In beef insulin, threonine 8 on the A chain is also replaced with alanine, and isoleucine 10 with valine. The cysteine residues, which form the disulfide bonds (shown in *blue*) holding the chains together, are invariant. In the bioengineered insulin Humalog (lispro insulin), the position of proline at B28 and lysine at B29 is switched. Insulin is synthesized as a longer precursor molecule, proinsulin, which is one polypeptide chain. Proinsulin is converted to insulin by proteolytic cleavage of certain peptide bonds (squiggly lines in the figure). The cleavage removes a few amino acids and the 31 amino acid C-peptide that connects the A and B chains. The active insulin molecule, thus, has two nonidentical chains.

## IV. MODIFIED AMINO ACIDS

After synthesis of a protein has been completed, a few amino acid residues in the primary sequence may be further modified in enzyme-catalyzed reactions that add a chemical group, oxidize, or otherwise modify specific amino acids in the protein. Because protein synthesis occurs by a process known as translation, these changes are called **posttranslational modification**. Over 100 different posttranslationally modified amino acid residues have been found in human proteins. These modifications change the structure of one or more specific amino acids on a protein in a way that may serve a regulatory function, target or anchor the protein in membranes, enhance a protein's association with other proteins, or target it for degradation (Fig. 4.9).

### A. Glycosylation

**Glycosylation** refers to the addition of carbohydrates to a molecule. In *O*-**glycosylation**, oligosaccharides (small carbohydrate chains) are bound to serine or threonine residues in proteins by *O*-linkages; in *N*-**glycosylation**, they are bound by *N*-linkages (see Fig. 4.9) to the amide group of asparagine. *N*-linked oligosaccharides are found attached to cell surface proteins, where they protect the cell from proteolysis or an immune attack. In contrast, an *O*-glycosidic link is a common way of attaching oligosaccharides to the serine or threonine hydroxyl groups in secreted or membrane-bound proteins.

### B. Fatty Acylation or Prenylation

The addition of lipids to a molecule is called **fatty acylation**. Many membrane proteins contain a covalently attached lipid group that interacts hydrophobically with lipids in the membrane. Palmitoyl groups (C16) are often attached to plasma membrane proteins (palmitoylation), and the myristoyl group (C14) is often attached to proteins in the lipid membranes of intracellular vesicles (myristoylation) (see Fig. 4.9). **Prenylation** involves the addition of farnesyl (C15) or geranylgeranyl groups (C20), which are synthesized from the five-carbon isoprene unit (isopentenyl pyrophosphate, see Fig. 3.1A). These are attached in thioether linkage to a specific cysteine residue of certain membrane proteins, particularly proteins involved in regulation.

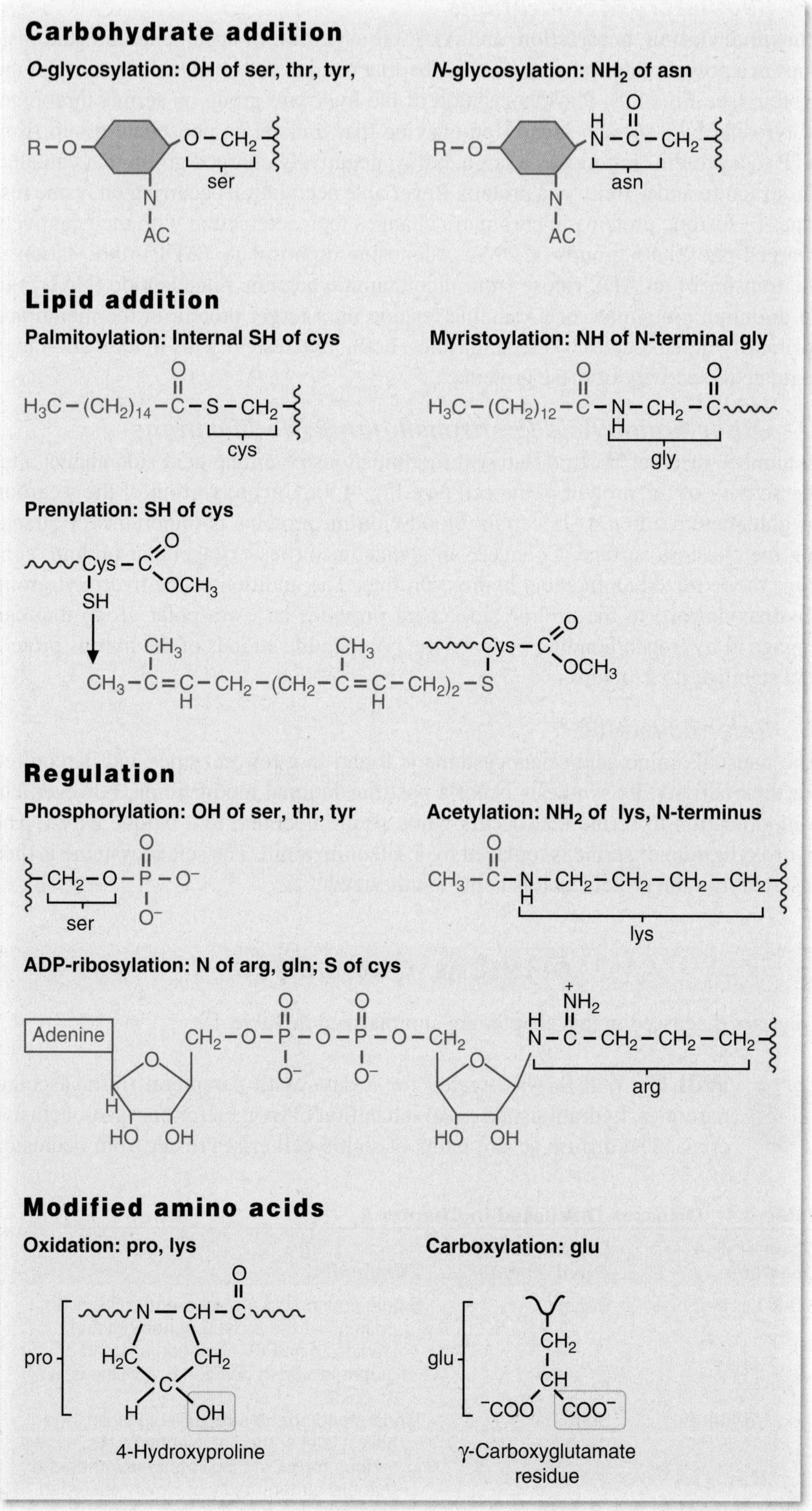
Carbohydrate addition
O-glycosylation: OH of ser, thr, tyr,
N-glycosylation: NH2 of asn
ser
asn
Lipid addition
Palmitoylation: Internal SH of cys
Myristoylation: NH of N-terminal gly
cys
gly
Prenylation: SH of cys
Regulation
Phosphorylation: OH of ser, thr, tyr
Acetylation: NH2 of lys, N-terminus
ser
lys
ADP-ribosylation: N of arg, gln; S of cys
Adenine
arg
Modified amino acids
Oxidation: pro, lys
Carboxylation: glu
pro
glu
4-Hydroxyproline
γ-Carboxyglutamate residue

*FIG. 4.9.* Posttranslational modifications of amino acids in proteins. Some of the common amino acid modifications and the sites of attachment are illustrated. The added group is shown in *red*. Because these modifications are enzyme-catalyzed, only a specific amino acid in the primary sequence is altered. R-O- represents additional carbohydrates attached to the first carbohydrate. In *N*-glycosylation, the attached sugar is usually *N*-acetylglucosamine (N-Ac).

A number of pathogenic bacteria produce bacterial toxins that are ADP-ribosyl transferases ($NAD^+$-glycohydrolases). These enzymes hydrolyze the *N*-glycosidic bond of $NAD^+$ and transfer the ADP-ribose portion to a specific amino acid residue on a protein in the affected human cell. Cholera A-B toxin, a pertussis toxin, and a diphtheria toxin are both ADP-ribosyl transferases.

## C. Regulatory Modifications

**Phosphorylation**, **acetylation**, and **ADP-ribosylation** of specific amino acid residues in a polypeptide can alter bonding by that residue and change the activity of the protein (see Fig. 4.9). Phosphorylation of the hydroxyl group on serine, threonine, or tyrosine by a protein kinase (an enzyme that transfers a phosphate group from ATP to a protein) introduces a large, bulky, negatively charged group that can alter the structure and activity of a protein. Reversible acetylation occurring on lysine residues of histone proteins in chromatin changes their interaction with the negatively charged phosphate groups of DNA. Adenosine diphosphate (ADP)-ribosylation is the transfer of an ADP-ribose from nicotinamide adenine dinucleotide ($NAD^+$) to an arginine, glutamine, or a cysteine residue on a target protein in the membrane (primarily in leukocytes, skeletal muscles, brain, and testes). This modification may regulate the activity of these proteins.

## D. Other Amino Acid Posttranslational Modifications

A number of other posttranslational modifications of amino acid side chains alter the activity of the protein in the cell (see Fig. 4.9). **Carboxylation** of the γ carbon of glutamate (carbon 4) in certain blood clotting proteins is important for attaching the clot to a surface. Collagen, an abundant fibrous extracellular protein, contains the oxidized amino acid hydroxyproline. The addition of the hydroxyl group (**hydroxylation**) to the proline side chain provides an extra polar group that can engage in hydrogen bonding between the polypeptide strands of the fibrous protein and stabilize its structure.

## E. Selenocysteine

The unusual amino acid selenocysteine is found in a few enzymes and is required for their activity. Its synthesis is not a posttranslational modification, however, but a modification to serine that occurs while serine is bound to a unique tRNA. The hydroxyl group of serine is replaced by a selenium atom. The selenocysteine is then inserted into the protein as it is being synthesized.

## CLINICAL COMMENTS

Diseases discussed in this chapter are summarized in Table 4.1.

 **Will S.** Will S. was treated for 3 days with parenteral (intravascular) narcotics, hydration, and nasal inhalation of oxygen for his vaso-occlusive crisis. The diffuse severe pains of sickle cell crises result from occlusion

**Table 4.1   Diseases Discussed in Chapter 4**

| Disorder or Condition | Genetic or Environmental | Comments |
|---|---|---|
| Sickle cell anemia | Genetic | Single amino acid replacement at the sixth position of the β chain of hemoglobin, leading to an E6V alteration (instead of glutamic acid at position 6, a valine is in its place). |
| Type 1 diabetes | Both | Understanding the structure of insulin, and how it is absorbed at injection sites, allows various forms of insulin to be synthesized that are either rapidly or slowly absorbed. This provides type 1 diabetic patients with a variety of treatment options. |
| Myocardial infarction | Both | Caused primarily by environmental factors, which can be exacerbated by genetic conditions. The release of heart-specific isozymes into the circulation is diagnostic for a heart attack. |

of small vessels in a variety of tissues, thereby causing damage to cells from ischemia (low blood flow) or hypoxia (low levels of oxygen). Vaso-occlusion occurs when HbS molecules in red blood cells polymerize in the capillaries where the partial pressure of $O_2$ ($pO_2$) is low. This polymerization causes the red blood cells to change from a biconcave disc to a sickle shape that cannot deform in order to pass through the narrow capillary lumen. The cells aggregate in the capillaries and occlude blood flow.

In addition, once he recovered from his sickle cell crisis, **Will** was treated with hydroxyurea therapy, which increases the production of red blood cells containing fetal hemoglobin. HbF molecules cannot participate in sickling and can decrease the frequency at which sickle crises occur.

**Will S.**'s acute symptoms gradually subsided. Patients with sickle cell anemia periodically experience sickle cell crises, and **Will**'s physician urged him to seek medical help whenever symptoms reappeared. He also counseled him to try to avoid triggers of sickle cell crisis: overexertion, dehydration, extremely cold weather, and exposure to tobacco.

**Di A.** Di A.'s treatment was initially changed from beef insulin to Humulin (synthetic human insulin). Humulin is mass produced by recombinant DNA techniques that insert the human DNA sequences for the insulin A and B chains into the *Escherichia coli* or yeast genome (see Chapter 14). The insulin chains that are produced are then extracted from the media and treated to form the appropriate disulfide bonds between the chains. As costs have fallen for production of the synthetic human insulins, they have replaced pork insulin and the highly antigenic beef insulin.

**Di**'s physician recommended that she take Humalog, an insulin preparation containing lispro, an ultrafast acting bioengineered insulin analogue in which lysine at position B29 has been moved to B28 and proline at B28 has been moved to B29 (hence lispro) (see Fig. 4.8). With lispro, **Di** will be able to time her injections of this rapidly acting insulin minutes before her consumption of carbohydrate-containing meals rather than having to remember to give herself an insulin injection 1 hour before a meal. **Di** will also take a long-acting insulin shot once a day (Lantus), along with her Humalog shots prior to meals each day.

**Anne J.** Mrs. J. continued to be monitored in the cardiac care unit. Her total creatine kinase (CK) continued to rise (228 units/L 12 hours after admission and 266 units/L at 24 hours), as did her muscle-brain (MB) fraction (8% at 12 hours and 10.8% at 24 hours). Within 2 hours of the onset of an acute myocardial infarction, the MB form of CK begins leaking from heart cells that were injured by the ischemic process. These rising serum levels of the MB fraction (and, therefore, of the total CK) reach their peak 12 to 36 hours later and usually return to normal within 3 to 5 days from the onset of the infarction (Fig. 4.10). In addition to the CK measurements, her blood levels were also analyzed for the heart isoform of troponin-T, a protein involved in muscle contraction (see Chapter 5). The levels of these myocardial proteins were elevated in her blood as well.

The switch in position of amino acids in lispro does not affect the action of this synthetic insulin on cells because it is not in a critical invariant region, but it does affect the ability of insulin to bind zinc. Normally, human insulin is secreted from the pancreas as a zinc hexamer in which six insulin molecules are bound to the zinc atom. When zinc insulin is injected, the binding to zinc slows the absorption from the subcutaneous (under the skin) injection site. Lispro cannot bind zinc to form a hexamer, and thus it is absorbed much more quickly than other insulins.

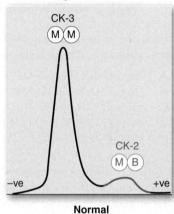

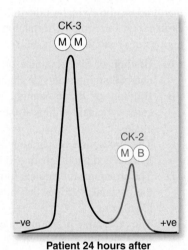

***FIG. 4.10.*** Electrophoretic separation of serum CK enzymes from a normal healthy adult and from a patient who had a myocardial infarction 24 hours previously. CK catalyzes the reversible transfer of a phosphate from ATP to creatine to form phosphocreatine and ADP. The reaction is an important part of energy metabolism in heart muscle, skeletal muscle, and brain. Three different forms of the dimer exist: BB (or CK-1) found in brain, MB (or CK-2) found only in heart, and MM (or CK-3), found only in skeletal and heart muscle (cathode, −ve; anode, +ve).

# REVIEW QUESTIONS-CHAPTER 4

1.  In a polypeptide at physiological pH, hydrogen bonding may occur between which one of the following?

    A.  The side chains of a leucine residue and a lysine residue
    B.  The side chains of an aspartyl residue and a glutamyl residue
    C.  The amide group in the peptide bond and an aspartyl side chain
    D.  The terminal α-amino group and the terminal α-carboxyl group
    E.  The SH groups of two cysteine residues

2.  Which one of the following shows the linear sequence of atoms joined by covalent bonds in a peptide backbone?

    A.  –N-C-O-N-C-O-N-C-O-
    B.  –N-C-C-O-N-C-C-O-N-C-C-O-
    C.  –N-H-C-C-N-H-C-C-N-H-C-C-
    D.  –N-H-C-O-H-N-H-C-O-H-N-H-C-C-
    E.  –N-C-C-N-C-C-N-C-C

3.  A patient's different preparations of insulin contain some insulin complexed with protamine that is absorbed slowly after injection. Protamine is a protein preparation from rainbow trout sperm containing arginine-rich peptides that bind insulin. Which of the following provides the best explanation for complex formation between arginine-rich regions of protamine and insulin?

    A.  Binding of the protamine preparation to negatively charged amino acid side chains in insulin
    B.  Binding of the protamine preparation to the α-carboxylic acid groups at the N-terminals of insulin chains
    C.  The protamine preparation forms complexes with leucine and phenylalanine in insulin.
    D.  The protamine preparation forms disulfide bonds with the cysteine residues that hold the A and B chains together.
    E.  The protamine preparation contains side chains that form peptide bonds with the carboxyl terminals of the insulin chains.

4.  Protein kinases phosphorylate proteins only at certain hydroxyl groups on amino acid side chains. Which one of the following groups of amino acids all contain potential targets for such protein kinases?

    A.  Aspartate, glutamate, and serine
    B.  Serine, threonine, and tyrosine
    C.  Threonine, phenylalanine, and arginine
    D.  Lysine, arginine, and proline
    E.  Alanine, asparagine, and serine

5.  In the human, endogenously produced opioid peptides serve many functions. Most of these opioids have an *N*-terminal sequence that ends in the following amino acids, as represented by the single-letter code: -Y-G-G-F-G-. In some of the opioids, an internal **L** is replaced by an **M** with little difference in activity. However, in one novel class of endogenous opioids, the *N*-terminal **Y** is replaced by an **F**, thereby abolishing certain of its classical opioid functions. Which one of the following best explains the differences between these two amino acid replacements?

    A.  Substitution of an F for a Y replaces an aliphatic amino acid with an aromatic amino acid, but M and L are both aliphatic.
    B.  Substitution of an F for a Y replaces a small amino acid with a much larger amino acid, but M and L have about the same size.
    C.  Substitution of an F for a Y changes the charge on the peptide, but M and L have the same charge.
    D.  Substitution of an F for a Y replaces a more polar amino acid with a very nonpolar amino acid, but M and L are both nonpolar.
    E.  Substitution of an F for a Y increases the hydrophilicity of that amino acid, whereas substitution of M by L has no effect on the hydrophilicity of that position in the amino acid chain.

# 5 Structure–Function Relationships in Proteins

## CHAPTER OUTLINE

## KEY POINTS

- There are four levels of protein structure:
  - The primary structure (linear sequence of amino acids within the protein)
  - The secondary structure (a regular, repeating pattern of hydrogen bonds stabilizing a particular structure)
  - The tertiary structure (the folding of the secondary structure elements into a three-dimensional conformation)
  - The quaternary structure (the association of subunits within a protein)
- The primary structure of a protein determines the way a protein folds into a unique three-dimensional structure, called its **native conformation.**
- When globular proteins fold, the tertiary structure generally forms a densely packed hydrophobic core with polar amino acid side chains on the outside, facing the aqueous environment.

continued

■ The tertiary structure of a protein consists of structural domains, which may be similar between different proteins, and performs similar functions for the different proteins.

■ Certain structural domains are binding sites for specific molecules, called a ligand, or for other proteins.

■ The affinity of a binding site for its ligand is quantitatively characterized by an association or affinity constant, $K_a$ (or dissociation constant, $K_d$).

■ Protein denaturation is the loss of tertiary (and/or secondary) structure within a protein, which can be caused by heat, acid, or other agents that interfere with hydrogen bonding, and usually causes a decrease in solubility (precipitation).

## THE WAITING ROOM

**Will S.**, who has sickle cell anemia, was readmitted to the hospital with symptoms indicating that he was experiencing another sickle cell crisis (see Chapter 4). Sickle cell disease is a result of improper aggregation of hemoglobin within the red blood cell.

**Anne J.** is a 54-year-old woman who arrived in the hospital 4 days ago, about 5 hours after she began to feel chest pain (see Chapter 4). In the emergency department, the physician drew blood for the measurement of creatine kinase, muscle-brain fraction (CK-MB) and cardiac troponin-T subunit (cTN-T). The results from these tests had supported the diagnosis of an acute myocardial infarction (MI), and Mrs. J. was hospitalized. Subtle differences in the structures of similar proteins in different tissues were used diagnostically to come to this conclusion.

**Di A.** returned to her physician's office for a routine visit to monitor her treatment (see Chapters 2 to 4). Her physician drew blood for an HbA$_{1c}$ (pronounced hemoglobin A-1-c) determination. The laboratory reported a value of 8.5%, compared to a normal reference range of less than 6%.

## I. GENERAL CHARACTERISTICS OF THREE-DIMENSIONAL STRUCTURE

The overall conformation of a protein, the particular position of the amino acid side chains in three-dimensional space, gives a protein its function.

### A. Descriptions of Protein Structure

Proteins are generally grouped into major structural classifications: globular proteins, fibrous proteins, transmembrane proteins, and DNA-binding proteins (Fig. 5.1). **Globular proteins** are usually soluble in aqueous medium and resemble irregular balls. The **fibrous proteins** are long and narrow polymers such as silk and collagen. They are geometrically linear, arranged around a single axis, and have a repeating unit structure. **Transmembrane proteins** consist of proteins that have one or more regions aligned to cross the lipid membrane. **DNA-binding proteins**, although members of the globular protein family, are usually classified separately and are considered in Chapter 13.

The structure of these proteins is often described according to levels called primary, secondary, tertiary, and quaternary structure (Fig. 5.2). The **primary structure**

**Globular**

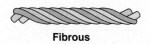

**Fibrous**

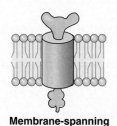

**Membrane-spanning**

 *FIG 5.1.* General shapes of proteins. DNA-binding proteins will be discussed in a later chapter.

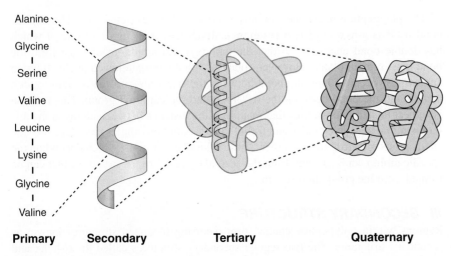

Alanine
|
Glycine
|
Serine
|
Valine
|
Leucine
|
Lysine
|
Glycine
|
Valine

**Primary          Secondary          Tertiary          Quaternary**

*FIG. 5.2.* Levels of structure in a protein.

is the linear sequence of amino acid residues joined through peptide bonds to form a polypeptide chain. The **secondary structure** refers to recurring structures (such as the regular structure of the α-helix) that form in short localized regions of the polypeptide chain. The overall three-dimensional conformation of a protein is its **tertiary structure**, the summation of its secondary structural units. The **quaternary structure** is the association of polypeptide subunits in a geometrically specific manner. The forces involved in a protein folding into its final conformation are primarily noncovalent interactions. These interactions include the attraction between positively and negatively charged molecules (ionic interactions), the hydrophobic effect, hydrogen bonding, and van der Waals interactions (the nonspecific attraction between closely packed atoms).

## B. Requirements of the Three-dimensional Structure

The overall three-dimensional structure of a protein must meet certain requirements to enable the protein to function in the cell or extracellular medium of the body. The first requirement is the creation of a binding site that is specific for just one molecule or a group of molecules with similar structural properties. The specific binding sites of a protein usually define its role. The three-dimensional structure must also exhibit the degrees of flexibility and rigidity appropriate to its function. Some rigidity is essential for the creation of binding sites and for a stable structure (i.e., a protein that flops all over the place cannot carry out its function). However, flexibility and mobility in structure enable the protein to fold as it is synthesized and to adapt as it binds other proteins and small molecules. The three-dimensional structure must have an external surface appropriate for its environment (e.g., cytoplasmic proteins need to keep polar amino acids on the surface to remain soluble in an aqueous environment). In addition, the conformation must also be stable, with little tendency to undergo refolding into a form that cannot fulfill its function or that precipitates in the cell. Finally, the protein must have a structure that can be degraded when it is damaged or no longer needed in the cell.

## II. THE THREE-DIMENSIONAL STRUCTURE OF THE PEPTIDE BACKBONE

The amino acids in a polypeptide chain are sequentially joined by peptide bonds between the carboxyl group of one amino acid and amide group of the next amino acid in the sequence (Fig. 5.3). Usually, the peptide bond assumes a *trans* **config-uration** in which successive α-carbons and their R groups are located on opposite sides of the peptide bond.

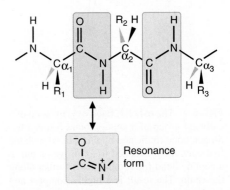

*FIG 5.3.* The peptide backbone. Because of the resonance nature of the peptide bond, the C and N of the peptide bonds form a series of rigid planes. Rotation within allowed torsion angles can occur around the bonds attached to the α-carbon. The side chains are *trans* to each other, and alternate above and below the peptide chain. The actual peptide bond is a hybrid between the resonance forms shown, resulting in a partial negative charge on the carbonyl oxygen, a partial positive charge on the nitrogen, and partial double bond character for the peptide bond itself.

The polypeptide backbone can only bend in a very restricted way. The peptide bond itself is a hybrid of two **resonance structures** (see Fig. 5.3), one of which has double bond character, so that the carboxyl and amide groups that form the bond must remain planar. However, rotation within certain allowed angles (torsion angles) can occur around the bond between the α-carbon and the α-amino group and around the bond between the α-carbon and the carbonyl group. This rotation is subject to steric constraints that maximize the distance between atoms in the different amino acid side chains and forbid torsion (rotation) angles that place the side chain atoms too close to each other. These folding constraints, which depend on the specific amino acids present, limit the secondary and tertiary structures that can be formed from the polypeptide chain.

## III. SECONDARY STRUCTURE

Regions within polypeptide chains form recurring localized structures known as secondary structures. The two regular secondary structures called the α-helix and the β-sheet contain repeating elements formed by hydrogen bonding between atoms of the peptide bonds. Other regions of the polypeptide chain form nonregular, nonrepetitive secondary structures, such as loops and coils.

### A. The α-Helix

The **α-helix** is a common secondary structural element of globular proteins, membrane-spanning domains, and DNA-binding proteins. It has a stable rigid conformation that maximizes hydrogen bonding while staying within the allowed rotation angles of the polypeptide backbone. The peptide backbone of the α-helix is formed by strong hydrogen bonds between each carbonyl oxygen atom and the amide hydrogen (N–H) of an amino acid residue located four residues further down the chain (Fig. 5.4). Thus, each peptide bond is connected by hydrogen bonds to the peptide bond four amino acid residues ahead of it and four amino acid residues behind it in the amino acid sequence. The core of the helix is tightly packed, thereby maximizing association energies between atoms. The *trans* side chains of the amino acids project backward and outward from the helix, thereby avoiding steric hindrance with the polypeptide backbone and with each other (Fig. 5.5). The amino acid proline, because of its ring structure, cannot form the necessary bond angles to fit within an α-helix. Thus, proline is known as a "helix breaker" and is not found in α-helical regions of proteins.

### B. β-Sheets

**β-Sheets** are a second type of regular secondary structure that maximizes hydrogen bonding between the peptide backbones while maintaining the allowed torsion angles. In β-sheets, the hydrogen bonding usually occurs between regions of separate neighboring polypeptide strands aligned parallel to each other (Fig. 5.6). Thus, the carbonyl oxygen of one peptide bond is hydrogen-bonded to the amide nitrogen of a peptide bond on an adjacent strand. This pattern contrasts with the α-helix, in which the peptide backbone hydrogen bonds are within the same strand. Optimal hydrogen bonding occurs when the sheet is bent (pleated) to form β-pleated sheets.

The β-pleated sheet is described as parallel if the polypeptide strands run in the same direction (as defined by their amino and carboxy terminals), and antiparallel if they run in opposite directions. Antiparallel strands are often the same polypeptide chain folded back on itself, with simple hairpin turns or long runs of polypeptide chain connecting the strands. The amino acid side chains of each polypeptide strand alternate between extending above and below the plane of the β-sheet (see Fig. 5.6). Parallel sheets tend to have hydrophobic residues on both sides of the sheets; antiparallel sheets usually have a hydrophobic side and a hydrophilic side. Frequently, sheets twist in one direction.

The hydrogen-bonding pattern is slightly different depending on whether one examines a parallel or antiparallel β-sheet (see Fig. 5.6B). In an antiparallel sheet,

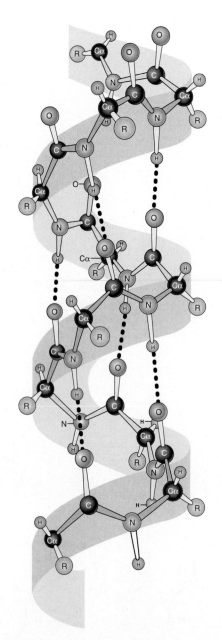

**FIG. 5.4.** The α-helix. Each oxygen atom of a carbonyl group of a peptide bond forms a hydrogen bond (indicated by *black dots*) with the hydrogen atom attached to a nitrogen atom in a peptide bond four amino acids further along the chain. The result is a highly compact and rigid structure.

the atoms involved in hydrogen bonding are directly opposite each other; in a parallel β-sheet, the atoms involved in hydrogen bonding are slightly skewed from one another, such that one amino acid is hydrogen bonded to two others in the opposite strand.

### C. Nonrepetitive Secondary Structures

α-Helices and β-pleated sheets are patterns of regular structure with a repeating element, the turn of a helix or a pleat. In contrast, bends, loops, and turns are nonregular secondary structures that do not have a repeating element. They are characterized by an abrupt change of direction and are often found on the protein surface. For example, β-turns are short regions usually involving four successive amino acid residues. They often connect strands of antiparallel β-sheets (Fig. 5.7).

## IV. TERTIARY STRUCTURE

The tertiary structure of a protein is the pattern of the secondary structural elements folding into a three-dimensional conformation. The three-dimensional structure is flexible and dynamic, with rapidly fluctuating movement in the exact position of amino acid side chains and domains. These fluctuating movements take place without unfolding of the protein. They allow ions and water to diffuse through the structure and provide alternative conformations for ligand binding. As illustrated with examples later in the chapter, this three-dimensional structure is designed to serve all aspects of the protein's function. It creates specific and flexible binding sites for **ligands** (the compound that binds), illustrated with actin and myoglobin. The tertiary structure also maintains residues on the surface appropriate for the protein's cellular location, polar residues for cytosolic proteins, and hydrophobic

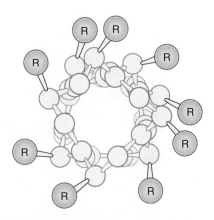

**FIG. 5.5.** A view down the axis of an α-helix. The side chains *(R)* jut out from the helix. Steric hindrance occurs if they come within their van der Waals radii of each other and a stable helix cannot form.

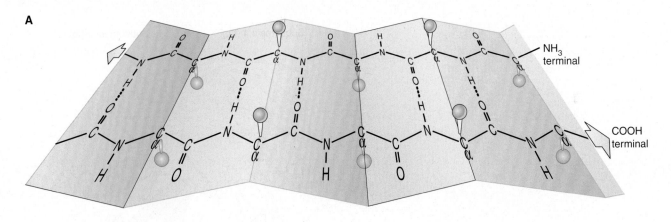

**A**

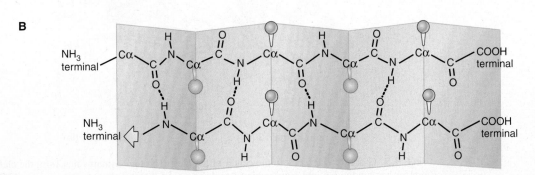

**B**

**FIG. 5.6. A.** A β-pleated sheet. In this case, the chains are oriented in opposite directions (antiparallel). The *large arrows* show the direction of the carboxy terminal. The amino acid side chains (R, designated by the *spherical balls* in the figure) in one strand are *trans* to each other, and alternate above and below the plane of the sheet, which can have a hydrophobic face and a polar face that engages in hydrogen bonding. **B.** Hydrogen-bonding patterns with parallel β-strands.

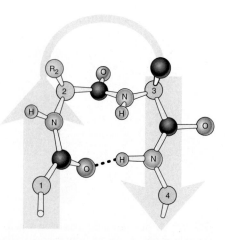

**FIG. 5.7.** β-turn. The four amino acid residues that form the β-turn (also called a hairpin loop) are held together by hydrogen bonds, which make this an extremely stable structure. The C α-carbons of the amino acids are numbered in the figure.

residues for transmembrane proteins (illustrated with the β₂-adrenergic receptor). The forces that maintain tertiary structure are hydrogen bonds, ionic bonds, van der Waals interactions, the hydrophobic effect, and disulfide bond formation.

## A. Domains in the Tertiary Structure

The tertiary structure of large, complex proteins is often described in terms of physically independent regions called **structural domains**. You can usually identify domains from visual examination of a three-dimensional figure of a protein, such as the three-dimensional figure of G-actin shown in Figure 5.8. Each domain is formed from a continuous sequence of amino acids in the polypeptide chain that are folded into a three-dimensional structure independently of the rest of the protein, and two domains are connected through a simpler structure like a loop (e.g., the hinge region of Fig. 5.8). The structural features of each domain can be discussed independently of another domain in the same protein, and the structural features of one domain may not match that of other domains in the same protein.

## B. Folds in Globular Proteins

**Folds** are relatively large patterns of three-dimensional structure that have been recognized in many proteins, including proteins from different branches of the phylogenetic tree. Over 1,000 folds have now been recognized, and it is predicted that there are only a few thousand different folds for all the proteins that have ever existed. A characteristic activity is associated with each fold, such as adenosine triphosphate (ATP) binding and hydrolysis (the actin fold) or $NAD^+$ (oxidized nicotinamide adenine dinucleotide) binding (the nucleotide binding fold).

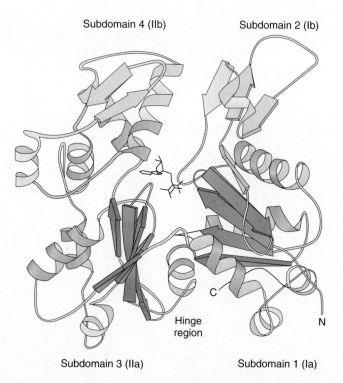

**FIG. 5.8.** G-actin. ATP binds in the center of the cleft. The two domains that form the cleft are further subdivided into subdomains 1 to 4. The overall structure is found in many ATP-binding proteins and is called the actin fold. The conformations of the regions shown in *green* are nearly superimposable among the proteins that contain the actin fold. The *arrows* represent regions of β-sheet, whereas the *coils* represent α-helical regions of the protein. (From Kabsch W, Holmes KC. The actin fold. *Faseb J* 1995;9:167–174.)

## C. The Solubility of Globular Proteins in an Aqueous Environment

Most globular proteins are soluble in the cell. In general, the core of a globular domain has a high content of amino acids with nonpolar side chains (valine, leucine, isoleucine, methionine, and phenylalanine), out of contact with the aqueous medium. This hydrophobic core is densely packed to maximize attractive van der Waals forces, which exert themselves over short distances. The charged polar amino acid side chains (arginine, histidine, lysine, aspartic acid, and glutamic acid) are generally located on the surface of the protein, where they form ion pairs (salt bridges) or are in contact with aqueous solvent. Charged side chains often bind inorganic ions (e.g., $K^+$, $PO_4^{3-}$, or $Cl^-$) to decrease repulsion between like charges. When charged amino acids are located on the interior, they are generally involved in forming specific binding sites. The polar uncharged amino acid side chains of serine, threonine, asparagine, glutamine, tyrosine, and tryptophan are also usually found on the surface of the protein but may occur in the interior, hydrogen-bonded to other side chains. Cystine disulfide bonds (the bond formed by two cysteine sulfhydryl groups) are sometimes involved in the formation of tertiary structure, where they add stability to the protein. However, their formation in soluble, globular proteins is infrequent.

## D. Tertiary Structure of Transmembrane Proteins

Transmembrane proteins, such as the $\beta_2$-adrenergic receptor, contain membrane-spanning domains and intra- and extracellular domains on either side of the membrane (Fig. 5.9). Many ion channel proteins, transport proteins, neurotransmitter receptors, and hormone receptors contain similar membrane-spanning segments that are $\alpha$-helices with hydrophobic residues exposed to the lipid bilayer. These rigid

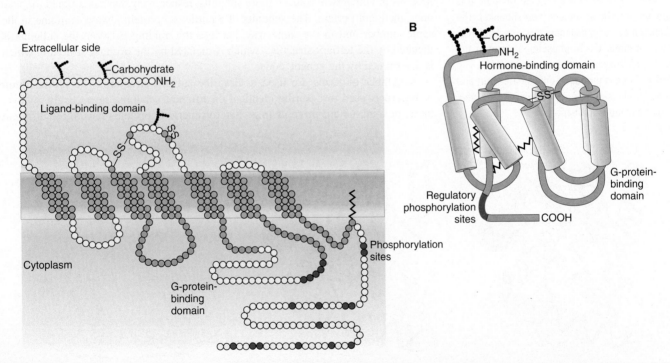

**FIG. 5.9.** $\beta_2$-Adrenergic receptor. The receptor has seven $\alpha$-helical domains that span the membrane and is therefore a member of the heptahelical class of receptors. **A.** The transmembrane domains are drawn in an extended form. The amino terminus (residues 1 through 34) extends out of the membrane and has branched high-mannose oligosaccharides linked through N-glycosidic bonds to the amide of asparagine. Part of the receptor is anchored in the lipid plasma membrane by a palmitoyl group (shown as a squiggle) that forms a thioester with the -SH residue of a cysteine. The -COOH terminus, which extends into the cytoplasm, has several serine and threonine phosphorylation sites (shown as *red circles*). **B.** The seven transmembrane helices (shown as *tubes*) form a cylindrical structure. Loops connecting helices form the hormone binding site on the external side of the plasma membrane, and a binding site for a G protein is on the intracellular side.

helices are connected by loops containing hydrophilic amino acid side chains that extend into the aqueous medium on both sides of the membrane. In the $\beta_2$-adrenergic receptor, the helices clump together so that the extracellular loops form a surface that acts as a binding site for the hormone adrenaline (epinephrine), our fight or flight hormone. The binding site is sometimes referred to as a binding domain (a functional domain), even though it is not formed from a continuous segment of the polypeptide chain. Once adrenaline binds to the receptor, a conformational change in the arrangement of rigid helical structures is transmitted to the intracellular domains that form a binding site for another signaling protein, a heterotrimeric G protein (a guanosine triphosphate [GTP] binding protein composed of three different subunits). Thus, receptors require both rigidity and flexibility in order to transmit signals across the cell membrane.

As discussed in Chapter 4, transmembrane proteins usually have a number of posttranslational modifications that provide additional chemical groups to fulfill requirements of the three-dimensional structure. The amino terminus (residues 1 to 34) extends out of the membrane and has branched high mannose oligosaccharides linked through $N$-glycosidic bonds to the amide of asparagine (see Fig. 5.9). It is anchored in the lipid plasma membrane by a palmitoyl group that forms a thioester with the SH residue of a cysteine. The COOH terminus, which extends into the cytoplasm, has a number of serine and threonine phosphorylation sites (shown as red circles) that regulate receptor activity.

## V. QUATERNARY STRUCTURE

The quaternary structure of a protein refers to the association of individual polypeptide chain subunits in a geometrically and stoichiometrically specific manner (Fig. 5.10). Many proteins function in the cell as dimers, tetramers, or oligomers, proteins in which two, four, or more subunits, respectively, have combined to make one functional protein. The subunits of a particular protein always combine in the same number and in the same way, because the binding between the subunits is dictated by the tertiary structure, which is dictated by the primary structure, which is determined by the genetic code.

A number of terms are used to describe subunit structure. The prefix **homo** or **hetero** is used to describe identical or different subunits, respectively, of two, three, or four subunit proteins (e.g., heterotrimeric G proteins have three different

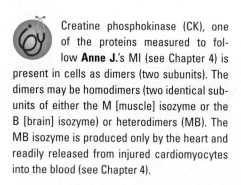 Creatine phosphokinase (CK), one of the proteins measured to follow **Anne J.**'s MI (see Chapter 4) is present in cells as dimers (two subunits). The dimers may be homodimers (two identical subunits of either the M [muscle] isozyme or the B [brain] isozyme) or heterodimers (MB). The MB isozyme is produced only by the heart and readily released from injured cardiomyocytes into the blood (see Chapter 4).

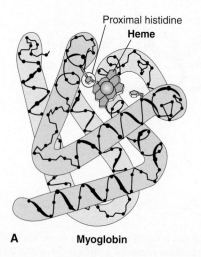 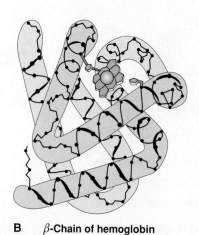 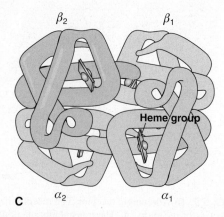

**A** Myoglobin  **B** $\beta$-Chain of hemoglobin  **C**

**FIG. 5.10.** Myoglobin and hemoglobin. Myoglobin (**panel A**) consists of a single polypeptide chain, which is similar in structure to the $\alpha$ and $\beta$ subunits of hemoglobin (**panel B**). In all of the subunits, heme is tightly bound in a hydrophobic binding pocket. The proximal histidine extends down from a helix to bind to the $Fe^{2+}$ atom. The $O_2$ binds between the distal histidine and the heme. **Panel C** displays the quaternary structure of hemoglobin (which consists of two $\alpha$- and two $\beta$-chains). (From Enzyme Structure and Mechanism by Fersht. Copyright © 1977 by WH Freeman and Company. Used with permission.)

subunits). A **protomer** is a unit structure composed of nonidentical subunits. In contrast, F-actin is an oligomer, a multisubunit protein composed of identical G-actin subunits. **Multimer** is sometimes used as a more generic term to designate a complex with many subunits of more than one type.

The contact regions between the subunits of globular proteins resemble the interior of a single subunit protein; they contain closely packed nonpolar side chains, hydrogen bonds involving the polypeptide backbones and their side chains, and occasional ionic bonds or salt bridges. The subunits of globular proteins are very rarely held together by interchain disulfide bonds and never by other covalent bonds. In contrast, fibrous and other structural proteins may be extensively linked to other proteins through covalent bonds.

Assembly into a multisubunit structure increases the stability of a protein. The increase in size increases the number of possible interactions between amino acid residues and therefore makes it more difficult for a protein to unfold and refold. As a result, many soluble proteins are composed of two or four identical or nearly identical subunits with an average size of about 200 amino acids. The forming of multisubunit proteins also aids in the function of the protein.

A multisubunit structure has many advantages besides increased stability. It may enable the protein to exhibit cooperativity between subunits in binding ligands (illustrated later with hemoglobin) or to form binding sites with a high affinity for large molecules. An additional advantage of a multisubunit structure is that the different subunits can have different activities and cooperate in a common function. Examples of enzymes that have regulatory subunits or exist as multiprotein complexes are provided in Chapter 7.

## VI. QUANTITATION OF LIGAND BINDING

In the examples of tertiary structure just discussed, the folding of a protein creates a three-dimensional binding site for a ligand (ATP for G-actin or adrenaline for the $\beta_2$-adrenergic receptor). The binding affinity of a protein for a ligand is quantitatively described by its **association constant**, $K_a$, which is the equilibrium constant for the binding reaction of a ligand (L) with a protein (P) (Equation 5.1). $K_a$ is equal to the rate constant ($k_1$) for association of the ligand with its binding site divided by the rate constant ($k_2$) for dissociation of the ligand–protein complex (LP). $K_d$, the **dissociation constant** for ligand–protein binding, is the reciprocal of $K_a$. The tighter the binding of the ligand to the protein, the higher is the $K_a$ and the lower is the $K_d$. The $K_a$ is useful for comparing proteins produced by different alleles or for describing the affinity of a receptor for different drugs.

## VII. STUCTURE–FUNCTION RELATIONSHIPS IN MYOGLOBIN AND HEMOGLOBIN

Myoglobin and hemoglobin are two oxygen ($O_2$)-binding proteins with a very similar primary structure (see Fig. 5.10). However, myoglobin is a globular protein composed of a single polypeptide chain that has one $O_2$ binding site. Hemoglobin is a tetramer composed of two different types of subunits ($2\alpha$ and $2\beta$ polypeptide chains, referred to as two $\alpha\beta$ protomers). Each subunit has a strong sequence homology to myoglobin and contains an $O_2$ binding site. A comparison between myoglobin and hemoglobin illustrates some of the advantages of a multisubunit quaternary structure.

The tetrameric structure of hemoglobin facilitates saturation with $O_2$ in the lungs and release of $O_2$ as it travels through the capillary beds (Fig. 5.11). When the amount of $O_2$ bound to myoglobin or hemoglobin is plotted against the partial pressure of oxygen ($pO_2$), a hyperbolic curve is obtained for myoglobin, whereas that for hemoglobin is sigmoidal. These curves show that when the $pO_2$ is high, as in the lungs, both myoglobin and hemoglobin are saturated with $O_2$. However, at the lower levels of $pO_2$ in $O_2$-using tissues, hemoglobin cannot bind $O_2$ as well as myoglobin (i.e., its percent saturation is much lower). Myoglobin, which is present in heart and

*Equation 5.1. The association constant, $K_a$ for a binding site on a protein*

Consider a reaction in which a ligand (L) binds to a protein (P) to form a ligand–protein complex (LP) with a rate constant of $k_1$. LP dissociates with a rate constant of $k_2$:

$$L + P \underset{k_2}{\overset{k_1}{\rightleftharpoons}} LP$$

then,

$$K_{eq} = \frac{k_1}{k_2} = \frac{[LP]}{[L][P]} = K_a = \frac{1}{K_d}$$

The equilibrium constant, $K_{eq}$, is equal to the association constant ($K_a$) or $1/K_d$, the dissociation constant. Unless otherwise given, the concentrations of L, P, and LP are expressed as mol/L, and $K_a$ has the units of $(mol/L)^{-1}$.

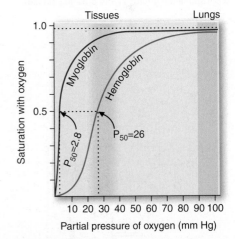

*FIG. 5.11.* $O_2$ saturation curves for myoglobin and hemoglobin. Note that the curve for myoglobin is hyperbolic, whereas that for hemoglobin is sigmoidal. The effect of the tetrameric structure of hemoglobin is to inhibit $O_2$ binding at low $O_2$ concentrations. $P_{50}$ is the partial pressure of $O_2$ ($pO_2$) at which the protein is half-saturated with $O_2$. $P_{50}$ for myoglobin is 2.8 torrs, and that for hemoglobin is 26 torrs, where 1 torr is equal to 1 mm Hg.

Myoglobin is readily released from skeletal muscle or cardiac tissue when the cell is damaged. It has a small molecular weight, 17,000 Da, and is not complexed to other proteins in the cell. (Da is the abbreviation for Dalton, which is a unit of mass approximately equal to 1 H atom. Thus, a molecular weight of 17,000 Da [equivalent to 17 kDa] is approximately equal to 17,000 g/mole.) Large injuries to skeletal muscle that result from physical crushing or lack of ATP production result in cellular swelling and the release of myoglobin and other proteins into the blood. Myoglobin passes into the urine (myoglobinuria) and turns the urine red because the heme (which is red) remains covalently attached to the protein. During an acute MI, myoglobin is one of the first proteins released into the blood from damaged cardiac tissue; however, the amount released is not high enough to cause myoglobinuria. Laboratory measurements of serum myoglobin were used in the past for early diagnosis in patients like **Anne J**. Because myoglobin is not present in skeletal muscle and the heart as tissue-specific isozymes, and the amount released from the heart is much smaller than the amount that can be released from a large skeletal muscle injury, myoglobin measurements are not specific for an MI. Due to the lack of specificity in myoglobin measurements, the cardiac markers of choice for detection of MIs are the heart isozymes of the troponins (I and/or T) and creatine kinase.

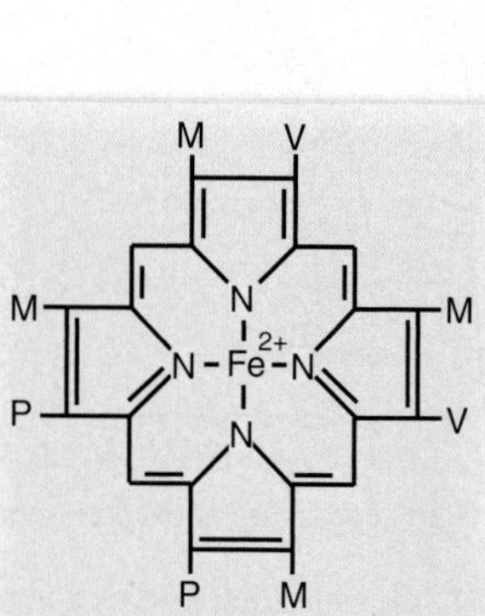

**Heme**

*FIG. 5.12.* Heme. The $Fe^{2+}$ is bound to four nitrogen atoms in the center of the heme porphyrin ring. Methyl (M, $CH_3$), vinyl (V, $-CH=CH_2$), and propionate (P, $CH_2CH_3COO^-$) side chains extend out from the four pyrrole rings that comprise the porphyrin ring.

skeletal muscle, can bind the $O_2$ released by hemoglobin, which it stores to meet the demands of contraction. As $O_2$ is used in the muscle cell for generation of ATP during contraction, it is released from myoglobin and picked up by cytochrome oxidase, a heme-containing enzyme in the electron transport chain that has an even higher affinity for $O_2$ than myoglobin.

### A. Oxygen Binding and Heme

The tertiary structure of myoglobin consists of eight α-helices connected by short coils, a structure that is known as the **globin fold** (see Fig. 5.10). This structure is unusual for a globular protein in that it has no β-sheets. The helices create a hydrophobic $O_2$-binding pocket containing tightly bound **heme** with an iron ($Fe^{2+}$) atom in its center.

Heme consists of a planar porphyrin ring composed of four pyrrole rings that lie with their nitrogen atoms in the center binding a $Fe^{2+}$ atom (Fig. 5.12). Negatively charged propionate groups on the porphyrin ring interact with arginine and histidine side chains from the hemoglobin, and the hydrophobic methyl and vinyl groups that extend out from the porphyrin ring interact with hydrophobic amino acid side chains from hemoglobin. Altogether, there are about 16 different interactions between myoglobin amino acids and different groups in the porphyrin ring.

Organic ligands that are tightly bound to proteins, such as the heme of myoglobin, are called **prosthetic groups**. A protein with its attached prosthetic group is called a **holoprotein**; without the prosthetic group, it is called an **apolipoprotein**. The tightly bound prosthetic group is an intrinsic part of the protein and does not dissociate until the protein is degraded.

Within the binding pocket of myoglobin and hemoglobin, $O_2$ binds directly to the $Fe^{2+}$ atom on one side of the planar porphyrin ring (Fig. 5.13). The $Fe^{2+}$ atom is able to chelate (bind to) six different ligands; four of the ligand positions are in a plane and taken by the central nitrogens in the planar porphyrin ring. There are two ligand positions perpendicular to this plane. One of these positions is taken by the nitrogen atom on a histidine, called the **proximal histidine**, which extends down from a myoglobin or hemoglobin helix. The other position is taken by $O_2$.

The proximal histidine of myoglobin and hemoglobin is sterically repelled by the heme porphyrin ring. Thus, when the histidine binds to the $Fe^{2+}$ in the middle of the ring, it pulls the $Fe^{2+}$ above the plane of the ring. When $O_2$ binds on the other side of the ring, it pulls the $Fe^{2+}$ back into the plane of the ring. The pull of $O_2$ binding moves the proximal histidine toward the porphyrin ring, which moves the helix containing the proximal histidine. This conformational change has no effect on the function of myoglobin. However, in hemoglobin, the movement of one helix leads to the movement of other helices in that subunit, including one in a corner of the subunit that is in contact with a different subunit through salt bridges. The loss of these salt bridges then induces conformational changes in all other subunits, and all four subunits may change in a concerted manner from their original conformation to a new conformation.

### B. Cooperativity of Oxygen Binding in Hemoglobin

The cooperativity in $O_2$ binding in hemoglobin comes from conformational changes in tertiary structure that take place when $O_2$ binds. The conformational change of hemoglobin is usually described as changing from a T (tense) state with low affinity for $O_2$ to an R (relaxed) state with a high affinity for $O_2$. Breaking the salt bridges in the contacts between subunits is an energy-requiring process, and consequently, the binding rate for the first $O_2$ is very low. When the next $O_2$ binds, many of the hemoglobin molecules containing one $O_2$ will already have all four subunits in the R state, and therefore, the rate of binding is much higher. With two $O_2$ molecules bound, an even higher percentage of the hemoglobin molecules will have all four subunits in the R state. This phenomenon, known as positive cooperativity, is responsible for the sigmoidal $O_2$ saturation curve of hemoglobin (see Fig. 5.11).

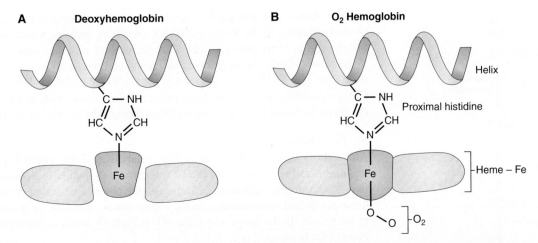

**FIG. 5.13. A.** $O_2$ binding to the $Fe^{2+}$ of heme in hemoglobin. A histidine residue called the proximal histidine binds to the $Fe^{2+}$ on one side of the porphyrin ring and slightly pulls the $Fe^{2+}$ out of the plane of the ring; $O_2$ binds to $Fe^{2+}$ on the other side. **B.** $O_2$ binding causes a conformational change that pulls the $Fe^{2+}$ back into the plane of the ring. As the proximal histidine moves, it moves the helix that contains it.

Sickle cell anemia is really a disease caused by an abnormal quaternary structure. The painful vaso-occlusive crises experienced by **Will S.** are caused by the polymerization of sickle cell hemoglobin (HbS) molecules into long fibers that distort the shape of the red blood cells into sickle cells. The substitution of a hydrophobic valine for a glutamate in the $\beta_2$-chain of hemoglobin creates a knob on the surface of deoxygenated hemoglobin that fits into a hydrophobic binding pocket on the $\beta_1$-subunit of a different hemoglobin molecule. A third hemoglobin molecule, which binds to the first and second hemoglobin molecules through aligned polar interactions, binds a fourth hemoglobin molecule through its valine knob. Thus, the polymerization continues until long fibers are formed.

Polymerization of the hemoglobin molecules is highly dependent on the concentration of HbS and is promoted by the conformation of the deoxygenated molecules. At 100% $O_2$ saturation, even high concentrations of HbS will not polymerize. A red blood cell spends the longest amount of time at the lower $O_2$ concentrations of the venous capillary bed, where polymerization is most likely initiated.

$$HbO_2 \longrightarrow Hb + O_2$$

① Hydrogen ions

② 2,3-Bisphosphoglycerate

③ Covalent binding of $CO_2$

**FIG. 5.14.** Agents that affect $O_2$ binding by hemoglobin. Binding of hydrogen ions, 2,3-bisphosphoglycerate, and carbon dioxide to hemoglobin decrease its affinity for $O_2$.

## C. Agents that Affect Oxygen Binding

The major agents that affect $O_2$ binding to hemoglobin are shown in Figure 5.14.

### 1. 2,3-BISPHOSPHOGLYCERATE

2,3-Bisphosphoglycerate (2,3-BPG) is formed in red blood cells from the glycolytic intermediate 1,3-bisphosphoglycerate (see Chapter 19). 2,3-BPG binds to hemoglobin in the central cavity formed by the four subunits, increasing the energy required for the conformational changes that facilitate the binding of $O_2$. Thus, 2,3-BPG lowers the affinity of hemoglobin for $O_2$. Therefore, $O_2$ is less readily bound (i.e., more readily released in tissues) when hemoglobin has bound 2,3-BPG. Red blood cells can modulate $O_2$ affinity for hemoglobin by altering the rate of synthesis or degradation of 2,3-BPG.

### 2. PROTON BINDING (BOHR EFFECT)

The binding of protons by hemoglobin lowers its affinity for $O_2$ (Fig. 5.15), contributing to a phenomenon known as the Bohr effect (Fig. 5.16). The pH of the blood decreases as it enters the tissues (and the proton concentration rises) because the $CO_2$ produced by metabolism is converted to carbonic acid by the reaction catalyzed by carbonic anhydrase in red blood cells. Dissociation of carbonic acid produces protons that react with several amino acid residues in hemoglobin, causing conformational changes that promote the release of $O_2$.

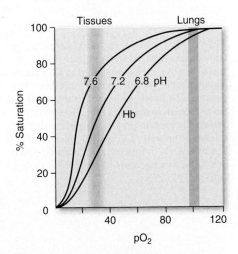

**FIG. 5.15.** Effect of pH on $O_2$ saturation curves. As the pH decreases, the affinity of hemoglobin for $O_2$ decreases, producing the Bohr effect.

**A**

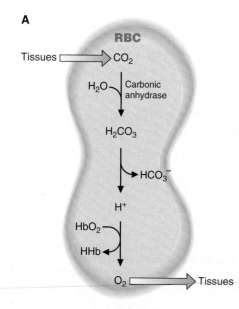

**B**

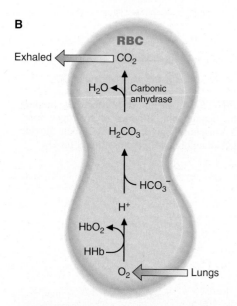

*FIG. 5.16.* Effect of $H^+$ on $O_2$ binding by hemoglobin (Hb). **A.** In the tissues, $CO_2$ is released. In the red blood cell, this $CO_2$ forms carbonic acid, which releases protons. The protons bind to Hb, causing it to release $O_2$ to the tissues. **B.** In the lungs, the reactions are reversed. $O_2$ binds to protonated Hb, causing the release of protons. The protons bind to bicarbonate ($HCO_3^-$), forming carbonic acid which is cleaved to water and $CO_2$, which is exhaled. *RBC,* red blood cell.

In the lungs, this process is reversed. $O_2$ binds to hemoglobin (due to the high $O_2$ concentration in the lung), causing a release of protons, which combine with bicarbonate to form carbonic acid. This decrease of protons causes the pH of the blood to rise. Carbonic anhydrase cleaves the carbonic acid to $H_2O$ and $CO_2$, and the $CO_2$ is exhaled. Thus, in tissues where the pH of the blood is low because of the $CO_2$ produced by metabolism, $O_2$ is released from hemoglobin. In the lungs, where the pH of the blood is higher because $CO_2$ is being exhaled, $O_2$ binds to hemoglobin.

### 3. CARBON DIOXIDE

Although most of the $CO_2$ produced by metabolism in the tissues is carried to the lungs as bicarbonate, some of the $CO_2$ is covalently bound to hemoglobin. In the tissues, $CO_2$ forms carbamate adducts with the N-terminal amino groups of deoxyhemoglobin and stabilizes the deoxy conformation, resulting in more $O_2$ delivery to the tissues. In the lungs where the $pO_2$ is high, $O_2$ binds to hemoglobin and this bound $CO_2$ is released (Fig. 5.17).

## VIII. PROTEIN FOLDING

Although the peptide bonds in a protein are rigid, flexibility around the other bonds in the peptide backbone allow an enormous number of possible conformations for each protein. However, every molecule of the same protein folds into the same stable three-dimensional structure. This shape is known as the **native conformation**.

### A. Primary Structure Determines Folding

The primary structure of a protein determines its three-dimensional conformation. More specifically, the sequence of amino acid side chains dictates the fold pattern of the three-dimensional structure and the assembly of subunits into quaternary structure. Proteins become denatured when they lose their overall structure. However, under certain conditions, denatured proteins can refold into their native conformation, regaining their original function. This indicates that the primary structure essentially specifies the folding pattern. In some cases, proteins are assisted in folding by heat shock proteins (some of which are also called chaperonins), which use the energy provided by ATP hydrolysis to assist in the folding process.

A ***cis-trans* isomerase** and a **protein disulfide isomerase** also participate in folding. The *cis-trans* isomerase converts a *trans* peptide bond preceding a proline into the *cis* conformation, which is well suited for making hairpin turns. The disulfide isomerase breaks and reforms disulfide bonds between the -SH groups of two cysteine residues in transient structures formed during the folding process. After the protein has folded, cysteine-SH groups in close contact in the tertiary structure can react to form the final disulfide bonds.

It is important to note that there is very little difference in the energy state of the native conformation and a number of other stable conformations that a protein might assume. This enables the protein to have the flexibility to change conformation when modifiers are bound to the protein, which enables a protein's activity to be regulated (similar to 2,3-bisphosphoglycerate binding to hemoglobin and stabilizing the deoxy form of hemoglobin).

### B. Fibrous Proteins

### 1. COLLAGEN

**Collagen**, a family of fibrous proteins, is produced by a variety of cell types, but principally by fibroblasts (cells found in interstitial connective tissue), muscle cells, and epithelial cells. Type I collagen, or collagen(I), the most abundant protein in mammals, is a fibrous protein that is the major component of connective tissue. It is found in the extracellular matrix (ECM) of loose connective tissue, bone, tendons, skin, blood vessels, and the cornea of the eye. Collagen(I) contains about 33% glycine and 21% proline and hydroxyproline. Hydroxyproline is an amino acid produced by posttranslational modification of peptidyl proline residues (see Fig. 4.9).

Procollagen(I), the precursor of collagen(I), is a triple helix composed of three polypeptide (pro-α) chains that are twisted around each other, forming a ropelike structure. Polymerization of collagen(I) molecules forms collagen fibrils, which provide great tensile strength to connective tissues (see Fig. 5.1; the representation of a fibrous protein). The individual polypeptide chains each contain about 1,000 amino acid residues. The three polypeptide chains of the triple helix are linked by interchain hydrogen bonds. Each turn of the triple helix contains three amino acid residues, such that every third amino acid is in close contact with the other two strands in the center of the structure. Only glycine, which lacks a side chain, can fit in this position, and indeed, every third amino acid residue of collagen is glycine. Thus, collagen is a polymer of (Gly-X-Y) repeats, where Y is frequently proline and/ or hydroxyproline and X is any other amino acid found in collagen.

Procollagen(I) is an example of a protein that undergoes extensive posttranslational modifications. Hydroxylation reactions produce hydroxyproline residues from proline residues and hydroxylysine from lysine residues. These reactions occur after the protein has been synthesized and require vitamin C (ascorbic acid) as a cofactor of the enzymes, which are prolyl hydroxylase and lysyl hydroxylase. Hydroxyproline residues are involved in hydrogen bond formation that helps to stabilize the triple helix, whereas hydroxylysine residues are the sites of attachment of disaccharide moieties (galactose-glucose).

The side chains of lysine residues may also be oxidized to form the aldehyde allysine. These aldehyde residues produce covalent cross-links between collagen molecules to further stabilize the triple helix. An allysine residue on one collagen molecule reacts with the amino group of a lysine residue on another molecule, forming a covalent Schiff base (a nitrogen-carbon double bond) that is converted to more stable covalent cross-links. Aldol condensation may also occur between two allysine residues, which forms the structure lysinonorleucine.

## 2. TYPES OF COLLAGEN

At least 28 different types of collagen have been characterized (Table A5.1) . Although each type of collagen is found only in particular locations in the body, more than one type may be present in the extracellular matrix at a given location. There are various types of collagen (fibril-forming, network-forming, those that associate with fibril surfaces, transmembrane proteins, endostatin-forming, and those that form periodic beaded filaments), but this text will focus on the fibril-forming collagens (types I, II, III, V, XI, XXIV, and XXVII). These collagen molecules form fibrils that assemble into large insoluble fibers. The fibrils are strengthened through covalent cross-links between lysine residues on adjacent fibrils. The arrangement of the fibrils gives individual tissues their distinct characteristics. Tendons, which attach muscles to bones, contain collagen fibrils aligned parallel to the long axis of the tendon, thus giving the tendon tremendous tensile strength.

## 3. SYNTHESIS AND SECRETION OF COLLAGEN

Collagen is synthesized within the endoplasmic reticulum as a precursor known as preprocollagen. The presequence acts as the signal sequence for the protein and is cleaved, forming procollagen within the endoplasmic reticulum. From there, it is transported to the Golgi apparatus (Table 5.1). Three procollagen molecules associate through formation of inter- and intrastrand disulfide bonds at the carboxy terminus; once these disulfides are formed, the three molecules can align properly to initiate formation of the triple helix. The triple helix forms from the carboxy end toward the amino end, forming tropocollagen. The tropocollagen contains a triple helical segment between two globular ends, the amino and carboxy terminal extensions. The tropocollagen is secreted from the cell, the extensions are removed using

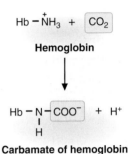

**FIG. 5.17.** Binding of $CO_2$ to hemoglobin. $CO_2$ forms carbamates with the N-terminal amino groups of hemoglobin chains. Approximately 15% of the $CO_2$ in blood is carried to the lungs bound to hemoglobin. The reaction releases protons, which contribute to the Bohr effect. The overall effect is the stabilization of the deoxy form of hemoglobin.

The hydroxyproline residues in collagen are required for stabilization of the triple helix via hydrogen bond formation. In the absence of vitamin C (scurvy), the melting temperature of collagen can drop from 42°C to 24°C as a result of the loss of interstrand hydrogen bond formation from the lack of hydroxyproline residues.

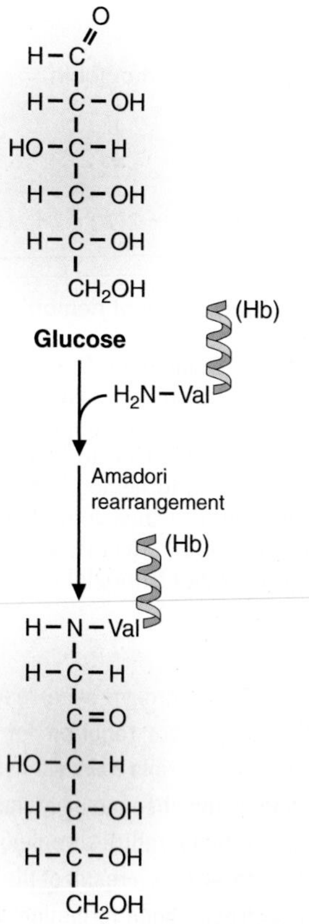

**FIG. 5.18.** Nonenzymatic glycosylation of hemoglobin (*Hb*). Glucose forms a Schiff base with the N-terminal amino group of the protein, which rearranges to form a stable glycosylated product. Similar nonenzymatic glycosylation reactions occur on other proteins.

Di A.'s physician used her glycosylated hemoglobin levels, specifically the HbA$_{1c}$ fraction, to determine whether she had sustained hyperglycemia over a long period of time. The rate of irreversible nonenzymatic glycosylation of hemoglobin and other proteins is directly proportional to the glucose concentration to which they are exposed over the last 4 months (the life span of the red blood cell). The danger of sustained hyperglycemia is that, over time, many proteins become glycosylated and subsequently oxidized, affecting their solubility and ability to function. The glycosylation of collagen in the heart, for example, is believed to result in a cardiomyopathy in patients with chronic uncontrolled diabetes mellitus. In contrast, glycosylation of hemoglobin has little effect on its function.

**Table 5.1  Steps in Collagen Biosynthesis**

| Location | Process |
|---|---|
| Rough endoplasmic reticulum (ER) | Synthesis of preprocollagen; insertion of the procollagen molecule into the lumen of the ER |
| Lumen of ER | Hydroxylation of proline and lysine residues; glycosylation of selected hydroxylysine residues |
| Lumen of ER and Golgi apparatus | Self-assembly of the tropocollagen molecule, initiated by disulfide bond formation in the carboxy terminal extensions; triple helix formation |
| Secretory vesicle | Procollagen prepared for secretion from cell |
| Extracellular | Cleavage of the propeptides, removing the amino and carboxy terminal extensions, and self-assembly of the collagen molecules into fibrils and then fibers |

extracellular proteases, and the mature collagen takes its place within the extracellular matrix. The individual fibrils of collagen line up in a highly ordered fashion to form the collagen fiber.

## C. Protein Denaturation

A protein's quaternary, tertiary, and secondary structures can be destroyed by a number of processes; when this occurs, the protein is said to be denatured.

### 1. DENATURATION THROUGH NONENZYMATIC MODIFICATION OF PROTEINS

Amino acids on proteins can undergo a wide range of chemical modifications that are not catalyzed by enzymes, such as nonenzymatic glycosylation or oxidation. Such modifications usually lead to a loss of function and denaturation of the protein, sometimes to a form that cannot be degraded in the cell. In nonenzymatic glycosylation, glucose that is present in blood, interstitial or intracellular fluid, binds to an exposed amino group on a protein (Fig. 5.18). The two-step process forms an irreversibly glycosylated protein. Proteins that turn over very slowly in the body, like collagen or hemoglobin, exist with a significant fraction present in the glycosylated form. Because the reaction is nonenzymatic, the rate of glycosylation is proportionate to the concentration of glucose present, and individuals with hyperglycemia have much higher levels of glycosylated proteins than individuals with normal blood glucose levels. Collagen and other glycosylated proteins in tissues are further modified by nonenzymatic oxidation and form additional cross-links. The net result is the formation of large protein aggregates referred to as AGEs (advanced glycosylation end products). AGE is a meaningful acronym because AGEs accumulate with age, even in individuals with normal blood glucose levels.

### 2. PROTEIN DENATURATION BY TEMPERATURE, pH, AND SOLVENT

Proteins can be denatured by changes of pH, temperature, or solvent that disrupt ionic, hydrogen, and hydrophobic bonds. At a low pH, ionic bonds and hydrogen bonds formed by carboxylate groups are disrupted; at a very alkaline pH, hydrogen and ionic bonds formed by the basic amino acids are disrupted. Thus, the pH of the body must be maintained within a range compatible with three-dimensional structure. Temperature increases vibrational and rotational energies in the bonds, thereby affecting the energy balance that goes into making a stable three-dimensional conformation. Thermal denaturation is often illustrated by the process of cooking an egg. With heat, the protein albumin converts from its native translucent state to a denatured white precipitate.

Hydrophobic molecules can also denature proteins by disturbing hydrophobic interactions in the protein. For example, long-chain fatty acids can inhibit many enzyme-catalyzed reactions by binding nonspecifically to hydrophobic pockets in proteins and disrupting hydrophobic interactions. Thus, long-chain fatty acids and other highly hydrophobic molecules have their own binding proteins in the cell.

## D. Protein Misfolding and Prions

Prion proteins are believed to cause a neurodegenerative disease by acting as a template to misfold other cellular prion proteins into a form that cannot be degraded. The word "prion" stands for proteinaceous infectious agent. The prion diseases may be acquired either through infection (mad cow disease) or from sporadic or inherited mutations (e.g., Creutzfeldt-Jakob disease [CJD]). Although the infectious prion diseases represent a small proportion of human cases, their link to mad cow disease in the United Kingdom (new variant CJD), to growth hormone inoculations in the United States and France (iatrogenic or "doctor-induced" CJD), and to ritualistic cannibalism in the Fore tribespeople (Kuru) have received the most publicity.

The prion protein is normally found in the brain and is encoded by a gene that is a normal component of the human genome. The disease-causing form of the prion protein has the same amino acid composition but is folded into a different conformation that aggregates into multimeric protein complexes resistant to proteolytic degradation (Fig. 5.19). The normal conformation of the prion protein has been designated PrP$^c$ and the disease-causing form PrP$^{Sc}$ (sc for the prion disease scrapie in sheep). Although PrP$^{Sc}$ and PrP$^c$ have the same amino acid composition, the PrP$^{Sc}$ conformer is substantially enriched in β-sheet structure compared to the normal PrP$^c$ conformer, which has little or no β-sheet structure and is about 40% α-helix. This difference favors the aggregation of PrP$^{Sc}$ into multimeric complexes. These two conformations presumably have similar energy levels. Fortunately, spontaneous refolding of PrP proteins into the PrP$^{Sc}$ conformation is prevented by a large activation energy barrier that makes this conversion extremely slow. Thus, very few molecules of PrP$^{Sc}$ are normally formed during a lifetime.

The infectious disease occurs with the ingestion of PrP$^{Sc}$ dimers in which the prion protein is already folded into the high β structure. These PrP$^{Sc}$ proteins are thought to act as a template to lower the activation energy barrier for the conformational change, causing native proteins to refold into the PrP$^{Sc}$ conformation much more rapidly (much like the role of chaperonins). The refolding initiates a cascade as each new PrP$^{Sc}$ formed acts as a template for the refolding of other molecules.

Familial prion diseases are caused by point mutations in the gene encoding the Pr protein (point mutations are changes in one base in the DNA nucleotide sequence). The diseases have various names related to the different mutations and the clinical syndrome (e.g., Gerstmann-Sträussler-Scheinker disease and familial Creutzfeldt-Jakob disease [fCJD]). fCJD arises from an inherited mutation and has an autosomal dominant pedigree. It typically presents in the fourth decade of life. The mutation lowers the energy required for the protein to fold into the PrP$^{Sc}$ conformation; thereby, the conversion occurs more readily. It is estimated that the rate of generating prion disease by refolding of PrP$^c$ in the normal cell is about 3,000 to 4,000 years. Lowering of the activation energy for refolding by mutation presumably decreases this time to the observed 30- to 40-year prodromal period. Sporadic CJD may arise from somatic cell mutation or rare spontaneous refolding that initiates a cascade of refolding into the PrP$^{Sc}$ conformation. The sporadic form of the disease accounts for 85% of all cases of CJD.

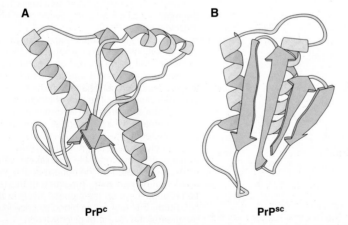

**A**    **B**

**PrP$^c$**    **PrP$^{Sc}$**

*FIG. 5.19.* The conformation of PrP$^c$ (normal) and PrP$^{Sc}$ (disease form). **A.** The prion proteins have two domains, an N-terminal region that binds four Cu$^{2+}$ per chain, and a C-terminal region. In PrP$^c$, the C-terminal regions contain three substantial helices and two three-residue β strands joined by two to three hydrogen bonds (about 40% α-helix and almost no β-sheet structure). It exists as a monomer. **B.** In PrP$^{Sc}$, the C-terminal region is folded into an extensive β-sheet. The overall structure is about 40% to 50% β-sheet and 20% to 30% α-helices. This conformation promotes aggregation.

As the number of PrP$^{Sc}$ molecules increases in the cell, they aggregate into a multi-meric assembly that is resistant to proteolytic digestion. Once an aggregate begins to form, the concentration of free PrP$^{Sc}$ decreases, thereby shifting the equilibrium between PrP and PrP$^{Sc}$ to produce more PrP$^{Sc}$. This leads to further aggregate formation through the shift in equilibrium.

## CLINICAL COMMENTS

Diseases discussed in this chapter are summarized in Table 5.2.

**Will S.** Will S. continues to experience severe low back and lower extremity pain for many hours after admission. The diffuse pains of sickle cell crises are believed to result from occlusion of small vessels in a variety of tissues, thereby depriving cells of $O_2$ and causing ischemic or anoxic damage to the tissues. In a *sickle cell crisis*, long hemoglobin polymers form, causing the red blood cells to become distorted and change from a biconcave disc to an irregular shape, such as a sickle (for which the disease was named) or a stellate structure. The aggregating hemoglobin polymers damage the red blood cell membrane and promote aggregation of membrane proteins leading to increased permeability of the red blood cell and dehydration. Surface charge and antigens of red blood cells are carried on the transmembrane proteins glycophorin and Band 3 (the erythrocyte anion exchange channel). Hemoglobin S binds tightly to the cytoplasmic portion of Band 3, contributing to further polymer aggregation and uneven distribution of negative charge on the sickle cell surface. As a result, the affected cells adhere to endothelial cells in capillaries, occluding the vessel and decreasing blood flow to the distal tissues. The subsequent hypoxia in these tissues causes cellular damage and even death.

**Table 5.2 Diseases Discussed in Chapter 5**

| Disorder or Condition | Genetic or Environmental | Comments |
|---|---|---|
| Myocardial infarction | Both | Specific heart proteins analyzed include CK-MB (heart-specific isozyme) and cardiac troponin (cTN-T, cardiac-specific isozyme). Myoglobin release is also evident after a heart attack, but it is the least specific marker, whereas cTN-T is the most specific marker for evidence of heart muscle damage. |
| Sickle cell disease | Genetic | Hemoglobin S polymerization under deoxygenated conditions, due to hydrophobic interactions caused by the valine in position 6 of the β-chain, instead of glutamic acid. This leads to alterations in red blood cell shape, which causes occluded capillaries. The lack of blood flow through the capillaries will lead to hypoxia and tissue damage, which generates some of the pain endured during a sickle cell crisis. |
| Diabetes types 1 and 2 | Both | The use of glycosylated hemoglobin (HbA$_{1c}$) to determine glycemic control in the diabetic patient. HbA$_{1c}$ is generated by the nonenzymatic glycosylation of hemoglobin. The extent of this reaction is dependent on the glucose levels in the circulation. The higher the blood glucose levels, the greater the extent of glycosylation. |
| Prion diseases | Both | Protein aggregation diseases due to altered tertiary structure for proteins with the same, or slightly altered, primary structure. The aggregates which form precipitate in the brain, leading to eventual neural degeneration and loss of function. |

CK-MB, creatine kinase, muscle-brain fraction; cTN-T, cardiac troponin-T.

The sickled cells are sequestered and destroyed mainly by phagocytic cells, particularly those in the spleen. An anemia results as the number of circulating red blood cells decreases and bilirubin levels rise in the blood as hemoglobin is degraded.

After a few days of treatment, **Will S.**'s crisis was resolved. In the future, should Will S. suffer a cerebrovascular accident as a consequence of vascular occlusion of a large cerebral artery or have recurrent life-threatening episodes of generalized vaso-occlusion in microvessels, a course of long-term maintenance blood transfusions to prevent cerebrovascular accident may be indicated. Iron chelation would have to accompany such a program to prevent or delay the development of iron overload. Although a few individuals with this disease have survived into the sixth decade, mean survival is probably into the fourth decade. Death usually results from infection, renal failure, and/or cardiopulmonary disease.

**Anne J.** Mrs. J.'s diagnosis of an acute MI was partly based on measurements of CK-MB and cTN-T (the cardiac isozyme of troponin-T, a subunit of the regulatory protein troponin). Early diagnosis is critical for a decision on the type of therapeutic intervention to be used. Serum cardiac troponin-T is a relatively late, but highly specific, marker of myocardial injury. It is typically detected in an acute MI within 3 to 5 hours after onset of symptoms, is positive in most cases within 8 hours, and approaches 100% sensitivity at 10 to 12 hours. It remains elevated for 5 to 10 days.

Mrs. J. stayed in the hospital until she had recovered from her catheterization and was stable on her medications. She was discharged on a low fat diet and medications for her heart disease and was asked to participate in the hospital's cardiac rehabilitation program for patients recovering from a recent heart attack. Her physician scheduled her for regular examinations.

**Dianne A.** Di A.'s HbA$_{1c}$ of 8.5% was above the normal level of less than 6% of total hemoglobin. Glycosylation is a nonenzymatic reaction that occurs with a rate directly proportionate to the concentration of glucose in the blood. In the normal range of blood glucose concentrations (about 80 to 140 mg/dL, depending on time after a meal), up to 6% of the hemoglobin is glycosylated to form HbA$_{1c}$. Hemoglobin turns over in the blood as red blood cells are phagocytosed and their hemoglobin degraded and new red blood cells enter the blood from the bone marrow. The average life span of a red blood cell is 120 days. Thus, the extent of hemoglobin glycosylation is a direct reflection of the average serum glucose concentration to which the cell has been exposed over its 120-day life span. **Di A.**'s elevated HbA$_{1c}$ indicates that her average blood glucose level has been elevated over the preceding 3 to 4 months. An increase of Di A.'s insulin dosage would decrease her hyperglycemia and, over time, decrease her HbA$_{1c}$ level as well.

Troponin is a heterotrimeric protein involved in the regulation of striated and cardiac muscle contraction. Most troponin in the cell is bound to the actin–tropomyosin complex in the muscle fibril. The three different subunits of troponin consist of troponin-C, troponin-T, and troponin-I, each with a specific function in the regulatory process. Troponin-T and troponin-I exist as different isoforms in cardiac and skeletal muscle (sequences with a different amino acid composition), thus allowing the development of specific antibodies against each form. As a consequence, either cardiac troponin-T or cardiac troponin-I may be rapidly measured in blood samples by immunoassay with a good degree of specificity.

Four minor components of adult hemoglobin (HbA) result from post-translational, nonenzymatic glycosylation of different amino acid residues (HbA$_{1a1}$, HbA$_{1a2}$, HbA$_{1b1}$, and HbA$_{1c}$). In HbA$_{1c}$, the fraction that is usually measured, the glycosylation occurs on an N-terminal valine.

## REVIEW QUESTIONS-CHAPTER 5

1.  Which one of the following best characterizes α-helical regions of proteins?

    A.  They require a high content of proline and glycine.
    B.  They are formed by hydrogen bonding between two adjacent amino acids in the primary sequence.
    C.  They are formed principally by hydrogen bonds between a carbonyl atom in one peptide bond and the hydrogen atoms on the side chain of another amino acid.
    D.  They all have the same primary structure.
    E.  They are formed principally by hydrogen bonds between a carbonyl oxygen atom in one peptide bond and the amide hydrogen from a different peptide bond.

2.  Which one of the following is a characteristic of globular proteins?

    A.  Hydrophilic amino acids tend to be on the inside.
    B.  Tertiary structure is formed by hydrophobic and electrostatic interactions between amino acid side chains and by hydrogen bonds between peptide bonds.
    C.  Hydrophobic amino acids tend to be on the exterior of the protein.
    D.  Secondary structures are formed principally by hydrophobic interactions between amino acid side chains and backbone atoms.
    E.  Covalent disulfide bonds are necessary to hold the protein in a rigid conformation.

3.  A protein has one transmembrane domain composed entirely of α-helical secondary structure. Which one of the following amino acids would you expect to find in the transmembrane domain?

    A.  Glutamate
    B.  Lysine
    C.  Leucine
    D.  Proline
    E.  Arginine

4.  While studying a novel pathway in a remote species of bacteria, you discover a new globular protein that phosphorylates a substrate using ATP as the phosphate donor. This protein most likely contains which one of the following structures?

    A.  A β-barrel
    B.  A globin fold
    C.  A nucleotide-binding fold
    D.  An actin fold
    E.  An immunoglobulin fold

5.  An increase in pH from 7 to 13 usually results in protein denaturation due to which one of the following?

    A.  Loss of tertiary structure caused by deprotonation of basic groups
    B.  Loss of tertiary structure caused by protonation of carboxylic acid groups
    C.  Loss of secondary structure caused by protonation of basic groups
    D.  Loss of quaternary structure caused by deprotonation of carboxylic acid groups
    E.  Loss of primary structure caused by base-induced cleavage of the peptide bonds

# 6 Enzymes as Catalysts

## CHAPTER OUTLINE

## KEY POINTS

- Enzymes are proteins that act as catalysts—molecules that can accelerate the rate of a reaction.
- Enzymes are specific for various substrates because of the selective nature of the binding sites on the enzyme.
- The catalytic (active) site is the portion of the enzyme molecule at which the reaction occurs.
- Enzymes accelerate reaction rates by decreasing the amount of energy required to reach a high-energy intermediate stage of the reaction known as the transition state complex. This is referred to as lowering the energy of activation.
- Enzymes utilize functional groups at the active site provided by coenzymes, metals, or amino acid residues to perform catalysis.
- Enzymes utilize general acid-base catalysis, formation of covalent intermediates, and transition state stabilization as various mechanisms to accelerate reaction rates.
- Many drugs and toxins act by inhibiting enzymes.
- Enzymes can be regulated to control reaction rates through a variety of mechanisms.

# THE WAITING ROOM

 A year after recovering from salicylate poisoning (see Chapter 2), **Dennis V.** was playing in his grandfather's basement. Dennis drank an unknown amount of the insecticide malathion, sometimes used for killing fruit flies and other insects. Sometime later when he was not feeling well, Dennis told his grandfather what he had done. Mr. V. retrieved the bottle and rushed Dennis to the emergency room of the local hospital. On the way, Dennis vomited repeatedly and complained of abdominal cramps. At the hospital, he began salivating and had an uncontrollable defecation.

In the emergency room, physicians passed a nasogastric tube for stomach lavage, started intravenous fluids, and recorded vital signs. Dennis' pulse rate was 48 beats per minute (slow), and his blood pressure was 78/48 mm Hg (low). The physicians noted involuntary twitching of the muscles in his extremities.

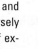 **Lotta T.** was diagnosed with acute gouty arthritis involving her right great toe (see Chapter 3). The presence of insoluble urate crystals within the joint space confirmed the diagnosis. Several weeks after her acute gout attack subsided, Ms. T. was started on allopurinol in an oral dose of 150 mg twice a day. Allopurinol therapy is effective because it inhibits the activity of a specific enzyme.

**Al M.**, a 44-year-old man who has been an alcoholic for the past 5 years, has a markedly diminished appetite for food. One weekend, he became unusually irritable and confused after drinking two-fifths of scotch and eating very little. His landlady convinced him to visit his doctor. Physical examination revealed a heart rate of 104 beats per minute. His blood pressure was slightly low, and he was in early congestive heart failure. He was poorly oriented to time, place, and person.

## I. THE ENZYME-CATALYZED REACTION

**Enzymes**, in general, provide speed, specificity, and regulatory control to reactions in the body. Enzymes are usually proteins that act as catalysts, compounds that increase the rate of chemical reactions. Enzyme-catalyzed reactions have three basic steps:

1. Binding of substrate: **E + S ↔ ES**
2. Conversion of bound substrate to bound product: **ES ↔ EP**
3. Release of product: **EP ↔ E + P**

An enzyme binds the substrates of the reaction it catalyzes and brings them together at the right orientation to react very efficiently. The enzyme then participates in the making and breaking of bonds required for product formation, releases the products, and returns to its original state once the reaction is completed.

Enzymes do not invent new reactions; they just make reactions occur faster. The catalytic power of an enzyme (the rate of the catalyzed reaction divided by the rate of the uncatalyzed reaction) is usually in the range of $10^6$ to $10^{14}$. Without the catalytic power of enzymes, reactions such as those involved in nerve conduction, heart contraction, and digestion of food would occur too slowly for life to exist.

Each enzyme usually catalyzes a specific biochemical reaction. The ability of an enzyme to select just one substrate and distinguish this substrate from a group of very similar compounds is referred to as **specificity**. The enzyme converts this substrate to just one product. The specificity, as well as the speed, of enzyme-catalyzed reactions results from the unique sequence of amino acids that form the three-dimensional structure of the enzyme.

 Most, if not all, of the tissues and organs in the body are adversely affected by chronic ingestion of excessive amounts of alcohol, including the liver, pancreas, heart, reproductive organs, central nervous system, and the fetus. Some of the effects of alcohol ingestion, such as the psychotropic effects on the brain or inhibition of vitamin transport, are direct effects caused by ethanol itself. However, many of the acute and chronic pathophysiological effects of alcohol relate to the pathways of ethanol metabolism.

## A. The Active Site

To catalyze a chemical reaction, the enzyme forms an enzyme-substrate complex in its active catalytic site (Fig. 6.1). The **active site** is usually a cleft or crevice in the enzyme formed by one or more regions of the polypeptide chain. Within the active site, cofactors and functional groups from the polypeptide chain participate in transforming the bound substrate molecules into products.

Initially, the substrate molecules bind to their substrate binding sites, also called the substrate **recognition sites** (see Fig. 6.1B). The three-dimensional arrangement of binding sites in a crevice of the enzyme allows the reacting portions of the substrates to approach each other from the appropriate angles. The proximity of the bound substrate molecules and their precise orientation toward each other contribute to the catalytic power of the enzyme.

The active site also contains functional groups that directly participate in the reaction (see Fig. 6.1C). The functional groups are donated by the polypeptide chain or by bound cofactors (nonprotein complexes which aid in catalysis; see Section III of this chapter). As the substrate binds, it induces conformational changes in the enzyme that promote further interactions between the substrate molecules and the enzyme functional groups. (For example, a coenzyme might form a covalent intermediate with the substrate, or an amino acid side chain might abstract a proton from the reacting substrate.) The activated substrates and the enzyme form a **transition state complex**, an unstable high-energy complex with a strained electronic configuration that is intermediate between substrate and product. Additional bonds with the enzyme stabilize the transition state complex and decrease the energy required for its formation.

The transition state complex decomposes to products, which dissociate from the enzyme (see Fig. 6.1D). The enzyme generally returns to its original form. The free enzyme then binds another set of substrates and repeats the process.

## B. Substrate Binding Sites

Enzyme specificity (the enzyme's ability to react with just one substrate) results from the three-dimensional arrangement of specific amino acid residues in the enzyme that form binding sites for the substrates and activate the substrates during

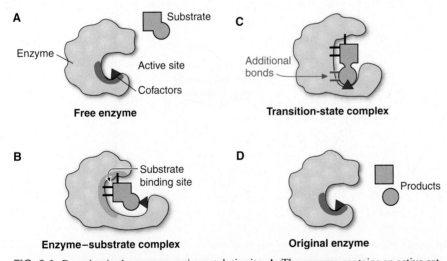

**FIG. 6.1.** Reaction in the enzyme active catalytic site. **A.** The enzyme contains an active catalytic site, shown in *dark red*, with a region or domain where the substrate binds. The active site also may contain cofactors, nonprotein components that assist in catalysis. **B.** The substrate forms bonds with amino acid residues in the substrate binding site. Substrate binding induces a conformational change in the active site. **C.** Functional groups of amino acid residues and cofactors in the active site participate in forming the transition state complex, which is stabilized by additional noncovalent bonds with the enzyme, shown in *red*. **D.** Because the products of the reaction dissociate, the enzyme returns to its original conformation.

the course of the reaction. The lock-and-key and the induced-fit models for substrate binding describe two aspects of the binding interaction between the enzyme and substrate.

### 1. LOCK-AND-KEY MODEL FOR SUBSTRATE BINDING

The substrate binding site contains amino acid residues arranged in a complementary three-dimensional surface that "recognizes" the substrate and binds it through multiple hydrophobic interactions, electrostatic interactions, or hydrogen bonds (Fig. 6.2). The amino acid residues that bind the substrate can come from very different parts of the linear amino acid sequence of the enzyme, as seen in glucokinase. The binding of compounds with a structure that differs from the substrate even to a small degree may be prevented by steric hindrance and charge repulsion. In the lock-and-key model, the complementarity between the substrate and its binding site is compared to that of a key fitting into a rigid lock.

### 2. INDUCED-FIT MODEL FOR SUBSTRATE BINDING

Complementarity between the substrate and the binding site is only part of the picture. As the substrate binds, enzymes undergo a conformational change ("induced fit") that repositions the side chains of the amino acids in the active site and increases the number of binding interactions (see Fig. 6.1). The induced-fit model for substrate binding recognizes that the substrate binding site is not a rigid lock, but a dynamic surface created by the flexible overall three-dimensional structure of the enzyme.

The function of the conformational change induced by substrate binding, the induced fit, is usually to reposition functional groups in the active site in a way that promotes the reaction, improves the binding site of a cosubstrate, or activates an adjacent subunit through cooperativity. For example, large conformational changes

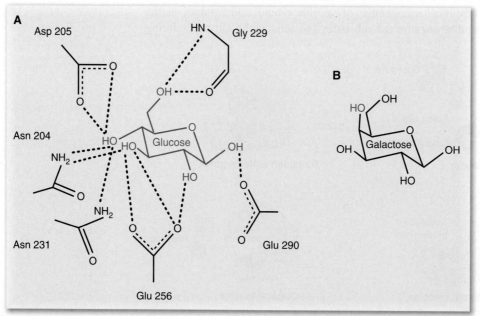

**_FIG. 6.2._** Glucose-binding site in glucokinase. Glucokinase catalyzes the transfer of a phosphate group from ATP to glucose, producing ADP and glucose-6-phosphate. **A.** Glucose, shown in *red*, is held in its binding site by multiple hydrogen bonds between each hydroxyl group and polar amino acids from different regions of the enzyme amino acid sequence in the actin fold (see Chapter 5). The position of the amino acid residue in the linear sequence is given by its number. The multiple interactions enable glucose to induce large conformational changes in the enzyme (induced fit). (Modified from Pilkis SJ, Weber IT, Harrison RW, et al. Glucokinase: structural analysis of a protein involved in susceptibility to diabetes. *J Biol Chem.* 1994;269:21925–21928.) **B.** Enzyme specificity is illustrated by the comparison of galactose and glucose. Galactose differs from glucose only in the position of the −OH group shown in *red*. However, due to its structural difference from glucose, it is not phosphorylated at a significant rate by the enzyme. Cells therefore require a separate galactokinase for the metabolism of galactose.

occur in the actin fold of glucokinase when glucose binds. The induced fit involves changes in the conformation of the whole enzyme that close the cleft of the fold, thereby improving the binding site for ATP and excluding water (which might interfere with the reaction) from the active site. Thus, the multiple interactions between the substrate and the enzyme in the catalytic site serve both for substrate recognition and for initiating the next stage of the reaction, formation of the transition state complex.

## C.  The Transition State Complex

In order for a reaction to occur, the substrates undergoing the reaction need to be activated. If the energy levels of a substrate are plotted as the substrate is progressively converted to product, the curve will exhibit a maximum energy level that is higher than that of either the substrate or the product (Fig. 6.3). This high energy level occurs at the transition state. For some enzyme-catalyzed reactions, the transition state is a condition in which bonds in the substrate are maximally strained. For other enzyme-catalyzed reactions, the electronic configuration of the substrate becomes very strained and unstable as it enters the transition state. The highest energy level corresponds to the most unstable substrate configuration, and the condition in which the changing substrate molecule is most tightly bound to participating functional groups in the enzyme. The difference in energy between the substrate and the transition state complex is called the **activation energy**.

According to transition state theory, the overall rate of the reaction is determined by the number of molecules acquiring the activation energy necessary to form the transition state complex. Enzymes increase the rate of the reaction by decreasing this activation energy. They use various catalytic strategies, such as electronic stabilization of the transition state complex or acid-base catalysis, to obtain this decrease.

Once the transition state complex is formed, it can collapse back to substrates or decompose to form products. The enzyme does not change the initial energy level of the substrates or the final energy level of the products.

## II.  CATALYTIC MECHANISM OF CHYMOTRYPSIN

The enzyme chymotrypsin provides a good example of the strategies and amino acid side chains used by enzymes to lower the amount of activation energy required. Chymotrypsin is a digestive enzyme released into the intestine that catalyzes the hydrolysis of specific peptide bonds in denatured proteins. **Hydrolysis** is the use of

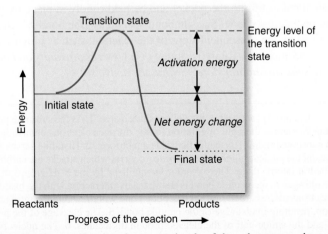

*FIG. 6.3.* Energy diagram showing the energy levels of the substrates as they progress toward products in the absence of enzyme. The substrates must pass through the high-energy transition state during the reaction. Although a favorable loss of energy occurs during the reaction, the energy barrier necessary to form the transition state slows the rate of the reaction. The energy barrier is referred to as the activation energy.

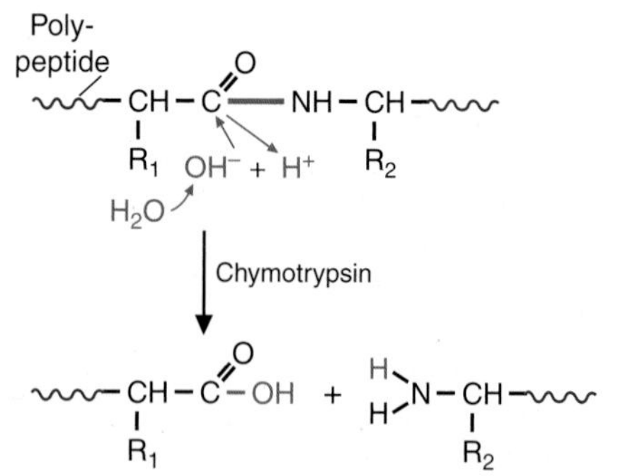

**FIG. 6.4.** Chymotrypsin hydrolyzes certain peptide bonds in proteins. The scissile bond (the bond which is cleaved) is shown in *red*. The carbonyl carbon, which carries a partial positive charge, is attacked by a hydroxyl group from water. An unstable tetrahedral oxyanion intermediate is formed, which is the transition state complex. As the electrons return to the carbonyl carbon, it becomes a carboxylic acid, and the remaining proton from water adds to the leaving group to form an amine.

water to lyse (break) a bond. **Proteolysis** is the hydrolysis of a peptide bond in a protein, a reaction catalyzed by enzymes called **proteases**. Chymotrypsin is a member of the serine protease superfamily, enzymes that utilize a serine in the active site to form a covalent intermediate during proteolysis. In the overall hydrolysis reaction, an $OH^-$ from water is added to the carbonyl carbon of the peptide bond, and an $H^+$ to the N, thereby cleaving the bond (Fig. 6.4). The bond that is cleaved is called the **scissile bond**.

## A. The Reaction in the Absence of Enzyme

In the reaction carried out in the absence of enzyme, the electrons of the negatively charged hydroxyl group of water attack the carbonyl carbon, which carries a partial positive charge. An unstable oxyanion tetrahedral transition state complex is formed in which the oxygen atom carries a full negative charge. The rate of the chemical reaction in the absence of chymotrypsin is slow because there are too few $OH^-$ molecules in $H_2O$ with enough energy to form the transition state complex and too few $OH^-$ molecules colliding with the substrate at the appropriate orientation.

## B. Catalytic Strategies in the Reaction Catalyzed by Chymotrypsin

In the reaction catalyzed by chymotrypsin, the same oxyanion intermediate is formed using the electrons of the hydroxyl group of a serine residue for the attack instead of electrons from a free hydroxyl anion. The rate of the chymotrypsin-catalyzed reaction is faster because functional groups in the enzyme active site activate the attacking hydroxyl group, stabilize the oxyanion transition state complexes, form a covalent intermediate, and destabilize the leaving group. The reaction takes place in two stages: (a) cleavage of the peptide bond in the denatured substrate protein and formation of a covalent acyl–enzyme intermediate (Fig. 6.5, steps 1 to 5) and (b) hydrolysis of the acyl–enzyme intermediate to release the remaining portion of the substrate protein (Fig. 6.5, steps 6 to 9). *The names of the catalytic strategies employed in the various steps are in italics in the following paragraphs.*

### 1. SPECIFICITY OF BINDING TO CHYMOTRYPSIN

Chymotrypsin hydrolyzes the peptide bond on the carbonyl side of a phenylalanine, tyrosine, or tryptophan in a denatured protein. The substrate recognition site consists of a hydrophobic binding pocket that holds the hydrophobic amino acid contributing the carbonyl group of the scissile bond (see Fig. 6.5, step 1). The substrate protein must be denatured to fit into the pocket and be held rigidly in place by glycines in the enzyme peptide backbone. Scissile bond specificity (the bond which is broken) is also provided by the subsequent steps of the reaction, such as moving serine 195 into attacking position (this catalytic strategy is known as *proximity and orientation; orienting the substrate appropriately within the active site*).

**FIG. 6.5.** Catalytic mechanism of chymotrypsin. The substrate (a denatured protein) is in the yellow shaded area. **1.** As the substrate protein binds to the active site, serine 195 and histidine 57 are moved closer together and at the right orientation for the nitrogen electrons on histidine to attract the hydrogen of serine. Without this change of conformation on substrate binding, the catalytic triad cannot form. **2.** Histidine serves as a general base catalyst because it abstracts a proton from the serine, increasing the nucleophilicity of the serine–oxygen, which attacks the carbonyl carbon. **3.** The electrons of the carbonyl group form the oxyanion tetrahedral intermediate. The oxyanion is stabilized by the N–H groups of serine-195 and glycine in the chymotrypsin peptide backbone. **4.** The amide nitrogen in the peptide bond is stabilized by interaction with the histidine proton. Here, the histidine acts as a general acid catalyst. Because the electrons of the carbon–nitrogen peptide bond withdraw into the nitrogen, the electrons of the carboxy anion return to the substrate carbonyl carbon, resulting in cleavage of the peptide bond. **5.** The cleavage of the peptide bond results in formation of the covalent acyl–enzyme intermediate, and the amide half of the cleaved protein dissociates. **6.** The nucleophilic attack by $H_2O$ on the carbonyl carbon is activated by histidine, whose nitrogen electrons attract a proton from water. **7.** The second tetrahedral oxyanion intermediate (the transition state complex) is formed. It is again stabilized by hydrogen bonds with the peptide backbone bonds of glycine and serine. **8.** Because the histidine proton is donated to the electrons of the bond between the serine oxygen and the substrate carbonyl group, the electrons from the oxyanion return to the substrate carbon to form the carboxylic acid, and the acyl–enzyme bond is broken. **9.** The enzyme, as it releases substrate, returns to its original state.

1. **Substrate binding**

2. **Histidine activates serine for nucleophilic attack**

3. **The oxyanion tetrahedral intermediate is stabilized by hydrogen bonds**

4. **Cleavage of the peptide bond**

5. **The covalent acyl–enzyme intermediate**

6. **Water attacks the carbonyl carbon**

7. **Second oxyanion tetrahedral intermediate**

8. **Acid catalysis breaks the acyl–enzyme covalent bond**

9. **The product is free to dissociate**

**Q:** In the stomach, gastric acid decreases the pH to 1 to 2 to denature proteins through disruption of hydrogen bonding. The protease in the stomach, pepsin, is a member of the aspartate protease superfamily, enzymes that utilize two aspartate residues in the active site for acid-base catalysis of the peptide bond. Why can they not use histidine like chymotrypsin?

## 2. FORMATION OF THE ACYL–ENZYME INTERMEDIATE IN CHYMOTRYPSIN

In the first stage of the reaction, the peptide bond of the denatured protein substrate is cleaved as an active-site serine hydroxyl group attacks the carbonyl carbon of the scissile bond (this catalytic strategy is *nucleophilic catalysis*; a nucleophile is a chemical group that is attracted to a positively charged nucleus) (see Fig. 6.5, step 2). Aspartate and histidine cooperate in converting this hydroxyl group (with a partial negative charge on the oxygen) into a better nucleophilic attacking group by giving it a more negative charge. An active-site histidine acts as a base and abstracts a proton from the serine hydroxyl (an example of *acid-base catalysis*). The protonated histidine is stabilized by the negative charge of a nearby aspartate.

The aspartate-histidine-serine combination, referred to as the catalytic triad, is an example of cooperative interactions between amino acid residues in the active site. The strong nucleophilic attacking group created by this charge-relay system has the same general effect on reaction rate as increasing the concentration of hydroxyl ions available for collision in the uncatalyzed reaction.

In the next step of the reaction sequence, an oxyanion tetrahedral transition state complex is formed that is stabilized by hydrogen bonds with −NH groups in the peptide backbone (see Fig. 6.5, step 3). The original view of the way enzymes form transition state complexes was that they stretched the bonds or distorted the bond angles of the reacting substrates. However, most transition state complexes, like the oxyanion tetrahedral complex, are better described as exhibiting *electronic strain*, an electrostatic state that would be highly improbable if it were not stabilized by bonds with functional groups on the enzyme. *Stabilization of the transition state complex* lowers its energy level and increases the number of molecules that reach this energy level.

Subsequently, the serine in the active site forms a full covalent bond with the carbon of the carbonyl group as the peptide bond is cleaved (an example of *covalent catalysis*). The formation of a stable covalent intermediate is a catalytic strategy employed by many enzymes, and often involves serine or cysteine residues. The covalent intermediate is subsequently hydrolyzed (*acid-base catalysis*). The dissociating products of an enzyme-catalyzed reaction are often destabilized by some degree of charge repulsion in the active site. In the case of chymotrypsin, the amino group formed after peptide bond cleavage is destabilized or "uncomfortable" in the presence of the active site histidine (*destabilization of developing product*).

## 3. HYDROLYSIS OF THE ACYL–CHYMOTRYPSIN INTERMEDIATE

The next sequence of events hydrolyzes the acyl–enzyme intermediate to release the bound carbonyl-side peptide (Fig. 6.5, steps 6 to 9). The active site histidine activates water to form an $OH^-$ for a nucleophilic attack, resulting in a second oxyanion transition state complex. When the histidine adds the proton back to serine, the reaction is complete and the product dissociates.

## C. Energy Diagram in the Presence of Chymotrypsin

The number of steps in real enzymatic reactions results in a multibump energy diagram (Fig. 6.6). At the initial stage of the reaction, a dip occurs because energy is provided by formation of the initial multiple weak bonds between the substrate and enzyme. As the reaction progresses, the curve rises because additional energy is required for formation of the transition state complex. This energy is provided by the subsequent steps in the reaction replacing the initial weak bonds with progressively tighter bonds. Semistable covalent intermediates of the reaction have lower energy levels than do the transition state complexes and are present in the reaction diagram as dips in the energy curve. The final transition state complex has the highest energy level in the reaction and is therefore the most unstable state. It can collapse back to substrates or decompose to form products.

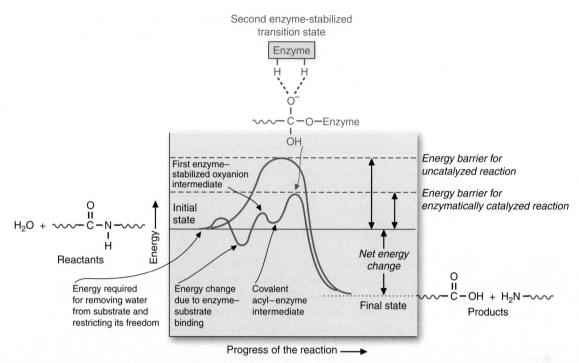

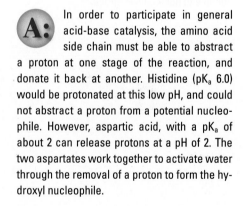

**FIG. 6.6.** A postulated energy diagram for the reaction catalyzed by chymotrypsin. In the presence of enzyme *(red)*; in the absence of enzyme *(blue)*. The energy barrier to the transition state is lowered in the enzyme-catalyzed reaction by the formation of additional bonds between the substrate and enzyme in the transition state complex. The energy is provided by substrate binding to the enzyme. The enzyme does not, however, change the energy levels of the substrate or product.

## III. FUNCTIONAL GROUPS IN CATALYSIS

The catalytic strategies employed by chymotrypsin to increase the reaction rate are common to many enzymes. One of these catalytic strategies, *proximity and orientation*, is an intrinsic feature of substrate binding and part of the catalytic mechanism of all enzymes. All enzymes also stabilize the transition state by electrostatic interactions, but not all enzymes form covalent intermediates.

A variety of functional groups are employed by different enzymes to carry out these catalytic strategies. Some enzymes, like chymotrypsin, rely on amino acid residues within the active site. Other enzymes increase their repertoire by employing cofactors to provide a functional group with the right size, shape, and properties. **Cofactors** are nonprotein compounds that participate in the catalytic process. They are generally divided into three categories: coenzymes, metal ions (e.g., $Fe^{2+}$, $Mg^{2+}$, or $Zn^{2+}$), and metallocoenzymes (similar to the $Fe^{2+}$ heme in hemoglobin; see Chapter 5).

### A. Functional Groups on Amino Acid Side Chains

Almost all of the polar amino acids participate directly in catalysis in one or more enzymes (Table 6.1). Serine, cysteine, lysine, and histidine can participate in covalent catalysis. Histidine, because it has a $pK_a$ that can donate and accept a proton at neutral pH, often participates in acid-base catalysis. Most of the polar amino acid side chains are nucleophilic and participate in nucleophilic catalysis by stabilizing more positively charged groups that develop during the reaction.

### B. Coenzymes in Catalysis

Coenzymes are complex nonprotein organic molecules that participate in catalysis by providing functional groups, much like the amino acid side chains. In humans, they are usually (but not always) synthesized from vitamins. Each coenzyme is involved in catalyzing a specific type of reaction for a class of substrates with certain structural features.

**A:** In order to participate in general acid-base catalysis, the amino acid side chain must be able to abstract a proton at one stage of the reaction, and donate it back at another. Histidine ($pK_a$ 6.0) would be protonated at this low pH, and could not abstract a proton from a potential nucleophile. However, aspartic acid, with a $pK_a$ of about 2 can release protons at a pH of 2. The two aspartates work together to activate water through the removal of a proton to form the hydroxyl nucleophile.

**Q:** Although coenzymes look like they should be able to catalyze reactions autonomously (on their own), they have almost no catalytic power when not bound to the enzyme. Why?

**Table 6.1   Some Functional Groups in the Active Site**

| Function of Amino Acid | Enzyme Example |
|---|---|
| *Covalent intermediates* | |
| Cysteine–SH | Glyceraldehyde 3–phosphate dehydrogenase |
| Serine–OH | Acetylcholinesterase |
| Lysine–NH$_2$ | Aldolase |
| Histidine–NH | Phosphoglucomutase |
| | |
| *Acid-base catalysis* | |
| Histidine–NH | Chymotrypsin |
| Aspartate–COOH | Pepsin |
| | |
| *Stabilization of anion formed during the reaction* | |
| Peptide backbone–NH | Chymotrypsin |
| Arginine–NH | Carboxypeptidase A |
| Serine–OH | Alcohol dehydrogenase |

**A:** In order for a substrate to react with a coenzyme, it must collide with a coenzyme at exactly the right angle. The probability of the substrate and coenzyme in free solution colliding in exactly the right place at the exactly right angle is very small. In addition to providing this proximity and orientation, enzymes contribute in other ways, such as activating the coenzyme by abstracting a proton (e.g., thiamine pyrophosphate and CoA) or polarizing the substrate to make it more susceptible to nucleophilic attack.

Many alcoholics like **Al M.** develop thiamine deficiency because alcohol inhibits the transport of thiamine through the intestinal mucosal cells. In the body, thiamine is converted to thiamine pyrophosphate (TPP). TPP acts as a coenzyme in the decarboxylation of α-keto acids such as pyruvate and α-ketoglutarate and in the utilization of pentose phosphates in the pentose phosphate pathway. As a result of thiamine deficiency, the oxidation of α-keto acids is impaired. Dysfunction occurs in the central and peripheral nervous system, the cardiovascular system, and other organs that require a large amount of energy.

Because most vitamins function as coenzymes, the symptoms of vitamin deficiencies reflect the loss of specific enzyme activities dependent on the coenzyme form of the vitamin. Thus, drugs and toxins that inhibit proteins required for coenzyme synthesis (e.g., vitamin transport proteins or biosynthetic enzymes) can cause the symptoms of a vitamin deficiency. This type of deficiency is called a **functional deficiency**, whereas an inadequate intake is called a **dietary deficiency**.

Most coenzymes are tightly bound to their enzymes and do not dissociate during the course of the reaction. However, a functional or dietary vitamin deficiency that decreases the level of a coenzyme will result in the presence of the apoenzyme in cells (an enzyme devoid of cofactor).

Coenzymes can be divided into two general classes: activation-transfer coenzymes and oxidation-reduction coenzymes.

## 1.   ACTIVATION-TRANSFER COENZYMES

**Activation-transfer coenzymes** usually participate directly in catalysis by forming a covalent bond with a portion of the substrate; the tightly held substrate moiety is then activated for transfer, addition of water, or some other reaction. The portion of the coenzyme that forms a covalent bond with the substrate is its functional group. A separate portion of the coenzyme binds tightly to the enzyme. In general, coenzymes are nonprotein organic cofactors that participate in reactions. They may be covalently bound to enzymes (like biotin), dissociate during deficiency (thiamine pyrophosphate), or freely dissociate at the end of the reaction (coenzyme A). Cofactors that are covalently or very tightly bound to nonenzyme proteins are usually called **prosthetic groups**. A prosthetic group, such as the heme in hemoglobin, usually does not dissociate from a protein until the protein is degraded.

Thiamine pyrophosphate provides a good illustration of the manner in which coenzymes participate in catalysis (Fig. 6.7A). It is synthesized in human cells from the vitamin thiamine by the addition of a pyrophosphate. This pyrophosphate provides negatively charged oxygen atoms that attract Mg$^{2+}$, which then binds tightly to the enzyme. The functional group that extends into the active site is the reactive carbon atom with a dissociable proton (see Fig. 6.7A). In all of the enzymes that use thiamine pyrophosphate, this reactive thiamine carbon forms a covalent bond with a substrate keto group while cleaving the adjacent carbon-carbon bond. However, each thiamine-containing enzyme catalyzes the cleavage of a different substrate (or group of substrates with very closely related structures).

Coenzymes have very little activity in the absence of the enzyme and very little specificity. The enzyme provides specificity, proximity, and orientation in the substrate recognition site, as well as other functional groups for stabilization of the transition state, acid-base catalysis, and so on. For example, thiamine is made into a better nucleophilic attacking group by a basic amino acid residue in the enzyme that

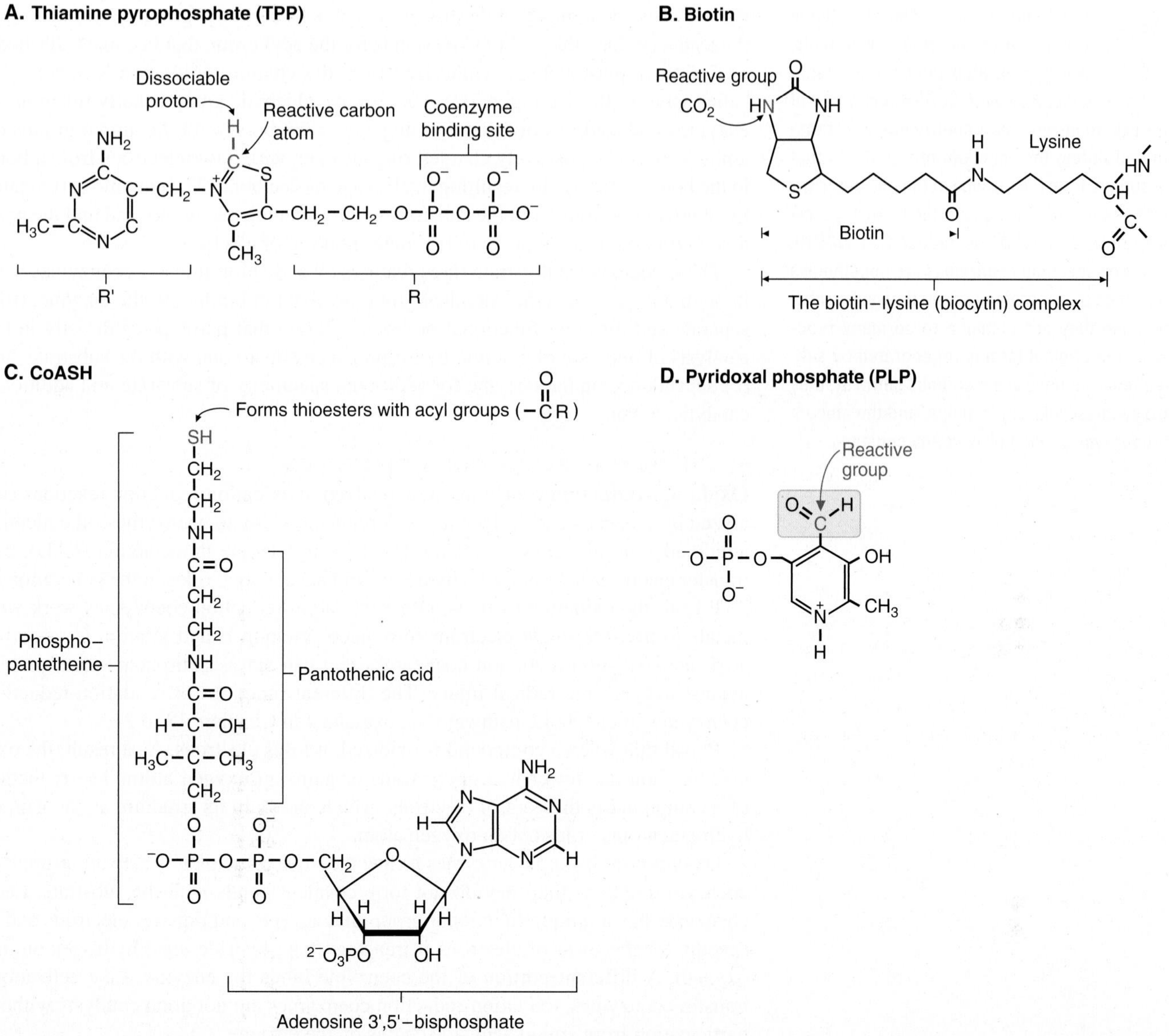

**A. Thiamine pyrophosphate (TPP)**

**B. Biotin**

The biotin–lysine (biocytin) complex

**C. CoASH**

Adenosine 3',5'–bisphosphate

**D. Pyridoxal phosphate (PLP)**

*FIG. 6.7.* Activation-transfer coenzymes. **A.** Thiamine pyrophosphate. Thiamine pyrophosphate is used for breaking carbon-carbon bonds. **B.** Biotin activates and transfers $CO_2$ to compounds in carboxylation reactions. The reactive N is shown in *red*. Biotin is covalently attached to a lysine residue in the carboxylase enzyme. **C.** Coenzyme A (CoA or CoASH) and phosphopantetheine are synthesized from the vitamin pantothenate (pantothenic acid). The active sulfhydryl group, shown in *red*, binds to acyl groups (e.g., acetyl, succinyl, or fatty acyl) to form thioesters. **D.** Reactive sites of pyridoxal phosphate. The functional group of pyridoxal phosphate is a reactive aldehyde (shown in *red*) that forms a covalent intermediate with amino groups of amino acids (a Schiff base). The positively charged pyridine ring is a strong electron-withdrawing group that can pull electrons into it (electrophilic catalysis).

removes the dissociable proton, thereby generating a negatively charged thiamine carbon anion. Later in the reaction, the enzyme returns the proton.

Biotin, coenzyme A (CoA), and pyridoxal phosphate are also activation-transfer coenzymes synthesized from vitamins. Biotin, which does not contain a phosphate group, is covalently bound to a lysine in enzymes called **carboxylases** (see Fig. 6.7B). Its functional group is a nitrogen atom that covalently binds a $CO_2$ group in an energy-requiring reaction. This bound $CO_2$ group is activated for addition to another molecule. In the human, biotin functions only in carboxylation reactions. CoA (CoASH), which is synthesized from the vitamin pantothenate, contains an adenosine 3',5'-bisphosphate, which binds reversibly, but tightly, to a site on an enzyme (see Fig. 6.7C). Its functional group, a sulfhydryl group at the other end of

Most coenzymes, like functional groups on the enzyme amino acids, are regenerated during the course of the reaction. However, CoASH and a few of the oxidation-reduction coenzymes are transformed during the reaction into products that dissociate from the enzyme at the end of the reaction (e.g., CoASH is converted to an acyl CoA derivative, and $NAD^+$ is reduced to NADH). These dissociating coenzymes are nonetheless classified as coenzymes rather than substrates because they are common to so many reactions, the original form is regenerated by subsequent reactions in a metabolic pathway, they are synthesized from vitamins, and the amount of coenzyme in the cell is nearly constant.

the molecule, is a nucleophile that always attacks carbonyl groups and forms acyl thioesters (in fact, the "A" in CoA stands for the acyl group that becomes attached).

Pyridoxal phosphate is synthesized from the vitamin pyridoxine, which is also called vitamin $B_6$ (see Fig. 6.7D). The reactive aldehyde group usually functions in enzyme-catalyzed reactions by forming a covalent bond with the amino groups on amino acids. The positively charged ring nitrogen withdraws electrons from a bond in the bound amino acid, resulting in cleavage of that bond. The enzyme participates by removing protons from the substrate and by keeping the amino acid and the pyridoxal group in a single plane to facilitate shuttling of electrons.

These coenzymes illustrate three features all activation-transfer coenzymes have in common: (a) a specific chemical group involved in binding to the enzyme, (b) a separate and different functional or reactive group that participates directly in the catalysis of one type of reaction by forming a covalent bond with the substrate, and (c) dependence on the enzyme for additional specificity of substrate and additional catalytic power.

## 2. OXIDATION-REDUCTION COENZYMES

**Oxidation-reduction** coenzymes are involved in oxidation-reduction reactions catalyzed by enzymes categorized as oxidoreductases. Some coenzymes, like nicotinamide adenine dinucleotide ($NAD^+$) and flavin adenine dinucleotide (FAD), can transfer electrons together with hydrogen and have unique roles in the generation of ATP from the oxidation of fuels. Other oxidation-reduction coenzymes work with metals to transfer single electrons to oxygen. Vitamin E and vitamin C (ascorbic acid) are oxidation-reduction coenzymes that can act as antioxidants and protect against oxygen free radical injury. The different functions of oxidation-reduction coenzymes in metabolic pathways are explained in Chapters 18 to 21.

Recall that when a compound is oxidized, it loses electrons. As a result, the oxidized carbon has fewer hydrogen atoms or gains an oxygen atom. The reduction of a compound is the gain of electrons, which shows in its structure as the gain of hydrogen atoms or loss of an oxygen atom.

Oxidation-reduction coenzymes follow the same principles as activation-transfer coenzymes, except that they do not form covalent bonds with the substrate. Each coenzyme has a unique functional group that accepts and donates electrons and is specific for the form of electrons it transfers (e.g., hydride ions, hydrogen atoms, oxygen). A different portion of the coenzyme binds the enzyme. Like activation-transfer coenzymes, oxidation-reduction coenzymes are not good catalysts without participation from amino acid side chains on the enzyme.

The enzyme lactate dehydrogenase, which catalyzes the transfer of electrons from lactate to $NAD^+$, illustrates these principles (Fig. 6.8). In the oxidation of lactate to pyruvate, lactate loses two electrons as a hydride ion, and a proton ($H^+$) is released. $NAD^+$, which accepts the hydride ion, is reduced to NADH. The carbon atom with the keto group in pyruvate is now at a higher oxidation state than in lactate because both of the electrons in bonds between carbon and oxygen are counted as belonging to oxygen, whereas the two electrons in the C—H bond are shared equally between carbon and hydrogen.

The coenzyme nicotinamide adenine dinucleotide ($NAD^+$) is synthesized from the vitamin niacin (which forms the nicotinamide ring) and from ATP (which contributes an AMP). The ADP portion of the molecule binds tightly to the enzyme and causes conformational changes in the enzyme. The functional group of $NAD^+$ is the carbon on the nicotinamide ring opposite the positively charged nitrogen. This carbon atom accepts the hydride ion (a hydrogen atom that has two electrons) transferred from a specific carbon atom on the substrate. The $H^+$ from the substrate alcohol (OH) group then dissociates, and a keto group (C=O) is formed. One of the roles of the enzyme is to contribute a histidine nitrogen that can bind the dissociable proton on lactate, thereby making it easier for $NAD^+$ to pull off the other hydrogen with both electrons. Finally, NADH dissociates.

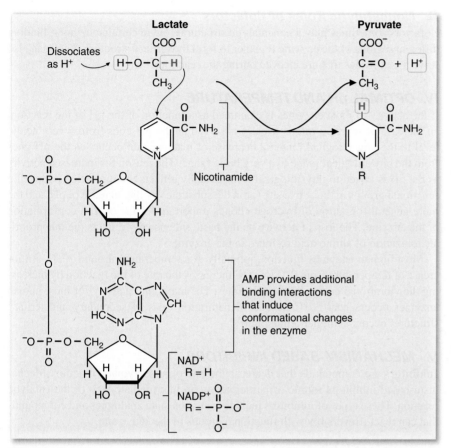

**FIG. 6.8.** The coenzyme $NAD^+$ accepting a hydride ion, shown in *red*, from lactate. $NAD^+$-dependent dehydrogenases catalyze the transfer of a hydride ion ($H^-$) from a carbon to $NAD^+$ in oxidation reactions such as the oxidation of alcohols to ketones or aldehydes to acids. The positively charged pyridine ring nitrogen of $NAD^+$ increases the electrophilicity of the carbon opposite it in the ring. This carbon then accepts the negatively charged hydride ion. The proton from the alcohol group is released into water. $NADP^+$ functions by the same mechanism but is usually involved in pathways of reductive synthesis.

## C. Metal Ions in Catalysis

Metal ions, which have a positive charge, contribute to the catalytic process by acting as **electrophiles** (electron-attracting groups). They assist in binding of the substrate, or they stabilize developing anions in the reaction. They can also accept and donate electrons in oxidation-reduction reactions.

The ability of certain metals to bind multiple ligands enables them to participate in binding substrates or coenzymes to enzymes. For example, $Mg^{2+}$ plays a role in the binding of the negatively charged phosphate groups of thiamine pyrophosphate to anionic or basic amino acids in the enzyme (see Fig. 6.7A). The phosphate groups of ATP are usually bound to enzymes through $Mg^{2+}$ chelation.

The metals of some enzymes bind anionic substrates or intermediates of the reaction to alter their charge distribution, thereby contributing to catalytic power. The enzyme alcohol dehydrogenase, which transfers electrons from ethanol to $NAD^+$ to generate acetaldehyde and NADH, illustrates this role (Fig. 6.9). In the active site of alcohol dehydrogenase, an activated serine pulls a proton off the ethanol $-OH$ group, leaving a negative charge on the oxygen that is stabilized by zinc. This electronic configuration allows the transfer of a hydride ion to $NAD^+$. Zinc is essentially fulfilling the same function in alcohol dehydrogenase that histidine fulfills in lactate dehydrogenase.

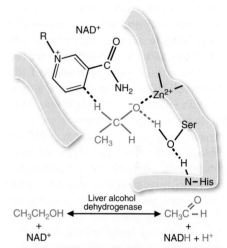

**FIG. 6.9.** Liver alcohol dehydrogenase (ADH) catalyzes the oxidation of ethanol (shown in *red*) to acetaldehyde. The active site of liver ADH contains a bound zinc atom, a serine side chain $-OH$, and histidine nitrogen that participate in the reaction. The histidine pulls an $H^+$ off the active site serine, which pulls the $H^+$ off of the substrate $-OH$ group, leaving the oxygen with a negative charge that is stabilized by zinc.

 In humans, most of ingested ethanol is oxidized to acetaldehyde in the liver by alcohol dehydrogenase (ADH):

**Ethanol + NAD$^+$ ↔ Acetaldehyde + NADH + H$^+$**

ADH is active as a dimer, with an active site containing zinc present in each subunit. The human has at least seven genes that encode isozymes of ADH, each with a slightly different range of specificities for the alcohols it oxidizes.

The acetaldehyde produced from ethanol is highly reactive, toxic, and immunogenic. In **Al M.** and other patients with chronic alcoholism, acetaldehyde is responsible for much of the liver injury associated with chronic alcoholism.

### D. Noncatalytic Roles of Cofactors

Cofactors sometimes play a noncatalytic structural role in certain enzymes, binding different regions of the enzyme together to form the tertiary structure. They can also serve as substrates that are cleaved during the reaction.

## IV. OPTIMAL pH AND TEMPERATURE

If the activity of most enzymes is examined as a function of the pH of the reaction, an increase of reaction rate is usually observed as the pH goes from a very acidic level to the physiological range; a decrease of reaction rate occurs as the pH goes from the physiological range to a very basic range. The reason for increased activity as the pH is raised to physiological levels usually reflects the ionization of specific functional groups in the active site (or in the substrate) by the increase of pH, and the more general formation of hydrogen bonds important for the overall conformation of the enzyme. The loss of activity on the basic side usually reflects the inappropriate ionization of amino acid residues in the enzyme.

Most human enzymes function optimally at a temperature around 37°C. An increase of temperature from 0°C to 37°C increases the rate of the reaction by increasing the vibrational energy of the substrates. The maximum activity for most human enzymes occurs near 37°C because denaturation (loss of secondary and tertiary structure) occurs at higher temperatures.

## V. MECHANISM-BASED INHIBITORS

**Inhibitors** are compounds that decrease the rate of an enzymatic reaction. Mechanism-based inhibitors mimic or participate in an intermediate step of the catalytic reaction. These types of inhibitors include transition state analogues and compounds that can react irreversibly with functional groups in the active site.

### A. Covalent Inhibitors

**Covalent inhibitors** form covalent or extremely tight bonds with functional groups in the catalytic active site. These functional groups are activated by their interactions with other amino acid residues and are therefore far more likely to be targeted by drugs and toxins than amino acid residues outside the active site.

The lethal compound diisopropyl phosphofluoridate (DFP, or diisopropylfluorophosphate) is an organophosphorus compound that served as a prototype for the development of the nerve gas Sarin and other organophosphorus toxins, such as the insecticides malathion and parathion (Fig. 6.10). DFP exerts its toxic effect by forming a covalent intermediate in the active site of acetylcholinesterase, thereby preventing the enzyme from degrading the neurotransmitter, acetylcholine. Once the covalent bond is formed, the inhibition by DFP is essentially irreversible and activity can only be recovered as new enzyme is synthesized. DFP also inhibits many other enzymes that utilize serine for hydrolytic cleavage, but the inhibition is not as lethal.

Aspirin (acetylsalicylic acid) provides an example of a pharmacological drug that exerts its effect through the covalent acetylation of an active site serine in the enzyme prostaglandin endoperoxide synthase (cyclo-oxygenase). Aspirin resembles a portion of the prostaglandin precursor that is a physiological substrate for the enzyme.

### B. Transition State Analogues and Compounds that Resemble Intermediate Stages of the Reaction

**Transition state analogues** are extremely potent and specific inhibitors of enzymes because they bind so much more tightly to the enzyme than do substrates or products. Drugs cannot be designed that precisely mimic the transition state because of its highly unstable structure. However, substrates undergo progressive

The symptoms experienced by **Dennis V.** resulted from inhibition of acetylcholinesterase. Acetylcholinesterase cleaves the neurotransmitter acetylcholine to acetate and choline in the postsynaptic terminal, thereby terminating the transmission of the neural signal (see Fig. 6.10). Malathion is metabolized in the liver to a toxic derivative (malaoxon) that binds to the active-site serine in acetylcholinesterase and other enzymes, an action similar to that of DFP. As a result, acetylcholine accumulates and overstimulates the autonomic nervous system (the involuntary nervous system, including heart, blood vessels, glands), thereby accounting for Dennis' vomiting, abdominal cramps, salivation, and sweating. Acetylcholine is also a neurotransmitter for the somatic motor nervous system, where its accumulation resulted in Dennis' involuntary muscle twitching (muscle fasciculations).

Because the transition state complex binds more tightly to the enzyme than does the substrate, compounds that resemble its electronic and three-dimensional surface (transition state analogues) are more potent inhibitors of an enzyme than are substrate analogues. Consequently, a drug developed as a transition state analogue would be highly specific for the enzyme it is designed to inhibit. However, transition state analogues are highly unstable when not bound to the enzyme and would have great difficulty making it from the digestive tract or injection site to the site of action. Some of the approaches in drug design that are being used to deal with the instability problem include designing drugs that are almost transition state analogues but have a stable modification, designing a prodrug that is converted to a transition state analogue at the site of action, and using the transition state analogue to design a complementary antibody.

**A. Normal reaction of acetylcholinesterase**

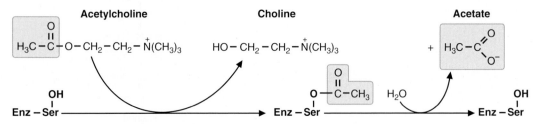

**B. Reaction with organophosphorus inhibitors**

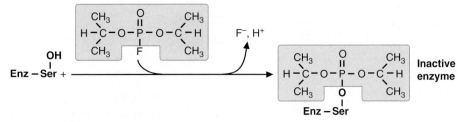

**FIG. 6.10.** **A.** Acetylcholinesterase normally catalyzes inactivation of the neurotransmitter acetylcholine in a hydrolysis reaction. The active-site serine forms a covalent intermediate with a portion of the substrate during the course of the reaction (similar to the mechanism of chymotrypsin). **B.** Diisopropyl phosphofluoridate (DFP), the ancestor of current organophosphorus nerve gases and pesticides, inactivates acetylcholinesterase by forming a covalent complex with the active-site serine that cannot be hydrolyzed by water. The result is that the enzyme cannot carry out its normal reaction and acetylcholine accumulates.

changes in their overall electrostatic structure during the formation of a transition state complex, and effective drugs often resemble an intermediate stage of the reaction more closely than they resemble the substrate. Medical literature often refers to such compounds as substrate analogues, even though they bind more tightly than substrates.

### 1. PENICILLIN

The antibiotic penicillin is a transition state analogue that binds very tightly to glycopeptidyl transferase, an enzyme required by bacteria for synthesis of the cell wall (Fig. 6.11). Glycopeptidyl transferase catalyzes a partial reaction with penicillin that covalently attaches penicillin to its own active-site serine. The reaction is favored by the strong resemblance between the peptide bond in the β-lactam ring of penicillin and the transition state complex of the natural transpeptidation reaction. Active-site inhibitors like penicillin that undergo partial reaction to form irreversible inhibitors in the active site are sometimes termed "suicide inhibitors."

### 2. ALLOPURINOL

Allopurinol, a drug used to treat gout, decreases urate production by inhibiting xanthine oxidase. This inhibition provides an example of an enzyme that commits suicide by converting a drug to a transition state analogue. The normal physiological function of xanthine oxidase is the oxidation of hypoxanthine to xanthine and xanthine to uric acid (urate) in the pathway for degradation of purines (Fig. 6.12). The enzyme contains a molybdenum-sulfide (Mo-S) complex that binds the substrates and transfers the electrons required for the oxidation reactions. Xanthine oxidase oxidizes the drug allopurinol to oxypurinol, a compound that binds very tightly to the Mo-S complex in the active site. As a result, the enzyme has committed suicide and is unable to carry out its normal function, the generation of uric acid (urate).

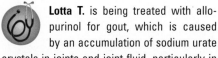 **Lotta T.** is being treated with allopurinol for gout, which is caused by an accumulation of sodium urate crystals in joints and joint fluid, particularly in the ankle and great toe. Allopurinol is a suicide inhibitor of the enzyme xanthine oxidase, which is involved in the degradation of purine nucleotides AMP and GMP to uric acid (urate). Although hypoxanthine levels increase in the presence of allopurinol, hypoxanthine does not participate in urate crystal formation and precipitation at this concentration. It is excreted in the urine.

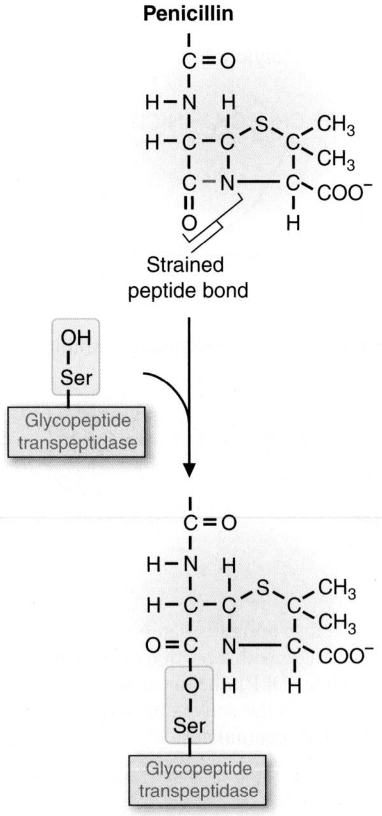

*FIG. 6.11.* The antibiotic penicillin inhibits the bacterial enzyme glycopeptidase transpeptidase. The transpeptidase is a serine protease involved in cross-linking components of bacterial cell walls and is essential for bacterial growth and survival. It normally cleaves the peptide bond between two D-alanine residues in a polypeptide. Penicillin contains a strained peptide bond within the β-lactam ring that resembles the transition state of the normal cleavage reaction, and thus, penicillin binds very readily in the enzyme active site. As the bacterial enzyme attempts to cleave this penicillin peptide bond, penicillin becomes irreversibly covalently attached to the enzyme's active-site serine, thereby inactivating the enzyme.

## C. Heavy Metals

Heavy metal toxicity is caused by tight binding of a metal such as mercury (Hg), lead (Pb), aluminum (Al), or iron (Fe) to a functional group in an enzyme. Heavy metals are relatively nonspecific for the enzymes they inhibit, particularly if the metal is associated with high-dose toxicity. Mercury, for example, binds to so many enzymes, often at reactive sulfhydryl groups in the active site, that it has been difficult to determine which of the inhibited enzymes is responsible for mercury toxicity. Lead provides an example of a metal that inhibits through replacing the normal functional metal in an enzyme. Its developmental and neurological toxicity may be caused by its ability to replace $Ca^{2+}$ in two regulatory proteins important in the central nervous system and other tissues, $Ca^{2+}$-calmodulin and protein kinase C.

## VI. BASIC REACTIONS AND CLASSES OF ENZYMES

In the following chapters of the text, students will be introduced to a wide variety of reaction pathways and enzyme names. Although it may seem that the number of reactions is infinite, many of these reactions are similar and occur frequently in different pathways. Recognition of the type of reaction can aid in remembering the pathways and enzyme names, thereby reducing the amount of memorization

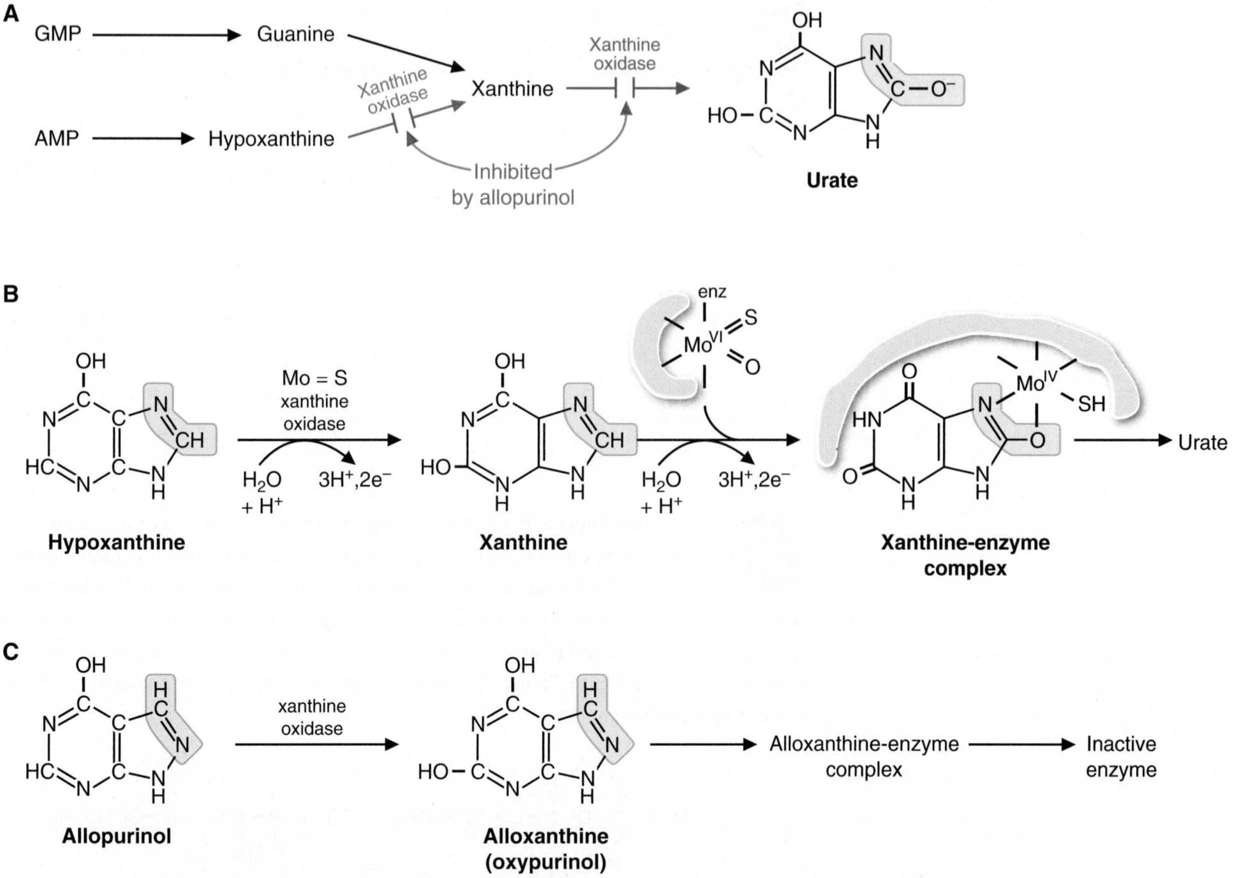

**FIG. 6.12.** Allopurinol is a suicide inhibitor of xanthine oxidase. **A.** Xanthine oxidase catalyzes the oxidation of hypoxanthine to xanthine, and xanthine to uric acid (urate) in the pathway for degradation of purine nucleotides. **B.** The oxidations are performed by a molybdenum–oxo–sulfide coordination complex in the active site that complexes with the group being oxidized. Oxygen is donated from water. The enzyme can work either as an oxidase ($O_2$ accepts the $2e^-$ and is reduced to $H_2O_2$) or as a dehydrogenase ($NAD^+$ accepts the $2e^-$ and is reduced to NADH). The figure only indicates that $2e^-$ are generated during the course of the reactions. **C.** Xanthine oxidase is able to perform the first oxidation step and convert allopurinol to alloxanthine (oxypurinol). As a result, the enzyme has committed suicide; the oxypurinol remains bound in the molybdenum coordination sphere, where it prevents the next step of the reaction. The portion of the purine ring in *green* indicates the major structural differences between hypoxanthine, xanthine, and allopurinol.

required. For those interested, these reaction types are discussed online in Section A6.1 @, along with the formal classification of enzymes.

## CLINICAL COMMENTS

Diseases discussed in this chapter are summarized in Table 6.2.

**Dennis V.** Dennis V. survived his malathion intoxication because he had ingested only a small amount of the chemical, vomited shortly after the agent was ingested, and was rapidly treated in the emergency room. Lethal doses of oral malathion are estimated at 1 g/kg of body weight for humans. Emergency room physicians used a drug (an oxime) to reactivate the acetylcholinesterase in Dennis before an aged irreversible complex formed. They also used intravenous atropine, an anticholinergic (antimuscarinic) agent, to antagonize the action of the excessive amounts of acetylcholine accumulating in cholinergic receptors throughout his body.

After several days of intravenous therapy, the signs and symptoms of acetylcholine excess abated and therapy was slowly withdrawn. Dennis made an uneventful recovery.

**Table 6.2    Diseases Discussed in Chapter 6**

| Disorder or Condition | Genetic or Environmental | Comments |
| --- | --- | --- |
| Malathion poisoning | Environmental | Inhibition of acetylcholinesterase at neuromuscular junctions. This leads to acetylcholine accumulation at the junction and overstimulation of the autonomic nervous system. |
| Gout | Both | Accumulation of uric acid in blood, leading to precipitation in joints, accompanied by severe pain and discomfort. |
| Thiamin deficiency (beriberi heart disease) | Environmental | Leads to lack of energy production due to reduced activity of key enzymes and can lead to the Wernicke-Korsakoff syndrome. Brought about by alcoholism, as manifest by a poor diet, and ethanol inhibition of thiamine transport through the intestinal mucosa. |

Once malathion is ingested, the liver converts it to the toxic reactive compound malaoxon by converting the phosphate–sulfur double bond to a phosphate–oxygen double bond. Malaoxon then binds to the active site of acetylcholinesterase and reacts to form the covalent intermediate. Unlike the complex formed between DFP and acetylcholinesterase, this initial acyl–enzyme intermediate is reversible. However, with time, the enzyme inhibitor complex "ages" (dealkylation of the inhibitor and enzyme modification) to form an irreversible complex.

**Malathion**          **Malaoxon**

**Lotta T.** Within several days of starting allopurinol therapy, Ms. T.'s serum uric acid level began to fall. Several weeks later, the level in her blood was normal. However, while Lotta was adapting to allopurinol therapy, she experienced a mild gout attack, which was treated with a low dose of colchicine (see Chapter 8).

At low concentrations of ethanol, liver alcohol dehydrogenase is the major route of ethanol oxidation to form acetaldehyde, a highly toxic chemical. Acetaldehyde not only damages the liver, it can enter the blood and potentially damage the heart and other tissues. At low ethanol intakes, much of the acetaldehyde produced is safely oxidized to acetate in the liver by aldehyde dehydrogenases.

**Al M.** Al M. was admitted to the hospital after intravenous thiamine was initiated at a dose of 100 mg/day (compared to an RDA of 1.4 mg/day). His congestive heart failure was believed to be the result, in part, of the cardiomyopathy (heart muscle dysfunction) of acute thiamine deficiency known as beriberi heart disease. This cardiac dysfunction and the peripheral nerve dysfunction that result from this nutritional deficiency usually respond to thiamine replacement. However, an alcoholic cardiomyopathy can also occur in well-nourished patients with adequate thiamine levels. Exactly how ethanol, or its toxic metabolite acetaldehyde, causes alcoholic cardiomyopathy in the absence of thiamine deficiency is not completely understood.

## REVIEW QUESTIONS-CHAPTER 6

1. A patient was born with a congenital mutation in an enzyme severely affecting its ability to bind an activation-transfer coenzyme. As a consequence, which one of the following would you expect to occur?

   A. The enzyme would be unable to bind the substrate of the reaction.
   B. The enzyme would be unable to form the transition state complex.
   C. The enzyme would normally use a different activation-transfer coenzyme.
   D. The enzyme would normally substitute the functional group of an active site amino acid residue for the coenzyme.
   E. The reaction could be carried out by the free coenzyme, provided the diet carried an adequate amount of its vitamin precursor.

2. An individual had a congenital mutation in glucokinase in which a proline was substituted for a leucine on a surface helix far from the active site, but within the hinge region of the actin fold. This mutation would be expected to do which one of the following?

   A. Probably affect the binding of ATP or a subsequent step in the reaction sequence.
   B. Have no effect on the rate of the reaction because it is not in the active site.
   C. Have no effect on the rate of the reaction because proline and leucine are both nonpolar amino acids.
   D. Have no effect on the number of substrate molecules reaching the transition state.
   E. Probably cause the reaction to proceed through an alternate mechanism.

3. A patient developed a bacterial overgrowth in his intestine that decreased the pH of the luminal contents from their normal pH of about 6.5 down to 5.5. This decrease of pH is likely to lead to which one of the following?

   A. Inhibit intestinal enzymes dependent on an active site lysine for binding substrate.
   B. Have little effect on intestinal hydrolases.
   C. Denature proteins reaching the intestine with their native structure intact.
   D. Disrupt hydrogen bonding essential for maintenance of tertiary structure.
   E. Inhibit intestinal enzymes dependent on histidine for acid-base catalysis.

4. Enzymes accelerate reaction rates due to which one of the following?

   A. Increase the effective concentration of the substrate.
   B. Reduce the frequency of collisions between the substrate molecules.
   C. Lower the energy of activation required to reach a transition state.
   D. Increase the free energy level of the final state of the reaction.
   E. Decrease the free energy level of the initial state of the reaction.

5. The enzyme alcohol dehydrogenase catalyzes the conversion of ethanol to acetaldehyde. Which one of the following occurs during the course of this reaction?

   A. The substrate, ethanol, is oxidized.
   B. An active site serine residue is oxidized.
   C. The coenzyme, NAD, is oxidized.
   D. An active site zinc atom is oxidized.
   E. Thiamine pyrophosphate is oxidized.

# 7 Regulation of Enzymes

## CHAPTER OUTLINE

## KEY POINTS

- Enzyme activity is regulated to reflect the physiological state of the organism.
- The rate of an enzyme-catalyzed reaction is dependent on substrate concentration and can be represented mathematically by the Michaelis-Menten equation.
- Allosteric activators or inhibitors are compounds that bind at sites other than the active catalytic site and regulate the enzyme through conformational changes affecting the catalytic site.
- A number of different mechanisms are available to regulate enzyme activity. These include:
  - Feedback inhibition, which often occurs at the first committed step of a metabolic pathway
  - Covalent modification of an amino acid residue (or residues) within the protein

continued

- Interactions with modulator proteins, which when bound to the enzyme, alter the conformation of the enzyme, and hence activity
- Altering the primary structure of the protein via proteolysis
- Increasing or decreasing the amount of enzyme available in the cell via alterations in the rate of synthesis or degradation of the enzyme
■ Metabolic pathways are frequently regulated at the slowest, or rate-limiting, step of the pathway.

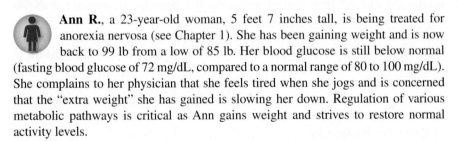

## THE WAITING ROOM

 **Al M.** is a 44-year-old man who has been an alcoholic for the past 5 years. He was recently admitted to the hospital for congestive heart failure (see Chapter 6). After being released from the hospital, he continued to drink. One night, he arrived at a friend's house at 7 PM. Between his arrival and 11 PM, he drank four beers and five martinis (for a total ethanol consumption of 9.5 oz). His friends encouraged him to stay an additional hour and drink coffee to sober up. Nevertheless, he ran his car off the road on his way home. He was taken to the emergency department of the local hospital and arrested for driving under the influence of alcohol. His blood alcohol concentration at the time of his arrest was 240 mg/dL, compared to the legal limit of ethanol for driving of 80 mg/dL (0.08% blood alcohol).

**Ann R.**, a 23-year-old woman, 5 feet 7 inches tall, is being treated for anorexia nervosa (see Chapter 1). She has been gaining weight and is now back to 99 lb from a low of 85 lb. Her blood glucose is still below normal (fasting blood glucose of 72 mg/dL, compared to a normal range of 80 to 100 mg/dL). She complains to her physician that she feels tired when she jogs and is concerned that the "extra weight" she has gained is slowing her down. Regulation of various metabolic pathways is critical as Ann gains weight and strives to restore normal activity levels.

 **Al M.** was not able to clear his blood ethanol rapidly enough to stay within the legal limit for driving. Ethanol is cleared from the blood at about half ounce per hour (15 mg/dL/hour). Liver metabolism accounts for over 90% of ethanol clearance from the blood. The major route of ethanol metabolism in the liver is the enzyme liver alcohol dehydrogenase (ADH), whereas the multienzyme complex MEOS (**m**icrosomal **e**thanol **o**xidizing **s**ystem), which is also called cytochrome P450-2E1, provides an additional route for ethanol oxidation to acetaldehyde in the liver and is utilized when ethanol levels are elevated.

## I. REGULATION BY SUBSTRATE AND PRODUCT CONCENTRATION

### A. Velocity and Substrate Concentration

The velocity (rate of formation of product per unit time) of all enzymes is dependent on the concentration of substrate. This dependence is reflected in conditions such as starvation, in which a number of pathways are deprived of substrate. In contrast, storage pathways (e.g., glucose conversion to glycogen in the liver) and toxic waste disposal pathways (e.g., the urea cycle, which prevents $NH_3$ toxicity by converting $NH_3$ to urea) are normally regulated to speed up when more substrate is available. In the following sections, we use the **Michaelis-Menten equation** to describe the response of an enzyme to changes in substrate concentration and use glucokinase to illustrate the role of substrate supply in regulation of enzyme activity.

### 1. MICHAELIS-MENTEN EQUATION

The equations of enzyme kinetics provide a quantitative way of describing the dependence of enzyme rate on substrate concentration. The simplest of these equations, the Michaelis-Menten equation, relates the initial velocity ($v_i$) to the

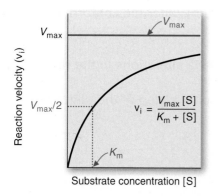

**FIG. 7.1.** A graph of the Michaelis-Menten equation. $V_{max}$ *(solid red line)* is the initial velocity extrapolated to infinite [S]. $K_m$ *(dotted red line)* is the concentration of S at which $v_i = V_{max}/2$.

Patients with maturity onset diabetes of the young (MODY) have a rare genetic form of diabetes mellitus in which the amount of insulin being secreted from the pancreas is too low, resulting in hyperglycemia. There are several forms of the disease, all caused by a mutation in a single gene. One of the mutations is in the pancreatic glucokinase (a closely related isozyme of liver glucokinase) gene that affects its kinetic properties ($K_m$ or $V_{max}$). Glucokinase is part of the mechanism controlling release of insulin from the pancreas. Decreased glucokinase activity results in lower insulin secretion for a given blood glucose level.

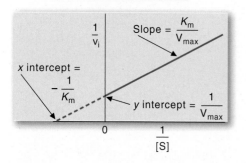

**FIG. 7.2.** The Lineweaver-Burk transformation (shown in the *green box*) for the Michaelis-Menten equation converts it to a straight line of the form $y = mx + b$. When [S] is infinite, $1/[S] = 0$, and the line crosses the ordinate (y-axis) at $1/v_i = 1/V_{max}$. The slope of the line is $K_m/V_{max}$. Where the line intersects the abscissa (x-axis), $1/[S] = -1/K_m$.

concentration of substrate [S] (the brackets denote concentration) and the two parameters $K_m$ and $V_{max}$ (Equation 7.1). The $V_{max}$ of the enzyme is the maximal velocity that can be achieved at an infinite concentration of substrate, and the $K_m$ of the enzyme for a substrate is the concentration of substrate required to reach one-half $V_{max}$. The Michaelis-Menten model of enzyme kinetics applies to a simple reaction in which the enzyme and substrate form an enzyme-substrate complex (ES) that can dissociate back to the free enzyme and substrate. The initial velocity of product formation, $v_i$, is proportionate to the concentration of ES. As substrate concentration is increased, the concentration of ES increases, and the reaction rate increases proportionally.

***Equation 7.1. The Michaelis-Menten equation***

For the reaction,

$$E + S \underset{k_2}{\overset{k_1}{\rightleftharpoons}} ES \overset{k_3}{\longrightarrow} E + P$$

the Michaelis-Menten equation is given by

$$v_i = \frac{V_{max}[S]}{K_m + [S]}$$

where $K_m = (k_2 + k_3)/k_1$ and $V_{max} = k_3 [E_T]$

The graph of the Michaelis-Menten equation ($v_i$ as a function of substrate concentration) is a rectangular hyperbola that approaches a finite limit, $V_{max}$, as the fraction of total enzyme present as ES increases (Fig. 7.1). At a hypothetical infinitely high substrate concentration, all of the enzyme molecules contain bound substrate, and the reaction rate is at $V_{max}$. The approach to the finite limit of $V_{max}$ is called **saturation kinetics** because velocity cannot increase any further once the enzyme is saturated with substrate. Saturation kinetics is a characteristic property of all rate processes dependent on the binding of a compound to a protein.

The $K_m$ of the enzyme for a substrate is defined as the concentration of substrate at which $v_i$ equals one-half $V_{max}$. The velocity of an enzyme is most sensitive to changes in substrate concentration over a concentration range below its $K_m$ (see Fig. 7.1). As an example, at substrate concentrations less than one-tenth of the $K_m$, a doubling of substrate concentration nearly doubles the velocity of the reaction; at substrate concentrations 10 times the $K_m$, doubling the substrate concentration has little effect on the velocity.

The $K_m$ of an enzyme for a substrate is related to the **dissociation constant**, $K_d$, which is the rate of substrate release divided by the rate of substrate binding. For example, a genetic mutation that decreases the rate of substrate binding to the enzyme decreases the affinity of the enzyme for the substrate and increases the $K_d$ and $K_m$ of the enzyme for that substrate. The higher the $K_m$, the higher is the substrate concentration required to reach one-half $V_{max}$.

## 2. THE LINEWEAVER-BURK TRANSFORMATION

The $K_m$ and $V_{max}$ for an enzyme can be visually determined from a plot of $1/v_i$ versus $1/[S]$, called a **Lineweaver-Burk** or a **double reciprocal plot**. The reciprocal of both sides of the Michaelis-Menten equation generates an equation that has the form of a straight line, $y = mx + b$ (Fig. 7.2). $K_m$ and $V_{max}$ are equal to the reciprocals of the intercepts on the x-axis and y-axis, respectively. The purpose of this transformation makes extrapolation easier so one can obtain accurate assessments of the $K_m$ and $V_{max}$.

The Michaelis-Menten equation was derived for the reaction in which one substrate is converted to one product (see Equation 7.1). For the reaction in which an enzyme forms a complex with two or more substrates, the $K_m$ for one substrate can vary with the concentration of cosubstrate (Fig. 7.3). At each constant concentration of cosubstrate, the plot of $1/v_i$ versus $1/[S]$ is a straight line. To obtain

$V_{max}$, the graph must be extrapolated to saturating concentrations of both substrates, which is equivalent to the intersection point of these lines for different cosubstrate concentrations.

### 3. HEXOKINASE ISOZYMES HAVE DIFFERENT $K_m$ VALUES FOR GLUCOSE

A comparison between the isozymes of hexokinase found in red blood cells and in the liver illustrates the significance of the $K_m$ of an enzyme for its substrate. Hexokinase catalyses the first step in glucose metabolism in most cells, the transfer of a phosphate from adenosine triphosphate (ATP) to glucose to form glucose-6-phosphate. Glucose-6-phosphate may then be metabolized in glycolysis, which generates energy in the form of ATP, or converted to glycogen, a storage polymer of glucose. Hexokinase I, the isozyme in red blood cells (erythrocytes), has a $K_m$ for glucose of about 0.05 mM (Fig. 7.4). The isozyme of hexokinase called **glucokinase** that is found in the liver and pancreas has a much higher $K_m$ of about 5 to 6 mM. The red blood cell is totally dependent on glucose metabolism to meet its needs for ATP. At the low $K_m$ of the erythrocyte hexokinase, blood glucose could fall drastically below its normal fasting level of about 5 mM, and the red blood cell could still phosphorylate glucose at rates near $V_{max}$. The liver, however, stores large amounts of "excess" glucose as glycogen or converts it to fat. Because glucokinase has a $K_m$ of about 5 mM, which is similar to the concentration of glucose in the blood under normal fasting conditions, the rate of glucose phosphorylation in the liver tends to increase as blood glucose increases after a high-carbohydrate meal and tends to decrease as blood glucose levels fall. The high $K_m$ of hepatic glucokinase thus promotes the storage of glucose as liver glycogen or as fat, but only when glucose is in excess supply.

### 4. VELOCITY AND ENZYME CONCENTRATION

The rate of a reaction is directly proportional to the concentration of enzyme; if you double the amount of enzyme, you will double the amount of product produced per minute, whether you are at low or at saturating concentrations of substrate. This important relationship between velocity and enzyme concentration is not immediately apparent in the Michaelis-Menten equation because the concentration of total enzyme present ($E_t$) has been incorporated into the term $V_{max}$ (i.e., $V_{max}$ is equal to

*For the reaction:* A + B ⟶ C + D

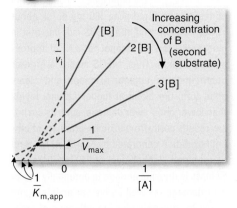

When the enzyme forms a complex with both substrates

**FIG. 7.3.** A Lineweaver-Burk plot for a two-substrate reaction in which A and B are converted to products. In the graph, 1/[A] is plotted against $1/v_i$ for three different concentrations of the cosubstrate, [B], 2[B], and 3[B]. As the concentration of B is increased, the intersection on the abscissa, equal to $1/K_{m,app}$ is increased. The "app" represents "apparent" as the $K_{m,app}$ is the $K_m$ at whatever concentration of cosubstrate, inhibitor, or other factor is present during the experiment.

**Q:** As **Ann R.** eats a high-carbohydrate meal, her blood glucose will rise to about 20 mM in the portal vein, and much of the glucose from her carbohydrate meal will enter the liver. How will the activity of glucokinase in the liver change as glucose is increased from 4 mM to 20 mM? (Hint: Calculate $v_i$ as a fraction of $V_{max}$ for both conditions using a $K_m$ for glucose of 5 mM and the Michaelis-Menten equation.)

The use of $V_{max}$ in the medical literature to describe the maximal rate at which a certain amount of tissue converts substrate to product can be confusing. The best way to describe an increase in enzyme activity in a tissue is to say that the maximal capacity of the tissue has increased. In contrast, the term $k_{cat}$ has been developed to clearly describe the speed at which an enzyme can catalyze a reaction under conditions of saturating substrate concentration. The rate constant $k_{cat}$, the turnover number of the enzyme, has the units of $min^{-1}$ (micromoles of product formed per minute divided by the micromoles of active site).

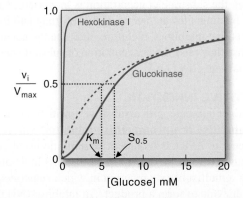

**FIG. 7.4.** A comparison between hexokinase I and glucokinase. The initial velocity ($v_i$) as a fraction of $V_{max}$ is graphed as a function of glucose concentration. The plot for glucokinase *(heavy blue line)* is slightly sigmoidal (S-shaped) possibly because the rate of an intermediate step in the reaction is so slow that the enzyme does not follow Michaelis-Menten kinetics. The *dashed blue line* has been derived from the Michaelis-Menten equation fitted to the data for concentrations of glucose greater than 5mM. For S-shaped curves, the concentration of substrate required to reach half $V_{max}$, or half-saturation, is sometimes called the $S_{0.5}$ or $K_{0.5}$, rather than $K_m$. At $v_i/V_{max}$ = 0.5, for glucokinase, the $K_m$ is 5mM, and the $S_{0.5}$ is 6.7 mM.

The liver alcohol dehydrogenase that is most active in oxidizing ethanol has a very low $K_m$ for ethanol, approximately 0.04 mM, and is at more than 99% of its $V_{max}$ at the legal limit of blood alcohol concentration for driving (80 mg/dL or about 17 mM). In contrast, the MEOS isozyme that is most active toward ethanol has a $K_m$ of approximately 11 mM. Thus, MEOS makes a greater contribution to ethanol oxidation and clearance from the blood at higher ethanol levels than lower ones. Liver damage, such as cirrhosis, results partly from toxic by-products of ethanol oxidation generated by MEOS. **Al M.**, who has a blood alcohol level of 240 mg/dL (about 52 mM), is drinking enough to potentially cause liver damage, as well as his car accident and arrest for driving under the influence of alcohol. The various isozymes and polymorphisms of alcohol dehydrogenase and MEOS are discussed further in Chapter 24.

**A:** Glucokinase, which has a high $K_m$ for glucose, phosphorylates glucose to glucose-6-phosphate about twice as fast after a carbohydrate meal than during fasting. Substitute the values for S and $K_m$ into the Michaelis-Menten equation, and solve for $v_i$ as a function of $V_{max}$. The initial velocity will be 0.44 times $V_{max}$ when blood glucose is at 4 mM and about 0.80 times $V_{max}$ when blood glucose is at 20 mM. In the liver, glucose-6-phosphate is a precursor for both glycogen and fat synthesis. Thus, these storage pathways are partially regulated through a direct effect of substrate supply. They are also partially regulated through an increase of insulin and a decrease of glucagon, two hormones that signal the supply of dietary fuel.

Some of **Al M.**'s problems have arisen from product inhibition of liver alcohol dehydrogenase by NADH. As ethanol is oxidized in liver cells, $NAD^+$ is reduced to NADH and the $NADH/NAD^+$ ratio rises. NADH is an inhibitor of alcohol dehydrogenase, competitive with respect to $NAD^+$, so the increased $NADH/NAD^+$ ratio slows the rate of ethanol oxidation and ethanol clearance from the blood.

NADH is also a product inhibitor of enzymes in the pathway that oxidizes fatty acids. Consequently, these fatty acids accumulate in the liver, eventually contributing to the alcoholic fatty liver.

the rate constant $k_3$ times $E_t$). However, $V_{max}$ is most often expressed as product produced per minute per milligram of enzyme and meant to reflect a property of the enzyme that is not dependent on its concentration.

## 5. MULTISUBSTRATE REACTIONS

Most enzymes have more than one substrate, and the substrate binding sites overlap in the catalytic (active) site. When an enzyme has more than one substrate, the sequence of substrate binding and product release affects the rate equation. As a consequence, there is an apparent value of $K_m$ ($K_{m,app}$) that depends on the concentration of cosubstrate or product present.

## 6. RATES OF ENZYME-CATALYZED REACTIONS IN THE CELL

Equations for the initial velocity of an enzyme-catalyzed reaction, such as the Michaelis-Menten equation, can provide useful parameters for describing or comparing enzymes. However, many multisubstrate enzymes, such as glucokinase, have kinetic patterns that do not fit the Michaelis-Menten model (or do so under nonphysiological conditions). The Michaelis-Menten model is also inapplicable to enzymes present in higher concentrations than their substrates. Nonetheless, the term "$K_m$" is still used for these enzymes to describe the approximate concentration of substrate at which velocity equals one-half $V_{max}$.

### B. Reversible Inhibition Within the Active Site

One of the ways of altering enzyme activity is through compounds binding in the active site. If these compounds are not part of the normal reaction, they inhibit the enzyme. An **inhibitor** of an enzyme is defined as a compound that decreases the velocity of the reaction by binding to the enzyme. It is a **reversible inhibitor** if it is not covalently bound to the enzyme and can dissociate at a significant rate. Reversible inhibitors are generally classified as competitive, noncompetitive, or uncompetitive with respect to their relationship to a substrate of the enzyme. In most reactions, the products of the reaction are reversible inhibitors of the enzyme producing them.

### A. COMPETITIVE INHIBITION

A **competitive inhibitor** "competes" with a substrate for binding at the enzyme's substrate recognition site and is usually, therefore, a close structural analogue of the substrate (Fig. 7.5A). An increase of substrate concentration can overcome competitive inhibition; when the substrate concentration is increased to a sufficiently high level, the substrate binding sites are occupied by substrate and inhibitor molecules cannot bind. Competitive inhibitors, therefore, increase the apparent $K_m$ of the enzyme ($K_{m,app}$) because they raise the concentration of substrate necessary to saturate the enzyme. They have no effect on $V_{max}$.

### B. NONCOMPETITIVE INHIBITION

If an inhibitor does not compete with a substrate for its binding site, the inhibitor is either a **noncompetitive** or **uncompetitive inhibitor** with respect to that particular substrate (see Fig. 7.5B). Uncompetitive inhibition is almost never encountered in medicine and will not be discussed further. To illustrate noncompetitive inhibition, consider a multisubstrate reaction in which substrates A and B react in the presence of an enzyme to form a product. An inhibitor (NI) that is a structural analogue of substrate B would fit into substrate B's binding site, but the inhibitor would be a noncompetitive inhibitor with regard to the other substrate, substrate A. An increase of A will not prevent the inhibitor from binding to substrate B's binding site. The inhibitor in effect lowers the concentration of the active enzyme and therefore changes the $V_{max}$ of the enzyme. If the inhibitor has absolutely no effect on the binding of substrate A, it will not change the $K_m$ for A (a pure noncompetitive inhibitor).

Lineweaver-Burk plots provide a good illustration of competitive inhibition and pure noncompetitive inhibition (Fig. 7.6.) In competitive inhibition, plots of $1/v_i$ versus $1/[S]$ at a series of inhibitor concentrations intersect on the y-axis. Thus, at infinite substrate concentration, or $1/[S] = 0$, there is no effect of the inhibitor. In pure noncompetitive inhibition, the inhibitor decreases the velocity even when $[S]$ has been extrapolated to an infinite concentration. However, if the inhibitor has no effect on the binding of the substrate, the $K_m$ is the same for every concentration of inhibitor, and the lines intersect on the x-axis.

Some inhibitors, such as metals, might not bind at either substrate recognition site. In this case, the inhibitor is noncompetitive with respect to both substrates.

### 3. SIMPLE PRODUCT INHIBITION IN METABOLIC PATHWAYS

All products are reversible inhibitors of the enzymes that produce them and may be competitive, noncompetitive, or uncompetitive relative to a particular substrate. **Simple product inhibition**, a decrease in the rate of an enzyme caused by the accumulation of its own product, plays an important role in metabolic pathways; it prevents one enzyme in a sequence of reactions from generating a product faster than it can be used by the next enzyme in that sequence. As an example, product inhibition of hexokinase by glucose-6-phosphate conserves blood glucose for tissues that need it. Tissues take up glucose from the blood and phosphorylate it to glucose-6-phosphate, which can then enter several different pathways (including glycolysis and glycogen synthesis). As these pathways become more active, the glucose-6-phosphate concentration decreases and the rate of hexokinase increases. When these pathways are less active, the glucose-6-phosphate concentration increases, hexokinase is inhibited, and glucose remains in the blood for other tissues to use.

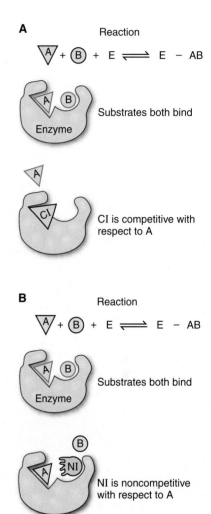

*FIG. 7.5.* **A.** Competitive inhibition with respect to substrate A. A and B are substrates for the reaction that forms the enzyme-substrate complex (E-AB). The enzyme has separate binding sites for each substrate, which overlap in the active site. The competitive inhibitor (CI) competes for the binding site of A, the substrate it most closely resembles. **B.** NI is a noncompetitive inhibitor with respect to substrate A. A can still bind to its binding site in the presence of NI. However, NI is competitive with respect to B because it binds to the B-binding site. In contrast, an inhibitor that is uncompetitive with respect to A might also resemble B, but it could only bind to the B site after A is bound.

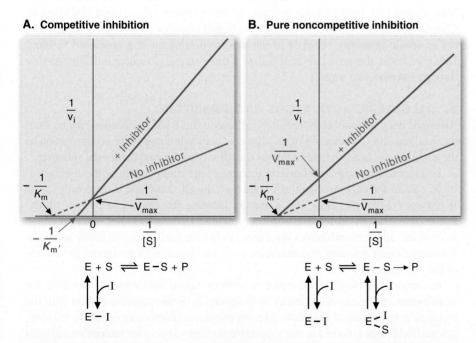

*FIG. 7.6.* Lineweaver-Burk plots of competitive and pure noncompetitive inhibition. **A.** $1/v_i$ versus $1/[S]$ in the presence of a competitive inhibitor. The competitive inhibitor alters the intersection on the x-axis. The new intersection is $1/K_{m,app}$ (also called $1/K'_m$). A competitive inhibitor does not affect $V_{max}$. **B.** $1/v_i$ versus $1/[S]$ in the presence of a pure noncompetitive inhibitor. The noncompetitive inhibitor alters the intersection on the x-axis, $1/V_{max,app}$ or $1/V'_{max}$ but does not affect $1/K_m$. A pure noncompetitive inhibitor binds to E and ES with the same affinity. If the inhibitor has different affinities for E and ES, the lines will intersect to either side of the y-axis, and the noncompetitive inhibitor will change both the $K'_m$ and the $V'_m$.

## II.  *REGULATION THROUGH CONFORMATIONAL CHANGES*

In substrate response and product inhibition, the rate of the enzyme is affected principally by the binding of a substrate or a product within the catalytic site. Most rate-limiting enzymes are also controlled through regulatory mechanisms that change the conformation of the enzyme in a way that affects the catalytic site. These regulatory mechanisms include (a) allosteric activation and inhibition, (b) phosphorylation or other covalent modification, (c) protein-protein interactions between regulatory and catalytic subunits or between two proteins, and (d) proteolytic cleavage. These types of regulation can rapidly change an enzyme from an inactive form to a fully active conformation.

### A.  *Conformational Changes in Allosteric Enzymes*

**Allosteric activators** and **inhibitors (allosteric effectors)** are compounds that bind to the **allosteric site** (a site separate from the catalytic site) and cause a conformational change that affects the affinity of the enzyme for the substrate. Usually, an allosteric enzyme has multiple interacting subunits that can exist in active and inactive conformations and the allosteric effector promotes or hinders conversion from one conformation to another.

### 1.  COOPERATIVITY IN SUBSTRATE BINDING TO ALLOSTERIC ENZYMES

Allosteric enzymes usually contain two or more subunits and exhibit positive cooperativity; the binding of substrate to one subunit facilitates the binding of substrate to another subunit. The first substrate molecule has difficulty in binding to the enzyme because all of the subunits are in the conformation with a low affinity for substrate (the taut "T" conformation). The first substrate molecule to bind changes its own subunit and at least one adjacent subunit to the high affinity conformation (the relaxed "R" state). In the example of the tetramer hemoglobin discussed in Chapter 6, the change in one subunit facilitated changes in all four subunits, and the molecule generally changed to the new conformation in a concerted fashion. However, most allosteric enzymes follow a more stepwise (sequential) progression through intermediate stages.

### 2.  ALLOSTERIC ACTIVATORS AND INHIBITORS

Allosteric enzymes bind activators at the allosteric site, a site physically separate from the catalytic site. The binding of an allosteric activator changes the conformation of the catalytic site in a way that increases the affinity of the enzyme for the substrate.

In general, activators of allosteric enzymes bind more tightly to the high affinity R state of the enzyme than the T state (i.e., the allosteric site is open only in the R enzyme) (Fig. 7.7). Thus, the activators increase the amount of enzyme in the active state, thereby facilitating substrate binding in their own and other subunits. In contrast, allosteric inhibitors bind more tightly to the T state, so either substrate concentration or activator concentration must be increased to overcome the effects of the allosteric inhibitor.

In the absence of activator, a plot of velocity versus substrate concentration for an allosteric enzyme usually results in a sigmoid or S-shaped curve (rather than the rectangular hyperbola of Michaelis-Menten enzymes; allosteric enzymes do not obey Michaelis-Menten kinetics) as the successive binding of substrate molecules activates additional subunits (see Fig. 7.7). In plots of velocity versus substrate concentration, the effect of an allosteric activator generally makes the sigmoidal S-shaped curve more like the rectangular hyperbola, with a substantial decrease in the $S_{0.5}$ ($K_m$) of the enzyme, because the activator changes all of the subunits to the high affinity state. These allosteric effectors alter the $K_m$ but not the $V_{max}$ of the enzyme. An allosteric inhibitor makes it more difficult for substrate or activators to convert the subunits to the most active conformation, and therefore, inhibitors generally shift the curve to the right, either increasing the $S_{0.5}$ alone or increasing it together with a decrease in the $V_{max}$.

**A model of an allosteric enzyme**

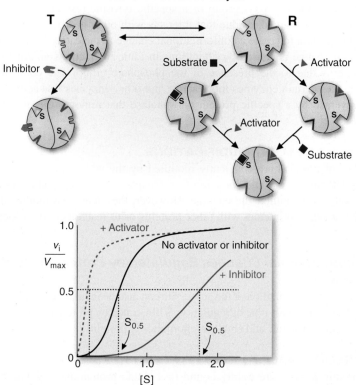

**FIG. 7.7.** Activators and inhibitors of an allosteric enzyme (simplified model). This enzyme has two identical subunits, each containing three binding sites: one for the substrate (s), one for the allosteric activator *(green triangle)*, and one for the allosteric inhibitor *(two-pronged red shape)*. The enzyme has two conformations, a relaxed active conformation (R) and an inactive conformation (T). The activator binds only to its activator site when the enzyme is in the R configuration. The inhibitor-binding site is open only when the enzyme is in the T state. A plot of velocity ($v_i$/Vmax) versus substrate concentration reveals that binding of the substrate at its binding site stabilizes the active conformation so that the second substrate binds more readily, resulting in an S (sigmoidal)-shaped curve. The graph of $v_i$/Vmax becomes hyperbolic in the presence of activator (which stabilizes the high affinity R form) and more sigmoidal with a higher $S_{0.5}$ in the presence of inhibitor (which stabilizes the low affinity form).

## C. ALLOSTERIC ENZYMES IN METABOLIC PATHWAYS

Regulation of enzymes by allosteric effectors provides several advantages over other methods of regulation. Allosteric inhibitors usually have a much stronger effect on enzyme velocity than competitive, noncompetitive, and uncompetitive inhibitors in the active catalytic site. Because allosteric effectors do not occupy the catalytic site, they may function as activators. Thus, allosteric enzymes are not limited to regulation through inhibition. Furthermore, the allosteric effector need not bear any resemblance to substrate or product of the enzyme. Finally, the effect of an allosteric effector is rapid, occurring as soon as its concentration changes in the cell. These features of allosteric enzymes are often essential for feedback regulation of metabolic pathways by end products of the pathway or by signal molecules that coordinate multiple pathways.

## B. Conformational Changes from Covalent Modification

### 1. PHOSPHORYLATION

The activity of many enzymes is regulated through **phosphorylation** by a protein kinase or dephosphorylation by a protein phosphatase (Fig. 7.8). Serine/threonine protein kinases transfer a phosphate from ATP to the hydroxyl group of a specific

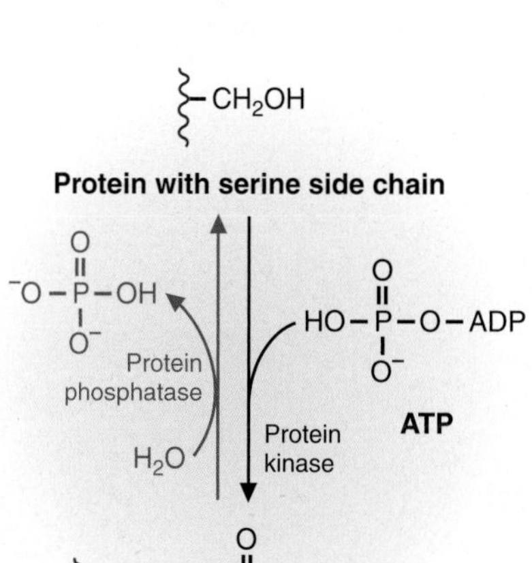

**FIG. 7.8.** Protein kinases and protein phosphatases.

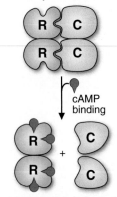

*FIG. 7.9.* **A.** Structure of cAMP (3′,5′-cyclic AMP). The phosphate group is attached to hydroxyl groups on both the third (3′) and fifth (5′) carbons of ribose, forming a cyclic structure. **B.** Protein kinase A. When the regulatory subunits (R) of protein kinase A bind the allosteric activator, cAMP, they dissociate from the enzyme, thereby releasing active catalytic subunits (C).

serine (and sometimes threonine) on the target enzyme; tyrosine kinases transfer a phosphate to the hydroxyl group of a specific tyrosine residue. Phosphate is a bulky, negatively charged residue that interacts with other nearby amino acid residues of the protein to create a conformational change at the catalytic site. The conformational change is caused by alterations in ionic interactions and/or hydrogen bond patterns due to the presence of the phosphate group. The conformational change makes certain enzymes more active and other enzymes less active. The effect is reversed by a specific protein phosphatase that removes the phosphate by hydrolysis.

### 2. OTHER COVALENT MODIFICATIONS

A number of proteins are covalently modified by the addition of groups such as acetyl, ADP-ribose, or lipid moieties (see Chapter 4). These modifications may directly activate or inhibit the enzyme. However, they may also modify the ability of the enzyme to interact with other proteins or to reach its correct location in the cell.

## C. Conformational Changes Regulated by Protein-Protein Interactions

Changes in the conformation of the active site can also be regulated by direct protein-protein interaction. This type of regulation is illustrated by protein kinase A, calcium ($Ca^{2+}$)-binding proteins, and small (monomeric) G proteins.

### 1. PROTEIN KINASE A

Some protein kinases are tightly bound to a single protein and regulate only the protein to which they are tightly bound. However, other protein kinases and protein phosphatases will simultaneously regulate a number of rate-limiting enzymes in a cell to achieve a coordinated response. For example, **protein kinase A**, a serine/threonine protein kinase, phosphorylates a number of enzymes that regulate different metabolic pathways.

Protein kinase A provides a means for hormones to control metabolic pathways. Epinephrine (adrenaline) and many other hormones increase the intracellular concentration of the allosteric regulator 3′,5′-cyclic AMP (cAMP), which is referred to as a hormonal second messenger (Fig. 7.9A). cAMP binds to regulatory subunits of protein kinase A, which dissociate and release the activated catalytic subunits (see Fig. 7.9B). Dissociation of inhibitory regulatory subunits is a common theme in enzyme regulation. The active catalytic subunits phosphorylate proteins at serine and threonine residues.

### 2. THE CALCIUM-CALMODULIN FAMILY OF MODULATOR PROTEINS

Modulator proteins bind to other proteins and regulate their activity by causing a conformational change at the catalytic site or by blocking the catalytic site (steric hindrance). They are protein allosteric effectors that can either activate of inhibit the enzyme or protein to which they bind.

$Ca^{2+}$-calmodulin is an example of a dissociable modulator protein that binds to several different proteins and regulates their function in either a positive or negative manner. It also exists in the cytosol and functions as a $Ca^{2+}$-binding protein (Fig. 7.10). The center of the symmetric molecule is a hinge region that bends as $Ca^{2+}$-calmodulin folds over the protein it is regulating.

### 3. G PROTEINS

The masters of regulation through reversible protein association in the cell are the **monomeric G proteins**, small single subunit proteins that bind and hydrolyze guanosine triphosphate (GTP). GTP is a purine nucleotide which, like ATP, contains

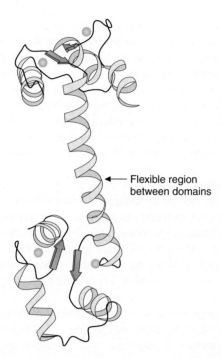

**FIG. 7.10.** $Ca^{2+}$-calmodulin has four binding sites for $Ca^{2+}$ (shown in *green*). Each $Ca^{2+}$ forms a multiligand coordination sphere by simultaneously binding several amino acid residues on calmodulin. Thus, calmodulin can create large conformational changes in proteins to which it is bound when $Ca^{2+}$ binds. Calmodulin has a flexible region in the middle connecting the two domains.

high-energy phosphoanhydride bonds that release energy when hydrolyzed. When G proteins bind GTP, their conformation changes so that they can bind to a target protein, which is then either activated or inhibited in carrying out its function (Fig. 7.11, *circle 1*).

G proteins are said to possess an internal clock because they are GTPases that slowly hydrolyze their own bound GTP to GDP and phosphate. As they hydrolyze GTP, their conformation changes and the complex they have formed with the target protein disassembles (see Fig. 7.11, *circle 2*). The bound GDP on the inactive G protein is eventually replaced by GTP, and the process can begin again (see Fig. 7.11, *circle 3*).

The activity of many G proteins is regulated by accessory proteins (GAPs, GEFs, and GDIs), which may, in turn, be regulated by allosteric effectors. GAPs (**G**TPase **a**ctivating **p**roteins) increase the rate of GTP hydrolysis by the G protein and, therefore, the rate of dissociation of the G protein–target protein complex (see Fig. 7.11, *circle 2*). When a GEF protein (**g**uanine nucleotide **e**xchange **f**actor) binds to a G protein, it increases the rate of GTP exchange for a bound GDP and therefore activates the G protein (see Fig. 7.11, *circle 3*). GDI proteins (**G**DP **d**issociation **i**nhibitor) bind to the GDP–G protein complex and inhibit dissociation of GDP, thereby keeping the G protein inactive. G proteins are discussed in more detail in Chapter 8.

## D. Proteolytic Cleavage

Although many enzymes undergo some cleavage during synthesis, others enter lysosomes or secretory vesicles or are secreted as proenzymes, which are precursor proteins that must undergo proteolytic cleavage to become fully functional. Unlike most other forms of regulation, proteolytic cleavage is irreversible.

The precursor proteins of proteases (enzymes that cleave specific peptide bonds) are called **zymogens**. To denote the inactive zymogen form of an enzyme, the

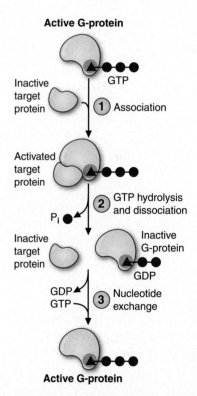

**FIG. 7.11.** Monomeric G proteins. **Step 1:** When GTP is bound, the conformation of the G protein allows it to bind target proteins, which are then activated (as shown) or inhibited. **Step 2:** The G protein hydrolyzes a phosphate from GTP to form guanosine diphosphate (GDP), which changes the G-protein conformation and causes it to dissociate from the target protein. **Step 3:** GDP is exchanged for GTP, which reactivates the G protein.

name is modified by addition of the suffix "-ogen" or the prefix "pro-." The synthesis of zymogens as inactive precursors prevents them from cleaving proteins prematurely at their sites of synthesis or secretion. Chymotrypsinogen, for example, is stored in vesicles within pancreatic cells until secreted into ducts leading to the intestinal lumen. In the digestive tract, chymotrypsinogen is converted to chymotrypsin by the proteolytic enzyme trypsin, which cleaves off a small peptide from the N-terminal region (and two internal peptides). This cleavage activates chymotrypsin by causing a conformational change in the spacing of amino acid residues around the binding site for the denatured protein substrate and around the catalytic site.

An excellent example of zymogen activation is in the mechanism of blood clotting. It is critical for individuals to maintain a constant blood volume (hemostasis), so injuries to the integrity of blood vessels must be repaired and closed before a significant amount of blood is lost. When damage to the circulatory system is found, a cascade of zymogen activation is initiated in order to form a clot (consisting of the protein fibrin), which seals the damaged area. Fibrin is initially synthesized as an inactive precursor, fibrinogen, which is converted to fibrin by the serine protease thrombin.

Thrombin activation is mediated by the complex interaction which comprises the blood coagulation cascade. This cascade (Fig. 7.12) consists primarily of proteins that serve as enzymes or cofactors, which function to accelerate thrombin

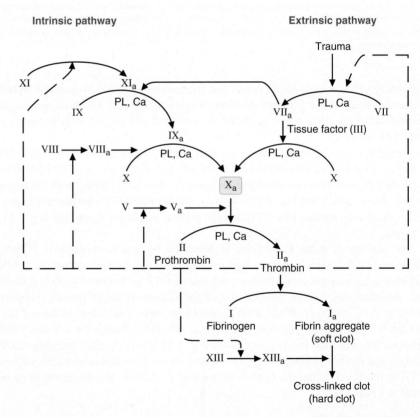

**FIG. 7.12.** The blood coagulation cascade. Activation of clot formation occurs through interlocking pathways, termed the intrinsic and extrinsic pathways. The intrinsic pathway is activated when factor XI is converted to factor XIa (the active form) by thrombin. The extrinsic pathway (external damage, such as a cut) is activated by tissue factor. The reactions designated by "PL, Ca" are occurring via cofactors bound to phospholipids (PL) on the platelet and blood vessel endothelial cell surface in a $Ca^{2+}$-coordination complex. Factors XIa, IXa, VIIa, Xa, and thrombin are serine proteases. Note the positive feedback regulation of thrombin on the activation of proteases earlier in the cascade sequence (indicated by the *dashed lines*).

**Table 7.1  Proteins of Blood Coagulation**

| Factor | Descriptive Name | Function/Active Form |
|---|---|---|
| *Coagulation factors* | | |
| I | Fibrinogen | Fibrin |
| II | Prothrombin | Serine protease |
| III | Tissue factor | Receptor and cofactor |
| IV | $Ca^{2+}$ | Cofactor |
| V | Proaccelerin, labile factor | Cofactor |
| VII | Proconvertin | Serine protease |
| VIII | Antihemophilia factor A | Cofactor |
| IX | Antihemophilia factor B, Christmas factor | Serine protease |
| X | Stuart-Prower factor | Serine protease |
| XI | Plasma thromboplastin antecedent | Serine protease |
| XIII | Fibrin-stabilizing factor | $Ca^{2+}$-dependent trans-glutaminase |
| *Regulatory proteins* | | |
| Thrombomodulin | Endothelial cell receptor, binds thrombin | |
| Protein C | Activated by thrombomodulin-bound thrombin | |
| Protein S | Protease cofactor; binds activated protein C | |

formation and localize it at the site of injury. These proteins are listed in Table 7.1. All of these proteins are present in the plasma as proproteins (zymogens). These precursor proteins are activated by cleavage of the polypeptide chain at one or more sites. The key to successful and appropriate clot (thrombus) formation is the regulation of the proteases, which activate these zymogens.

The proenzymes (factors VII, IX, X, XI, and prothrombin) are serine proteases that, when activated by cleavage, cleave the next proenzyme in the cascade. Because of the sequential activation, great acceleration and amplification of the response is achieved. That cleavage and activation have occurred is indicated by the addition of an "a" to the name of the proenzyme (e.g., factor IX is cleaved to form the active factor IXa).

The cofactor proteins (tissue factor, factors V and VIII) serve as binding sites for other factors. Tissue factor is not related structurally to the other blood coagulation cofactors and is an integral membrane protein that does not require cleavage for active function. Factors V and VIII serve as pro-cofactors, which, when activated by cleavage, function as binding sites for other factors.

Two additional proteins that are considered part of the blood coagulation cascade, protein S and protein C, are regulatory proteins. Only protein C is regulated by proteolytic cleavage, and when activated, is itself a serine protease. These proteins are critical to stopping clot formation when the damage has been repaired. A more detailed discussion of blood clotting can be found online in Section A7.1. @

## III. REGULATION THROUGH CHANGES IN AMOUNT OF ENZYME

Tissues continuously adjust the rate at which proteins are synthesized to vary the amount of different enzymes present. The expression for $V_{max}$ in the Michaelis-Menten equation incorporates the concept that the rate of a reaction is proportional to the amount of enzyme present. Thus, the maximal capacity of a tissue can change with increased protein synthesis or with increased protein degradation.

### A. Regulated Enzyme Synthesis

Protein synthesis begins with the process of gene transcription, transcribing the genetic code for that protein from DNA into messenger RNA. The code in messenger RNA is then translated into the primary amino acid sequence of the protein. Generally, the rate of enzyme synthesis is regulated by increasing or decreasing the rate of gene transcription, processes generally referred to as induction (increase) and repression (decrease). However, the rate of enzyme synthesis is sometimes regulated through stabilization of the messenger RNA. (These processes are covered in Section III of this text.) Compared to the more immediate types of regulation

 The maximal capacity of MEOS (cytochrome P450-2E1) is increased in the liver with continued ingestion of ethanol through a mechanism involving induction of gene transcription. Thus, **AI M.** has a higher capacity to oxidize ethanol to acetaldehyde than a naive drinker (a person not previously subjected to alcohol). Nevertheless, the persistence of his elevated blood alcohol level shows he has saturated his capacity for ethanol oxidation (i.e., the enzyme is always running at $V_{max}$). Once his enzymes are operating near $V_{max}$, any additional ethanol he drinks will not appreciably increase the rate of ethanol clearance from his blood.

discussed earlier, regulation by means of induction or repression of enzyme synthesis is usually slow in the human, occurring over hours to days.

### B. Regulated Protein Degradation

The content of an enzyme in the cell can be altered through selective regulated degradation as well as through regulated synthesis. For example, during fasting or infective stress, protein degradation in skeletal muscle is activated to increase the supply of amino acids in the blood for gluconeogenesis or for the synthesis of antibodies and other components of the immune response. Under these conditions, synthesis of ubiquitin, a protein that targets proteins for degradation in proteosomes, is increased by the steroid hormone cortisol. Although all proteins in the cell can be degraded with a characteristic half-life within lysosomes, protein degradation via two specialized systems, proteosomes and caspases, is highly selective and regulated.

## IV. REGULATION OF METABOLIC PATHWAYS

The different means of regulating enzyme activity described earlier are utilized to control metabolic pathways, cellular events, and physiological processes to match the body's requirements. Although there are hundreds of metabolic pathways in the body, there are a few common themes or principles involved in their regulation.

Metabolic pathways are a series of sequential reactions in which the product of one reaction is the substrate of the next reaction (Fig. 7.13). Each step or reaction is usually catalyzed by a separate enzyme. The enzymes of a pathway have a common function, conversion of substrate to the final end products of the pathway. A pathway may also have a branch point at which an intermediate becomes the precursor for another pathway.

### A. Role of the Rate-limiting Step in Regulation

Pathways are principally regulated at one key enzyme, the regulatory enzyme, which catalyzes the rate-limiting step in the pathway. This is the slowest step and is usually not readily reversible. Thus, changes in the rate-limiting step can influence flux through the rest of the pathway. The rate-limiting step is usually the first committed step in a pathway or a reaction that is related to or influenced by the first committed step. Additional regulated enzymes occur after each metabolic branchpoint to direct flow into the branch. (For example, in Fig. 7.13, feedback inhibition of enzyme 2 results in accumulation of B, which enzyme 5 then uses for synthesis of compound G.) Inhibition of the rate-limiting enzyme in a pathway usually leads to accumulation of the pathway precursor.

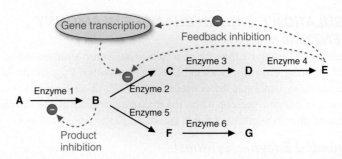

**FIG. 7.13.** A common pattern for feedback inhibition of metabolic pathways. The letters represent compounds formed from different enzymes in the reaction pathway. *Compound B* is at a metabolic branchpoint: it can go down one pathway to *E*, or down an alternate pathway to *G*. The end product of the pathway, *E*, might control its own synthesis by allosterically inhibiting *enzyme 2*, the first committed step of the pathway, or inhibiting transcription of the gene for *enzyme 2*. As a result of the feedback inhibition, *B* accumulates and more *B* enters the pathway for conversion to *G*, which could be a storage, or disposal pathway. In this hypothetical pathway, *B* is a product inhibitor of *enzyme 1*, competitive with respect to *A*. *Precursor A* might induce the synthesis of *enzyme 1*, which would allow more *A* to go to *G*.

## B. Feedback Regulation

**Feedback regulation** refers to a situation in which the end product of a pathway controls its own rate of synthesis (see Fig. 7.13). Feedback regulation usually involves allosteric regulation of the rate-limiting enzyme by the end product of a pathway (or a compound that reflects changes in the concentration of the end product). The end product of a pathway may also control its own synthesis by inducing or repressing the gene for transcription of the rate-limiting enzyme in the pathway. This type of regulation is much slower to respond to changing conditions than allosteric regulation.

## C. Feed-forward Regulation

Certain pathways, such as those involved in the disposal of toxic compounds, are feed-forward regulated. **Feed-forward regulation** may occur through an increased supply of substrate to an enzyme with a high $K_m$, allosteric activation of a rate-limiting enzyme through a compound related to substrate supply, substrate-related induction of gene transcription (e.g., induction of cytochrome P450-2E1 by ethanol), or increased concentration of a hormone that stimulates a storage pathway by controlling enzyme phosphorylation state.

## D. Tissue Isozymes of Regulatory Proteins

The human is composed of a number of different cell types that perform specific functions unique to that cell type and synthesize only the proteins consistent with their functions. Because regulation matches function, regulatory enzymes of pathways usually exist as tissue-specific isozymes with somewhat different regulatory properties unique to their function in different cell types. For example, hexokinase and glucokinase are tissue-specific isozymes with different kinetic properties.

## E. Counter-regulation of Opposing Pathways

A pathway for the synthesis of a compound usually has one or more enzymatic steps that differ from the pathway for degradation of that compound. A biosynthetic pathway can therefore have a different regulatory enzyme from that of the opposing degradative pathway, and one pathway can be activated while the other is inhibited (e.g., glycogen synthesis is activated while glycogen degradation is inhibited).

## F. Substrate Channeling through Compartmentation

In the cell, compartmentation of enzymes into multienzyme complexes or organelles provides a means of regulation, either because the compartment provides unique conditions or because it limits or channels access of the enzymes to substrates. Enzymes or pathways with a common function are often assembled into organelles. For example, enzymes of the TCA cycle are all located within the mitochondrion. The enzymes catalyze sequential reactions, and the product of one reaction is the substrate for the next reaction. The concentration of the pathway intermediates remains much higher within the mitochondrion than in the surrounding cellular cytoplasm.

Another type of compartmentation involves the assembly of enzymes catalyzing sequential reactions into multienzyme complexes so that intermediates of the pathway can be directly transferred from the active site on one enzyme to the active site on another enzyme, thereby preventing loss of energy and information.

When **Ann R.** jogs, the increased use of ATP for muscle contraction results in an increase of AMP, which allosterically activates both the key enzyme phosphofructokinase-1, the rate-limiting enzyme of glycolysis, and muscle glycogen phosphorylase, the rate-limiting enzyme of glycogenolysis. These pathways both provide for a means to increase ATP production. This is an example of feedback regulation by the ATP/AMP ratio. Unfortunately, her low caloric consumption has not allowed feed-forward activation of the rate-limiting enzymes in her fuel storage pathways, and she has very low glycogen stores. Consequently, she has inadequate fuel stores to supply the increased energy demands of exercise.

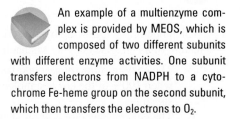

An example of a multienzyme complex is provided by MEOS, which is composed of two different subunits with different enzyme activities. One subunit transfers electrons from NADPH to a cytochrome Fe-heme group on the second subunit, which then transfers the electrons to $O_2$.

## CLINICAL COMMENTS

A summary of the diseases discussed in this chapter can be found in Table 7.2.

**Al M.** In the emergency department, Al M. was evaluated for head injuries. From the physical examination and blood alcohol levels, it was determined that his change in mental status resulted from his alcohol consumption. Although his chronic ethanol consumption had increased his level of microsomal

**Table 7.2    Diseases Discussed in Chapter 7**

| Disorder or Condition | Genetic or Environmental | Comments |
|---|---|---|
| Alcoholism | Both | Both alcohol dehydrogenase and the micro-somal ethanol oxidizing system (MEOS) are active in detoxifying ethanol. High NADH can inhibit alcohol dehydrogenase, allowing toxic metabolites to accumulate. |
| Anorexia nervosa | Both | Effects of malnutrition on energy production were discussed. |
| Maturity onset diabetes of the young (MODY) | Genetic | Mutations in various proteins can lead to this form of diabetes, which is manifest by hyperglycemia, without, however, other complications associated with either type 1 or 2 diabetes. Specifically, mutations in pancreatic glucokinase were discussed. |

The hormones epinephrine (released during stress and exercise) and glucagon (released during fasting) activate the synthesis of cAMP in a number of tissues. cAMP activates protein kinase A. Because protein kinase A is able to phosphorylate key regulatory enzymes in many pathways, these pathways can be regulated coordinately. In muscle, for example, glycogen degradation is activated while glycogen synthesis is inhibited. At the same time, fatty acid release from adipose tissue is activated to provide more fuel for muscle. The regulation of glycolysis, glycogen metabolism, and other pathways of metabolism is much more complex than has been illustrated here and is discussed in many subsequent chapters of this text.

ethanol oxidizing system (MEOS) (and, therefore, rate of ethanol oxidation in his liver), his excessive drinking resulted in a blood alcohol level greater than the legal limit of 80 mg/dL. He suffered bruises and contusions but was otherwise uninjured. He left in the custody of the police officer and his driving license was suspended.

 **Ann R.** Ann R.'s physician explains that she has inadequate fuel stores for her exercise program. In order to jog, her muscles require an increased rate of fuel oxidation to generate the ATP for muscle contraction. The fuels utilized by muscles for exercise include glucose from muscle glycogen, fatty acids from adipose tissue triacylglycerols, and blood glucose supplied by liver glycogen. These fuel stores were depleted during her prolonged bout of starvation. In addition, starvation resulted in the loss of muscle mass as muscle protein was being degraded to supply amino acids for other processes, including gluconeogenesis (the synthesis of glucose from amino acids and other noncarbohydrate precursors). Therefore, Ann will need to increase her caloric consumption to rebuild her fuel stores. Her physician helps her calculate the additional amount of calories her jogging program will need and they discuss which foods she will eat to meet these increased caloric requirements. He also helps her visualize the increase of weight as an increase in strength.

## REVIEW QUESTIONS–CHAPTER 7

1.  Which one of the following best describes a characteristic feature of an enzyme obeying Michaelis-Menten kinetics?

    A.  The enzyme velocity is at one-half the maximal rate when 100% of the enzyme molecules contain bound substrate.

    B.  The enzyme velocity is at one-half the maximal rate when 50% of the enzyme molecules contain bound substrate.

    C.  The enzyme velocity is at its maximal rate when 50% of the enzyme molecules contain bound substrate.

    D.  The enzyme velocity is at its maximal rate when all of the substrate molecules in solution are bound by the enzyme.

    E.  The velocity of the reaction is independent of the concentration of enzyme.

2.  The pancreatic glucokinase of a patient with MODY contained an amino acid substitution (due to a mutation) in which a leucine was replaced with a proline. The result was that the $K_m$ for glucose was decreased from a normal value of 6 mM to a value of 2.2 mM, and the $V_{max}$ was changed from 93 units/mg protein to 0.2 units/mg protein. Which one of the following best describes the patient's glucokinase as compared to the normal enzyme?

    A.  The patient's enzyme requires a lower concentration of glucose to reach one-half $V_{max}$.

    B.  The patient's enzyme is faster than the normal enzyme at concentrations of glucose below 2.2 mM.

    C.  The patient's enzyme is faster than the normal enzyme at concentrations of glucose above 2.2 mM.

D. At near saturating glucose concentration, the patient would need 90 to 100 times more enzyme than normal to achieve normal rates of glucose phosphorylation.

E. As blood glucose levels increase after a meal from a fasting value of 5 mM to 10 mM, the rate of the patient's enzyme will increase more than the rate of the normal enzyme.

3. Methanol ($CH_3OH$) is converted by alcohol dehydrogenases to formaldehyde (CHO), a compound that is highly toxic in the human. Patients who have ingested toxic levels of methanol are sometimes treated with ethanol ($CH_3CH_2OH$) to inhibit methanol oxidation by alcohol dehydrogenase. Which one of the following statements provides the best rationale for this treatment?

A. Ethanol would be expected to alter the $V_{max}$ of alcohol dehydrogenase for the oxidation of methanol to formaldehyde.

B. Ethanol is a structural analogue of methanol and might therefore be an effective noncompetitive inhibitor.

C. Ethanol would be an effective inhibitor of methanol oxidation regardless of the concentration of methanol.

D. Ethanol would be expected to inhibit the enzyme by binding to the formaldehyde binding site on the enzyme, even though it cannot bind at the substrate binding site for methanol.

E. Ethanol is a structural analogue of methanol that would be expected to compete with methanol for its binding site on the enzyme.

4. Which one of the following describes a characteristic of most allosteric enzymes?

A. They are composed of single subunits.

B. In the absence of effectors, they generally follow Michaelis-Menten kinetics.

C. They have allosteric activators that bind in the catalytic site.

D. They show cooperativity in substrate binding.

E. They have irreversible allosteric inhibitors that bind at allosteric sites.

5. A mutation in a guanine nucleotide exchange protein decreased its ability to bind to the monomeric G protein it is supposed to regulate. As a consequence, the monomeric G protein would exhibit which one of the following?

A. Retain bound GDP for a longer period of time.

B. Retain bound GTP for a longer period of time.

C. Exchange GDP for bound GTP at a faster rate.

D. Bind its target enzyme for a longer period of time.

E. Hydrolyze bound GTP at a faster rate.

# 8 Cell Structure and Signaling by Chemical Messengers

## CHAPTER OUTLINE

### I. COMPARTMENTATION IN CELLS
A. Plasma membrane
1. Structure of the plasma membrane
2. Lipids in the plasma membrane
3. Proteins in the plasma membrane
4. Transport of molecules across the plasma membrane
B. Mitochondria
C. Lysosomes
D. Peroxisomes
E. Nucleus
F. Endoplasmic reticulum
G. Golgi complex
H. Cytoskeleton

### II. GENERAL FEATURES OF CHEMICAL MESSENGERS
A. General features of chemical messenger systems applied to the nicotinic acetylcholine receptor
B. Endocrine, paracrine, and autocrine actions
C. Types of chemical messengers

### III. INTRACELLULAR TRANSCRIPTION FACTOR RECEPTORS
A. Intracellular versus plasma membrane receptors
B. The steroid hormone/thyroid hormone superfamily of receptors

### IV. PLASMA MEMBRANE RECEPTORS AND SIGNAL TRANSDUCTION
A. Major classes of plasma membrane receptors
1. Ion channel receptors
2. Receptors that are kinases or bind kinases
3. Heptahelical receptors
   a. Heterotrimeric G proteins
   b. Adenylyl cyclase and cAMP phosphodiesterase
B. Changes in response to signals

### V. SIGNAL TERMINATION

## KEY POINTS

- The cell is the basic unit of living organisms.
- Unique features of each cell type define tissue specificity and function.
- Despite the variety of cell types, cells share many common features, which include a plasma membrane and intracellular organelles.
- In eukaryotes, the intracellular organelles consist of lysosomes, the nucleus, ribosomes, the endoplasmic reticulum, the Golgi apparatus, mitochondria, peroxisomes, and the cytoplasm. Some cells may lack one or more of these internal organelles.
- In order to integrate cellular function with the needs of the organism, cells communicate with each other via chemical messengers. Chemical messengers include neurotransmitters (for the nervous system), hormones (for the endocrine system), cytokines (for the immune system), retinoids, eicosanoids, and growth factors.

continued

■ Chemical messengers transmit their signals by binding to receptors on target cells. When a messenger binds to a receptor, a signal transduction pathway is activated which generates second messengers within the cell.

■ Receptors can be either plasma membrane proteins or intracellular binding proteins.

■ Intracellular receptors act primarily as transcription factors, which regulate gene expression in response to a signal being released.

■ Plasma membrane receptors fall into different classes, such as ion channel receptors, tyrosine kinase receptors, tyrosine kinase–associated receptors, serine-threonine kinase receptors, or G-protein–coupled receptors (GPCR).

# THE WAITING ROOM

Two years after **Dennis V.** successfully recovered from his malathion poisoning, he once again visited his grandfather, **Percy V.** Mr. V. took Dennis with him to a picnic at the shore, where they ate steamed crabs. Later that night, Dennis experienced episodes of vomiting and watery diarrhea, and Mr. V. rushed him to the hospital emergency department. Dennis' hands and feet were cold, he appeared severely dehydrated, and he was approaching hypovolemic shock (a severe drop in blood pressure). He was diagnosed with cholera, caused by the bacteria *Vibrio cholerae*. Dennis was placed on intravenous rehydration therapy, followed by oral rehydration therapy with high glucose- and sodium ($Na^+$)-containing fluids. *V. cholerae* epidemics are associated with unsanitary conditions affecting the drinking water supply and are rare in the United States. However, these bacteria grow well under the alkaline conditions found in seawater and attach to chitin in shellfish. Thus, sporadic cases occur in the southeast United States associated with the ingestion of contaminated shellfish.

**Mia S.** is a 37-year-old woman who complains of increasing muscle fatigue. If she rests for 5 to 10 minutes, her strength returns to normal. She also notes that if she talks on the phone, her ability to form words gradually decreases because of fatigue of the muscles of speech. By evening, her upper eyelids droop to the point that she has to mechanically pull her upper lids back in order to see normally. These symptoms are becoming increasingly severe. When Mia is asked to sustain an upward gaze, her upper eyelids eventually drift downward involuntarily. When she is asked to hold both arms straight out in front of her for as long as she is able, both arms begin to drift downward within minutes. Her physician suspects that **Mia** has myasthenia gravis and orders a test to determine if she has antibodies in her blood directed against the acetylcholine receptor. Acetylcholine is released by neurons and acts on acetylcholine receptors at neuromuscular junctions to stimulate muscular contraction. Myasthenia gravis is an acquired autoimmune disease in which the patient has developed pathogenic antibodies against these receptors. **Mia**'s decreasing ability to form words and her other symptoms of muscle weakness may be caused by the inability of acetylcholine to stimulate repeated muscle contraction when the numbers of effective acetylcholine receptors at neuromuscular junctions are greatly reduced.

**Ann R.**, who suffers from anorexia nervosa, has increased her weight to 102 lb from a low of 85 lb (see Chapter 1). On the advice of her physician, she has been eating more to prevent fatigue during her daily jogging regimen. She runs about 10 miles before breakfast every second day and forces herself to drink a high-energy supplement immediately afterward.

Endocrine hormones enable **Ann R.** to mobilize fuels from her adipose tissue during her periods of fasting and during jogging. While she fasts overnight, α-cells of her pancreas increase secretion of the polypeptide hormone glucagon. The stress of prolonged fasting and chronic exercise stimulates release of cortisol, a steroid hormone, from her adrenal cortex. The exercise of jogging also increases secretion of the hormones epinephrine and norepinephrine from the adrenal medulla. Each of these hormones is being released in response to a specific signal and causes a characteristic response in a target tissue, enabling her to exercise. However, each of these hormones binds to a different type of receptor and works in a different way.

## I.   COMPARTMENTATION IN CELLS

The structure of a typical **eukaryotic** cell is shown in Figure 8.1. The cells of humans and other animals are classified as eukaryotes because the genetic material is organized into a membrane-enclosed **nucleus**. In contrast, bacteria are **prokaryotes**; they do not contain nuclei or other organelles found in eukaryotic cells.

**Membranes** are lipid structures that separate the contents of the compartment they surround from its environment. An outer **plasma membrane** separates the cell from the external aqueous environment. **Organelles** (such as the **nucleus**, **mitochondria**, **lysosomes**, and **peroxisosmes**) are also surrounded by a membrane system that separates the internal compartment of the organelle from the intracellular milieu, known as the **cytoplasm**. The function of these membranes is to collect or concentrate enzymes and other molecules serving a common function into a compartment with a localized environment. The transporters and receptors in each membrane system control this localized environment and communication of the cell or organelle with the surrounding milieu.

The following sections briefly describe various organelles and membrane systems found in most human cells and outline the relationship between their properties and function. Consult the cell biology texts listed within the online references for more detail on these topics.

### A.  Plasma Membrane

### 1.   STRUCTURE OF THE PLASMA MEMBRANE

All mammalian cells are enclosed by a plasma membrane composed of a **lipid bilayer** (two layers) containing embedded proteins (Fig. 8.2). The membrane layer facing the "inside" of the organelle or cell is termed the **inner leaflet**; the other layer is the **outer**, or **external**, **leaflet**. The membranes are continuous and sealed so that the hydrophobic lipid bilayer selectively restricts the exchange of polar compounds between the external fluid and the intracellular compartment. The membrane is referred to as a fluid mosaic because it consists of a mosaic of proteins and lipid molecules that can for the most part move laterally in the plane of the membrane.

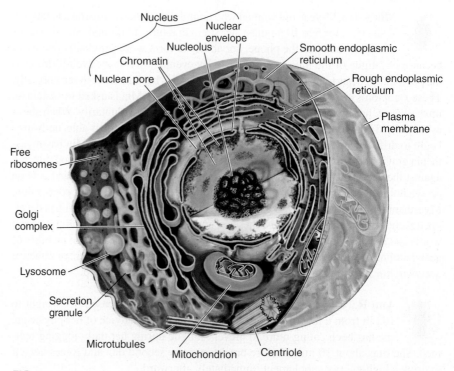

*FIG. 8.1.* Common components of human cells.

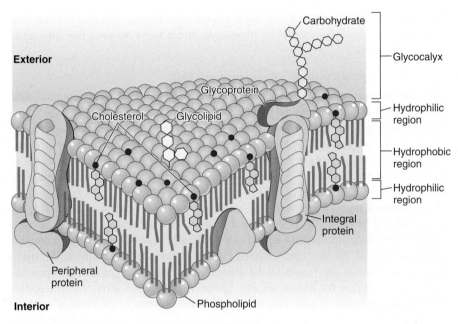

*FIG. 8.2.* Basic structure of a mammalian cell membrane.

The proteins are classified as **integral proteins**, which span the cell membrane, or **peripheral proteins**, which are attached to the membrane surface through electrostatic bonds to lipids or integral proteins. Many of the proteins and lipids on the external leaflet contain covalently bound carbohydrate chains and are therefore **glycoproteins** and **glycolipids**. This layer of carbohydrate on the outer surface of the cell is called the **glycocalyx**. The variable carbohydrate components of the glycolipids on the cell surface functions, in part, as cell recognition markers for small molecules or other cells.

## 2. LIPIDS IN THE PLASMA MEMBRANE

Each layer of the plasma membrane lipid bilayer is formed primarily by **phospholipids**, which are arranged with their hydrophilic head groups facing the aqueous medium and their fatty acyl tails forming a hydrophobic membrane core (see Fig. 8.2). The principle phospholipids in the membrane are the glycerol lipids **phosphatidylcholine** (also called lecithin), **phosphatidylethanolamine**, and **phosphatidylserine** and the **sphingolipid sphingomyelin**. The lipid composition varies among different cell types, with phosphatidylcholine being the major plasma membrane lipid in most cell types and glycosphingolipids being the most variable.

The lipid composition of the bilayer is asymmetrical, with a higher content of phosphatidylcholine and sphingomyelin in the outer leaflet and a higher content of phosphatidylserine and phosphatidylethanolamine in the inner leaflet. Phosphatidylinositol, which can function in the transfer of information from hormones and neurotransmitters across the cell membrane, is also only found in the inner leaflet. Phosphatidylserine contains a net negative charge that contributes to the membrane potential and may be important for binding positively charged molecules within the cell.

**Cholesterol**, which is interspersed between the phospholipids, maintains membrane fluidity. The presence of cholesterol and the *cis* unsaturated fatty acids of the phospholipids in the membrane prevent the hydrophobic chains from packing too closely together. As a consequence, lipid and protein molecules that are not bound to external or internal structural proteins can rotate and move laterally in the plane of the leaflet. This movement enables the plasma membrane to partition between daughter cells during cell division, to deform as cells pass through capillaries, and to form and fuse with vesicle membranes. Cholesterol can also stabilize very fluid membranes by increasing interactions between the fatty acids of phospholipids.

### 3.  PROTEINS IN THE PLASMA MEMBRANE

**Integral proteins** contain transmembrane domains with hydrophobic amino acid side chains that interact with the hydrophobic portions of the lipids to seal the membrane (see Fig. 8.2). Hydrophilic regions of the proteins protrude into the aqueous medium on both sides of the membrane. Many of these proteins function as either channels or transporters for the movement of compounds across the membrane, as receptors for the binding of hormones and neurotransmitters, or as structural proteins (Fig. 8.3).

**Peripheral membrane proteins**, which were originally defined as those proteins that can be released from the membrane by ionic solvents, are bound through weak electrostatic interactions with the polar head groups of lipids or with integral proteins. One of the best-characterized classes of peripheral proteins is the **spectrin** family, which are bound to the intracellular membrane surface and provide mechanical support for the membrane. Spectrin is bound to actin, which together forms a structure that is called the inner membrane skeleton or the corticol skeleton (see Fig. 8.3).

A third classification of membrane proteins consists of **lipid-anchored proteins** bound to the inner or outer surface of the membrane. The glycophosphatidylinositol glycan (GPI) anchor is a covalently attached lipid that anchors proteins to the external surface of the membrane. The prion protein (see Chapter 5) is an example of a GPI-anchored protein. Several proteins involved in hormonal regulation are anchored to the internal surface of the membrane through palmityl (C16) or myristyl (C14) fatty acyl groups or through geranylgeranyl (C20) or farnesyl (C15) isoprenyl groups. However, many integral proteins also contain attached lipid groups to increase their stability within the membrane.

All cells contain an inner membrane skeleton of spectrin-like proteins. Red blood cell spectrin was the first member of the spectrin family to be described. The protein dystrophin, present in skeletal muscle cells, is a member of the spectrin family. Genetic defects in the dystrophin gene are responsible for Duchenne and Becker muscular dystrophies.

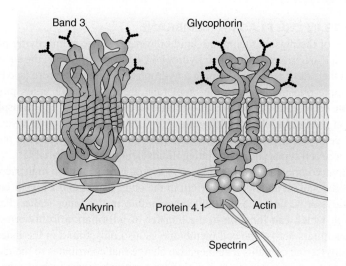

**FIG. 8.3.** Proteins in the red blood cell membrane. The proteins named Band 3 (the bicarbonate-chloride exchange transporter) and glycophorin (provides an external negative charge that repels other cells) both contain nonpolar α-helical segments spanning the lipid bilayer. These proteins contain a large number of polar and charged hydrophilic amino acids in the intracellular and extracellular domains. On the inside of the cell, they are attached to peripheral proteins comprising the inner membrane skeleton. Band 3 is connected to spectrin filaments via the protein ankyrin. Glycophorin is connected to short actin filaments and spectrin via protein 4.1. Band 3 allows the transport of bicarbonate into the red blood cell in exchange for chloride. This allows bicarbonate transport to the lung, where it is expired as carbon dioxide.

## 4. TRANSPORT OF MOLECULES ACROSS THE PLASMA MEMBRANE

Membranes form hydrophobic barriers around cells to control the internal environment by restricting the entry and exit of molecules. As a consequence, cells require **transport systems** to permit entry of small polar compounds that they need (e.g., glucose), to concentrate compounds inside the cell (e.g., potassium [$K^+$]), and to expel other compounds (e.g., calcium [$Ca^{2+}$] and $Na^+$). The transport systems for small organic molecules and inorganic ions generally fall into four categories: First is **simple diffusion** through the lipid bilayer (examples include gases such as oxygen and carbon dioxide, and lipid-soluble substances, such as steroid hormones). Second is **facilitative diffusion** (many sugars are transported by facilitative diffusion). Third is **gated channels** (transmembrane proteins form a pore for ions that is either opened or closed in response to a stimulus, whether it be voltage changes across the membrane, the binding of a compound, or a regulatory change in the intracellular domain). Fourth is **active transport pumps** (energy, usually in the form of ATP hydrolysis, is used to allow compounds to move against their concentration gradient) (Fig. 8.4). These transport mechanisms are classified as passive if energy is not required, or active if energy is required. Primary active transport occurs when a gradient is established across the membrane, using energy. The $Na^+$, $K^+$-ATPase creates both $Na^+$ and $K^+$ gradients across the membrane, by transporting three $Na^+$ ions out of the cell in exchange for two $K^+$ ions entering the cell, powered by the hydrolysis of ATP. The creation of the $Na^+$ gradient (the $Na^+$ concentration outside the cell is much greater than the $Na^+$ concentration inside the cell) leads to secondary active transport of glucose and amino acids. The transporter for these compounds binds $Na^+$ and the cosubstrate (either glucose or an amino acid), and then using the $Na^+$ gradient as a driving force, transports both the $Na^+$ and the cosubstrate into the cell. Thus, glucose and amino acids are concentrated within cells via the creation of the $Na^+$ gradient by the $Na^+$, $K^+$-ATPase.

In addition to these mechanisms for the transport of small individual molecules, cells engage in **endocytosis**. The plasma membrane extends or invaginates to surround a particle, a foreign cell, or extracellular fluid, which then closes into a vesicle that is released into the cytoplasm (see Fig. 8.4). **Receptor-mediated endocytosis** is the name given to the formation of **clathrin-coated vesicles** that mediate the internalization of membrane-bound receptors in vesicles coated on the intracellular side with subunits of the protein clathrin.

CFTR (**c**ystic **f**ibrosis **t**ransmembrane conductance **r**egulator) is a chloride channel that provides an example of a ligand-gated channel regulated through phosphorylation (phosphorylation gated). CFTR is a member of the ABC (**a**denine nucleotide **b**inding **c**assette, or ATP binding cassette) superfamily of transport proteins and is the protein mutated in cystic fibrosis. CFTR consists of two transmembrane domains that form a closed channel, each connected to an ATP binding site, and a regulatory domain that sits in front of the channel. When the regulatory domain is phosphorylated by a kinase, its conformation changes and it moves away from the ATP binding domains. As ATP binds and is hydrolyzed, the transmembrane domains change conformation and open the channel, and $Cl^-$ ions diffuse through. As the conformation reverts back to its original form, the channel closes. Individuals homozygous for mutations in CFTR display cystic fibrosis; heterozygotes for the mutated gene are thought to have protection against cholera. An inactive CFTR leads to an inability to release $Cl^-$ ions from cells into the extracellular space, with a concomitant reduced diffusion of water into the same space. Thus, a consequence of the CFTR mutation is the dehydration of respiratory and interstitial mucosal linings, leading to a plugging of airways and ducts with a thick mucus.

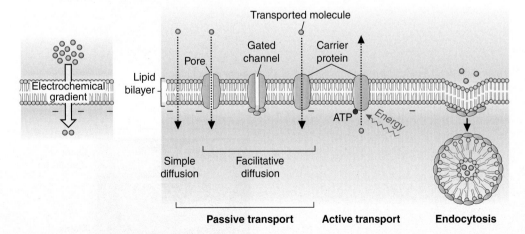

***FIG. 8.4.*** Common types of transport mechanisms for human cells. The electrochemical gradient consists of the concentration gradient of the compound and the distribution of charge on the membrane, which affects the transport of charged ions like $Cl^-$. Both protein amino acid residues and lipid polar head groups contribute to the net negative charge on the inside of the membrane. Generally, the diffusion of uncharged molecules (passive transport) is net movement from a region of high concentration to a low concentration, and active transport (energy-requiring) is net movement from a region of low concentration to high concentration.

**Dennis V.** has become dehydrated because he has lost so much water through vomiting and diarrhea (see Chapter 2). Cholera toxin increases the efflux of $Na^+$ and $Cl^-$ ions from his intestinal mucosal cells into the intestinal lumen. The increase of water in his stools results from the passive transfer of water from inside the cell and body fluids, where it is in high concentration (i.e., intracellular $Na^+$ and $Cl^-$ concentrations are low), to the intestinal lumen and bowel, where water is in lower concentration (relative to high $Na^+$ and $Cl^-$). The watery diarrhea is also high in $K^+$ ions and bicarbonate. All the signs and symptoms of cholera generally derive from this fluid loss.

## B. Mitochondria

**Mitochondria** contain most of the enzymes for the pathways of fuel oxidation and oxidative phosphorylation and thus generate most of the ATP required by mammalian cells. Each mitochondrion is surrounded by two membranes, an **outer membrane** and a highly impermeable **inner membrane**, separating the mitochondrial **matrix** from the cytosol (Fig. 8.5). The inner membrane forms invaginations known as **cristae** containing the electron transport chain and ATP synthase. Most of the enzymes for the Krebs tricarboxylic acid (TCA) cycle and other pathways for oxidation are located in the mitochondrial matrix, the compartment enclosed by the inner mitochondrial membrane. (The TCA cycle and electron transport chain are described in more detail in Chapters 17 and 18.)

The inner mitochondrial membrane is highly impermeable, and the proton gradient that is built up across the membrane during electron transfer through the electron transport chain is essential for ATP generation from adenosine diphosphate (ADP) and phosphate. The transport of ions and other small molecules across the inner mitochondrial membrane occurs principally through facilitative transporters in a form of secondary active transport powered by the proton gradient established by the electron transport chain. The outer membrane contains pores made from proteins called **porins** and is permeable to molecules with a molecular weight up to about 1,000 g.

Mitochondria can replicate by division; however, most of their proteins must be imported from the cytosol. Mitochondria contain a small amount of DNA, which encodes for only 13 different subunits of proteins involved in oxidative phosphorylation. Most of the enzymes and proteins in mitochondria are encoded by nuclear DNA and synthesized on cytoplasmic ribosomes. They are imported

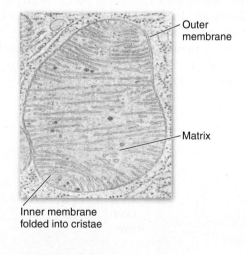

Outer membrane

Matrix

Inner membrane folded into cristae

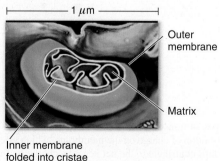

├─── 1 μm ───┤

Outer membrane

Matrix

Inner membrane folded into cristae

*FIG. 8.5.* Mitochondrion. Electron micrograph (**top**); three-dimensional drawing (**bottom**).

through membrane pores by a receptor-mediated process involving members of the heat shock family of proteins (proteins whose synthesis is induced by an elevation in temperature or other indicators of stress). Mutations in mitochondrial DNA result in a number of genetic diseases that affect skeletal muscle, neuronal, and renal tissues (known as **mitochondrial disorders**). Mitochondrial inheritance is maternal, as the sperm do not contribute mitochondria to the fertilized egg. Spontaneous mutations within mitochondrial DNA have been implicated with the mechanism of aging.

## C.  Lysosomes

**Lysosomes** are the intracellular organelles of digestion enclosed by a single membrane that prevents the release of its digestive enzymes into the cytosol. They are central to a wide variety of body functions that involve elimination of unwanted material and recycling their components, including destruction of infectious bacteria and yeast, recovery from injury, tissue remodeling, involution of tissues during development, and normal turnover of cells and organelles. The **lysosomal digestive enzymes** include **nucleases, phosphatases, glycosidases, esterases**, and **proteases** called **cathepsins**. These enzymes are all hydrolases, enzymes that cleave amide, ester, and other bonds through the addition of water. Many of the products of lysosomal digestion, such as the amino acids, return to the cytosol. Lysosomes are, therefore, involved in recycling compounds.

Most of these lysosomal hydrolases have their greatest activity near a pH of about 5.5 (the pH optimum). The intralysosomal pH is maintained near 5.5 principally by **v-ATPases (vesicular ATPases)**, which actively pump protons into the lysosome. The cytosol and other cellular compartments have a pH nearer 7.2 and are, therefore, protected from escaped lysosomal hydrolases.

## D.  Peroxisomes

**Peroxisomes** are cytoplasmic organelles, similar in size to lysosomes, that are involved in **oxidative reactions** using **molecular oxygen**. These reactions produce the toxic chemical **hydrogen peroxide** ($H_2O_2$), which is subsequently utilized or degraded within the peroxisome by catalase and other enzymes. Peroxisomes function in the oxidation of very long chain fatty acids (containing 20 or more carbons) to shorter chain fatty acids, the conversion of cholesterol to bile acids, and the synthesis of **ether lipids** called **plasmalogens**. They are bounded by a single membrane.

## E.  Nucleus

The largest of the subcellular organelles of animal cells is the **nucleus** (Fig. 8.6). Most of the genetic material of the cell is located in the chromosomes of the nucleus, which are composed of DNA, an equal weight of small, positively charged proteins called **histones**, and a variable amount of other proteins. The **nucleolus**, a substructure of the nucleus, is the site of **ribosomal RNA (rRNA) transcription and processing** and of **ribosome assembly**. Ribosomes are required for the synthesis of proteins. Replication, transcription, translation, and the regulation of these processes are the major focus of the molecular biology section of this text. The nucleus is separated from the rest of the cell (the cytoplasm) by the nuclear envelope, which consists of two membranes joined at **nuclear pores**. The outer nuclear membrane is continuous with the rough endoplasmic reticulum. Transport through the pores is bidirectional, certain molecules leave the nucleus and others can enter, through the pores.

## F.  Endoplasmic Reticulum

The **endoplasmic reticulum (ER)** is a network of membranous tubules within the cell consisting of **smooth endoplasmic reticulum (SER)**, which lacks ribosomes, and **rough endoplasmic reticulum (RER)**, which is studded with

Genetic defects in lysosomal enzymes, or in proteins such as the mannose-6-phosphate receptor required for targeting the enzymes to the lysosome, lead to an abnormal accumulation of undigested material in lysosomes that may be converted to residual bodies. The accumulation may be so extensive that normal cellular function is compromised, particularly in neuronal cells. Genetic diseases such as **Tay-Sachs disease** (an accumulation of partially digested gangliosides in lysosomes), and **Pompe disease** (an accumulation of glycogen particles in lysosomes) are caused by the absence or deficiency of specific lysosomal enzymes. Such diseases, in which a lysosomal function is compromised, are known as **lysosomal storage diseases**.

Several diseases are associated with peroxisomes. Peroxisomal diseases are caused by mutations that affect either the synthesis of functional peroxisomal enzymes or their incorporation into peroxisomes. For example, adrenoleukodystrophy involves a mutation that decreases the content of a fatty acid transporter in the peroxisomal membrane. Zellweger syndrome is caused by the failure to complete the synthesis of peroxisomes.

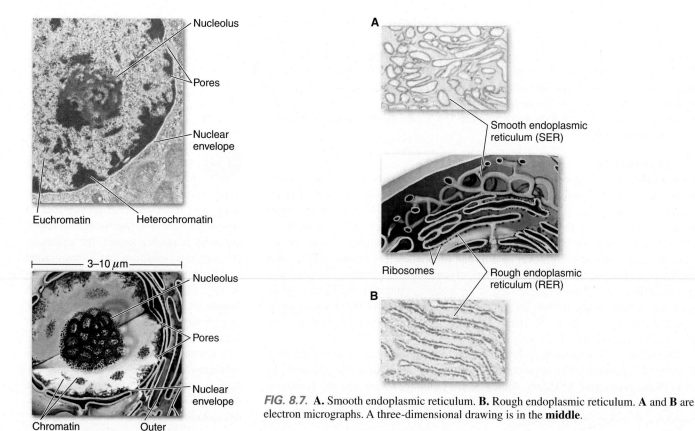

*FIG. 8.6.* Nucleus. Electron micrograph (**top**); three-dimensional drawing (**bottom**).

*FIG. 8.7.* **A.** Smooth endoplasmic reticulum. **B.** Rough endoplasmic reticulum. **A** and **B** are electron micrographs. A three-dimensional drawing is in the **middle**.

The dehydration of cholera is often treated with an oral rehydration solution containing Na$^+$, K$^+$, and glucose or a digest of rice (which contains glucose and amino acids). Glucose is absorbed from the intestinal lumen via the Na$^+$-dependent glucose cotransporters, which cotransport Na$^+$ into the cells together with glucose. Many amino acids are also absorbed by Na$^+$-dependent cotransport. With the return of Na$^+$ to the cytoplasm, water efflux from the cell into the intestinal lumen decreases.

ribosomes (Fig. 8.7). The SER has a number of functions. It contains enzymes for the synthesis of many lipids, such as triacylglycerols and phospholipids. It also contains the **cytochrome P450 oxidative enzymes** involved in metabolism of drugs and toxic chemicals like ethanol and the synthesis of hydrophobic molecules like steroid hormones. Glycogen is stored in regions of liver cells that are rich in SER.

The RER is involved in the synthesis of certain proteins. Ribosomes attached to the membranes of the RER give them their "rough" appearance. Proteins produced on these ribosomes enter the lumen of the RER, travel to another membrane system, the **Golgi complex** (see Section G, next) in vesicles, and are subsequently either secreted from the cell, sequestered within membrane-enclosed organelles such as lysosomes, or embedded in the plasma membrane. **Posttranslational modifications** of these proteins, such as the initiation of **N-linked glycosylation** and the addition of **lipid-based anchors**, and disulfide bond formation occur in the RER. In contrast, proteins encoded by the nucleus and found in the cytoplasm, peroxisomes, or mitochondria are synthesized on free ribosomes in the cytosol and are seldom modified by the attachment of oligosaccharides.

### G.  Golgi Complex

The **Golgi complex** is involved in modifying proteins produced in the RER and **in sorting and distributing** these proteins to the lysosomes, secretory vesicles, or the plasma membrane. It consists of a curved stack of flattened vesicles in the cytoplasm, which is generally divided into three compartments: the *cis* Golgi network, which is often convex and faces the nucleus; the *medial* Golgi stacks; and the *trans* Golgi network, which often faces the plasma membrane. Vesicles transport materials to and from the Golgi. The Golgi complex also participates in posttranslational modification of proteins, such as branched-chain complex carbohydrate addition, sulfation, and phosphorylation.

## H. Cytoskeleton

The structure of the cell, the shape of the cell surface, and the arrangement of subcellular organelles is organized by three major protein components: **microtubules** composed of **tubulin**, which move and position organelles and vesicles; **thin filaments** composed of **actin**, which form a cytoskeleton; and **intermediate filaments** composed of different fibrous proteins. Actin and tubulin, which are also involved in cell movement, are dynamic structures composed of continuously associating and dissociating globular subunits. Intermediate filaments, which play a structural role, are composed of stable fibrous proteins that turn over more slowly than do the components of microtubules and thin filaments.

## II. GENERAL FEATURES OF CHEMICAL MESSENGERS

There are certain universal characteristics of chemical messenger systems illustrated in Figure 8.8. Signaling generally follows the following sequence: (a) the chemical messenger is secreted from a specific cell in response to a stimulus; (b) the messenger diffuses or is transported through blood or other extracellular fluid to the target cell; (c) a molecule in the target cell, termed a receptor, (a plasma membrane receptor or intracellular receptor) specifically binds the messenger; (d) binding of the messenger to the receptor elicits a response; (e) the signal ceases and is terminated. Chemical messengers elicit their response in the target cell without being metabolized by the cell.

An additional feature of chemical messenger systems is that the specificity of the response is dictated by the type of receptor and its location. Generally, each receptor binds only one specific chemical messenger, and each receptor initiates a characteristic signal transduction pathway that will ultimately activate or inhibit certain processes in the cell. Only certain cells, the target cells, carry receptors for that messenger and are capable of responding to its message.

The means of signal termination is an exceedingly important aspect of cell signaling, and failure to terminate a message contributes to several diseases, such as cancer.

 **Lotta T.** (see Chapter 6) was given colchicine, a drug that is frequently used to treat gout in its initial stages. One of colchicine's actions is to prevent phagocytic activity by binding to dimers of the α- and β-subunits of tubulin. When the tubulin dimer-colchicine complexes bind to microtubules, further polymerization of the microtubule is inhibited, depolymerization predominates, and the microtubules disassemble. Microtubules are necessary for vesicular movement of urate crystals during phagocytosis and release of mediators that activate the inflammatory response. Thus, colchicine diminishes the inflammatory response, swelling, and pain caused by formation of the urate crystals.

**Ann R.**'s fasting is accompanied by high levels of the endocrine hormone glucagon, which is secreted in response to low blood glucose levels. It enters the blood and acts on the liver to stimulate a number of pathways, including the release of glucose from glycogen stores (glycogenolysis) (see Chapter 1). The specificity of its action is determined by the location of receptors. Although liver parenchymal cells have glucagon receptors, skeletal muscle and many other tissues do not. Therefore, glucagon cannot stimulate glycogenolysis in these tissues.

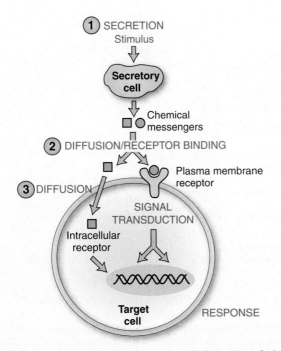

**FIG. 8.8.** General features of chemical messengers. *(1)* Secretion of chemical message. *(2)* Binding of message to cell surface receptor. *(3)* Diffusion of a hydrophobic message across the plasma membrane and binding to an intracellular receptor.

Acetylcholine works on two different types of receptors: nicotinic and muscarinic. Nicotinic receptors (for which nicotine is an activator) are found at the neuromuscular junction of skeletal muscle cells as well as in the parasympathetic nervous system. Muscarinic receptors (for which muscarine, a mushroom toxin, is an activator) are found at the neuromuscular junction of cardiac and smooth muscle cells as well as in the sympathetic nervous system. Curare (a paralyzing agent) is an inhibitor of nicotinic acetylcholine receptors, whereas atropine is an inhibitor of muscarinic acetylcholine receptors. Atropine may be used under conditions in which acetylcholinesterase has been inactivated by various nerve gases or chemicals such that atropine will block the effects of the excess acetylcholine present at the synapse.

## A. General Features of Chemical Messenger Systems Applied to the Nicotinic Acetylcholine Receptor

The individual steps involved in cell signaling by chemical messengers are illustrated with **acetylcholine (ACh)**, a neurotransmitter that acts on **nicotinic acetylcholine receptors** on the plasma membrane of certain muscle cells. This system exhibits the classical features of chemical messenger release and specificity of response.

**Neurotransmitters** are secreted from neurons in response to an electrical stimulus called the **action potential** (a voltage difference across the plasma membrane caused by changes in $Na^+$ and $K^+$ gradients that is propagated along a nerve). The neurotransmitters diffuse across a synapse to another excitable cell, where they elicit a response (Fig. 8.9). Acetylcholine is the neurotransmitter at neuromuscular junctions, where it transmits a signal from a motor nerve to a muscle fiber that elicits contraction of the fiber. Prior to release, acetylcholine is sequestered in vesicles clustered near an active zone in the **presynaptic membrane**. This membrane also has voltage-gated $Ca^{2+}$ channels, which open when the **action potential** reaches them, resulting in an influx of $Ca^{2+}$. $Ca^{2+}$ triggers fusion of the vesicles with the plasma membrane and acetylcholine is released into the synaptic cleft. Thus, the chemical messenger is released from a specific cell in response to a specific stimulus. The mechanism of vesicle fusion with the plasma membrane is common to the release of many second messengers.

Acetylcholine diffuses across the synaptic cleft to bind to the nicotinic acetylcholine receptor on the plasma membrane of the muscle cells. The subunits of the receptor are assembled around a channel, which has a funnel-shaped opening in the center. As acetylcholine binds to one of the subunits of the receptor, a conformational change opens the narrow portion of the channel (the gate), allowing $Na^+$ to diffuse in and $K^+$ to diffuse out (a uniform property of most receptors is that signal transduction begins with conformational changes in the receptor). The change in ion concentration activates a sequence of events that eventually triggers the cellular response–contraction of the fiber.

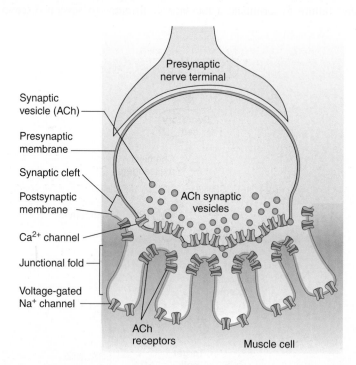

**FIG. 8.9.** Acetylcholine receptors at the neuromuscular junction. A motor nerve terminates in several branches; each branch terminates in a bulb-shaped structure called the presynaptic bouton. Each bouton synapses with a region of the muscle fiber that contains junctional folds. At the crest of each fold, there is a high concentration of acetylcholine receptors, which are gated ion channels.

**Mia S.** was tested with an inhibitor of acetylcholinesterase, edrophonium chloride, administered intravenously. After this drug inactivates acetylcholinesterase, acetylcholine that is released from the nerve terminal accumulates in the synaptic cleft. Even though **Mia** expresses fewer acetylcholine receptors on her muscle cells (due to the autoantibody-induced degradation of receptors) by increasing the local concentration of acetylcholine, these receptors have a higher probability of being occupied and activated. Therefore, acute intravenous administration of this short-acting drug briefly improves muscular weakness in patients with myasthenia gravis.

Once acetylcholine secretion stops, the message is rapidly terminated by **acetylcholinesterase**, an enzyme located on the postsynaptic membrane that cleaves acetylcholine. It is also terminated by diffusion of acetylcholine away from the synapse. Rapid termination of message is a characteristic of systems requiring a rapid response from the target cell.

### B. Endocrine, Paracrine, and Autocrine Actions

The actions of chemical messengers are often classified as endocrine, paracrine, or autocrine (Fig. 8.10). Each **endocrine hormone** (e.g., insulin) is secreted by a specific cell type (generally in an endocrine gland), enters the blood, and exerts its actions on specific target cells, which may be some distance away. In contrast to endocrine hormones, **paracrine actions** are those carried out on nearby cells and the location of the cells plays a role in specificity of the response. Synaptic transmission by acetylcholine and other neurotransmitters (sometimes called neurocrine signaling) is an example of paracrine signaling. Acetylcholine activates only those acetylcholine receptors located across the synaptic cleft from the signaling nerve, not every muscle cell with acetylcholine receptors. Paracrine actions are also very important in limiting the immune response to a specific location in the body, a feature that helps prevent the development of autoimmune disease. **Autocrine actions** involve a messenger acting on the cell from which it is secreted or on nearby cells that are the same type as the secreting cells.

### C. Types of Chemical Messengers

There are three types of major signaling systems in the body employing chemical messengers: the nervous system, the endocrine system, and the immune system. The major properties of these messengers are summarized in Table 8.1. It is important to realize that each of the hundreds of chemical messengers has its own specific receptor, which will usually bind no other messenger. There are also some

**A. Endocrine**

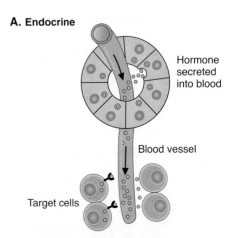

Hormone secreted into blood

Blood vessel

Target cells

**B. Paracrine**

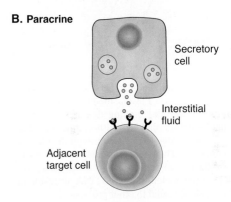

Secretory cell

Interstitial fluid

Adjacent target cell

**C. Autocrine**

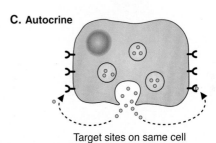

Target sites on same cell

Y Receptor    ∘ Hormone or other chemical messenger

**FIG. 8.10.** Endocrine (**A**), paracrine (**B**), and autocrine (**C**) actions of hormones and other chemical messengers.

**Table 8.1   Types of Chemical Messengers**

| System | Types of Messengers | Examples of Messengers |
|---|---|---|
| Nervous (neurotransmitters act as messengers) | Biogenic amines | Acetylcholine γ-Aminobutyric acid (GABA) |
| | Neuropeptides | Endorphins Neuropeptide-Y |
| Endocrine (molecule secreted by one organ but acts at another organ) | Polypeptide | Insulin Glucagon |
| | Catecholamines | Epinephrine Dopamine |
| | Steroid hormones (lipophilic) | Estrogen Cortisol |
| Immune (alters gene transcription in target cells) | Cytokines | Interleukins Colony-stimulating factors Interferons |
| Eicosanoids (control cellular function in response to injury) | Primarily 20 carbon lipids | Prostaglandins Leukotrienes |
| Growth factors (goes across all systems) | Proteins | Platelet-derived growth factor (PDGF) Epidermal growth factor (EGF) |

**Cell-surface receptors**

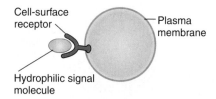

**Intracellular receptors**

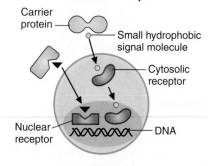

**FIG. 8.11.** Intracellular versus plasma membrane receptors. Plasma membrane receptors have extracellular binding domains. Intracellular receptors bind steroid hormones or other messengers able to diffuse through the plasma membrane. Their receptors may reside in the cytoplasm and translocate to the nucleus, reside in the nucleus bound to DNA, or reside in the nucleus bound to other proteins.

compounds normally considered hormones that are more difficult to categorize. For example, retinoids, which are derivatives of vitamin A (also called retinol) and vitamin D (which is also derived from cholesterol), are usually classified as hormones, although they are not synthesized in endocrine cells.

## III. INTRACELLULAR TRANSCRIPTION FACTOR RECEPTORS

### A. Intracellular versus Plasma Membrane Receptors

The structural properties of a messenger determine, to some extent, the type of receptor it binds. Most receptors fall into two broad categories: **intracellular receptors** or **plasma membrane receptors** (Fig. 8.11). Messengers using intracellular receptors must be hydrophobic molecules able to diffuse through the plasma membrane into cells. In contrast, polar molecules such as peptide hormones, cytokines, and catecholamines cannot rapidly cross the plasma membrane and must bind to a plasma membrane receptor.

Most of the intracellular receptors for lipophilic messengers are **gene-specific transcription factors**. A transcription factor is a protein that binds to a specific site on DNA and regulates the rate of transcription of a gene (i.e., synthesis of the mRNA, see Chapter 11). External signaling molecules bind to transcription factors that bind to a specific sequence on DNA and regulate the expression of only certain genes; they are thus called gene-specific or site-specific transcription factors.

### B. The Steroid Hormone/Thyroid Hormone Superfamily of Receptors

**Lipophilic hormones** that utilize intracellular gene-specific transcription factors include the steroid hormones (such as estrogen and cortisol), thyroid hormone, retinoic acid (active form of vitamin A), and vitamin D. Because these compounds are water-insoluble, they are transported in the blood bound to serum albumin, which has a hydrophobic binding pocket, or to a more specific transport protein, such as steroid hormone binding globulin (SHBG) and thyroid hormone binding globulin (TBG). The intracellular receptors for these hormones are structurally similar and referred to as the **steroid hormone/thyroid hormone superfamily** of receptors.

The steroid hormone/thyroid hormone superfamily of receptors reside primarily in the nucleus, although some are found in the cytoplasm. The glucocorticoid receptor, for example, exists as cytoplasmic multimeric complexes associated with heat shock proteins. When the hormone cortisol (a glucocorticoid) binds, the receptor undergoes a conformational change and dissociates from the heat shock proteins, exposing a nuclear translocation signal (a signal specifying its transport to the nucleus). The receptors dimerize and the complex (including bound hormone) translocates to the nucleus, where it binds to a portion of the DNA called the hormone response element (e.g., the glucocorticoid receptor binds to the glucocorticoid response element, GRE). The majority of the intracellular receptors, however, reside principally in the nucleus, and some of these are constitutively bound to their response element in DNA (e.g., the thyroid hormone receptor). Binding of the hormone changes their activity and their ability to associate with or disassociate from DNA. Regulation of gene transcription by these receptors is described in Chapter 13.

## IV. PLASMA MEMBRANE RECEPTORS AND SIGNAL TRANSDUCTION

All plasma membrane receptors are proteins with certain features in common: an **extracellular domain** that binds the chemical messenger, one or more **membrane-spanning domains** that are α-helices, and an **intracellular domain** that initiates signal transduction. As the ligand binds to the extracellular domain of its receptor, it causes a **conformational change** that is communicated to the intracellular domain through the rigid α-helix of the transmembrane domain. The activated intracellular domain initiates a characteristic **signal transduction pathway** that usually involves the binding of a specific intracellular signal transduction protein. Signal transduction pathways run in one direction. From a given point in a signal transduction, pathway events closer to the receptor are termed "upstream" and events closer to the response are termed "downstream."

The pathways of signal transduction for plasma membrane receptors have two major types of effects on the cell: (a) rapid and immediate effects on cellular ion levels or activation/inhibition of enzymes and/or (b) slower changes in the rate of gene expression for a specific set of proteins. Often, a signal transduction pathway will diverge to produce both kinds of effects.

## A. Major Classes of Plasma Membrane Receptors

Individual plasma membrane receptors are grouped into the categories of **ion channel receptors**, **receptor that are kinases or bind kinases**, and receptors that work through **second messengers**. This classification is based on the receptor's general structure and means of signal transduction.

### 1.  ION CHANNEL RECEPTORS

The ion channel receptors are similar in structure to the previously discussed nicotinic acetylcholine receptor. Signal transduction consists of the conformational change when ligand binds. Most small molecule neurotransmitters and some neuropeptides use ion channel receptors.

### 2.  RECEPTORS THAT ARE KINASES OR BIND KINASES

There are several types of receptors that are kinases or bind kinases. Protein kinases transfer a phosphate group from ATP to the hydroxyl group of a specific amino acid side chain in the target protein. Their common feature is that the intracellular kinase domain of the receptor (or the kinase domain of the associated protein) is activated when the messenger binds to the extracellular domain. The receptor kinase phosphorylates an amino acid residue (serine, threonine, tyrosine or, rarely, histidine) on the receptor (autophosphorylation) and/or an associated protein. The message is propagated downstream through signal transducer proteins that bind to the activated messenger-receptor complex. Several types of these receptors are outlined in Table 8.2. We will examine one of these receptors, the insulin receptor, in more detail.

The insulin receptor, a member of the tyrosine kinase family of receptors, provides a good example of divergence in the pathway of signal transduction. Unlike other

**Table 8.2  Types of Plasma Membrane–Associated Kinase Receptors**

| Type | Example | Summary |
|---|---|---|
| Tyrosine-kinase receptors | EGF receptor | Binding of the messenger to the receptor activates the kinase, which phosphorylates both the receptor and target proteins on tyrosine residues. Second messengers include ras and mitogen-activated protein kinases (MAP kinase) and, for some receptors, derivatives of phosphatidylinositol. Ras is a critical molecule for signal transduction and is activated through binding GTP. |
| JAK-STAT receptors | Cytokines | JAK is a kinase that binds to the receptor and is activated when the receptor binds the cytokine. Activated JAK phosphorylates STAT (signal transducer and activator of transcription), which acts as a gene-specific transcription factor after being translocated to the nucleus. |
| Serine/threonine receptor kinases | TGF-β | Activation of the receptor kinase by TGF-β binding to the receptor results in the phosphorylation and activation of SMAD proteins, which, like STAT, are gene-specific transcription factors and are translocated to the nucleus to alter gene expression. |

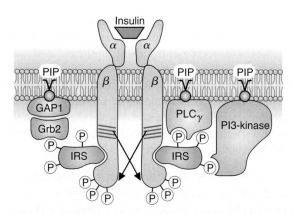

*FIG. 8.12.* Insulin receptor signaling. The insulin receptor is a dimer of two membrane-spanning α-β pairs. The tyrosine kinase domains are shown in *red*, and *arrows* indicate autocross-phosphorylation. The activated receptor binds IRS molecules (insulin receptor substrates) and phosphorylates IRS at multiple sites, thereby forming binding sites for proteins with SH2 domains (domains which recognize phosphotyrosine residues in proteins), examples being Grb2, PI 3-kinase, and phospholipase Cγ (PLCγ). Both PLCγ and PI 3-kinase are associated with various phosphatidylinositol phosphates (all designated with PIP) in the plasma membrane and are an important part of second messenger production. Grb2 associates with a protein known as GAP1 (Grb-associated protein), which has a pleckstrin homology domain that associates with phosphatidylinositol phosphates in the membrane.

growth factor receptors, the insulin receptor exists in the membrane as a preformed dimer, with each half containing an α and a β subunit (Fig. 8.12). The β-subunits auto-phosphorylate each other when insulin binds, thereby activating the receptor. The activated phosphorylated receptor binds a protein named IRS (**i**nsulin **r**eceptor **s**ubstrate). The activated receptor kinase phosphorylates IRS at multiple sites, creating multiple binding sites for different proteins with domains that recognize phosphotyrosine residues (termed SH2 domains). One of the sites binds the adapter protein Grb2, which leads to the activation of the GTP-binding protein Ras, which leads to the activation of a number of kinases known as the MAP kinases (the overall pathway is described as the MAP kinase pathway). Grb2 is anchored to a phosphatidylinositol derivative in the plasma membrane through a specific binding domain. At another phosphotyrosine site, phosphatidylinositol 3-kinase (PI 3-kinase) binds and is activated. This pathway will lead to the activation of protein kinase B. The insulin receptor can also transmit signals through a direct docking with other signal transduction intermediates. For example, the protein phospholipase Cγ (PLCγ) binds directly to the insulin receptor and is activated, which leads to activated lipid messengers being generated. Thus, insulin binding to its receptor can lead to the generation of many diverse signals, depending on which secondary signal transduction proteins are activated at the time.

### 3.  HEPTAHELICAL RECEPTORS

The **heptahelical receptors** (also known as **G-protein–coupled receptors, GPCR**) contain seven membrane-spanning α-helices (Fig. 8.13) and are the most common type of plasma membrane receptor. Although there are hundreds of hormones and neurotransmitters that work through heptahelical receptors, the extracellular binding domain of each receptor is specific for just one polypeptide hormone, catecholamine or neurotransmitter (or its close structural analogue). Heptahelical receptors have no intrinsic kinase activity, but initiate signal transduction through heterotrimeric G proteins (proteins which are activated upon binding GTP) composed of α-, β-, and γ-subunits. However, different types of heptahelical receptors bind different G proteins and different G proteins exert different effects on their target proteins. The activation of the G protein leads to second messenger production within the cell. Second messengers are present in low concentrations, so that modulation of their level, and hence the message, can be rapidly initiated and terminated.

**Heptahelical receptors**

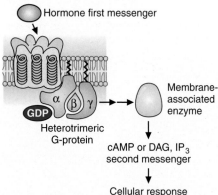

*FIG. 8.13.* G-protein–coupled receptors and second messengers. The secreted chemical messenger (hormone, cytokine, or neurotransmitter) is the first messenger, which binds to a plasma membrane receptor such as the heptahelical receptors. The activated hormone-receptor complex activates a heterotrimeric G protein (via an exchange of GTP for the bound GDP; see Fig. 8.14) and via stimulation of membrane-bound enzymes, different G proteins lead to generation of one or more intracellular second messengers, such as cAMP, diacylglycerol (DAG), or inositol trisphosphate ($IP_3$).

### a.  Heterotrimeric G proteins

The function of **heterotrimeric G proteins** is illustrated in Figure 8.14 using a hormone that activates adenylyl cyclase (e.g., glucagon or epinephrine). While the $\alpha$ subunit contains bound GDP, it remains associated with the $\beta$- and $\gamma$-subunits, either free in the membrane or bound to an unoccupied receptor (see Fig. 8.14, part 1). When the hormone binds, it causes a conformational change in the receptor that activates GDP dissociation and GTP binding. The exchange of GTP for bound GDP causes dissociation of the $\alpha$-subunit from the receptor and from the $\beta\gamma$-subunits (see Fig. 8.14, part 2). The $\alpha$- and $\gamma$-subunits are tethered to the intracellular side of the plasma membrane through lipid anchors but can still move around on the membrane surface. The GTP-$\alpha$-subunit binds its target enzyme in the membrane, thereby changing its activity. In this example, the $\alpha$-subunit binds and activates adenylyl cyclase, thereby increasing synthesis of cAMP (see Fig. 8.14, part 3).

With time, the G$\alpha$-subunit inactivates itself by hydrolyzing its own bound GTP to GDP and $P_i$. This action is unrelated to the number of cAMP molecules formed. When this occurs, the GDP-$\alpha$-subunit dissociates from its target protein, adenylyl cyclase (see Fig. 8.14, part 4). It reforms the trimeric G-protein complex, which may return to bind the empty hormone receptor. As a result of this GTPase "internal clock," sustained elevations of hormone levels are necessary for continued signal transduction and elevation of cAMP.

There are a large number of different heterotrimeric G-protein complexes, which are generally categorized according to the activity of the $\alpha$-subunit (see Table A8.1 of the online resources @ ). The 20 or more different isoforms of G$\alpha$ fall into five broad categories: G$\alpha_s$, G$\alpha_{i/0}$, G$\alpha_T$, G$\alpha_{q/11}$, and G$\alpha$12/13. G$\alpha_s$ refers to $\alpha$-subunits which, like the one in Figure 8.14, stimulate adenylyl cyclase (hence the "s").

The importance of signal termination is illustrated by the "internal clock" of G proteins, which is the rate of spontaneous hydrolysis of GTP to GDP. Mutations in *ras* (the gene encoding Ras) that decrease the rate of GTP hydrolysis are found in about 20% to 30% of all human cancers, including approximately 25% of lung cancers, 50% of colon cancers, and more than 90% of pancreatic cancers. In these mutations of Ras, GTP hydrolysis is decreased and Ras remains locked in the active GTP-bound form rather than alternating normally between the inactive and active state in response to extracellular signals. Consequently, MAP kinase pathways are continuously stimulated and drive cell proliferation, even in the absence of growth factors that would be required for *ras* activation in normal cells.

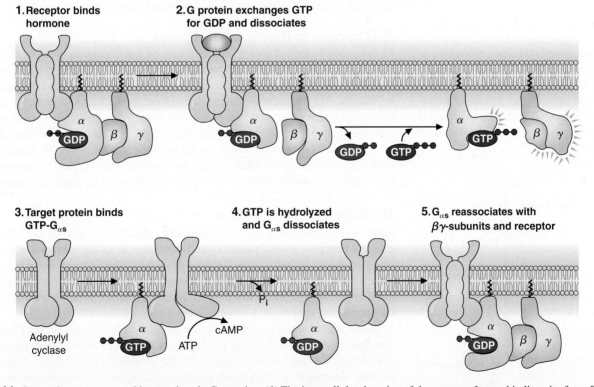

**FIG. 8.14.** Serpentine receptors and heterotrimeric G proteins. *(1)* The intracellular domains of the receptor form a binding site for a G protein containing GDP bound to the $\alpha$-subunit. *(2)* Hormone binding to the receptor promotes the exchange of GTP for GDP. As a result, the complex disassembles, releasing the G-protein $\alpha$-subunit from the $\beta\gamma$ complex. *(3)* The Gs $\alpha$-subunit binds to a target enzyme (in the example shown, the target is adenylyl cyclase), thereby changing its activity (for the G proteins, the activity is stimulated). The $\beta\gamma$ complex may simultaneously target another protein and change its activity. *(4)* Over time, bound GTP is hydrolyzed to GDP, causing dissociation of the $\alpha$-subunit from adenylyl cyclase. The GDP-$\alpha$-subunit reassociates with the $\beta\gamma$ subunit and the hormone receptor.

G$\alpha$-subunits that inhibit adenylyl cyclase are called G$\alpha_i$. The $\beta\gamma$-subunits likewise exist as different isoforms, which also transmit messages. G$\alpha$qs subunits activate phospholipase C$\beta$, which generates second messengers based on phosphatidylinositol. G$\alpha_T$ subunits activate cGMP phosphodiesterase. G$\alpha$12/13 activates a guanine nucleotide exchange factor (GEF), which activates the small GTP-binding protein rho, which is involved in cytoskeletal alterations.

### b. Adenylyl cyclase and cAMP phosphodiesterase

**cAMP** is referred to as a second messenger because changes in its concentration reflect changes in the concentration of the hormone (the first messenger). When a hormone binds and adenylyl cyclase is activated, it synthesizes cAMP from ATP. cAMP is hydrolyzed to AMP by cAMP phosphodiesterase, which also resides in the plasma membrane. The concentration of cAMP and other second messengers is kept at very low levels in cells by balancing the activity of these two enzymes so that cAMP levels can change rapidly when hormone levels change. Some hormones change the concentration of cAMP by targeting the phosphodiesterase enzyme rather than adenylyl cyclase. For example, insulin lowers cAMP levels by causing phosphodiesterase activation.

cAMP exerts diverse effects in cells. It is an allosteric activator of protein kinase A, which is a serine/threonine protein kinase that phosphorylates a large number of metabolic enzymes, thereby providing a rapid response to hormones like glucagon and epinephrine. It is also the enzyme which phosphorylates the cystic fibrosis transmembrane conductance regulator (CFTR), activating the channel. The catalytic subunits of protein kinase A also enter the nucleus and phosphorylate a gene-specific transcription factor called CREB (cyclic AMP response element binding protein). Thus, cAMP also activates a slower response pathway, gene transcription. In other cell types, cAMP directly activates ligand-gated channels.

## B. Changes in Response to Signals

Tissues vary in their ability to respond to a message through changes in receptor activity or number. Many receptors contain intracellular phosphorylation sites that alter their ability to transmit signals. Receptor number is also varied through downregulation. After a hormone binds to the receptor, the hormone-receptor complex may be taken into the cell by the process of endocytosis in clathrin-coated pits. The receptors may be degraded or recycled back to the cell surface. This internalization of receptors decreases the number available on the surface under conditions of constant high hormone levels when more of the receptors are occupied by hormones and results in decreased synthesis of new receptors. Hence, it is called **downregulation**.

## V. SIGNAL TERMINATION

Some signals, such as those that modify the metabolic responses of cells or that transmit neural impulses, need to turn off rapidly when the hormone is no longer being produced. Other signals, such as those that stimulate proliferation, turn off more slowly. In contrast, signals regulating differentiation may persist throughout our lifetime. Many chronic diseases are caused by failure to terminate a response at the appropriate time.

Signal transduction pathways can be terminated by various means (Fig. 8.15). The first level of termination is the chemical messenger itself. When the stimulus is no longer applied to the secreting cell, the messenger is no longer secreted, and existing messenger is catabolized. For example, many polypeptide hormones such as insulin are taken up into the liver and degraded. Termination of the acetylcholine signal by acetylcholinesterase has already been mentioned.

Within each pathway of signal transduction, the signal may be turned off at specific steps. For example, serpentine receptors can be desensitized to the messenger by phosphorylation, internalization, and degradation. G proteins, both monomeric and heterotrimeric, automatically terminate messages as they hydrolyze GTP via their

In myasthenia gravis, increased endocytosis and degradation of acetylcholine receptors leads to a signal transduction pathway that decreases synthesis of new receptors. Thus, downregulation of acetylcholine receptors is part of this disease.

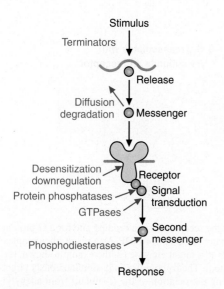

*FIG. 8.15.* Sites of signal termination. Processes that terminate signals are shown in *red*.

intrinsic GTPase activity. Although G proteins do contain intrinsic GTPase activity, this activity is relatively weak and can be accelerated through interaction with a class of proteins known as GAP, for GTPase-activating protein. Termination can also be achieved through degradation of the second messenger (e.g., phosphodiesterase cleavage of cAMP). Each of these terminating processes is also highly regulated.

Another important pathway for reversing the message typically used by receptor kinase pathways is through protein phosphatases, enzymes that reverse the action of kinases by removing phosphate groups from proteins. There are specific tyrosine or serine/threonine phosphatases for all of the sites phosphorylated by signal transduction kinases. There are even receptors that are protein phosphatases.

## CLINICAL COMMENTS

The clinical disorders discussed in this chapter are summarized in Table 8.3.

 **Mia S.** Mia S. has myasthenia gravis, an autoimmune disease caused by the production of antibodies directed against the nicotinic acetylcholine receptor in skeletal muscles. The diagnosis is made by history (presence of typical muscular symptoms), physical examination (presence of inability to do specific repetitive muscular activity over time), and tests such as the inhibition of acetylcholinesterase activity and antibodies against acetylcholine receptors. The diagnosis can be further confirmed with an electromyogram (EMG) demonstrating a partial blockade of ion flux across muscular membranes and a diagnostic procedure involving repetitive electrical nerve stimulation. The prognosis for this otherwise debilitating disease has improved dramatically with the advent of new therapies. Virtually all myasthenia patients can live full, productive lives with proper treatment. These therapies include anticholinesterase agents; immunosuppressive drugs, such as glucocorticoids, azathioprine, or mycophenolate; thymectomy (removal of the thymus gland, which offers long-term benefit which may eliminate the need for a continuing medical therapy by reducing immunoreactivity); and plasmapheresis (which reduces antiacetylcholine receptor antibody levels). Plasmapheresis is usually reserved as a means of rapidly helping the patient through a period of serious myasthenia signs and symptoms or prior to a surgical procedure.

**Table 8.3   Diseases Discussed in Chapter 8**

| Disorder or Condition | Genetic or Environmental | Comments |
|---|---|---|
| Cholera | Environmental | Watery diarrhea leading to dehydration and hypovolemic shock due to cholera toxin ADP-ribosylating a class of G proteins, altering their function and affecting water and salt transport across the intestinal mucosa. Treat with a glucose–electrolyte solution to increase coupled glucose–sodium uptake into the intestinal epithelial cells, reversing the loss of water from these cells. |
| Gout | Both | Treat by inhibiting xanthine oxidase, thereby reducing the production of uric acid, using the analogue allopurinol. Prior to allopurinol, the patient is treated with colchicine, which blocks microtubule formation and the migration of neutrophils to the affected area. |
| Myasthenia gravis | Environmental | Autoantibodies to the acetylcholine receptor, leading to neuromuscular dysfunction. |
| Cystic fibrosis | Genetic | Due to inherited mutations in the CFTR, which leads to reduced mucous secretion, and a drying of the mucus in the ducts of the lungs and leading from the pancreas to the small intestine (pancreatic duct). This leads to breathing and digestive problems. |
| Anorexia nervosa | Both | Effects of inadequate nutrition on hormone release and response. Cortisol, glucagon, and epinephrine levels are all increased under these conditions. |

CFTR, cystic fibrosis transmembrane conductance regulator.

**Ann R.** Anorexia nervosa presents as a distorted visual self-image often associated with compulsive exercise. Although Ann has been gaining weight, she is still relatively low on stored fuels needed to sustain the metabolic requirements of exercise. Her prolonged starvation has resulted in release of the steroid hormone cortisol and the polypeptide hormone glucagon, while levels of the polypeptide hormone insulin have decreased. Cortisol activates transcription of genes for some of the enzymes of gluconeogenesis (the synthesis of glucose from amino acids and other precursors; see Chapter 1). Glucagon binds to heptahelical receptors in liver and adipose tissue and, working through cAMP and protein kinase A, activates many enzymes involved in fasting fuel metabolism. Insulin, which is released when she drinks her high-energy supplement, works through a specialized tyrosine kinase receptor to promote fuel storage. Epinephrine, a catecholamine released when she exercises, promotes fuel mobilization.

**Dennis V.** *Vibrio cholerae* secrete a toxin whose A subunit is processed and transported in the cell in conjunction with the monomeric G-protein Arf (ADP-ribosylation factor). Cholera A toxin is a NAD-glycohydrolase, which cleaves $NAD^+$ and transfers the ADP-ribose portion to other proteins. The toxin ADP-ribosylates the $G_\alpha$-subunit of a class of heterotrimeric G proteins, thereby inhibiting their GTPase activity. The net result is activation of protein kinase A, which then phosphorylates the CFTR (cystic fibrosis transmembrane conductance regulator) chloride ($Cl^-$) channel so that it remains permanently open. The subsequent efflux of $Cl^-$, $Na^+$, and water into the bowel lumen is responsible for Dennis V.'s diarrhea and subsequent dehydration. The CFTR was named for its role in cystic fibrosis. A mutation in the gene encoding its subunits results in dried mucus accumulation in the airways and pancreatic ducts.

In the emergency room, Dennis received intravenous rehydration therapy (normal saline, 0.9% NaCl) and oral hydration therapy containing $Na^+$, $K^+$, and glucose or a digest of rice (which contains glucose and amino acids). Glucose is absorbed from the intestinal lumen via the $Na^+$-dependent glucose cotransporters, which cotransport $Na^+$ into the cells together with gluocuse. Many amino acids are also absorbed by $Na^+$-dependent cotransport. With the return of $Na^+$ to the cytoplasm, water efflux from the cell into the intestinal lumen decreases. Dennis quickly recovered from his bout of cholera. Cholera is self-limiting, possibly because the bacteria remain in the intestine where they are washed out of the system by the diffuse watery diarrhea. Antibiotics (tetracycline or doxycycline) can also be used to decrease the duration of the diarrhea and vibrio excretion.

## REVIEW QUESTIONS–CHAPTER 8

1. Transmembrane proteins are best described by which one of the following?

   A. They are classified as peripheral membrane proteins.
   B. They contain hydrophobic amino acid residues at their carboxy terminus.
   C. They contain hydrophilic amino acid residues extending into the lipid bilayer.
   D. They can usually be dissociated from membranes without disrupting the lipid bilayer.
   E. They contain membrane-spanning regions that are α-helices.

2. A patient had a sudden heart attack caused by a reduced blood flow through the vessels of the heart. As a consequence, there was an inadequate supply of oxygen to generate ATP in his cardiomyocytes. The compartment of the cardiomyocyte most directly involved in ATP generation is which one of the following?

   A. Lysosome
   B. Mitochondria
   C. Nucleus
   D. Peroxisome
   E. Golgi apparatus

3. Which one of the following is a general characteristic of all chemical messengers?

   A. Chemical messengers are metabolized to intracellular second messengers to transmit their message.
   B. Chemical messengers must enter cells to transmit their message.
   C. To achieve a coordinated response, each messenger is secreted by several types of cells.
   D. They are secreted by one cell, enter the blood, and act on a distant target cell.
   E. Each messenger binds to a specific protein receptor in a target cell.

4. Use the following case history for this question. Pseudohypoparathyroidism is a heritable disorder caused by target organ unresponsiveness to parathyroid hormone (a polypeptide hormone secreted by the parathyroid gland). One of the mutations causing this disease occurs in the gene encoding a $G\alpha_s$ in certain cells. The receptor for parathyroid hormone is most likely which one of the following?

   A. A heptahelical receptor
   B. An intracellular transcription factor
   C. A cytoplasmic guanylyl cyclase
   D. A receptor that must be endocytosed in clathrin-coated pits to transmit its signal.
   E. A tyrosine kinase receptor

5. Use the following case history for this question. Pseudohypoparathyroidism is a heritable disorder caused by target organ unresponsiveness to parathyroid hormone (a polypeptide hormone secreted by the parathyroid gland). One of the mutations causing this disease occurs in the gene encoding $G\alpha_s$ in certain cells. This mutation most likely is which one of the following?

   A. A gain-of-function mutation
   B. A decrease in the GTPase activity of the $G_{\alpha s}$ subunit
   C. A decrease in the generation of $IP_3$ in response to parathyroid hormone
   D. A decrease in the synthesis of cAMP in response to parathyroid hormone
   E. A decrease in the synthesis of phosphatidylinositol 3,4,5-trisphosphate in response to parathyroid hormone

# 9   Structure of the Nucleic Acids

## CHAPTER OUTLINE

**I. DNA STRUCTURE**
- A. Location of DNA
- B. Determination of the structure of DNA
- C. Concept of base pairing
- D. DNA strands are antiparallel
- E. The double helix
- F. Characteristics of DNA

**II. STRUCTURE OF CHROMOSOMES**
- A. Size of DNA molecules
- B. Packing of DNA
- C. The human genome

**III. STRUCTURE OF RNA**
- A. General features of RNA
- B. Structure of mRNA
- C. Structure of rRNA
- D. Structure of tRNA
- E. Other types of RNA

## KEY POINTS

- The central dogma of molecular biology is that DNA is transcribed to RNA, which is translated to protein.
- Nucleotides, consisting of a nitrogenous base, a five-carbon sugar, and phosphate, are the monomeric unit of the nucleic acids, DNA and RNA (see Chapter 3).
- DNA contains the sugar 2′-deoxyribose; RNA contains ribose.
- DNA and RNA contain the purine bases adenine (A) and guanine (G).
- DNA contains the pyrimidine bases cytosine (C) and thymine (T), whereas RNA contains C and uracil (U).
- DNA and RNA are linear sequences of nucleotides linked by phosphodiester bonds between the 3′ sugar of one nucleotide and the 5′ sugar of the next nucleotide.
- Genetic information is encoded by the sequence of the nucleotide bases in DNA.
- DNA is double stranded; one strand runs in the 5′ to 3′ direction, while the other is antiparallel and runs in the 3′ to 5′ direction.
- The two strands of DNA wrap about each other to form a double helix and are held together by hydrogen bonding between bases in each strand and hydrophobic interactions between the stacked bases in the core of the molecule.
- The base adenine hydrogen bonds to thymine, while cytosine hydrogen bonds to guanine.
- Transcription of a gene generates a single-stranded RNA; the three major types of RNA are messenger RNA (mRNA), ribosomal RNA (rRNA), and transfer RNA (tRNA).
- Eukaryotic mRNA is modified at both the 5′ and 3′ ends. In between it contains a coding region for the synthesis of a protein.
- Codons within the coding region dictate the sequence of amino acids in a protein. Each codon is three nucleotides long.

continued

- rRNA and tRNA are required for protein synthesis.
  - rRNA is complexed with proteins to form ribonucleoprotein particles called **ribosomes**, which bind mRNA and tRNAs during translation.
  - The tRNA contains an anticodon which binds to a complementary codon on mRNA, ensuring insertion of the correct amino acid into the protein being synthesized.

# THE WAITING ROOM

**Isabel S.** is a 26-year-old intravenous drug abuser who has shared needles with another addict for several years. Five months before presenting to the hospital emergency department with soaking night sweats, she experienced a 3-week course of a flulike syndrome with fever, malaise, and muscle aches. Four months ago, she noted generalized lymph node enlargement associated with chills, anorexia, and diarrhea, which led to a 22-lb weight loss. Tests were positive for antibodies to HIV. Because of her symptoms and a low CD4 count, a multidrug regimen was initiated.

**Clark T.** had intestinal polyps at age 50, which were removed via a colonoscope. However, he did not return for a 5-year colonoscopic examination as instructed. At age 59, he reappeared, complaining of maroon-colored stools, an indication of intestinal bleeding. The source of the blood loss was an adenocarcinoma growing from a colonic polyp of the large intestine. At surgery, it was found that the tumor had invaded the gut wall and penetrated the visceral peritoneum and several pericolic lymph nodes contained cancer cells. A computed tomography (CT) scan of the abdomen and pelvis showed several small nodules of metastatic cancer in the liver. Following resection of the tumor in both the colon and liver, the oncologist began treatment with 5-fluorouracil (5-FU) combined with other chemotherapeutic agents.

An adenoma is a mass of rapidly proliferating cells, called a neoplasm (neo = new; plasm = growth), that is formed from epithelial cells growing into a glandlike structure. The cells lining all the external and internal organs are epithelial cells, and most human tumors are adenocarcinomas. Adenomatous polyps are adenomas that grow into the lumen of the colon or rectum. The term malignant applied to a neoplasm refers to invasive unregulated growth. **Clark T.** has an adenocarcinoma, which is a malignant adenoma that has started to grow through the wall of the colon into surrounding tissues. Cells from adenocarcinomas can break away and spread through the blood or lymph to other parts of the body, where they form "colony" tumors. This process is called metastasis.

## I. DNA STRUCTURE
### A. Location of DNA

**DNA** and **RNA** serve as the genetic material for prokaryotic and eukaryotic cells, for viruses, and for plasmids, each of which stores it in a different arrangement or location. In prokaryotes, DNA is not separated from the rest of the cellular contents. In eukaryotes, however, DNA is located in the nucleus, where it is separated from the rest of the cell by the nuclear envelope and in the mitochondria. Eukaryotic nuclear DNA is bound to proteins, forming a complex called **chromatin**. During interphase (when cells are not dividing), some of the chromatin is diffuse (euchromatin) and some is dense (heterochromatin), but no distinct structures can be observed. However, before mitosis (when cells divide), the DNA is replicated, resulting in two identical chromosomes called **sister chromatids**. During metaphase (a period in mitosis), these condense into discrete, visible chromosomes.

Less than 0.1% of the total DNA in a eukaryotic cell is present in mitochondria. The genetic information in a mitochondrion is encoded in less than 20,000 base pairs of DNA; the information in a human haploid nucleus (i.e., an egg or a sperm cell) is encoded in about $3 \times 10^9$ (3 billion) base pairs. The DNA and protein synthesizing systems in mitochondria more closely resemble the systems in bacteria, which do not have membrane-enclosed organelles, than those in the eukaryotic nucleus and

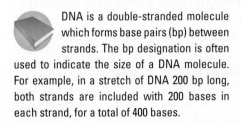

DNA is a double-stranded molecule which forms base pairs (bp) between strands. The bp designation is often used to indicate the size of a DNA molecule. For example, in a stretch of DNA 200 bp long, both strands are included with 200 bases in each strand, for a total of 400 bases.

cytoplasm. It has been suggested that mitochondria were derived from ancient bacterial invaders of primordial eukaryotic cells.

Viruses are small infectious particles consisting of a DNA or RNA genome (but not both), proteins required for pathogenesis or replication, and a protein coat. They lack, however, complete systems for DNA replication, production of RNA (transcription), and synthesis of proteins (translation). Consequently, viruses must invade other cells and commandeer their DNA, RNA, and protein-synthesizing machinery in order to reproduce. Both eukaryotes and prokaryotes can be infected by viruses. Viruses that infect bacteria are known as bacteriophages (or more simply as phages).

Plasmids are small, circular DNA molecules that can enter bacteria and replicate autonomously, that is, outside the host genome. In contrast to viruses, plasmids are not infectious; they do not convert their host cells into factories devoted to plasmid production. Genetic engineers use plasmids as tools for transfer of foreign genes into bacteria because segments of DNA can be readily incorporated into plasmids.

## B. Determination of the Structure of DNA

In 1865, Frederick Meischer first isolated DNA, obtaining it from pus scraped from surgical bandages. Initially, scientists speculated that DNA was a cellular storage form for inorganic phosphate, an important but unexciting function that did not spark widespread interest in determining its structure. Early in the 20th century, the **bases** of DNA were identified as the purines adenine (A) and guanine (G), and the pyrimidines cytosine (C) and thymine (T) (Fig. 9.1A). The sugar was found to be deoxyribose, a derivative of ribose, lacking a hydroxyl ($-OH$) group on carbon 2 (see Fig. 9.1B).

**Nucleotides**, composed of a base, a sugar, and phosphate, were found to be the monomeric units of the nucleic acids (Table 9.1). In nucleosides, the nitrogenous base is linked by an *N*-glycosidic bond to the anomeric carbon of the sugar, either ribose or deoxyribose. The atoms in the sugar are numbered using the prime symbol (′) to distinguish them from the numbering of the atoms in the nitrogenous base. A nucleotide is a nucleoside with an inorganic phosphate attached to a 5′-hydroxyl group of the sugar in ester linkage (Fig. 9.2). The names and abbreviations of nucleotides specify the base, the sugar, and the number of phosphates attached (MP, **m**ono**p**hosphate; DP, **d**i**p**hosphate; TP, **tri**phosphate). In deoxynucleotides, the prefix "d" precedes the abbreviation. For example, GDP is guanosine diphosphate (the base guanine attached to a ribose which has two phosphate groups) and dATP is deoxyadenosine triphosphate (the base adenine attached to a deoxyribose with three phosphate groups).

In 1944, after Oswald Avery's experiments establishing DNA as the genetic material were published, interest in determining the structure of DNA intensified. Digestion with enzymes of known specificity proved that inorganic phosphate joined the nucleotide monomers, forming a phosphodiester bond between the 3′-carbon of one sugar and the 5′-carbon of the next sugar along the polynucleotide chain (Fig. 9.3). Another key to DNA structure was provided by experiments performed

**Table 9.1   Names of Bases and Their Corresponding Nucleosides[a]**

| Base | Nucleoside |
|------|------------|
| Adenine (A) | Adenosine |
| Guanine (G) | Guanosine |
| Cytosine (C) | Cytidine |
| Thymine (T) | Thymidine |
| Uracil (U) | Uridine |
| Hypoxanthine (I) | Inosine[b] |

[a]If the sugar is deoxyribose rather than ribose, the nucleoside has "deoxy" as a prefix (e.g., deoxyadenosine). Nucleotides are given the name of the nucleoside plus mono-, di-, or triphosphate (e.g., adenosine triphosphate or deoxyadenosine triphosphate).
[b]The base hypoxanthine is not found in DNA but is produced during degradation of the purine bases. It is found in certain tRNA molecules. Its nucleoside, inosine, is produced during synthesis of the purine nucleotides (see Chapter 34).

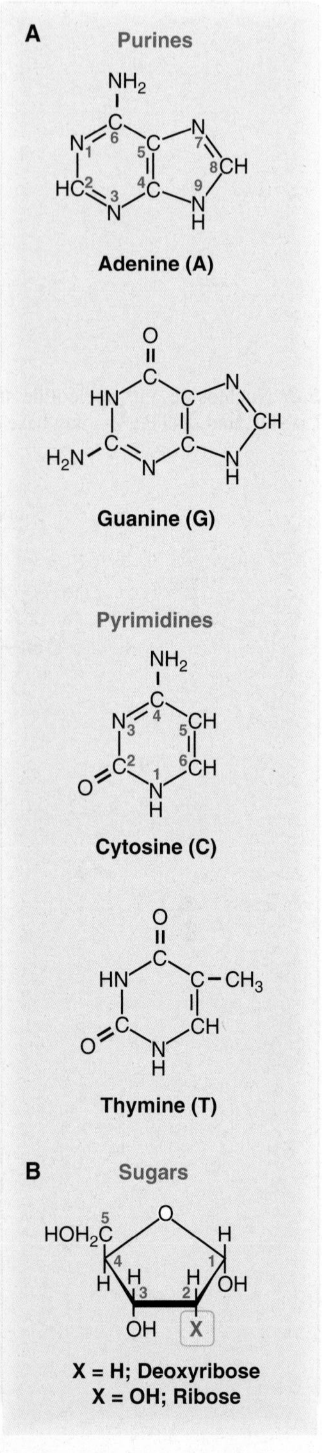

**FIG. 9.1. A.** Purine and pyrimidine bases in DNA. **B.** Deoxyribose and ribose, the sugars of DNA and RNA. The carbon atoms are numbered from 1 to 5. When the sugar is attached to a base, the carbon atoms are numbered from 1′ to 5′ to distinguish it from the base. In deoxyribose, the X = H; in ribose, the X = OH.

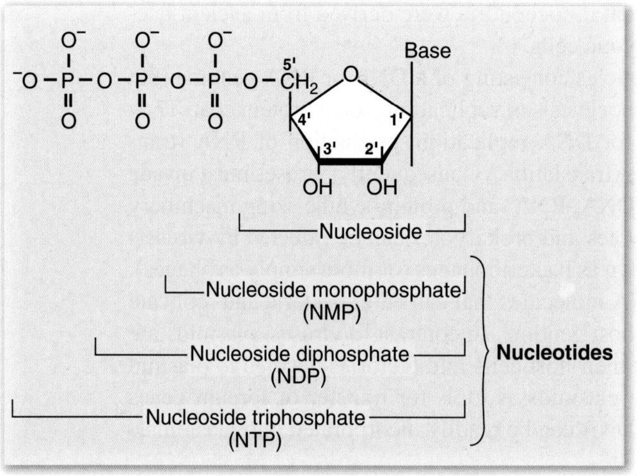

***FIG. 9.2.*** Nucleoside and nucleotide structures displayed with ribose as the sugar. The corresponding deoxyribonucleotides are abbreviated dNMP, dNDP, and dNTP. N = any base (A, G, C, U, or T).

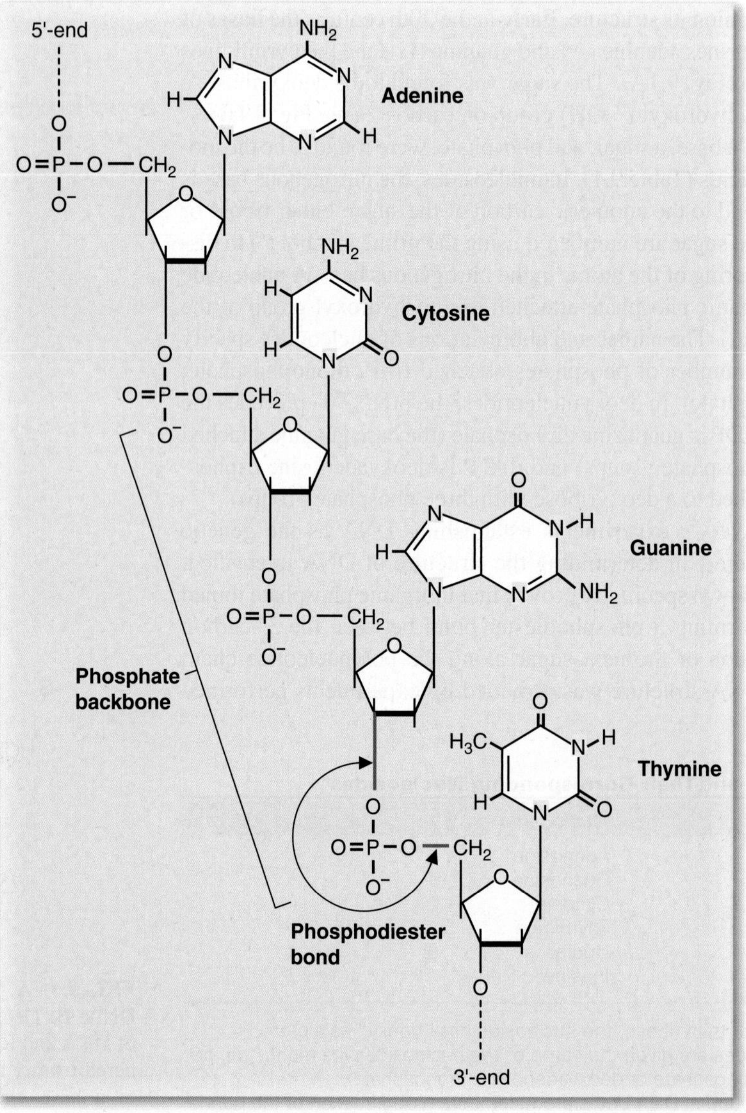

***FIG. 9.3.*** A segment of a polynucleotide chain of DNA. The *dashes* at the 5′ and 3′ ends indicate that the molecule contains more nucleotides than are shown. The hydrogen atoms (H) have been omitted from the sugar structures to increase the clarity of the figure.

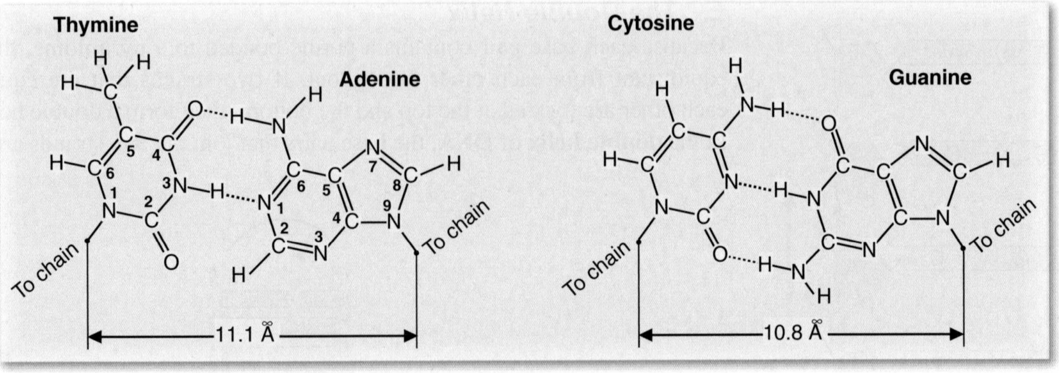

**FIG. 9.4.** Base pairs of DNA. Note that the purine bases are "flipped over" from the positions in which they are usually shown (see Fig. 9.3). The bases must be in this orientation to form base pairs. The *dotted lines* indicate hydrogen bonds between the bases. Although the hydrogen bonds participate in holding the bases and thus the two DNA strands together, they are weaker than covalent bonds and allow the DNA strands to separate during replication and transcription.

by Erwin Chargaff. He analyzed the base composition of DNA from various sources and concluded that on a molar basis, the amount of adenine was always equal to the amount of thymine and the amount of guanine was equal to the amount of cytosine.

During this era, James Watson and Francis Crick joined forces and, using the x-ray diffraction data of Maurice Wilkins and Rosalind Franklin, they incorporated the available information into a model for DNA structure. In 1953, they published a brief paper describing DNA as a double helix consisting of two polynucleotide strands joined by pairing between the bases (adenine with thymine and guanine with cytosine). The model of **base pairing** they proposed is the basis of modern molecular biology.

### C. Concept of Base Pairing

As proposed by Watson and Crick, each DNA molecule consists of two polynucleotide chains joined by hydrogen bonds between the bases. In each base pair, a purine on one strand forms hydrogen bonds with a pyrimidine on the other strand. In one type of base pair, adenine on one strand pairs with thymine on the other strand (Fig. 9.4). This base pair is stabilized by two hydrogen bonds. The other base pair, formed between guanine and cytosine, is stabilized by three hydrogen bonds. As a consequence of base pairing, the two strands of DNA are complementary, that is, adenine on one strand corresponds to thymine on the other strand, and guanine corresponds to cytosine.

The concept of base pairing proved to be essential for determining the mechanism of DNA replication (in which the copies of DNA are produced and distributed to daughter cells) and the mechanisms of transcription and translation (in which mRNA is produced from genes and used to direct the process of protein synthesis). As Watson and Crick suggested in their article, base pairing allows one strand of DNA to serve as a template for the synthesis of the other strand (Fig. 9.5). Base pairing also allows a strand of DNA to serve as a template for the synthesis of a complementary strand of RNA.

### D. DNA Strands Are Antiparallel

As concluded by Watson and Crick, the two complementary strands of DNA run in opposite directions (antiparallel). On one strand, the 5′-carbon of the sugar is above the 3′-carbon (Fig. 9.6). This strand is said to run in a 5′ to 3′ direction. On the other strand, the 3′-carbon is above the 5′-carbon. This strand is said to run in a 3′ to 5′ direction. Thus, the strands are antiparallel (i.e., they run in opposite directions.). This concept of directionality of nucleic acid strands is essential for understanding the mechanisms of replication and transcription.

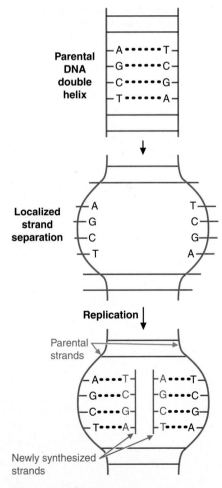

**FIG. 9.5.** DNA strands serve as templates. During replication, the strands of the helix separate in a localized region. Each parental strand serves as a template for the synthesis of a new DNA strand.

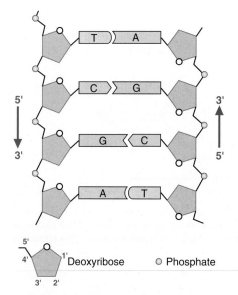

**5'** → **3'** (left strand)

**3'** → **5'** (right strand)

**5'**
**4'** **1'** Deoxyribose    ○ Phosphate
**3'** **2'**

*FIG. 9.6.* Antiparallel strands of DNA. For the strand on the left, the 5'-carbon of each sugar is above the 3'-carbon, so it runs 5' to 3'. For the strand on the right, the 3'-carbon of each sugar is above the 5'-carbon, so it runs 3' to 5'.

### E. The Double Helix

Because each base pair contains a purine bonded to a pyrimidine, the strands are equidistant from each other throughout. If two strands that are equidistant from each other are twisted at the top and the bottom, they form a double helix (Fig. 9.7). In the **double helix** of DNA, the base pairs that join the two strands are stacked like

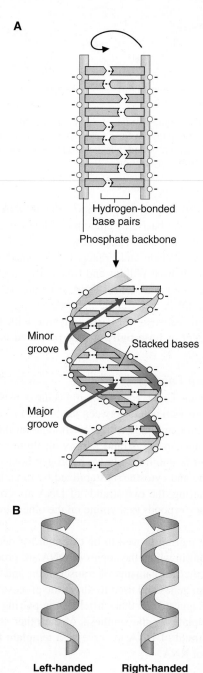

**A**

Hydrogen-bonded base pairs

Phosphate backbone

Minor groove

Stacked bases

Major groove

**B**

Left-handed     Right-handed

*FIG. 9.7.* **A.** Two DNA strands twist to form a double helix. The distance between the two phosphodiester backbones is about 11 Å. The hydrogen-bonded base pairs, shown bonded by *dotted lines*, create stacking forces with adjacent base pairs. Each phosphate group contains one negatively charged oxygen atom that provides the phosphodiester backbone with a negative charge. Because of the twisting of the helix grooves are formed along the surface, the larger one being the major groove, and the smaller one the minor groove. **B.** If you look up through the bottom of a helix along the central axis and the helix spirals away from you in a clockwise direction (toward the *arrowhead* in the drawing), it is a right-handed helix. If it spirals away from you in a counterclockwise direction, it is a left-handed helix.

a spiral staircase along the central axis of the molecule. The electrons of the adjacent base pairs interact, generating hydrophobic stacking forces that, in addition to the hydrogen bonding of the base pairs, help to stabilize the helix.

The phosphate groups of the sugar-phosphate backbones are on the outside of the helix. Each phosphate has two oxygen atoms forming the phosphodiester bonds that link adjacent sugars. However, the third $-OH$ group on the phosphate is free and dissociates a hydrogen ion at physiological pH. Therefore, each DNA helix has negative charges coating its surface that facilitate the binding of specific proteins.

The helix contains grooves of alternating size, known as the major and minor grooves (see Fig. 9.7). The bases in these grooves are exposed and, therefore, can interact with proteins or other molecules.

Watson and Crick described the B form of DNA, a right-handed helix, containing 3.4 Å (1 Å $= 10^{-8}$ cm) between base pairs and 10.4 base pairs per turn. Although this form predominates in vivo (in the cell), other forms also occur. The A form, which predominates in DNA-RNA hybrids, is similar to the B form but is more compact (2.3 Å between base pairs and 11 base pairs per turn). In the Z form, the bases of the two DNA strands are positioned toward the periphery of a left-handed helix. There are 3.8 Å between base pairs and 12 base pairs per turn in Z DNA.

### F. Characteristics of DNA

Both alkali and heat cause the two strands of the DNA helix to separate (denature). Many techniques employed to study DNA or to produce recombinant DNA molecules make use of this property. Although alkali causes the two strands of DNA to separate, it does not break the phosphodiester bonds. In contrast, the phosphodiester bonds of RNA are cleaved by alkali because of the hydroxyl group on the $3'$-carbon losing its proton, allowing the negatively charged oxygen to attack and break the phosphodiester linkage. Therefore, alkali is used to remove RNA from DNA and to separate DNA strands prior to or after electrophoresis on polyacrylamide or agarose gels.

Heat alone converts double-stranded DNA to single-stranded DNA. The separation of strands is called melting, and the temperature at which 50% of the DNA is separated is called the $T_m$. If the temperature is slowly decreased, complementary single strands can realign and base-pair, re-forming a double helix essentially identical to the original DNA. This process is known as renaturation, reannealing, or hybridization. The process by which a single-stranded DNA anneals with complementary strands of RNA is also called **hybridization** (Fig. 9.8). Hybridization is used extensively in research and clinical testing (see Chapter 14).

## II. STRUCTURE OF CHROMOSOMES
### A. Size of DNA Molecules

A prokaryotic cell generally contains a single **chromosome** composed of double-stranded DNA that forms a circle. These circular DNA molecules are extremely large. The entire chromosome of the bacterium *Escherichia coli*, composed of a single circular double-stranded DNA molecule, contains over $4 \times 10^6$ base pairs. Its molecular weight is over $2,500 \times 10^6$ g/mol (compared to the molecular weight for a glucose molecule of 180 g/mol). If this molecule were linear, its length would measure almost 2 mm. DNA from eukaryotic cells is about 1,000 times larger than that from bacterial cells. In eukaryotes, each chromosome contains one continuous linear DNA helix. The DNA of the longest human chromosome is over 7 cm in length. In fact, if the DNA from all 46 chromosomes in a diploid human cell were placed end to end, our total DNA would span a distance of about 2 m (over 6 feet). Our total DNA contains about $6 \times 10^9$ base pairs.

### B. Packing of DNA

DNA molecules require special packaging to enable them to reside within cells because the molecules are so large. In *E. coli*, the circular DNA is supercoiled and attached to an RNA-protein core. Packaging of eukaryotic DNA is much

Multidrug regimens used to treat cancers (e.g., lymphomas) sometimes include the drug doxorubicin (Adriamycin). It is a natural product with a complex multi-ring structure that intercalates or slips in between the stacked base pairs of DNA and inhibits replication and transcription. It will inhibit DNA synthesis in all cells but will preferentially affect rapidly growing cells (such as tumor cells) as compared to normal cells.

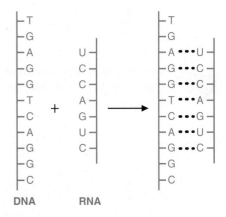

**FIG. 9.8.** Hybridization of DNA and complementary RNA.

DNA consists of a double helix, with the two strands of DNA wrapping around each other to form a helical structure. In order to compact, the DNA molecule coils about itself to form a structure called a supercoil. A telephone cord, which connects the handpiece to the phone displays supercoiling when the coiled cord wraps about itself. When the strands of a DNA molecule separate and unwind over a small local region (which occurs during DNA replication), supercoils are introduced into the remaining portion of the molecule, thereby increasing stress on this portion of the molecule. Enzymes known as topoisomerases relieve this stress so that unwinding of the DNA strands can occur.

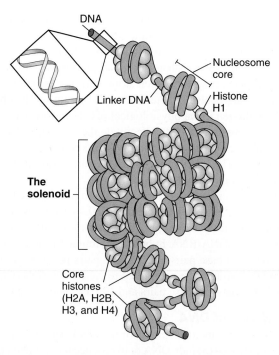

*FIG. 9.9.* A polynucleosome, indicating the histone cores and linker DNA. The DNA is depicted in *blue*, whereas the histones are depicted as *light brown spheres*.

 If histones contain large amounts of arginine and lysine, will their net charge be positive or negative?

more complex because it is larger and must be contained within the nucleus of the eukaryotic cell. Eukaryotic DNA binds to an equal weight of **histones**, which are small basic proteins containing large amounts of arginine and lysine. The complex of DNA and proteins is called **chromatin**. The organization of eukaryotic DNA into chromatin is essential for controlling transcription, as well as for packaging. When chromatin is extracted from cells, it has the appearance of beads on a string. The beads with DNA protruding from each end are known as nucleosomes, and the beads themselves are known as **nucleosome** cores (Fig. 9.9). Two molecules of each of four histone classes (histones H2A, H2B, H3, and H4) form the center of the core around which approximately 140 base pairs of double-stranded DNA are wound. The DNA wrapped around the nucleosome core is continuous and joins one nucleosome core to the next. The DNA joining the cores is complexed with the fifth type of histone, H1. Further compaction of chromatin occurs as the strings of nucleosomes wind into helical tubular coils called **solenoid** structures.

Although complexes of DNA and histones form the nucleosomal substructures of chromatin, other types of proteins are also associated with DNA in the nucleus. These proteins were given the unimaginative name of "nonhistone chromosomal proteins." The cells of different tissues contain different amounts and types of these proteins, which include enzymes that act on DNA and factors that regulate transcription.

### C. The Human Genome

The **genome**, or total genetic content, of a human **haploid** cell (a sperm or an egg) is distributed in 23 chromosomes. Haploid cells contain one copy of each chromosome. The haploid egg and haploid sperm cells combine to form the **diploid** zygote, which continues to divide to form our other cells (mitosis), also diploid. In diploid cells, there are thus 22 pairs of **autosomal chromosomes**, with each pair composed of two **homologous chromosomes** containing a similar series of genes (Fig. 9.10). In addition to the autosomal chromosomes, each diploid cell has two sex chromosomes, designated X and Y. A female has two X chromosomes, and a male has one X and one Y chromosome. The total number of chromosomes per diploid cell is 46.

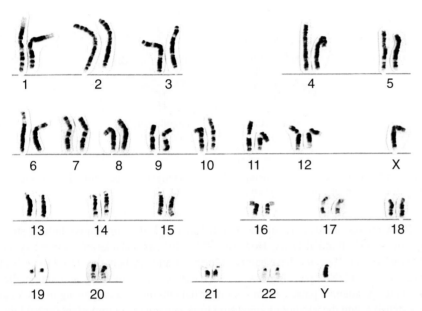

*FIG. 9.10.* Human chromosomes from a male diploid cell. Each diploid cell contains 22 pairs of autosomes (the numbered chromosomes 1–22) plus one X and one Y. Each female diploid cell contains two X chromosomes. Each haploid cell contains chromosomes 1 through 22 plus either an X or a Y. (From Gelehrter TD, Collins FS, Ginsburg D, eds. Structure and behavior of genes and chromosomes. In: *Principles of Medical Genetics.* 2nd ed. Baltimore, MD: Williams & Wilkins; 1998:18.)

Genes are arranged linearly along each chromosome. A **gene**, in genetic terms, is the fundamental unit of heredity. In structural terms, a gene encompasses the DNA sequence encoding the structural components of the gene product (whether it be a polypeptide chain or RNA molecule) along with the DNA sequences adjacent to the 5′ end of the gene which regulates its expression. A **genetic locus** is a specific position or location on a chromosome. Each gene on a chromosome in a diploid cell is matched by an alternate version of the gene at the same genetic locus on the homologous chromosome. These alternate versions of a gene are called **alleles**. We thus have two alleles of each gene, one from our mother and one from our father. If the alleles are identical in base sequence, we are homozygous for this gene. If the alleles differ, we are heterozygous for this gene and may produce two versions of the encoded protein that differ somewhat in primary structure.

The genomes of prokaryotic and eukaryotic cells differ in size. The genome of the bacterium *E. coli* contains about 3,000 genes. All of this bacterial DNA has a function; it either codes for proteins, rRNA, and tRNA, or it serves to regulate the synthesis of these gene products. In contrast, the genome of the human haploid cell contains approximately 20,000 to 25,000 genes, about seven to eight times the number in *E. coli*. The function of most of this extra DNA has not been determined (an issue considered in more detail in Chapter 13).

## III. STRUCTURE OF RNA

### A. General Features of RNA

RNA is similar to DNA. Like DNA, it is composed of nucleotides joined by 3′ to 5′-phosphodiester bonds, the purine bases adenine and guanine, and the pyrimidine base cytosine. However, its other pyrimidine base is uracil rather than thymine. Uracil and thymine are identical bases except that thymine has a methyl group at position 5 of the ring (Fig. 9.11). In RNA, the sugar is ribose, which contains a hydroxyl group on the 2′-carbon (see Fig. 9.1B; the prime refers to the position on the ribose ring—the presence of this hydroxyl group is what enables RNA to be cleaved to its constituent nucleotides in alkaline solutions).

**A:** At physiological pH, arginine and lysine carry positive charges on their side chains; therefore, histones have a net positive charge. The arginine and lysine residues are clustered in regions of the histone molecules. These positively charged regions of the histones interact with the negatively charged DNA phosphate groups.

**Clark T.** is being treated with 5-fluorouracil (5-FU), a pyrimidine base similar to uracil and thymine. 5-FU inhibits the synthesis of the thymine nucleotides required for DNA replication. Thymine is normally produced by a reaction catalyzed by thymidylate synthase, an enzyme that converts deoxyuridine monophosphate (dUMP) to deoxythymidine monophosphate (dTMP). 5-FU is converted in the body to F-dUMP, which binds tightly to thymidylate synthase in a transition state complex and inhibits the reaction (recall that thymine is 5-methyl uracil). Thus, thymine nucleotides cannot be generated for DNA synthesis, and the rate of cell proliferation decreases.

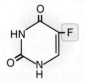

**5-Fluorouracil (5-FU),**
**an analogue of uracil or thymine**

5-FU → F-dUMP

dUMP ─┤► dTMP → dTTP → DNA

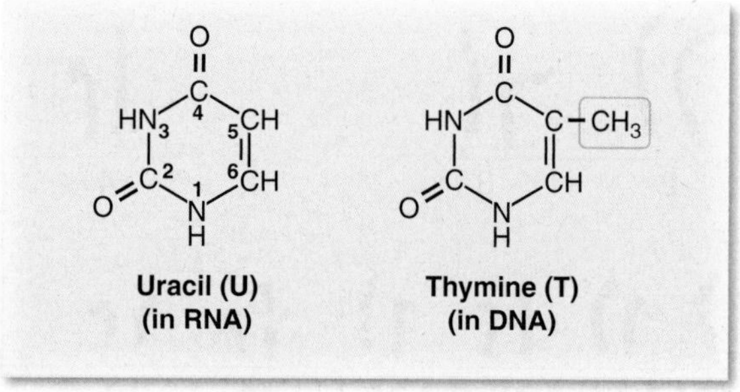

**FIG. 9.11.** Comparison of the structures of uracil and thymine. They differ in structure only by a methyl group at carbon 5, shown in the *yellow box.*

RNA chains are usually single-stranded and lack the continuous helical structure of double-stranded DNA. However, RNA still has considerable secondary and tertiary structure, because base pairs can form in regions where the strand loops back on itself. As in DNA, pairing between the bases is complementary and antiparallel. But in RNA, adenine pairs with uracil rather than thymine. Base pairing in RNA can be extensive, and the irregular looped structures generated are important for the binding of molecules, such as enzymes, that interact with specific regions of the RNA.

The three major types of RNA (mRNA, rRNA, and tRNA) participate directly in the process of protein synthesis. Other less abundant RNAs are involved in replication or in the processing of RNA, that is, in the conversion of RNA precursors to their mature forms.

Some RNA molecules are capable of catalyzing reactions. Thus, RNA, as well as protein, can have enzymatic activity. Certain rRNA precursors can remove internal segments of themselves, splicing the remaining fragments together. Because this RNA is changed by the reaction that it catalyzes, it is not truly an enzyme and therefore has been termed a "ribozyme." Other RNAs act as true catalysts, serving as ribonucleases that cleave other RNA molecules or as a peptidyl transferase, the enzyme in protein synthesis that catalyzes the formation of peptide bonds.

## B.  Structure of mRNA

Each **messenger RNA (mRNA)** molecule contains a nucleotide sequence that is converted into the amino acid sequence of a polypeptide chain in the process of translation. In eukaryotes, mRNA is transcribed from protein-coding genes as a long primary transcript that is processed in the nucleus to form mRNA. The various processing intermediates, which are mRNA precursors, are called pre-mRNA or hnRNA (**h**eterogenous **n**uclear RNA). mRNA travels through nuclear pores to the cytoplasm, where it binds to ribosomes and tRNAs and directs the sequential insertion of the appropriate amino acids into a polypeptide chain.

Eukaryotic mRNA consists of a leader sequence at the 5′ end, a coding region, and a trailer sequence at the 3′ end (Fig. 9.12). The leader sequence begins with a guanosine cap structure at its 5′ end. The coding region begins with a trinucleotide start codon that signals the beginning of translation, followed by the trinucleotide codons for amino acids and ending at a termination signal. The trailer terminates at its 5′ end with a poly(A) tail that may be up to 200 nucleotides long. Most of the leader sequence, all of the coding region, and most of the trailer are formed by transcription of the complementary nucleotide sequence in DNA. However, the terminal guanosine in the cap structure and the poly(A) tail do not have complementary sequences; they are added posttranscriptionally.

## C.  Structure of rRNA

**Ribosomes** are subcellular ribonucleoprotein complexes on which protein synthesis occurs. Different types of ribosomes are found in prokaryotes and in the cytoplasm

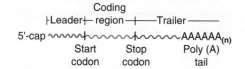

**FIG. 9.12.** The regions of eukaryotic mRNA. The *wavy line* indicates the polynucleotide chain of the mRNA and the As comprise the poly(A) tail. The 5′-cap consists of a guanosine residue linked at its 5′-hydroxyl group to three phosphates, which are linked to the 5′-hydroxyl group of the next nucleotide in the RNA chain (a 5′-5′ triphosphate linkage). The start and stop codons represent where protein synthesis is initiated and terminated from this mRNA.

RNA also serves as the genome for certain types of viruses, including retroviruses (HIV is the virus that causes AIDS). Viruses must invade host cells in order to reproduce. They are not capable of reproducing independently. Some viruses that are pathogenic to humans contain DNA as their genetic material. Others contain RNA as their genetic material. HIV invades cells of the immune system and prevents the affected individual from mounting an adequate immune response to combat infections.

According to the "central dogma" proposed by Francis Crick, information flows from DNA to RNA to proteins. For the most part, this concept holds true. However, retroviruses provide one violation of this rule. When retroviruses invade cells, their RNA genome is transcribed to produce a DNA copy. The enzyme that catalyzes this process is encoded in the viral RNA and is known as reverse transcriptase. This DNA copy integrates into the genome of the infected cell and enzymes of the host cell are used to produce many copies of the viral RNA, as well as viral proteins, which can be packaged into new viral particles.

The figure above depicts the life cycle of a retrovirus. The virus contains two identical RNA strands, only one of which is shown for clarity. After penetrating the plasma membrane, the single-stranded viral RNA genome is reverse-transcribed to a double-stranded DNA form. The viral DNA migrates to the nucleus and integrates into the chromosomal DNA, where it is transcribed to form a viral RNA transcript. The viral transcript can form the viral RNA genome for progeny viruses, or can be translated to generate viral structural proteins.

and mitochondria of eukaryotic cells (Fig. 9.13). Prokaryotic ribosomes contain three types of **ribosomal RNA (rRNA)** molecules with sedimentation coefficients of 16, 23, and 5S. The 30S ribosomal subunit contains the 16S rRNA complexed with proteins, and the 50S ribosomal subunit contains the 23S and 5S rRNAs complexed with proteins. The 30S and 50S ribosomal subunits join to form the 70S ribosome, which participates in protein synthesis.

Cytoplasmic ribosomes in eukaryotes contain four types of rRNA molecules of 18, 28, 5, and 5.8S. The 40S ribosomal subunit contains the 18S rRNA complexed with proteins, and the 60S ribosomal subunit contains the 28, 5, and 5.8S rRNAs complexed with proteins. In the cytoplasm, the 40S and 60S ribosomal subunits combine to form the 80S ribosomes that participate in protein synthesis.

Mitochondrial ribosomes, with a sedimentation coefficient of 55S, are smaller than cytoplasmic ribosomes. Their properties are similar to those of the 70S ribosomes of bacteria.

### D. Structure of tRNA

During protein synthesis, **tRNA** molecules carry amino acids to ribosomes and ensure that they are incorporated into the appropriate positions in the growing polypeptide chain (Fig. 9.14). This is done through base pairing in an antiparallel manner (see Chapter 12) of three bases of the tRNA (the anticodon) with the three base codons within the coding region of the mRNA. Therefore, cells contain at least 20 different tRNA molecules that differ somewhat in nucleotide sequence, one for each of the amino acids found in proteins. Many amino acids have more than one tRNA.

tRNA molecules contain not only the usual nucleotides but also derivatives of these nucleotides that are produced by posttranscriptional modifications.

A sedimentation coefficient is a measure of the rate of sedimentation of a macromolecule in a high-speed centrifuge (an ultracentrifuge). It is expressed in Svedberg units (S). Although larger macromolecules generally have higher sedimentation coefficients than do smaller macromolecules, sedimentation coefficients are not additive. Because frictional forces acting on the surface of a macromolecule slow its migration through the solvent, the rate of sedimentation depends not only on the density of the macromolecule but also on its shape.

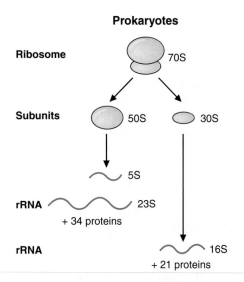

**Prokaryotes**

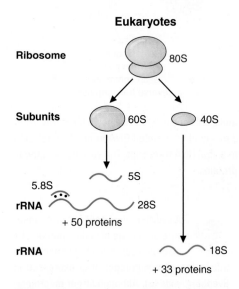

**Eukaryotes**

FIG. 9.13. Comparison of prokaryotic and eukaryotic ribosomes. The cytoplasmic ribosomes of eukaryotes are shown. Mitochondrial ribosomes are similar to prokaryotic ribosomes, but they are smaller (55S rather than 70S).

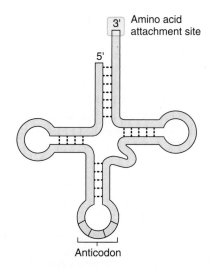

FIG. 9.14. The typical cloverleaf structure of tRNA.

In eukaryotic cells, 10% to 20% of the nucleotides of tRNA are modified. Most tRNA molecules contain ribothymidine (rT), in which a methyl group is added to uridine to form ribothymidine. They also contain dihydrouridine (D), in which one of the double bonds of the base is reduced; and pseudouridine (Ψ), in which uracil is attached to ribose by a carbon-carbon bond rather than a nitrogen-carbon bond. The base at the 5′ end of the anticodon of tRNA is frequently modified.

tRNA molecules are rather small compared to both mRNA and the large rRNA molecules. On average, tRNA molecules contain about 80 nucleotides and have a sedimentation coefficient of 4S. Because of their small size and high content of modified nucleotides, tRNAs were the first nucleic acids to be sequenced. Since 1965, when Robert Holley deduced the structure of the first tRNA, the nucleotide sequences of many different tRNAs have been determined. Although their primary sequences differ, all tRNA molecules can form a structure resembling a cloverleaf (discussed in more detail in Chapter 11).

## E.  Other Types of RNA

In addition to the three major types of RNA described earlier, other RNAs are present in cells. These RNAs include the **oligonucleotides** that serve as primers for DNA replication and the RNAs in the **small nuclear ribonucleoproteins** (**snRNPs** or **snurps**) that are involved in the splicing and modification reactions that occur during the maturation of RNA precursors (see Chapter 11). Also included are **microRNAs**, which participate in the regulation of gene expression (see Chapters 13 and 15).

### CLINICAL COMMENTS

Diseases discussed in this chapter are summarized in Table 9.2.

**Isabel S.** Isabel's clinical course was typical for the development of AIDS, in this case, caused by the use of needles contaminated with HIV. The progressive immunological deterioration that accompanies this disease ultimately results in life-threatening opportunistic infections with fungi (e.g., *Candida*, *Cryptococcus*, *Pneumocystis jiroveci* [formerly known as *Pneumocystis carinii*]), other viruses (e.g., cytomegalovirus, herpes simplex), and bacteria (e.g., *Mycobacterium* and *Salmonella*). The immunological incompetence also frequently results in the development of certain neoplasms (e.g., Kaposi sarcoma, non-Hodgkin lymphoma) as well as meningitis, neuropathies, and neuropsychiatric disorders

**Table 9.2   Diseases Discussed in Chapter 9**

| Disorder or Condition | Genetic or Environmental | Comments |
|---|---|---|
| AIDS | Environmental | AIDS is due to infection by the HIV, a retrovirus containing an RNA genome. Through its growth in immune cells, active infection by the virus leads to an immunocompromised state. Nucleoside analogues are one class of drug used to treat those with HIV infections. |
| Adenocarcinoma | Both | Use of nucleotide analogs as chemotherapeutic agents. Specifically, 5-fluorouracil is used to inhibit dTMP synthesis by the enzyme thymidylate synthase, which will lead to the death of rapidly proliferating cells. |

After **Isabel S.** was diagnosed with AIDS, she was treated with a mixture of drugs targeting different aspects of the viral life cycle, including zidovudine (ZDV), formerly called azidothymidine (AZT). This drug is an analogue of the thymine nucleotide found in DNA (the modified group is shown in the yellow box). ZDV is phosphorylated in the body by the kinases that normally phosphorylate nucleosides and nucleotides. As the viral DNA chain is being synthesized in a human cell, ZDV is then added to the growing 3′ end by viral reverse transcriptase. However, ZDV lacks a 3′ OH group and, therefore, no additional nucleotides can be attached through a 5′ → 3′ phosphodiester bond. Thus, chain elongation of the DNA is terminated. Reverse transcriptase has a higher affinity for ZDV than does normal human cellular DNA polymerases, enabling the drug to target viral replication more specifically than cellular replication.

**ZDV,
an analog of deoxythymidine**

causing cognitive dysfunction. Although recent advances in drug therapy can slow the course of the disease, no cure is yet available.

**Clark T.** Clark's original benign adenomatous polyp was located in the ascending colon, where about 30% of large bowel cancers eventually arise. Because Mr. T.'s father died from a cancer of the colon, his physician had warned him that his risk for developing colon cancer was three times higher than for the general population. Unfortunately, Mr. T. neglected to have his annual colonoscopic examinations as prescribed, and he developed an adenocarcinoma that metastasized.

The most malignant characteristic of neoplasms is their ability to metastasize, that is, form a new neoplasm at a noncontiguous site. The initial site of metastases for a tumor is usually at the first capillary bed encountered by the malignant cells once they are released. Thus, cells from tumors of the gastrointestinal tract often pass through the portal vein to the liver, which is Clark T.'s site of metastasis.

 **Clark T.** completed his first course of combined chemotherapy including intravenous 5-fluorouracil (5-FU) in the hospital. He tolerated the therapy with only mild anorexia and diarrhea and with only a mild leukopenia (a decreased white blood cell count; leuko = white). Thirty days after the completion of the initial course, these symptoms abated and he started his second course of chemotherapy with 5-FU as an outpatient.

Because 5-FU inhibits synthesis of thymine, DNA synthesis is affected in all cells in the human body that are rapidly dividing, such as the cells in the bone marrow that produce leukocytes and the mucosal cells lining the intestines. Inhibition of DNA synthesis in rapidly dividing cells contributes to the side effects of 5-FU and many other chemotherapeutic drugs.

1. For the following DNA sequence, determine the sequence and direction of the complementary strand.

    5′ – ATCGATCGATCGATCG – 3′

    A.  5′ – ATCTATCGATCGATCG – 3′
    B.  3′ – ATCGATCGATCGATCG – 5′
    C.  5′ – CGATCGATCGATCGAT – 3′
    D.  5′ – CGAUCGAUCAUCGAU – 3′
    E.  3′ – CGATCGATCGATCGAT – 5′

2. If the DNA strand shown below serves as a template for the synthesis of RNA, which one of the following choices gives the sequence and direction of the RNA which will be synthesized?

    5′ – GCTATGCATCGTGATCGAATTGCGT – 3′

    A.  5′ – ACGCAAUUCGAUCACGAUGCAUAGC – 3′
    B.  5′ – ACGCAATTCGATCACGATGCATAGC – 3′
    C.  5′ – UGCGUUAAGCUAGUGCUACGUAUCG – 3′
    D.  5′ – CGAUACGUAGCACUAGCUUAACGCA – 3′
    E.  5′ – GCTATGCATCGTGATCGAATTGCGT – 3′

3. In DNA, the bond between the deoxyribose sugar and the phosphate is best described as which one of the following?

    A.  A polar bond
    B.  An ionic bond
    C.  A hydrogen bond
    D.  A covalent bond
    E.  A van der Waals bond

4. How many double-stranded DNA molecules 8 base pairs long are theoretically possible?

    A.  12
    B.  32
    C.  64
    D.  256
    E.  65,536

5. A major difference between RNA and DNA, based on physical characteristics, is which one of the following?

    A.  The ability to form secondary structure due to base pairing
    B.  Hydrolysis of the phosphodiester bonds by alkali
    C.  The presence of negatively charged phosphate groups
    D.  The denaturation of secondary structure by heat
    E.  The presence of G-C base pairs, which are more stable than base pairs involving the base A

# 10   Synthesis of DNA

## CHAPTER OUTLINE

## KEY POINTS

- Replication of the genome requires DNA synthesis.
- During replication, each of the two parental strands of DNA serves as a template for the synthesis of a complementary strand.
- The site at which replication is occurring is called the replication fork.
- Helicases and topoisomerases are required to unwind the DNA helix of the parental strands.
- DNA polymerase is the major enzyme involved in replication.
- DNA polymerase copies each parental template strand in the 3′ to 5′ direction, producing new strands in a 5′ to 3′ direction.
- The precursors for replication are deoxyribonucleotide triphosphates.
- As DNA synthesis proceeds in the 5′ to 3′ direction, one parental strand is synthesized continuously, whereas the other exhibits discontinuous synthesis, creating small fragments named Okazaki fragments, which are subsequently joined. This is necessary because DNA polymerase can only synthesize DNA in the 5′ to 3′ direction.
- DNA polymerase requires a free 3′ hydroxyl group on a nucleotide primer in order to replicate DNA. The primer is synthesized by the enzyme primase, which provides an RNA primer.
- The enzyme telomerase synthesizes the replication of the ends of linear chromosomes (telomeres).
- Errors during replication can lead to mutations, so error checking and repair systems function to maintain the integrity of the genome.

# THE WAITING ROOM

 **Isabel S.** is having difficulty complying with her multidrug regimen. She often forgets to take her pills. When she returns for a checkup, she asks if it is that important to take her pills every day for treatment of AIDS.

**Calvin A.** is a 46-year-old man who noted a superficial, brownish-black, 5-mm nodule with irregular borders in the skin on his chest. He was scheduled for outpatient surgery, at which time a wide excision biopsy was performed (in an excision biopsy, the complete mole is removed and biopsied). Examination of the nodule revealed histological changes characteristic of a malignant melanoma reaching a thickness of only 0.7 mm (stage I).

**Michael T.** is a 62-year-old electrician who has smoked two packs of cigarettes a day for 40 years. He recently noted that his chronic cough had gotten worse. His physician ordered a chest radiograph, which showed a 2-cm nodule in the upper lobe of the right lung. A computed tomography (CT) scan was performed and confirmed a 2-cm nodule, very concerning for malignancy. The patient was taken for surgery and the nodule excised. The pathology showed a poorly differentiated adenocarcinoma of the lung. Malignant neoplasms (new growth, a tumor) of epithelial cell origin (including the intestinal lining, cells of the skin, and cells lining the airways of the lungs) are called **carcinomas**. If the cancer grows in a glandlike pattern, it is an adenocarcinoma.

## I. DNA SYNTHESIS IN PROKARYOTES

The basic features of the mechanism of DNA replication are illustrated by the processes occurring in the bacterium *Escherichia coli*. This bacillus grows symbiotically in the human colon. It has been extensively studied and serves as a model for the more complex and consequently less well-understood processes that occur in eukaryotic cells. As an overview, during replication, each of the two parental strands of DNA serves as a template for the synthesis of a complementary strand. Thus, each DNA molecule generated by the replication process contains one intact parental strand and one newly synthesized strand (Fig. 10.1).

### A. Bidirectional Replication

Replication of the circular double-stranded DNA of the chromosome of *E. coli* begins at a single point of origin (known as the origin of replication), designated *oriC* (Fig. 10.2). With the assistance of other proteins (e.g., a helicase, gyrase, and single-strand binding protein), the two parental strands separate within this region and both strands are copied simultaneously. Synthesis begins at the origin and occurs at two **replication forks** that move away from the origin bidirectionally (in both directions at the same time). Replication ends on the other side of the chromosome at a termination point. One round of synthesis, involving the incorporation of over 4 million nucleotides in each new strand of DNA, is completed in about 40 minutes. However, a second round of synthesis can begin at the origin before the first round is finished. These multiple initiations of replication allow bacterial multiplication to occur much more quickly than the time it takes to complete a single round of replication.

### B. Semiconservative Replication

Each daughter chromosome contains one of the parental DNA strands and one newly synthesized, complementary strand. Therefore, replication is said to be

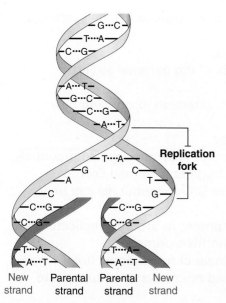

**Replication fork**

New strand | Parental strand | Parental strand | New strand

**FIG. 10.1.** A replicating DNA helix. The parental strands separate at the replication fork. Each parental strand serves as a template for the synthesis of a new strand.

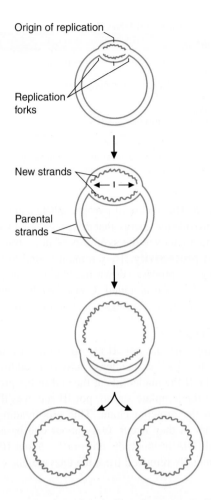

**FIG. 10.2.** Bidirectional replication of a circular chromosome. Replication begins at the point of origin (*oriC*) and proceeds in both directions at the same time. Parental strands are shown in *blue*; newly synthesized strands are shown in *red*.

**semiconservative**; that is, the parental strands are conserved but are no longer together. Each one is paired with a newly synthesized strand (see Figs. 10.1 and 10.2).

## C. DNA Unwinding

Replication requires separation of the parental DNA strands and unwinding of the helix ahead of the replication fork. **Helicases** (an example of which is the protein DnaB) separate the DNA strands and unwind the parental duplex. Single-strand binding proteins prevent the strands from reassociating and protect them from enzymes that cleave single-stranded DNA. **Topoisomerases**, enzymes that can break phosphodiester bonds and rejoin them, relieve the supercoiling of the parental duplex caused by unwinding. DNA gyrase is a major topoisomerase in bacterial cells.

## D. DNA Polymerase Action

Enzymes that catalyze the synthesis of DNA are known as **DNA polymerases**. *E. coli* has three DNA polymerases: pol I, pol II, and pol III. Pol III is the major replicative enzyme (Table 10.1). All DNA polymerases that have been studied copy a DNA template strand in its 3′ to 5′ direction, producing a new strand in the 5′ to 3′ direction (Fig. 10.3). Deoxyribonucleoside triphosphates (dATP, dGTP, dCTP, and dTTP) serve as substrates for the addition of nucleotides to the growing chain.

The incoming nucleotide forms a base pair with its complementary nucleotide on the template strand. Then, an ester bond is formed between the first 5′ phosphate of the incoming nucleotide and the free 3′ hydroxyl group at the end of the growing chain.

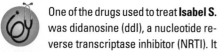

One of the drugs used to treat **Isabel S.** was didanosine (ddI), a nucleotide reverse transcriptase inhibitor (NRTI). It is a dideoxynucleoside, an example of which is shown in the following.

HOCH₂ — O — Base
H  H
H  H

**A dideoxynucleoside**

The dideoxynucleosides do not have a hydroxyl group on either the 2′- or 3′-carbon. They can be converted to dideoxynucleoside triphosphates in cells, and like zidovudine (ZDV), terminate chain growth when incorporated into DNA. In the case of the dideoxynucleosides, chain termination results from the absence of a hydroxyl group on the 3′-carbon. The HIV virus mutates very rapidly (mostly because reverse transcriptase lacks 3′ to 5′ exonuclease activity, the proofreading activity) and frequently develops resistance to one or more of these drugs. Therefore, it is recommended that AIDS patients take several drugs, including two NRTIs.

**Table 10.1   Functions of Bacterial DNA Polymerases**

| Polymerases | Functions[a] | Exonuclease Activity[b] |
|---|---|---|
| Pol I | Filling of gap after removal of RNA primer | 5′ to 3′ and 3′ to 5′ |
| | DNA repair | |
| | Removal of RNA primer in conjunction with RNAse H | |
| Pol II | DNA repair | 3′ to 5′ |
| Pol III | Replication—synthesis of DNA | 3′ to 5′ |

[a]Synthesis of new DNA strands always occurs 5′ to 3′.
[b]Exonucleases remove nucleotides from DNA strands and act at the 5′ end (cleaving 5′ to 3′) or at the 3′ end (cleaving 3′ to 5′). Endonucleases cleave bonds within polynucleotide chains.

Pyrophosphate is released. The release of pyrophosphate and its subsequent cleavage by a pyrophosphatase provide the energy that drives the polymerization process.

DNA polymerases that catalyze the synthesis of new strands during replication exhibit a feature called **processivity**. They remain bound to the parental template strand while continuing to "process" down the chain rather than dissociating and reassociating as each nucleotide is added. Consequently, synthesis is much more rapid than it would be with an enzyme that was not processive.

### E.  Base-Pairing Errors

In *E. coli*, the replicative enzyme pol III also performs a proofreading or editing function. This enzyme has 3′-5′ exonuclease activity in addition to its polymerase activity (see Table 10.1). If the nucleotide at the end of the growing chain is incorrectly base-paired with the template strand, pol III removes this nucleotide before continuing to lengthen the growing chain. This proofreading activity eliminates most base-pairing errors as they occur. Only about one base pair in a million is mismatched in the final DNA product; the error rate is about $10^{-6}$. If this proofreading activity is experimentally removed from the enzyme, the error rate increases to about $10^{-3}$.

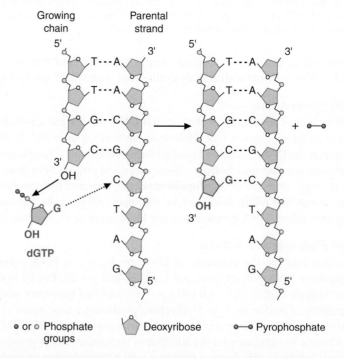

● or ○ Phosphate groups      Deoxyribose      ●—● Pyrophosphate

*FIG. 10.3.* Action of DNA polymerase. Deoxyribonucleoside triphosphates serve as precursors (substrates) used by DNA polymerase to lengthen the DNA chain. DNA polymerase copies the DNA template strand in the 3′ to 5′ direction. The new strand grows 5′ to 3′.

After replication, other mechanisms replace mismatched bases that escaped proofreading so that the fidelity of DNA replication is very high. The two processes of proofreading and postreplication mismatch repair result in an overall error rate of about $10^{-10}$, that is, less than one mismatched base pair in 10 billion.

## F. RNA Primer Requirement

DNA polymerase cannot initiate the synthesis of new strands; it requires the presence of a free 3′ OH group in order to function. Therefore, a **primer** is required to supply the free 3′ OH group. This primer is an RNA oligonucleotide. It is synthesized in a 5′ to 3′ direction by an RNA polymerase (primase) that copies the DNA template strand. DNA polymerase initially adds a deoxyribonucleotide to the 3′ hydroxyl group of the primer and then continues adding deoxyribonucleotides to the 3′ end of the growing strand (Fig. 10.4).

## G. The Replication Fork

Both parental strands are copied at the same time in the direction of the replication fork, an observation difficult to reconcile with the known activity of DNA polymerase, which can produce chains only in a 5′ to 3′ direction. Because the parental strands run in opposite directions relative to each other, synthesis should occur in a 5′ to 3′ direction *toward* the fork on one template strand and in a 5′ to 3′ direction *away* from the fork on the other template strand.

Okazaki resolved this dilemma by showing that synthesis on one strand, called the **leading strand**, is continuous in the 5′ to 3′ direction toward the fork. The other strand, called the **lagging strand**, is synthesized discontinuously in short fragments (see Fig. 10.4). These fragments, named for Okazaki, are produced in a 5′ to 3′ direction (away from the fork) but then joined together so that, overall, synthesis proceeds toward the replication fork.

## H. DNA Ligase

As replication progresses, the RNA primers are removed from Okazaki fragments, probably by the combined action of DNA polymerase I (pol I, using its 5′ to 3′ exonuclease activity) and RNase H, an enzyme that removes RNA from DNA-RNA hybrids. Pol I fills in the gaps produced by removal of the primers. Because DNA polymerases cannot join two polynucleotide chains together, an additional enzyme, **DNA ligase**, is required to perform this function. The 3′ hydroxyl group at the end of one fragment is ligated to the phosphate group at the 5′ end of the next fragment (Fig. 10.5).

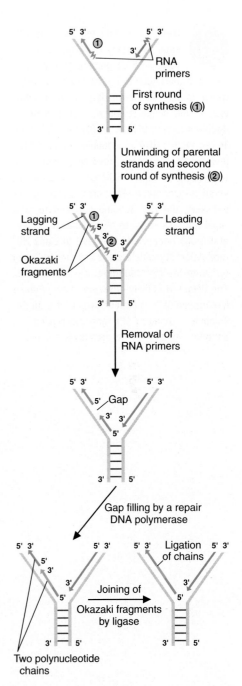

**FIG. 10.4.** Synthesis of DNA at the replication fork. (See Fig. 10.5 for the ligation reaction.)

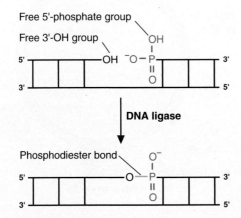

**FIG. 10.5.** Action of DNA ligase. Two polynucleotide chains, one with a free 3′ OH group and one with a free 5′ phosphate group, are joined by DNA ligase, which forms a phosphodiester bond.

**Isabel S.** is infected with the HIV virus. This virus (see Chapter 9) converts an RNA genome to a double-stranded DNA copy using the enzyme reverse transcriptase. An intermediate in the conversion of the single-stranded RNA genome to double-stranded DNA is an RNA–DNA hybrid. To remove the RNA so a double-stranded DNA molecule can be made, reverse transcriptase also contains RNase H activity. Because reverse transcriptase lacks error-checking capabilities, the HIV genome can mutate at a rapid rate. Isabel takes a combination of several drugs because of the need to block HIV replication at multiple steps in order to "keep up" with the high mutation rate of the virus. The RNase H activity of reverse transcriptase has proven to be a difficult target for drug development to block HIV genome replication, although research in this area is quite active.

## II. DNA SYNTHESIS IN EUKARYOTES

The process of replication in eukaryotes is similar to that in prokaryotes. Differences in the processes are related mainly to the vastly larger amount of DNA in eukaryotic cells (over 1,000 times the amount in *E. coli*) and the association of eukaryotic DNA with histones in nucleosomes. Enzymes with DNA polymerase, primase, ligase, helicase, and topoisomerase activity are all present in eukaryotes, although these enzymes differ in some respects from those of prokaryotes.

### A. Eukaryotic Cell Cycle

The **cell cycle** of eukaryotes consists of four phases (Fig. 10.6). The first three phases ($G_1$, S, $G_2$) constitute **interphase**. Cells spend most of their time in these three phases, carrying out their normal metabolic activities. The fourth phase is **mitosis**, the process of cell division. This phase is very brief.

The first phase of the cell cycle, $G_1$ (the first "gap" phase), is the most variable in length. Late in $G_1$, the cells prepare to duplicate their chromosomes (e.g., by producing nucleotide precursors). In the second or S phase, DNA replicates. Nucleosomes disassemble as the replication forks advance. Throughout S phase, the synthesis of histones and other proteins associated with DNA is markedly increased. The amount of DNA and histones both double and chromosomes are duplicated. Histones complex with DNA and nucleosomes are formed very rapidly behind the advancing replication forks.

During the third phase of the cell cycle, $G_2$ (the second gap phase), the cells prepare to divide and synthesize tubulin for construction of the microtubules of the spindle apparatus. Finally, nuclear and cellular division occurs in the brief mitotic or M phase.

Following mitosis, some cells reenter $G_1$, repeatedly going through the phases of the cell cycle and dividing. Other cells arrest in the cycle after mitosis, never to divide again, or they enter an extended $G_1$ phase (sometimes called $G_0$), in which they remain quiescent but metabolically active for long periods of time. Upon the appropriate signal, cells in $G_0$ are stimulated to reenter the cycle and divide.

### B. Points of Origin for Replication

In contrast to bacterial chromosomes (see Section I.A of this chapter), eukaryotic chromosomes have multiple points of origin at which replication begins. "Bubbles" appear at these points on the chromosomes. At each end of a bubble, a replication

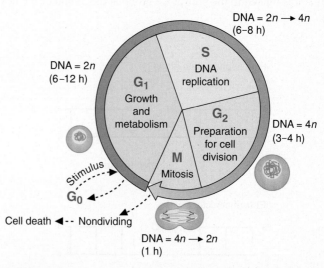

**FIG. 10.6.** Eukaryotic cell cycle. The times given for the length of each phase are for cells growing in culture. DNA content is expressed as 2N (diploid), and after DNA replication, as 4N (tetraploid).

fork forms; thus, each bubble has two forks. DNA synthesis occurs at each of these forks, as illustrated in Figure 10.7. As the bubbles enlarge, they eventually merge, and replication is completed. Because eukaryotic chromosomes contain multiple points of origin of replication (and thus multiple replicons or units of replication), duplication of such large chromosomes can occur within a few hours.

## C. Eukaryotic DNA Polymerases

Fifteen different DNA polymerases have been identified in eukaryotic cells. Examples of some of these polymerases, and their properties, are displayed in the online Table A10.1 @. To summarize the polymerases, polymerases δ (pol δ) and ε (pol ε) are the major replicative enzymes. Pol α is also involved in replication. Polymerases δ and ε, as well as pol α, appear to be involved in DNA repair. Pol γ is located in mitochondria and replicates the DNA of this organelle. Polymerases ζ, κ, η, and ι, which lack 5′-exonuclease activity, are used when DNA is damaged and are known as the bypass polymerases because they can bypass the damaged area of DNA and continue replication.

## D. The Eukaryotic Replication Complex

Many proteins bind at or near the replication fork and participate in the process of duplicating DNA (Fig. 10.8) (Table 10.2). Polymerases δ and ε are the major replicative enzymes. However, before the DNA polymerases can act, a primase associated with polymerase α (pol α) produces an RNA primer (about 10 nucleotides in length). Then, pol α adds about 20 deoxyribonucleotides to this RNA and dissociates from the template because of the low processivity of pol α. Pol α also lacks proofreading activity. On the leading strand, pol ε adds deoxyribonucleotides to this RNA-DNA primer, continuously producing this strand. Pol ε is a highly processive enzyme (the enzyme can synthesize many bases in a row before it falls off the template).

The lagging strand is produced from a series of Okazaki fragments (see Fig. 10.4). Synthesis of each Okazaki fragment is initiated by pol α and its associated primase,

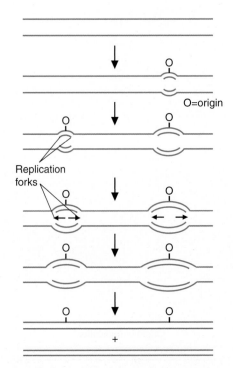

**FIG. 10.7.** Replication of a eukaryotic chromosome. Synthesis is bidirectional from each point of origin *(O)* and semiconservative. Each daughter DNA helix contains one intact parental strand *(blue line)* and one newly synthesized strand *(red line)*.

 Okazaki fragments are much smaller in eukaryotes than in prokaryotes (about 200 nucleotides vs. 1,000 to 2,000). Because the size of eukaryotic Okazaki fragments are equivalent to the size of the DNA found in nucleosomes, it seems likely that one nucleosome at a time may release its DNA for replication.

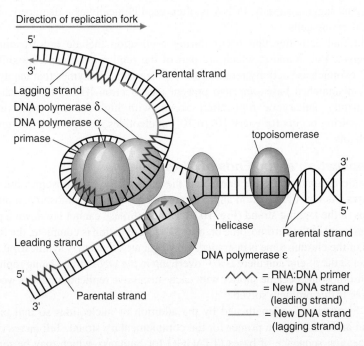

**FIG. 10.8.** Replication complex in eukaryotes. The lagging strand is shown looped around the replication complex to demonstrate that all DNA synthesis is in the 5′ to 3′ direction. Single-strand binding proteins (not shown) are bound to the unpaired, single-stranded DNA. Other proteins also participate in this complex (see text).

**Table 10.2   Major Proteins Involved in Replication**

| | |
|---|---|
| DNA polymerases | Add nucleotides to a strand growing 5' to 3', copying a DNA template 3' to 5' |
| Primase | Synthesizes RNA primers |
| Helicases | Separate parental DNA strands (i.e., unwind the double helix) |
| Single-strand binding proteins | Prevent single strands of DNA from reassociating |
| Topoisomerases | Relieve torsional strain on parental duplex caused by unwinding |
| Enzymes that remove primers | RNase H hydrolyzes RNA of DNA–RNA hybrids |
| | Flap endonuclease 1 (FEN1) recognizes "flap" (unannealed portion of RNA) near 5' end of primer and cleaves downstream in DNA region of primer; the flap is created by polymerase δ displacing the primer as the Okazaki fragment is synthesized |
| DNA ligase | Joins, by forming a phosphodiester bond, two adjacent DNA strands that are bound to the same template |
| PCNA | Enhances processivity of the DNA polymerases; binds to many proteins present at the replication fork |

PCNA, proliferating cell nuclear antigen.

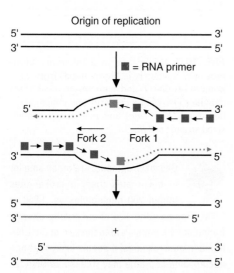

**FIG. 10.9.** The end replication problem in linear chromosomes. After replication and removal of the RNA primers, the telomeres have 3' overhangs. When these molecules are replicated, chromosome shortening will result. The figure depicts a linear chromosome with one origin of replication. At the origin, two replication forks are generated, each moving opposite directions, labeled as *Fork 1* and *Fork 2*. As *Fork 1* moves to the right, the bottom strand is read in the 3' to 5' direction, which means it is the template for the leading strand. The newly synthesized DNA complementary to the upper strand at *Fork 1* will be the lagging strand. Now, consider *Fork 2*. As this replication fork moves to the left, the upper strand is read in the 3' to 5' direction, so the newly synthesized DNA complementary to this strand will be the leading strand. For this fork, the newly synthesized DNA complementary to the bottom strand will be the lagging strand. The overhangs result from degradation of the RNA primers at the 5' end of the lagging strand, resulting in a 3' overhang.

as described earlier. After pol α dissociates, pol δ adds deoxyribonucleotides to the primer, producing an Okazaki fragment. Pol δ stops synthesizing one fragment when it reaches the start of the previously synthesized Okazaki fragment (see Fig. 10.4). The primer of the previously synthesized Okazaki fragment is removed by flap endonuclease 1 (FEN1) and RNase H. The gap left by the primer is filled by pol δ, using the parental DNA strand as its template and the newly synthesized Okazaki fragment as its primer. DNA ligase subsequently joins the Okazaki fragments together (see Fig. 10.5).

Obviously, eukaryotic replication requires many proteins. The complexity of the fork and the fact that it is not completely understood limits the detail shown in Figure 10.8. One protein (not shown) is proliferating cell nuclear antigen (PCNA), which is involved in organizing and orchestrating the replication process on both the leading and lagging strands. PCNA is often used clinically as a diagnostic marker for proliferating cells.

Additional activities that occur during replication include proofreading and DNA repair. Pols δ and ε, which are part of the replication complex, exhibit the 3' to 5' exonuclease activity required for proofreading. Enzymes that catalyze repair of mismatched bases are also present (see Section III.B.3 of this chapter). Consequently, eukaryotic replication occurs with high fidelity; approximately one mispairing occurs for every $10^9$ to $10^{12}$ nucleotides incorporated into growing DNA chains.

## E. Replication at the Ends of Chromosomes

Eukaryotic chromosomes are linear and the ends of the chromosomes are called **telomeres**. As DNA replication approaches the end of the chromosome, a problem develops in the lagging strand (Fig. 10.9). Either primase cannot lay down a primer at the very end of the chromosome or, after DNA replication is complete, the RNA at the end of the chromosome is degraded. Consequently, the newly synthesized strand is shorter at the 5' end and there is a 3' overhang in the DNA strand being replicated. If the chromosome became shorter with each successive replication, genes would be lost. How is this problem solved?

The 3' overhang is lengthened by the addition of nucleotides so that primase can bind and synthesize a primer for the complementary strand. Telomeres consist of a repeating sequence of bases (TTAGGG for humans), which may be repeated thousands of times. The enzyme telomerase contains both proteins and RNA and acts as an RNA-dependent DNA polymerase (just like reverse transcriptase). The RNA within telomerase contains the complementary copy of the repeating sequence

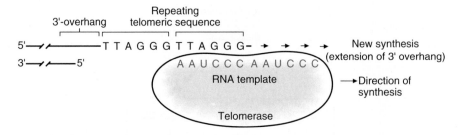

FIG. 10.10. Telomerase action. The RNA present in telomerase base-pairs with the overhanging 3′ end of telomeres and extends it by acting both as a template and a reverse transcriptase. After copying a small number of repeats, the complex moves down to the 3′-end of the overhang and repeats the process.

An inability to replicate telomeres has been linked to cell aging and death. Many somatic cells do not express telomerase; when they are placed in culture, they survive a fixed number of population doublings, enter senescence, and then die. Analysis has shown significant telomere shortening in those cells. In contrast, stem cells do express telomerase and appear to have an infinite lifetime in culture. Research is underway to understand the role of telomeres in cell aging, growth, and cancer.

in the telomeres and can base-pair with the existing 3′ overhang (Fig. 10.10). The polymerase activity of telomerase then uses the existing 3′ hydroxyl group of the overhang as a primer and its own RNA as a template and synthesizes new DNA that lengthens the 3′ end of the DNA strand. The telomerase moves down the DNA toward the new 3′ end and repeats the process many times. When the 3′ overhang is sufficiently long, primase binds and synthesis of the complementary strand is initiated. Even after this lengthening process, there is still a 3′ overhang that forms a complicated structure with telomere-binding proteins to protect the ends of the chromosomes from damage and nuclease attack once they have been lengthened.

## III. DNA REPAIR

### A. Actions of Mutagens

Despite proofreading and mismatch repair during replication, some mismatched bases do persist. Additional problems may arise from DNA damaged by **mutagens**, chemicals produced in cells, inhaled or absorbed from the environment that cause mutations. Mutagens that cause normal cells to become cancer cells are known as carcinogens. Unfortunately, mismatching of bases and DNA damage produce thousands of potentially mutagenic lesions in each cell every day. Without repair mechanisms, we could not survive these assaults on our genes.

DNA damage can be caused by radiation and by chemicals. These agents can directly affect the DNA or they can act indirectly. For example, x-rays, a type of ionizing radiation, act indirectly to damage DNA by exciting water in the cell and generating the hydroxyl radical, which reacts with DNA, thereby altering the structure of the bases or cleaving the DNA strands.

While exposure to x-rays is infrequent, it is more difficult to avoid exposure to cigarette smoke and virtually impossible to avoid exposure to sunlight. Cigarette smoke contains carcinogens such as the aromatic polycyclic hydrocarbon benzo[a] pyrene. When this compound is oxidized by cellular enzymes, which normally act to make foreign compounds more water soluble and easy to excrete, it becomes capable of forming bulky adducts with guanine residues in DNA. Ultraviolet rays from the sun, which also produce distortions in the DNA helix, excite adjacent pyrimidine bases on DNA strands, causing them to form covalent dimers, usually in the form of thymine dimers (Fig. 10.11).

### B. Repair Mechanisms

The mechanisms used for the repair of DNA have many similarities (Fig. 10.12). First, a distortion in the DNA helix is recognized and the region containing the distortion is removed. The gap in the damaged strand is replaced by the action of a DNA polymerase that uses the intact, undamaged strand as a template. Finally, a ligase seals the nick in the strand that has undergone repair. The one exception to this occurs in bacteria. Bacteria can remove thymine dimmers by photoactivating

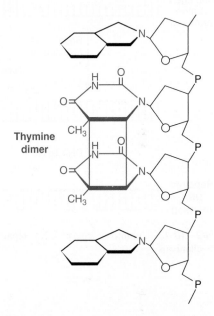

Thymine dimer

FIG. 10.11. A thymine dimer in a DNA strand. Ultraviolet light can cause two adjacent pyrimidines to form a covalent dimer.

**Michael T.** has been smoking for 40 years because of the highly addictive nature of nicotine in tobacco in spite of the warnings on cigarette packs that this habit can be dangerous and even deadly. The burning of tobacco—and for that matter, the burning of any organic material—produces many different carcinogens such as benzo[a] pyrene. These carcinogens coat the airways and lungs. They can cross cell membranes and interact with DNA, causing damage to bases that interferes with normal base-pairing. If these DNA lesions cannot be repaired or if they are not repaired rapidly enough, a permanent mutation can be produced when the cells replicate. Some mutations are silent, whereas other mutations can lead to abnormal cell growth and cancer results.

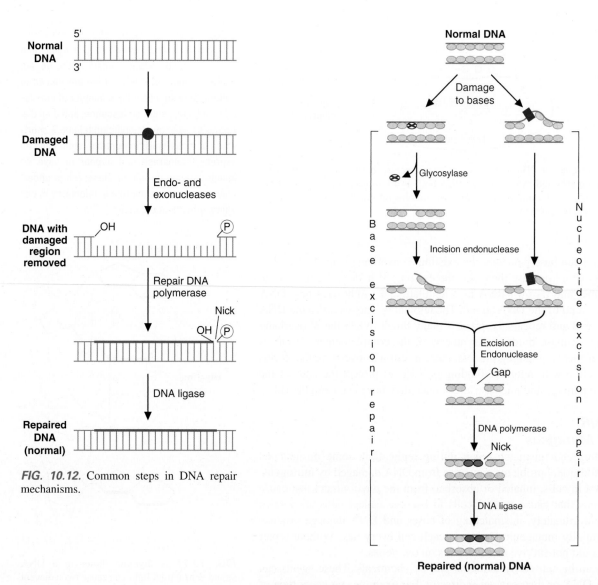

*FIG. 10.12.* Common steps in DNA repair mechanisms.

*FIG. 10.13.* Types of damage and various repair mechanisms. In base excision repair, the glycosylase cleaves the glycosidic bond between the altered base (shown with an *X*) and ribose. In NER, the entire nucleotide is removed at once. The gap formed by the incision (cut) and excision (removal) endonucleases is usually several nucleotides wider than that shown.

Melanomas develop from exposure of the skin to the ultraviolet rays of the sun. The ultraviolet radiation causes pyrimidine dimers to form in DNA. Mutations may result from nonrepair of the dimers that produce melanomas, appearing as dark brown growths on the skin.

Fortunately, **Calvin A.'s** malignant skin lesion was discovered at an early stage. Because there was no evidence of cancer in the margins of the resected mass, full recovery was expected. However, lifelong surveillance for return of the melanoma was recommended.

enzymes that cleave the bonds between the bases using energy from visible light. In this process, nucleotides are not released from the damaged DNA.

### 1. NUCLEOTIDE EXCISION REPAIR

Nucleotide excision repair (NER) involves local distortions of the DNA helix such as mismatched bases or bulky adducts (e.g., oxidized benzo[*a*]pyrene) (Fig. 10.13; see also Fig. 10.12). Endonucleases cleave the abnormal chain and remove the distorted region. The gap is then filled by a DNA polymerase that adds deoxyribonucleotides one at a time to the 3′ end of the cleaved DNA, using the intact complementary DNA strand as a template. The newly synthesized segment is joined to the 5′ end of the remainder of the original DNA strand by a DNA ligase.

### 2. BASE EXCISION REPAIR

DNA glycosylases recognize small distortions in DNA involving lesions caused by damage to a single base (e.g., the conversion of cytosine to uracil). A glycosylase cleaves the *N*-glycosidic bond that joins the damaged base to deoxyribose (see Fig. 10.13). The sugar-phosphate backbone of the DNA now lacks a base at this site (known as an apurinic or apyrimidinic site or an AP site). Then, an AP endonuclease cleaves the sugar-phosphate strand at this site. Subsequently, the same types of enzymes involved in other types of repair mechanisms restore this region to normal.

### 3. MISMATCH REPAIR

Mismatched bases (bases that do not form normal Watson-Crick base pairs) are recognized by enzymes of the mismatch repair system. Because neither of the bases in a mismatch is damaged, these repair enzymes must be able to determine which base of the mispair to correct.

The mismatch repair enzyme complex acts during replication when an incorrect but normal base (i.e., A, G, C, or T) is incorporated into the growing chain (Fig. 10.14). In bacteria, parental DNA strands contain methyl groups on adenine bases in specific sequences. During replication, the newly synthesized strands are not immediately methylated. Before methylation occurs, the proteins involved in mismatch repair can distinguish parental from newly synthesized strands. A region of the new unmethylated strand containing the mismatched base is removed and replaced.

Human enzymes can also distinguish parental from newly synthesized strands and repair mismatches. However, the mechanisms have not yet been as clearly defined as those in bacteria.

### 4. TRANSCRIPTION-COUPLED REPAIR

Genes that are actively transcribed to produce mRNA are preferentially repaired. The RNA polymerase that is transcribing a gene (see Chapter 11 for a description of the process) stalls when it encounters a damaged region of the DNA template. Excision repair proteins are attracted to this site and repair the damaged region, similar to the steps of NER. Subsequently, RNA polymerase can resume transcription.

## IV. REVERSE TRANSCRIPTASE

**Reverse transcriptase** is an enzyme that uses a single-stranded RNA template and makes a DNA copy (Fig. 10.15). The RNA template can be transcribed from DNA by RNA polymerase or obtained from another source, such as an RNA virus. The DNA copy of the RNA produced by reverse transcriptase is known as complementary DNA (since it is complementary to the RNA template) or cDNA.

 Spontaneous deamination occurs frequently in human DNA and converts cytosine bases to uracil. This base is not normally found in DNA and is potentially harmful because U pairs with A, forming U-A base pairs instead of the normal C-G pairs. To prevent this change from occurring, a uracil *N*-glycosylase removes uracil and it is replaced by a cytosine via base excision repair.

 Pyrimidine dimers occur frequently in the skin. Usually, repair mechanisms correct this damage and cancer rarely occurs. However, in individuals with xeroderma pigmentosum, cancers are extremely common. These individuals have defects in their DNA repair systems. The first defect to be identified was a deficiency of the endonuclease involved in removal of pyrimidine dimers from DNA. Because of the inability to repair DNA, the frequency of mutation increases. A cancer develops once protooncogenes or tumor suppressor genes mutate (see Chapter 15). By scrupulously avoiding sunlight, these individuals can reduce the number of skin cancers that develop.

 Hereditary nonpolyposis colorectal cancer (a human cancer that does not arise from intestinal polyps) is caused by mutations in genes for proteins involved in mismatch repair (*MLH1*, *MSH2*, *MSH6*, and *PMS2*, with *MLH1* and *MSH2* being the genes most often mutated). The inability to repair mismatches increases the mutation frequency, resulting in cancers from mutations in growth regulatory genes.

 Hereditary breast cancer is caused by mutations in genes for proteins involved, in part, in repairing single- and double-strand breaks in DNA. These genes, *BRCA1* and *BRCA2*, encode large proteins with a variety of functions in addition to their role in DNA strand break repair.

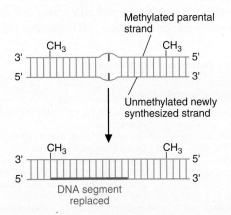

**FIG. 10.14.** Mismatch repair. Normal, undamaged but mismatched bases bind proteins of the mismatch repair system. In bacteria, these proteins recognize the older, parental strand because it is methylated and replace a segment of newly synthesized (and unmethylated) DNA containing the mismatched base. The mechanism for distinguishing between parental and newly synthesized strands in humans is not as well understood.

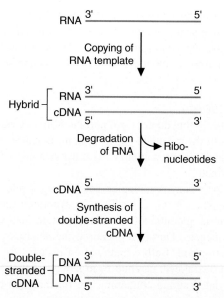

**FIG. 10.15.** Action of reverse transcriptase. This enzyme catalyzes the production of a DNA copy (cDNA) from an RNA template. The RNA of a DNA–RNA hybrid is degraded by an associated activity of reverse transcriptase (designated as RNase H), and the single DNA strand is used as a template to make double-stranded DNA. This figure is a simplified version of a more complex process.

Retroviruses (RNA viruses) contain a reverse transcriptase, which copies the viral RNA genome. A double-stranded cDNA is produced, which can become integrated into the human genome (see Chapter 9). After integration, the viral genes may be inactive, or they may be transcribed, sometimes causing diseases such as HIV/AIDS or cancer. The integration event may also disrupt an adjacent cellular gene, which may also lead to disease (see Chapter 15).

## CLINICAL COMMENTS

Diseases discussed in this chapter are summarized in Table 10.3.

**Isabel S.** Isabel S. contracted HIV when she used needles contaminated with HIV to inject drugs intravenously. Intravenous drug users account for about 10% of newly diagnosed HIV cases and about 15% of newly diagnosed AIDS cases in the United States. HIV mutates rapidly, and therefore,

**Table 10.3   Diseases Discussed in Chapter 10**

| Disorder or Condition | Genetic or Environmental | Comments |
|---|---|---|
| AIDS | Environmental | The rationale for the multidrug regime for AIDS patients is explained. |
| Melanoma | Both | Drugs used to treat cancer can inhibit DNA replication by a variety of mechanisms. |
| Lung cancer | Both | Drugs used to treat cancer can inhibit DNA replication. |
| Hereditary nonpolyposis colon cancer | Genetic | Mutations in enzymes required for DNA mismatch repair, which can lead to mutations in genes regulating cell proliferation. |
| Xeroderma pigmentosum | Genetic | Mutations involved in nucleotide excision repair, leading to a greatly elevated risk for the development of skin cancer. |
| Hereditary breast cancer | Genetic | Mutations in the genes *BRCA1* and *BRCA2*, which lead to defects in the repair of single-strand and double-strand breaks in DNA. |

current treatment involves a combination of drugs that affect different aspects of its life cycle. This multidrug therapy lowers the viral titer (the number of viral particles found in a given volume of blood), sometimes to undetectable levels. However, if treatment is not followed carefully (i.e., if the patient is not "compliant"), the titer increases rapidly. Therefore, Isabel's physician emphasized that she must carefully follow her drug regimen.

 **Calvin A.** The average person has about 30 moles on the body surface, yet only 20 to 30 people out of every 100,000 develop a malignant melanoma. The incidence of malignant melanoma, however, is rising rapidly. Because 12% to 15% of patients over age 40 years with malignant melanoma die as a result of this cancer, the physician's decision to biopsy a pigmented mole with an irregular border and variation of color probably saved **Calvin's** life.

**Michael T.** Lung cancer currently accounts for 15% of all cancers in men and women. The overall 5-year survival rate is approximately 15%. Thankfully, cigarette smoking has declined in the United States. Whereas 50% of men and 32% of women smoked in 1965, these figures have, in 2012, fallen to 21% and 17%, respectively.

## REVIEW QUESTIONS-CHAPTER 10

1. Reverse transcriptase, an RNA-dependent DNA polymerase, differs from DNA polymerase δ by which one of the following?

   A. Contains 3′ to 5′ exonuclease activity
   B. Synthesizes DNA in the 5′ to 3′ direction
   C. Follows Watson-Crick base-pair rules
   D. Synthesizes DNA in the 3′ to 5′ direction
   E. Can insert inosine into a growing DNA chain

2. If a 1,000 kilobase fragment of DNA has 10 evenly spaced and symmetrical replication origins and DNA polymerase moves at 1 kilobase per second, how many seconds will it take to produce two daughter molecules (ignore potential problems at the ends of this linear piece of DNA)? Assume that the 10 origins are evenly spaced from each other but not from the ends of the chromosome.

   A. 20
   B. 30
   C. 40
   D. 50
   E. 100

3. Primase is not required during DNA repair processes because of which one of the following?

   A. All of the primase is associated with replication origins.
   B. DNA pol I or III can use any 3′ OH for elongation.
   C. RNA would be highly mutagenic at a repair site.
   D. DNA pol I does not require a primer.
   E. DNA pol III does not require a primer.

4. The key mechanistic failure in patients with xeroderma pigmentosum involves which one of the following?

   A. An inactivating mutation in the primase gene
   B. An inactivating mutation of one of the mismatch repair components
   C. An inability to synthesize DNA across a damaged region
   D. The loss of proofreading capacity
   E. An inability to excise a section of ultraviolet (UV)-damaged DNA

5. The replication of DNA is best described by which one of the following?

   A. It progresses in both directions away from each origin of replication on the chromosome.
   B. It requires a DNA template that is copied in its 5′ to 3′ direction.
   C. It occurs during the M phase of the cell cycle.
   D. It produces one double helix consisting of the two newly synthesized strands.
   E. It requires a 3′ phosphate to initiate replication.

# 11 Transcription: Synthesis of RNA

## CHAPTER OUTLINE

## KEY POINTS

- Transcription is the synthesis of RNA from a DNA template.
- The enzyme RNA polymerase transcribes genes into a single-stranded RNA.
- The RNA produced is complementary to one of the strands of DNA, which is known as the template strand. The other DNA strand is the coding or sense strand.
- Bacteria contain a single RNA polymerase; eukaryotic cells utilize three different RNA polymerases.
- The DNA template is copied in the 3′ to 5′ direction and the RNA transcript is synthesized in the 5′ to 3′ direction.
- RNA polymerases do not require a primer to initiate transcription nor do they contain extensive error-checking capabilities.
- Promoter regions, specific sequences in DNA, determine where on the DNA template RNA polymerase binds to initiate transcription.
- Transcription initiation requires a number of protein factors to allow for efficient RNA polymerase binding to the promoter.
- Other DNA sequences, such as promoter-proximal elements and enhancers, affect the rate of transcription initiation through the interactions of DNA-binding proteins with RNA polymerase and other initiation factors.
- Eukaryotic genes contain exons and introns. Exons specify the coding region of proteins, whereas introns have no coding function.
- The primary transcript of eukaryotic genes is modified to remove the introns (splicing) before a final, mature mRNA is produced.

# THE WAITING ROOM

**Lisa N.** is a 4-year-old girl of Mediterranean ancestry whose height and body weight are below the 20th percentile for girls of her age. She tires easily and complains of loss of appetite and shortness of breath on exertion. A dull pain has been present in her right upper quadrant for the last 3 months and she appears pale. Initial laboratory studies reveal a severe anemia (decreased red blood cell count) with a hemoglobin of 7 g/dL (reference range = 12 to 16 g/dL). A battery of additional hematological tests reveals that Lisa has $\beta^+$-thalassemia, intermediate type.

**Isabel S.**, a patient with AIDS (see Chapters 9 and 10), has developed a cough that produces a gray, slightly blood-tinged sputum. A chest radiograph reveals an infiltrate around a cavity present in the right upper lung field (cavitary infiltrate). A stain of sputum reveals the presence of acid-fast bacilli, suggesting a diagnosis of pulmonary tuberculosis caused by *Mycobacterium tuberculosis*.

**Sarah L.**, a 28-year-old computer programmer, notes increasing fatigue, pleuritic chest pain, and a nonproductive cough. In addition, she complains of joint pains, especially in her hands. A rash on both cheeks and the bridge of her nose ("butterfly rash") has been present for the last 6 months. Initial laboratory studies reveal a subnormal white blood cell count and a mild reduction in hemoglobin. Tests result in a diagnosis of systemic lupus erythematosus (SLE) (frequently called lupus).

## I.   ACTION OF RNA POLYMERASE

**Transcription**, the synthesis of RNA from a DNA template, is carried out by **RNA polymerases** (Fig. 11.1). Like DNA polymerases, RNA polymerases catalyze the formation of ester bonds between nucleotides that base-pair with the complementary nucleotides on the DNA template. Unlike DNA polymerases, RNA polymerases can initiate the synthesis of new chains in the absence of primers. They also lack the 3′ to 5′ exonuclease activity found in DNA polymerases. A strand of DNA serves as the template for RNA synthesis and is copied in the 3′ to 5′ direction. Synthesis of the new RNA molecule occurs in the 5′ to 3′ direction. The ribonucleoside triphosphates ATP, GTP, CTP, and UTP serve as the precursors. Each nucleotide base sequentially pairs with the complementary deoxyribonucleotide base on the DNA template (A, G, C, and U pair with T, C, G and A, respectively). The polymerase forms an ester bond between the α-phosphate on the ribose 5′ hydroxyl of the nucleotide precursor and the ribose 3′ hydroxyl at the end of the growing RNA chain. The cleavage of a high-energy phosphate bond in the nucleotide triphosphate and release of pyrophosphate (from the β- and γ-phosphates) provides the energy for this polymerization reaction. Subsequent cleavage of the pyrophosphate by a pyrophosphatase also helps to drive the polymerization reaction forward by removing a product.

RNA polymerases must be able to recognize the start point for transcription of each gene and the appropriate strand of DNA to use as a template. A **gene** is a segment of DNA that functions as a unit to generate and regulate the expression of an RNA product or, through the processes of transcription and translation, a polypeptide chain (Fig. 11.2). RNA polymerase must also be sensitive to signals that reflect the need for the gene product and control the frequency of transcription. A region of regulatory sequences called the **promoter** (often composed of smaller sequences called **boxes** or **elements**), usually contiguous with the transcribed region, controls the binding of RNA polymerase to DNA and identifies the start point (see Fig. 11.2). The frequency of transcription is controlled by regulatory sequences within the

The thalassemias are a heterogenous group of hereditary anemias that constitute the most common gene disorder in the world, with a carrier rate of almost 7%. The disease was first discovered in countries around the Mediterranean Sea and was named for the Greek word "thalassa," meaning "sea." However, it is also present in areas extending into India and China that are near the equator.

The thalassemia syndromes are caused by mutations that decrease or abolish the synthesis of the α- or β-chains in the adult hemoglobin A tetramer. Individual syndromes are named according to the chain whose synthesis is affected and the severity of the deficiency. Thus, in $\beta^0$-thalassemia, the superscript 0 denotes none of the β-chain is present; in $\beta^+$-thalassemia, the + denotes a partial reduction in the synthesis of the β-chain. More than 170 different mutations have been identified that cause β-thalassemia; most of these interfere with the transcription of β-globin mRNA or its processing or translation.

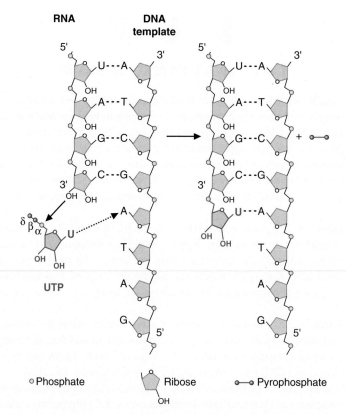

**FIG. 11.1.** RNA synthesis. The α-phosphate from the added nucleotide connects the ribosyl groups.

Patients with AIDS frequently develop tuberculosis. After **Isabel S.**'s sputum stain suggested that she had tuberculosis, a multidrug antituberculous regimen, which includes an antibiotic of the rifamycin family (rifampin), was begun. A culture of her sputum was taken to confirm the diagnosis.

Rifampin inhibits bacterial RNA polymerase, selectively killing the bacteria that cause the infection. The nuclear RNA polymerase from eukaryotic cells is not affected. Although rifampin can inhibit the synthesis of mitochondrial RNA, the concentration required is considerably higher than that used for treatment of tuberculosis.

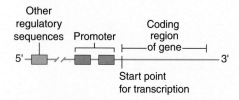

**FIG. 11.2.** Regions of a gene. A gene is a segment of DNA that functions as a unit to generate an RNA product or, through the processes of transcription and translation, a polypeptide chain. The transcribed region of a gene contains the template for synthesis of a RNA, which begins at the start point. A gene also includes regions of DNA that regulate production of the encoded product, such as a promoter region. In a structural gene, the transcribed region contains the coding sequences that dictate the amino acid sequence of a polypeptide chain.

promoter and nearby the promoter (promoter-proximal elements) and by other regulatory sequences, such as enhancers, that may be located at considerable distances, sometimes thousands of nucleotides, from the start point. Both the promoter-proximal elements and the enhancers interact with proteins, which stabilize RNA polymerase binding to the promoter.

## II.  TYPES OF RNA POLYMERASES

Bacterial cells have a single RNA polymerase that transcribes DNA to generate all the different types of RNA (mRNA, rRNA, and tRNA). The RNA polymerase of *Escherichia coli* contains five subunits ($\alpha_2\beta\beta'$), which form the core enzyme. Another protein called a σ (sigma) factor binds the core enzyme and directs binding of RNA polymerase to specific promoter regions of the DNA template. The σ factor dissociates shortly after transcription begins. *E. coli* has a number of different σ factors that recognize the promoter regions of different groups of genes. The major σ factor is $\sigma^{70}$, a designation related to its molecular weight of 70,000 daltons.

In contrast to prokaryotes, eukaryotic cells have three RNA polymerases. Polymerase I produces most of the rRNAs, polymerase II produces mRNA, and polymerase III produces small RNAs, such as tRNA and 5S rRNA. All of these RNA polymerases have the same mechanism of action. However, they recognize different types of promoters. A certain species of mushroom, *Amanita phalloides*, contains the toxin α-amanitin, which effectively blocks RNA polymerase II action and is fatal at low doses.

### A.  Sequences of Genes

Double-stranded DNA consists of a **coding strand** and a **template strand** (Fig. 11.3). The DNA template strand is the strand that is actually used by RNA polymerase

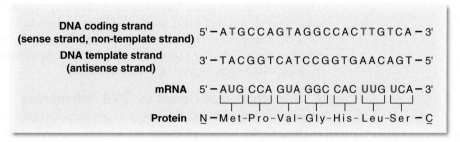

| | |
|---|---|
| **DNA coding strand** (sense strand, non-template strand) | 5′ − A T G C C A G T A G G C C A C T T G T C A − 3′ |
| **DNA template strand** (antisense strand) | 3′ − T A C G G T C A T C C G G T G A A C A G T − 5′ |
| **mRNA** | 5′ − AUG CCA GUA GGC CAC UUG UCA − 3′ |
| **Protein** | N − Met−Pro−Val−Gly−His−Leu−Ser − C |

*FIG. 11.3.* Relationship between the coding strand of DNA (also known as the sense strand or the nontemplate strand), the DNA template strand (also known as the antisense strand), the mRNA transcript, and the protein produced from the gene. The bases in mRNA are used in sets of three (called codons) to specify the order of the amino acids inserted into the growing polypeptide chain during the process of translation (see Chapter 12).

during the process of transcription. It is complementary and antiparallel both to the coding (nontemplate) strand of the DNA and to the RNA transcript produced from the template. Thus, the coding strand of the DNA is identical in base sequence and direction to the RNA transcript, except, of course, that wherever this DNA strand contains a T, the RNA transcript contains a U. By convention, the nucleotide sequence of a gene is represented by the letters of the nitrogenous bases of the coding strand of the DNA duplex. It is written from left to right in the 5′ to 3′ direction.

During translation, mRNA is read 5′ to 3′ in sets of three bases, called **codons**, that determine the amino acid sequence of the protein (see Fig. 11.3) Thus, the base sequence of the coding strand of the DNA can be used to determine the amino acid sequence of the protein. For this reason, when gene sequences are given, they refer to the coding strand.

An expanded view of a gene is shown in Figure 11.4. The base in the coding strand of the gene serving as the start point for transcription is numbered +1. This nucleotide corresponds to the first nucleotide incorporated into the RNA at the 5′ end of the transcript. Subsequent nucleotides within the transcribed region of the gene are numbered +2, +3, and so on, toward the 3′ end of the gene. Untranscribed sequences

The two strands of DNA are antiparallel, with complementary nucleotides at each position. Thus, each strand would produce a different mRNA, resulting in different codons for amino acids and a different protein product. Therefore, it is critical that RNA polymerase transcribe the correct strand.

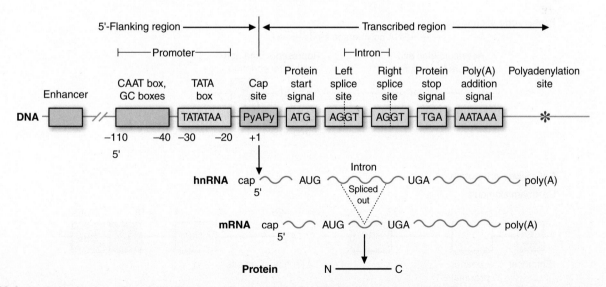

*FIG. 11.4.* A schematic view of a eukaryotic gene and steps required to produce a protein product. The gene consists of promoter and transcribed regions. The transcribed region contains introns, which do not contain coding sequence for proteins and exons, which do carry the coding sequences for proteins. The first RNA form produced is heterogenous nuclear RNA (hnRNA), which contains both intronic and exonic sequences. The hnRNA is modified such that a cap is added at the 5′ end (cap site), and a poly(A) tail added to the 3′ end. The introns are removed (a process called splicing) to produce the mature mRNA, which leaves the nucleus to direct protein synthesis in the cytoplasm. Py is pyrimidine (C or T). Although the TATA box is still included in this figure for historical reasons, only 12.5% of eukaryotic promoters contain this sequence.

to the left of the start point, known as the **5′ flanking region** of the gene, are numbered −1, −2, −3, and so on, starting with the nucleotide (−1) immediately to the left of the start point (+1) and moving from right to left. By analogy to a river, the sequences to the left of the start point are said to be **upstream** from the start point and those to the right are said to be **downstream**.

## B. Recognition of Genes by RNA Polymerase

For genes to be expressed, RNA polymerase must recognize the appropriate point on which to start transcription and the strand of the DNA to transcribe (the template strand). RNA polymerase also must recognize which genes to transcribe because transcribed genes are only a small fraction of the total DNA. The genes that are transcribed differ from one type of cell to another and can be altered with changes in physiological conditions. These signals in DNA that RNA polymerase recognizes are called **promoters**. Promoters are sequences in DNA (often composed of smaller sequences called boxes or elements) that determine the start point and the frequency of transcription. Because promoters are located on the same molecule of DNA and near the gene they regulate, they are said to be *cis* acting (i.e., "*cis*" refers to acting on the same side). Proteins that bind to these DNA sequences and facilitate or prevent the binding of RNA polymerase are said to be *trans* acting.

## C. Promoter Regions of Genes for mRNA

The binding of RNA polymerase and the subsequent initiation of gene transcription involves a number of **consensus sequences** in the promoter regions of the gene (Fig. 11.5). A consensus sequence is the sequence that is most commonly found in a given region when many genes are examined. In prokaryotes, an adenine- and thymine-rich consensus sequence in the promoter determines the start point of transcription by binding proteins that facilitate the binding of RNA polymerase. In the prokaryote *E. coli*, this consensus sequence is TATAAT, which is known as the TATA or Pribnow box. It is centered about −10 and is recognized by the sigma factor σ⁷⁰. A similar sequence in the −25 region of about 12.5% of eukaryotic genes has a consensus sequence of TATA(A/T)A. (The [A/T] in the fifth position indicates that either A or T occurs with equal frequency.) This eukaryotic sequence is also known as

**Q:** What property of an AT-rich region of a DNA double helix makes it suitable to serve as a recognition site for the start point of transcription?

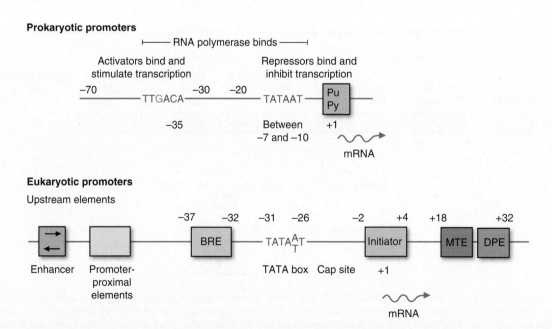

**FIG. 11.5.** Prokaryotic and eukaryotic promoters. The promoter-proximal region contains binding sites for transcription factors that can accelerate the rate at which RNA polymerase binds to the promoter. *BRE*, TFIIB recognition element; *DPE*, downstream promoter element; *Inr*, Initiation element; *MTE*, motif ten element; *Pu*, purine; *Py*, pyrimidine.

a TATA box but is sometimes named the Hogness or Hogness-Goldberg box after its discoverers. Other consensus sequences involved in binding of RNA polymerase are found further upstream in the promoter region (see Fig. 11.5) or downstream after the transcriptional start signal. Bacterial promoters contain a sequence TTGACA in the −35 region. Eukaryotes frequently have disparate sequences, such as the TFIIB recognition element (a GC-rich sequence, abbreviated as BRE), the initiator element, the downstream promoter element (DPE), and the motif ten element (MTE). The DPE and MTE are found downstream from the transcription start site. Eukaryotic genes also contain promoter-proximal elements (in the region of −100 to −200), which are sites that bind other gene regulatory proteins. Genes vary in the number of such sequences present (i.e., not all genes contain all of these initiating elements).

In bacteria, a number of protein-producing genes may be linked together and controlled by a single promoter. This genetic unit is called an **operon**. One mRNA is produced that contains the coding information for all of the proteins encoded by the operon. Proteins bind to the promoter and either inhibit or facilitate transcription of the operon. **Repressors** are proteins that bind to a region in the promoter known as the operator and inhibit transcription by preventing the binding of RNA polymerase to DNA. **Activators** are proteins that stimulate transcription by binding within the −35 region or upstream from it, facilitating the binding of RNA polymerase. (Operons are described in more detail in Chapter 13.)

In eukaryotes, proteins known as **general transcription factors** (or basal factors) bind to the TATA box (or other promoter elements, in the case of TATA-less promoters) and facilitate the binding of RNA polymerase II, the polymerase that transcribes mRNA (Fig. 11.6 ). This binding process involves at least six basal transcription factors (labeled as TFIIs, transcription factors for RNA polymerase II). The TATA-binding protein (TBP), which is a component of TFIID, initially binds to the TATA box. TFIID consists of both the TBP and a number of transcriptional coactivators. Components of TFIID will also recognize initiator and DPE boxes in the absence of a TATA box. TFIIA and TFIIB interact with TBP. RNA polymerase II binds to the complex of transcription factors and to DNA and is aligned at the start point for transcription. TFIIE, TFIIF, and TFIIH subsequently bind, cleaving ATP, and transcription of the gene is initiated.

With only these transcription (or basal) factors and RNA polymerase II attached (the basal transcription complex), the gene is transcribed at a low or basal rate.

 In regions where DNA is being transcribed, the two strands of the DNA must be separated. AT base pairs in DNA are joined by only two hydrogen bonds while GC pairs have three hydrogen bonds. Therefore, in AT-rich regions of DNA, the two strands can be separated more readily than in regions that contain GC base pairs.

 **Lisa N.** has a $\beta^+$-thalassemia classified clinically as β-thalassemia intermedia. She produces an intermediate amount of functional β-globin chains (her hemoglobin is 7 g/dL; normal is 12 to 16 g/dL). β-Thalassemia intermedia is usually the result of two different mutations (one that mildly affects the rate of synthesis of β-globin and one severely affecting its rate of synthesis) or, less frequently, homozygosity for a mild mutation in the rate of synthesis or a complex combination of mutations. For example, mutations within the promoter region of the β-globin gene could result in a significantly decreased rate of β-globin synthesis in an individual who is homozygous for the allele, without completely abolishing synthesis of the protein.

Two of the point mutations that result in a $\beta^+$ phenotype are within the TATA box (A → G or A → C in the −28 to −31 region) for the β-globin gene. These mutations reduce the accuracy of the start point of transcription so that only 20% to 25% of the normal amount of β-globin is synthesized. Other mutations that also reduce the frequency of β-globin transcription have been observed further upstream in the promoter region (−87 C → G and −88 C →T ).

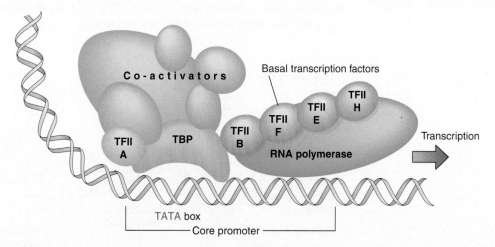

**FIG. 11.6.** Transcription apparatus. The TATA-binding protein (TBP), a component of TFIID, binds to the TATA box. Transcription factors TFII A and B bind to TBP. RNA polymerase binds, then TFII E, F, and H bind. This complex can transcribe at a basal level. Some coactivator proteins are present as a component of TFIID and these can bind to other regulatory DNA-binding proteins (called specific transcription factors or transcriptional activators). TFIID also recognizes the initiator element (Inr) and the DPE in the case of TATA-less promoters (see Fig. 11.5).

The rate of transcription can be further increased by binding of other regulatory DNA-binding proteins to additional gene regulatory sequences (such as the promoter-proximal or enhancer regions). These regulatory DNA-binding proteins are called **gene-specific transcription factors** (or transactivators) because they are specific to the gene involved (see Chapter 13). They interact with coactivators in the basal transcription complex. They are depicted in Figure 11.6 under the general term coactivators. Coactivators consist of transcription-associated factors (TAF) that interact with transcription factors through an activation domain on the transcription factor (which is bound to the DNA). The TAFs interact with other factors (described as the mediator proteins), which, in turn, interact with the RNA polymerase complex. These interactions will be further discussed in Chapter 14.

## III. TRANSCRIPTION OF BACTERIAL GENES

In bacteria, binding of RNA polymerase with a σ factor to the promoter region of DNA causes the two DNA strands to unwind and separate within a region about 10 to 20 nucleotides in length. As the polymerase transcribes the DNA, the untranscribed region of the helix continues to separate, while the transcribed region of the DNA template rejoins its DNA partner (Fig. 11.7). The σ factor is released when the growing RNA chain is about 10 nucleotides long. The elongation reactions continue until the RNA polymerase encounters a transcription **termination signal**. One type of termination signal involves the formation of a hairpin loop in the transcript, preceding a number of U residues. The second type of mechanism for termination involves the binding of a protein, the rho (ρ) factor, which causes release of the RNA transcript from the template. The signal for both termination processes is the sequence of bases in the newly synthesized RNA.

A **cistron** is a region of DNA that encodes a single polypeptide chain. In bacteria, mRNA is usually generated from an operon as a **polycistronic transcript** (one that contains the information to produce a number of different proteins). Because bacteria do not contain a nucleus, the polycistronic transcript is translated as it is being transcribed. This process is known as **coupled transcription-translation**. This transcript is not modified or trimmed, and it does not contain introns (regions within the coding sequence of a transcript that are removed before translation occurs). Several different proteins are produced during translation of the polycistronic transcript, one from each cistron.

In prokaryotes, rRNA is produced as a single, long transcript that is cleaved to produce the 16S, 23S, and 5S ribosomal RNAs. tRNA is also cleaved from larger transcripts. One of the cleavage enzymes, RNase P, is a protein containing an RNA molecule. This RNA actually catalyzes the cleavage reaction.

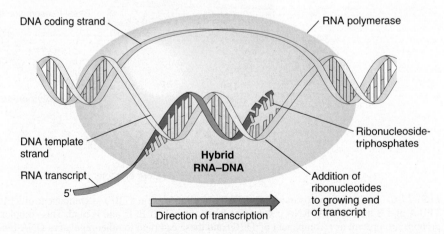

**FIG. 11.7.** An overview of transcription at the site of RNA synthesis.

## IV. TRANSCRIPTION OF EUKARYOTIC GENES

The process of transcription in eukaryotes is similar to that in prokaryotes: RNA polymerase binds to the transcription factor complex in the promoter region and to the DNA, the helix unwinds within a region near the start point of transcription, DNA strand separation occurs, synthesis of the RNA transcript is initiated, and the RNA transcript is elongated, copying the DNA template. The DNA strands separate as the polymerase approaches and rejoin as the polymerase passes.

One of the major differences between eukaryotes and prokaryotes is that eukaryotes have more elaborate mechanisms for processing the transcripts, particularly the precursors of mRNA (pre-mRNA). Eukaryotes also have three polymerases rather than just the one present in prokaryotes. Other differences include the fact that eukaryotic mRNA usually contains the coding information for only one polypeptide chain and that eukaryotic RNA is transcribed in the nucleus and migrates to the cytoplasm where translation occurs. Thus, coupled transcription-translation does not occur in eukaryotes.

### A. Synthesis of Eukaryotic mRNA

In eukaryotes, extensive processing of the primary transcript occurs before the mature mRNA is formed and can migrate to the cytosol where it is translated into a protein product. RNA polymerase II synthesizes a large primary transcript from the template strand that is capped at the 5′ end as it is transcribed (Fig. 11.8). The transcript also rapidly acquires a poly(A) tail at the 3′ end. Pre-mRNAs thus contain untranslated regions at both the 5′ and 3′ ends (the leader and trailing sequences, respectively). These untranslated regions are retained in the mature mRNA. The coding region of the pre-mRNA, which begins with the start codon for protein synthesis and ends with the stop codon, contains both exons and introns. **Exons** consist of the nucleotide codons that dictate the amino acid sequence of the eventual protein product. Between the exons, interspersing regions called **introns** contain nucleotide sequences that are removed by splicing reactions to form the mature RNA. The mature

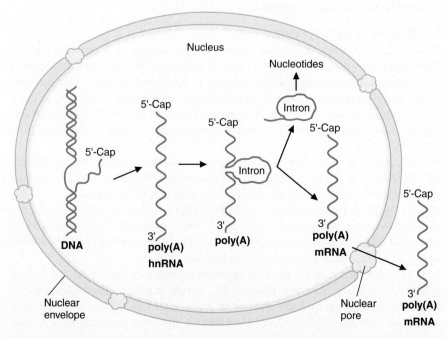

**FIG. 11.8.** Overview of mRNA synthesis. Transcription produces hnRNA (also known as pre-mRNA) from the DNA template. hnRNA processing involves addition of a 5′ cap and a poly(A) tail and splicing to join exons and remove introns. The product, mRNA, migrates to the cytoplasm in which it will direct protein synthesis.

Within about 4 weeks of initiation of treatment for tuberculosis, culture results of **Isabel S.**'s sputum confirmed the diagnosis of pulmonary tuberculosis caused by *M. tuberculosis*. Therefore, the multidrug therapy, which included the antibiotic rifampin, was continued. Rifampin binds to the RNA polymerases of several bacteria. *M. tuberculosis* rapidly develops resistance to rifampin through mutations that result in an RNA polymerase that cannot bind the complex structure. Simultaneous treatment with drugs that work through different mechanisms decreases the selective advantage of the mutation and the rate at which resistance develops.

The presence of a poly(A) tail on eukaryotic mRNA allows this form of RNA to be easily separated from the more abundant rRNA. After extracting all of the RNA from a cell, the total RNA is applied to a column of beads to which oligo-dT has been covalently attached. As the mRNA flows through the column, its poly(A) tail will basepair with the oligo-dT, and the mRNA will become bound to the column. All other types of RNA will flow through the column and not bind to the beads. The bound mRNA can then be eluted from the column by changing the ionic strength of the buffer.

RNA thus contains a leader sequence (that includes the cap), a coding region comprising exons, and a tailing sequence that includes the poly(A) tail.

This mature mRNA complexes with the poly(A)-binding protein and other proteins. It travels through pores in the nuclear envelope into the cytoplasm. There, it combines with ribosomes and directs the incorporation of amino acids into proteins.

## 1. TRANSCRIPTION AND CAPPING OF mRNA

Capping of the primary transcript synthesized by RNA polymerase II occurs at its 5′ end as it is being transcribed. The linkage formed is an unusual 5′-5′ triphosphate linkage between a guanosine residue and the 5′ termini of the original transcript. The now terminal guanine (part of the cap) is frequently methylated, and methylation can also occur on the 2′ hydroxyl of the terminal ribose sugar (and sometimes on the 2′ hydroxyl of the adjacent ribose). This cap seals the 5′ end of the primary transcript and decreases the rate of degradation. It also serves as a recognition site for the binding of the mature mRNA to a ribosome at the initiation of protein synthesis.

## 2. ADDITION OF A POLY(A) TAIL

After the RNA polymerase transcribes the stop codon for protein translation, it passes a sequence called the **polyadenylation signal (AAUAAA)**. It continues past the polyadenylation signal until it reaches an unknown and possibly unspecific termination signal many nucleotides later. However, as the primary transcript is released from the RNA polymerase elongation complex, an enzyme complex binds to the polyadenylation signal and cleaves the primary transcript approximately 10 to 20 nucleotides downstream, thereby forming the 3′ end. Following this cleavage, a poly(A) tail that can be greater than 200 nucleotides in length is added to the 3′ end. Thus, there is no poly(dT) sequence in the DNA template that corresponds to this tail; it is added posttranscription. ATP serves as the precursor for the sequential addition of the adenine nucleotides. They are added one at a time, with poly(A) polymerase catalyzing each addition. The poly(A) tail is a protein binding site that protects the mRNA from degradation.

## 3. REMOVAL OF INTRONS

Eukaryotic pre-mRNA transcripts contain regions known as exons and introns. Exons appear in the mature mRNA; introns are removed from the transcript and are not found in the mature mRNA (see Fig. 11.8). Therefore, introns do not contribute to the amino acid sequence of the protein. Some genes contain 50 or more introns. These introns are carefully removed from the pre-mRNA transcript and the exons are spliced together so that the appropriate protein is produced from the gene.

The consensus sequences at the intron/exon boundaries of the pre-mRNA are AGGU (AGGT in the DNA). The sequences vary to some extent on the exon side of the boundaries, but almost all introns begin with a 5′ GU and end with a 3′ AG (Fig. 11.9). These intron sequences at the left splice site and the right splice site are therefore invariant. Since every 5′ GU and 3′ AG combination does not result in a functional splice site, clearly, other features (still to be determined) within the exon or intron help to define the appropriate splice sites.

A complex structure known as a **spliceosome** ensures that exons are spliced together with great accuracy (Fig. 11.10). **Small nuclear ribonucleoproteins (snRNPs)**, called "snurps," are involved in formation of the spliceosome. Because snurps are rich in uracil, they are identified by numbers preceded by a U (see Fig. 11.10).

Exons frequently code for separate functional or structural domains of proteins. Proteins with similar functional regions (e.g., ATP- or NAD-binding regions) frequently have similar domains, although their overall structure and amino acid

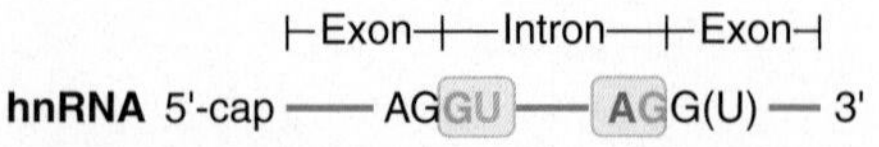

├─Exon─┤├──Intron──┤├─Exon─┤

**hnRNA** 5′-cap ── AG GU ── AG G(U) ── 3′

*FIG. 11.9.* Splice junctions in hnRNA. The intron sequences shown in the boxes are invariant. They always appear at this position in introns. The sequences on the exon side of the splice sites are more variable.

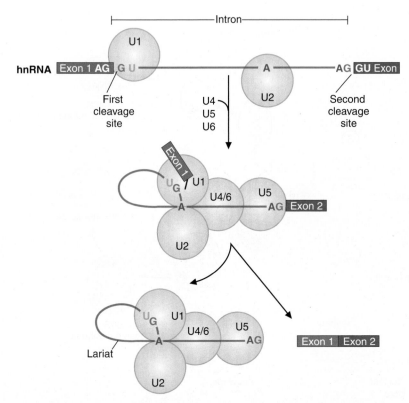

**FIG. 11.10.** Splicing process. Nuclear ribonucleoproteins (snurps U1 to U6) bind to the intron, causing it to form a loop. The complex is called a spliceosome. The U1 snurp binds near the first exon/intron junction, and U2 binds within the intron in a region containing an adenine nucleotide residue. Another group of snurps, U4, U5, and U6, binds to the complex and the loop is formed. The phosphate attached to the G residue at the 5′ end of the intron forms a 2′ to 5′ linkage with the 2′ hydroxyl group of the adenine nucleotide residue. Cleavage occurs at the end of the first exon, between the AG residues at the 3′ end of the exon and the GU residues at the 5′ end of the intron. The complex continues to be held in place by the spliceosome. A second cleavage occurs at the 3′ end of the intron after the AG sequence. The exons are joined together. The intron, shaped like a lariat, is released and degraded to nucleotides.

sequence is quite different. A process known as **exon shuffling** has probably occurred throughout evolution, allowing new proteins to develop with functions similar to those of other proteins.

## B. Synthesis of Eukaryotic rRNA

Ribosomal RNAs (rRNAs) form the ribonucleoprotein complexes on which protein synthesis occurs. In eukaryotes, the rRNA gene exists as many copies in the nucleolar organizer region of the nucleus (Fig. 11.11, *circle 1*). Each gene produces a large, 45S transcript (synthesized by RNA polymerase I) that is cleaved to produce the 18S, 28S, and 5.8S rRNAs. About 1,000 copies of this gene are present in the human genome. The genes are linked in tandem, separated by spacer regions that contain the termination signal for one gene and the promoter for the next. Promoters for rRNA genes are located in the 5′ flanking region of the genes and extend into the region surrounding the start point. rRNA genes caught in the act of transcription by electron micrographs show that many RNA polymerase I molecules can be attached to a gene at any given time, all moving toward the 3′ end as the 45S rRNA precursors are synthesized.

As the 45S rRNA precursors are released from the DNA, they complex with proteins, forming ribonucleoprotein particles that generate the granular regions of the nucleolus (see Fig. 11.11, *circle 2*). Processing of the transcript occurs in the

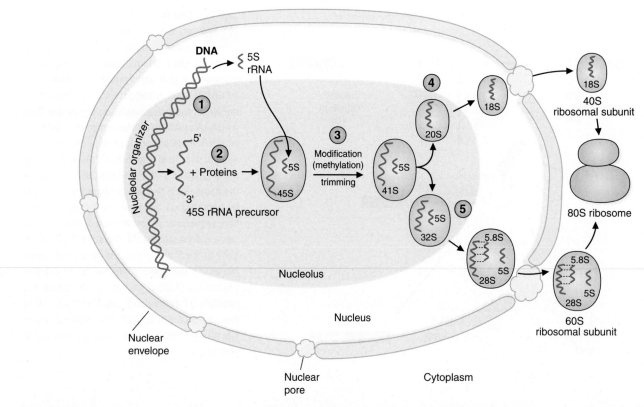

**FIG. 11.11.** rRNA and ribosome synthesis. The 5S rRNA is transcribed in the nucleoplasm and moves into the nucleolus. The other rRNAs are transcribed from DNA and mature in the nucleolus, forming the 40S and 60S ribosomal subunits, which migrate to the cytoplasm. See the text for a detailed explanation.

granular regions. 5S rRNA, produced by RNA polymerase III from genes located outside the nucleolus in the nucleoplasm, migrates into the nucleolus and joins the ribonucleoprotein particles.

One to two percent of the nucleotides of the 45S precursor become methylated, primarily on the 2′ hydroxyl groups of ribose moieties (see Fig. 11.11, *circle 3*). These methyl groups may serve as markers for cleavage of the 45S precursors and are conserved in the mature rRNA. A series of cleavages in the 45S transcripts occur to produce the mature rRNAs.

In the production of cytoplasmic ribosomes in human cells, one portion of the 45S rRNA precursor becomes the 18S rRNA that, complexed with proteins, forms the small 40S ribosomal subunit (see Fig. 11.11, *circle 4*). Another segment of the precursor folds back on itself and is cleaved, forming 28S rRNA, hydrogen-bonded to the 5.8S rRNA. The 5S rRNA, transcribed from nonnucleolar genes, and several proteins complex with the 28S and 5.8S rRNAs to form the 60S ribosomal subunit (see Fig. 11.11, *circle 5*). The ribosomal subunits migrate through the nuclear pores. In the cytoplasm, the 40S and 60S ribosomal subunits interact with mRNA, forming the 80S ribosomes on which protein synthesis occurs.

## C. Synthesis of Eukaryotic tRNA

A transfer RNA has one binding site for a specific sequence of three nucleotides in mRNA (the anticodon site) and another binding site for the encoded amino acid. Thus, tRNAs ensure that the genetic code is translated into the correct sequence of amino acids. At least 20 types of tRNAs occur in cells, one for every amino acid that is incorporated into growing polypeptide chains during the synthesis of proteins. tRNAs have a cloverleaf structure that folds into a three-dimensional L shape and contains a number of bases, which are modified posttranscriptionally

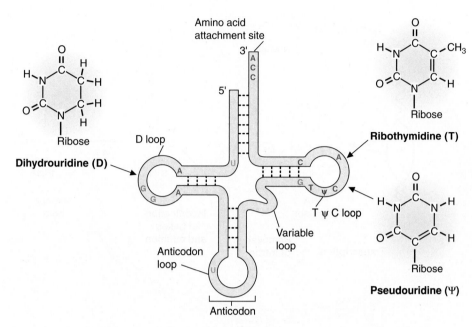

*FIG. 11.12.* The tRNA cloverleaf. Bases that commonly occur in a particular position are indicated by letters. Base pairing in stem regions is indicated by lines between the strands. The locations of the modified bases dihydrouridine (D), ribothymidine (T), and pseudouridine (ψ) are indicated.

(Fig. 11.12). The loop closest to the 5′ end is known as the **D-loop** because it contains dihydrouridine (D). The second, or **anticodon loop**, contains the trinucleotide anticodon that base-pairs with the codon on mRNA. The third loop (the **TΨC loop**) contains both ribothymidine (T) and pseudouridine (Ψ). A fourth loop, known as the **variable loop** because it varies in size, is frequently found between the anticodon and TΨC loops. Base pairing occurs in the stem regions of tRNA and a three-nucleotide sequence (e.g., CCA) at the 3′ end is the attachment site for the specific amino acid carried by each tRNA. Different tRNAs bind different amino acids.

tRNA precursors of about 100 nucleotides in length are generated (Fig. 11.13, *circle 1*) by transcription of the gene by RNA polymerase III. The pre-tRNA assumes a cloverleaf shape and is subsequently cleaved at the 5′ and 3′ ends (see Fig. 11.13, *circle 2*). The enzyme that acts at the 5′ end is RNase P, similar to the RNase P of bacteria. Both enzymes contain a small RNA (M1) that has catalytic activity and serves as an endonuclease. Some tRNA precursors contain introns that are removed by endonucleases. To close the opening, a 2′ or 3′ phosphate group from one end is ligated to a 5′ hydroxyl on the other end by an RNA ligase.

The bases are modified at the same time the endonucleolytic cleavage reactions are occurring (see Fig. 11.13, *circles 2* and *3*). Three modifications occur in most tRNAs: (a) uracil is methylated by *S*-adenosylmethionine (SAM) to form thymine, (b) one of the double bonds of uracil is reduced to form dihydrouracil, and (c) a uracil residue (attached to ribose by an *N*-glycosidic bond) is rotated to form pseudouridine, which contains uracil linked to ribose by a carbon–carbon bond (see Fig. 11.12). Other less common but more complex modifications also occur and involve bases other than uracil. Of particular note is the deamination of adenosine to form the base inosine.

The final step in forming the mature tRNA is the addition of a CCA sequence at its 3′ end (see Fig 11.13, *circle 3*). These nucleotides are added one at a time by nucleotidyltransferase. The tRNA then migrates to the cytoplasm. The terminal

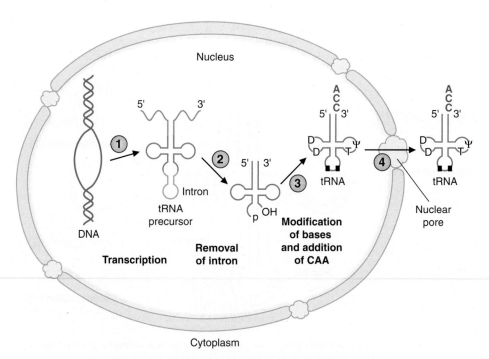

**FIG. 11.13.** Overview of tRNA synthesis. D, T, Ψ, and ■ indicate modified bases. D, dihydrouracil; T, ribothymine; ψ, pseudouridine; ■, other modified bases.

adenosine at the 3' end is the site where the specific amino acid for each tRNA is bound and activated for incorporation into a protein.

## V. DIFFERENCES IN SIZE BETWEEN EUKARYOTIC AND PROKARYOTIC DNA

### A. Diploid versus Haploid

Except for the germ cells, most normal human cells are diploid. Therefore, they contain two copies of each chromosome, and each chromosome contains genes that are alleles of the genes on the homologous chromosome. Since one chromosome in each set of homologous chromosomes is obtained from each parent, the alleles can be identical, containing the same DNA sequence, or they can differ. A diploid human cell contains 2,000 times more DNA than the genome of the bacterium in the haploid *E. coli* cell (about $4 \times 10^6$ base pairs).

### B. Introns

Eukaryotic introns contribute to the DNA size difference between bacteria and human cells. In eukaryotic genes, introns (noncoding regions) occur within sequences that code for proteins. Consequently, the primary transcript (heterogeneous nuclear RNA or hnRNA) averages about 10 times longer than the mature mRNA produced by removal of the introns. In contrast, bacterial genes do not contain introns.

### C. Repetitive Sequences in Eukaryotic DNA

Although being diploid, and containing introns account for some of the difference between the DNA content of humans and bacteria, a large difference remains that is related to the greater complexity of the human organism. Bacterial cells have a single copy of each gene, called **unique DNA**, and they contain very little DNA that does not produce functional products. Eukaryotic cells contain substantial amounts of DNA that does not code for functional products (i.e., proteins or rRNA and

**Q:** Calculate the number of different proteins, 300 amino acids in length, which could be produced from the *E. coli* genome ($4 \times 10^6$ base pairs of DNA).

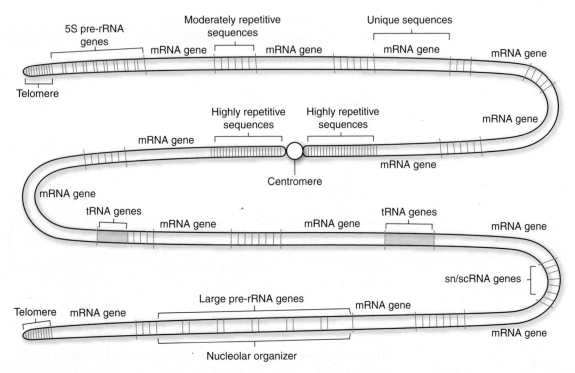

*FIG. 11.14.* Distribution of unique, moderately repetitive, and highly repetitive sequences in a hypothetical human chromosome. Unique genes encode mRNA. These genes occur in single copies. The genes for the large rRNA and the tRNA precursors occur in multiple copies that are clustered in the genome. The large rRNA genes form the nucleolar organizer. Moderately repetitive sequences are dispersed throughout the genome, and highly repetitive sequences are clustered around the centromere and at the ends of the chromosome (the telomeres). Small nuclear RNA (snRNA) and small cytoplasmic RNA (scRNA) are usually found in ribonucleoprotein particles. (From Wolfe SL. *Mol Cell Biol* 1993:761.)

tRNA). In addition, some genes that encode functional products are present in multiple copies, called **highly repetitive** or **moderately repetitive DNA**. About 64% of the DNA in the human genome is unique, consisting of DNA sequences present in one or a very few copies in the genome (Fig. 11.14). Some of the unique DNA sequences are transcribed to generate mRNA, which is translated to produce proteins.

Highly repetitive DNA consists of sequences about 6 to 100 base pairs in length that are present in hundreds of thousands to millions of copies, clustered within a few locations in the genome (see Fig. 11.14). It occurs in centromeres (which join sister chromatids during mitosis) and in telomeres (the ends of chromosomes). This DNA represents about 10% of the human genome. It is not transcribed.

Moderately repetitive DNA is present in a few to tens of thousands of copies in the genome (see Fig. 11.14). This fraction constitutes about 25% of the human genome. It contains DNA that is functional and transcribed to produce rRNA, tRNA, and also some mRNA. The histone genes, present in a few hundred copies in the genome, belong to this class. Moderately repetitive DNA also includes some gene sequences that are functional but not transcribed. Promoters and enhancers (which are involved in regulating gene expression) are examples of gene sequences in this category. Other groups of moderately repetitive gene sequences that have been found in human are called the **Alu sequences** (about 300 base pairs in length). Alu sequences are also examples of short interspersed elements (SINEs). The long interspersed elements (LINE) sequences are 6,000 to 7,000 base pairs in length. The function of the Alu and LINE sequences has not been determined.

Major differences between prokaryotic and eukaryotic DNA and RNA are summarized in Table 11.1.

**A:** Four million base pairs contain $4 \times 10^6/3$ or 1.33 million codons. If each protein contained about 300 amino acids, *E. coli* could produce about 4,000 different proteins ($1.33 \times 10^6/300$).

**Table 11.1   Differences Between Eukaryotes and Prokaryotes**

| | Eukaryotes (Human) | Prokaryotes (E. coli) |
|---|---|---|
| Nucleus | Yes | No |
| Chromosomes | | |
|    Number | 23 per haploid cell | 1 per haploid cell |
|    DNA | Linear | Circular |
|    Histones | Yes | No |
| Genome | | |
|    Diploid | Somatic cells | No |
|    Haploid | Germ cells | All cells |
|    Size | $3 \times 10^9$ base pairs per haploid cell | $4 \times 10^6$ base pairs |
| Genes | | |
|    Unique | 64% | 100% |
|    Repetitive | | |
|    Moderately | 25% | None |
|    Highly | 10% | None |
| Operons | No | Yes |
| mRNA | | |
|    Polycistronic | No | Yes |
|    Introns (hnRNA) | Yes | No |
| Translation | Separate from transcription | Coupled with transcription |

## CLINICAL COMMENTS

The diseases discussed in this chapter are summarized in Table 11.2.

 The mutations that cause the thalassemias affect the synthesis of either the α- or the β-chain of adult hemoglobin, causing an anemia. They are classified by the chain affected (α- or β-chain) and by the amount of chain synthesized (0 for no synthesis and + for synthesis of some functional chains). They are also classified as major, intermediate, or minor, according to the severity of the clinical disorder. β-Thalassemia major (also called homozygous β-thalassemia) is a clinically severe disorder requiring frequent blood transfusions. It is caused by the inheritance of two alleles for a severe mutation. In β-thalassemia intermedia, the patient exhibits a less severe clinical phenotype and is able to maintain hemoglobin levels above 6 g/dL. It is usually the result of two different mild mutations or homozygosity for a mild mutation. β-Thalassemia minor (also known as β-thalassemia trait) is a heterozygous disorder involving a single mutation that is often clinically asymptomatic.

During embryonic and fetal life, the β-chain is replaced by the ε-and γ-chains, respectively. As a result, patients with severe mutations in the α-chain tend to die in utero, while those with mutations in the β-chains exhibit symptoms postnatally as hemoglobin F ($\alpha_2\gamma_2$) is normally replaced with adult hemoglobin A ($\alpha_2\beta_2$) after birth.

**Lisa N.** Patients with $\beta^+$-thalassemia who maintain their hemoglobin levels above 6.0 to 7.0 g/dL are usually classified as having thalassemia intermedia. In the β-thalassemias, the α-chains of adult hemoglobin A ($\alpha_2\beta_2$) continue to be synthesized at a normal rate. These chains accumulate in the bone marrow in which the red blood cells are synthesized during the process of erythropoiesis (generation of red blood cells). The accumulation of α-chains diminishes erythropoiesis, resulting in an anemia. Individuals who are homozygous for a severe mutation require constant transfusions.

Individuals with thalassemia intermedia, such as **Lisa N.**, could have inherited two different defective alleles, one from each parent. One parent may be a "silent" carrier, with one normal allele and one mildly affected allele. This parent produces enough functional β-globin so few or no clinical symptoms of thalassemia appear. (However, they generally have a somewhat decreased amount of hemoglobin, resulting in microcytic hypochromic red blood cells.) When this parent contributes the mildly defective allele and the other heterozygous parent contributes a more severely defective allele, thalassemia intermedia occurs in the child. The child is thus heterozygous for two different defective alleles.

**Table 11.2   Diseases Discussed in Chapter 11**

| Disorder or Condition | Genetic or Environmental | Comments |
|---|---|---|
| β-Thalassemia | Genetic | An anemia due to an imbalance in β- and α-globin chain synthesis. For a β-thalassemia, more α-chain is synthesized than functional β-chain. |
| Tuberculosis, a complication of AIDS | Environmental | The drug rifampin, amongst others, is used to treat tuberculosis via inhibition of bacterial RNA polymerase. |
| Mushroom poisoning (α-amanitin poisoning) | Environmental | Inhibition of RNA polymerase II by α-amanitin. There is no effective antidote for this poison. |
| Systemic lupus erythematosus (SLE) | Both | The development of autoantibodies directed against various cellular proteins, including those involved in RNA processing (such as complexes involved in RNA splicing, the snRNPs). |

**Isabel S.** Isabel S. was treated with a multidrug regimen for tuberculosis because the microbes that cause the disease frequently become resistant to the individual drugs. As with patients with a normal immune system, the current approach in patients with AIDS who develop opportunistic infection with *Mycobacterium tuberculosis* is to initiate antimycobacterial therapy with four agents because the mycobacteria frequently become resistant to one or more of the particular antitubercular drugs. **Isabel S.** was started on isoniazid (INH), rifampin, pyrazinamide, and ethambutol. INH inhibits the biosynthesis of mycolic acids, which are important constituents of the mycobacterial cell wall. Rifampin binds to and inhibits bacterial RNA polymerase, which selectively kills the bacteria that cause the infection. Pyrazinamide, a synthetic analogue of nicotinamide, targets the mycobacterial fatty acid synthase I gene involved in mycolic acid biosynthesis in *M. tuberculosis*. Ethambutol blocks arabinosyl transferases that are involved in cell wall biosynthesis.

Just as bacteria can become resistant to drugs, so can HIV. Because of this concern, patients with HIV are no longer treated with a single-drug regimen. Multidrug regimens usually include two nucleoside reverse transcriptase inhibitors (NRTIs), such as dideoxyinosine (didanosine, formerly called ddI) and dideoxycytidine (zalcitabine, formerly called ddC), as well as nonnucleoside reverse transcriptase inhibitors (NNRTIs) (e.g., efavirenz) or protease inhibitors (PIs) (e.g., indinavir). PIs prevent the HIV polyprotein from being cleaved into its mature products. (When the HIV mRNA is translated, a polyprotein is formed, which must be cleaved by HIV protease in order to form the mature proteins needed for the assembly of the virus. An inability to cleave the proprotein will block viral maturation and further infection of other cells.) There are also integrase strand transfer inhibitors (INSTIs), which block integration of the viral genome into the host genome, and entry inhibitors (EIs), which block viral entry into target cells.

**Isabel S.** was started on efavirenz (an NNRTI) as her third drug and was counseled on not getting pregnant because the drug is teratogenic.

**Sarah L.** Systemic lupus erythematosus (SLE) is a multisystem disease of unknown origin characterized by inflammation related to the presence of autoantibodies in the blood. These autoantibodies react with antigens normally found in the nucleus, cytoplasm, and plasma membrane of the cell. Such "self" antigen–antibody (autoimmune) interactions initiate an inflammatory cascade that produces the broad symptom profile of multiorgan dysfunction found in **Sarah L**.

Pharmacological therapy for SLE involves anti-inflammatory drugs and immunosuppressive agents. It can include nonsteroidal anti-inflammatory drugs (NSAIDs), corticosteroids, antimalarials, or several newer agents that cause immunosuppression. Plaquenil is an antimalarial drug used to treat skin and joint symptoms in SLE, although its exact mechanism of action in these patients is not fully understood. **Sarah** was placed on such a drug regimen.

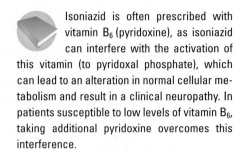

Isoniazid is often prescribed with vitamin B$_6$ (pyridoxine), as isoniazid can interfere with the activation of this vitamin (to pyridoxal phosphate), which can lead to an alteration in normal cellular metabolism and result in a clinical neuropathy. In patients susceptible to low levels of vitamin B$_6$, taking additional pyridoxine overcomes this interference.

Studies have indicated that a failure to properly dispose of cellular debris, a normal byproduct of cell death, may lead to the induction of autoantibodies directed against chromatin in patients with SLE. Normal cells have a finite lifetime and are programmed to die (apoptosis) through a distinct biochemical mechanism. One of the steps in this mechanism is the stepwise degradation of cellular DNA (and other cellular components). If the normal intracellular components are exposed to the immune system, autoantibodies against them may be generated. The enzyme in cells that degrades DNA is deoxyribonuclease I (DNase I), and individuals with SLE have reduced serum activity levels of DNase I, compared to individuals who do not have the disease. Through an understanding of the molecular mechanism whereby autoantibodies are generated, it may be possible to develop therapies to combat this disorder.

## REVIEW QUESTIONS–CHAPTER 11

1. The short transcript AUCCGUACG would be derived from which one of the following template DNA sequences? (Note all sequences are written from 5′ to 3′.)

    A. ATCCGTACG
    B. AUCCGUACG
    C. TAGGCATGC
    D. GCATGCCTA
    E. CGTACGGAT

2. Which one of the following eukaryotic DNA control sequences does not need to be in a fixed location and is most responsible for high rates of transcription of particular genes?

    A. Promoter
    B. Enhancer
    C. Promoter-proximal elements
    D. Operator
    E. Splice donor site

3. Which one of the following is true of both eukaryotic and prokaryotic gene expression?

    A. Translation of mRNA can begin before transcription is complete.
    B. mRNA is synthesized in the 3′ to 5′ direction.
    C. RNA polymerase binds at a promoter region upstream of the gene.
    D. After transcription, a 3′ poly(A) tail and a 5′ cap are added to mRNA.
    E. Mature mRNA is always precisely colinear to the gene from which it was transcribed.

4. In a segment of a transcribed gene, the nontemplate strand of DNA has the following sequence:

    5′...AGCTCACTG...3′

    What will be the corresponding sequence in the RNA produced from this segment of the gene?

    A. AGCUCACUG
    B. CAGUGAGCU
    C. CAGTGAGCT
    D. UCGAGUGAC
    E. GTCACTCGA

5. A single nucleotide mutation in a promoter-proximal element led to increased expression of an associated eukaryotic gene. This effect is best explained by which one of the following?

    A. A more efficient splice site recognition
    B. Less energy required to melt the helix at this location
    C. Beneficial amino acid replacement derived from the missense mutation
    D. Increased amount of sigma factor binding
    E. Additional opportunity for hydrogen-bonding to a *trans* acting factor

# 12 Translation: Synthesis of Proteins

## CHAPTER OUTLINE

## KEY POINTS

- Translation is the process of translating the sequence of nucleotides in mRNA to an amino acid sequence of a protein.
- Translation proceeds from the amino to carboxy terminal, reading the mRNA in the 5′ to 3′ direction.
- Protein synthesis occurs on ribosomes.
- The mRNA is read in codons, sets of three nucleotides that specify individual amino acids.
- AUG, which specifies methionine, is the start codon for all protein synthesis.
- Specific stop codons (UAG, UGA, and UAA) signal when the translation of the mRNA is to end.
- Amino acids are covalently linked to tRNA by the enzyme aminoacyl-tRNA synthetase, creating charged tRNA.
- Charged tRNAs base-pair with the codon via the anticodon region of the tRNA.
- Protein synthesis is divided into three stages: initiation, elongation, and termination.
- Multiprotein factors are required for each stage of protein synthesis.
- Proteins fold as they are synthesized.
- Specific amino acid side chains may be modified after translation in a process known as posttranslational modification.
- Mechanisms within eukaryotic cells specifically target newly synthesized proteins to different compartments in the cell.

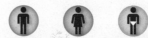

# THE WAITING ROOM

**Lisa N.**, a 4-year-old patient with $\beta^+$-thalassemia intermedia (see Chapter 11), showed no improvement in her symptoms at her second visit. Her hemoglobin level was 7.3 g/dL (reference range for females = 12 to 16 g/dL).

**Jay S.** is a 9-month-old male infant of Ashkenazi Jewish parentage. His growth and development were normal until age 5 months when he began to exhibit mild, generalized muscle weakness. By 7 months, he had poor head control, slowed development of motor skills, and was increasingly inattentive to his surroundings. His parents also noted unusual eye movements and staring episodes. On careful examination of his retinae, his pediatrician observed a "cherry red" spot within a pale macula. The physician suspected Tay-Sachs disease and, after confirming the disease by measuring $\beta$-hexosaminidase A and B activity, sent whole blood samples to the molecular biology–genetics laboratory. The results of molecular genetic tests indicated that **Jay S.** has an insertion in exon 11 of the $\beta$-chain of the hexosaminidase A gene, the most common mutation found in patients of Ashkenazi Jewish background who have Tay-Sachs disease.

## I.    THE GENETIC CODE

**Transcription**, the transfer of the genetic message from DNA to RNA, and **translation**, the transfer of the genetic message from the nucleotide language of nucleic acids to the amino acid language of proteins, both depend on base pairing. In the late 1950s and early 1960s, molecular biologists attempting to decipher the process of translation recognized two problems. The first involved decoding the relationship between the language of the nucleic acids and the language of the proteins, and the second involved determining the molecular mechanism by which translation between these two languages occurs.

Twenty different amino acids are commonly incorporated into proteins and, therefore, the protein alphabet has 20 characters. The nucleic acid alphabet, however, has only four characters, corresponding to the four nucleotides of mRNA (A, G, C, and U). If two nucleotides constituted the code for an amino acid, then only $4^2$, or 16, amino acids could be specified. Therefore, the number of nucleotides that code for an amino acid has to be three, providing $4^3$ or 64 possible combinations or **codons**, more than required but not excessive.

Scientists set out to determine the specific codons for each amino acid. In 1961, Marshall Nirenberg produced the first crack in the genetic code (the collection of codons that specify all the amino acids found in proteins). He showed that poly(U), a polynucleotide in which all the bases are uracil, produced polyphenylalanine in a cell-free protein-synthesizing system. Thus, UUU must be the codon for phenylalanine. As a result of experiments using synthetic polynucleotides in place of mRNA, other codons were identified.

The pioneering molecular biologists recognized that because amino acids cannot bind directly to the sets of three nucleotides that form their codons, adapters are required. The adapters were found to be **transfer RNA (tRNA)** molecules. Each tRNA molecule contains an **anticodon** and covalently binds a specific amino acid at its 3' end (see Chapters 9 and 11). The anticodon of a tRNA molecule is a set of three nucleotides that can interact with a codon on **messenger RNA (mRNA)** (Fig. 12.1). In order to interact, the codon and anticodon must be complementary (i.e., they must be able to form base pairs in an antiparallel orientation). Thus, the

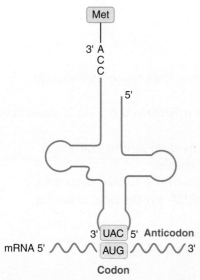

**FIG. 12.1.** Binding of tRNA to a codon on mRNA. The tRNA contains an amino acid at its 3' end that corresponds to the codon on mRNA with which the anticodon of the tRNA can base-pair. Note that the codon-anticodon pairing is complementary and antiparallel.

**Table 12.1  The Genetic Code**

| First Base | Second Base | | | | Third Base |
|---|---|---|---|---|---|
| (5') | U | C | A | G | (3') |
| U | Phe | Ser | Tyr | Cys | U |
|  | Phe | Ser | Tyr | Cys | C |
|  | Leu | Ser | Stop | Stop | A |
|  | Leu | Ser | Stop | Trp | G |
| C | Leu | Pro | His | Arg | U |
|  | Leu | Pro | His | Arg | C |
|  | Leu | Pro | Gln | Arg | A |
|  | Leu | Pro | Gln | Arg | G |
| A | Ile | Thr | Asn | Ser | U |
|  | Ile | Thr | Asn | Ser | C |
|  | Ile | Thr | Lys | Arg | A |
|  | Met | Thr | Lys | Arg | G |
| G | Val | Ala | Asp | Gly | U |
|  | Val | Ala | Asp | Gly | C |
|  | Val | Ala | Glu | Gly | A |
|  | Val | Ala | Glu | Gly | G |

anticodon of a tRNA serves as the link between an mRNA codon and the amino acid that the codon specifies.

Obviously, each codon present within mRNA must correspond to a specific amino acid. Nirenberg found that trinucleotides of known base sequence could bind to ribosomes and induce the binding of specific aminoacyl-tRNAs (i.e., tRNAs with amino acids covalently attached). As a result of these and the earlier experiments, the relationship between all 64 codons and the amino acids they specify (the entire genetic code) was determined by the mid-1960s (Table 12.1).

Three of the 64 possible codons (UGA, UAG, and UAA) terminate protein synthesis and are known as **stop** or **nonsense codons**. The remaining 61 codons specify amino acids. Two amino acids each have only one codon (AUG for methionine; UGG for tryptophan). The remaining amino acids have multiple codons.

## A.  The Code Is Degenerate yet Unambiguous

Because many amino acids are specified by more than one codon, the genetic code is described as degenerate, which means that an amino acid may have more than one codon. However, each codon specifies only one amino acid and the genetic code is thus unambiguous.

Inspection of a codon table shows that in most instances of multiple codons for a single amino acid, the variation occurs in the third base of the codon (see Table 12.1). Crick noted that the pairing between the 3' base of the codon and the 5' base of the anticodon does not always follow the strict base-pairing rules that he and Watson had previously discovered (i.e., A pairs with U and G with C). This observation resulted in the wobble hypothesis.

At the third base of the codon (the 3' position of the codon and the 5' position of the anticodon), the base pairs can wobble. For example, G can pair with U; and A, G, or U can pair with the unusual base hypoxanthine (I) found in tRNA. Thus, three of the four codons for alanine (GCU, GCC, and GCA) can pair with a single tRNA that contains the anticodon 5'-IGC-3' (Fig. 12.2). If each of the 61 codons for amino acids required a distinct tRNA, cells would contain 61 tRNAs. However, because of wobble between the codon and anticodon, fewer than 61 tRNAs are required to translate the genetic code.

All organisms studied so far use the same genetic code, with some rare exceptions. One exception occurs in human mitochondrial mRNA, where UGA codes for tryptophan instead of serving as a stop codon, AUA codes for methionine instead of isoleucine, and CUA codes for threonine instead of leucine.

Hypoxanthine is the base attached to ribose in the nucleoside inosine. The single-letter abbreviation for hypoxanthine is I, in reference to the nucleoside inosine. (In other cases, the first letter of the base is also the first letter of the nucleoside and the single-letter abbreviation. For example, A is the base adenine and the nucleoside adenosine.)

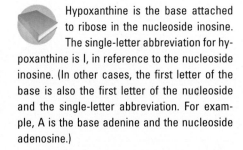

**A. Codons for alanine**

5' — G  C  U — 3'
      G  C  C
      G  C  A
      G  C  G

**B. Base pairing of three alanine codons with anticodon IGC**

```
                U
5' — G  C  C — 3'   Codon
            A       on mRNA
     :  :  :
3' — C  G  I — 5'   Anticodon
                    on tRNA
```

**FIG. 12.2.**  Base pairing of codons for alanine with 5'-IGC-3'. **A.** The variation is in the third base. **B.** The first three of these codons can pair with a tRNA that contains the anticodon 5'-IGC-3'. Hypoxanthine (I) is an unusual base found in tRNA that can form base pairs with U, C, or A. It is formed by the deamination of adenine. Hypoxanthine is the base attached to ribose in the nucleoside inosine.

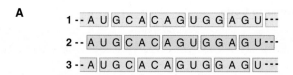

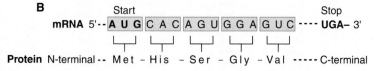

*FIG. 12.3.* Reading frame of mRNA. **A.** For any given mRNA sequence, there are three possible reading frames (1, 2, and 3). **B.** An AUG near the 5′ end of the mRNA (the start codon) sets the reading frame for translation of a protein from the mRNA. The codons are read in linear order, starting with this AUG. (The other potential reading frames are not used. They would give proteins with different amino acid sequences.)

### B. The Code Is Nonoverlapping

mRNA does not contain "extra nucleotides," or punctuation, to separate one codon from the next, and the codons do not overlap. Each nucleotide is read only once. Beginning with a start codon (AUG) near the 5′ end of the mRNA, the codons are read sequentially, ending with a stop codon (UGA, UAG, or UAA) near the 3′ end of the mRNA.

### C. Relationship Between mRNA and the Protein Product

The start codon (AUG) sets the reading frame, the order in which the sequence of bases in the mRNA is sorted into codons (Fig. 12.3). The order of the codons in the mRNA determines the sequence in which amino acids are added to the growing polypeptide chain. Thus, the order of the codons in the mRNA determines the linear sequence of amino acids in the protein.

## II. EFFECTS OF MUTATIONS

Mutations that result from damage to the nucleotides of DNA molecules or from unrepaired errors during replication (see Chapter 10) can be transcribed into mRNA and therefore can result in the translation of a protein with an abnormal amino acid sequence. Various types of mutations can occur that have different effects on the encoded protein (Table 12.2).

### A. Point Mutations

**Point mutations** occur when only one base in DNA is altered, producing a change in a single base of an mRNA codon. There are three basic types of point mutations: silent mutations, missense mutations, and nonsense mutations. Point mutations are said to be "silent" when they do not affect the amino acid sequence of the protein. For example, a codon change from CGA to CGG does not affect the protein because both of these codons specify arginine (see Table 12.1). In missense mutations, one amino acid in the protein is replaced by a different amino acid. For example, a change from CGA to CCA causes arginine to be replaced by proline. A nonsense

Sickle cell anemia is caused by a missense mutation. In each of the alleles for β-globin, **Will S.**'s DNA has a single base change (see Chapter 5). In the sickle cell gene, GTG replaces the normal GAG. Thus, in the mRNA, the codon GUG replaces GAG and a valine residue replaces a glutamate residue in the protein. The amino acid change is indicated as E6V; the normal glutamate (E) at position 6 of the β-chain has been replaced by valine (V).

**Table 12.2 Types of Mutations**

| Type | Description | Example |
|---|---|---|
| Point | A single base change | |
| Silent | A change that specifies the same amino acid | CGA → CGG Arg → Arg |
| Missense | A change that specifies a different amino acid | CGA → CCA Arg → Pro |
| Nonsense | A change that produces a stop codon | CGA → UGA Arg → Stop |
| Insertion | An addition of one or more bases | |
| Deletion | A loss of one or more bases | |

mutation causes the premature termination of a polypeptide chain. For example, a codon change from **CGA** to **UGA** causes a codon for arginine to be replaced by a stop codon, and synthesis of the mutant protein terminates at this point.

### B. Insertions, Deletions, and Frameshift Mutations

An **insertion** occurs when one or more nucleotides are added to DNA. If the insertion does not generate a stop codon, a protein with more amino acids than normal could be produced.

When one or more nucleotides are removed from DNA, the mutation is known as a **deletion**. If the deletion does not affect the normal start and stop codons, a protein with fewer than the normal number of amino acids could be produced.

A **frameshift mutation** occurs when the number of inserted or deleted nucleotides is not a multiple of three (Fig. 12.4). The reading frame shifts at the point where the insertion or deletion begins. Beyond that point, the amino acid sequence of the protein translated from the mRNA differs from the normal protein.

### III. FORMATION OF AMINOACYL-tRNA

tRNA that contains an amino acid covalently attached to its 3′ end is called an **aminoacyl-tRNA** and is said to be charged. Aminoacyl-tRNAs are named both for the amino acid and the tRNA that carries the amino acid. For example, the tRNA for alanine (tRNA$^{Ala}$) acquires alanine to become alanyl-tRNA$^{Ala}$. A particular tRNA recognizes only the AUG start codon that initiates protein synthesis and not other AUG codons that specify insertion of methionine within the polypeptide chain. This initiator methionyl-tRNA$^{Met}$ is denoted by the subscript "i" in methionyl-tRNA$_i^{Met}$.

Amino acids are attached to their tRNAs by highly specific enzymes known as aminoacyl-tRNA synthetases. Twenty different synthetases exist, one for each amino acid. Each synthetase recognizes a particular amino acid and all of the tRNAs that carry that amino acid.

The formation of the ester bond that links the amino acid to the tRNA by an aminoacyl-tRNA synthetase is an energy-requiring process that occurs in two steps. The amino acid is activated in the first step when its carboxyl group reacts with adenosine triphosphate (ATP) to form an enzyme-aminoacyl-adenosine monophosphate (AMP) complex and pyrophosphate (Fig. 12.5). The cleavage of a high-energy bond of ATP in this reaction provides energy, and the subsequent cleavage of pyrophosphate by a pyrophosphatase helps to drive the reaction by removing one of the products. In the second step, the activated amino acid is transferred to the 2′ or 3′ hydroxyl group (depending on the type of aminoacyl-tRNA synthetase catalyzing the reaction) of the ribose connected to the 3′ terminal A residue of the tRNA, and AMP is released (recall that all tRNAs have a CCA added to their 3′ end posttranscriptionally). The energy in the aminoacyl-tRNA ester bond is subsequently used in the formation of a peptide bond during the process of protein synthesis. The aminoacyl tRNA synthetase provides the first error-checking step in preserving the fidelity of translation. The enzymes check their work, and if the incorrect amino acid

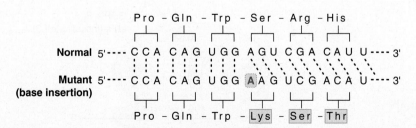

**FIG. 12.4.** A frameshift mutation. The insertion of a single nucleotide (the *A* in the *dotted red box*) causes the reading frame to shift so that the amino acid sequence of the protein translated from the mRNA is different after the point of insertion. A similar effect can result from the insertion or deletion of nucleotides if the number inserted or deleted is not a multiple of three.

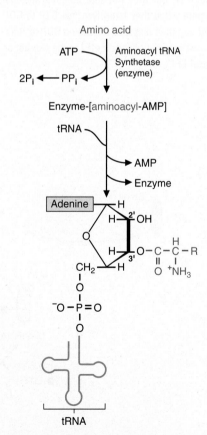

**FIG. 12.5.** Formation of aminoacyl-tRNA. The amino acid is first activated by reacting with ATP. The amino acid is then transferred from the aminoacyl-AMP to tRNA.

**A:** A nonsense mutation at codon 17 would cause premature termination of translation. A nonfunctional peptide containing only 16 amino acids would result, producing a $\beta^0$-thalassemia if the mutation occurred in both alleles. A large deletion in the coding region of the gene could also produce a truncated protein. If **Lisa N.** has a nonsense mutation or a large deletion, it could only be in one allele. The mutation in the other allele must be milder because she produces some normal $\beta$-globin. Her hemoglobin is 7 g/dL, typical of thalassemia intermedia (a $\beta^+$-thalassemia).

has been linked to a particular tRNA, the enzyme will remove the amino acid from the tRNA and try again using the correct amino acid.

Some aminoacyl-tRNA synthetases use the anticodon of the tRNA as a recognition site as they attach the amino acid to the hydroxyl group at the 3′ end of the tRNA. However, other synthetases do not use the anticodon but recognize only bases located at other positions in the tRNA. Nevertheless, insertion of the amino acid into a growing polypeptide chain depends solely on the bases of the anticodon, through complementary base pairing with the mRNA codon.

## IV. PROCESS OF TRANSLATION

Translation of a protein involves three steps: **initiation, elongation,** and **termination**. It begins with the formation of the initiation complex. Subsequently, synthesis of the polypeptide occurs by a series of elongation steps that are repeated as each amino acid is added to the growing chain. Termination occurs where the mRNA contains an in-frame stop codon and the completed polypeptide chain is released.

### A. Initiation of Translation

In eukaryotes, initiation of translation involves formation of an **initiation complex** composed of methionyl-tRNA$_i^{Met}$, mRNA, and a ribosome (Fig. 12.6). Methionyl-tRNA$_i^{Met}$ (also known as Met-tRNA$_i^{Met}$) initially forms a complex with the protein eukaryotic initiation factor 2 (eIF2), which binds guanosine triphosphate (GTP). This complex then binds to the small (40S) ribosomal subunit with the participation of eukaryotic initiation factor 3 (eIF3). The cap at the 5′ end of the mRNA binds to components of the eIF4 complex, known as the cap-binding complex. The mRNA, in association with the cap-binding complex, then binds to the eIFs-Met-tRNA$_i^{Met}$ −40S ribosome complex. In a reaction that requires ATP hydrolysis (due to the helicase activity of an eIF subunit), this complex unwinds a hairpin loop in the mRNA and scans the mRNA until it locates the AUG start codon (usually the first AUG in the mRNA). GTP is hydrolyzed, the initiation factors (IFs) are released, and the large ribosomal (60S) subunit binds. The ribosome is now complete. It contains one small and one large subunit, and it has three binding sites for tRNA, known as the **P (peptidyl)**,

Eukaryotic initiation factor 2 (eIF2) and also elongation factor 1 (EF1) are types of heterotrimeric G proteins. They dramatically change their conformation and actively form complexes when they bind GTP, but they become inactive and dissociate when they hydrolyze this GTP to GDP. GTP can then displace the bound GDP to reactivate the initiation factor eIF2 or the elongation factor EF1.

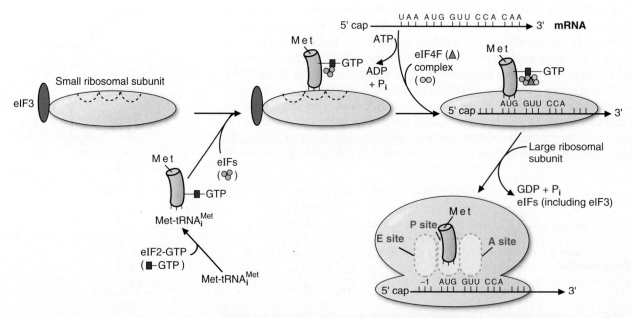

**FIG. 12.6.** Initiation of protein synthesis. *P site,* peptidyl site on the ribosome; *A site,* aminoacyl site on the ribosome; *E site,* free tRNA rejection site on the ribosome. The A, P, and E sites or portions of them are indicated by *dashed lines.* The figure depicts a simplified view of translation initiation because many more initiation steps and factors are required than shown. *eIF,* eukaryotic initiation factor.

**A (aminoacyl)**, and **E (ejection) sites**. During initiation, Met-tRNA$_i$$^{Met}$ binds to the ribosome at the P site, which is located initially at the start site for translation.

The initiation process differs for prokaryotes and eukaryotes. In bacteria, the initiating methionyl-tRNA is formylated on the amino group, producing a formyl-methionyl-tRNA$_f$$^{Met}$ that only participates in formation of the initiation complex. Only three IFs are required to generate this complex in prokaryotes, compared to the dozen or more required by eukaryotes. The ribosomes also differ in size. Prokaryotes have 70S ribosomes, composed of 30S and 50S subunits, and eukaryotes have 80S ribosomes, composed of 40S and 60S subunits. Unlike eukaryotic mRNA, bacterial mRNA is not capped. Identification of the initiating AUG triplet in prokaryotes occurs when a sequence in the mRNA (known as the Shine-Dalgarno sequence) binds to a complementary sequence near the 3′ end of the 16S rRNA of the small ribosomal subunit.

## B. Elongation of Polypeptide Chains

After the initiation complex is formed, addition of each amino acid to the growing polypeptide chain involves binding of an aminoacyl-tRNA to the A site on the ribosome, formation of a peptide bond, and translocation of the peptidyl-tRNA to the P site (Fig. 12.7). The peptidyl-tRNA contains the growing polypeptide chain.

### 1. BINDING OF AMINOACYL-tRNA TO THE A SITE

When Met-tRNA$_i$ (or a peptidyl-tRNA) is bound to the P site, the mRNA codon in the A site determines which aminoacyl-tRNA will bind to that site. An aminoacyl-tRNA binds when its anticodon is antiparallel and complementary to the mRNA

Many antibiotics that are used to combat bacterial infections in humans take advantage of the differences between the mechanisms for protein synthesis in prokaryotes and eukaryotes. For example, streptomycin binds to the 30S ribosomal subunit of prokaryotes. It interferes with initiation of protein synthesis and causes misreading of mRNA. Streptomycin, however, can cause permanent hearing loss and its use is therefore confined mainly to the treatment of nontuberculous mycobacteria or additional infections that do not respond adequately to other antibiotics. Other examples include tetracycline, which binds to the 30S ribosomal subunit of prokaryotes and inhibits binding of aminoacyl-tRNA to the A site of the ribosome; chloramphenicol, which binds to the 50S ribosomal subunit and inhibits peptidyltransferase activity; and erythromycin, which also binds to the 50S subunit but acts by preventing translocation from occurring.

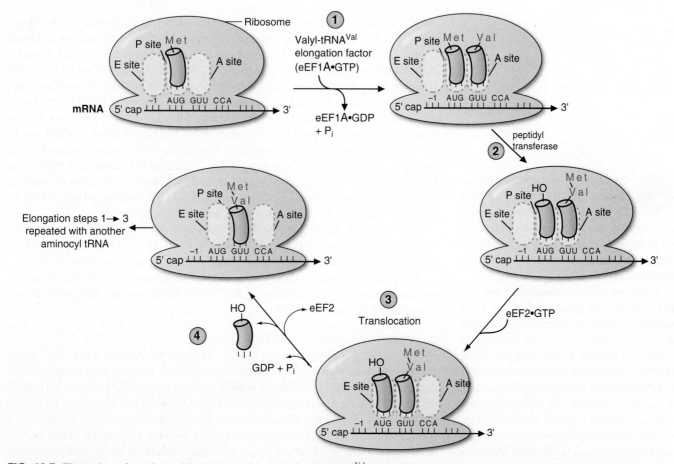

**FIG. 12.7.** Elongation of a polypeptide chain. *(1)* Binding of valyl-tRNA$^{Val}$ to the A site. *(2)* Formation of a peptide bond. *(3)* Translocation. *(4)* Ejection of the free tRNA. After step *4*, step *1* is repeated using the aminoacyl-tRNA for the new codon in the A site. Steps *2*, *3*, and *4* follow. These four steps keep repeating until termination occurs. *EF*, elongation factor.

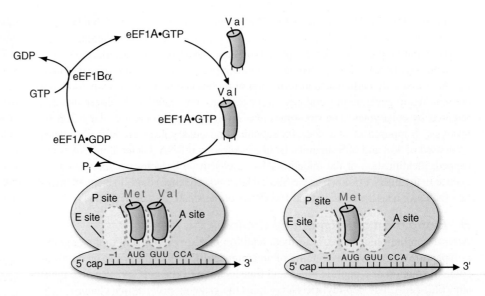

**FIG. 12.8.** Recycling of eEF1A in eukaryotes. eEF1A contains GTPase activity, which is activated upon binding to the ribosome. GTP is hydrolyzed, and eEF1A is released from the ribosome binding to eEF1Bα—a guanine nucleotide exchange factor—and accelerates the substitution of GTP for the GDP on eEF1A. Once this occurs, eEF1A is ready for another round of translation. In prokaryotes, eEF1A is EF-Tu and the protein complex corresponding to eEF1Bα is EF-Ts.

codon. In eukaryotes, the incoming aminoacyl-tRNA first combines with elongation factor eEF1A containing bound GTP before binding to the mRNA-ribosome complex. eEFA is similar to the α-subunit of a heterotrimeric G protein, in that it contains GTPase activity (see Chapter 9). When the aminoacyl-tRNA-eEF1A-GTP complex binds to the A site, GTP is hydrolyzed to GDP as the ribosome activates the GTPase activity of eEF1A. This prompts dissociation of eEF1A-GDP from the aminoacyl-tRNA ribosomal complex, thereby allowing protein synthesis to continue (Fig. 12.8). The binding of the appropriate aminoacyl-tRNA to the A site of the ribosome comprises the second error-checking step in protein synthesis. If an improper aminoacyl-tRNA is brought to the A site, the ribosomal activation of the GTPase activity of eEF1A does not occur, and the complex will leave the binding site, along with the aminoacyl-tRNA. Only when GTP is hydrolyzed can eEF1A release the aminoacyl-tRNA and dissociate from the complex.

Once released, the free eEF1A-GDP binds with eEFB1α, which accelerates the replacement of bound GDP with GTP (see Fig. 12.8). Thus, eEF1A-GTP is ready to bind another aminoacyl-tRNA molecule and to continue protein synthesis.

The process of elongation is very similar in prokaryotes, except that the corresponding factor for eEF1A is named EF-Tu and the associating elongation factors are called EF-Ts instead of eEFB1α.

## 2. FORMATION OF A PEPTIDE BOND

In the first round of elongation, the amino acid on the tRNA in the A site forms a peptide bond with the methionine on the tRNA in the P site. In subsequent rounds of elongation, the amino acid on the tRNA in the A site forms a peptide bond with the peptide on the tRNA in the P site (see Fig. 12.7). Peptidyltransferase, which is not a protein but the rRNA of the large ribosomal subunit, catalyzes the formation of the peptide bond. The tRNA in the A site now contains the growing polypeptide chain, and the tRNA in the P site is uncharged (i.e., it no longer contains an amino acid or peptide). The antibiotic chloramphenicol interferes with the peptidyltransferase activity of the 50S bacterial ribosomal subunit. Its use is limited in humans, however, because it also inhibits mitochondrial protein synthesis and can cause serious side effects.

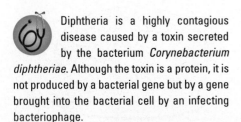

Diphtheria is a highly contagious disease caused by a toxin secreted by the bacterium *Corynebacterium diphtheriae*. Although the toxin is a protein, it is not produced by a bacterial gene but by a gene brought into the bacterial cell by an infecting bacteriophage.

Diphtheria toxin is composed of two protein subunits. The B-subunit binds to a cell surface receptor, facilitating the entry of the A-subunit into the cell. In the cell, the A-subunit catalyzes a reaction in which the ADP-ribose (ADPR) portion of $NAD^+$ is transferred to eEF2 (ADP-ribosylation). In this reaction, the ADPR is covalently attached to a posttranslationally modified histidine residue, known as diphthamide. ADP-ribosylation of eEF2 inhibits protein synthesis leading to cell death. Diphtheria toxoid vaccine is part of the standard vaccination schedule for children, preventing an often fatal disease.

## 3. TRANSLOCATION

Translocation in eukaryotes involves another G protein, elongation factor eEF2 (EF-G in prokaryotes) that complexes with GTP and binds to the ribosome, causing a conformational change that moves the mRNA and its base-paired tRNAs with respect to the ribosome. The uncharged tRNA moves from the P site to the E site. It is released from the ribosome when the next charged tRNA enters the A site. The peptidyl-tRNA moves into the P site and the next codon of the mRNA occupies the A site. During translocation, GTP is hydrolyzed to GDP, which is released from the ribosome along with the elongation factor (see Fig. 12.7).

## 4. TERMINATION OF TRANSLATION

The three elongation steps are repeated until a termination (stop) codon moves into the A site on the ribosome. Because no tRNAs with anticodons that can pair with stop codons normally exist in cells, release factors bind to the ribosome instead, causing peptidyltransferase to hydrolyze the bond between the peptide chain and tRNA. The newly synthesized polypeptide is released from the ribosome, which dissociates into its individual subunits, releasing the mRNA.

Protein synthesis requires a considerable amount of energy. Formation of each aminoacyl-tRNA requires the equivalent of two high-energy phosphate bonds because ATP is converted to AMP and pyrophosphate, which is cleaved to form two inorganic phosphates. As each amino acid is added to the growing peptide chain, two GTPs are hydrolyzed, one at the step involving eEF1A and the second at the translocation step. Thus, four high-energy bonds are cleaved for each amino acid of the polypeptide. In addition, energy is required for initiation of synthesis of a polypeptide chain and for synthesis from nucleotide triphosphate precursors of the mRNA, tRNA, and rRNA involved in translocation.

## V. POLYSOMES

As one ribosome moves along the mRNA, producing a polypeptide chain, a second ribosome can bind to the vacant 5′ end of the mRNA. Many ribosomes can simultaneously translate a single mRNA, forming a complex known as a **polysome** (or **polyribosome**). A single ribosome covers about 80 nucleotides of mRNA. Therefore, ribosomes are positioned on mRNA at intervals of about 100 nucleotides. The growing polypeptide chains attached to the ribosomes become longer as each ribosome moves from the 5′ end toward the 3′ end of the mRNA.

## VI. PROCESSING OF PROTEINS

Nascent polypeptide chains (i.e., polypeptides that are in the process of being synthesized) are processed. As they are being produced, they travel through a tunnel in the ribosome, which can hold roughly 30 amino acid residues. As polymerization of the chain progresses, the amino acid residues at the N-terminal end begin to emerge from this protected region within the ribosome and to fold and refold into the three-dimensional conformation of the polypeptide. Proteins bind to the nascent polypeptide and mediate the folding process. These mediators are called **chaperones** because they prevent improper interactions from occurring. Disulfide bond formation between cysteine residues is catalyzed by protein disulfide isomerases and may also be involved in producing the three-dimensional structure of the polypeptide.

## VII. POSTTRANSLATIONAL MODIFICATIONS

After proteins emerge from the ribosome, they may undergo **posttranslational modifications**. The initial methionine is removed by specific proteases, so methionine is not the N-terminal amino acid of all mature proteins. Subsequently, other specific cleavages may also occur that convert proteins to more active forms (e.g., the conversion of proinsulin to insulin). In addition, amino acid residues within the peptide chain can be modified enzymatically to alter the activity or stability of the proteins, direct it to a subcellular compartment, or prepare it for secretion from the cell.

The macrolide antibiotics (e.g., erythromycin, clarithromycin, azithromycin) bind to the 50S ribosomal subunit of bacteria and inhibit translocation. Azithromycin has less serious side effects than many other antibiotics and can be used as an alternative drug in patients who are allergic to penicillin.

**Table 12.3    Posttranslational Modifications of Proteins**

Acetylation
ADP-ribosylation
Carboxylation
Fatty acylation
Glycosylation
Hydroxylation
Methylation
Phosphorylation
Prenylation

Amino acid residues are modified enzymatically by the addition of various types of functional groups, as outlined in Table 12.3. For example, the N-terminal amino acid is sometimes **acetylated**, and methyl groups can be added to lysine residues (**methylation**). These changes alter the charge on the protein. Proline and lysine residues can be modified by **hydroxylation**. In collagen, hydroxylations lead to stabilization of the protein. **Carboxylations** are important, especially for the function of proteins involved in blood coagulation. Formation of γ-carboxyglutamate allows these proteins to chelate $Ca^{2+}$, a step in clot formation. Fatty acids or other hydrophobic groups (e.g., prenyl groups) anchor the protein in membranes (**fatty acylation and prenylation**). An adenosine diphosphate (ADP)-ribose group can be transferred from $NAD^+$ to certain proteins (**ADP-ribosylation**). The addition and removal of phosphate groups (**phosphorylation**), which bind covalently to serine, threonine, or tyrosine residues, serve to regulate the activity of many proteins (e.g., the enzymes of glycogen degradation and regulators of gene transcription). **Glycosylation**, the addition of carbohydrate groups, is a common modification that occurs mainly on proteins that are destined to be secreted or incorporated into lysosomes or cellular membranes.

## VIII. TARGETING OF PROTEINS TO SUBCELLULAR AND EXTRACELLULAR LOCATIONS

Many proteins are synthesized on polysomes in the cytosol. After they are released from ribosomes, they remain in the cytosol where they carry out their functions. Other proteins synthesized on cytosolic ribosomes enter organelles, such as mitochondria or nuclei. These proteins contain amino acid sequences called **targeting sequences** or **signal sequences** that facilitate their transport into a certain organelle. Another group of proteins are synthesized on ribosomes bound to the rough endoplasmic reticulum (RER). These proteins are destined for secretion or for incorporation into various subcellular organelles (e.g., lysosomes, endoplasmic reticulum [ER], Golgi complex) or cellular membranes, including the plasma membrane.

Proteins that enter the RER as they are being synthesized have signal peptides near their N-termini, which do not have a common amino acid sequence. However, they do contain several hydrophobic residues and are 15 to 30 amino acids in length (Fig. 12.9). A **signal recognition particle (SRP)** binds to the ribosome and to the signal peptide as the nascent polypeptide emerges from the tunnel in the ribosome and translation ceases. When the SRP subsequently binds to an SRP receptor (docking protein) on the RER, translation resumes, and the polypeptide begins to enter the lumen of the RER. The signal peptide is removed by the signal peptidase and the remainder of the newly synthesized protein enters the lumen of the RER. These proteins are transferred in small vesicles to the Golgi complex.

The Golgi complex serves to process the proteins it receives from the RER and to sort them so that they are delivered to their appropriate destinations. Processing, which can be initiated in the ER, involves glycosylation, the addition of carbohydrate groups, and modification of existing carbohydrate chains. Sorting signals permit delivery of proteins to their target locations. For example, glycosylation of enzymes destined to become lysosomal enzymes results in the presence of a mannose 6-phosphate residue on an oligosaccharide attached to the enzyme. This residue is recognized by the mannose 6-phosphate receptor protein, which incorporates the enzyme into a clathrin-coated vesicle. The vesicle travels to endosomes and is eventually incorporated into lysosomes. Other proteins containing a KDEL (lys-asp-glu-leu) sequence at their carboxyl terminal are returned to the ER from the Golgi. Proteins with hydrophobic regions can embed in various membranes. Some proteins, whose sorting signals have not yet been determined, enter secretory vesicles and travel to the cell membrane where they are secreted by the process of exocytosis.

I-cell disease (mucolipidosis II) is an inherited recessive disorder of protein targeting. Lysosomal proteins are not sorted properly from the Golgi to the lysosomes, and lysosomal enzymes end up secreted from the cell. This is due to a mutation in the enzyme N-acetylglucosamine phosphotransferase, which is a required first step for attaching the lysosomal targeting signal, mannose 6-phosphate, to lysosomal proteins. Thus, lysosomal proteins cannot be targeted to the lysosomes, and these organelles become clogged with materials that cannot be digested, destroying overall lysosomal function. This leads to a lysosomal storage disease of severe consequence, with death before the age of 8 years.

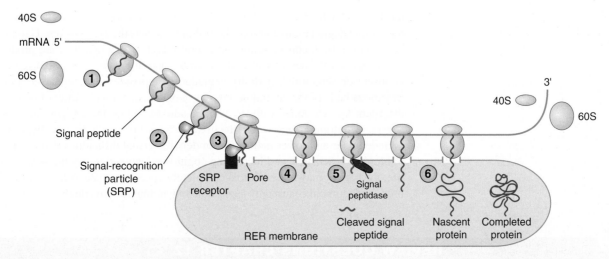

**FIG. 12.9.** Synthesis of proteins on the RER. *(1)* Translation of the protein begins in the cytosol. *(2)* As the signal peptide emerges from the ribosome, an SRP binds to it and to the ribosome and inhibits further synthesis of the protein. *(3)* The SRP binds to the SRP receptor in the RER membrane, docking the ribosome on the RER. *(4)* The SRP is released and protein synthesis resumes. *(5)* As the signal peptide moves through a pore into the RER, a signal peptidase removes the signal peptide. *(6)* Synthesis of the nascent protein continues, and the completed protein is released into the lumen of the RER.

## CLINICAL COMMENTS

Diseases discussed in this chapter are summarized in Table 12.4.

 **Lisa N.** Lisa N. has a $\beta^+$-thalassemia classified clinically as β-thalassemia intermedia. She produces an intermediate amount of functional β-globin chains (her hemoglobin is 7 g/dL; normal is 12 to 16 g/dL). In $\beta^0$-thalassemia, little or none of the hemoglobin β-chain is produced. β-Thalassemia intermedia is usually the result of two different mutations (one that mildly affects the rate of synthesis of β-globin and one that severely affects its rate of synthesis), or, less frequently, homozygosity for a mild mutation in the rate of synthesis or a complex combination of mutations. The mutations that cause the thalassemias have been studied extensively and some of these are summarized in Table A12.1 of the online material @.

**Jay S.** The molecular biology–genetics laboratory's report on **Jay S.'s** white blood cells revealed that he had a deficiency of hexosaminidase A caused by a defect in the gene encoding the α-subunit of this enzyme (vari-

**Table 12.4   Diseases Discussed in Chapter 12**

| Disorder or Condition | Genetic or Environmental | Comments |
|---|---|---|
| β-Thalassemia | Genetic | Lisa N. has β-thalassemia intermedia, indicating that the β-globin gene product is produced at reduced levels as compared to the α-globin gene product. This can happen by a variety of mutations. |
| Tay-Sachs disease | Genetic | Mutation in a gene encoding a lysosomal enzyme, leading to loss of lysosomal function and death at an early age for the patient. |
| Diphtheria | Environmental | Diphtheria toxin catalyzes the ADP-ribosylation of eEF2, a necessary factor for eukaryotic protein synthesis. This results in cell death. Vaccination against diphtheria toxin will prevent the enzymatic actions of the toxin. |
| I-cell disease | Genetic | Mutation in posttranslational processing that leads to mistargeting of enzymes destined for the lysosomes. Disease leads to lysosomal dysfunction and early death. |

ant B, Tay-Sachs disease). Hexosaminidases are lysosomal enzymes necessary for the normal degradation of glycosphingolipids such as the gangliosides. Gangliosides are found in high concentrations in neural ganglia, although they are produced in many areas of the nervous system. When the activity of these degradative enzymes is absent or subnormal, partially degraded gangliosides accumulate in lysosomes in various cells of the central nervous system, causing a wide array of neurological disorders known collectively as gangliosidoses. When the enzyme deficiency is severe, symptoms appear within the first 3 to 5 months of life. Eventually, symptoms include upper and lower motor neuron deficits, visual difficulties that can progress to blindness, seizures, and increasing cognitive dysfunction. By the second year of life, the patient may regress into a completely vegetative state, often succumbing to bronchopneumonia caused by aspiration and an inability to cough.

## REVIEW QUESTIONS-CHAPTER 12

1. In the readout of the genetic code in prokaryotes, which one of the following processes acts before any of the others?

   A. tRNA$_i$ alignment with mRNA
   B. Termination of transcription
   C. Movement of the ribosome from one codon to the next
   D. Recruitment of termination factors to the A site
   E. Export of mRNA from the nucleus

2. tRNA charged with cysteine can be chemically treated so that the amino acid changes its identity to alanine. If some of this charged tRNA is added to a protein-synthesizing extract that contains *all* the normal components required for translation, which of the following statements represents *the most likely outcome* after adding a sample of mRNA that has both Cys and Ala codons in the normal reading frame?

   A. Cysteine would be added each time the alanine codon was translated.
   B. Alanine would be added each time the cysteine codon was translated.
   C. The protein would have a deficiency of cysteine residues.
   D. The protein would have a deficiency of alanine residues.
   E. The protein would be entirely normal.

3. The genetic code is said to be degenerate because of which one of the following?

   A. All triplets seem to have at least one uracil.
   B. There is wobble in the bond between the first base of the anticodon and the third base of the codon.
   C. Some triplets are made up of repeating purines or pyrimidines.
   D. Many codons have pairs of identical bases next to each other.
   E. Many of the amino acids have more than one triplet code.

4. The reason there are 64 possible codons is most likely which one of the following?

   A. There are 64 aminoacyl tRNA synthetases.
   B. There are four possible bases at each of three codon positions
   C. Each base is able to participate in wobbling.
   D. All possible reading frames can be used this way.
   E. The more codons, the faster protein synthesis can be accomplished.

5. Repeating dinucleotide sequences are very common in eukaryotic genomes (e.g., . . . ACACACACACACACACA-CACAC . . . ). Based on what you know, which one of the following statements is likely to be correct?

   A. When occurring within genes, they will give rise to a monotonous run of a single amino acid.
   B. Irrespective of reading frame, they will produce a run of the same two alternating amino acids.
   C. Depending on the reading frame, they will give rise to repetitive runs of 1, 2, or 3 amino acids.
   D. Ribosomes will rapidly dissociate from mRNAs containing such sequences.
   E. If located within introns, they will initiate alternative splicing events.

# 13 Regulation of Gene Expression

## CHAPTER OUTLINE

## KEY POINTS

- Prokaryotic gene expression is primarily regulated at the level of initiation of gene transcription. In general, there is one protein per gene.
  - Sets of genes encoding proteins with related functions are organized into operons.
  - Each operon is under the control of a single promoter.
  - Repressors bind to the promoter to inhibit RNA polymerase binding.
  - Activators facilitate RNA polymerase binding to the promoter.
- Eukaryotic gene regulation occurs at several levels.
  - At the DNA structural level, chromatin must be remodeled to allow access for RNA polymerase.
  - Transcription is regulated by transcription factors, which either enhance or restrict RNA polymerase access to the promoter.
  - RNA processing (including alternative splicing), transport from the nucleus to the cytoplasm, mRNA stability, and translation are also regulated in eukaryotes.

# THE WAITING ROOM

**Mannie W.** is a 56-year-old male who complains of weight loss related to a decreased appetite and increased fatigue. He notes discomfort in the left upper quadrant of his abdomen. On physical examination, he is noted to be pale and to have ecchymoses (bruises) on his arms and legs. His spleen is markedly enlarged.

Initial laboratory studies show a hemoglobin of 10.4 g/dL (normal, 13.5 to 17.5 g/dL) and a leukocyte (white blood cell) count of 86,000 cells/mm$^3$ (normal, 4,500 to 11,000 cells/mm$^3$). The majority of the leukocytes are granulocytes (white blood cells arising from the myeloid lineage), some of which have an "immature" appearance. The percentage of lymphocytes in the peripheral blood is decreased. A bone marrow aspiration and biopsy show the presence of an abnormal chromosome (the Philadelphia chromosome) in dividing marrow cells.

**Ann R.**, who has anorexia nervosa, has continued on an almost meat-free diet (see Chapters 1, 7, and 8). She now appears emaciated and pale. Her hemoglobin is 9.7 g/dL (normal, 12 to 16 g/dL), her hematocrit (volume of packed red cells) is 31% (reference range for women, 36% to 46%), and her mean corpuscular volume (the average volume of a red cell) is 70 femtoliters (fl, 1 fl is equal to $10^{-15}$ L) (reference range, 80 to 100 fl). These values indicate an anemia that is microcytic (small red cells) and hypochromic (light in color, indicating a reduced amount of hemoglobin per red cell). Her serum ferritin (the cellular storage form of iron) was also subnormal. Her plasma level of transferrin (the iron transport protein in plasma) was greater than normal, but its percent saturation with iron was below normal. This laboratory profile is consistent with changes that occur in an iron deficiency state.

## I.   OVERVIEW OF GENE EXPRESSION

Virtually all cells of an organism contain identical sets of genes. However, at any given time, only a small number of the total genes in each cell are expressed (i.e., generate a protein or RNA product). The remaining genes are inactive. Organisms gain a number of advantages by regulating the activity of their genes. For example, both prokaryotic and eukaryotic cells adapt to changes in their environment by turning the expression of genes on and off. Because the processes of RNA transcription and protein synthesis consume a considerable amount of energy, cells conserve fuel by making proteins only when they are needed.

In addition to regulating gene expression to adapt to environmental changes, eukaryotic organisms alter expression of their genes during development. As a fertilized egg becomes a multicellular organism, different kinds of proteins are synthesized in varying quantities. As the human child progresses through adolescence and into adulthood, physical and physiological changes result from variations in gene expression and, therefore, of protein synthesis. Even after an organism has reached the adult stage, regulation of gene expression enables certain cells to undergo differentiation to assume new functions.

## II.   REGULATION OF GENE EXPRESSION IN PROKARYOTES

Prokaryotes are single-celled organisms and therefore require less complex regulatory mechanisms than the multicellular eukaryotes. The most extensively studied prokaryote is the bacterium *Escherichia coli*, an organism that thrives in the human colon, usually enjoying a symbiotic relationship with its host. Based on the size

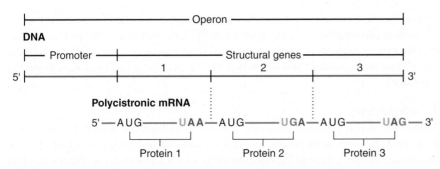

*FIG. 13.1.* An operon. The structural genes of an operon are transcribed as one long polycistronic mRNA. During translation, different start (AUG) and stop (UAA, UGA, or UAG) codons lead to several distinct proteins being produced from this single mRNA.

of its genome ($4.6 \times 10^6$ base pairs), *E. coli* should be capable of making several thousand proteins. However, under normal growth conditions, they synthesize much fewer than that. Thus, many genes are inactive and only those genes that generate the proteins required for growth in that particular environment are expressed.

All *E. coli* cells of the same strain are morphologically similar and contain an identical circular chromosome. As in other prokaryotes, DNA is not complexed with histones, no nuclear envelope separates the genes from the contents of the cytoplasm, and gene transcripts do not contain the noncoding intervening sequences known as introns. In fact, as mRNA is being synthesized, ribosomes bind and begin to produce proteins, so that transcription and translation occur simultaneously (known as coupled transcription–translation). The mRNA molecules in *E. coli* have a very short half-life and are degraded within a few minutes. mRNA molecules must be constantly generated from transcription to maintain synthesis of its proteins. Thus, regulation of transcription, principally at the level of initiation, is sufficient to regulate the level of proteins within the cell.

## A. Operons

The genes encoding proteins are called **structural genes**. In the bacterial genome, the structural genes for proteins involved in performing a related function (such as the enzymes of a biosynthetic pathway) are often grouped sequentially into units called **operons** (Fig. 13.1). The genes in an operon are coordinately expressed; that is, they are either all turned on or all turned off. When an operon is expressed, all of its genes are transcribed. A single polycistronic mRNA is produced that codes for all the proteins of the operon. This polycistronic mRNA contains multiple sets of start and stop codons that allow a number of different proteins to be produced from this single transcript at the translational level. Transcription of the genes in an operon is regulated by its **promoter**, which is located in the operon at the 5′ end, upstream from the structural genes.

## B. Regulation of RNA Polymerase Binding by Repressors

In bacteria, the principle means of regulating gene transcription is through **repressors**, which are regulatory proteins that prevent the binding of RNA polymerase to the promoter and thus act on initiation of transcription (Fig. 13.2). In general, regulatory mechanisms, such as repressors, that work through inhibition of gene transcription are referred to as **negative control**, and mechanisms that work through stimulation of gene transcription are called **positive control**.

The repressor is encoded by a regulatory gene (see Fig. 13.2). Although this gene is considered part of the operon, it is not always located near the remainder of the operon. Its product, the **repressor protein**, diffuses to the promoter and binds to a region of the operon called the **operator**. The operator is located within the promoter or near its 3′ end, just upstream from the transcription start point. When a

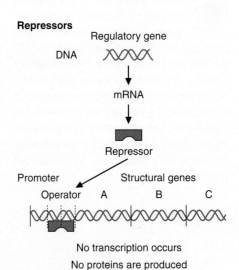

*FIG. 13.2.* Regulation of operons by repressors. When the repressor protein is bound to the operator (a DNA sequence adjacent to or within the promoter), RNA polymerase cannot bind, and transcription therefore does not occur.

**Inducers**

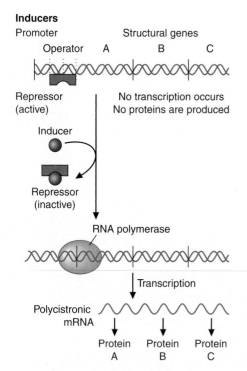

*FIG. 13.3.* An inducible operon. In the absence of an inducer, the repressor binds to the operator, preventing the binding of RNA polymerase. When the inducer is present, the inducer binds to the repressor, inactivating it. The inactive repressor no longer binds to the operator. Therefore, RNA polymerase can bind to the promoter region and transcribe the structural genes.

If one of the *lac* operon enzymes induced by lactose is lactose permease (which increases lactose entry into the cell), how does lactose initially get into the cell to induce these enzymes? A small amount of the permease exists even in the absence of lactose, and a few molecules of lactose enter the cell and are metabolized to allolactose, which begins the process of inducing the operon. As the amount of the permease increases, more lactose can be transported into the cell.

repressor is bound to the operator, the operon is not transcribed because the repressor protein physically blocks the binding of RNA polymerase to the promoter. Two regulatory mechanisms work through controlling repressors: induction (an inducer inactivates the repressor) and repression (a corepressor is required to activate the repressor).

## 1. INDUCERS

**Induction** involves a small molecule, known as an **inducer**, which stimulates expression of the operon by binding to the repressor and changing its conformation so that it can no longer bind to the operator (Fig. 13.3). The inducer is either a nutrient or a metabolite of the nutrient. In the presence of the inducer, RNA polymerase can therefore bind to the promoter and transcribe the operon. The key to this mechanism is that *in the absence of the inducer, the repressor is active, transcription is repressed, and the genes of the operon are not expressed.*

Consider, for example, induction of the *lac* **operon** of *E. coli* by lactose (Fig. 13.4). The enzymes for metabolizing glucose by glycolysis are produced constitutively; that is, they are constantly being made. If the milk sugar lactose is available, the cells adapt and begin to produce the three additional enzymes required for lactose metabolism, which are encoded by the *lac* operon. A metabolite of lactose (allolactose) serves as an inducer, binding to the repressor and inactivating it. Because the inactive repressor no longer binds to the operator, RNA polymerase can bind to the promoter and transcribe the structural genes of the *lac* operon, producing a polycistronic mRNA that encodes for the three additional proteins. However, the presence of glucose can prevent activation of the *lac* operon (discussed in Section II.C).

## 2. COREPRESSORS

In a regulatory model called **repression**, the repressor is inactive until a small molecule called a **corepressor** (a nutrient or its metabolite) binds to the repressor,

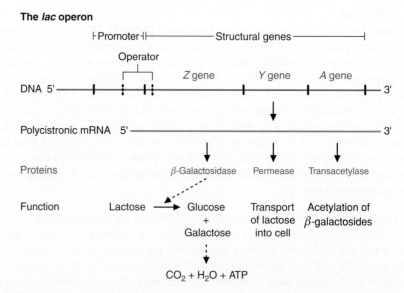

*FIG. 13.4.* The protein products of the *lac* operon. Lactose is a disaccharide that is hydrolyzed to glucose and galactose by β-galactosidase (the *Z* gene). Both glucose and galactose can be oxidized by the cell for energy. The permease (*Y* gene) enables the cell to take up lactose more readily. The *A* gene produces a transacetylase that acetylates β-galactosides. The function of this acetylation is not clear. The promoter binds RNA polymerase and the operator binds a repressor protein. Lactose is converted to allolactose, an inducer that binds the repressor protein and prevents it from binding to the operator. Transcription of the *lac* operon also requires activator proteins that are inactive when glucose levels are high.

**Co-repressors**

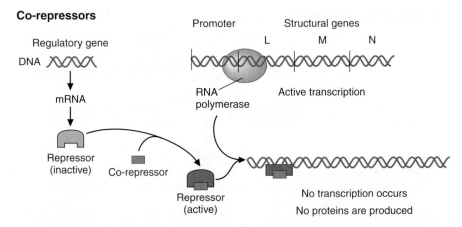

**FIG. 13.5.** A repressible operon. The repressor is inactive until a small molecule, the co-repressor, binds to it. The repressor-corepressor complex binds to the operator and prevents transcription.

activating it (Fig. 13.5). The repressor–corepressor complex then binds to the operator, preventing binding of RNA polymerase and gene transcription. Consider, for example, the **trp operon**, which encodes the five enzymes required for the synthesis of the amino acid tryptophan. When tryptophan is available, *E. coli* cells save energy by no longer making these enzymes. Tryptophan is a corepressor that binds to the inactive repressor, causing it to change conformation and bind to the operator, thereby inhibiting transcription of the operon. *Thus, in the repression model, the repressor is inactive without a corepressor; in the induction model, the repressor is active unless an inducer is present.*

### C. Stimulation of RNA Polymerase Binding

In addition to regulating transcription by means of repressors that inhibit RNA polymerase binding to promoters (negative control), bacteria regulate transcription by means of activating proteins that bind to the promoter and stimulate the binding of RNA polymerase (positive control). Transcription of the *lac* operon, for example, can be induced by allolactose only if glucose is absent. The presence or absence of glucose is communicated to the promoter by a regulatory protein called the **cyclic adenosine monophosphate** (cAMP) **receptor protein** (CRP) (Fig. 13.6). This regulatory protein is also called a **catabolite activator protein** (CAP). A decrease in glucose levels increases levels of the intracellular second messenger cAMP by a mechanism that is not well understood. cAMP binds to CRP and the cAMP-CRP complex binds to a regulatory region of the operon, stimulating binding of RNA polymerase to the promoter and transcription. When glucose is present, cAMP levels decrease, CRP assumes an inactive conformation that does not bind to the operon, and transcription is inhibited. Thus, the enzymes encoded by the *lac* operon are not produced if cells have an adequate supply of glucose, even if lactose is present at very high levels.

### III. REGULATION OF GENE EXPRESSION IN EUKARYOTES

Multicellular eukaryotes are much more complex than single-celled prokaryotes. As the human embryo develops into a multicellular organism, different sets of genes are turned on and different groups of proteins are produced, resulting in differentiation into morphologically distinct cell types that perform different functions. Even beyond development, certain cells within the organism continue to differentiate, such as those that produce antibodies in response to an infection, renew the population of red blood cells, and replace digestive cells that have been sloughed into the intestinal lumen. All of these physiological changes are dictated by complex alterations in gene expression.

**A. In the presence of lactose and glucose**

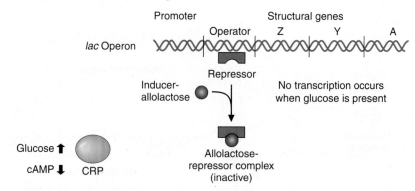

**B. In the presence of lactose and absence of glucose**

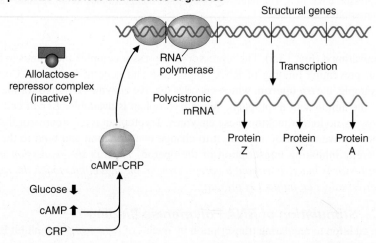

*FIG. 13.6.* Catabolite repression of stimulatory proteins. The *lac* operon is used as an example. **A.** The inducer allolactose (a metabolite of lactose) inactivates the repressor. However, because of the absence of the required coactivator, cAMP-CRP, no transcription occurs unless glucose is absent. **B.** In the absence of glucose, cAMP levels rise. cAMP forms a complex with the CRP. The binding of the cAMP-CRP complex to a regulatory region of the operon permits the binding of RNA polymerase to the promoter. Now, the operon is transcribed and the proteins are produced.

## A. Regulation at Multiple Levels

Differences between eukaryotic and prokaryotic cells result in different mechanisms for regulating gene expression. DNA in eukaryotes is organized into the nucleosomes of chromatin, and genes must be in an active structure to be expressed in a cell. Furthermore, operons are not present in eukaryotes, and the genes encoding proteins that function together are usually located on different chromosomes. Thus, each gene needs its own promoter. In addition, the processes of transcription and translation are separated in eukaryotes by intracellular compartmentation (nucleus and cytosol or endoplasmic reticulum [ER]) and by time (eukaryotic heteronuclear RNA [hnRNA] must be processed and translocated out of the nucleus before it is translated). Thus, regulation of eukaryotic gene expression occurs at multiple levels:

- DNA and the chromosome, including chromosome remodeling and gene rearrangement
- Transcription, primarily through transcription factors affecting binding of RNA polymerase
- Processing of transcripts, including alternative splicing
- Initiation of translation and stability of mRNA

The globin chains of hemoglobin provide an example of functionally related proteins that are on different chromosomes. The gene for the α-globin chain is on chromosome 16, whereas the gene for the β-globin chain is on chromosome 11. As a consequence of this spatial separation, each gene must have its own promoter. This situation is different from that of bacteria, in which genes encoding proteins that function together are often sequentially arranged in operons controlled by a single promoter.

Once a gene is activated through chromatin remodeling, the major mechanism of regulating expression affects initiation of transcription at the promoter.

## B. Regulation of Availability of Genes for Transcription

Once a haploid sperm and egg combine to form a diploid cell, the number of genes in human cells remains approximately the same. As cells differentiate, different genes are available for transcription. A typical nucleus contains chromatin that is condensed (**heterochromatin**) and chromatin that is diffuse (**euchromatin**). The genes in heterochromatin are inactive, whereas those in euchromatin produce mRNA. Long-term changes in the activity of genes occur during development as chromatin goes from a diffuse to a condensed state or vice versa.

The cellular genome is packaged together with histones into nucleosomes, and initiation of transcription is prevented if the promoter region is part of a nucleosome. Thus, activation of a gene for transcription requires changes in the state of the chromatin, called **chromatin remodeling**. The availability of genes for transcription also can be affected in certain cells, or under certain circumstances, by **gene rearrangements**, **amplification**, or **deletion**. For example, during lymphocyte maturation, genes are rearranged to produce a variety of different antibodies. The term *epigenetics* is used to refer to changes in gene expression without altering the sequence of the DNA. Chromatin remodeling and DNA methylation are such changes that can be inherited and which contribute to the regulation of gene expression.

### 1. CHROMATIN REMODELING

The remodeling of chromatin generally refers to displacement of the nucleosome from specific DNA sequences so that transcription of the genes in that sequence can be initiated. This occurs through two different mechanisms. The first mechanism is by an adenosine triphosphate (ATP)-driven chromatin remodeling complex, which uses energy from ATP hydrolysis to unwind certain sections of DNA from the nucleosome core. The second mechanism is by covalent modification of the histone tails through acetylation (Fig. 13.7). Histone acetyltransferases (HAT) transfer an acetyl group from acetyl CoA to lysine residues in the histone tails (the amino terminal ends of histones H2A, H2B, H3, and H4). This reaction removes a positive charge from the ε-amino group of the lysine, thereby reducing the electrostatic interactions between the histones and the negatively charged DNA, making it easier for DNA to unwind from the histones. The acetyl groups can be removed by histone deacetylases (HDAC). Each histone has a number of lysine residues that may be acetylated, and through a complex mixing of acetylated and nonacetylated sites, different segments of DNA can be freed from the nucleosome. A number of transcription factors and coactivators also exhibit histone acetylase activity, which facilitates the binding of these factors to the DNA and simultaneous activation of the gene and initiation of its transcription.

### 2. METHYLATION OF DNA

Cytosine residues in DNA can be methylated to produce 5-methylcytosine. The methylated cytosines are located in GC-rich sequences (called GC islands), which are often near or in the promoter region of a gene. In certain instances, genes that are methylated are less readily transcribed than those that are not methylated. For example, globin genes are more extensively methylated in nonerythroid cells (cells which are not a part of the erythroid or red blood cell lineage) than in the cells in which these genes are expressed (such as the erythroblast and reticulocyte). Methylation is a mechanism for regulating gene expression during differentiation, particularly in fetal development.

### 3. GENE REARRANGEMENT

Segments of DNA can move from one location to another in the genome, associating with each other in various ways so that different proteins are produced.

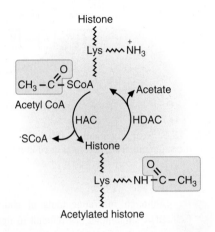

**FIG. 13.7.** Histone acetylation. *HAT,* histone acetyltransferase; *HDAC,* histone deacetylase.

 Methylation has been implicated in genomic imprinting, a process that occurs during the formation of the eggs or sperm that blocks the expression of the gene in the fertilized egg. Males methylate a different set of genes than females. This sex-dependent differential methylation has been most extensively studied in two human disorders, Prader-Willi syndrome and Angelman syndrome. Both syndromes, which have very different symptoms, result from deletions of the same region of chromosome 15 (a microdeletion of less than 5 megabases in size). If the deletion is inherited from the father, Prader-Willi syndrome is seen in the child. If the deletion is inherited from the mother, Angelman syndrome is observed. A disease occurs when a gene that is in the deleted region of one chromosome is methylated on the other chromosome. The mother methylates different genes than the father, so different genes are expressed depending on which parent transmitted the intact chromosome.

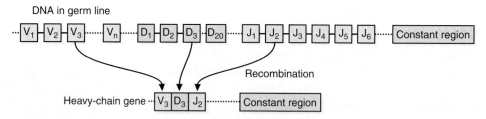

**FIG. 13.8.** Rearrangement of DNA. The heavy-chain gene from which lymphocytes produce immunoglobulins is generated by combining specific segments from among a large number of potential sequences in the DNA of precursor cells.

Although rearrangements of short DNA sequences are difficult to detect, microscopists have observed major rearrangements for many years. Such major rearrangements, known as translocations, can be observed in metaphase chromosomes under the microscope.

**Mannie W.** has such a translocation, known as the Philadelphia chromosome because it was first observed in that city. The Philadelphia chromosome is produced by a balanced exchange between chromosomes 9 and 22. In this translocation, most of a gene from chromosome 9, the *c-abl* gene, is transferred to the *BCR* gene on chromosome 22. This creates a fused *BCR-abl* gene. The *abl* gene is a tyrosine kinase (see Chapter 8) and its regulation by the BCR promoter results in uncontrolled growth stimulation rather than differentiation in cells containing this translocation.

In fragile X syndrome, a GCC triplet is amplified on the 5' side of a gene (fragile X mental retardation 1 [*FMR-1*]) associated with the disease. This gene is located on the X chromosome. The disease is named for the finding that when cells containing this triplet repeat expansion are cultured in the absence of folic acid (which impairs nucleotide production and hence the replication of DNA) the X chromosome develops single- and double-stranded breaks in its DNA. These were termed fragile sites. It was subsequently determined that the *FMR-1* gene was located in one of these fragile sites. A nonaffected person has about 30 copies of the GCC triplet, but in affected individuals, thousands of copies can be present. This syndrome, which is a common form of inherited mental retardation, affects about 1 in 3,600 males and 1 in 4,000 to 1 in 6,000 females worldwide.

The most thoroughly studied example of gene rearrangement occurs in cells that produce antibodies. Antibodies contain two light chains and two heavy chains, each of which contains both a variable and a constant region. Cells called B cells make antibodies. In the precursors of B cells, the variable region of the heavy chain is composed of sequences derived from $V_H$, $D_H$, and $J_H$ areas of the chromosome (Fig. 13.8). During the production of the immature B cells, a series of recombinational events occur that join one $V_H$, one $D_H$, and one $J_H$ sequence into a single exon. This exon now encodes the variable region of the heavy chain of the antibody. Given the large number of immature B cells that are produced, virtually every recombinational possibility occurs, such that all VDJ combinations are represented within this cell population. Later in development, during differentiation of mature B cells, recombinational events join a VDJ sequence to one of the nine heavy chain elements. When the immune system encounters an antigen, the one immature B cell that can bind to that antigen (because of its unique manner of forming the VDJ exon) is stimulated to proliferate (clonal expansion) and to produce antibodies against the antigen.

## 4. GENE AMPLIFICATION

Gene amplification is not the usual physiological means of regulating gene expression in normal cells, but it does occur in response to certain stimuli if the cell can obtain a growth advantage by producing large amounts of a protein. In gene amplification, certain regions of a chromosome undergo repeated cycles of DNA replication. The newly synthesized DNA is excised and forms small, unstable chromosomes called **double minutes**. The double minutes integrate into other chromosomes throughout the genome, thereby amplifying the gene. Normally, gene amplification occurs through errors during DNA replication and cell division, and if the environmental conditions are correct, cells containing amplified genes may have a growth advantage over those without the amplification.

## 5. GENE DELETIONS

With a few exceptions, the deletion of genetic material is likewise not a normal means of controlling transcription, although such deletions do result in disease. Gene deletions can occur through errors in DNA replication and cell division and are usually only noticed if a disease results. For example, various types of cancers result from the loss of a good copy of a tumor suppressor gene, leaving the cell with a mutated copy of the gene (see Chapter 15).

## C. Regulation at the Level of Transcription

The transcription of active genes is regulated by controlling assembly of the basal transcription complex containing RNA polymerase and its binding to distinct elements of the promoter such as the TATA box (see Chapter 11). The basal transcription complex contains TFIID (which binds to elements within the promoter such as the TATA box) and other proteins called **general (basal) transcription factors** (such as TFIIA) that form a complex with RNA polymerase II.

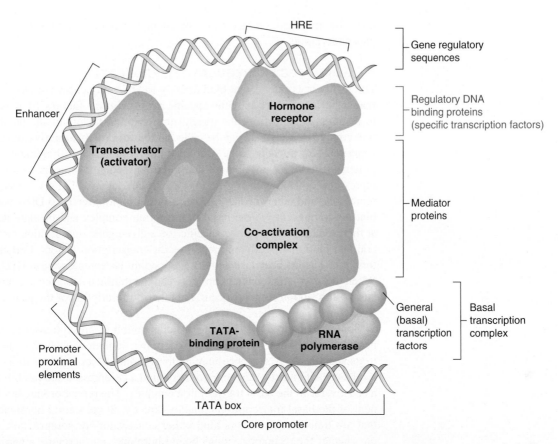

**FIG. 13.9.** The gene regulatory control region consists of the promoter region and additional gene regulatory sequences, including enhancers and hormone response elements *(HRE)*. In this case, a promoter containing a TATA box is shown. Gene regulatory proteins that bind directly to DNA (regulatory DNA-binding proteins) are usually called specific transcription factors or transactivators; they may be either activators or repressors of the transcription of specific genes. The specific transcription factors bind mediator proteins (coactivators or corepressors) that interact with the general transcription factors of the basal transcription complex. The basal transcription complex contains RNA polymerase and associated general transcription factors (TFII factors) and binds, in this case, to the TATA box of the promoter, initiating gene transcription.

Additional transcription factors that are ubiquitous to all promoters bind upstream at various sites in the promoter region. They increase the frequency of transcription and are required for a promoter to function at an adequate level. Genes that are regulated solely by these consensus elements in the promoter region are said to be constitutively expressed.

The control region of a gene also contains DNA regulatory sequences that are specific for that gene and may increase its transcription 1,000-fold or more (Fig. 13.9). Gene-specific transcription factors (also called transactivators or activators) bind to these regulatory sequences and interact with mediator proteins, such as coactivators. By forming a loop in the DNA, coactivators interact with the basal transcription complex and can activate its assembly at the initiation site on the promoter. These DNA regulatory sequences might be some distance from the promoter and may be either upstream or downstream of the initiation site.

Depending on the system, the terminology used to describe components of gene-specific regulation varies somewhat. For example, in the original terminology, DNA regulatory sequences called **enhancers** bound transactivators, which bound coactivators. Similarly, silencers bound corepressors. Hormones bound to hormone receptors, which bound to hormone response elements in DNA. Although these terms are still used, they are often replaced by more general terms, such as DNA regulatory sequences and specific transcription factors, in recognition of the fact that many transcription factors activate one gene while inhibiting another or that a specific transcription factor may be changed from a repressor to an activator by phosphorylation.

## 1. GENE-SPECIFIC REGULATORY PROTEINS

The regulatory proteins that bind directly to DNA sequences are most often called **transcription factors** or **gene-specific transcription factors** (if it is necessary to distinguish them from the general transcription factors of the basal transcription complex). They also can be called **activators** (or **transactivators**), **inducers**, **repressors**, or **nuclear receptors**. In addition to their DNA-binding domain, these proteins usually have a domain that binds to mediator proteins (coactivators, corepressors, or TATA binding protein–associated factors [TAFs]). Coactivators, corepressors, and other mediator proteins do not bind directly to DNA but generally bind to components of the basal transcription complex and mediate its assembly at the promoter. They can be specific for a given gene transcription factor or general and bind many different gene-specific transcription factors. Certain coactivators have histone acetylase activity and certain corepressors have HDAC activity. When the appropriate interactions between the transactivators, coactivators, and the basal transcription complex occur, the rate of transcription of the gene is increased (induction).

Some regulatory DNA-binding proteins inhibit (repress) transcription and may be called **repressors**. Repression can occur in a number of ways. A repressor bound to its specific DNA sequence may inhibit binding of an activator to its regulatory sequence. Alternately, the repressor may bind a corepressor that inhibits binding of a coactivator to the basal transcription complex. The repressor may bind a component of the basal transcription complex directly. Some steroid hormone receptors that are transcription factors bind either coactivators or corepressors, depending on whether the receptor contains bound hormone. Furthermore, a particular transcription factor may induce transcription when bound to the regulatory sequence of one gene and may repress transcription when bound to the regulatory sequence of another gene.

## 2. TRANSCRIPTION FACTORS THAT ARE STEROID HORMONE/THYROID HORMONE RECEPTORS

In a condition known as androgen insensitivity, patients produce androgens (the male sex steroids), but target cells fail to respond to these steroid hormones because they lack the appropriate intracellular transcription factor receptors (androgen receptors). Therefore, the transcription of the genes responsible for masculinization is not activated. A patient with this condition has an XY (male) karyotype (set of chromosomes) but has external characteristics of a female. External male genitalia do not develop, but testes are present, usually in the inguinal region or abdomen.

In the human, steroid hormones and other lipophilic hormones activate or inhibit transcription of specific genes through binding to nuclear receptors that are gene-specific transcription factors (Fig. 13.10A). The nuclear receptors bind to DNA regulatory sequences called **hormone response elements** and induce or repress transcription of target genes. The receptors contain a hormone (ligand)-binding domain, a DNA-binding domain, and a dimerization domain that permits two receptor molecules to bind to each other, forming characteristic homodimers or heterodimers. A transactivation domain binds the coactivator proteins that interact with the basal transcription complex. The receptors also contain a nuclear localization signal domain that directs them to the nucleus at various times after they are synthesized.

Various members of the steroid hormone/thyroid hormone receptor family work in different ways. The **glucocorticoid receptor**, which binds the steroid hormone cortisol, resides principally in the cytosol bound to heat shock proteins. As cortisol binds, the receptor dissociates from the heat shock proteins, exposing the nuclear localization signal (see Fig. 13.10B). The receptors form homodimers that are translocated to the nucleus, where they bind to the hormone response elements (glucocorticoid response elements [GREs]) in the DNA control region of certain genes. The transactivation domains of the receptor dimers bind mediator proteins, thereby activating transcription of specific genes and inhibiting transcription of others.

Other members of the steroid hormone/thyroid hormone family of receptors are also gene-specific transactivation factors but generally form heterodimers that

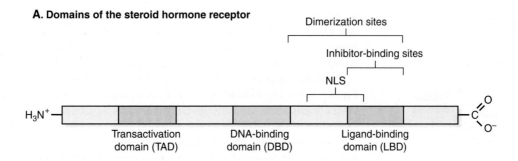

**A. Domains of the steroid hormone receptor**

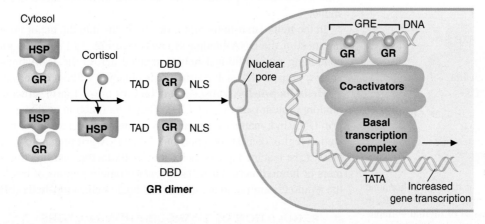

**B. Transcriptional regulation by steroid hormone receptors**

*FIG. 13.10.* Steroid hormone receptors. **A.** Domains of the steroid hormone receptor. The transactivation domain (TAD) binds coactivators; DNA-binding domain (DBD) binds to the hormone response element in DNA; ligand-binding domain (LBD) binds hormone; NLS is the nuclear localization signal; the dimerization sites are the portions of the protein involved in forming a dimer. The inhibitor-binding site binds heat shock proteins and masks the nuclear localization signal. **B.** Transcriptional regulation by steroid hormone receptors. *HSP*, heat shock proteins; *GRE*, glucocorticoid response element; *GR*, glucocorticoid receptor.

bind constitutively to a DNA regulatory sequence in the absence of their hormone ligand and repress gene transcription (Fig. 13.11). For example, the **thyroid hormone receptor** forms a heterodimer with the **retinoid X receptor** (RXR) that binds to thyroid hormone response elements and to corepressors (including one with deacetylase activity), thereby inhibiting expression of certain genes. When thyroid hormone binds, the receptor dimer changes conformation and the transactivation domain binds coactivators, thereby initiating transcription of the genes.

The RXR receptor, which binds the retinoid 9-*cis* retinoic acid, can form heterodimers with at least eight other nuclear receptors. Each heterodimer has a different DNA-binding specificity. This allows the RXR to participate in the regulation of a wide variety of genes and to regulate gene expression differently, depending on the availability of other active receptors.

### 3.  STRUCTURE OF DNA-BINDING PROTEINS

Several unique structural motifs have been characterized for specific transcription factors. Each of these proteins has a distinct recognition site (DNA-binding domain) that binds to the bases of a specific sequence of nucleotides in DNA. Four of the best characterized structural motifs are zinc fingers, b-zip proteins (including leucine zippers), helix-turn-helix, and helix-loop-helix.

**Zinc finger motifs** (commonly found in the DNA-binding domain of steroid hormone receptors) contain a bound zinc chelated at four positions with either histidine or cysteine in a sequence of approximately 20 amino acids. The result is a relatively small, tight, autonomously folded domain. The zinc is required to maintain

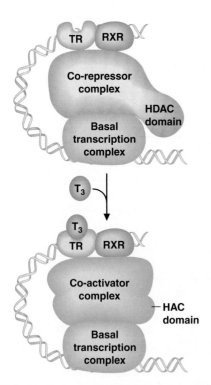

*FIG. 13.11.* Activity of the thyroid hormone receptor–retinoid receptor dimer (TR-RXR) in the presence and absence of thyroid hormone (T$_3$). *HAC*, histone acetylase; *HDAC*, histone deacetylase.

the tertiary structure of this domain. Eukaryotic transcription factors generally have two to six zinc finger motifs that function independently. At least one of the zinc fingers forms an α-helix containing a nucleotide recognition signal, a sequence of amino acids that specifically fits into the major groove of DNA (Fig. 13.12A).

**Leucine zippers** also function as dimers to regulate gene transcription (see Fig. 13.12B). The leucine zipper motif is an α-helix of 30 to 40 amino acid residues that contains a leucine every seven amino acids, positioned so that they align on the same side of the helix. Two helices dimerize so that the leucines of one helix align with the other helix through hydrophobic interactions to form a coiled coil. The portions of the dimer adjacent to the zipper grip the DNA through basic amino acid residues (arginine and lysine) that bind to the negatively charged phosphate groups. This DNA-binding portion of the molecule also contains a nucleotide recognition signal.

In the **helix-turn-helix** motif, one helix fits into the major groove of DNA, making most of the DNA-binding contacts (see Fig. 13.12C). It is joined to a segment containing two additional helices that lie across the DNA-binding helix at right angles. Thus, a very stable structure is obtained without dimerization.

**Helix-loop-helix transcription factors** are a fourth structural type of DNA-binding protein (see Fig. 13.12D). They also function as dimers that fit around and grip DNA in a manner geometrically similar to leucine zipper proteins. The dimerization region consists of a portion of the DNA-gripping helix and a loop to another helix. Like leucine zippers, helix-loop-helix factors can function as either heterodimers or homodimers. These factors also contain regions of basic amino acids near the amino terminus and are also called **basic helix-loop-helix** (bHLH) proteins.

## 4. REGULATION OF TRANSCRIPTION FACTORS

The activity of transcription factors is regulated in a number of different ways. Because transcription factors must interact with a variety of coactivators to stimulate transcription (see Fig. 13.9), the availability of coactivators or other mediator proteins is critical for transcription factor function. If a cell upregulates or downregulates its synthesis of coactivators, the rate of transcription can also be increased or decreased. Transcription factor activity can be modulated by changes in the amount of transcription factor synthesized (see Section III.C.5 in this chapter), by binding a stimulatory or inhibitory ligand (such as steroid hormone binding to the steroid hormone receptors) (see Fig. 13.10), and by stimulation of nuclear entry (illustrated

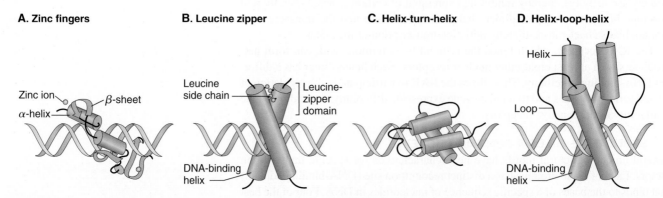

*FIG. 13.12.* Interaction of DNA-binding proteins with DNA. **A.** Zinc finger motifs consist of an α-helix and a β-sheet in which four cysteine and/or histidine residues coordinately bind a zinc ion. The nucleotide recognition signal (contained within the α-helix) of at least one zinc finger binds to a specific sequence of bases in the major groove of DNA. **B.** Leucine zipper motifs form from two distinct polypeptide chains. Each polypeptide contains a helical region in which leucine residues are exposed on one side. These leucines form hydrophobic interactions with each other, causing dimerization. The remaining helices interact with DNA. **C.** Helix-turn-helix motifs contain three (or sometimes four) helical regions, one of which binds to DNA, whereas the others lie on top and stabilize the interaction. **D.** Helix-loop-helix motifs contain helical regions that bind to DNA like leucine zippers. However, their dimerization domains consist of two helices, each of which is connected to its DNA-binding helix by a loop.

by the glucocorticoid receptor). The ability of a transcription factor to influence the transcription of a gene is also augmented or antagonized by the presence of other transcription factors. For example, the thyroid hormone receptor is critically dependent on the concentration of the retinoid receptor to provide a dimer partner. Another example is provided by the phosphoenolpyruvate (PEP) carboxykinase gene, which is induced or repressed by a variety of hormone-activated transcription factors. Frequently, transcription factor activity is regulated through phosphorylation.

Growth factors, cytokines, polypeptide hormones, and a number of other signaling molecules regulate gene transcription through phosphorylation of specific transcription factors by receptor kinases (see Chapter 8).

Nonreceptor kinases, such as protein kinase A, also regulate transcription factors through phosphorylation. Many hormones generate the second messenger **cAMP**, which activates protein kinase A. Activated protein kinase A enters the nucleus and phosphorylates the transcription factor cAMP response element binding (CREB) protein. CREB is constitutively bound to the DNA response element cAMP response element (CRE) and is activated by phosphorylation. Other hormone signaling pathways, such as the mitogen-activated protein (MAP) kinase pathway, also lead to the phosphorylation of CREB (as well as many other transcription factors).

## 5. MULTIPLE REGULATORS OF PROMOTERS

The same transcription factor inducer can activate transcription of many different genes if the genes each contain a common response element. Furthermore, a single inducer can activate sets of genes in an orderly, programmed manner (Fig. 13.13). The inducer initially activates one set of genes. One of the protein products of this set of genes can then act as a specific transcription factor for another set of genes.

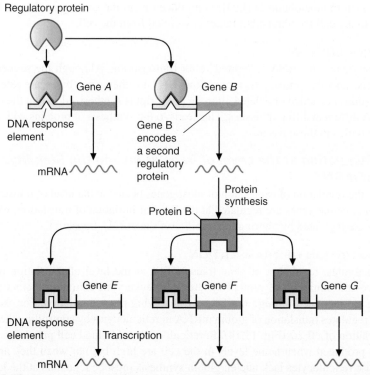

**FIG. 13.13.** Activation of sets of genes by a single inducer. Each gene in a set has a common DNA regulatory element, so one regulatory protein can activate all the genes in the set. In the example shown, the first regulatory protein stimulates the transcription of genes *A* and *B*, which have a common DNA regulatory sequence in their control regions. The protein product of gene *B* is itself a transcriptional activator, which in turn stimulates the transcription of genes *E*, *F*, and *G*, which likewise contain common response elements.

 Interferons, cytokines produced by cells that have been infected with a virus, bind to the cytokine family of cell surface receptors. When an interferon binds, JAK (a receptor-associated tyrosine kinase) phosphorylates a STAT transcription factor (see Chapter 8). The phosphorylated STAT proteins are released from the JAK–receptor complex, dimerize, enter the nucleus, and bind to specific gene regulatory sequences. Different combinations of phosphorylated STAT proteins bind to different sequences and activate transcription of a different set of genes. One of the genes activated by interferon produces the oligonucleotide 2′-5′-oligo(A), which is an activator of a ribonuclease. This RNase degrades mRNA, thus inhibiting synthesis of the viral proteins required for its replication. In addition to stimulating degradation of mRNA, interferon also leads to the phosphorylation of eIF2$\alpha$ (a necessary factor for protein synthesis), which inactivates the eIF2$\alpha$ complex. This enables interferons to prevent the synthesis of viral proteins.

In addition to antiviral effects, interferons were shown to have antitumor effects. The mechanisms of the antitumor effects are not well understood but are probably likewise related to stimulation of specific gene expression by STAT proteins. Interferon-$\alpha$, produced by recombinant DNA technology, has been used to treat patients, such as **Mannie W.**, who has CML. As targeted therapy became available to reduce the side effects of treatments, interferon therapy was reduced in scope.

 An example of a transcriptional cascade of gene activation is observed during adipocyte (fat cell) differentiation. Fibroblast-like cells can be induced to form adipocytes by the addition of dexamethasone (a steroid hormone), cAMP-elevating agents, and insulin to the cells. These factors induce the transient expression of two similar transcription factors named C/EPB-$\beta$ and C/EPB-$\delta$. The names stand for CCAAT enhancer binding protein, and $\beta$ and $\delta$ are two forms of these factors that recognize CCAAT sequences in DNA. The C/EPB transcription factors then induce the synthesis of yet another transcription factor, named the peroxisome proliferator-activated receptor-$\gamma$ (PPAR-$\gamma$), which forms heterodimers with RXR to regulate the expression of yet another transcription factor, C/EPB-$\alpha$. The combination of PPAR-$\gamma$ and C/EPB-$\alpha$ then leads to the expression of adipocyte-specific genes.

The enzyme PEP carboxykinase (PEPCK) is required for the liver to produce glucose from amino acids and lactate. **Ann R.**, who has an eating disorder, needs to maintain a certain blood glucose level in order to keep her brain functioning normally. When her blood glucose levels drop, cortisol (a glucocorticoid) and glucagon (a polypeptide hormone) are released. In the liver, glucagon increases intracellular cAMP levels, resulting in activation of protein kinase A and subsequent phosphorylation of CREB. Phosphorylated CREB binds to its response element in DNA, as does the cortisol receptor. Both transcription factors enhance transcription of the PEPCK gene. Insulin, which is released when blood glucose levels rise after a meal, can inhibit expression of this gene, in part by leading to the dephosphorylation of CREB.

If this process is repeated, the net result is that one inducer can set off a series of events that result in the activation of many different sets of genes.

An individual gene contains many different response elements and enhancers, and genes that encode different protein products contain different combinations of response elements and enhancers. Thus, each gene does not have a single, unique protein that regulates its transcription. Rather, as different proteins are stimulated to bind to their specific response elements and enhancers in a given gene, they act cooperatively to regulate expression of that gene. Overall, a relatively small number of response elements and enhancers and a relatively small number of regulatory proteins generate a wide variety of responses from different genes.

## D. Posttranscriptional Processing of RNA

After the gene is transcribed (i.e., posttranscription), regulation can occur during processing of the RNA transcript (hnRNA) into the mature mRNA. The use of alternative splice sites or sites for addition of the poly(A) tail (polyadenylation sites) can result in the production of different mRNAs from a single hnRNA and, consequently, in the production of different proteins from a single gene.

### 1. ALTERNATIVE SPLICING AND POLYADENYLATION SITES

Processing of the primary transcript involves the addition of a cap to the 5′ end, removal of introns, and polyadenylation (the addition of a poly(A) tail to the 3′ end) to produce the mature mRNA (see Chapter 11). In certain instances, the use of alternative splicing and polyadenylation sites causes different proteins to be produced from the same gene. For example, genes that code for antibodies are regulated by alterations in the splicing and polyadenylation sites, in addition to undergoing gene rearrangement. At an early stage of maturation, pre-B lymphocytes produce immunoglobulin M (IgM) antibodies that are bound to the cell membrane. Later, a shorter protein (immunoglobulin D [IgD]) is produced from the same gene that no longer binds to the cell membrane but rather is secreted from the cell.

### 2. RNA EDITING

In some instances, RNA is "edited" after transcription. Although the sequence of the gene and the primary transcript (hnRNA) are the same, bases are altered or nucleotides are added or deleted after the transcript is synthesized so that the mature mRNA differs in different tissues. This leads to the synthesis of proteins with different activities in those tissues.

## E. Regulation at the Level of Translation and the Stability of mRNA

While the regulation of expression of most genes occurs at the level of transcription initiation, some genes are regulated at the level of initiation of translation, whereas others are regulated by altering the stability of the mRNA transcript.

### 1. INITIATION OF TRANSLATION

In eukaryotes, regulation of gene transcription at the level of translation usually involves the initiation of protein synthesis by eukaryotic initiation factors (eIFs), which are regulated through mechanisms involving phosphorylation. For example, heme regulates translation of globin mRNA in reticulocytes by controlling the phosphorylation of eIF2α (Fig. 13.14). In reticulocytes (red blood cell precursors), globin is produced when heme levels in the cell are high but not when they are low. Because reticulocytes lack nuclei, globin synthesis must be regulated at the level of translation rather than transcription. Heme acts by preventing phosphorylation of eIF2α by a specific kinase (heme-regulated inhibitor kinase) that is inactive when heme is bound. Thus, when heme levels are high, eIF2α is not phosphorylated and is active, resulting in globin synthesis. Similarly, in other cells, conditions such as starvation, heat shock, or viral infections may result in activation of a specific kinase

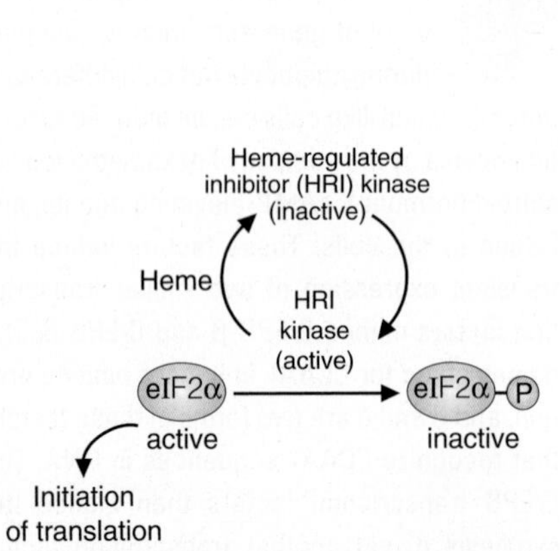

*FIG. 13.14.* Heme prevents inactivation of eIF2α. When eIF2α is phosphorylated by heme-regulated inhibitor kinase, it is inactive, and protein synthesis cannot be initiated. Heme inactivates the heme-regulated inhibitor kinase, thereby preventing phosphorylation of eIF2α and activating translation of the globin mRNA.

that phosphorylates eIF2α to an inactive form. Another example is provided by insulin, which stimulates general protein synthesis by inducing the phosphorylation of 4E-BP, a binding protein for eIF4E. When 4E-BP, in its nonphosphorylated state, binds eIF4E, the initiating protein is sequestered from participating in protein synthesis. When 4E-BP is phosphorylated, as in response to insulin binding to its receptor on the cell surface, the 4E-BP dissociates from eIF4E, leaving eIF4E in the active form, and protein synthesis is initiated.

A different mechanism for regulation of translation is illustrated by iron regulation of ferritin synthesis (Fig. 13.15). Ferritin, the protein involved in the storage of iron within cells, is synthesized when iron levels increase. The mRNA for ferritin has an iron response element (IRE), consisting of a hairpin loop near its 5′ end, which can bind a regulatory protein called the **iron response element-binding protein** (IRE-BP). When IRE-BP does not contain bound iron, it binds to the IRE and prevents initiation of translation. When iron levels increase and IRE-BP binds iron, it changes to a conformation that can no longer bind to the IRE on the ferritin mRNA. Therefore, the mRNA is translated and ferritin is produced.

## 2. microRNAs

microRNAs (miRNAs) are small RNA molecules which regulate protein expression at a posttranscriptional level. A miRNA can either induce the degradation of a target mRNA or block translation of the target mRNA. In either event, the end result is reduced expression of the target mRNA.

miRNAs were first discovered in nematodes and have since been shown to be present in plant and animal cells. There are believed to be approximately 1,000 miRNA genes in the human genome, some of which are located within the introns of the genes they regulate. Other miRNA genes are organized into operons, such that certain miRNA families are produced at the same time. It is also evident that one miRNA can regulate multiple mRNA targets and that a particular mRNA may be regulated by more than one miRNA.

The biogenesis of miRNA is shown in Figure 13.16. miRNA is transcribed by RNA polymerase II and is capped and polyadenylated in the same manner as mRNA. The initial RNA product is designated the primary miRNA (pri-miRNA). The pri-miRNA is modified in the nucleus by an RNA-specific endonuclease named Drosha, in concert with a double-stranded RNA binding protein named DGCR8/

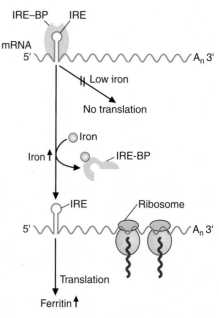

**Ferritin synthesis**

*FIG. 13.15.* Translational regulation of ferritin synthesis. The mRNA for ferritin has an IRE. When the IRE-BP does not contain bound iron, it binds to IRE, preventing translation. When IRE-BP binds iron, it dissociates and the ferritin mRNA is translated.

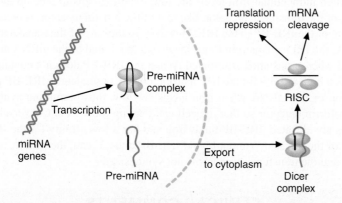

*FIG. 13.16.* miRNA synthesis and action. miRNA genes are transcribed in the nucleus by RNA polymerase II, generating the pri-miRNA, processed to a pre-miRNA, and then exported to the cytoplasm. In the cytoplasm, the pre-miRNA is further processed by a ribonuclease (Dicer), and resulting double-stranded miRNA is strand selected, with the guide strand (designated in *black*) entering the RISC. The guide strand of RISC targets the complex to the 3′ untranslated region of the target mRNA, leading to either degradation of the mRNA or an inhibition of translation.

Pasha. The action of Drosha is to create a stem-loop RNA structure of about 70 to 80 nucleotides in length, which is the precursor-miRNA (pre-miRNA). The pre-miRNA is exported form the nucleus to the cytoplasm (via the protein exportin 5), where it interacts with another RNA endonuclease named Dicer and Dicer's binding partner TRBP. Dicer cleaves the pre-miRNA to mature miRNA (a double-stranded RNA with a two nucleotide overhang at the ends). One of the strands of the miRNA (known as the guide strand) is incorporated into the RNA-induced silencing complex (RISC) while the other RNA strand (the passenger strand) is degraded. The major protein in RISC is known as Argonaute. It is the RISC that will block translation of the target mRNA.

The guide strand leads the RISC to the target mRNA, as the guide strand forms base pairs within a section of the 3′ untranslated region of the mRNA. If there is a high homology in base-pairing, then Argonaute, a ribonuclease, will degrade the mRNA. However, if the homology between the guide strand and the target mRNA is poor (due to mismatches), then translation of the mRNA will be blocked.

The net result of miRNA expression is the loss of target mRNA translation. As miRNAs have multiple targets and these targets will vary from tissue to tissue, an alteration in miRNA expression will have profound effects on gene expression within cells. As will be discussed in Chapter 15, tumors can result from the loss or overexpression of miRNA genes.

### 3. TRANSPORT AND STABILITY OF mRNA

Stability of an mRNA also plays a role in regulating gene expression, because mRNAs with long half-lives can generate a greater amount of protein than can those with shorter half-lives. The mRNA of eukaryotes is relatively stable (with half-lives measured in hours to days), although it can be degraded by nucleases in the nucleus or cytoplasm before it is translated. To prevent degradation during transport from the nucleus to the cytoplasm, mRNA is bound to proteins that help to prevent its degradation. Sequences at the 3′ end of the mRNA appear to be involved in determining its half-life and binding proteins that prevent degradation. One of these is the poly(A) tail, which protects the mRNA from attack by nucleases. As mRNA ages, its poly(A) tail becomes shorter.

An example of the role of mRNA degradation in control of translation is provided by the transferrin receptor mRNA (Fig. 13.17). The transferrin receptor is a protein located in cell membranes that permits cells to take up transferrin, the protein that transports iron in the blood. The rate of synthesis of the transferrin receptor increases when intracellular iron levels are low, enabling cells to take up more iron. Synthesis of the transferrin receptor, like that of the ferritin receptor, is regulated by the binding of the IRE-BP to the IRE. However, in the case of the transferrin receptor mRNA, the IREs are hairpin loops located at the 3′ end of the mRNA and not at the 5′ end where translation is initiated. When the IRE-BP does not contain bound iron, it has a high affinity for the IRE hairpin loops. Consequently, IRE-BP prevents degradation of the mRNA when iron levels are low, thus permitting synthesis of more transferrin receptor so that the cell can take up more iron. Conversely, when iron levels are elevated, IRE-BP binds iron and has a low affinity for the IRE hairpin loops of the mRNA. Without bound IRE-BP at its 3′ end, the mRNA is rapidly degraded and the transferrin receptor is not synthesized.

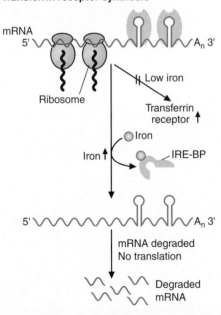

**Transferrin receptor synthesis**

*FIG. 13.17.* Regulation of degradation of the mRNA for the transferrin receptor (TfR). Degradation of the TfR mRNA is prevented by binding of the IRE-BP to IRE, which are hairpin loops located at the 3′ end of the TfR mRNA. When iron levels are high, IRE-BP binds iron and is not bound to the TfR mRNA. The TfR mRNA is rapidly degraded, preventing synthesis of the TfR.

## CLINICAL COMMENTS

Diseases discussed in this chapter are summarized in Table 13.1.

**Mannie W.** Mannie W. has CML (chronic myelogenous leukemia), a hematological disorder in which the proliferating leukemic cells are believed to originate from a single line of precursor myeloid cells. It is

**Table 13.1.   Diseases Discussed in Chapter 13**

| Disorder or Condition | Genetic or Environmental | Comments |
|---|---|---|
| Chronic myelogenous leukemia (CML) | Both | More than 90% of CML arises due to the generation of the Philadelphia chromosome, which is created by an exchange of genetic material between chromosomes 9 and 22. This translocation creates a unique fusion protein (BCR-abl), which facilitates uncontrolled proliferation of cells that express this fusion protein. |
| Anorexia nervosa | Both | The patient's poor diet has led to a hypochromic anemia due to low iron levels. This leads to a reduction of expression of serum and tissue ferritin but an increase of expression of the transferrin protein and the transferrin receptor. |
| Angelman and Prader-Willi syndromes | Genetic | The use of base methylation, within promoter regions, to regulate gene expression. The methylation of key bases within the promoter leads to nonexpression of the gene and forms the basis for imprinting. This is an example of epigenetic modification of gene expression. |
| Fragile X disease | Genetic | A significant number of triplet repeat expansions within a gene may lead to dysfunction of the protein product, leading to disease. In fragile X, mental retardation is the primary symptom due to expansions in the *FMR-1* gene on the X chromosome. |
| Androgen insensitivity | Genetic | Lack of androgen receptors, leading to default female sexual characteristics. The patient produces androgens but cannot respond to them. These patients have an XY genotype but female sexual characteristics. |

Omnipotent stem cells in the bone marrow normally differentiate and mature in a highly selective and regulated manner, becoming red blood cells, white blood cells, or platelets. Cytokines stimulate differentiation of the stem cells into the lymphoid and myeloid lineages. The lymphoid lineage gives rise to B and T lymphocytes, which are white blood cells that work together to generate antibodies for the immune response. The myeloid lineage gives rise to three types of progenitor cells: erythroid, granulocytic–monocytic, and megakaryocytic. The erythroid progenitor cells differentiate into red blood cells (erythrocytes), and the other myeloid progenitors give rise to nonlymphoid white blood cells and platelets. Various medical problems can affect this process. In **Mannie W.**, who has CML, a single line of primitive myeloid cells undergo the event which leads to the Philadelphia chromosome being generated. This produces leukemic cells that proliferate abnormally, causing a large increase in the number of white blood cells in the circulation. The Philadelphia chromosome is a somatic translocation, not found in the germ line. In **Lisa N.**, who has a deficiency of red blood cells caused by her $\beta^+$-thalassemia (see Chapter 12), differentiation of precursor cells into mature red blood cells is stimulated to compensate for the anemia.

classified as one of the myeloproliferative disorders, and CML is distinguished by the presence of a specific cytogenetic abnormality of the dividing marrow cells known as the Philadelphia chromosome, found in more than 90% of cases. In most instances, the cause of CML is unknown, but the disease occurs with an incidence of around 1.5 per 100,000 population in Western societies.

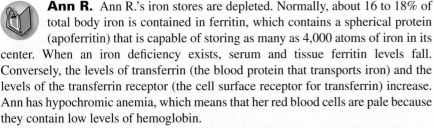

**Ann R.**   Ann R.'s iron stores are depleted. Normally, about 16 to 18% of total body iron is contained in ferritin, which contains a spherical protein (apoferritin) that is capable of storing as many as 4,000 atoms of iron in its center. When an iron deficiency exists, serum and tissue ferritin levels fall. Conversely, the levels of transferrin (the blood protein that transports iron) and the levels of the transferrin receptor (the cell surface receptor for transferrin) increase. Ann has hypochromic anemia, which means that her red blood cells are pale because they contain low levels of hemoglobin.

Why does anemia result from iron deficiency? When an individual is deficient in iron, the reticulocytes do not have sufficient iron to produce heme, the required prosthetic group of hemoglobin. When heme levels are low, the eukaryotic initiation factor eIF2α (see Fig. 13.13) is phosphorylated and inactive. Thus, globin mRNA cannot be translated because of the lack of heme. This results in red blood cells with inadequate levels of hemoglobin for oxygen delivery and an anemia.

1.  In *E. coli*, under high-lactose, high-glucose conditions, which one of the following could lead to maximal transcription activation of the *lac* operon?

    A.  A mutation in the CRP binding site leading to enhanced binding
    B.  A mutation in the *lac I* gene (which encodes the repressor)
    C.  A mutation in the operator sequence
    D.  A mutation leading to lower binding of repressor
    E.  A mutation leading to enhanced cAMP levels

2.  A mutation in the *I* (repressor) gene of a "noninducible" strain of *E. coli* resulted in an inability to synthesize any of the proteins of the *lac* operon. Which one of the following provides a rational explanation?

    A.  The repressor has lost its affinity for operator.
    B.  The repressor has lost its affinity for inducer.
    C.  A *trans*-acting factor can no longer bind to the promoter.
    D.  The CAP protein is no longer made.
    E.  Lactose feedback inhibition becomes constitutive.

3.  Which one of the following double-stranded DNA sequences shows perfect dyad symmetry (the same sequence of bases on both strands)?

    A.  TGACCGGTGACCGG
    B.  GCAGATTTTAGACG
    C.  GAACTGCTAGTCGC
    D.  GGCATCGCGATGCC
    E.  TAATCGGAACCAAT

4.  Which one of the following describes a common theme in the structure of DNA-binding proteins?

    A.  The presence of a specific helix that lies across the major groove of DNA
    B.  The ability to form dimers with disulfide linkages
    C.  The presence of zinc
    D.  The ability to form multiple hydrogen bonds between the protein peptide backbone and the DNA phosphodiester backbone
    E.  The ability to recognize RNA molecules with the same sequence

5.  Proteins recognize specific DNA sequences through which one of the following mechanisms?

    A.  Base pairing through the major groove
    B.  Efficient codon-anticodon interactions
    C.  Selective hydrogen bonding from amino acid side chains to nucleotide bases
    D.  Aminoacyl linkages
    E.  Preferential displacement of one strand from the double helix

# 14 Use of Recombinant DNA Techniques in Medicine

## CHAPTER OUTLINE

I. RECOMBINANT DNA TECHNIQUES
   A. Strategies for obtaining fragments of DNA and copies of genes
      1. Restriction fragments
      2. DNA produced by reverse transcriptase
      3. Chemical synthesis of DNA
   B. Techniques for identifying DNA sequences
      1. Probes
      2. Gel electrophoresis
      3. Detection of specific DNA sequences
      4. DNA sequencing
   C. Techniques for amplifying DNA sequences
      1. Cloning of DNA
      2. Polymerase chain reaction

II. USE OF RECOMBINANT DNA TECHNIQUES FOR DIAGNOSIS OF DISEASE
   A. DNA polymorphisms
   B. Detection of polymorphisms
      1. Restriction fragment length polymorphisms
      2. Detection of mutations by allele-specific oligonucleotide probes
      3. Testing for mutations by polymerase chain reaction
      4. Detection of polymorphisms caused by repetitive DNA
      5. DNA chips (microarrays)

III. USE OF RECOMBINANT DNA TECHNIQUES FOR THE PREVENTION AND TREATMENT OF DISEASE
   A. Vaccines
   B. Production of therapeutic proteins
      1. Insulin and growth hormone
      2. Complex human proteins
   C. Genetic counseling
   D. Gene therapy

IV. PROTEOMICS

## KEY POINTS

- Techniques for isolating and amplifying genes and studying and manipulating DNA sequences are currently being used in the diagnosis, prevention, and treatment of disease.
- These techniques require an understanding of the following tools and processes:
  - Restriction enzymes
  - Cloning vectors
  - Polymerase chain reaction
  - Dideoxy DNA sequencing
  - Gel electrophoresis
  - Nucleic acid hybridization
  - Expression vectors
- Recombinant DNA molecules produced by these techniques can be used as diagnostic probes, in gene therapy, or for the large-scale production of proteins for the treatment of disease.

continued

- Identified genetic polymorphisms, inherited differences in DNA base sequences between individuals, can be utilized for both diagnosis of disease, and the generation of an individual's molecular fingerprint.
- Genetic treatment of disease is possible, using either gene therapy or gene ablation techniques. Technical difficulties currently restrict the widespread use of these treatments.
- Proteomics is the study of proteins expressed by a cell. Differences in protein expression between normal and cancer cells can be used to identify potential targets for future therapy.

# THE WAITING ROOM

Cystic fibrosis is a disease caused by an inherited deficiency in the cystic fibrosis transmembrane conductance regulator (CFTR) protein, which is a chloride channel (see Chapter 8). In the absence of chloride secretion, thick mucus blocks the pancreatic duct, resulting in decreased secretion of digestive enzymes into the intestinal lumen. The resulting malabsorption of fat and other foodstuffs decreases growth and may lead to varying degrees of small bowel obstruction. Liver and gallbladder secretions may be similarly affected. Eventually, atrophy of the secretory organs or ducts may occur. Thick mucus also blocks the airways, markedly diminishing air exchange and predisposing the patient to stasis of secretions, diminished immune defenses, and increased secondary infections. Defects in the CFTR chloride channel also affect sweat composition, increasing the sodium and chloride contents of the sweat, thereby providing a diagnostic tool.

**Susan F.** is a 3-year-old Caucasian girl who has been diagnosed with cystic fibrosis. Her growth rate has been in the 30th percentile over the last year. Since birth, she has had occasional episodes of spontaneously reversible and minor small bowel obstruction. These episodes are superimposed on gastrointestinal symptoms that suggest a degree of dietary fat malabsorption, such as bulky, glistening, foul-smelling stools two or three times a day. She has experienced recurrent flare-ups of bacterial bronchitis/bronchiolitis in the last 10 months, each time caused by *Pseudomonas aeruginosa*. A quantitative sweat test was unequivocally positive (excessive sodium and chloride were found in her sweat on two occasions.). Based on these findings, the pediatrician informed Susan's parents that Susan probably has cystic fibrosis (CF). A sample of her blood was sent to a DNA testing laboratory to confirm the diagnosis and to determine specifically which one of the many potential genetic mutations known to cause CF was present in her cells.

**Carrie S., Will S.**'s 19-year-old sister, is considering marriage. Her growth and development have been normal and she is free of symptoms of sickle cell anemia. Because a younger sister, Amanda, was tested and found to have sickle trait and because of Will's repeated sickle crises, Carrie wants to know whether she also has sickle trait (see Chapters 4 and 5 for **Will S.**'s history). A hemoglobin electrophoresis is performed that reveals the composition of her hemoglobin to be 58% HbA, 39% HbS, 1% HbF, and 2% HbA$_2$, a pattern consistent with the presence of sickle cell trait. The hematologist who saw her in the clinic on her first visit is studying the genetic mutations of sickle cell trait and asks Carrie for permission to draw additional blood for more sophisticated analysis of the genetic disturbance that causes her to produce HbS. Carrie informed her fiancé that she has sickle cell trait and that she wants to delay their marriage until he is tested.

**Victoria T.** was a 21-year-old female who was the victim of rape and murder. Her parents told police she had left her home and drove to the local convenience store. When she had not returned home an hour later, her father drove to the store, looking for Victoria. He had found her car still parked in front of the store and called the police. They searched the area around the store and found Victoria's body in a wooded area behind the building. She had been sexually assaulted and strangled. Medical technologists from the police laboratory collected a semen sample from vaginal fluid and took samples of dried blood from under the victim's fingernails. Witnesses identified three men who spoke to Victoria while she was at the convenience store. DNA samples were obtained from these suspects to determine whether any of them was the perpetrator of the crime.

# I.  RECOMBINANT DNA TECHNIQUES

Techniques for joining DNA sequences into new combinations (**recombinant DNA**) were originally developed as research tools to explore and manipulate genes and to produce the gene products (proteins). Now, they are also being used to identify mutated genes associated with disease and to correct genetic defects. These techniques will soon replace many current clinical testing procedures. A basic appreciation of recombinant DNA techniques is required to understand how genetic variations among individuals are determined and how these differences can be used to diagnose disease. The first steps in determining individual variations in genes involve isolating the genes (or fragments of DNA) that contain variable sequences and obtaining adequate quantities for study. The human genome project has succeeded in sequencing the 3 billion bases of the human genome and can now be used as a template to discover and understand the molecular bases of disease.

## A.  Strategies for Obtaining Fragments of DNA and Copies of Genes

### 1.  RESTRICTION FRAGMENTS

Enzymes called **restriction endonucleases** enable molecular biologists to cleave segments of DNA from the genome of various types of cells or to fragment DNA obtained from other sources. A **restriction enzyme** is an endonuclease that specifically recognizes a short sequence of DNA, usually four to six base pairs (bp) in length, and cleaves a phosphodiester bond in both DNA strands within this sequence (Fig. 14.1). A key feature of restriction enzymes is their specificity. A restriction enzyme always cleaves at the same DNA sequence and only cleaves at that particular sequence. Most of the DNA sequences recognized by restriction enzymes are palindromes, that is, both strands of DNA have the same base sequence when read in a 5′ to 3′ direction. The cuts made by these enzymes are usually sticky; that is, the products are single stranded at the ends with one strand overhanging the other, so they anneal with complementary sequences to the overhang. However, sometimes, they are blunt (the products are double stranded at the ends, with no overhangs). Hundreds of restriction enzymes with different specificities have been isolated (see Table A14.1 of the online supplement @ ).

Restriction fragments of DNA can be used to identify variations in base sequence in a gene. However, they also can be used to synthesize a **recombinant DNA** (also called **chimeric DNA**), which is composed of molecules of DNA from different sources that have been recombined in vitro (outside the organism, e.g., in a test tube). The sticky ends of two unrelated DNA fragments can be joined to each other if they have sticky ends that are complementary. Complementary ends are obtained by cleaving the unrelated DNAs with the same restriction enzyme (Fig. 14.2). After the sticky ends of the fragments base-pair with each other, the fragments can be covalently attached by the action of DNA ligase.

### 2.  DNA PRODUCED BY REVERSE TRANSCRIPTASE

If messenger RNA (mRNA) transcribed from a gene is isolated, this mRNA can be used as a template by the enzyme reverse transcriptase, which produces a DNA copy (cDNA, for complementary DNA) of the RNA. In contrast to DNA fragments cleaved from the genome by restriction enzymes, DNA produced by reverse transcriptase does not contain introns because mRNA, which has no introns, is used as a template. cDNA also lacks the regulatory regions of a gene, as those sequences (promoter, promoter-proximal elements, and enhancers) are not transcribed into mRNA.

### 3.  CHEMICAL SYNTHESIS OF DNA

Automated machines can synthesize **oligonucleotides** (short molecules of single-stranded DNA) up to 150 nucleotides in length. These machines can be programmed to produce oligonucleotides with a specified base sequence. Although entire genes cannot yet be synthesized in one piece, appropriate overlapping of pieces of genes can

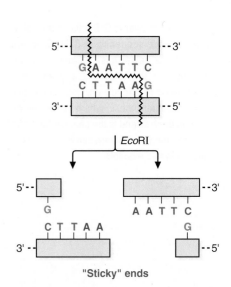

**FIG. 14.1.** Action of restriction enzymes. Note that the DNA sequence shown is a palindrome; each strand of the DNA when read in a 5′ to 3′ direction has the same sequence. Cleavage of this sequence by *Eco*RI produces single-stranded (or "sticky") ends or tails. Not shown is an example of an enzyme that generates blunt ends (see Table A14.1 of the online supplement @ ).

**Q:** Which **ONE** of the following sequences is most likely to be a restriction enzyme recognition sequence? All sequences are written in standard notation, with the top strand going 5′ to 3′, left to right.

A.  G T C C T G
    C A G G A C
B.  T A C G A T
    A T G C T A
C.  C T G A G
    G A C T C
D.  A T C C T A
    T A G G A T

 In sickle cell anemia, the point mutation that converts a glutamate residue to a valine residue (**GA**G to **GT**G) occurs in a site that is cleaved by the restriction enzyme *Mst*II (recognition sequence CCTNAGG, where N can be any base) within the normal β-globin gene. The sickle cell mutation causes the β-globin gene to lose this *Mst*II restriction site. Therefore, because **Will S.** is homozygous for the sickle cell gene, neither of the two alleles of his β-globin gene will be cleaved at this site.

**A:** The answer is C. C follows the palindromic sequence of CTNAG, where N can be any base. None of the other sequences are this close to a palindrome. Although most restriction enzymes recognize a "perfect" palindrome, in which the sequence of bases in each strand is the same, others can have intervening bases between the regions of identity, as in this example.

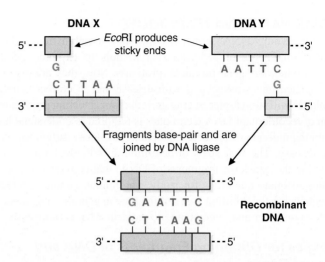

**FIG. 14.2.** Production of recombinant DNA molecules with restriction enzymes and DNA ligase. The *broken lines* at the 5' and 3' ends indicate that this sequence is part of a longer DNA molecule.

be made and then ligated together to produce a fully synthetic gene. Additionally, oligonucleotides can be prepared that will base-pair with segments of genes. These oligonucleotides can be used in the process of identifying, isolating, and amplifying genes.

## B. Techniques for Identifying DNA Sequences

### 1. PROBES

A **probe** is a single-stranded polynucleotide of DNA or RNA that is used to identify a complementary sequence on a larger single-stranded DNA or RNA molecule (Fig. 14.3). Formation of base-pairs with a complementary strand is called **annealing** or **hybridization**. Probes can be composed of cDNA, fragments of genomic DNA (cleaved by restriction enzymes from the genome), chemically synthesized oligonucleotides or, occasionally, RNA.

To identify the target sequence, the probe must carry a **label** (see Fig. 14.3). If the probe has a radioactive label such as $^{32}$P, it can be detected by autoradiography. An autoradiogram is produced by covering the material containing the probe with a sheet of x-ray film. Electrons (β-particles) emitted by disintegration of the radioactive atoms expose the film in the region directly over the probe. Several techniques can be used to introduce labels into these probes. Not all probes are radioactive. Some are chemical adducts (compounds that bind covalently to DNA) that can be identified by, for example, fluorescence.

### 2. GEL ELECTROPHORESIS

**Gel electrophoresis** is a technique that uses an electrical field to separate molecules on the basis of size. Because DNA contains negatively charged phosphate groups, it

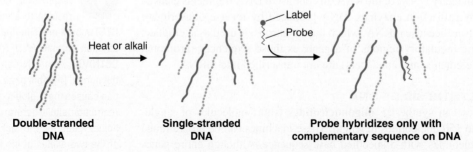

**FIG. 14.3.** Use of probes to identify DNA sequences. The probe can be either DNA or RNA.

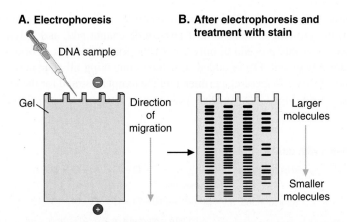

**A. Electrophoresis**

**B. After electrophoresis and treatment with stain**

DNA sample

Gel

Direction of migration

Larger molecules

Smaller molecules

**FIG. 14.4.** Gel electrophoresis of DNA. **A.** DNA samples are placed into depressions ("wells") at one end of a gel, and an electrical field is applied. The DNA migrates toward the positive electrode at a rate that depends on the size of the DNA molecules. As the gel acts as a sieve, shorter molecules migrate more rapidly than longer molecules. **B.** The gel is removed from the apparatus. The bands are not visible until techniques are performed to visualize them (see Fig. 14.6).

will migrate in an electrical field toward the positive electrode (Fig. 14.4). Shorter molecules migrate more rapidly through the pores of a gel than do longer molecules, so separation is based on length. Gels composed of polyacrylamide, which can separate DNA molecules that differ in length by only one nucleotide, are used to determine the base sequence of DNA. Agarose gels are used to separate longer DNA fragments that have larger size differences.

The bands of DNA in the gel can be visualized by various techniques. Staining with dyes such as ethidium bromide allows direct visualization of DNA bands under ultraviolet light. Specific sequences are generally detected by means of a labeled probe.

### 3.  DETECTION OF SPECIFIC DNA SEQUENCES

To detect specific sequences, DNA is usually transferred to a solid support, such as a sheet of nitrocellulose paper. For example, if bacteria are growing on an agar plate, cells from each colony will adhere to a nitrocellulose sheet pressed against the agar, and an exact replica of the bacterial colonies can be transferred to the nitrocellulose paper (Fig. 14.5). A similar technique is used to transfer bands of DNA from electrophoretic gels to nitrocellulose sheets. After bacterial colonies or bands of DNA are transferred to nitrocellulose paper, the paper is treated with an alkaline solution and then heated. Alkaline solutions denature DNA (i.e., separate the two strands of each double helix), and the heating fixes the DNA on the filter paper such that it will not move from its position during the rest of the blotting procedure. The single-stranded DNA is then hybridized with a probe, and the regions on the nitrocellulose blot containing DNA that base-pairs with the probe are identified.

E. M. Southern developed the technique, which bears his name, for identifying DNA sequences on gels. **Southern blots** are produced when DNA on a nitrocellulose blot of an electrophoretic gel is hybridized with a DNA probe. Molecular biologists decided to continue with this geographic theme as they named two additional techniques. **Northern blots** are produced when RNA on a nitrocellulose blot is hybridized with a DNA probe. A slightly different but related technique, known as a **Western blot**, involves separating proteins by gel electrophoresis and probing with labeled antibodies for specific proteins (Fig. 14.6).

### 4.  DNA SEQUENCING

The most common procedure for determining the sequence of nucleotides in a DNA strand was developed by Frederick Sanger and involves the use of dideoxynucleotides. Dideoxynucleotides lack a 3′ hydroxyl group (in addition to lacking the 2′ hydroxyl

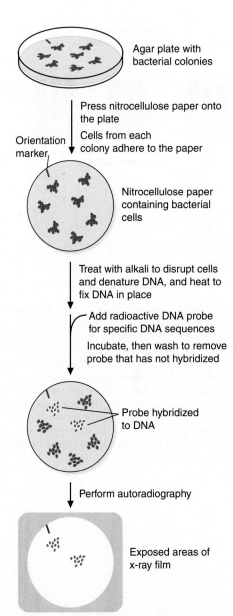

Agar plate with bacterial colonies

Orientation marker

Press nitrocellulose paper onto the plate

Cells from each colony adhere to the paper

Nitrocellulose paper containing bacterial cells

Treat with alkali to disrupt cells and denature DNA, and heat to fix DNA in place

Add radioactive DNA probe for specific DNA sequences

Incubate, then wash to remove probe that has not hybridized

Probe hybridized to DNA

Perform autoradiography

Exposed areas of x-ray film

**FIG. 14.5.** Identification of bacterial colonies containing specific DNA sequences. The autoradiogram can be used to identify bacterial colonies on the original agar plate that contain the desired DNA sequence. Note that an orientation marker is placed on the nitrocellulose and the agar plate so the results of the autoradiogram can be properly aligned with the original plate of bacteria.

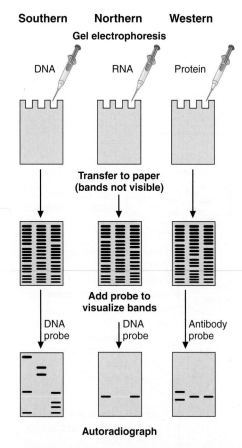

**Southern　　Northern　　Western**

group normally absent from DNA deoxynucleotides). Thus, once they are incorporated into the growing chain, the next nucleotide cannot add, and polymerization is terminated. In this procedure, only one of the four dideoxynucleotides (ddATP, ddTTP, ddGTP, or ddCTP) is added to a tube containing all four normal deoxynucleotides, DNA polymerase, a primer, and the template strand for the DNA that is being sequenced (Fig. 14.7). As DNA polymerase catalyzes the sequential addition

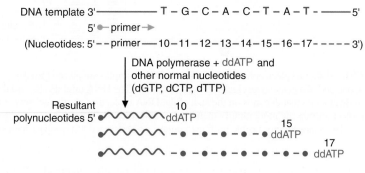

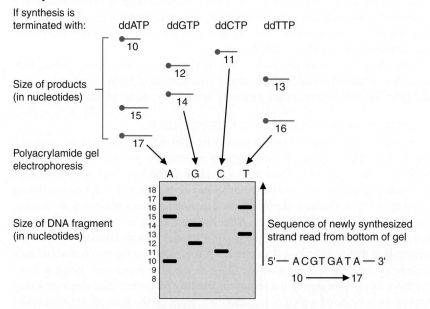

**FIG. 14.6.** Southern, Northern, and Western blots. For Southern blots, DNA molecules are separated by electrophoresis, denatured, transferred to nitrocellulose paper (by "blotting"), and hybridized with a DNA probe. For Northern blots, RNA is electrophoresed and treated similarly except that alkali is not used (first, because alkali hydrolyzes RNA, and second, because RNA is already single stranded). For Western blots, proteins are electrophoresed, transferred to nitrocellulose, and probed with a specific antibody.

**FIG. 14.7.** The Sanger method of DNA sequencing. **A.** Reaction mixtures contain one of the dideoxynucleotides, such as ddATP, and some of the normal nucleotide, dATP, which compete for incorporation into the growing polypeptide chain. When a T is encountered on the template strand (position 10), some of the molecules will incorporate a ddATP, and the chain will be terminated. Those that incorporate a normal dATP will continue growing until position 15 is reached, where they will incorporate either a ddATP or the normal dATP. Only those that incorporate a dATP will continue growing to position 17. Thus, strands of different length from the 5' end are produced, corresponding to the position of a T in the template strand. **B.** DNA sequencing by the dideoxynucleotide method. Four tubes are used. Each one contains DNA polymerase, a DNA template hybridized to a primer, plus dATP, dGTP, dCTP, and dTTP. Either the primer or the nucleotides must have a radioactive label, so bands can be visualized on the gel by autoradiography. Only one of the four dideoxyribonucleotides (ddNTPs) is added to each tube. Termination of synthesis occurs where the ddNTP is incorporated into the growing chain. The template is complementary to the sequence of the newly synthesized strand. Automated DNA sequencers use fluorescent-labeled ddNTPs and a column to separate the oligonucleotides by size. As samples leave the column, their fluorescence is analyzed to determine which base has terminated synthesis of that fragment.

of complementary bases to the 3′ end, the dideoxynucleotide competes with its corresponding normal nucleotide for insertion. Whenever the dideoxynucleotide is incorporated, further polymerization of the strand cannot occur, and synthesis is terminated. Some of the chains will terminate at each of the locations in the template strand that is complementary to the dideoxnucleotide. Consider, for example, a growing polynucleotide strand in which adenine (A) should add at positions 10, 15, and 17. Competition between ddATP and dATP for each position results in some chains terminating at position 10, some at 15, and some at 17. Thus, DNA strands of varying lengths are produced from a template. The shortest strands are closest to the 5′ end of the growing DNA strand because the strand grows in a 5′ to 3′ direction.

Four separate reactions are performed, each with only one of the dideoxynucleotides present (ddATP, ddTTP, ddGTP, ddCTP) plus a complete mixture of normal nucleotides (see Fig. 14.7B). In each tube, some strands are terminated whenever the complementary base for that dideoxynucleotide is encountered. If these strands are subjected to gel electrophoresis, the sequence 5′ to 3′ of the DNA strand complementary to the template can be determined by "reading" from the bottom to the top of the gel, that is, by noting the lanes (A, G, C, or T) in which bands appear, starting at the bottom of the gel and moving sequentially toward the top.

## C. Techniques for Amplifying DNA Sequences

To study genes or other DNA sequences, adequate quantities of material must be obtained. It is often difficult to isolate significant quantities of DNA from the original source. For example, an individual cannot usually afford to part with enough tissue to provide the amount of DNA required for clinical testing. Therefore, the available quantity of DNA has to be amplified.

### 1. CLONING OF DNA

The first technique developed for amplifying the quantity of DNA is known as **cloning** (Fig. 14.8). The DNA that you want amplified (the "foreign" DNA) is attached to a **vector** (a carrier DNA), which is introduced into a host cell that makes multiple copies of the DNA. The foreign DNA and the vector DNA are usually cleaved with the same restriction enzyme, which produces complementary sticky ends in both DNAs. The foreign DNA is then added to the vector. Base-pairs form between the complementary single-stranded regions, and DNA ligase joins the molecules to produce a chimera, or recombinant DNA. As the host cells divide, they replicate their own DNA, and they also replicate the DNA of the vector, which includes the foreign DNA.

If the host cells are bacteria, commonly used vectors are **bacteriophage** (viruses that infect bacteria), **plasmids** (extrachromosomal pieces of circular DNA that are taken up by bacteria), or **cosmids** (plasmids that contain DNA sequences from the bacteriophage lambda). When eukaryotic cells are used as the host, the vectors are often retroviruses, adenoviruses, free DNA, or DNA coated with a lipid layer (liposomes). The foreign DNA sometimes integrates into the host cell genome or it exists as episomes (extrachromosomal fragments of DNA).

Host cells that contain recombinant DNA are called **transformed cells** if they are bacteria, or **transfected** (or **transduced**, if the vector is a virus) **cells** if they are eukaryotes. Markers in the vector DNA are used to identify cells that have been transformed, and probes for the foreign DNA can be used to determine that the host cells actually contain the foreign DNA. If the host cells containing the foreign DNA are incubated under conditions in which they replicate rapidly, large quantities of the foreign DNA can be isolated from the cells. With the appropriate vector and growth conditions that permit expression of the foreign DNA, large quantities of the protein produced from this DNA can be isolated.

A **genomic "library"** in molecular biologists' terms is a set of host cells that collectively contain all of the DNA sequences from the genome of another organism. Thus, a genomic library contains promoter and intron sequences of every gene. A **cDNA library** is a set of host cells that collectively contain all the DNA sequences

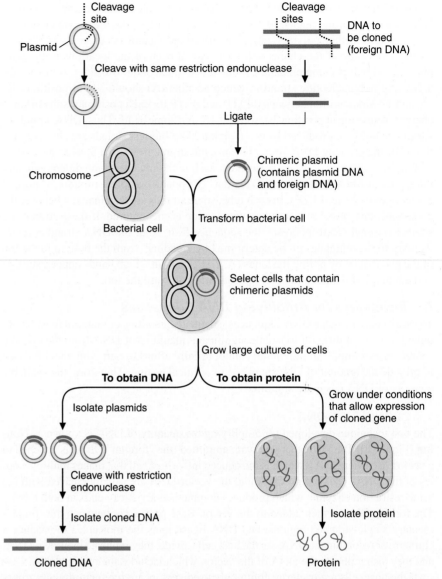

*FIG. 14.8.* Simplified scheme for cloning of DNA in bacteria. A plasmid is a specific type of vector, or carrier, which can contain inserts of foreign DNA of up to 2.0 kb in size. For clarity, the sizes of the pieces of DNA are not drawn to scale (e.g., the bacterial chromosomal DNA should be much larger than the plasmid DNA).

produced by reverse transcriptase from the mRNA obtained from cells of a particular type. Thus, a cDNA library contains all the genes expressed in that cell type, at the stage of differentiation when the mRNA was isolated. Since cDNA libraries are generated by reverse transcription of mRNA, promoter and intron sequences of genes are not present in those libraries.

## 2. POLYMERASE CHAIN REACTION

The polymerase chain reaction (PCR) is an in vitro method that can be used for rapid production of very large amounts of specific segments of DNA. It is particularly suited for amplifying regions of DNA for clinical or forensic testing procedures because only a very small sample of DNA is required as the starting material. Regions of DNA can be amplified by PCR from a single strand of hair or a single drop of blood or semen.

First, a sample of DNA containing the segment to be amplified must be isolated. Large quantities of primers, the four deoxyribonucleoside triphosphates, and

Although only small amounts of semen were obtained from **Victoria T.**'s body, the quantity of DNA in these specimens could be amplified by PCR. This technique provided sufficient amounts of DNA for comparison with DNA samples from the three suspects.

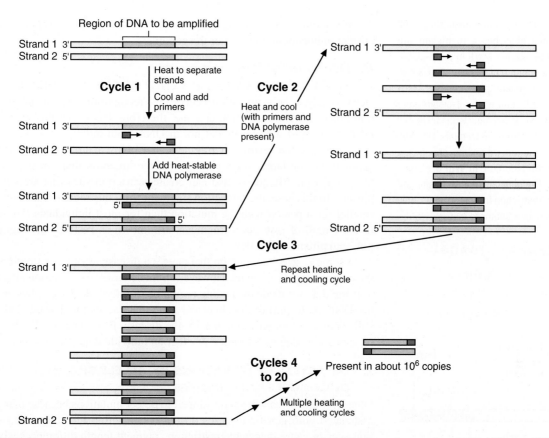

*FIG. 14.9.* PCR. Strand 1 and strand 2 are the original DNA strands. The short *dark blue* fragments are the primers. After multiple heating and cooling cycles, the original strands remain, but most of the DNA consists of amplified copies of the segment (shown in *lighter blue*) synthesized by the heat-stable DNA polymerase.

a heat-stable DNA polymerase are added to a solution in which the DNA is heated to separate the strands (Fig. 14.9). The primers are two synthetic oligonucleotides; one oligonucleotide is complementary to a short sequence in one strand of the DNA to be amplified, and the other is complementary to a sequence in the other DNA strand. As the solution is cooled, the oligonucleotides form base-pairs with the DNA and serve as primers for the synthesis of DNA strands by the heat-stable DNA polymerase (this polymerase is isolated from the bacterium *Thermus aquaticus*, which grows in hot springs). The process of heating, cooling, and new DNA synthesis is repeated many times until a large number of copies of the DNA is obtained. The process is automated, so that each round of replication takes only a few minutes, and in 20 heating and cooling cycles, the DNA is amplified over a millionfold.

## II.  USE OF RECOMBINANT DNA TECHNIQUES FOR DIAGNOSIS OF DISEASE

### A.  DNA Polymorphisms

**Polymorphisms** are variations among individuals of a species in DNA sequences of the genome. They serve as the basis for using recombinant DNA techniques in the diagnosis of disease. The human genome probably contains millions of different polymorphisms. Some polymorphisms involve **point mutations**, the substitution of one base for another. **Deletions** and **insertions** are also responsible for variations in DNA sequences. Some polymorphisms occur within the coding region of genes. Others are found in noncoding regions closely linked to genes involved in the cause of inherited disease, in which case, they can be used as a marker for the disease.

The mutation that causes sickle cell anemia abolishes a restriction site for the enzyme *Mst*II in the β-globin gene. The consequence of this mutation is that the restriction fragment produced by *Mst*II that includes the 5′ end of the β-globin gene is larger (1.3 kb) for individuals with sickle cell anemia than for normal individuals (1.1 kb). Analysis of restriction fragments provides a direct test for the mutation. In **Will S.**'s case, both alleles for β-globin lack the *Mst*II site and produce 1.3-kb restriction fragments; thus, only one band is seen in a Southern blot.

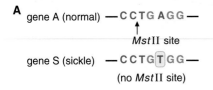

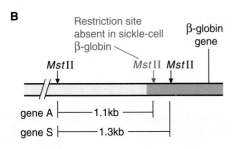

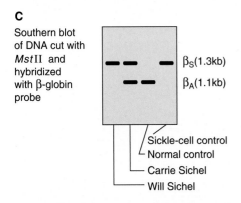

Carriers have both a normal and a mutant allele. Therefore, their DNA will produce both the larger and the smaller *Mst*II restriction fragments. When **Will S.**'s sister **Carrie S.** was tested, she was found to have both the small and the large restriction fragments, and her status as a carrier of sickle cell anemia, initially made on the basis of protein electrophoresis, was confirmed.

As only about 1.5% of the human genome codes for genes, most polymorphisms are present in noncoding regions of the genome.

### B. Detection of Polymorphisms

#### 1. RESTRICTION FRAGMENT LENGTH POLYMORPHISMS

Occasionally, a point mutation occurs in a recognition site for one of the restriction enzymes. The restriction enzyme, therefore, can cut at this restriction site in DNA from most individuals but not in DNA from individuals with this mutation. Consequently, the restriction fragment that binds a probe for this region of the genome will be larger for a person with the mutation than for most members of the population. Mutations also can create restriction sites that are not commonly present. In this case, the restriction fragment from this region of the genome will be smaller for a person with the mutation than for most individuals. These variations in the length of restriction fragments are known as **restriction fragment length polymorphisms** (**RFLPs**).

In some cases, the mutation that causes a disease affects a restriction site within the coding region of a gene. However, in many cases, the mutation affects a restriction site that is outside the coding region but tightly linked (i.e., physically close on the DNA molecule) to the abnormal gene that causes the disease. This RFLP can still serve as a biological marker for the disease. Both types of RFLPs can be used for genetic testing to determine whether an individual has the disease.

#### 2. DETECTION OF MUTATIONS BY ALLELE-SPECIFIC OLIGONUCLEOTIDE PROBES

Other techniques have been developed to detect mutations because many mutations associated with genetic diseases do not occur within restriction enzyme recognition sites or cause detectable restriction fragment length differences when digested with restriction enzymes. For example, oligonucleotide probes (containing 15 to 20 nucleotides) can be synthesized that are complementary to a DNA sequence that includes a mutation. Different probes are produced for alleles that contain mutations and for those that have a normal DNA sequence. The region of the genome that contains the abnormal gene is amplified by PCR, and the samples of DNA are placed in narrow bands on nitrocellulose paper ("slot blotting"). The paper is then treated with the radioactive probe for either the normal or the mutant sequence. Appropriate manipulation of the hybridization conditions (e.g., high temperature and low salt concentration) will allow probes with only a one-base difference to distinguish between normal and mutant alleles, making this a very sensitive technique. Autoradiograms indicate whether the normal or mutant probe has preferentially base-paired (hybridized) with the DNA, that is, whether the alleles are normal or mutated. Carriers have two different alleles, one that binds to the normal probe and one that binds to the mutant probe.

#### 3. TESTING FOR MUTATIONS BY POLYMERASE CHAIN REACTION

If an oligonucleotide that is complementary to a DNA sequence containing a mutation is used as a primer for PCR, the DNA sample used as the template will be amplified only if it contains the mutation. If the DNA is normal, the primer will not hybridize because of the one-base difference, and the DNA will not be amplified. This concept is extremely useful for clinical testing. In fact, several oligonucleotides, each specific for a different mutation and each containing a different label, can be used as primers in a single PCR reaction. This procedure results in rapid and relatively inexpensive testing for multiple mutations.

#### 4. DETECTION OF POLYMORPHISMS CAUSED BY REPETITIVE DNA

Human DNA contains many sequences that are repeated in tandem a variable number of times at certain loci in the genome. These regions are called **highly variable regions** because they contain a **variable number of tandem repeats**

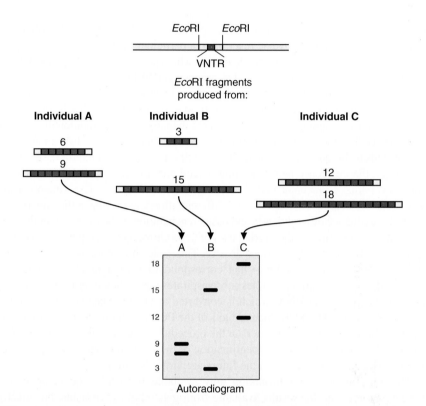

*FIG. 14.10.* Restriction fragments produced from a gene with a VNTR. Each individual has two homologs of every somatic chromosome and thus two genes each containing this region with a VNTR. Cleavage of each individual's genomic DNA with a restriction enzyme produces two fragments containing this region. The length of the fragments depends on the number of repeats they contain. Electrophoresis separates the fragments, and a labeled probe that binds to the fragments allows them to be visualized. Each short *blue* block represents one repeat.

(**VNTR**). Digestion with restriction enzymes that recognize sites that flank the VNTR region produces fragments containing these loci, which differ in size from one individual to another, depending on the number of repeats that are present. Probes used to identify these restriction fragments bind to or near the sequence that is repeated (Fig. 14.10).

The restriction fragment patterns produced from these loci can be used to identify individuals as accurately as the traditional fingerprint. In fact, this restriction fragment technique has been called "DNA fingerprinting" and has gained widespread use in forensic analysis. Family relationships can be determined by this method, and it can be used to help acquit or convict suspects in criminal cases.

Individuals who are closely related genetically will have restriction fragment patterns (DNA fingerprints) that are more similar than those who are more distantly related. Only monozygotic twins will have identical patterns.

## 5.  DNA CHIPS (MICROARRAYS)

Over the past 10 years, a powerful technique has been developed that permits screening many genes simultaneously to determine which alleles of these genes are present in samples obtained from patients. The surface of a small chip is dotted with thousands of pieces of single-stranded DNA, each representing a different gene or segment of a gene. The chip is then incubated with a sample of a patient's DNA, and the pattern of hybridization is determined by computer analysis. The results of the hybridization analysis can be used, for example, to determine which one of the many known mutations for a particular genetic disease is the specific defect underlying a patient's problem. An individual's gene chip also may be used to determine which

DNA samples were obtained from each of the three suspects in **Victoria T.**'s rape and murder case, and these samples were compared with the victim's DNA by using DNA fingerprinting. Because **Victoria T.**'s sample size was small, PCR was used to amplify the regions containing the VNTRs. The results, using a probe for one of the repeated sequences in human DNA, are shown below to illustrate the process. For more positive identification, a number of different restriction enzymes and probes were used. The DNA from suspect 2 produced the same restriction pattern as the DNA from the semen obtained from the victim (indicated as evidence in the blot below). If the other restriction enzymes and probes corroborate this finding, suspect 2 can be identified by DNA fingerprinting as the rapist and murderer.

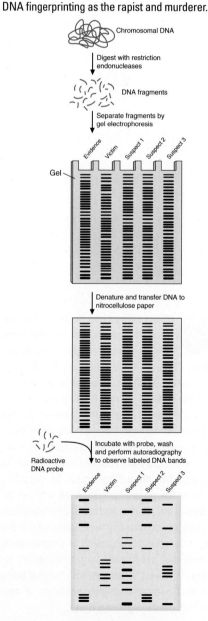

alleles of drug-metabolizing enzymes are present and, therefore, the likelihood of that individual having an adverse reaction to a particular drug.

Another use for a DNA chip is to determine which genes are being expressed. If the mRNA from a tissue specimen is used to produce cDNA by reverse transcriptase, the cDNA will hybridize with only those genes being expressed in that tissue. In the case of a cancer patient, this technique could be used to determine the classification of the cancer much more rapidly and more accurately than the methods traditionally used by pathologists. The treatment then could be more specifically tailored to the individual patient. This technique also can be used to identify the genes required for tissue specificity (e.g., the difference between a muscle cell and a liver cell) and differentiation (the conversion of precursor cells into the different cell types). Experiments using gene chips are helping us to understand differentiation and may open the opportunity to artificially induce differentiation and tissue regeneration in the treatment of disease.

As another example of the myriad uses of gene chips, a gene chip has been developed for the diagnosis of infectious disease. This gene chip contains 29,445 distinct oligonucleotides (60 bases long) that correspond to vertebrate viruses, bacteria, fungi, and parasites. Patient samples (nose aspirates, urine, blood, or tissue samples) are used as a source of RNA, which is converted to cDNA. Specific regions of the cDNA are amplified by PCR (the products of the PCR are fluorescent because of the incorporation of fluorescent primers in the procedure). Hybridization of the fluorescent probe with the chip allows identification of the infectious agent. The possibilities for gene chip applications in the future are virtually limitless.

The huge amount of information now available from the sequencing of the human genome, and the results available from gene chip experiments, has greatly expanded the field of bioinformatics. Bioinformatics can be defined as the gathering, processing, data storage, data analysis, information extraction, and visualization of biological data. Bioinformatics also provides scientists with the capability to organize vast amounts of data in a manageable form that allows easy access and retrieval. Powerful computers are required to perform these analyses. As an example of an experiment that requires these tools, suppose you want to compare the effects of two different immunosuppressant drugs on gene expression in lymphocytes. Lymphocytes would be treated with either nothing (the control) or with the drugs individually (experimental samples). RNA would be isolated from the cells during drug treatment and the RNA converted to fluorescent cDNA using the enzyme reverse transcriptase and a fluorescent nucleotide analogue. The cDNA produced from your three samples would be used as probes for a gene chip containing DNA fragments from more than 5,000 human genes. The samples would be allowed to hybridize to the chips, and you would then have 15,000 results to interpret (the extent of hybridization of each cDNA sample with each of the 5,000 genes on the chip). Computers are used to analyze the fluorescent spots on the chips and to compare the levels of fluorescent intensity from one chip to another. In this way, you could group genes showing similar levels of stimulation or inhibition in the presence of the drugs and compare the two drugs with respect to which genes have had their levels of expression altered by drug treatment.

## III. USE OF RECOMBINANT DNA TECHNIQUES FOR THE PREVENTION AND TREATMENT OF DISEASE

### A. Vaccines

Before the advent of recombinant DNA technology, vaccines were made exclusively from infectious agents that had been either killed or attenuated (altered so that they can no longer multiply in an inoculated individual). Both types of vaccines were potentially dangerous because they could be contaminated with the live, infectious agent. In fact, in a small number of instances, disease has actually been caused by vaccination. For the vaccine to be successful in preventing future infections, the human immune system must respond to the antigenic proteins on the surface of an infectious

Gene chips have been used to answer the question of whether there are changes in gene expression during dieting. Gene chips containing approximately 47,000 unique genes were used, and the probes were cDNA prepared from adipose tissue of control and calorie-restricted overweight women. On caloric restriction, 334 transcripts were upregulated, whereas 342 transcripts were reduced in expression as compared to the control group. As expected, many of the genes corresponded to those involved in metabolism and metabolic regulation. Increased use of these techniques will, in the future, enable development of pharmaceutic agents that specifically target transcripts involved in weight regulation, with the goal being the development and implementation of new and improved weight loss drugs.

agent. The immune system is then prepared if the body is exposed to the infectious agent in the future. By recombinant DNA techniques, these antigenic proteins can be solely produced, in large quantities, completely free of the infectious agent, and used in a vaccine. Thus, any risk of infection by the vaccine is eliminated. The first successful recombinant DNA vaccine to be produced was for the hepatitis B virus.

## B. Production of Therapeutic Proteins

### 1. INSULIN AND GROWTH HORMONE

Recombinant DNA techniques are used to produce proteins that have therapeutic properties. One of the first such proteins to be produced was human **insulin**. Recombinant DNA corresponding to the A chain of human insulin was prepared and inserted into plasmids that were used to transform *E. coli* cells. The bacteria then synthesized the insulin chain, which was purified. A similar process was used to obtain B chains. The A and B chains were then mixed and allowed to fold and form disulfide bonds, producing active insulin molecules. Insulin is not glycosylated, so there was no problem with differences in glycosyltransferase activity between *E. coli* and human cell types.

**Human growth hormone** has also been produced in *E. coli* and is used to treat children with growth hormone deficiencies. Before production of recombinant growth hormone, only a small supply of growth hormone isolated from cadaver pituitary tissue was used, which was in short supply.

### 2. COMPLEX HUMAN PROTEINS

More complex proteins have been produced in mammalian cell culture using recombinant DNA techniques. Three examples will be discussed. The gene for **factor VIII**, a protein involved in blood clotting, is defective in individuals with hemophilia. Before genetically engineered factor VIII became available, several hemophiliac patients died of AIDS or hepatitis that they contracted from transfusions of contaminated blood or from factor VIII isolated from contaminated blood.

**Tissue plasminogen activator** (**TPA**) is a protease in blood that converts plasminogen to plasmin. Plasmin is a protease that cleaves fibrin (a major component of blood clots), and thus, administered TPA dissolves blood clots. Recombinant TPA, produced in mammalian cell cultures, can be administered during or immediately after a heart attack to dissolve the thrombi that occlude coronary arteries and prevent oxygen from reaching the heart muscle. It can also be used to treat other serious conditions caused by blood clots including stroke and pulmonary embolus.

**Hematopoietic growth factors** also have been produced in mammalian cell cultures by recombinant DNA techniques. Erythropoietin can be used in certain types of anemias to stimulate the production of red blood cells. Colony-stimulating factors (CSFs) and interleukins (ILs) can be used after bone marrow transplants and after chemotherapy to stimulate white blood cell production and decrease the risk of infection. Recombinant β-interferon is the first drug known to decrease the frequency and severity of episodes resulting from the effects of demyelination in patients with multiple sclerosis.

## C. Genetic Counseling

One means of preventing disease is to avoid passing defective genes to offspring. If individuals are tested for genetic diseases, particularly in families known to carry a defective allele, genetic counselors can inform them of their risks and options. With this information, individuals can decide in advance whether to have children.

Screening tests based on the recombinant DNA techniques outlined in this chapter have been developed for many inherited diseases. Although these tests are currently rather expensive, particularly, if entire families have to be screened, the cost may be trivial compared with the burden of raising children with severe disabilities. Obviously, cost and ethical considerations must be taken into account, but recombinant DNA technology has provided individuals with the opportunity to make choices.

**Dianne A.** is using a recombinant human insulin called lispro (Humalog) (see Chapter 4, Fig. 4.8). Lispro was genetically engineered so that lysine is at position 28 and proline is at position 29 of the B chain (the reverse of their positions in normal human insulin). Dianne injects lispro right before each meal to help keep her blood sugars controlled. The switch of position of the two amino acids leads to a faster acting insulin homolog. The lispro is absorbed from the site of injection much more quickly than other forms of insulin, and it acts to lower blood glucose levels much more rapidly than the other insulin forms.

**Carrie S.**'s fiancé decided to be tested for the sickle cell gene. He was found to have both the 1.3-kb and the 1.1-kb *Mst*II restriction fragments that include a portion of the β-globin gene. Therefore, like Carrie, he also is a carrier for the sickle cell gene.

Screening can be performed on the prospective parents before conception. If they decide to conceive, the fetus can be tested for the genetic defect. In some cases, if the fetus has the defect, treatment can be instituted at an early stage, even in utero. For certain diseases, early therapy leads to a more positive outcome.

### D. Gene Therapy

The ultimate cure for genetic diseases is to introduce normal genes into individuals who have defective genes. Currently, gene therapy is being attempted in animals, cell cultures, and human subjects. It is not possible at present to replace a defective gene with a normal gene at its usual location in the genome of the appropriate cells. However, as long as the gene is expressed at the appropriate time and produces adequate amounts of the protein to return the person to a normal state, the gene does not have to integrate into the precise place in the genome. Sometimes, the gene does not even have to be in the cells that normally contain it.

Retroviruses were the first vectors used to introduce genes into human cells. Normally, retroviruses enter target cells, their RNA genome is copied by reverse transcriptase, and the double-stranded DNA copy is integrated into the host cell genome. If the retroviral genes (e.g., *gag*, *pol*, and *env*) are first removed and replaced with the therapeutic gene, the retroviral genes integrated into the host cell genome will produce the therapeutic protein rather than the viral proteins. This process works only when the human host cells are undergoing division, so it has limited applicability. Other problems with this technique are that it can only be used with small genes ($\leq 8$ kilobases [kb]) and it may disrupt other genes because the insertion point is random, thereby possibly resulting in cancer.

Adenoviruses, which are natural human pathogens, can also be used as vectors. As in retroviral gene therapy, the normal viral genes required for synthesis of viral particles are replaced with the therapeutic genes. The advantages to using an adenovirus are that the introduced gene can be quite large ($\sim 36$ kb) and infection does not require division of host cells. The disadvantage is that genes carried by the adenovirus do not stably integrate into the host genome, resulting in only transient expression of the therapeutic proteins (but preventing disruption of host genes and the complications that may arise from it). Thus, the treatment must be repeated periodically. Another problem with adenoviral gene therapy is that the host can mount an immune response to the pathogenic adenovirus, causing complications including death.

To avoid the problems associated with viral vectors, researchers are employing treatment with DNA alone or with DNA coated with a layer of lipid (i.e., in liposomes). Adding a ligand for a receptor located on the target cells could aid delivery of the liposomes to the appropriate host cells. Many problems still plague the field of gene therapy. In many instances, the therapeutic genes must be targeted to the cells where they normally function—a difficult task at present. Deficiencies in dominant genes are more difficult to treat than those in recessive genes, and the expression of the therapeutic genes often needs to be carefully regulated. Although the field is moving forward, progress is slow.

Another approach to gene therapy involves the use of antisense oligonucleotides rather than vectors. These oligonucleotides are designed to hybridize either with the target gene to prevent transcription or with mRNA to prevent translation. Again technical problems have plagued the development of therapy based on this theoretically promising idea, although the discovery of microRNAs has renewed interest in this approach.

### IV. PROTEOMICS

The techniques described previously have concentrated on nucleic acid identification, but there have also been rapid advances in analyzing all proteins expressed by a cell at a particular stage of development. The techniques are sophisticated enough to allow comparisons between two different samples, such as normal cells and cancer cells

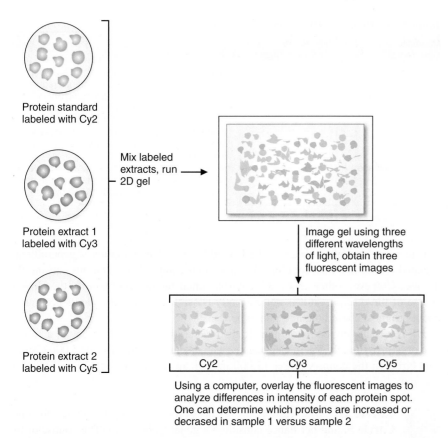

Protein standard labeled with Cy2

Mix labeled extracts, run 2D gel

Protein extract 1 labeled with Cy3

Protein extract 2 labeled with Cy5

Image gel using three different wavelengths of light, obtain three fluorescent images

Cy2        Cy3        Cy5

Using a computer, overlay the fluorescent images to analyze differences in intensity of each protein spot. One can determine which proteins are increased or decreased in sample 1 versus sample 2

*FIG. 14.11.* Using proteomics to determine if a protein is upregulated or downregulated; see text for more details.

from the same tissue. An abbreviated view of this technique is shown in Figure 14.11. Proteins from the two different cell types (A and B) are isolated and labeled with different fluorescent dyes. The proteins are then separated by two-dimensional gel electrophoresis (the first dimension, or separation, is by charge, and the second dimension is by size), which generates a large number of spots that can be viewed under a fluorescent imaging device, each of these spots corresponding to an individual protein. A computer aligns the spots from the two samples and can determine, by the level of fluorescence expressed at each protein spot, if a protein has been up- or downregulated in one sample compared to the other. Proteins whose expression levels change can then be identified by sensitive techniques involving protein mass spectrometry.

The proteomics approach holds great promise in molecularly fingerprinting particular tumors and for discovering novel targets for drug development that are only expressed in the cancerous state. A physician's knowledge of the markers expressed by a particular tumor should allow for specific drug regimes to be used; no longer will one treatment be the norm for a particular tumor. Depending on a patient's proteome, treatments for the patient's specific tumor can be devised and prescribed.

## CLINICAL COMMENTS

Diseases discussed in this chapter are summarized in Table 14.1.

**Susan F.** Cystic fibrosis (CF) is a genetically determined autosomal recessive disease that can be caused by a variety of mutations within the CF gene located on chromosome 7. **Susan F.** was found to have a 3-bp deletion at residue 508 of the CF gene (the mutation present in approximately 70%

**Q:** Testing for CF by DNA sequencing is time consuming and expensive. Therefore, another technique that uses allele-specific oligonucleotide probes has been developed. **Susan F.** and her family were tested by this method. Oligonucleotide probes, complementary to the region where the 3-bp deletion is located, have been synthesized. One probe binds to the mutant ($\Delta F_{508}$) gene and the other to the normal gene.

DNA was isolated from Susan, her parents, and two siblings and amplified by PCR. Samples of the DNA were spotted on nitrocellulose paper, treated with the oligonucleotide probes, and the following results were obtained. (Dark spots indicate binding of the probe.)

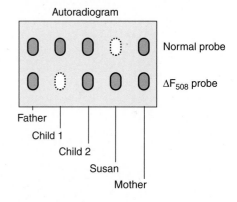

Autoradiogram

Normal probe

$\Delta F_{508}$ probe

Father
Child 1
Child 2
Susan
Mother

Which members of Susan's family have CF, which are normal, and which are carriers?

The most common CF mutation is a 3-bp deletion that causes the loss of phenylalanine at position 508 ($\Delta$508; the $\Delta$ signifies deletion). This mutation is present in more than 70% of CF patients. The defective protein is synthesized in the endoplasmic reticulum but is misfolded. It is therefore not transported to the Golgi but is degraded by a proteolytic enzyme complex called the proteosome. Other mutations responsible for CF generate an incomplete mRNA because of premature stop signals, frameshifts, or abnormal splice sites or create a CFTR channel in the membrane that does not function properly.

**A:** Individuals to which both probes hybridize are carriers (as they contain one normal allele and one mutant allele). Thus, both the father and mother are both carriers of the defective allele, as is one of the two siblings (child 2). Susan has the disease (expressing only the mutant allele), and the other sibling (child 1) is genetically normal (expressing only the normal allele).

**Table 14.1    Diseases Discussed in Chapter 14**

| Disorder or Condition | Genetic or Environmental | Comments |
| --- | --- | --- |
| Cystic fibrosis | Genetic | Cystic fibrosis is due to a mutation in the cystic fibrosis transmembrane conductance regulator (CFTR) protein, which is a chloride channel. The most common mutation in the CFTR gene is Δ508, a triplet deletion which removes codon 508 from the primary sequence. The disease leads to pancreatic duct blockage as well as clogged airways. |
| Sickle cell disease | Genetic | The development of genetic testing for sickle cell disease based on understanding the base change in DNA which leads to the disease. |

of Caucasian patients with CF in the United States). This mutation is generally associated with a more severe clinical course than many other mutations causing the disease. However, other genes and environmental factors may modify the clinical course of the disease, so it is not currently possible to counsel patients accurately about prognosis based on their genotype.

CF is a relatively common genetic disorder in the United States, with a carrier rate of approximately 5% in Caucasians. The disease occurs in 1 per 3,000 Caucasian births in the country (1 per 15,000 in African Americans and 1 per 30,000 in Asians).

 **Carrie S.** After learning the results of their tests for the sickle cell gene, **Carrie S.** and her fiancé consulted a genetic counselor. The counselor informed them that, because they were both carriers of the sickle cell gene, their chance of having a child with sickle cell anemia was fairly high (approximately 1 in 4). She told them that prenatal testing was available with fetal DNA obtained from cells by amniocentesis or chorionic villus sampling. If these tests indicated that the fetus had sickle cell disease, abortion was a possibility. Carrie, because of her religious background, was not sure that abortion was an option for her. But having witnessed her brother's sickle cell crises for many years, she also was not sure that she wanted to risk having a child with the disease. Her fiancé also felt that, at 25 years of age, he was not ready to deal with such difficult problems. They mutually agreed to cancel their marriage plans.

 **Victoria T.** DNA fingerprinting represents an important advance in forensic medicine. Before development of this technique, identification of criminals was far less scientific. The suspect in the rape and murder of **Victoria T.** was arrested and convicted mainly on the basis of the results of DNA fingerprint analysis.

This technique has been challenged in some courts on the basis of technical problems in statistical interpretation of the data and sample collection. It is absolutely necessary for all of the appropriate controls to be run, including samples from the victim's DNA as well as the suspect's DNA. Another challenge to the fingerprinting procedure has been raised because PCR is such a powerful technique that it can amplify minute amounts of contaminating DNA from a source unrelated to the case.

## REVIEW QUESTIONS-CHAPTER 14

1. Electrophoresis resolves double-stranded DNA fragments based on which one of the following?

    A. Sequence
    B. Molecular weight
    C. Isoelectric point
    D. Frequency of CTG repeats
    E. Secondary structure

2. If a restriction enzyme recognizes a six-base sequence, how frequently, on average, will this enzyme cut a large piece of DNA?

    A. Once every 16 bases
    B. Once every 64 bases
    C. Once every 256 bases
    D. Once every 1,024 bases
    E. Once every 4,096 bases

3. Which one of the following statements correctly describes a feature of DNA electrophoresis?

    A. Larger DNA fragments migrate farther in the gel.
    B. DNA fragments migrate toward the negative charge (anode).

    C. DNA can be visualized using UV light and the dye ethidium bromide.
    D. Total human genomic DNA cut by a specific restriction endonuclease will generate three distinctly separable bands.
    E. DNA must be denatured before it can be run in the gel.

4. The best method to determine whether albumin is transcribed in the liver of a mouse model of hepatocarcinoma is which one of the following?

    A. Tissue Northern blot
    B. Genomic library screening
    C. Genomic Southern blot
    D. Tissue Western blot
    E. VNTR analysis

5. Which one of the following would be used to examine hybridization of a radiolabeled nucleic acid probe to a nitrocellulose-bound cDNA?

    A. Southern blot
    B. Northern blot
    C. Western blot

# 15  The Molecular Biology of Cancer

## CHAPTER OUTLINE

## KEY POINTS

- Cancer is the term applied to a group of diseases in which cells no longer respond to normal constraints on growth.
- Cancer arises due to mutations in the genome (either inherited or formed in somatic cells).
- The mutations that lead to cancer occur in certain classes of genes, including
  - Those that regulate cellular proliferation and differentiation
  - Those that suppress growth
  - Those that target cells for apoptosis
  - Those that repair damaged DNA
- Mutations that lead to cancer can be either gain-of-function mutations or loss-of-function mutations within a protein.
  - Gain-of-function mutations occur in protooncogenes, resulting in oncogenes.
  - Loss-of-function mutations occur in tumor suppressor genes.

continued

- Examples of protooncogenes are those involved in signal transduction and cell cycle progression:
  - Growth factors and growth factor receptors
  - Ras (a GTP-binding protein)
  - Transcription factors
  - Cyclins and proteins that regulate them
  - microRNAs that regulate growth-inhibitory proteins
- Examples of tumor suppressor genes include
  - Retinoblastoma (Rb) gene product, which regulates the $G_1$-to-S phase of the cell cycle
  - p53, which monitors DNA damage and arrests cell cycle progression until the damage has been repaired
  - Regulators of *ras*
  - microRNAs, which regulate growth-promoting signals
- Apoptosis, programmed cell death, leads to the destruction of damaged cells that cannot be repaired and consists of three phases:
  - Initiation phase (external signals or mitochondrial release of cytochrome c)
  - Signal integration phase
  - Execution phase
- Apoptosis is regulated by a group of proteins of the Bcl-2 family, which consists of both pro- and antiapoptotic factors.
- Cancer cells have developed mechanisms to avoid apoptosis.
- Multiple mutations are required for a tumor to develop in a patient, acquired over a number of years.
- Both RNA and DNA viruses can cause a normal cell to become transformed.
- Exploitation of DNA repair mechanisms may provide novel means for regulating tumor cell growth.

# THE WAITING ROOM

**Mannie W.** has chronic myelogenous leukemia (CML), a disease in which a single line of myeloid cells in the bone marrow proliferates abnormally, causing a large increase in the number of nonlymphoid white blood cells (see Chapter 13). His myeloid cells contain the abnormal Philadelphia chromosome, which increases their proliferation. He has recently complained of pain and tenderness in various areas of his skeleton, possibly stemming from the expanding mass of myeloid cells within his bone marrow. He also reports a variety of hemorrhagic signs, including bruises (ecchymoses), bleeding gums, and the appearance of small red spots (petechiae caused by release of red cells into the skin).

Determination of abnormal chromosome structures is done by karyotype analysis (see Fig. 9.10). Karyotypes are created by arresting cells in mitotic metaphase, a stage at which the chromosomes are condensed and visible under the light microscope. Nuclei are isolated, placed on a microscope slide, and the chromosomes stained. Pictures of the chromosomes through the microscope are obtained, and the homologous chromosomes are paired. Through this type of analysis, translocations between chromosomes can be determined, as can trisomies and monosomies. As seen in the figure, this karyotype indicates a translocation between chromosomes 9 and 22 (a piece of chromosome 22 is now attached to chromosome 9; note the *arrows* in the figure). This is known as the Philadelphia chromosome, and it gives rise to CML, the disease exhibited by **Mannie W**.

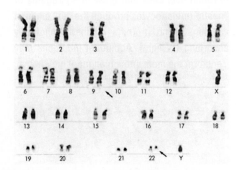

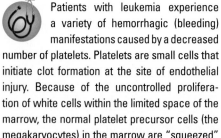 Patients with leukemia experience a variety of hemorrhagic (bleeding) manifestations caused by a decreased number of platelets. Platelets are small cells that initiate clot formation at the site of endothelial injury. Because of the uncontrolled proliferation of white cells within the limited space of the marrow, the normal platelet precursor cells (the megakaryocytes) in the marrow are "squeezed" or crowded and fail to develop into mature platelets. Consequently, the number of mature platelets (thrombocytes) in the circulation falls, and a thrombocytopenia develops. Because there are fewer platelets to contribute to clot formation, bleeding problems are common.

Malignant neoplasms (new growth, a tumor) of epithelial cell origin (including the intestinal lining, cells of the skin, and cells lining the airways of the lungs) are called carcinomas. If the cancer grows in a glandlike pattern, it is an adenocarcinoma. Thus, **Michael T.** and **Clark T.** have adenocarcinomas. **Calvin A.** had a carcinoma arising from melanocytes, which is technically a melanocarcinoma but is usually referred to as a melanoma. Moles (also called nevi) are tumors of the skin. They are formed by melanocytes that have been transformed from highly dendritic single cells interspersed among other skin cells to round oval cells that grow in aggregates or "nests" (melanocytes produce the dark pigment melanin, which protects against sunlight by absorbing UV light). Additional mutations may transform the mole into a malignant melanoma.

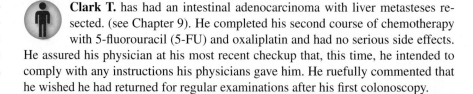 **Michael T.** was diagnosed with a poorly differentiated adenocarcinoma of the lung (see Chapter 10). He underwent a computed tomography (CT) scan to determine the location and severity of the tumor. As a result of these tests, he was considered a candidate for surgical resection of the primary tumor, aimed at cure. He survived the surgery and was recovering uneventfully until 6 months later, when he complained of an increasingly severe right temporal headache. A CT scan of his brain was performed. Results indicated that the cancer, which had originated in his lungs, had metastasized to his brain.

**Clark T.** has had an intestinal adenocarcinoma with liver metasteses resected. (see Chapter 9). He completed his second course of chemotherapy with 5-fluorouracil (5-FU) and oxaliplatin and had no serious side effects. He assured his physician at his most recent checkup that, this time, he intended to comply with any instructions his physicians gave him. He ruefully commented that he wished he had returned for regular examinations after his first colonoscopy.

**Calvin A.** returned to his physician after observing a brownish-black, irregular mole on his forearm (see Chapter 10). His physician thought the mole looked suspiciously like a malignant melanoma and so performed an excision biopsy (surgical removal for cytologic analysis).

## I. CAUSES OF CANCER

The term *cancer* applies to a group of diseases in which cells grow abnormally and form a malignant tumor. Malignant cells can invade nearby tissues and metastasize (i.e., travel to other sites in the body where they establish secondary areas of growth). This aberrant growth pattern results from mutations in genes that regulate proliferation, differentiation, and survival of cells in a multicellular organism. Because of these genetic changes, cancer cells no longer respond to the signals that govern growth of normal cells (Fig. 15.1)

Normal cells in the body respond to signals, such as cell–cell contact (contact inhibition), that direct them to stop proliferating. Cancer cells do not require growth-stimulatory signals and they are resistant to growth-inhibitory signals. They are also resistant to apoptosis, the programmed cell death process whereby unwanted or irreparably damaged cells self-destruct. They have an infinite proliferative capacity and do not become senescent (i.e., they are immortalized). Furthermore, they can grow independent of structural support, such as the extracellular matrix (loss of anchorage dependence).

The study of cells in culture was, and continues to be, a great impetus for the study of cancer. Tumor development in animals can take months, and it was difficult to do experiments with tumor growth in animals. Once cells could be removed from an animal and propagated in a tissue culture dish, the onset of transformation (the normal cell becoming a cancer cell) could be seen in days.

Drs. Michael Bishop and Harold Varmus demonstrated that cancer is not caused by unusual and novel genes, but rather, by mutation within existing cellular genes; and that for every gene that causes cancer (an oncogene), there is a corresponding cellular gene, called the **protooncogene**. Although this concept seems straightforward today, it was a significant finding when it was first announced and, in 1989, Drs. Bishop and Varmus were awarded the Nobel Prize in Medicine.

A single cell that divides abnormally eventually forms a mass called a **tumor**. A tumor can be benign and harmless; the common wart is a benign tumor formed from a slowly expanding mass of cells. In contrast, a malignant neoplasm (malignant tumor) is a proliferation of rapidly growing cells that progressively infiltrate, invade, and destroy surrounding tissue. Tumors develop angiogenic potential, which is the capacity to form new blood vessels and capillaries. Thus, tumors can generate their own blood supply to bring in oxygen and nutrients. Cancer cells also can metastasize, separating from the growing mass of the tumor and traveling through the blood or lymph to unrelated organs, where they establish new growths of cancer cells.

The transformation of a normal cell to a cancer cell begins with damage to DNA (base changes or strand breaks) caused by chemical carcinogens, ultraviolet (UV) light, viruses, or replication errors (see Chapter 10). Mutations result from the damaged DNA if it is not repaired properly or if it is not repaired before replication occurs. A mutation that can lead to transformation also may be inherited. When a cell with one mutation proliferates, this clonal expansion (proliferation of cells arising from a single cell) results in a substantial population of cells containing this one mutation from which one cell may acquire a second mutation relevant to control of cell growth or death. With each clonal expansion, the probability of another transforming mutation increases. As mutations accumulate in genes that control proliferation, subsequent mutations occur even more rapidly until the cells acquire the multiple mutations (in the range of four to seven) necessary for full transformation.

The transforming mutations occur in genes that regulate cellular proliferation and differentiation (protooncogenes), suppress growth (tumor suppressor genes), target irreparably damaged cells for apoptosis, or repair damaged DNA. The genes that regulate cellular growth are called protooncogenes, and their mutated forms are called oncogenes. The term **oncogene** is derived from the Greek word "onkos," meaning bulk or tumor. A transforming mutation in a protooncogene increases the activity or amount of the gene product (a gain-of-function mutation). Tumor suppressor genes (normal growth suppressor genes) and repair enzymes protect against uncontrolled cell proliferation. A transforming mutation in these protective genes results in a loss of activity or a decreased amount of the gene product.

In summary, cancer is caused by the accumulation of mutations in the genes involved in normal cellular growth and differentiation. These mutations give rise to cancer cells that are capable of unregulated, autonomous, and infinite proliferation. As these cancer cells proliferate, they impinge on normal cellular functions, leading to the symptoms exhibited by individuals with the tumors.

## II.  DAMAGE TO DNA LEADING TO MUTATIONS

### A.  Chemical and Physical Alterations in DNA

An alteration in the chemical structure of DNA, or of the sequence of bases in a gene, is an absolute requirement for the development of cancer. The function of DNA depends on the presence of various polar chemical groups in DNA bases, which are capable of forming hydrogen bonds between DNA strands or other chemical reactions. The oxygen and nitrogen atoms in DNA bases are targets for a variety of electrophiles (electron-seeking chemical groups). Chemical carcinogens (compounds that can cause transforming mutations) found in the environment and ingested in foods are generally stable lipophilic compounds that must be activated by metabolism in the body to react with DNA. Many chemotherapeutic agents, which are designed to kill proliferating cells by interacting with DNA, may also act as carcinogens and cause new mutations and tumors while eradicating the old. Structural alterations in DNA also occur through radiation and through UV light, which causes the formation of pyrimidine dimers. More than 90% of skin cancers occur in sunlight-exposed areas. UV rays derived from the sun induce an increased incidence of all skin cancers, including squamous cell carcinoma, basal cell carcinoma, and malignant melanoma of the skin. The wavelength of UV light that is most associated with skin cancer is UVB (280 to 320 nm), which forms pyrimidine dimers in DNA. This type of DNA damage is repaired by nucleotide excision repair pathways that require products of at least 20 genes. With excessive exposure to the sun, the nucleotide excision repair pathway is overwhelmed, and some damage remains unrepaired.

 The first experiments to show that oncogenes were mutant forms of protooncogenes in human tumors involved cells cultured from a human bladder carcinoma. The DNA sequence of the *ras* oncogene cloned from these cells differed from the normal *c-ras* protooncogene. Similar mutations were subsequently found in the *ras* gene of lung and colon tumors. **Clark T.**'s malignant polyp had a mutation in the *ras* protooncogene.

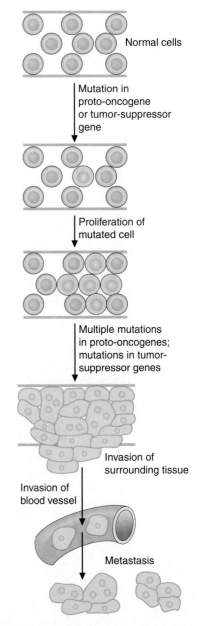

Normal cells

Mutation in proto-oncogene or tumor-suppressor gene

Proliferation of mutated cell

Multiple mutations in proto-oncogenes; mutations in tumor-suppressor genes

Invasion of surrounding tissue

Invasion of blood vessel

Metastasis

*FIG. 15.1.* Development of cancer. Accumulation of mutations in several genes results in transformation. Cancer cells change morphologically, proliferate, invade other tissues, and metastasize.

Each chemical carcinogen or reactant creates a characteristic modification in a DNA base. The DNA damage, if not repaired, introduces a mutation into the next generation when the cell proliferates.

## B.  Gain-of-Function Mutations in Protooncogenes

Protooncogenes are converted to oncogenes by mutations in the DNA that cause a gain in function; that is, the protein can now function better in the absence of the normal activating events. Several mechanisms that lead to the conversion of protooncogenes to oncogenes are known:

- Radiation and chemical carcinogens act (a) by causing a mutation in the regulatory region of a gene, increasing the rate of production of the protooncogene protein; or, (b) by producing a mutation in the coding portion of the oncogene that results in the synthesis of a protein of slightly different amino acid composition capable of transforming the cell (Fig. 15.2A).
- The entire protooncogene or a portion of it may be transposed or translocated, that is, moved from one position in the genome to another (see Fig. 15.2B). In its new location, the protooncogene may be under the control of a promoter that is regulated differently than the promoter that normally regulates this gene. This

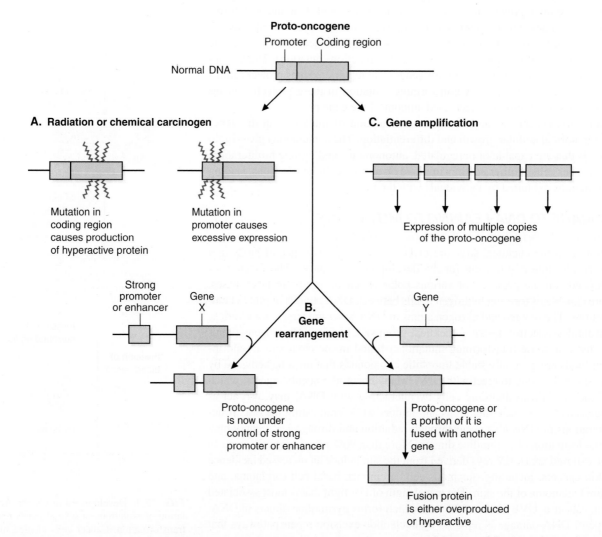

**FIG. 15.2.** Transforming mutations in protooncogenes. **A.** Effect of radiation or chemical carcinogens on protooncogenes or their promoters. The mutations may be point mutations, deletions, or insertions. **B.** Gene rearrangements as caused by transposition or translocation of a protooncogene or protooncogene fragment. **C.** Amplification of a protooncogene allows more protein to be produced.

may allow the gene to be expressed in a tissue where it is not normally expressed or at higher than normal levels of expression. If only a portion of the protooncogene is translocated, it may be expressed as a truncated protein with altered properties, or it may fuse with another gene and produce a fusion protein containing portions of what are normally two separate proteins. The truncated or fusion protein may be hyperactive and cause inappropriate cell growth.

- The protooncogene may be amplified (see Fig. 15.2C), so that multiple copies of the gene are produced in a single cell. If more genes are active, more protooncogene protein will be produced, increasing the growth rate of the cells. As examples, the oncogene N-*myc* (a cell proliferation transcription factor related to c-*myc*) is amplified in some neuroblastomas, and amplification of the *erb*-B2 oncogene (a growth factor receptor) is associated with several breast carcinomas.
- If an oncogenic virus infects a cell, its oncogene may integrate into the host cell genome, permitting production of the abnormal oncogene protein. The cell may be transformed and exhibit an abnormal pattern of growth. Rather than inserting an oncogene, a virus may simply insert a strong promoter into the host cell genome. This promoter may cause increased or untimely expression of a normal protooncogene.

The important point to remember is that transformation results from abnormalities in the normal growth regulatory program caused by gain-of-function mutations in protooncogenes. However, loss-of-function mutations also occur in the tumor suppressor genes, repair enzymes, or activators of apoptosis, and a combination of both types of mutations is usually required for full transformation to a cancer cell.

### C. Mutations in Repair Enzymes

Repair enzymes are the first line of defense preventing conversion of chemical damage in DNA to a mutation (see Chapter 10, Section III.B). DNA repair enzymes are tumor suppressor genes in the sense that errors repaired before replication do not become mutagenic. DNA damage is constantly occurring from exposure to sunlight, background radiation, toxins, and replication errors. If DNA repair enzymes are absent, mutations accumulate much more rapidly, and once a mutation develops in a growth regulatory gene, a cancer may arise. As an example, inherited mutations in the tumor suppressor genes *brca1* and *brca2* predispose women to the development of breast cancer. The protein products of these genes play roles in DNA repair, recombination, and regulation of transcription. A second example, HNPCC (**h**ereditary **n**on**p**olyposis **c**olorectal **c**ancer), was introduced in Chapter 10. It results from inherited mutations in enzymes involved in the DNA mismatch repair system.

### III. ONCOGENES

Protooncogenes control normal cell growth and division. These genes encode proteins that are growth factors, growth factor receptors, signal transduction proteins, transcription factors, cell cycle regulators, and regulators of apoptosis (examples of such proteins are detailed in Table A15.1, which can be found in the online materials associated with the text) @. (The name representing the gene of an oncogene is referred to in lowercase letters and italics [e.g., *myc*], but the name of the protein product is capitalized and italics are not used [e.g., Myc]). The mutations in oncogenes that give rise to transformation are usually gain-of-function mutations; either a more active protein is produced or an increased amount of the normal protein is synthesized.

MicroRNAs (miRNA) can also behave as oncogenes. If a miRNA is overexpressed (increased function), it can act as an oncogene if its target (which would exhibit reduced expression under these conditions) is a protein which is involved in inhibiting or antagonizing cell proliferation.

### A. Oncogenes and Signal Transduction Cascades

All of the proteins in growth factor signal transduction cascades are protooncogenes (Fig. 15.3).

Burkitt lymphoma is a B-cell malignancy, which usually results from a translocation between chromosomes 8 and 14. The translocation of genetic material moves the protooncogene transcription factor c-*myc* (normally found on chromosome 8) to another chromosome, usually chromosome 14. The translocated gene is now under the control of the promoter region for the immunoglobulin heavy chain gene, which leads to inappropriate and overexpression of c-*myc*. The result may be uncontrolled cell proliferation and tumor development. All subtypes of Burkitt lymphoma contain this translocation. EBV infection of B-cells is also associated with certain types of Burkitt lymphoma.

**Mannie W.**'s bone marrow cells contain the Philadelphia chromosome, typical of CML. The Philadelphia chromosome results from a reciprocal translocation between the long arms of chromosome 9 and 22. As a consequence, a fusion protein is produced that contains the N-terminal region of the Bcr protein from chromosome 22 and the C-terminal region of the Abl protein from chromosome 9. *Abl* is a protooncogene, and the resulting fusion protein (Bcr-Abl) has lost its regulatory region and is constitutively active, resulting in deregulated tyrosine kinase activity. When it is active, Abl stimulates the Ras pathway of signal transduction, leading to cell proliferation.

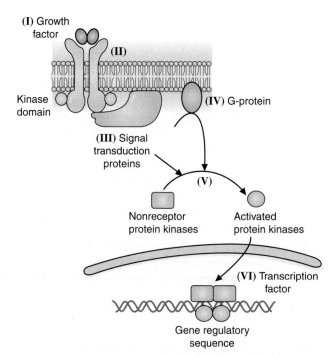

**FIG. 15.3.** Protooncogene sites for transforming mutations in growth factor signaling pathways. *(I)* The amount of growth factor. *(II)* The receptor, which normally must bind the growth factor to dimerize and activate a kinase domain. *(III)* Signal transduction proteins. Some, such as PI-3 kinase, form second messengers. *(IV)* G proteins, and their regulators, which are also signal transduction proteins. *(V)* Nonreceptor protein kinase cascades, which lead to phosphorylation of transcription factors. *(VI)* Nuclear transcription factors that are normally activated through phosphorylation or binding of a ligand.

 The gene for the human epidermal growth factor receptor (*HER2, c-erbB-2*) is overexpressed in 18% to 20% of breast cancer cases. Several drugs have been developed that recognize and block the receptor's action. The drug most studied is trastuzumab (Herceptin), which has been shown to have survival benefit in patients when used in combination with other chemotherapy. However, some tumors that overexpress *HER2* show resistence to Herceptin. Thus, it appears that more complete testing of breast cancer cells may be necessary (using the microarray techniques described in Chapter 14) to develop an effective therapy for each patient with the disease, leading to individualized therapy.

## 1. GROWTH FACTORS AND GROWTH FACTOR RECEPTORS

The genes for both growth factors and growth factor receptors are protooncogenes.

Growth factors generally regulate growth by serving as ligands that bind to cellular receptors located on the plasma membrane (cell surface receptors) (see Chapter 8). Binding of ligands to these receptors stimulates a signal transduction pathway in the cell that activates the transcription of certain genes. If too much of a growth factor or a growth factor receptor is produced, the target cells may respond by proliferating inappropriately. Growth factor receptors may also become oncogenic through translocation or point mutations in domains that affect binding of the growth factor, dimerization, kinase activity, or some other aspect of their signal transmission. In such cases, the receptor transmits a proliferative signal even though the growth factor normally required to activate the receptor is absent. In other words, the receptor is stuck in the "on" position.

## 2. SIGNAL TRANSDUCTION PROTEINS

The genes that encode proteins involved in growth factor signal transduction cascades may also be protooncogenes. Consider, for example, the monomeric G protein Ras. Binding of growth factor leads to the activation of Ras (see Chapter 8). When Ras binds guanosine triphosphate (GTP), it is active, but Ras slowly inactivates itself by hydrolyzing its bound GTP to guanosine diphosphate (GDP) and inorganic phosphate ($P_i$). This controls the length of time that Ras is active. Ras is converted to an oncogenic form by point mutations that decrease the activity of the GTPase domain of Ras, thereby increasing the length of time it remains in the active form.

Ras, when it is active, activates the serine–threonine kinase Raf (a mitogen-activated protein [MAP] kinase kinase kinase), which activates MEK (a MAP kinase kinase), which activates MAP kinase (Fig. 15.4). Activation of MAP kinase results in the phosphorylation of cytoplasmic and nuclear proteins, followed by increased

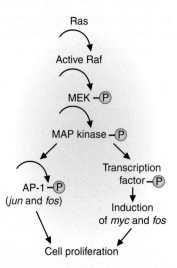

**FIG. 15.4.** Phosphorylation cascade leading to activation of protooncogene transcription factors *myc*, *fos*, and *jun*.

transcription of the transcription factor protooncogenes *myc* and *fos* (see below). Note that mutations in the genes for any of the proteins that regulate MAP kinase activity, as well as those proteins induced by MAP kinase activation, can lead to uncontrolled cell proliferation.

### 3. TRANSCRIPTION FACTORS

Many transcription factors, such as Myc and Fos, are proto-oncoproteins (the products of protooncogenes). MAP kinase, in addition to inducing *myc* and *fos*, also directly activates the activator protein-1 (AP-1) transcription factor through phosphorylation (see Fig. 15.4). AP-1 is a heterodimer formed by the protein products of the *fos* and *jun* families of protooncogenes. The targets of AP-1 activation are genes involved in cellular proliferation and progression through the cell cycle as are the targets of the *myc* transcription factor. The synthesis of the transcription factor c-*myc* is tightly regulated in normal cells, and it is expressed only during the S phase of the cell cycle. In a large number of tumor types, this regulated expression is lost and c-*myc* becomes inappropriately expressed or overexpressed throughout the cell cycle, driving cells continuously to proliferate.

The net result of alterations in the expression of transcription factors is the increased production of the proteins that carry out the processes required for proliferation.

### B. Oncogenes and the Cell Cycle

The growth of human cells involving DNA replication and cell division in the cell cycle is activated by growth factors, hormones, and other messengers. These activators work through cyclins and cyclin-dependent kinases (CDKs) that control progression from one phase of the cycle to another (Fig. 15.5). For quiescent cells to proliferate, they must leave $G_0$ and enter the $G_1$ phase of the cell cycle (see Chapter 10, Fig. 10.6). If the proper sequence of events occurs during $G_1$, the cells enter the S phase and are committed to DNA replication and cell division. Similarly, during $G_2$, cells make a commitment to mitotic division. CDKs are made constantly throughout the cell cycle but require binding of a specific cyclin to be active. Different cyclins made at different times in the cell cycle control each of the transitions ($G_1$/S, S/$G_2$, $G_2$/M).

The activity of the cyclin-CDK complex is further regulated through phosphorylation and through inhibitory proteins called **cyclin-dependent kinase inhibitors** **(CKIs)** (Fig. 15.6). CKIs slow cell cycle progression by binding and inhibiting the cyclin-CDK complexes. CDKs are also controlled through activating phosphorylation by CAK (cyclin-activating kinases) and inhibitory hyperphosphorylation kinases.

### IV. TUMOR SUPPRESSOR GENES

Like the oncogenes, the tumor suppressor genes encode molecules involved in the regulation of cell proliferation. Table A15.2 in the online supplement to the text provides several examples. @ The normal function of tumor suppressor proteins is generally to inhibit proliferation in response to certain signals such as DNA damage. The signal is removed when the cell is fully equipped to proliferate; the effect of the elimination of tumor suppressor genes is to remove the brakes on cell growth. They affect cell cycle regulation, signal transduction, transcription, and cell adhesion. The products of tumor suppressor genes frequently modulate pathways that are activated by the products of protooncogenes.

Tumor suppressor genes contribute to the development of cancer when both copies of the gene are inactivated. This is different from the case of protooncogene mutations because only one allele of a protooncogene needs to be converted to an oncogene to initiate transformation. As with the oncogenes, this is also applicable to miRNAs. If the expression of a particular miRNA is lost, the mRNA it regulates would be overexpressed, which could lead to enhanced cellular proliferation. Thus, miRNAs can be classified as either oncogenes (overexpression) or tumor suppressors (loss of function), depending on the genes which they regulate.

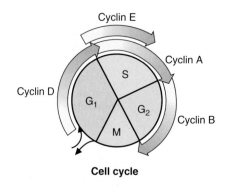

**FIG. 15.5.** Cyclin synthesis during different phases of the cell cycle.

 In addition to sunlight and a preexisting nevus, hereditary factors also play a role in the development of malignant melanoma. Ten percent of melanomas tend to run in families. Some of the suspected melanoma-associated genes include the tumor suppressor gene *p16* (an inhibitor of cdk 4) and CDK4. **Calvin A.** was the single child of parents who had died of a car accident in their 50s, and thus, a familial tendency could not be assessed.

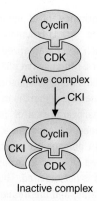

**FIG. 15.6.** CKI inhibition of cyclin-CDK activity.

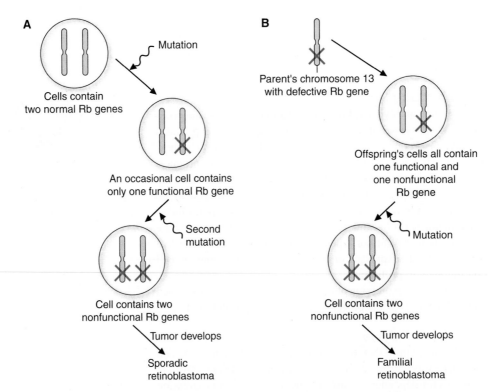

*FIG. 15.7.* Mutations in the retinoblastoma (*rb*) gene. **A.** Sporadic retinoblastoma. **B.** Familial retinoblastoma.

## A. Tumor Suppressor Genes That Regulate the Cell Cycle Directly

The two best understood cell cycle regulators that are also tumor suppressors are the retinoblastoma (*rb*) and *p53* genes.

### 1. THE RETINOBLASTOMA GENE

The retinoblastoma gene product, Rb, functions in the transition from G$_1$ to S phase and regulates the activation of members of the E2F family of transcription factors, which are necessary for this transition to occur. If an individual inherits a mutated copy of the *rb* allele, there is a 100% chance of that individual developing retinoblastoma, because of the high probability that the second allele of *rb* will gain a mutation (Fig.15.7). This is considered familial retinoblastoma. Individuals who do not inherit mutations in *rb*, but who develop retinoblastoma, are said to have sporadic retinoblastoma, and acquire two specific mutations, one in each *rb* allele of the retinoblast, during their lifetime.

### 2. p53, THE GUARDIAN OF THE GENOME

The p53 protein is a transcription factor that regulates the cell cycle and apoptosis—programmed cell death. Loss of both *p53* alleles is found in more than 50% of human tumors. The p53 acts as the "guardian of the genome" by halting replication in cells that have suffered DNA damage and targeting unrepaired cells to apoptosis.

In response to DNA-damaging mutagens, ionizing radiation, or UV light, the level of p53 rises (Fig. 15.8, *circle 1*). The p53, acting as a transcription factor, stimulates transcription of p21 (a member of the Cip/Kip family of CKIs), as shown in Figure 15.8, *circle 2*. The p21 gene product inhibits the cyclin-CDK complexes, which prevents the phosphorylation of Rb and release of E2F proteins. The cell is thus prevented from entering S phase. The p53 also stimulates the transcription of a number of DNA repair enzymes (including **g**rowth **a**rrest and **DNA d**amage 45 [GADD45]) (Fig. 15.8, *circle 3*). If the DNA is successfully repaired, p53 induces its own downregulation through the activation of the *mdm2* gene. If the DNA repair was not successful, p53

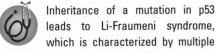

Inheritance of a mutation in p53 leads to Li-Fraumeni syndrome, which is characterized by multiple types of tumors. Mutations in p53 are present in more than 50% of human tumors. These are secondary mutations within the cell, and if p53 is mutated, the overall rate of cellular mutation will increase, because there is no p53 to check for DNA damage, to initiate the repair of the damaged DNA, or to initiate apoptosis if the damage is not repaired. Thus, damaged DNA is replicated, and the frequency of additional mutations within the same cell increases remarkably.

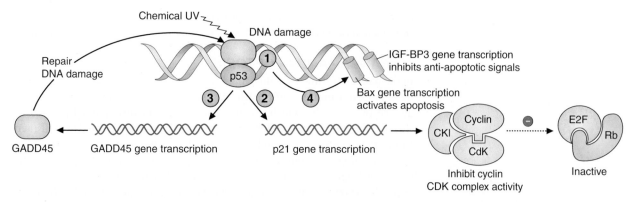

**FIG. 15.8.** The p53 and cell cycle arrest. Mechanisms that recognize DNA damage stop p53 degradation and modify the p53 protein *(circle 1)*. The p53 stimulates the transcription of p21 *(circle 2)* and GADD45 *(circle 3)*. The p21 blocks the cyclin/CDK phosphorylation of Rb, which continues to inhibit the E2F family of transcription factors, thereby blocking cell progression through the cell cycle. GADD45 allows the DNA damage to be repaired. If the damage is not repaired, apoptotic genes are activated *(circle 4)*.

activates a number of genes involved in apoptosis, including *bax* (discussed in the following text) and insulin-like growth factor–binding protein 3 (IGF-BP3) (Fig. 15.8, *circle 4*). The IGF-BP3 protein product binds the receptor for insulin-like growth factor, which presumably induces apoptosis by blocking the antiapoptotic signaling by growth factors, and the cell enters a growth factor deprivation mode.

## B. Tumor Suppressor Genes That Affect Receptors and Signal Transduction

Tumor suppressor genes may encode receptors, components of the signaling transduction pathway, or transcription factors.

### 1. REGULATORS OF RAS

The Ras family of proteins is involved in signal transduction for many hormones and growth factors (see previous discussion) and is, therefore, oncogenic. The activity of these pathways is interrupted by GAPs (**G**TPase-**a**ctivating **p**roteins), which vary among cell types. Neurofibromin, the product of the tumor suppressor gene *NF-1*, is a nervous system–specific GAP that regulates the activity of Ras in neuronal tissues. The growth signal is transmitted so long as the Ras protein binds GTP. Binding of NF-1 to Ras activates the GTPase domain of Ras, which hydrolyzes GTP to GDP, thereby inactivating Ras. Without a functional neurofibromin molecule, Ras is perpetually active.

### 2. PATCHED AND SMOOTHENED

A good example of tumor suppressors and oncogenes working together is provided by the coreceptor genes *patched* and *smoothened*, which encode the receptor for the hedgehog class of signaling peptides (the strange names of some of the tumor suppressor genes arose because they were first discovered in *Drosophila* [fruit fly], and the names of *Drosophila* mutations are often based on the appearance of a fly that expresses the mutation. Once the human homolog is found, it is given the same name as the *Drosophila* gene). These coreceptors normally function to control growth during embryogenesis and illustrate the importance of maintaining a balance between oncogenes and tumor suppressor genes. The patched receptor protein inhibits smoothened, its coreceptor protein. Binding of a hedgehog ligand to patched releases the inhibition of smoothened, which then transmits an activating signal to the nucleus, stimulating new gene transcription. *Smoothened* is a proto-oncogene, and *patched* is a tumor suppressor gene. If *patched* loses its function (definition of a tumor suppressor), then smoothened can signal the cell to proliferate, even in the absence of a hedgehog signal. Conversely, if *smoothened* undergoes a gain-of-function mutation (definition of an oncogene), it can signal in the absence of

An inherited mutation in *NF-1* can lead to neurofibromatosis, a disease primarily of numerous benign, but painful, tumors of the nervous system. The movie *Elephant Man* was based on an individual who was believed to have this disease. Recent analysis of the patient's remains, however, indicates that he may have suffered from the rare Proteus syndrome, not neurofibromatosis.

the hedgehog signal, even in the presence of patched. Inherited mutations in either *smoothened* or *patched* will lead to an increased incidence of basal cell carcinoma.

## V.  CANCER AND APOPTOSIS

In the body, superfluous or unwanted cells are destroyed by a pathway called **apoptosis** or **programmed cell death**. Apoptosis is a regulated energy-dependent sequence of events by which a cell self-destructs. In this suicidal process, the cell shrinks, the chromatin condenses, and the nucleus fragments. The cell membrane forms blebs (outpouches), and the cell breaks up into membrane-enclosed apoptotic vesicles (apoptotic bodies) containing varying amounts of cytoplasm, organelles, and DNA fragments. Phosphatidylserine, a lipid on the inner leaflet of the cell membrane, is exposed on the external surface of these apoptotic vesicles. It is one of the phagocytic markers recognized by macrophages and other nearby phagocytic cells that engulf the apoptotic bodies.

Apoptosis is a normal part of multiple processes in complex organisms: embryogenesis, the maintenance of proper cell number in tissues, the removal of infected or otherwise injured cells, the maintenance of the immune system, and aging. It can be initiated by injury, radiation, free radicals or other toxins, withdrawal of growth factors or hormones, binding of proapoptotic cytokines, or interactions with cytotoxic T-cells in the immune system. Apoptosis can protect organisms from the negative effects of mutations by destroying cells with irreparably damaged DNA before they proliferate. Just as an excess of a growth signal can produce an excess of unwanted cells, the failure of apoptosis to remove excess or damaged cells can contribute to the development of cancer.

### A.  Normal Pathways to Apoptosis

Apoptosis can be divided into three general phases: an initiation phase, a signal integration phase, and an execution phase. Apoptosis can be initiated by external signals that work through death receptors, such as tumor necrosis factor (TNF), or deprivation of growth hormones (Fig. 15.9). It can also be initiated by intracellular events that affect mitochondrial integrity (e.g., oxygen deprivation, radiation) and irreparably damaged DNA. In the signal integration phase, these proapoptotic signals are balanced against antiapoptotic cell survival signals by several pathways including members of the Bcl-2 family of proteins. The execution phase is carried out by proteolytic enzymes called **caspases**.

### 1.  CASPASES

Caspases are cysteine proteases that cleave peptide bonds next to an aspartate residue. They are present in the cell as procaspases, zymogen-type enzyme precursors that are activated by proteolytic cleavage of the inhibitory portion of their polypeptide chain. The different caspases are generally divided into two groups according to their function: initiator caspases, which specifically cleave other procaspases; and execution caspases, which cleave other cellular proteins involved in maintaining cellular integrity (see Fig. 15.9). The initiator caspases are activated through two major signaling pathways: the death receptor pathway and the mitochondrial integrity pathway. They activate the execution caspases, which cleave protein kinases involved in cell adhesion, lamins that form the inner lining of the nuclear envelope, actin and other proteins required for cell structure, and DNA repair enzymes. They also cleave an inhibitor protein of the endonuclease CAD (**c**aspase-**a**ctivated **D**Nase), thereby activating CAD to initiate the degradation of cellular DNA. With destruction of the nuclear envelope, additional endonucleases ($Ca^{2+}$- and $Mg^{2+}$-dependent) also become activated.

### 2.  THE DEATH RECEPTOR PATHWAY TO APOPTOSIS

The death receptors are a subset of TNF-1 receptors, which includes Fas/CD95, TNF-receptor 1 (TNF-R1) and death receptor 3 (DR3). These receptors form a trimer that binds TNF-1 or another death ligand on its external domain and binds

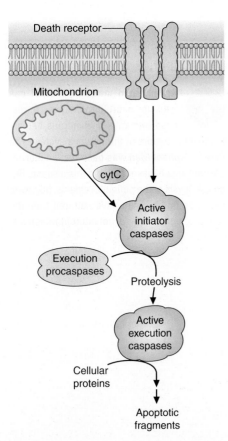

**FIG. 15.9.** Major components in apoptosis. The release of cytochrome c from mitochondria or activation of death receptors can both lead to the initiation of apoptosis.

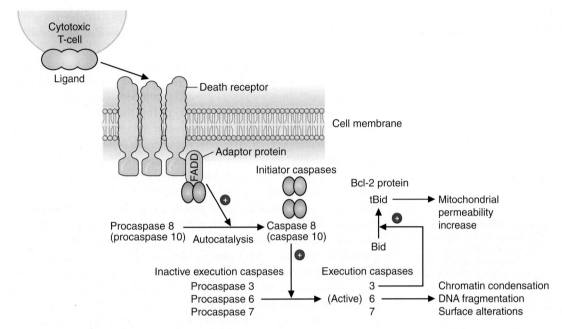

**FIG. 15.10.** The death receptor pathway to apoptosis. The ligand (either a free ligand or a cell surface-associated protein from another cell) binds to the death receptor, which makes a scaffold for autocatalytic activation of caspases 8 (and sometimes 10). Active caspases 8 (and sometimes 10) cleave apoptotic execution caspases directly. However, the pathway also activates Bid, which acts on mitochondrial membrane integrity.

adaptor proteins to its intracellular domain (Fig.15.10). The activated TNF-receptor complex forms the scaffold for binding two molecules of procaspase 8 (or procaspase 10), which autocatalytically cleave each other to form active caspase 8 (or caspase 10). Caspases 8 and 10 are initiator caspases that activate execution caspases 3, 6, and 7. Caspase 3 also cleaves a Bcl-2 protein, Bid, to a form that activates the mitochondrial integrity pathway to apoptosis.

### 3. THE MITOCHONDRIAL INTEGRITY PATHWAY TO APOPTOSIS

Apoptosis is also induced by intracellular signals indicating that cell death should occur. Examples of these signals include growth factor withdrawal, cell injury, the release of certain steroids, and an inability to maintain low levels of intracellular calcium. All of these treatments, or changes, lead to release of cytochrome c from the mitochondria (Fig. 15.11). Cytochrome c is a necessary protein component of the mitochondrial electron transport chain that is loosely bound to the outside of the inner mitochondrial membrane. Its release initiates apoptosis.

In the cytosol, cytochrome c binds Apaf (pro**a**poptotic **p**rotease-**a**ctivating **f**actor). The Apaf–cytochrome c complex binds caspase 9, an initiator caspase, to form an active complex called the **apoptosome**. The apoptosome, in turn, activates execution caspases (3, 6, and 7) by zymogen cleavage.

### 4. INTEGRATION OF PRO- AND ANTIAPOPTOTIC SIGNALS BY THE BCL-2 FAMILY OF PROTEINS

The Bcl-2 family members are decision makers that integrate prodeath and antideath signals to determine whether the cell should commit suicide. Both proapoptotic and antiapoptotic members of the Bcl-2 family exist (Table 15.1). Bcl-2 family members contain regions of homology, known as Bcl-2 homology (BH) domains. There are four such domains. The antiapoptotic factors contain all four domains (BH1 to BH4). The channel forming proapoptotic factors contain just three domains (BH1 to BH3), whereas the proapoptotic BH3-only family members contain just one BH domain, BH3.

The antiapoptotic Bcl-2–type proteins (including Bcl-2, Bcl-L, and Bcl-w) have at least two ways of antagonizing death signals. They insert into the outer

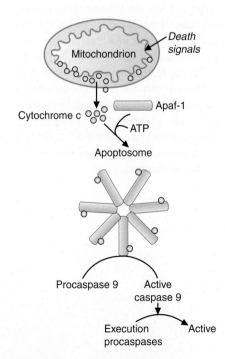

**FIG. 15.11.** The mitochondrial integrity pathway releases cytochrome c, which binds to Apaf and forms a multimeric complex called the apoptosome. The apoptosome converts procaspase 9 to active caspase 9, an initiator caspase, which is released by the apoptosome into the cytosol.

**Table 15.1   Examples of Bcl-2 Family Members**

Antiapoptotic
   Bcl-2
   Bcl-x
   Bcl-w
Proapoptotic
Channel-forming
   Bax
   Bak
   Bok
Proapoptotic
BH3-only
   Bad
   Bid
   Bim

Roughly 30 Bcl-2 family members are currently known. These proteins play tissue-specific as well as signal pathway–specific roles in regulating apoptosis. The tissue specificity is overlapping. For example, Bcl-2 is expressed in hair follicles, kidney, small intestines, neurons, and the lymphoid system, whereas Bcl-x is expressed in the nervous system and hemato-poietic cells.

When Bcl-2 is mutated and onco-genic, it is usually overexpressed, for example, in follicular lymphoma and CML. Overexpression of Bcl-2 disrupts the normal regulation of pro- and antiapoptotic factors and tips the balance to an antiapop-totic stand. This leads to an inability to destroy cells with damaged DNA, such that mutations can accumulate within the cell. Bcl-2 is also a multidrug-resistant transport protein and if it is overexpressed, it will block the induction of apoptosis by antitumor agents by rapidly re-moving them from the cell. Thus, strategies are being developed to reduce Bcl-2 levels in tu-mors that overexpress it before initiating drug or radiation treatment.

mitochondrial membrane to antagonize channel-forming proapoptotic factors, thereby decreasing cytochrome c release. They may also bind cytoplasmic Apaf so that it cannot form the apoptosome complex (Fig. 15.12).

These antiapoptotic Bcl-2 proteins are opposed by proapoptotic family members that fall into two categories: ion-channel–forming members and BH3-only mem-bers. The prodeath ion-channel–forming members, such as Bax, are very similar to the antiapoptotic family members, except that they do not contain the binding do-main for Apaf. They have the other structural domains, however, and when they di-merize with proapoptotic BH3-only members in the outer mitochondrial membrane, they form an ion channel that promotes cytochrome c release rather than inhibiting it (see Fig. 15.12). The prodeath BH3-only proteins (e.g., Bim and Bid) contain only the structural domain that allows them to bind to other Bcl-2 family members (the BH3 domain) and not the domains for binding to the membrane, forming ion channels, or binding to Apaf. Their binding activates the prodeath family members and inactivates the antiapoptotic members. When the cell receives a signal from a prodeath agonist, a BH3 protein such as Bid is activated (see Fig. 15.12). The BH3 protein activates Bax (an ion-channel–forming proapoptotic channel member), which stimulates release of cytochrome c. Normally, Bcl-2 acts as a death antagonist by binding Apaf and keeping it in an inactive state. However, at the same time that Bid is activating Bax, Bid also binds to Bcl-2, thereby disrupting the Bcl-2–Apaf complex and freeing Apaf to bind to released cytochrome c to form the apoptosome.

## B.   Cancer Cells Bypass Apoptosis

Apoptosis should be triggered by a number of stimuli, such as withdrawal of growth factors, elevation of p53 in response to DNA damage, monitoring of DNA damage by repair enzymes, or release of TNF or other immune factors. However, mutations in oncogenes can create apoptosis-resistant cells primarily by continuously stimulat-ing the growth promoting pathways.

## C.   MicroRNAs and Apoptosis

Recent work has identified a number of miRNAs which regulate apoptotic factors. Bcl-2, for example, is regulated by at least 2 miRNAs, designated as miR-15 and miR-16. Expression of these miRNAs will control Bcl-2 (an antiapoptotic factor) levels in the cell. If, for any reason, the expression of these miRNAs is altered, Bcl-2 levels will also be altered, promoting either apoptosis (if Bcl-2 levels decrease) or cell proliferation (if Bcl-2 levels increase). Loss of both of these miRNAs is found in 68% of chronic lymphocytic leukemia (CLL) cells, most often due to a deletion on

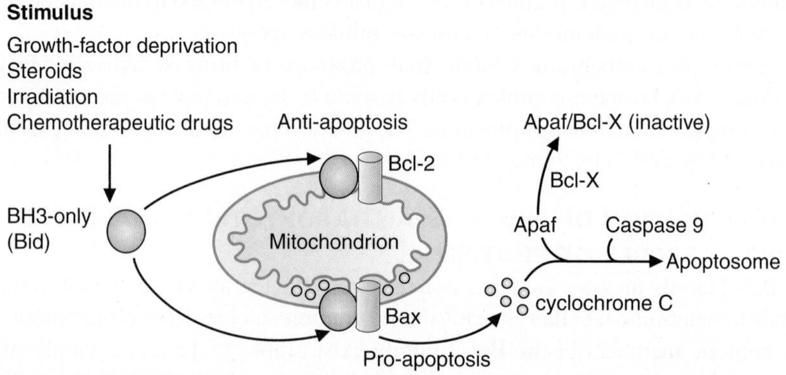

**Stimulus**

Growth-factor deprivation
Steroids
Irradiation
Chemotherapeutic drugs

FIG. 15.12.   Roles of the Bcl-2 family members in regulating apoptosis. Bcl-2, which is anti-apoptotic, binds Bid (or tBid) and blocks formation of channels that allow cytochrome c release from the mitochondria. Death signals result in activation of a BH3-only protein such as Bid, which can lead to mitochondrial pore formation, swelling, and release of cytochrome c. Bid binds to and activates the membrane ion-channel proapoptotic protein Bax, activating cyto-chrome c release, which binds to Apaf and leads to formation of the apoptosome.

chromosome 13q14. Loss of miR-15 and -16 expression would lead to an increase in Bcl-2 levels, favoring increased cell proliferation.

Other miRNA species have been identified, which regulate factors involved in apoptosis. For example, miR-21 regulates the expression of the programmed cell death 4 (PDCD4) gene. PDCD4 is upregulated during apoptosis and functions to block translation. Loss of miR-21 activity would lead to cell death, as PDCD4 would be overexpressed. However, overexpression of miR-21 would be antiapoptotic, as PDCD4 expression would be ablated.

## VI. CANCER REQUIRES MULTIPLE MUTATIONS

Cancer takes a long time to develop in humans because multiple genetic alterations are required to transform normal cells into malignant cells (see Fig. 15.1). A single change in one oncogene or tumor suppressor gene in an individual cell is not adequate for transformation. For example, if cells derived from biopsy specimens of normal cells are not already "immortalized," that is, able to grow in culture indefinitely, addition of the *ras* oncogene to the cells is not sufficient for transformation. However, additional mutations in a combination of oncogenes, for example, *ras* and *myc*, can result in transformation. Epidemiologists have estimated that four to seven mutations are required for normal cells to be transformed.

Cells accumulate multiple mutations through clonal expansion. When DNA damage occurs in a normally proliferative cell, a population of cells with that mutation is produced. Expansion of the mutated population enormously increases the probability of a second mutation in a cell containing the first mutation. After one or more mutations in protooncogenes or tumor suppressor genes, a cell may proliferate more rapidly in the presence of growth stimuli and with further mutations grow autonomously, that is, independent of normal growth controls. Enhanced growth increases the probability of further mutations. Some families have a strong predisposition to cancer. Individuals in these families have inherited a mutation or deletion of one allele of a tumor suppressor gene, and as progeny of that cell proliferate, mutations can occur in the second allele, leading to a loss of control of cellular proliferation. These familial cancers include familial retinoblastoma, familial adenomatous polyps of the colon, and multiple endocrine neoplasia (MEN), one form of which involves tumors of the thyroid, parathyroid, and adrenal medulla (MEN type II).

Studies of benign and malignant polyps of the colon show that these tumors have a number of different genetic abnormalities. The incidence of these mutations increases with the level of malignancy. In the early stages, normal cells of the intestinal epithelium proliferate, develop mutations in the APC gene, and polyps develop (Fig. 15.13). This change is associated with a mutation in the *ras* protooncogene that converts it to an active oncogene. Progression to the next stage is associated with a deletion or alteration of a tumor suppressor gene on chromosome 5. Subsequently, mutations occur in chromosome 18, inactivating a gene that may be involved in cell adhesion, and in chromosome 17, inactivating the *p53* tumor suppressor gene. The cells become malignant, and further mutations result in growth that is more aggressive and metastatic. This sequence of mutations is not always followed precisely, but an accumulation of mutations in these genes is found in a large percentage of colon carcinomas.

## VII. AT THE MOLECULAR LEVEL, CANCER IS MANY DIFFERENT DISEASES

More than 20% of the deaths in the United States each year are caused by cancer, with tumors of the lung, large intestine, and the breast being the most common. Different cell types typically use different mechanisms through which they lose the ability to control their own growth. An examination of the genes involved in the development of cancer shows that a particular type of cancer can arise in multiple ways. For example, patched and smoothened are the receptor and coreceptor for the

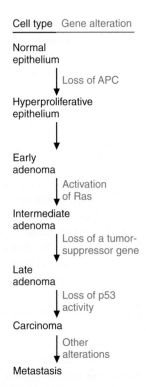

**FIG. 15.13.** Possible steps in the development of colon cancer. The changes do not always occur in this order, but the most benign tumors have the lowest frequency of mutations, and the most malignant have the highest frequency.

**Michael T.** had been smoking for 40 years before he developed lung cancer. The fact that cancer takes so long to develop has made it difficult to prove that the carcinogens in cigarette smoke cause lung cancer. Studies in England and Wales show that cigarette consumption by men began to increase in the early 1900s. Followed by a 20-year lag, the incidence in lung cancer in men also began to rise. Women began smoking later, in the 1920s. Again the incidence of lung cancer began to increase after a 20-year lag.

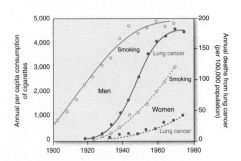

A treatment for CML based on rational drug design has been developed. The fusion protein Bcr-Abl is found only in transformed cells that express the Philadelphia chromosome and not in normal cells. Once the structure of Bcr-Abl was determined, the drug imatinib (Gleevec) was designed to specifically bind to and inhibit only the active site of the fusion protein and not the normal protein. Imatinib was successful in blocking Bcr-Abl function, thereby stopping cell proliferation, and in some cells inducing apoptosis, so the cells would die. Because normal cells do not express the hybrid protein, they were not affected by the drug. The problem with this treatment is that some patients suffered relapses, and when their Bcr-Abl proteins were studied, it was found that in some patients, the fusion protein had a single amino acid substitution near the active site that prevented imatinib from binding to the protein. Other patients had an amplification of the Bcr-Abl gene product. Other tyrosine kinase inhibitors (such as dasatinib and nilotinib) can also be used in treating CML if a resistance to imatinib is encountered.

signaling peptide, sonic hedgehog. Either mutation of *smoothened*, an oncogene, or inactivation of *patched*, a tumor suppressor gene, can give rise to basal cell carcinoma. Similarly, transforming growth factor β and its signal transduction proteins SMAD4/DPC are part of the same growth-inhibiting pathway and either may be absent in colon cancer. Thus, treatments that are successful for one patient with colon cancer may not be successful in a second patient with colon cancer because of the differences in the molecular basis of each individual's disease (this now appears to be the case with other cancers as well). Cancer treatment is advancing to include targeted therapies, which require identifying the molecular lesions involved in a particular disease and using appropriate treatments accordingly. The use of proteomics and gene chip technology (see Chapter 14) to genotype tumor tissues and to understand which proteins they express will aid greatly in allowing patient-specific treatments to be developed.

## VIII. VIRUSES AND HUMAN CANCER

Three RNA retroviruses are associated with the development of cancer in humans: human T-lymphotrophic virus type 1 (HTLV-1), HIV, and hepatitis C. There are also DNA viruses associated with cancer, such as hepatitis B, Epstein–Barr virus (EBV), human papillomavirus (HPV), and human herpesvirus 8 (HHV-8).

HTLV-1 causes adult T-cell leukemia. The HTLV-1 genome encodes a protein Tax, which is a transcriptional coactivator. The cellular protooncogenes *c-sis* and *c-fos* are activated by Tax, thereby altering the normal controls on cellular proliferation and leading to malignancy. Thus, *tax* is a viral oncogene without a counterpart in the host cell genome.

Infection with HIV, the virus that causes AIDS, leads to the development of neoplastic disease through several mechanisms. HIV infection leads to immunosuppression and, consequently, loss of immune-mediated tumor surveillance. HIV-infected individuals are predisposed to non-Hodgkin lymphoma, which results from an overproduction of T-cell lymphocytes. The HIV genome encodes a protein, Tat, a transcription factor that activates transcription of the *interleukin-6* (IL-6) and *interleukin-10* (IL-10) genes in infected T-cells. IL-6 and IL-10 are growth factors that promote proliferation of T-cells, and thus, their increased production may contribute to the development of non-Hodgkin lymphoma. Tat can also be released from infected cells and act as an angiogenic (blood vessel forming) growth factor. This property is thought to contribute to the development of Kaposi sarcoma.

DNA viruses also cause human cancer but by different mechanisms. Chronic hepatitis B infections will lead to hepatocellular carcinoma. A vaccine currently is available to prevent hepatitis B infections. EBV is associated with B- and T-cell lymphomas, Hodgkin disease, and other tumors. The EBV encodes a Bcl-2 protein that restricts apoptosis of the infected cell. HHV-8 has been associated with Kaposi sarcoma. Certain strains of papillomavirus have been shown to be the major cause of cervical cancer, and a vaccine has been developed against the specific papillomavirus strains that often lead to cancer development.

### CLINICAL COMMENTS

Diseases discussed in this chapter are summarized in Table 15.2.

**Mannie W.** The treatment of a symptomatic patient with CML whose white blood cell count is in excess of 50,000 cells/mL is usually initiated with a tyrosine kinase inhibitor. If the patient is intolerant to all tyrosine kinase inhibitors, then busulfan, a DNA-alkylating agent, may be used. Other alkylating agents, such as cyclophosphamide, have also been used alone or in combination with busulfan. Purine and pyrimidine antagonists and hydroxyurea

**Table 15.2   Diseases Discussed in Chapter 15**

| Disease or Disorder | Environmental or Genetic | Comments |
|---|---|---|
| Chronic myelogenous leukemia | Environmental | Chromosomal translocation leading to the novel Bcr-Abl protein being produced, leading to uncontrolled cell growth. Rational drug design has led to Bcr-Abl targeted agents, such as imatinib, which have a high rate of initial success in controlling tumor cell proliferation. |
| Lung adenocarcinoma | Environmental | Lung tumor, due to inhalation of mutagenic compounds over a number of years. Longitudinal data indicates a 20-year lag from the initiation of smoking and a rise in cancer incidence in such individuals. |
| Intestinal adenocarcinoma | Both | Colon tumors may result from environmental insult, leading to mutations, or an inherited mutation in a tumor suppressor gene, such as APC. Hereditary nonpolyposis colon cancer (HNPCC) is due to inherited mutations in proteins involved in DNA mismatch repair. |
| Melanoma | Environmental | Tumor of the melanocyte, leading to uncontrolled cell growth. Mutations associated with malignant melanomas include ras, p53, p16 (a regulator of cdk4), cdk4, and cadherin–β-catenin regulation. |
| Burkitt lymphoma | Environmental | Disorder due to a chromosomal translocation, usually chromosomes 8 and 14, leading to the transcription factor *myc* being moved from chromosome 8 to 14. This leads to inappropriate and overexpression of c-*myc*, leading to uncontrolled cell proliferation. |
| Li-Fraumeni syndrome | Genetic | An inherited mutation in the protein p53, which is responsible for protecting the genome against environmental damage. Lose of p53 activity will lead to an increased mutation rate, eventually leading to a mutation in a gene which regulates cell proliferation. |
| Neurofibromatosis (NF-1) | Genetic | A mutation in a protein (neurofibromin-1) which regulates the GTPase activity of *ras*, which leads to numerous, benign tumors of the nervous system. |

(an inhibitor of the enzyme ribonucleotide reductase, which converts ribonucleotides to deoxyribonucleotides for DNA synthesis) are sometimes effective in CML as well. In addition, past experience with both γ- and β-interferon has shown promise in increasing survival in these patients, if they are intolerant to the tyrosine kinase ihibitors. Interestingly, the interferons have been associated with the disappearance of the Philadelphia chromosome in dividing marrow cells of some patients treated in this way.

 **Michael T.** Surgical resection of the primary lung cancer with an attempt at cure was justified in **Michael T.**, who had a good prognosis with a $T_1,N_0,M_0$ staging classification preoperatively. Without any evidence of metastases at that time, a preoperative CT scan of the brain would not have been justified. This conservative approach would require scanning of all of the potential sites for metastatic disease from a non–small cell cancer of the lung in all patients who present in this way. In an era of runaway costs of health care delivery, such an approach could not be considered cost-effective.

Unfortunately, Michael developed a metastatic lesion in the right temporal cortex of his brain. Because metastases were almost certainly present in other organs, Michael's brain tumor was not treated surgically. In spite of palliative radiation therapy to the brain, **Michael T.** succumbed to his disease just 9 months after its discovery, an unusually virulent course for this malignancy. On postmortem examination, it was found that his body was riddled with metastatic disease.

**Clark T.** requires regular colonoscopies to check for new polyps in his intestinal tract. Because the development of a metastatic adenoma requires a number of years (because of the large numbers of mutations that must occur), frequent checks will enable new polyps to be identified and removed before malignant tumors develop.

**Calvin A.** The biopsy of Calvin's excised mole showed that it was not malignant. Important clinical signs of a malignant melanoma are change in color or variation in color and irregular borders. Unlike benign (nondysplastic)

 The TNM system standardizes the classification of tumors. The T stands for the stage of tumor (the higher the number, the worse the prognosis), the N stands for the number of lymph nodes that are affected by the tumor (again, the higher the number, the worse the prognosis), and M stands for the presence of metastasis (0 for none, 1 for the presence of metastatic cells).

 Mutations associated with malignant melanomas include *ras* (gain of function in growth signal transduction oncogene), p53 (loss of function of tumor suppressor gene), p16 (loss of function in Cdk inhibitor tumor suppressor gene), Cdk4 (gain of function in a cell cycle progression oncogene), and cadherin–β-catenin regulation (loss of regulation that requires attachment).

nevi, melanomas exhibit striking variations in pigmentation, appearing in shades of black, brown, red, dark blue, and gray. Additional clinical warning signs of a melanoma are enlargement of a preexisting mole, itching or pain in a preexisting mole, and development of a new pigmented lesion during adult life. **Calvin A.** was advised to conduct a monthly self-examination, to have a clinical skin examination once or twice yearly, to avoid sunlight, and to use appropriate sunscreens.

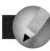

## REVIEW QUESTIONS-CHAPTER 15

1. The *ras* oncogene in **Clark T.**'s malignant polyp differs from the *c-ras* protooncogene only in the region that encodes the N-terminus of the protein. This portion of the normal and mutant sequences is

```
              10          20          30
Normal  ATGACGGAATATAAGCTGGTGGTGGTGGGCGCCGGCGGT
Mutant  ATGACGGAATATAAGCTGGTGGTGGTGGGCGCCGTCGGT
```

This mutation is similar to the mutation found in the *ras* oncogene in various tumors. What type of mutation converts the *ras* protooncogene to an oncogene?

A. An insertion that disrupts the reading frame of the protein
B. A deletion that disrupts the reading frame of the protein
C. A missense mutation that changes one amino acid within the protein
D. A silent mutation that produces no change in amino acid sequence of the protein
E. An early termination that creates a stop codon in the reading frame of the protein

2. The mechanism through which Ras becomes an oncogenic protein is which one of the following?

A. Ras remains bound to GAP.
B. Ras can no longer bind cAMP.
C. Ras has lost its GTPase activity.
D. Ras can no longer bind GTP.
E. Ras can no longer be phosphorylated by MAP kinase.

3. Which one of the following statements best describes a characteristic of oncogenes?

A. All retroviruses contain at least one oncogene.
B. Retroviral oncogenes were originally obtained from a cellular host chromosome.
C. Protooncogenes are genes found in retroviruses, which have the potential to transform normal cells when expressed inappropriately.
D. The oncogenes that lead to human disease are different from those that lead to tumors in animals.
E. Oncogenes are mutated versions of normal viral gene products.

4. When p53 increases in response to DNA damage, which one of the following events occurs?

A. p53 induces transcription of cdk4.
B. p53 induces transcription of cyclin D.
C. p53 binds E2F to activate transcription.
D. p53 induces transcription of p21.
E. p53 directly phosphorylates the transcription factor *jun*.

5. A tumor suppressor gene is best described by which one of the following?

A. A gain-of-function mutation leads to uncontrolled proliferation.
B. A loss-of-function mutation leads to uncontrolled proliferation.
C. When it is expressed, the gene suppresses viral genes from being expressed.
D. When it is expressed, the gene specifically blocks the $G_1$/S checkpoint.
E. When it is expressed, the gene induces tumor formation.

# 16   Cellular Bioenergetics: ATP and $O_2$

## CHAPTER OUTLINE

## KEY POINTS

- Bioenergetics refers to cellular energy transformations.
- The high-energy phosphate bonds of ATP are a cell's primary source of energy.
- ATP is generated through cellular respiration; the oxidation of fuels to carbon dioxide and water.
- The electrons captured from fuel oxidation regenerate ATP via the process of oxidative phosphorylation.
- The energy available from ATP hydrolysis can be used for
  - Mechanical work (muscle contraction)
  - Transport work (establishment of ion gradients across membranes)
  - Biochemical work (energy-requiring chemical reactions)
- Energy released from fuel oxidation that is not used for work is transformed into and released as heat.
- Fuel oxidation is regulated to maintain ATP homeostasis.
- $\Delta G^{0'}$ is the change in Gibbs free energy at pH 7.0 under standard conditions.
- Fuel oxidation has a negative $\Delta G^{0'}$; the products formed have a lower chemical energy than the reactants (an exergonic reaction pathway).
- ATP synthesis has a positive $\Delta G^{0'}$ and is endergonic; the reaction requires energy.
- Metabolic pathways have an overall negative $\Delta G^{0'}$.

# THE WAITING ROOM

**Otto S.** is a 26-year-old medical student who has completed his first year of medical school. He is 5 feet 10 inches tall and began medical school weighing 154 lb, within his ideal weight range (see Chapter 1). By the time he finished his last examination in his first year, he weighed 187 lb. He had calculated his basal metabolic rate (BMR) at approximately 1,680 kcal, and his energy expenditure for physical exercise equal to 30% of his BMR. He planned on returning to his pre–medical school weight in 6 weeks over the summer by eating 576 kcal less each day and playing 7 hours of tennis every day. However, he did a summer internship instead of playing tennis. When Otto started his second year of medical school, he weighed 210 lb.

**Cora N.** is a 64-year-old female who had a myocardial infarction (MI; often referred to as a "coronary") 8 months ago. Although she managed to lose 6 lb since the MI, she remains overweight and has not reduced the fat content of her diet adequately. The graded aerobic exercise program she started 5 weeks after her infarction is now followed irregularly, falling far short of the cardiac conditioning intensity prescribed by her cardiologist. She is readmitted to the hospital's cardiac care unit (CCU) after experiencing a severe "viselike pressure" in the midchest area while cleaning ice from the windshield of her car. The electrocardiogram (ECG) shows evidence of a new posterior wall MI. Signs and symptoms of left ventricular failure are present.

**Cora N.** suffered a heart attack 8 months ago and had a significant loss of functional heart muscle. She occasionally gets pain while walking. The pain she is experiencing is called angina (or angina pectoris) and is a crushing or constricting pain located in the center of the chest, often radiating to the neck or arms (see Ann J., Chapters 4 and 5). The most common cause of angina is partial blockage of coronary arteries from atherosclerosis. The heart muscle cells beyond the block receive an inadequate blood flow and oxygen and they die when ATP production falls too low.

## I.  ENERGY AVAILABLE TO DO WORK

The central role of the high-energy bonds of ATP is summarized in the adenosine triphosphate–adenosine diphosphate (**ATP-ADP**) **cycle** (Fig. 16.1). The basic principle of the cycle is that fuel oxidation generates ATP, and hydrolysis of ATP to ADP provides the energy to perform most of the work required in the cell. ATP has therefore been called the energy currency of our cells. To keep up with the demand, we must constantly replenish our ATP supply through the use of oxygen ($O_2$) for fuel oxidation.

The amount of energy from ATP cleavage available to do useful work is related to the difference in energy levels between the products and substrates of the reaction and is called the change in **Gibbs free energy** ($\Delta G$) ($\Delta$, difference; G, Gibbs free energy). In cells, the $\Delta G$ for energy production from fuel oxidation must be greater than the $\Delta G$ of energy-requiring processes, such as protein synthesis and muscle contraction, for life to continue.

The heart is a specialist in the transformation of ATP chemical bond energy into mechanical work. Each single heartbeat uses approximately 2% of the ATP in the heart. If the heart were not able to regenerate ATP, all its ATP would be hydrolyzed in less than 1 minute. Because the amount of ATP required by the heart is so high, it must rely on the pathway of oxidative phosphorylation for generation of this ATP. In **Cora N.'s** heart, hypoxia (lack of oxygen) is affecting her ability to generate ATP.

### A.  The High-Energy Phosphate Bonds of ATP

The amount of energy released or required by bond cleavage or formation is determined by the chemical properties of the substrates and products. The bonds between the phosphate groups in ATP are called phosphoanhydride bonds (Fig. 16.2). When these bonds are hydrolyzed, energy is released because the products of the reaction (ADP and phosphate) are more stable, with lower bond energies, than the reactants (ATP and water [$H_2O$]). The instability of the phosphoanhydride bonds arises from their negatively charged phosphate groups, which repel each other and strain the bonds between them. It takes energy to make the phosphate groups stay together. In contrast, there are fewer negative charges in ADP to repel each other. The phosphate group as a free anion is more stable than it is in ATP because of an increase in resonance structures (i.e., the electrons of the oxygen double bond are shared by all the oxygen atoms). As a consequence, ATP hydrolysis is energetically favorable and proceeds with release of energy as heat.

In the cell, ATP is not directly hydrolyzed. Energy released as heat from ATP hydrolysis cannot be transferred efficiently into energy-requiring processes such as

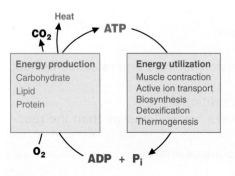

*FIG. 16.1.* The ATP-ADP cycle.

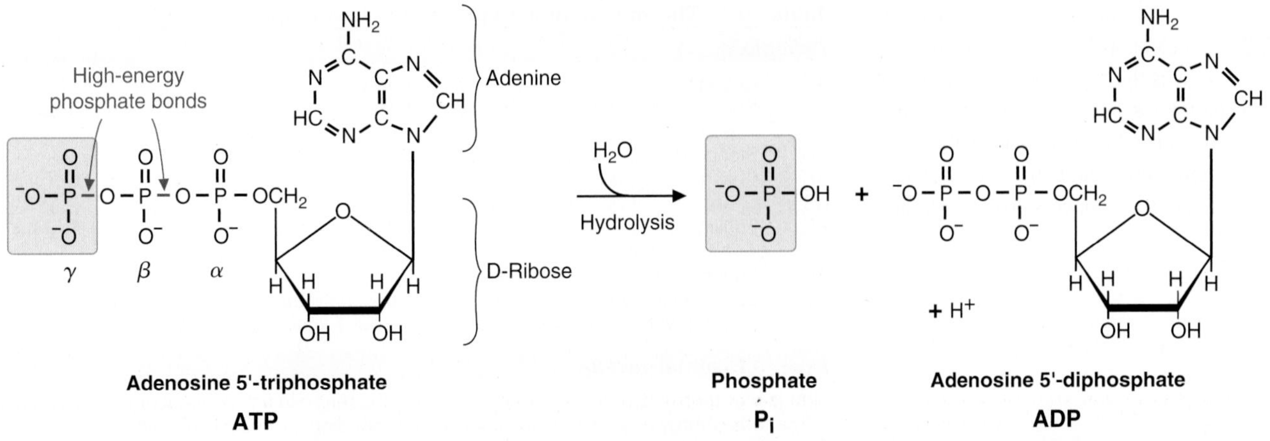

**FIG. 16.2.** Hydrolysis of ATP to ADP and Pi. Cleavage of the phosphoanhydride bonds between either the β- and γ-phosphates or the α- and β-phosphates releases the same amount of energy, approximately −7.3 kcal/mole. However, hydrolysis of the phosphate-adenosine bond (a phosphoester bond) releases less energy (~3.4 kcal/mole), and consequently, this bond is not considered a high-energy phosphate bond. During ATP hydrolysis, the change in disorder during the reaction is small and so $\Delta G$ values at physiological temperature (37°C) are similar to those at standard temperature (25°C). $\Delta G$ is affected by pH, which alters the ionization state of the phosphate groups of ATP and by the intracellular concentration of $Mg^{2+}$ ions, which bind to the β- and γ-phosphate groups of ATP.

biosynthetic reactions or maintenance of an ion gradient. Instead, cellular enzymes directly transfer the phosphate group to a metabolic intermediate or protein that is part of the energy-requiring process (a phosphoryl transfer reaction).

### B. Change in Free Energy (ΔG) during a Reaction

How much energy can be obtained from ATP hydrolysis to do the work required in the cell? The maximum amount of useful energy that can be obtained from a reaction is called $\Delta G$, the change in Gibbs free energy. The value of $\Delta G$ for a reaction can be influenced by the initial concentration of substrates and products, by temperature, pH, and pressure. The $\Delta G^0$ for a reaction refers to the energy change for a reaction starting at 1 M substrate and product concentrations and proceeding to equilibrium (equilibrium by definition occurs when there is no change in substrate and product concentrations with time). $\Delta G^{0'}$ is the value for $\Delta G^0$ under standard conditions (pH = 7.0, [H₂O] = 55 M, and 25°C) as well as standard concentrations (Table 16.1).

$\Delta G^{0'}$ is equivalent to the chemical bond energy of the products minus that of the reactants, corrected for energy that has gone into entropy (an increase in amount of molecular disorder). This correction for change in entropy is very small for most reactions occurring in cells, and thus, the $\Delta G^{0'}$ for hydrolysis of various chemical bonds reflects the amount of energy available from that bond.

The value of −7.3 kcal/mole (−30.5 kJ/mole) that is generally used for the $\Delta G^{0'}$ of ATP hydrolysis is thus the amount of energy available from hydrolysis of ATP under standard conditions that can be spent on energy-requiring processes; it defines the "monetary value" of our "ATP currency." Although the difference between cellular conditions (pH 7.3, 37°C) and standard conditions is very small, the difference between cellular concentrations of ATP, ADP, and inorganic phosphate (Pi) and the standard 1-M concentrations is huge and greatly affects the availability of energy in the cell.

### C. Exothermic and Endothermic Reactions

The value of $\Delta G^{0'}$ tells you whether the reaction requires or releases energy, the amount of energy involved, and the ratio of products to substrates at equilibrium. The negative value for the $\Delta G^{0'}$ of ATP hydrolysis indicates that, if you begin with equimolar (1 M) concentrations of substrates and products, the reaction proceeds in the forward direction with the release of energy. From initial concentrations of 1 M, the ATP concentration will decrease, and ADP and Pi will increase until equilibrium is reached.

**Q:** The reaction catalyzed by phosphoglucomutase (PGM) is reversible and functions in the synthesis of glycogen from glucose as well as the degradation of glycogen back to glucose. If the $\Delta G^0$ for conversion of G6P to G1P is +1.65 kcal/mole, what is the $\Delta G^{0'}$ of the reverse reaction?

**A:** The $\Delta G^{0'}$ for the reverse reaction is $-1.65$ kcal. The change in free energy is the same for the forward and reverse directions but has an opposite sign. Because negative $\Delta G^{0'}$ values indicate favorable reactions, this reaction under standard conditions favors the conversion of G1P to G6P.

**Table 16.1  Thermodynamic Expressions, Laws, and Constants**

### Definitions

| | |
|---|---|
| $\Delta G$ | Change in free energy or Gibbs free energy |
| $\Delta G^0$ | Standard free energy change, $\Delta G$ starting with 1 M concentrations of substrates and products |
| $\Delta G^{0'}$ | Standard free energy change at 25°C, pH 7.0 |
| $\Delta H$ | Change in enthalpy or heat content |
| $\Delta S$ | Change in entropy or increase in disorder |
| $K'_{eq}$ | Equilibrium constant at 25°C, pH 7.0, incorporating $[H_2O] = 55.5$ M and $[H^+] = 10^{-7}$ M in the constant |
| $\Delta E^{0'}$ | Change in reduction potential |
| ~P | Biochemical symbol for a high-energy phosphate bond (i.e., a bond which is hydrolyzed with the release of more than about 7 kcal/mole of heat) |

### Laws of Thermodynamics

First law of thermodynamics, the conservation of energy: In any physical or chemical change, the total energy of a system, including its surroundings, remains constant.
Second law of thermodynamics: The universe tends toward disorder. In all natural processes, the total entropy of a system always increases.

### Constants

Units of $\Delta G$ and $\Delta H$ = cal/mole or J/mole: 1 cal = 4.18 J
T, absolute temperature: K, Kelvin = 273 + °C (25°C = 298°K)
R, universal gas constant: 1.98 cal/mole-K or 8.31 J/mole-K
F, Faraday constant: F = 23 kcal/mole-volt or 96,500 J/V·mole
Units of $E_0'$, volts

### Formulas

$\Delta G = \Delta H - T\Delta S$
$\Delta G^{0'} = -RT\ln K'_{eq}$
$\Delta G^{0'} = -nF\Delta E^{0'}$
$\ln = 2.303 \log_{10}$

For a reaction in which a substrate S is converted to a product P, the ratio of the product concentration to the substrate concentration at equilibrium is given by:

**Equation 16.1.**

$$\Delta G^{0'} = -RT \ln[P]/[S]$$

Table 16.2 has a more general form of this equation; R is equal to the gas constant (1.98 calories/mole-degree Kelvin), and T is equal to the temperature in degrees Kelvin.

Thus, the difference in chemical bond energies of the substrate and product ($\Delta G^{0'}$) determines the concentration of each at equilibrium.

Reactions such as ATP hydrolysis are **exergonic** (release energy) or **exothermic** (release heat). Both exergonic and exothermic reactions have a negative $\Delta G^{0'}$ and release energy while proceeding in the forward direction to equilibrium.

**Table 16.2  A General Expression for $\Delta G$**

To generalize the expression for $\Delta G$, consider a reaction in which

$$aA + bB \rightarrow cC + dD$$

The lowercase letters denote that a moles of A will combine with b moles of B to produce c moles of C and d moles of D.

$$\Delta G^{0'} = -RT \ln K_{eq} = -RT \ln \frac{[C]_{eq}^c [D]_{eq}^d}{[A]_{eq}^a [B]_{eq}^b}$$

and

$$\Delta G^0 = \Delta G^{0'} + RT \ln \frac{[C]^c [D]^d}{[A]^a [B]^b}$$

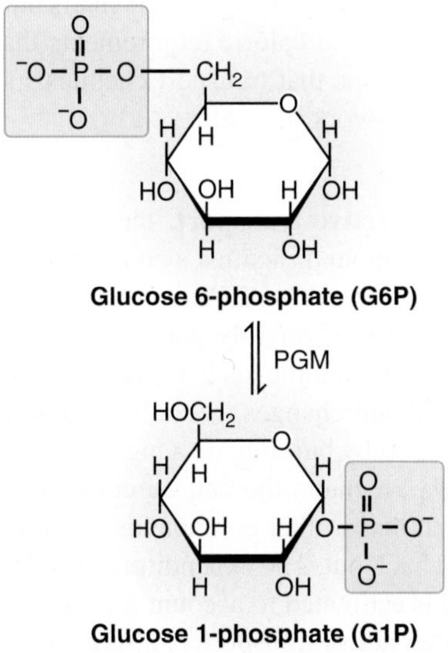

**Glucose 6-phosphate (G6P)**

PGM

**Glucose 1-phosphate (G1P)**

For G6P → G1P:

$\Delta G^{0\prime} = +1.6$ kcal/mol

$\Delta G^{0\prime} = -RT \ln \dfrac{[G1P]}{[G6P]}$

*FIG. 16.3.* The phosphoglucomutase reaction. The forward direction (formation of G1P) is involved in converting glucose to glycogen and the reverse direction in converting glycogen to G6P. *PGM,* phosphoglucomutase.

Endergonic, or endothermic, reactions have a positive $\Delta G^{0\prime}$ for the forward direction (the direction shown), and the backward direction is favored. For example, in the pathway of glycogen synthesis, phosphoglucomutase converts glucose-6-phosphate (G6P) to glucose-1-phosphate (G1P). G1P has a higher phosphate bond energy than G6P because the phosphate is on the aldehyde carbon (Fig. 16.3). The $\Delta G^{0\prime}$ for the forward direction (G1P → G6P) is therefore positive. Beginning at equimolar concentrations of both compounds, there is a net conversion of G1P back to G6P and, at equilibrium, the concentration of G6P is higher than G1P. The exact ratio is determined by the $\Delta G^{0\prime}$ for the reaction.

It is often said that a reaction with a negative $\Delta G^{0\prime}$ proceeds spontaneously in the forward direction, meaning that products accumulate at the expense of reactants. However, $\Delta G^{0\prime}$ is not an indicator of the velocity of the reaction or the rate at which equilibrium can be reached. In the cell, the velocity of the reaction depends on the efficiency and amount of enzyme available to catalyze the reaction (see Chapter 7), and therefore, "spontaneously" in this context can be misleading.

## II.  ENERGY TRANSFORMATIONS TO DO MECHANICAL AND TRANSPORT WORK

For work in the cell to be done, a mechanism must be available for converting the chemical bond energy of ATP into another form, such as an Na⁺ gradient across a membrane. These energy transformations usually involve intermediate steps in which ATP is bound to a protein, and cleavage of the bound ATP results in a conformational change of the protein.

### A.  Mechanical Work

In **mechanical work**, the high-energy phosphate bond of ATP is converted into movement by changing the conformation of a protein. For example, in contracting muscle fibers, the hydrolysis of ATP while it is bound to myosin ATPase changes the conformation of myosin so that it is in a "cocked" position, ready to associate with

**Otto S.** has not followed his proposed diet and exercise regimen and has been gaining weight. He has a positive caloric balance because his daily energy expenditure is less than his daily energy intake (see Chapter 1). Although the energy expenditure for physical exercise is only approximately 30% of the BMR in a sedentary individual, it can be 100% or more of the BMR in a person who exercises strenuously for several hours or more. The large increase in ATP utilization for muscle contraction during exercise accounts for its contribution to the daily energy expenditure.

The equations for calculating ΔG are based on the first law of thermodynamics (see Table 16.1). The change in chemical bond energy that occurs during a reaction is ΔH, the change in enthalpy of the reaction. At constant temperature and pressure, ΔH is equivalent to the chemical bond energy of the products minus that of the reactants. ΔG, the maximum amount of useful work available from a reaction, is equal to ΔH minus TΔS. TΔS is a correction for the amount of energy that has gone into an increase in the entropy (disorder in arrangement of molecules) of the system.

$$\Delta G = \Delta H - T \Delta S$$

where ΔH is the change in enthalpy, T is the temperature of the system in Kelvin, and ΔS is the change in entropy or increased disorder of the system. ΔS is often negligible in reactions such as ATP hydrolysis in which the number of substrates ($H_2O$, ATP) and products (ADP, $P_i$) are equal and no gas is formed. Under these conditions, the values for ΔG at physiological temperature (37°C) are similar to those at standard temperature (25°C).

Approximately 70% of our resting daily energy requirement arises from work carried out by our largest organs: the heart, brain, kidneys, and liver. Using their rate of $O_2$ consumption and an assumption that for each oxygen atom consumed 2.5 moles of ATP are synthesized (see Chapter 18), it can be estimated that each of these organs is using and producing several times its own weight in ATP each day. The heart, which rhythmically contracts, is using this ATP for mechanical work. In contrast, skeletal muscles in a resting individual use far less ATP per gram of tissue. The kidney has an ATP consumption per gram of tissue similar to that of the heart and is using this ATP largely for transport work to recover usable nutrients and maintain pH and electrolyte balance. The brain, likewise, uses most of its ATP for transport work, maintaining the ion gradients necessary for conduction of the nerve impulse. The liver, in contrast, has a high rate of ATP consumption and utilization to carry out metabolic work (biosynthesis and detoxification).

**Estimated Daily Use of ATP (g ATP/g tissue)**

| | |
|---|---|
| Heart | 16 |
| Brain | 6 |
| Kidneys | 24 |
| Liver | 6 |
| Skeletal muscle (rest) | 0.3 |
| Skeletal muscle (running) | 23.6 |

the sliding actin filament. Thus, exercising muscle fibers have almost a hundred-fold higher rate of ATP utilization and caloric requirements than resting muscle fibers. Motor proteins, such as kinesins that transport chemicals along fibers, provide another example of mechanical work in a cell.

### B. Transport Work

In **transport work**, called **active transport**, the high-energy phosphate bond of ATP is used to transport compounds against a concentration gradient. In P-ATPases (plasma membrane ATPases) and V-ATPases (vesicular ATPases), the chemical bond energy of ATP is used to reversibly phosphorylate the transport protein and change its conformation. For example, as $Na^+$, $K^+$-ATPase binds and cleaves ATP, it becomes phosphorylated and changes its conformation to release three $Na^+$ ions to the outside of the cell, thereby building up a higher extracellular than intracellular concentration of $Na^+$. $Na^+$ reenters the cell on cotransport proteins that drive the uptake of amino acids and many other compounds into the cell. Thus, $Na^+$ must be continuously transported back out. The expenditure of ATP for $Na^+$ transport occurs even while we sleep and is estimated to account for 10% to 30% of our BMR.

A large number of other active transporters also convert ATP chemical bond energy into an ion gradient (membrane potential). Vesicular ATPases pump protons into lysosomes. $Ca^{2+}$ATPases in the plasma membrane move $Ca^{2+}$ out of the cell against a concentration gradient. Similarly, $Ca^{2+}$ATPases pump $Ca^{2+}$ into the lumen of the endoplasmic reticulum and the sarcoplasmic reticulum (in muscle). Thus, a considerable amount of energy is expended in maintaining a low cytoplasmic $Ca^{2+}$ level.

## III. BIOCHEMICAL WORK

The high-energy phosphate bonds of ATP are also used for **biochemical work**. Biochemical work occurs in **anabolic pathways**, which are pathways that synthesize large molecules (e.g., DNA, glycogen, triacylglycerols, and proteins) from smaller compounds. Biochemical work also occurs when toxic compounds are converted to nontoxic compounds that can be excreted (e.g., the liver converts $NH_4^+$ ions to urea in the urea cycle). In general, formation of chemical bonds between two organic molecules (e.g., C—C bonds in fatty acid synthesis or C—N bonds in protein synthesis) requires energy and is therefore biochemical work. How do our cells get these necessary energy-requiring reactions to occur?

To answer this question, the next sections consider how energy is used to synthesize glycogen from glucose (Fig. 16.4). Glycogen is a storage polysaccharide consisting of glucosyl units linked together through glycosidic bonds. If an anabolic pathway, such as glycogen synthesis, were to have an overall positive $\Delta G^{0'}$, the cell would be full of glucose and intermediates of the pathway but very little glycogen would be formed. To avoid this, cells do biochemical work and spend enough of their ATP currency to give anabolic pathways an overall negative $\Delta G^{0'}$.

### A. Adding $\Delta G^0$ Values

Reactions in which chemical bonds are formed between two organic molecules are usually catalyzed by enzymes that transfer energy from cleavage of ATP in a phosphoryl transfer reaction or by enzymes that cleave a high-energy bond in an activated intermediate of the pathway. Because the $\Delta G^{0'}$ values in a reaction sequence are additive, the pathway acquires an overall negative $\Delta G^{0'}$, and the reactions in the pathway will occur to move toward an equilibrium state in which the concentration of final products is greater than that of the initial reactants.

#### 1. PHOSPHORYL TRANSFER REACTIONS

One of the characteristics of Gibbs free energy is that $\Delta G^0$ values for consecutive steps or reactions in a sequence can be added together to obtain a single value for the overall process. Thus, the high-energy phosphate bonds of ATP can be used to

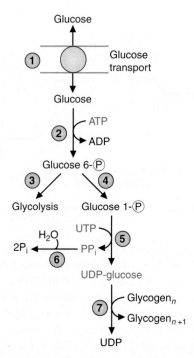

***FIG. 16.4.*** Energetics of glycogen synthesis. Compounds containing high-energy bonds are shown in *red.* *(1)* Glucose is transported into the cell. *(2)* Glucose phosphorylation uses the high-energy phosphate bond ($\sim$P) of ATP in a phosphoryl transfer step. *(4)* Conversion of G6P to G1P by phosphoglucomutase. *(5)* UDP-glucose pyrophosphorylase cleaves a $\sim$P bond in UTP, releasing pyrophosphate and forming UDP-glucose, an activated intermediate. *(6)* The pyrophosphate is hydrolyzed, releasing additional energy. *(7)* The phosphoester bond of UDP-glucose is cleaved during the addition of a glucosyl unit to the end of a glycogen polysaccharide chain. The UDP-glucose acts as the leaving group in this reaction. G6P also can be metabolized via glycolysis *(3)* when energy is required.

drive a reaction forward that would otherwise be highly unfavorable energetically. Consider, for example, synthesis of G6P from glucose, the first step in glycolysis and glycogen synthesis (see Fig.16.4, *circle 2*). If the reaction were to proceed by addition of $P_i$ to glucose, G6P synthesis would have a positive $\Delta G^{0\prime}$ value of 3.3 kcal/mole (Table 16.3). However, when this reaction is coupled to cleavage of the high-energy ATP bond through a phosphoryl transfer reaction, the $\Delta G^{0\prime}$ for G6P synthesis acquires a net negative value of $-4.0$ kcal/mole, which can be calculated from the sum of the two reactions. G6P cannot be transported back out of the cell, and therefore, the net negative $\Delta G^{0\prime}$ for G6P synthesis helps the cell to trap glucose for its own metabolic needs.

The net value for synthesis of G6P from glucose and ATP will be the same whether the two reactions are catalyzed by the same enzyme, are catalyzed by two separate enzymes, or are not catalyzed by an enzyme at all because the net value of G6P synthesis is dictated by the amount of energy in the chemical bonds being broken and formed.

## 2.  ACTIVATED INTERMEDIATES IN GLYCOGEN SYNTHESIS

To synthesize glycogen from glucose, energy is provided by the cleavage of three high-energy phosphate bonds in ATP, uridine triphosphate (UTP), and pyrophosphate

**Q:** Given a $\Delta G^{0\prime}$ of $+1.65$ kcal/mole for the conversion of G6P to G1P, and a $\Delta G^{0\prime}$ of $-4.0$ kcal/mole for the conversion of glucose + ATP to G6P + ADP, what is the value of $\Delta G^{0\prime}$ for the conversion of glucose to G1P?

**Table 16.3   $\Delta G^{0\prime}$ for the Transfer of a Phosphate from ATP to Glucose**

| | |
|---|---|
| Glucose + $P_i$ → glucose-6-P + $H_2O$ | $\Delta G^{0\prime} = +3.3$ kcal/mole |
| ATP + $H_2O$ → ADP + $P_i$ | $\Delta G^{0\prime} = -7.3$ kcal/mole |
| Sum: glucose + ATP → glucose-6-P + ADP | $\Delta G^{0\prime} = -4.0$ kcal/mole |

$\Delta G^{0'}$ for the overall reaction is the sum of the individual reactions and is −2.35 kcal. The individual reactions are

$$Glucose + ATP \rightarrow G6P + ADP$$
$$\Delta G^{0'} = -4.0 \, kcal/mole$$
$$G6P \rightarrow G1P$$
$$\Delta G^{0'} = +1.65 \, kcal/mole$$

Sum: Glucose + ATP → G1P + ADP,
$\Delta G^{0'} = -2.35 \, kcal/mole$

Thus, the cleavage of ATP has made the synthesis of G1P from glucose energetically favorable.

**Uridine diphosphate glucose
(UDP-glucose)**

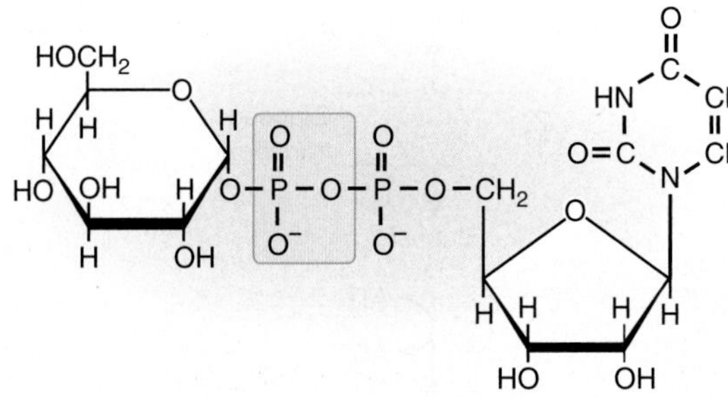

FIG. 16.5. UDP-glucose contains a high-energy pyrophosphate bond, shown in the *green box*.

(PPi) (see Fig. 16.4, steps 2, 5, and 6). Energy transfer is facilitated by phosphoryl group transfer and by formation of an activated intermediate (uridine diphosphate [UDP]-glucose). Step 4, the conversion of G6P to G1P, has a positive $\Delta G^{0'}$. This step is pulled and pushed in the desired direction by the accumulation of substrate and removal of product in reactions that have a negative $\Delta G^{0'}$ from cleavage of high-energy bonds. In step 5, the UTP high-energy phosphate bond is cleaved to form the activated sugar, UDP-glucose (Fig. 16.5). This reaction is further facilitated by cleavage of the high-energy bond in the pyrophosphate (step 6) that is released in step 5 (approximately −7.7 kcal). In step 7, cleavage of the bond between UDP and glucose in the activated intermediate provides the energy for attaching the glucose moiety to the end of the glycogen molecule (approximately −3.3 kcal). In general, the amount of ATP phosphate bond energy used in an anabolic pathway or detoxification pathway must provide the pathway with an overall negative $\Delta G^{0'}$, so that the concentration of products is favored over that of reactants.

## B. ΔG Depends on Substrate and Product Concentrations

$\Delta G^{0'}$ reflects the energy difference between reactants and products at specific concentrations (each at 1 M) and standard conditions (pH 7.0, 25°C). However, these are not the conditions prevailing in cells, where variations from "standard conditions" are relevant to determining actual free energy changes and hence the direction in which reactions are likely to occur. One aspect of free energy changes contributing to the forward direction of anabolic pathways is the dependence of $\Delta G$, the free energy change of a reaction, on the initial substrate and product concentrations. Reactions in the cell with a positive $\Delta G^{0'}$ can proceed in the forward direction if the concentration of substrate is raised to high enough levels or if the concentration of product is decreased to very low levels. Product concentrations can be very low if, for example, the product is rapidly used in a subsequent energetically favorable reaction or if the product diffuses or is transported away.

### 1. THE DIFFERENCE BETWEEN ΔG AND ΔG⁰'

The driving force toward equilibrium starting at any concentration of substrate and product is expressed by $\Delta G$, and not by $\Delta G^{0'}$, which is the free energy change to reach equilibrium starting with 1 M concentrations of substrate and product. For a reaction in which the substrate S is converted to the product P

***Equation 16.2.***

$$\Delta G = \Delta G^{0'} + RT \ln [P]/[S]$$

(See Table 16.2 for the general form of this equation.)

The expression for $\Delta G$ has two terms: $\Delta G^{0'}$, the energy change to reach equilibrium starting at equal and 1 M concentrations of substrates and products, and the second term, the energy change to reach equal concentrations of substrate and product starting from any initial concentration. (When [P] = [S] and [P]/[S] = 1, the ln of [P]/[S] is 0, and $\Delta G = \Delta G^{0'}$). The second term will be negative for all concentrations of substrate greater than product, and the greater the substrate concentration, the more negative this term will be. Thus, if the substrate concentration is suddenly raised high enough or the product concentration decreased low enough, $\Delta G$ (the sum of the first and second terms) will also be negative, and conversion of substrate to product becomes thermodynamically favorable.

## 2. THE REVERSIBILITY OF THE PHOSPHOGLUCOMUTASE REACTION IN THE CELL

The effect of substrate and product concentration on $\Delta G$ and the direction of a reaction in the cell can be illustrated with conversion of G6P to G1P, the reaction catalyzed by phosphoglucomutase in the pathway of glycogen synthesis (see Fig. 16.3). The reaction has a small positive $\Delta G^{0'}$ for G1P synthesis (+1.65 kcal/mole) and, at equilibrium, the ratio of [G1P]/[G6P] is approximately 6 to 94. However, if another reaction uses G1P such that this ratio suddenly becomes 3 to 94, there is now a driving force for converting more G6P to G1P and restoring the equilibrium ratio. Substitution in Equation 16.2 gives $\Delta G$, the driving force to equilibrium, as + 1.65 + RT ln [G1P]/[G6P] = 1.65 + (−2.06) = −0.41, which is a negative value. Thus, a decrease in the ratio of product to substrate has converted the synthesis of G1P from a thermodynamically unfavorable to a thermodynamically favorable reaction that will proceed in the forward direction until equilibrium is reached.

## C. Activated Intermediates with High-Energy Bonds

Many biochemical pathways form activated intermediates containing high-energy bonds to facilitate biochemical work. The term "high-energy bond" is a biological term defined by the $\Delta G^{0'}$ for ATP hydrolysis; any bond that can be hydrolyzed with the release of approximately as much or more energy than ATP is called a high-energy bond. The high-energy bond in activated intermediates, such as UDP-glucose in glycogen synthesis, facilitates energy transfer.

Cells use guanosine triphosphate (GTP) and cytidine triphosphate (CTP), as well as UTP and ATP, to form activated intermediates. Different anabolic pathways generally use different nucleotides as their direct source of high-energy phosphate bond: UTP is used for combining sugars, CTP in lipid synthesis, and GTP in protein synthesis.

The high-energy phosphate bonds of UTP, GTP, and CTP are energetically equivalent to ATP and are synthesized from ATP by nucleoside diphosphokinases and nucleoside monophosphokinases. For example, UTP is formed from UDP by a nucleoside diphosphokinase in the reaction:

$$ATP + UDP \leftrightarrow UTP + ADP$$

ADP is converted back to ATP by the process of oxidative phosphorylation, using energy supplied by fuel oxidation.

Energy-requiring reactions often generate the nucleoside diphosphate ADP. Adenylate kinase, an important enzyme in cellular energy balance, is a nucleoside monophosphate kinase that transfers a phosphate from one ADP to another ADP to form ATP and AMP:

$$ADP + ADP \leftrightarrow AMP + ATP$$

This enzyme thus can regenerate ATP under conditions in which ATP utilization is required.

In addition to the nucleoside triphosphates, other compounds containing high-energy bonds are formed to facilitate energy transfer in anabolic and catabolic pathways. A common feature of these molecules is that all of these high-energy bonds are "unstable," and their hydrolysis yields substantial free energy because the products are much more stable as a result of electron resonance within their structures.

## IV. THERMOGENESIS

According to the first law of thermodynamics, energy cannot be destroyed. Thus, energy from oxidation of a fuel (its caloric content) must be equal to the amount of heat released, the work performed against the environment, and the increase in order of molecules in our bodies. Some of the energy from fuel oxidation is converted into heat as the fuel is oxidized, and some heat is generated as ATP is used to do work. If we become less efficient in converting energy from fuel oxidation into ATP or if we use an additional amount of ATP for muscular contraction, we will oxidize an additional amount of fuel to maintain ATP homeostasis (constant cellular ATP levels). With the oxidation of additional fuel, we release additional heat. Thus, heat production is a natural consequence of "burning fuel."

The term **thermogenesis** refers to energy expended for the purpose of generating heat in addition to that expended for ATP production. To maintain our body at 37°C despite changes in environmental temperature, it is necessary to regulate fuel oxidation and its efficiency (as well as heat dissipation). In shivering thermogenesis, we respond to sudden cold with asynchronous muscle contractions (shivers) that increase ATP utilization and therefore fuel oxidation and the release of energy as heat. In nonshivering thermogenesis (adaptive thermogenesis), the efficiency of converting energy from fuel oxidation into ATP is decreased. More fuel needs to be oxidized to maintain constant ATP levels and thus more heat is generated.

## V. ENERGY FROM FUEL OXIDATION

Fuel oxidation provides energy for bodily processes principally through generation of the reduced coenzymes, nicotinamide adenine dinucleotide (NADH) and flavin adenine dinucleotide (FAD[2H]). They are used principally to generate ATP in oxidative phosphorylation. However, fuel oxidation also generates nicotinamide adenine dinucleotide phosphate (NADPH), which is most often used directly in energy-requiring processes. Carbohydrates also may be used to generate ATP through a nonoxidative pathway called anaerobic glycolysis.

### A. Energy Transfer from Fuels through Oxidative Phosphorylation

Fuel oxidation is our major source of ATP and our major means of transferring energy from the chemical bonds of the fuels to cellular energy-requiring processes. The amount of energy available from a fuel is equivalent to the amount of heat that is generated when a fuel is burned. To conserve this energy for the generation of ATP, the process of cellular respiration transforms the energy from the chemical bonds of fuels into the reduction state of electron-accepting coenzymes, $NAD^+$ and FAD (Fig. 16.6, *circle 1*). As these compounds transfer electrons to $O_2$ in the electron transport chain, most of this energy is transformed into an electrochemical gradient across the inner mitochondrial membrane (Fig. 16.6, *circle 2*). Much of the energy in the electrochemical gradient is used to regenerate ATP from ADP in oxidative phosphorylation (phosphorylation that requires $O_2$).

### 1. OXIDATION–REDUCTION REACTIONS

**Oxidation–reduction reactions** always involve a pair of chemicals: an electron donor, which is oxidized in the reactions, and an electron acceptor, which is reduced in the reaction. In fuel metabolism, the fuel donates electrons and is oxidized, and $NAD^+$ and FAD accept electrons and are reduced.

When is $NAD^+$, rather than FAD, used in a particular oxidation–reduction reaction? It depends on the chemical properties of the electron donor and the enzyme catalyzing the reaction. In oxidation reactions, $NAD^+$ accepts two electrons as a hydride ion to form NADH, and a proton ($H^+$) is released into the medium (Fig. 16.7). It is generally used for metabolic reactions involving oxidation of alcohols and aldehydes. In contrast, FAD accepts two electrons as hydrogen atoms, which are

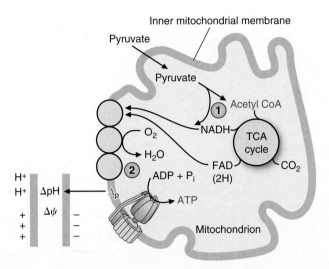

***FIG. 16.6.*** Overview of energy transformations in oxidative phosphorylation. The electrochemical potential gradient across the mitochondrial membrane ($\Delta$p) is represented by two components: the $\Delta$pH, the proton gradient, and $\Delta\psi$, the membrane potential. The role of the electrochemical potential in oxidative phosphorylation is discussed in more depth in Chapter 18.

donated singly from separate atoms (e.g., formation of a double bond or a disulfide) (Fig. 16.8).

As the reduced coenzymes donate these electrons to $O_2$ through the electron transport chain, they are reoxidized. The energy derived from reoxidation of NADH and FAD(2H) is available for the generation of ATP by oxidative phosphorylation. In our analogy of ATP as currency, the reduced coenzymes are our paychecks for oxidizing fuels. Because our cells spend ATP so fast, we must immediately convert our paychecks into ATP cash.

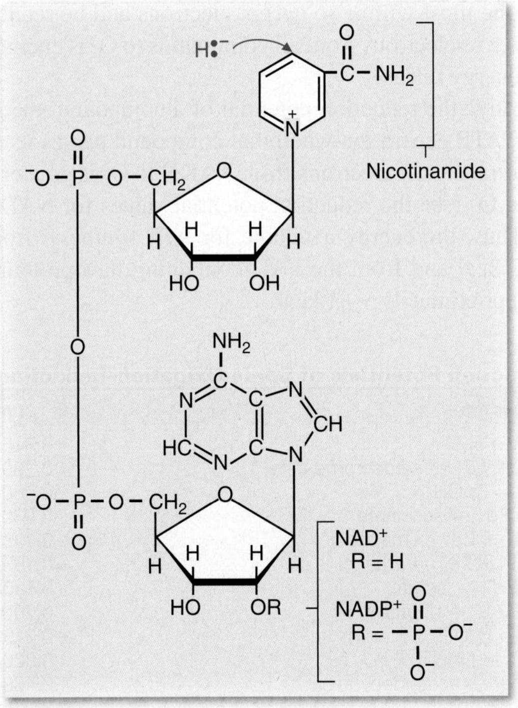

***FIG. 16.7.*** Reduction of $NAD^+$ and $NADP^+$. These structurally related coenzymes are reduced by accepting two electrons as $H:^-$, the hydride ion.

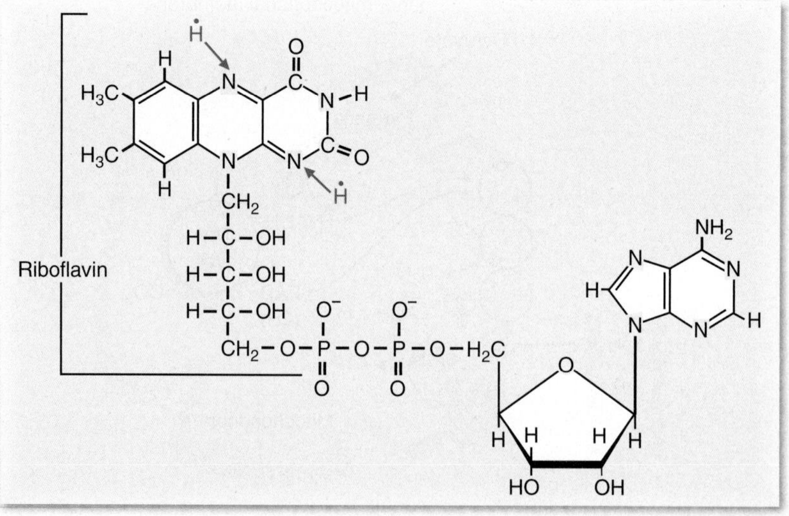

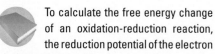

**FIG. 16.8.** Reduction of FAD. FAD accepts two electrons as two hydrogen atoms and is reduced. The reduced coenzyme is denoted in this text as FAD(2H) because it often accepts a total of two electrons one at a time, never going to the fully reduced form, FADH$_2$. FMN (flavin mononucleotide) consists of riboflavin with one phosphate group attached.

## 2. REDUCTION POTENTIAL

Each oxidation–reduction reaction makes or takes a fixed amount of energy, $(\Delta G^{0'})$, which is directly proportional to the $\Delta E^{0'}$ (the difference in reduction potentials of the oxidation–reduction pair). The **reduction potential** of a compound, $E^{0'}$, is a measure in volts of the energy change when that compound accepts electrons (becomes reduced); $-E^{0'}$ is the energy change when the compound donates electrons (becomes oxidized). $E^{0'}$ can be considered an expression of the willingness of the compound to accept electrons. Some examples of reduction potentials are shown in Table 16.4. $O_2$, which is the best electron acceptor, has the largest positive reduction potential (i.e., is the most willing to accept electrons and be reduced). As a consequence, the transfer of electrons from all compounds to $O_2$ is energetically favorable and occurs with energy release.

The more negative the reduction potential of a compound, the greater is the energy available for ATP generation when that compound passes its electrons to oxygen. The $\Delta G^{0'}$ for transfer of electrons from NADH to $O_2$ is greater than the transfer from FAD(2H) to $O_2$ (see the reduction potential values for NADH and FAD[2H] in Table 16.4). Thus, the energy available for ATP synthesis from NADH is approximately $-53$ kcal and from the FAD-containing flavoproteins in the electron transport chain approximately $-41$ kcal.

To calculate the free energy change of an oxidation-reduction reaction, the reduction potential of the electron donor (NADH) is added to that of the acceptor ($O_2$). The $\Delta E^{0'}$ for the net reaction is calculated from the sum of the half reactions. For NADH donation of electrons, it is $+0.320$ volts, opposite of that shown in Table 16.4 (remember, Table 16.4 shows the $E^{0'}$ for accepting electrons), and for $O_2$ acceptance, it is $+0.816$. The number of electrons being transferred is two (so, n = 2). The direct relationship between the energy changes in oxidation-reduction reactions and $\Delta G^{0'}$ is expressed by the Nernst equation

$$\Delta G^{0'} = -n\,F\,\Delta E^{0'}$$

where n is the number of electrons transferred and F is Faraday constant (23 kcal/mole − volt). Thus, a value of approximately $-53$ kcal/mole is obtained for the energy available for ATP synthesis by transferring two electrons from NADH to $O_2$.

**Table 16.4   Reduction Potentials of Some Oxidation–Reduction Half-Reactions**

| Reduction Half-Reactions | $E^{0'}$ at pH 7.0 |
|---|---|
| ½ $O_2$ + 2H$^+$ + 2$e^-$ → $H_2O$ | 0.816 |
| Cytochrome a-Fe$^{3+}$ + 1$e^-$ → cytochrome a-Fe$^{2+}$ | 0.290 |
| CoQ + 2H$^+$ + 2$e^-$ → CoQH$_2$ | 0.060 |
| Fumarate + 2H$^+$ + 2$e^-$ → succinate | 0.030 |
| Oxaloacetate + 2H$^+$ + 2$e^-$ → malate | −0.102 |
| Acetaldehyde + 2H$^+$ + 2$e^-$ → ethanol | −0.163 |
| Pyruvate + 2H$^+$ + 2$e^-$ → lactate | −0.190 |
| Riboflavin + 2H$^+$ + 2$e^-$ → riboflavin-H$_2$ | −0.200 |
| FAD + 2H$^+$ + 2$e^-$ → FAD(2H) | −0.219[a] |
| NAD$^+$ + 2H$^+$ + 2$e^-$ → NADH + H$^+$ | −0.320 |
| Acetate + 2H$^+$ + 2$e^-$ → acetaldehyde | −0.468 |

[a]This is the value for free FAD; when FAD is bound to a protein, its value can be altered in either direction.

## 3. CALORIC VALUES OF FOODS

The caloric value of a food is directly related to its oxidation state, which is a measure of $\Delta G^{0'}$ for transfer of electrons from that fuel to $O_2$. The electrons donated by the fuel are from its C—H and C—C bonds. Fatty acids such as palmitate $(CH_3[CH_2]_{14}COOH)$ have a caloric value of roughly 9 kcal/g. Glucose is already partially oxidized and has a caloric value of only about 4 kcal/g. The carbons, on an average, contain fewer C—H bonds from which to donate electrons.

The caloric value of a food is applicable in humans only if our cells have enzymes that can oxidize that fuel by transferring electrons from the fuel to $NAD^+$, $NADP^+$, or FAD. When we burn wood in a fireplace, electrons are transferred from cellulose and other carbohydrates to $O_2$, releasing energy as heat. However, wood has no caloric content for humans; we cannot digest it and convert cellulose to a form that can be oxidized by our enzymes. Cholesterol, although a lipid, also has no caloric value for us because we cannot oxidize the carbons in its complex ring structure in reactions that generate NADH, FAD(2H), or NADPH.

### B. NADPH in Oxidation–Reduction Reactions

$NADP^+$ is similar to $NAD^+$ and has the same reduction potential. However, $NADP^+$ has an extra phosphate group on the ribose, which affects its enzyme binding (see Fig. 16.7). Consequently, most enzymes use either $NAD^+$ or $NADP^+$ but seldom both. In certain reactions, fuels are oxidized by transfer of electrons to $NADP^+$ to form NADPH. For example, G6P dehydrogenase, in the pentose phosphate pathway, transfers electrons from G6P to $NADP^+$ instead of $NAD^+$. NADPH usually donates electrons to biosynthetic reactions such as fatty acid synthesis and to detoxification reactions that use oxygen directly. Consequently, the energy in its reduction potential is usually used in energy-requiring reactions without first being converted to ATP currency.

### C. Anaerobic Glycolysis

Not all ATP is generated by fuel oxidation. In **anaerobic glycolysis**, glucose is degraded in reactions that form high-energy phosphorylated intermediates of the pathway. These activated high-energy intermediates provide the energy for the generation of ATP from ADP without involving electron transfer to $O_2$. Therefore, this pathway is called anaerobic glycolysis, and ATP is generated from substrate-level phosphorylation rather than oxidative phosphorylation (see Chapter 19). Anaerobic glycolysis is a critical source of ATP for cells that have a decreased $O_2$ supply, either because they are physiologically designed that way (e.g., cells in the kidney medulla) or because their supply of $O_2$ has been pathologically decreased (e.g., coronary artery disease).

## VI. OXYGENASES AND OXIDASES NOT INVOLVED IN ATP GENERATION

Approximately 90% to 95% of the oxygen we consume is used by the terminal oxidase in the electron transport chain for ATP generation via oxidative phosphorylation. The remainder of the $O_2$ is used directly by oxygenases and other oxidases, enzymes that oxidize a compound in the body by transferring electrons directly to $O_2$ (Fig. 16.9). The large positive reduction potential of $O_2$ makes all of these reactions extremely favorable thermodynamically, but the electronic structure of $O_2$ slows the speed of electron transfer. These enzymes, therefore, contain a metal ion that facilitates reduction of $O_2$.

### A. Oxidases

**Oxidases** transfer electrons from the substrate to $O_2$, which is reduced to $H_2O$ or to hydrogen peroxide $(H_2O_2)$. The terminal protein complex in the electron transport chain, called cytochrome oxidase, is an oxidase because it accepts electrons donated to the chain by NADH and FAD(2H) and uses these to reduce $O_2$ to $H_2O$. Most of

**Oxidases**

$$O_2 + 4e^-, 4H^+ \longrightarrow 2H_2O$$

$$O_2 + SH_2 \longrightarrow S + H_2O_2$$

**Monooxygenases**

$$O_2 + S + \text{Electron} \longrightarrow \text{donor–}XH_2$$

$$H_2O + \text{Electron} + S-OH$$
$$\text{donor–}X$$

**Dioxygenases**

$$S + O_2 \longrightarrow SO_2$$

**FIG. 16.9.** Oxidases and oxygenases. The fate of $O_2$ is shown in *red*. S represents an organic substrate.

the other oxidases in the cell form $H_2O_2$ instead of $H_2O$ and are called peroxidases. Peroxidases are generally confined to peroxisomes to protect DNA and other cellular components from toxic free radicals (compounds containing single electrons in an outer orbital) generated by $H_2O_2$.

### B. Oxygenases

**Oxygenases**, in contrast to oxidases, incorporate one or both of the atoms of oxygen into the organic substrate (see Fig. 16.9). Monooxygenases, enzymes that incorporate one atom of oxygen into the substrate and the other into $H_2O$, are often named hydroxylases (e.g., phenylalanine hydroxylase, which adds a hydroxyl group to phenylalanine to form tyrosine) or mixed-function oxidases. Monooxygenases require an electron donor substrate, such as NADPH; a coenzyme such as FAD, which can transfer single electrons; and a metal or similar compound that can form a reactive oxygen complex. They are usually found in the endoplasmic reticulum and occasionally in mitochondria. Dioxygenases, enzymes that incorporate both atoms of oxygen into the substrate, are used in the pathways for converting arachidonate into prostaglandins, thromboxanes, and leukotrienes.

## VII. ENERGY BALANCE

Our total energy expenditure is equivalent to our oxygen consumption. The **resting metabolic rate** accounts for approximately 60% to 70% of our total energy expenditure and $O_2$ consumption, and physical exercise accounts for the remainder. Of the resting metabolic rate, approximately 90% to 95% of $O_2$ consumption is used by the mitochondrial electron transport chain, and only 5% to 10% is required for nonmitochondrial oxidases and oxygenases and is not related to ATP synthesis. Approximately 20% to 30% of the energy from this mitochondrial $O_2$ consumption is lost by proton leak back across the mitochondrial membrane, which dissipates the electrochemical gradient without ATP synthesis. The remainder of our $O_2$ consumption is used for ATPases that maintain ion gradients and for biosynthetic pathways.

**ATP homeostasis** refers to the ability of our cells to maintain constant levels of ATP despite fluctuations in the rate of utilization. Thus, increased utilization of ATP for exercise or biosynthetic reactions increases the rate of fuel oxidation. The major mechanism employed is feedback regulation; all of the pathways of fuel oxidation leading to generation of ATP are feedback-regulated by ATP levels or by compounds related to the concentration of ATP. In general, the less ATP used, the less fuel will be oxidized to generate ATP.

According to the first law of thermodynamics, the energy (calories) in our consumed fuel can never be lost. Consumed fuel is either oxidized to meet the energy demands of the basal metabolic rate plus exercise or it is stored as fat. Thus, an intake of calories in excess of those expended results in weight gain. The simple statement, "If you eat too much and don't exercise, you will gain weight," is really a summary of the bioenergetics of the ATP-ADP cycle.

### CLINICAL COMMENTS

Diseases discussed in this chapter are summarized in Table 16.5.

**Otto S.** Otto S. visited his physician, who noted the increased weight. He recommended several diet modifications to Otto that would decrease the caloric content of his diet and pointed out the importance of exercise for weight reduction. He reminded Otto that the American Heart Association recommended 30 minutes of moderate exercise 5 days per week. He also reminded Otto that he should be a role model for his patients. Otto decided to begin an exercise regimen that includes an hour of running and tennis at least 5 days a week.

**Table 16.5  Diseases Discussed in Chapter 16**

| Disease or Disorder | Environmental or Genetic | Comments |
|---|---|---|
| Obesity | Both | Understanding daily caloric needs can enable one to gain or lose weight through alterations in exercise and eating habits. |
| Heart attack (myocardial infarction) | Both | The heart requires a constant level of energy, derived primarily from lactate, glucose, and fatty acids. This is necessary so that the rate of contraction can remain constant or increase during appropriate periods. Interference of oxygen flow to certain areas of the heart will reduce energy generation, leading to a myocardial infarction. |

 **Cora N.** Cora N. was in left ventricular failure (LVF) when she presented to the hospital with her second heart attack in 8 months. The diagnosis of LVF was suspected, in part, by her rapid heart rate (104 beats per minute) and respiratory rate. On examining her lungs, her physician heard respiratory rales (or crackles) caused by inspired air bubbling in fluid that had filled her lung air spaces secondary to LVF. This condition is referred to as congestive heart failure.

**Cora N.'s** rapid heart rate (tachycardia) resulted from a reduced capacity of her ischemic, failing left ventricular muscle to eject a normal amount of blood into the arteries leading away from the heart with each contraction. The resultant drop in intra-arterial pressure signaled a reflex response in the central nervous system that, in turn, caused an increase in heart rate in an attempt to bring the total amount of blood leaving the left ventricle each minute (the cardiac output) back toward a more appropriate level to maintain systemic blood pressure.

Initial treatment of Cora's congestive heart failure will include efforts to reduce the workload of the heart by decreasing blood volume (preload) with diuretics and decreasing her blood pressure, and the administration of oxygen by nasal cannula to improve the oxygen levels in her blood. It may also include attempts to improve the force of left ventricular contraction with digitalis.

 Congestive heart failure occurs when the weakened pumping action of the left ventricular heart muscle, usually from ischemia, leads to a reduced blood flow from the heart to the rest of the body. This leads to an increase in blood volume in the vessels that bring oxygenated blood from the lungs to the left side of the heart. The pressure inside these pulmonary vessels eventually reaches a critical level, above which water from the blood moves down a "pressure gradient" from the capillary lumen into alveolar air spaces of the lung (transudation). The patient experiences shortness of breath as the fluid in the air spaces interferes with oxygen exchange from the inspired air into arterial blood, causing hypoxia. The hypoxia then stimulates the respiratory center in the central nervous system, leading to a more rapid respiratory rate in an effort to increase the oxygen content of the blood. As the patient inhales deeply, the physician hears gurgling or crackling sounds (known as inspiratory rales or crackles) with a stethoscope placed over the posterior lung bases. These sounds represent the bubbling of inspired air as it enters the fluid-filled pulmonary alveolar air spaces.

## REVIEW QUESTIONS-CHAPTER 16

1. The highest energy phosphate bond in ATP is located between which of the following groups?

    A. Two phosphate groups
    B. Adenosine and phosphate
    C. Ribose and phosphate
    D. Ribose and adenine
    E. Two hydroxyl groups in the ribose ring

2. Which one of the following bioenergetic terms or phrases is correctly defined?

    A. The first law of thermodynamics states that the universe tends toward a state of increased order.
    B. The second law of thermodynamics states that the total energy of a system remains constant.
    C. The $\Delta G^{0'}$ of a reaction is the standard free energy change measured at 37°C and a pH of 7.4.

    D. The change in enthalpy of a reaction is a measure of the total amount of heat that can be released from changes in the chemical bonds.
    E. A high-energy bond is a bond that releases more than 3 kcal/mole of heat when it is hydrolyzed.

3. Which statement best describes the direction a chemical reaction will follow?

    A. The enzyme for the reaction must be working at better than 50% of its maximum efficiency for the reaction to proceed in the forward direction.
    B. A reaction with a positive free energy will proceed in the forward direction if the substrate concentration is raised high enough.
    C. Under standard conditions, a reaction will proceed in the forward direction if the free energy ($\Delta G^{0'}$) is positive.

D. The direction of a reaction is independent of the initial substrate and product concentrations because the direction is determined by the change in free energy.

E. The concentration of all of the substrates must be higher than all of the products to proceed in the forward direction.

4. A patient, Mr. Perkins, has just suffered a heart attack. As a consequence, his heart would display which one of the following changes?

A. An increased intracellular $O_2$ concentration
B. An increased intracellular ATP concentration
C. An increased intracellular $H^+$ concentration

D. A decreased intracellular $Na^+$ concentration
E. A decreased intracellular $Ca^{2+}$ concentration

5. Which one of the following statements correctly describes reduction of one of the electron carriers, $NAD^+$ or FAD?

A. FAD must accept two electrons at a time.
B. $NAD^+$ accepts two electrons as a hydride ion to form NADH.
C. $NAD^+$ accepts two electrons as hydrogen atoms to form $NADH_2$.
D. $NAD^+$ accepts two electrons that are each donated from a separate atom of the substrate.
E. FAD releases a proton as it accepts two electrons.

# 17 Tricarboxylic Acid Cycle

## CHAPTER OUTLINE

## KEY POINTS

- The TCA cycle accounts for over two-thirds of the ATP generated from fuel oxidation.
- Acetyl CoA, generated from fuel oxidation, is the substrate for the TCA cycle.
- Acetyl CoA, when oxidized via the cycle, generates $CO_2$, reduced electron carriers, and guanosine triphosphate (GTP).
- The reduced electron carriers (NADH, FAD[2H]) donate electrons to $O_2$ via the electron transport chain, which leads to ATP generation from oxidative phosphorylation.
- The cycle requires a number of cofactors to function properly, some of which are derived from vitamins. These include thiamine pyrophosphate (derived from vitamin $B_1$), FAD (derived from vitamin $B_2$) and coenzyme A (derived from pantothenic acid).
- Intermediates of the TCA cycle are used for many biosynthetic reactions and are replaced by anaplerotic (refilling) reactions within the cell.
- The cycle is carefully regulated within the mitochondria by energy and the levels of reduced electron carriers.
- Impaired functioning of the TCA cycle leads to an inability to generate ATP from fuel oxidation and an accumulation of TCA cycle precursors.

# THE WAITING ROOM

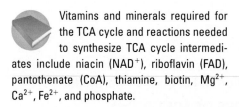

**Otto S.**, a 26-year-old medical student, has faithfully followed his diet and aerobic exercise program of daily tennis and jogging (see Chapter 16). He has lost a total of 33 lb and is just 23 lb from his college weight of 154 lb. His exercise capacity has markedly improved; he can run for a longer time at a faster pace before noting shortness of breath or palpitations of his heart. Even his test scores in his medical school classes have improved.

Vitamins and minerals required for the TCA cycle and reactions needed to synthesize TCA cycle intermediates include niacin ($NAD^+$), riboflavin (FAD), pantothenate (CoA), thiamine, biotin, $Mg^{2+}$, $Ca^{2+}$, $Fe^{2+}$, and phosphate.

**Ann R.** suffers from anorexia nervosa (see Chapters 1 and 7). In addition to a low body weight and decreased muscle mass, glycogen, and fat stores, she has iron deficiency anemia (see Chapter 14). She has started to gain weight and is trying a daily exercise program. However, she constantly feels weak and tired. When she walks, she feels pain in her calf muscles. On this visit to her nutritionist, they discuss the vitamin content of her diet and its role in energy metabolism.

**Al M.** has been hospitalized for congestive heart failure (see Chapter 6) and for head injuries sustained while driving under the influence of alcohol (Chapters 7 and 8). He completed an alcohol detoxification program, enrolled in a local Alcoholics Anonymous (AA) group, and began seeing a psychologist. During this time, his alcohol-related neurological and cardiac manifestations of thiamine deficiency partially cleared. However, in spite of the support he was receiving, he began drinking excessive amounts of alcohol again while eating poorly. Three weeks later, he was readmitted with symptoms of "high-output" heart failure, sometimes referred to as wet beriberi or as the beriberi heart.

## I. REACTIONS OF THE TRICARBOXYLIC ACID CYCLE

In the tricarboxylic acid (TCA) cycle, the two-carbon acetyl group of **acetyl coenzyme A (CoA)** is oxidized to two $CO_2$ molecules (Fig. 17.1). The function of the cycle is to conserve the energy from this oxidation, which it accomplishes principally by transferring electrons from intermediates of the cycle to $NAD^+$ and **FAD**. The eight electrons donated by the acetyl group (four from each carbon) eventually end up in three molecules of NADH and one of flavin adenine dinucleotide (FAD[2H]). As a consequence, adenosine triphosphate (ATP) can be generated from oxidative phosphorylation when NADH and FAD(2H) donate these electrons to $O_2$ via the electron transport chain. The TCA cycle is frequently called the **Krebs cycle** because Sir Hans Krebs first formulated its reactions into a cycle. It is also called the **citric acid cycle** because citrate was one of the first compounds known to participate. The most common name for this pathway, the tricarboxylic acid or TCA cycle, denotes the involvement of the tricarboxylates citrate and isocitrate.

Initially, the acetyl group is incorporated into **citrate**, an intermediate of the TCA cycle (Fig. 17.2). As citrate progresses through the cycle to **oxaloacetate**, it is oxidized by four dehydrogenases (isocitrate dehydrogenase, α-ketoglutarate dehydrogenase, succinate dehydrogenase, and malate dehydrogenase), which transfer electrons to $NAD^+$ or FAD. The isomerase aconitase rearranges electrons in citrate, thereby forming isocitrate, to facilitate an electron transfer to $NAD^+$.

The overall yield of energy-containing compounds from the TCA cycle is three NADH, one FAD(2H), and one guanosine triphosphate (GTP). The high-energy phosphate bond of GTP is generated from substrate-level phosphorylation (see Section I.C) catalyzed by succinate thiokinase (succinyl CoA synthetase). As the NADH and FAD(2H) are reoxidized in the electron transport chain, approximately

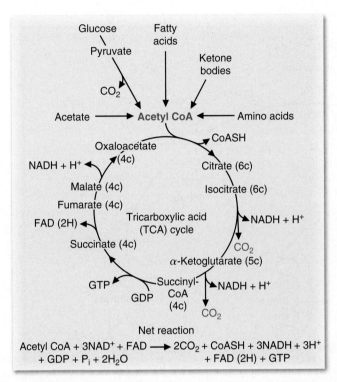

**FIG. 17.1.** Summary of the TCA cycle. The major pathways of fuel oxidation generate acetyl CoA, which is the substrate for the TCA cycle. The number of carbons in each intermediate of the cycle is indicated in parentheses by the name of the compound.

2.5 ATP are generated for each NADH and 1.5 ATP for the FAD(2H). Consequently, the net energy yield from the TCA cycle and oxidative phosphorylation is about 10 high-energy phosphate bonds for each acetyl group oxidized.

## A. Formation and Oxidation of Isocitrate

The TCA cycle begins with condensation of the activated acetyl group and oxaloacetate to form the six-carbon intermediate citrate, a reaction catalyzed by the enzyme citrate synthase (see Fig. 17.2). Because oxaloacetate is regenerated with each turn of the cycle, it is not really considered a substrate of the cycle or a source of electrons or carbon.

In the next step of the TCA cycle, the hydroxyl (alcohol) group of citrate is moved to an adjacent carbon so that it can be oxidized to form a keto group. The isomerization of citrate to isocitrate is catalyzed by the enzyme aconitase, which is named for an intermediate of the reaction. The enzyme isocitrate dehydrogenase catalyzes the oxidation of the alcohol group and the subsequent cleavage of the carboxyl group to release $CO_2$ (an oxidation followed by a decarboxylation), forming α-ketoglutarate.

## B. α-Ketoglutarate to Succinyl CoA

The next step of the TCA cycle is the oxidative decarboxylation of α-ketoglutarate to succinyl CoA, catalyzed by the α-ketoglutarate dehydrogenase complex (see Fig. 17.2). The dehydrogenase complex contains the coenzymes thiamine pyrophosphate (TPP), lipoic acid, and FAD.

In this reaction, one of the carboxyl groups of α-ketoglutarate is released as $CO_2$, and the adjacent keto group is oxidized to the level of an acid, which then combines with the sulfhydryl group of coenzyme A (CoASH) to form succinyl CoA (see Fig. 17.2). Energy from the reaction is conserved principally in the reduction state of NADH, with a smaller amount present in the high-energy thioester bond of succinyl CoA.

 **Otto S.'s** exercise program increases his rate of ATP utilization and his rate of fuel oxidation in the TCA cycle. The TCA cycle generates NADH and FAD(2H), and the electron transport chain transfers electrons from NADH and FAD(2H) to $O_2$, thereby creating the electrochemical potential that drives ATP synthesis from ADP. As ATP is used in the cell, the rate of the electron transport chain increases. The TCA cycle and other fuel oxidative pathways respond by increasing their rates of NADH and FAD(2H) production.

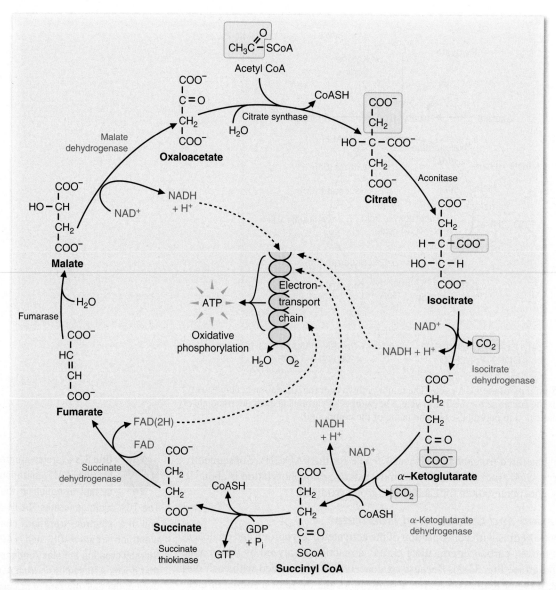

**FIG. 17.2.** Reactions of the TCA cycle. The oxidation–reduction enzymes and coenzymes are shown in *red*. Entry of the two carbons of acetyl CoA into the TCA cycle are indicated with the *green box*. The carbons released as $CO_2$ are shown with *yellow boxes*.

## C. Generation of GTP

Energy from the succinyl CoA thioester bond is used to generate GTP from guanosine diphosphate (GDP) and inorganic phosphate ($P_i$) in the reaction catalyzed by succinate thiokinase (see Fig. 17.2). This reaction is an example of **substrate-level phosphorylation**. By definition, substrate-level phosphorylation is the formation of a high-energy phosphate bond where none previously existed without the use of molecular $O_2$ (in other words, not oxidative phosphorylation). The high-energy phosphate bond of GTP is energetically equivalent to that of ATP and can be used directly for energy-requiring reactions like protein synthesis.

## D. Oxidation of Succinate to Oxaloacetate

Up until this stage of the TCA cycle, two carbons have been stripped of their available electrons and released as $CO_2$. Two pairs of these electrons have been transferred to two $NAD^+$, and one GTP has been generated. However, two additional pairs of electrons arising from acetyl CoA still remain in the TCA cycle as part of succinate. The remaining steps of the TCA cycle transfer these two pairs of electrons to FAD and $NAD^+$ and add $H_2O$, thereby regenerating oxaloacetate.

The sequence of reactions converting succinate to oxaloacetate begins with the oxidation of succinate to fumarate (see Fig. 17.2). Single electrons are transferred from the two adjacent—$CH_2$—methylene groups of succinate to an FAD bound to succinate dehydrogenase, thereby forming the double bond of fumarate. From the reduced enzyme-bound FAD, the electrons are passed into the electron transport chain. A hydroxyl group and a proton from water add to the double bond of fumarate, converting it to malate. In the last reaction of the TCA cycle, the alcohol group of malate is oxidized to a keto group through the donation of electrons to $NAD^+$.

With regeneration of oxaloacetate, the TCA cycle is complete; the chemical bond energy, carbon, and electrons donated by the acetyl group have been converted to $CO_2$, NADH, FAD(2H), GTP, and heat.

## II. COENZYMES OF THE TCA CYCLE

The enzymes of the TCA cycle rely heavily on coenzymes for their catalytic function. Isocitrate dehydrogenase and malate dehydrogenase use $NAD^+$ as a coenzyme, and succinate dehydrogenase uses FAD. Citrate synthase catalyzes a reaction that uses a CoA derivative, acetyl CoA. The α-ketoglutarate dehydrogenase complex uses TPP, lipoate and FAD as bound coenzymes, and $NAD^+$ and CoASH as substrates. Each of these coenzymes has unique structural features that enable it to fulfill its role in the TCA cycle.

### A. FAD and $NAD^+$

Both FAD and $NAD^+$ are electron-accepting coenzymes. Why is FAD used in some reactions and $NAD^+$ in others? Their unique structural features enable FAD and $NAD^+$ to act as electron acceptors in different types of reactions and play different physiological roles in the cell. FAD is able to accept single electrons (H•) and forms a half-reduced single electron intermediate (Fig. 17.3). It thus participates in reactions in which single electrons are transferred independently from two different atoms, which occurs in double-bond formation (e.g., succinate to fumarate) and disulfide bond formation (e.g., lipoate to lipoate disulfide in the α-ketoglutarate dehydrogenase reaction). In contrast, $NAD^+$ accepts a pair of electrons as the hydride ion ($H^-$), which is attracted to the carbon opposite the positively charged pyridine ring (Fig. 17.4). This occurs, for example, in the oxidation of alcohols to ketones by malate dehydrogenase and isocitrate dehydrogenase. The nicotinamide ring accepts a $H^-$ from the C—H bond, and the alcoholic hydrogen is released into the medium as a positively charged proton, $H^+$.

The free radical, single-electron forms of FAD are very reactive, and FADH can lose its electron through exposure to water or the initiation of chain reactions. As a consequence, FAD must remain very tightly, sometimes covalently, attached to its enzyme while it accepts and transfers electrons to another group bound on the enzyme. Because FAD interacts with many functional groups on amino acid side chains in the active site, the $E^{0'}$ for enzyme-bound FAD varies greatly and can be greater or much less than that of $NAD^+$. In contrast, $NAD^+$ and NADH are more like substrate and product than coenzymes.

NADH plays a regulatory role in balancing energy metabolism that FAD(2H) cannot because FAD(2H) remains attached to its enzyme. Free $NAD^+$ binds to a dehydrogenase and is reduced to NADH, which is then released into the medium, where it can bind and inhibit a different dehydrogenase. Consequently, oxidative enzymes are controlled by the NADH/$NAD^+$ ratio and do not generate NADH faster than it can be reoxidized in the electron transport chain. The regulation of the TCA cycle and other pathways of fuel oxidation by the NADH/$NAD^+$ ratio is part of the mechanism for coordinating the rate of fuel oxidation to the rate of ATP utilization.

### B. Role of Coenzyme A in the TCA Cycle

Coenzyme A (CoASH), the acylation coenzyme, participates in reactions through the formation of a thioester bond between the sulfur (S) of CoASH and an acyl group

**Ann R.** has been malnourished for some time and has developed subclinical deficiencies of many vitamins, including riboflavin. The coenzymes FAD and flavin mononucleotide (FMN) are synthesized from the vitamin riboflavin. Riboflavin is actively transported into cells where the enzyme flavokinase adds a phosphate to form FMN. FAD synthetase then adds AMP to form FAD. FAD is the major coenzyme in tissues and is generally found tightly bound to proteins, with about 10% being covalently bound. Its turnover in the body is very slow, and people can live for long periods on low intakes without displaying any signs of a riboflavin deficiency.

**Q:** One of **Otto S.'s** tennis partners told him that he had heard about a health food designed for athletes that contained succinate. The advertisement made the claim that succinate would provide an excellent source of energy during exercise because it could be metabolized directly without oxygen. Do you see anything wrong with this statement?

CoASH is synthesized from the vitamin pantothenate in a sequence of reactions that phosphorylate pantothenate, add the sulfhydryl portion of CoA from cysteine, and then add AMP and an additional phosphate group from ATP (see Fig. 6.7). Pantothenate is widely distributed in foods ("pantos" means everywhere), so it is unlikely that **Ann R.** has developed a pantothenate deficiency. Although CoA is required in approximately 100 different reactions in mammalian cells, no recommended daily allowance (RDA) has been established for pantothenate, in part because indicators have not yet been found that specifically and sensitively reflect a deficiency of this vitamin in the human. The reported symptoms of pantothenate deficiency (fatigue, nausea, and loss of appetite) are characteristic of vitamin deficiencies in general.

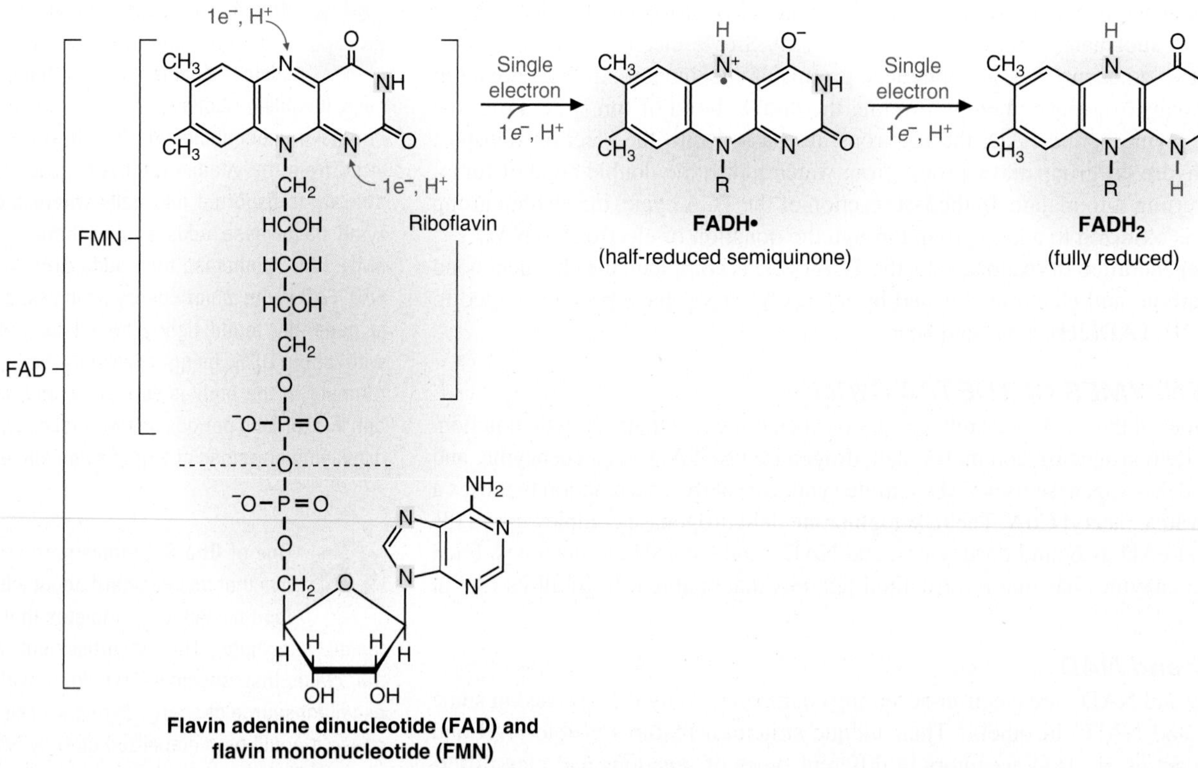

Flavin adenine dinucleotide (FAD) and
flavin mononucleotide (FMN)

*FIG. 17.3.* One-electron steps in the reduction of FAD. When FAD and FMN accept single electrons, they are converted to the half-reduced semiquinone, a semistable free radical form. They can also accept two electrons to form the fully reduced form, $FADH_2$. However, in most dehydrogenases, $FADH_2$ is never formed. Instead, the first electron is shared with a group on the protein as the next electron is transferred. Therefore, in this text, overall acceptance of two electrons by FAD has been denoted by the more general abbreviation, FAD(2H).

**A:** The claim that succinate oxidation could produce energy without oxygen is wrong. It was probably based on the fact that succinate is oxidized to fumarate by the donation of electrons to FAD. However, ATP can be generated from this process only when these electrons are donated to oxygen in the electron transport chain. The energy generated by the electron transport chain is used for ATP synthesis in the process of oxidative phosphorylation. After the covalently bound FAD(2H) is oxidized back to FAD by the electron transport chain, succinate dehydrogenase can oxidize another succinate molecule. If oxygen was not present, the FAD(2H) would remain reduced, and the enzyme could no longer convert succinate to fumarate.

(e.g., acetyl CoA, succinyl CoA) (Fig. 17.5). The complete structure of CoASH and its vitamin precursor, pantothenate, is shown in Figure 6.7. A thioester bond differs from a typical oxygen ester bond because S, unlike $O_2$, does not share its electrons and participate in resonance formations. One of the consequences of this feature of sulfur chemistry is that the thioester bond is a high-energy bond that has a large negative $\Delta G^{0'}$ of hydrolysis (approximately $-13$ kcal/mole).

The energy from cleavage of the high-energy thioester bonds of succinyl CoA and acetyl CoA is used in two different ways in the TCA cycle. When the succinyl

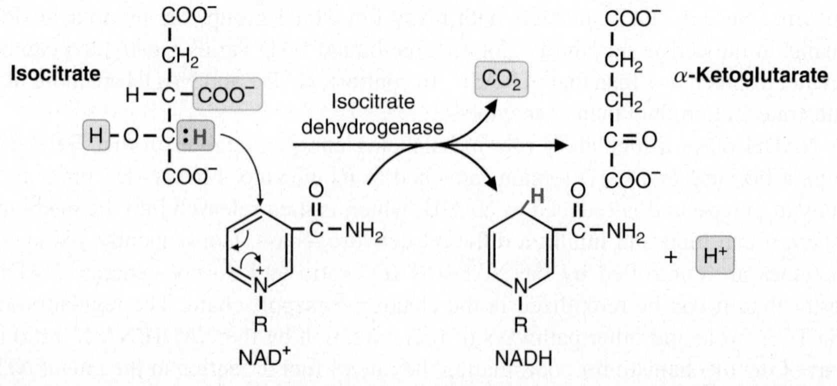

*FIG. 17.4.* Oxidation and decarboxylation of isocitrate. The alcohol group (C—OH) is oxidized to a ketone, with the C—H electrons donated to $NAD^+$ as the $H^-$. Subsequent electron shifts in the pyridine ring remove the positive charge. The H of the —OH group dissociates into water as a proton, $H^+$. $NAD^+$, the electron acceptor, is reduced.

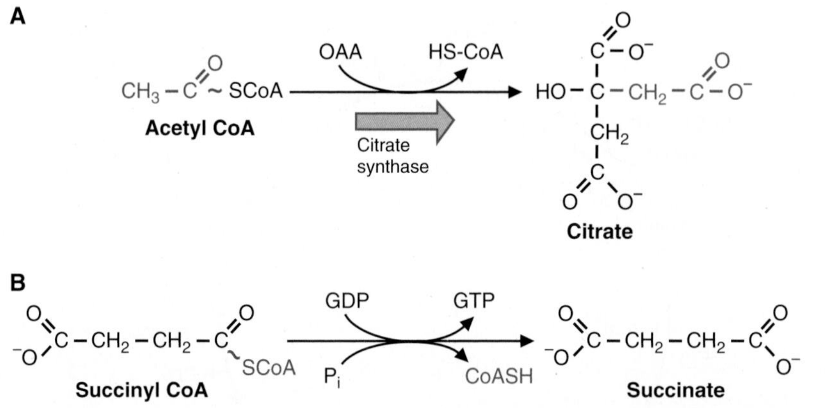

**A**

CH$_3$ – C $\sim$ SCoA
**Acetyl CoA**

OAA    HS-CoA

Citrate synthase

HO – C – CH$_2$ – C – O$^-$

Citrate

**B**

$^-$O–C – CH$_2$ – CH$_2$ – C $\sim$ SCoA
**Succinyl CoA**

GDP    GTP

P$_i$    CoASH

$^-$O–C – CH$_2$ – CH$_2$ – C – O$^-$
**Succinate**

**FIG. 17.5.** Utilization of the high-energy thioester bond of acyl CoAs. Energy transformations are shown in *red*. **A.** The energy released by hydrolysis of the thioester bond of acetyl CoA in the citrate synthase reaction contributes a large negative $\Delta G^{0'}$ to the forward direction of the TCA cycle. **B.** The energy of the succinyl CoA thioester bond is used for the synthesis of the high-energy phosphate bond of GTP.

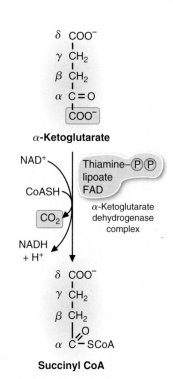

$\alpha$-Ketoglutarate

NAD$^+$    Thiamine—$\text{P}$$\text{P}$ lipoate FAD

CoASH    $\alpha$-Ketoglutarate dehydrogenase complex

CO$_2$

NADH + H$^+$

**Succinyl CoA**

**FIG. 17.6.** Oxidative decarboxylation of $\alpha$-ketoglutarate. The $\alpha$-ketoglutarate dehydrogenase complex oxidizes $\alpha$-ketoglutarate to succinyl CoA. The carboxyl group is released as CO$_2$. The keto group on the $\alpha$-carbon is oxidized and then forms the acyl CoA thioester, succinyl CoA. The $\alpha$, $\beta$, $\gamma$, and $\delta$ on succinyl CoA refer to the sequence of atoms in $\alpha$-ketoglutarate.

CoA thioester bond is cleaved by succinate thiokinase, the energy is used directly for activating an enzyme-bound phosphate that is transferred to GDP (see Fig. 17.5B). In contrast, when the thioester bond of acetyl CoA is cleaved in the citrate synthase reaction, the energy is released, giving the reaction a large negative $\Delta G^{0'}$ of $-7.7$ kcal/mole. The large negative $\Delta G^{0'}$ for citrate formation helps to keep the TCA cycle going in the forward direction.

## C.  The $\alpha$-Keto Acid Dehydrogenase Complexes

The **$\alpha$-ketoglutarate dehydrogenase complex** is one of a three-member family of similar **$\alpha$-keto acid dehydrogenase complexes**. The other members of this family are the **pyruvate dehydrogenase complex (PDC)** and the **branched-chain amino acid $\alpha$-keto acid dehydrogenase complex**. Each of these complexes is specific for a different $\alpha$-keto acid structure. In the sequence of reactions catalyzed by the complexes, the $\alpha$-keto acid is decarboxylated (i.e., releases the carboxyl group as CO$_2$) (Fig.17.6). The keto group is oxidized to the level of a carboxylic acid and then combined with CoASH to form an acyl CoA thioester (e.g., succinyl CoA).

All of the $\alpha$-keto acid dehydrogenase complexes are huge enzyme complexes composed of multiple subunits of three different enzymes, E$_1$, E$_2$, and E$_3$. E$_1$ is an $\alpha$-keto acid decarboxylase, which contains TPP; it cleaves off the carboxyl group of the $\alpha$-keto acid. E$_2$ is a transacylase containing lipoate; it transfers the acyl portion of the $\alpha$-keto acid from thiamine to CoASH. E$_3$ is dihydrolipoyl dehydrogenase, which contains FAD; it transfers electrons from reduced lipoate to FAD, which then transfers the electrons to NAD$^+$. The collection of three enzyme activities into one huge complex enables the product of one enzyme to be transferred to the next enzyme without loss of energy. Complex formation also increases the rate of catalysis because the substrates for E$_2$ and E$_3$ remain bound to the enzyme complex.

## III.  ENERGETICS OF THE TCA CYCLE

Like all metabolic pathways, the TCA cycle operates with an overall net negative $\Delta G^{0'}$ (Fig 17.7). The conversion of substrates to products is therefore energetically favorable. However, some of the reactions, such as the malate dehydrogenase reaction, have a positive value.

## A.  Overall Efficiency of the TCA Cycle

The reactions of the TCA cycle are extremely efficient in converting energy in the chemical bonds of the acetyl group to other forms. The total amount of energy

In **Al M.'s** heart failure, which is caused in part by a dietary deficiency of the vitamin thiamine, pyruvate dehydrogenase, $\alpha$-ketoglutarate dehydrogenase, and the branched-chain $\alpha$-keto acid dehydrogenase complexes are less functional than normal. Because heart muscle, skeletal muscle, and nervous tissue have high rates of ATP production from the NADH produced by the oxidation of pyruvate to acetyl CoA and of acetyl CoA to CO$_2$ in the TCA cycle, these tissues present with the most obvious signs of thiamine deficiency.

In Western societies, gross thiamine deficiency is most often associated with alcoholism. The mechanism for active absorption of thiamine is strongly and directly inhibited by alcohol. Subclinical deficiency of thiamine from malnutrition or anorexia may be common in the general population and is usually associated with multiple vitamin deficiencies.

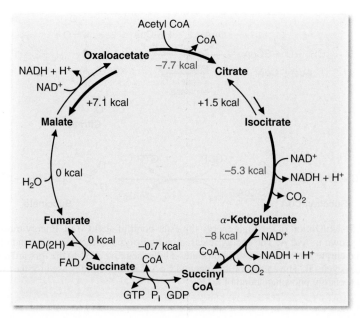

**FIG. 17.7.** Approximate $\Delta G^{0'}$ values for the reactions in the TCA cycle, given for the forward direction. The reactions with large negative $\Delta G^{0'}$ values are shown in *red*. The standard free energy ($\Delta G^{0'}$) refers to the free energy change for conversion of 1 mole of substrate to 1 mole of product under standard conditions (see Chapter 16).

**Otto S.** had difficulty losing weight because human fuel utilization is too efficient. His adipose tissue fatty acids are being converted to acetyl CoA, which is being oxidized in the TCA cycle, thereby generating NADH and FAD(2H). The energy in these compounds is used for ATP synthesis from oxidative phosphorylation. If his fuel utilization were less efficient and his ATP yield were lower, he would have to oxidize much greater amounts of fat to get the ATP he needs for exercise.

available from the acetyl group is about 228 kcal/mole (the amount of energy that could be released from complete combustion of 1 mole of acetyl groups to $CO_2$ in an experimental chamber). The products of the TCA cycle (NADH, FAD[2H], and GTP) contain about 207 kcal. Thus, the TCA cycle reactions are able to conserve about 90% of the energy available from the oxidation of acetyl CoA. The net standard free energy change for the TCA cycle, $\Delta G^{0'}$, can be calculated from the sum of the $\Delta G^{0'}$ values for the individual reactions. The $\Delta G^{0'}$, $-13$ kcal, is the amount of energy lost as heat. It can be considered the amount of energy spent to ensure that oxidation of the acetyl group to $CO_2$ goes to completion. This value is surprisingly small. However, oxidation of NADH and FAD(2H) in the electron transport chain helps to make acetyl oxidation more energetically favorable and pull the TCA cycle forward.

### B. Thermodynamically and Kinetically Reversible and Irreversible Reactions

Three reactions in the TCA cycle have large negative values for $\Delta G^{0'}$ that strongly favor the forward direction: the reactions catalyzed by citrate synthase, isocitrate dehydrogenase, and $\alpha$-ketoglutarate dehydrogenase (see Fig. 17.7). Within the TCA cycle, these reactions are physiologically irreversible for two reasons: The products do not rise to high enough concentrations under physiological conditions to overcome the large negative $\Delta G^{0'}$ values, and the enzymes involved catalyze the reverse reaction very slowly. These reactions make the major contribution to the overall negative $\Delta G^{0'}$ for the TCA cycle and keep it going in the forward direction.

In contrast to these irreversible reactions, the reactions catalyzed by aconitase and malate dehydrogenase have a positive $\Delta G^{0'}$ for the forward direction and are thermodynamically and kinetically reversible. Because aconitase is rapid in both directions, equilibrium values for the concentration ratio of products to substrates are maintained, and the concentration of citrate is about 20 times that of isocitrate. The accumulation of citrate instead of isocitrate facilitates transport of excess citrate to the cytosol, where it can provide a source of acetyl CoA for pathways like fatty acid and cholesterol synthesis. It also allows citrate to serve as an inhibitor of citrate synthase when flux through isocitrate dehydrogenase is decreased. Likewise, the equilibrium constant of the malate dehydrogenase reaction favors the accumulation of malate over oxaloacetate, resulting in a low oxaloacetate concentration that is influenced by the NADH/NAD$^+$ ratio. Thus, there is a net flux of oxaloacetate toward malate in the liver during fasting (due to fatty acid oxidation, which raises the NADH/NAD$^+$ ratio), and malate can then be transported out of the mitochondria to provide a substrate for gluconeogenesis.

## IV. REGULATION OF THE TCA CYCLE

The oxidation of acetyl CoA in the TCA cycle and the conservation of this energy as NADH and FAD(2H) is essential for generation of ATP in almost all tissues in the body. In spite of changes in the supply of fuels, type of fuels in the blood, or rate of ATP utilization, cells maintain ATP homeostasis (a constant level of ATP). The rate of the TCA cycle, like that of all fuel oxidation pathways, is principally regulated to correspond to the rate of the electron transport chain, which is regulated by the ATP/ADP ratio and the rate of ATP utilization (see Chapter 18). The major sites of regulation are shown in Figure 17.8.

Two major messengers feed information on the rate of ATP utilization back to the TCA cycle: (a) the phosphorylation state of ATP, as reflected in ATP and ADP

As **Otto S.** exercises, his myosin ATPase hydrolyzes ATP to provide the energy for movement of myofibrils. The decrease of ATP and increase of ADP stimulates the electron transport chain to oxidize more NADH and FAD(2H). The TCA cycle is stimulated to provide more NADH and FAD(2H) to the electron transport chain. The activation of the TCA cycle occurs through a decrease of the NADH/NAD$^+$ ratio, an increase of ADP concentration, and an increase of Ca$^{2+}$. Although regulation of the transcription of genes for TCA cycle enzymes is too slow to respond to changes of ATP demands during exercise, the number and size of mitochondria increase during training. Thus, **Otto S.** is increasing his capacity for fuel oxidation as he trains.

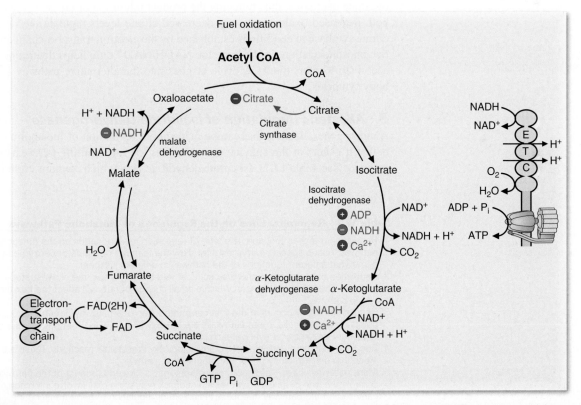

**FIG. 17.8.** Major regulatory interactions in the TCA cycle. The rate of ATP hydrolysis controls the rate of ATP synthesis, which controls the rate of NADH oxidation in the electron transport chain (ETC). All NADH and FAD(2H) produced by the cycle donate electrons to this chain (shown on the **right**). Thus, oxidation of acetyl CoA in the TCA cycle can go only as fast as electrons from NADH enter the ETC, which is controlled by the ATP and ADP content of the cells. The ADP and NADH concentrations feed information on the rate of oxidative phosphorylation back to the TCA cycle. Isocitrate dehydrogenase (DH), α-ketoglutarate DH, and malate DH are inhibited by increased NADH concentration. The NADH/NAD$^+$ ratio changes the concentration of oxaloacetate. Citrate is a product inhibitor of citrate synthase. ADP is an allosteric activator of isocitrate dehydrogenase. During muscular contraction, increased Ca$^{2+}$ concentrations activate isocitrate DH and α-ketoglutarate dehydrogenase (as well as pyruvate dehydrogenase).

levels, and (b) the reduction state of $NAD^+$, as reflected in the ratio of $NADH/NAD^+$. Within the cell, even within the mitochondrion, the total adenine nucleotide pool (AMP, ADP, plus ATP) and the total NAD pool ($NAD^+$ plus NADH) are relatively constant. Thus, an increased rate of ATP utilization results in a small decrease of ATP concentration and an increase of ADP. Likewise, increased NADH oxidation to $NAD^+$ by the electron transport chain increases the rate of pathways producing NADH. Under normal physiological conditions, the TCA cycle and other oxidative pathways respond so rapidly to increased ATP demand that the ATP concentration does not significantly change.

### A. Regulation of Citrate Synthase

The principles of pathway regulation are summarized in Table 17.1. In pathways subject to feedback regulation, the first step of the pathway must be regulated so that precursors flow into alternative pathways if product is not needed. Citrate synthase, which is the first enzyme of the TCA cycle, is a simple enzyme that has no allosteric regulators. Its rate is controlled principally by the concentration of oxaloacetate, its substrate, and by the concentration of citrate, a product inhibitor competitive with oxaloacetate (see Fig. 17.8). The malate-oxaloacetate equilibrium favors malate, so the oxaloacetate concentration is very low inside the mitochondrion and is below the $K_{m,app}$ (apparent Michaelis constant; see Chapter 7) of citrate synthase. When the $NADH/NAD^+$ ratio decreases, the ratio of oxaloacetate to malate increases. When isocitrate dehydrogenase is activated, the concentration of citrate decreases, thus relieving the product inhibition of citrate synthase. Thus, both increased oxaloacetate and decreased citrate levels regulate the response of citrate synthase to conditions established by the electron transport chain and oxidative phosphorylation. In the liver, the $NADH/NAD^+$ ratio helps determine whether acetyl CoA enters the TCA cycle or goes into the alternative pathway for ketone body synthesis.

### B. Allosteric Regulation of Isocitrate Dehydrogenase

Another generalization that can be made about regulation of metabolic pathways is that it occurs at the enzyme that catalyzes the rate-limiting (slowest) step in a pathway (see Table 17.1). Isocitrate dehydrogenase, which contains eight subunits,

---

**Table 17.1   Generalizations on the Regulation of Metabolic Pathways**

1. Regulation matches function. The type of regulation used depends on the function of the pathway. Tissue-specific isozymes may allow the features of regulatory enzymes to match somewhat different functions of the pathway in different tissues.
2. Regulation of metabolic pathways occurs at rate-limiting steps, the slowest steps, in the pathway. These are reactions in which a small change of rate will affect the flux through the whole pathway.
3. Regulation usually occurs at the first committed step of a pathway or at metabolic branch points. In human cells, most pathways are interconnected with other pathways and have regulatory enzymes for every branch point.
4. Regulatory enzymes often catalyze physiologically irreversible reactions. These are also the steps that differ in biosynthetic and degradative pathways.
5. Many pathways have "feedback" regulation, that is, the end product of the pathway controls the rate of its own synthesis. Feedback regulation may involve inhibition of an early step in the pathway (feedback inhibition) or regulation of gene transcription.
6. Human cells use compartmentation to control access of substrate and activators or inhibitors to different enzymes.
7. Hormonal regulation integrates responses in pathways requiring more than one tissue. Hormones generally regulate fuel metabolism by
    a. Changing the phosphorylation state of enzymes
    b. Changing the amount of enzyme present by changing its rate of synthesis (often induction or repression of mRNA synthesis) or degradation
    c. Changing the concentration of an activator or inhibitor

is considered one of the rate-limiting steps of the TCA cycle and is allosterically activated by ADP and inhibited by NADH. In the absence of ADP, the enzyme exhibits positive cooperativity; as isocitrate binds to one subunit, other subunits are converted to an active conformation. In the presence of ADP, all of the subunits are in their active conformation, and isocitrate binds more readily. Consequently, the $K_{m,app}$ (the $S_{0.5}$) shifts to a much lower value. Thus, at the concentration of isocitrate found in the mitochondrial matrix, a small change in the concentration of ADP can produce a large change in the rate of the isocitrate dehydrogenase reaction. Small changes in the concentration of the product, NADH, and of the cosubstrate, $NAD^+$, also affect the rate of the enzyme more than they would a nonallosteric enzyme.

### C. Regulation of α-Ketoglutarate Dehydrogenase

The α-ketoglutarate dehydrogenase complex, although not an allosteric enzyme, is product-inhibited by NADH and succinyl CoA and may also be inhibited by GTP (see Fig. 17.8). Thus, both α-ketoglutarate dehydrogenase and isocitrate dehydrogenase respond directly to changes in the relative levels of ADP and hence the rate at which NADH is oxidized by electron transport. Both of these enzymes are also activated by $Ca^+$. In contracting heart muscle and possibly other muscle tissues, the release of $Ca^+$ from the sarcoplasmic reticulum during muscle contraction may provide an additional activation of these enzymes when ATP is being rapidly hydrolyzed.

### D. Regulation of TCA Cycle Intermediates

Regulation of the TCA cycle serves two functions: It ensures that NADH is generated fast enough to maintain ATP homeostasis and it regulates the concentration of TCA cycle intermediates. For example, in the liver, a decreased rate of isocitrate dehydrogenase increases citrate concentration, which stimulates citrate efflux to the cytosol. A number of regulatory interactions occur in the TCA cycle, in addition to those mentioned earlier, that control the levels of TCA intermediates and their flux into pathways that adjoin the TCA cycle.

## V. PRECURSORS OF ACETYL CoA

Compounds enter the TCA cycle as acetyl CoA or as an intermediate that can be converted to malate or oxaloacetate. Compounds that enter as acetyl CoA are oxidized to $CO_2$. Compounds that enter as TCA cycle intermediates replenish intermediates that have been used in biosynthetic pathways, such as gluconeogenesis or heme synthesis, but cannot be fully oxidized to $CO_2$.

### A. Sources of Acetyl CoA

Acetyl CoA serves as a common point of convergence for the major pathways of fuel oxidation. It is generated directly from the β-oxidation of fatty acids and degradation of the ketone bodies β-hydroxybutyrate and acetoacetate (Fig. 17.9). It is also formed from acetate, which can arise from the diet or from ethanol oxidation. Glucose and other carbohydrates enter glycolysis, a pathway common to all cells, and are oxidized to pyruvate. The amino acids alanine and serine are also converted to pyruvate. Pyruvate is oxidized to acetyl CoA by the PDC. A number of amino acids, such as leucine and isoleucine, are also oxidized to acetyl CoA. Thus, the final oxidation of acetyl CoA to $CO_2$ in the TCA cycle is the last step in all the major pathways of fuel oxidation.

### B. Pyruvate Dehydrogenase Complex

The **PDC** oxidizes pyruvate to acetyl CoA, thus linking glycolysis and the TCA cycle. In the brain, which is dependent on the oxidation of glucose to $CO_2$ to fulfill its ATP needs, regulation of the PDC is a life-and-death matter.

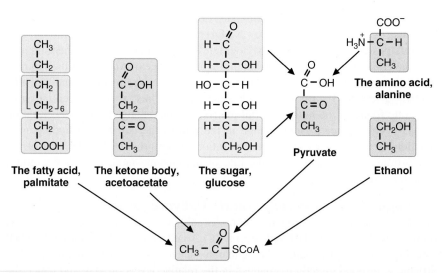

**FIG. 17.9.** Origin of the acetyl group from various fuels. Acetyl CoA is derived from the oxidation of fuels. The portions of fatty acids, ketone bodies, glucose, pyruvate, the amino acid alanine, and ethanol that are converted to the acetyl group of acetyl CoA are shown in *boxes*.

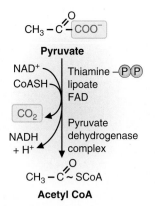

**FIG. 17.10.** The PDC catalyzes the oxidation of the α-keto acid pyruvate to acetyl CoA.

## 1. STRUCTURE OF THE PDC

PDC belongs to the α-keto acid dehydrogenase complex family and thus shares structural and catalytic features with the α-ketoglutarate dehydrogenase complex and the branched-chain α-keto acid dehydrogenase complex (Fig. 17.10). It contains the same three basic types of catalytic subunits: (a) pyruvate decarboxylase subunits that bind thiamine pyrophosphate ($E_1$), (b) transacetylase subunits that bind lipoate ($E_2$), and (c) dihydrolipoyl dehydrogenase subunits that bind FAD ($E_3$). Although the $E_1$ and $E_2$ enzymes in PDC are relatively specific for pyruvate, the same dihydrolipoyl dehydrogenase participates in all of the α-keto acid dehydrogenase complexes. In addition to these three types of subunits, the PDC complex contains one additional subunit, an $E_3$-binding protein ($E_3$-BP). Each functional component of the PDC complex is present in multiple copies (e.g., bovine heart PDC has 30 subunits of $E_1$, 60 subunits of $E_2$, and 6 subunits each of $E_3$ and $E_3$-BP). The $E_1$ enzyme is itself a tetramer of two different types of subunits, α and β.

Deficiencies of the PDC are among the most common inherited diseases leading to lactic acidemia and, similar to pyruvate carboxylase deficiency, are grouped into the category of Leigh disease (subacute necrotizing encephalopathy). When PDC is defective, pyruvate will accumulate and ATP production will drop. The low ATP will stimulate glycolysis (see Chapter 19) to proceed anaerobically, and to do so, pyruvate is reduced to lactate. In its severe form, PDC deficiency presents with overwhelming lactic acidosis at birth, with death in the neonatal period. In a second form of presentation, the lactic acidemia is moderate, but there is profound psychomotor retardation with increasing age. In many cases, concomitant damage to the brain stem and basal ganglia lead to death in infancy. The neurological symptoms arise because the brain has a very limited ability to use fatty acids as a fuel and is, therefore, dependent on glucose metabolism for its energy supply.

The most common PDC genetic defects are in the gene for the α-subunit of $E_1$. The $E_1$ α-gene is X-linked. Because of its importance in central nervous system metabolism, pyruvate dehydrogenase deficiency is a problem in both males and females, even if the female is a carrier. For this reason, it is classified as an X-linked dominant disorder.

## 2. REGULATION OF THE PDC

PDC activity is controlled principally through phosphorylation by pyruvate dehydrogenase kinase, which inhibits the enzyme and dephosphorylation by pyruvate dehydrogenase phosphatase, which activates it (Fig. 17.11). Pyruvate dehydrogenase kinase and pyruvate dehydrogenase phosphatase are regulatory subunits within the PDC complex and act only on the complex. PDC kinase transfers a phosphate from ATP to specific serine hydroxyl (ser-OH) groups on pyruvate decarboxylase ($E_1$). PDC phosphatase removes these phosphate groups by hydrolysis. Phosphorylation of just one serine on the PDC $E_1$ α-subunit can decrease its activity by over 99%. PDC kinase is present in complexes as tissue-specific isozymes that vary in their regulatory properties.

PDC kinase is itself inhibited by ADP and pyruvate. Thus, when rapid ATP utilization results in an increase of ADP or when activation of glycolysis increases pyruvate levels, PDC kinase is inhibited and PDC remains in an active, nonphosphorylated form. PDC phosphatase requires $Ca^{2+}$ for full activity. In the heart, increased intramitochondrial $Ca^{2+}$ during rapid contraction activates the phosphatase, thereby increasing the amount of active, nonphosphorylated PDC.

PDC is also regulated through inhibition by its products, acetyl CoA and NADH. This inhibition is stronger than regular product inhibition because their binding to PDC stimulates its phosphorylation to the inactive form. The substrates of the enzyme, CoASH and $NAD^+$, antagonize this product inhibition. Thus, when an ample supply of acetyl CoA for the TCA cycle is already available from fatty acid oxidation, acetyl CoA and NADH build up and dramatically decrease their own further synthesis by PDC.

PDC can also be activated rapidly through a mechanism involving insulin, which plays a prominent role in adipocytes. In many tissues, insulin may, over time, slowly increase the amount of PDC present.

The rate of other fuel oxidation pathways that feed into the TCA cycle is also increased when ATP utilization increases. Insulin, other hormones, and diet control the availability of fuels for these oxidative pathways.

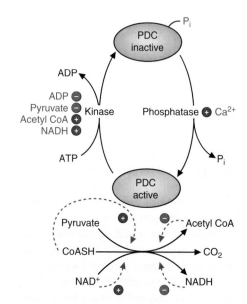

**FIG. 17.11.** Regulation of PDC. PDC kinase, a subunit of the enzyme, phosphorylates PDC at a specific serine residue, thereby converting PDC to an inactive form. The kinase is inhibited by ADP and pyruvate. PDC phosphatase, another subunit of the enzyme, removes the phosphate, thereby activating PDC. The phosphatase is activated by $Ca^{2+}$. When the substrates pyruvate and CoASH are bound to PDC, the kinase activity is inhibited and PDC is active. When the products acetyl CoA and NADH bind to PDC, the kinase activity is stimulated, and the enzyme is phosphorylated to the inactive form. $E_1$ and the kinase exist as tissue-specific isozymes with overlapping tissue specificity and somewhat different regulatory properties.

## VI. TCA CYCLE INTERMEDIATES AND ANAPLEROTIC REACTIONS

### A. TCA Cycle Intermediates as Biosynthetic Precursors

The intermediates of the TCA cycle serve as precursors for a variety of different pathways present in different cell types (Fig. 17.12). This is particularly important in the central metabolic role of the liver. The TCA cycle in the liver is often called an **open cycle** because there is such a high efflux of intermediates. After a high-carbohydrate meal, citrate efflux and cleavage to acetyl CoA provides acetyl units for cytosolic fatty acid synthesis. During fasting, gluconeogenic precursors are converted to malate, which leaves the mitochondria for cytosolic gluconeogenesis. The liver also uses TCA cycle intermediates to synthesize carbon skeletons of amino acids. Succinyl CoA may be removed from the TCA cycle to form heme in cells of the liver and bone marrow. In the brain, α-ketoglutarate is converted to glutamate and then to γ-aminobutyric acid (GABA), a neurotransmitter. In skeletal muscle, α-ketoglutarate is converted to glutamine, which is transported through the blood to other tissues.

### B. Anaplerotic Reactions

Removal of any of the intermediates from the TCA cycle removes the four carbons that are used to regenerate oxaloacetate during each turn of the cycle. With depletion of oxaloacetate, it is impossible to continue oxidizing acetyl CoA. To enable the TCA cycle to keep running, cells have to supply enough four-carbon intermediates from degradation of carbohydrate or certain amino acids to compensate for the rate

Pyruvate, citrate, α-ketoglutarate and malate, ADP, ATP, and phosphate (as well as many other compounds) have specific transporters in the inner mitochondrial membrane that transport compounds between the mitochondrial matrix and cytosol in exchange for a compound of similar charge. In contrast, CoASH, acetyl CoA, other CoA derivatives, $NAD^+$ and NADH, and oxaloacetate are not transported at a metabolically significant rate. To obtain cytosolic acetyl CoA, many cells transport citrate to the cytosol, where it is cleaved to acetyl CoA and oxaloacetate by citrate lyase.

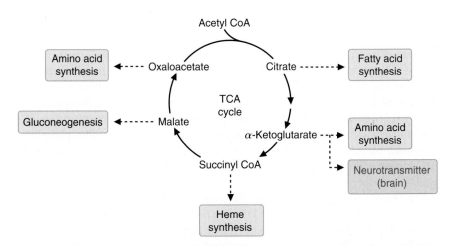

FIG. 17.12. Efflux of intermediates from the TCA cycle. In the liver, TCA cycle intermediates are continuously withdrawn into the pathways of fatty acid synthesis, amino acid synthesis, gluconeogenesis, and heme synthesis. In the brain, α-ketoglutarate is converted to glutamate and GABA, both neurotransmitters.

Pyruvate carboxylase deficiency is one of the genetic diseases grouped together under the clinical manifestations of Leigh disease. In the mild form, the patient presents early in life with delayed development and a mild to moderate lactic acidemia (similar to PDC defects, pyruvate will accumulate when pyruvate carboxylase is defective). Patients who survive are severely mentally retarded, and there is a loss of cerebral neurons. In the brain, pyruvate carboxylase is present in the astrocytes, which use TCA cycle intermediates to synthesize glutamine. This pathway is essential for neuronal survival. The major cause of the lactic acidemia is that cells dependent on pyruvate carboxylase for an anaplerotic supply of oxaloacetate cannot oxidize pyruvate in the TCA cycle (because of low oxaloacetate levels), and the liver cannot convert pyruvate to glucose (because the pyruvate carboxylase reaction is required for this pathway to occur), so the excess pyruvate is converted to lactate.

of removal. Pathways or reactions that replenish the intermediates of the TCA cycle are referred to as **anaplerotic** ("filling up").

### 1. PYRUVATE CARBOXYLASE

Pyruvate carboxylase is one of the major anaplerotic enzymes in the cell. It catalyzes the addition of $CO_2$ to pyruvate to form oxaloacetate (Fig. 17.13). Like most carboxylases, pyruvate carboxylase contains the vitamin biotin, which forms a covalent intermediate with $CO_2$ in a reaction requiring ATP and $Mg^{2+}$ (see Fig. 6.7). The activated $CO_2$ is then transferred to pyruvate to form the carboxyl group of oxaloacetate.

Pyruvate carboxylase is found in many tissues, such as liver, brain, adipocytes, and fibroblasts, where its function is anaplerotic. Its concentration is high in liver and kidney cortex, where there is a continuous removal of oxaloacetate and malate from the TCA cycle to enter the gluconeogenic pathway.

Pyruvate carboxylase is activated by acetyl CoA and inhibited by high concentrations of many acyl CoA derivatives. As the concentration of oxaloacetate is depleted through the efflux of TCA cycle intermediates, the rate of the citrate synthase reaction decreases and acetyl CoA concentration rises. The acetyl CoA then activates pyruvate carboxylase to synthesize more oxaloacetate.

### 2. AMINO ACID DEGRADATION

The pathways for oxidation of many amino acids convert their carbon skeletons into five- and four-carbon intermediates of the TCA cycle that can regenerate oxaloacetate (Fig. 17.14). Alanine and serine carbons can enter through pyruvate carboxylase (see Fig.17.14, *circle 1*). In all tissues with mitochondria (except for, surprisingly, the liver), oxidation of the two branched-chain amino acids isoleucine and valine to succinyl CoA forms a major anaplerotic route (see Fig.17.14, *circle 3*). In the liver, other compounds forming propionyl CoA (e.g., methionine, threonine, and odd chain length or branched fatty acids) also enter the TCA cycle as succinyl CoA. In most tissues, glutamine is taken up from the blood, converted to glutamate, and then oxidized to α-ketoglutarate, forming another major anaplerotic route (see Fig. 17.14, *circle 2*). However, the TCA cycle cannot be resupplied with intermediates of fatty acid oxidation of even chain length or ketone body oxidation, both of which only form acetyl CoA. In the TCA cycle, two carbons are lost from citrate before succinyl CoA is formed, and therefore, there is no net conversion of acetyl carbon to oxaloacetate.

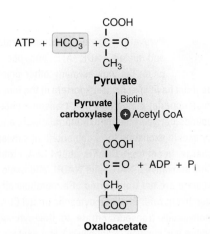

FIG. 17.13. Pyruvate carboxylase reaction. Pyruvate carboxylase adds a carboxyl group from bicarbonate (which is in equilibrium with $CO_2$) to pyruvate to form oxaloacetate. Biotin is used to activate and transfer the $CO_2$. The energy to form the covalent biotin-$CO_2$ complex is provided by the high-energy phosphate bond of ATP, which is cleaved in the reaction. The enzyme is activated by acetyl CoA.

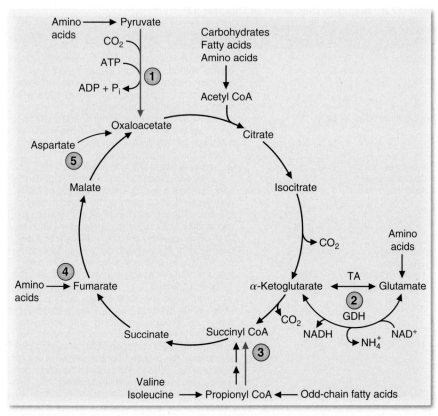

**FIG. 17.14.** Major anaplerotic pathways of the TCA cycle. *1* and *3 (red arrows)* are the two major anabolic pathways. *(1)* Pyruvate carboxylase. *(2)* Glutamate is reversibly converted to α-ketoglutarate by transaminases *(TA)* and glutamate dehydrogenase *(GDH)* in many tissues. *(3)* The carbon skeletons of valine and isoleucine, a three-carbon unit from odd-chain fatty acid oxidation, and a number of other compounds enter the TCA cycle at the level of succinyl CoA. Other amino acids are also degraded to fumarate *(4)* and oxaloacetate *(5)*, principally in the liver.

## CLINICAL COMMENTS

Diseases discussed in this chapter are summarized in Table 17.2.

**Otto S.** Otto S. is experiencing the benefits of physical conditioning. A variety of functional adaptations in the heart, lungs, vascular system, and skeletal muscle occur in response to regular graded exercise. The pumping efficiency of the heart increases, allowing a greater cardiac output with fewer beats per minute and at a lower rate of oxygen utilization. The lungs extract a greater percentage of oxygen from the inspired air, allowing fewer respirations per unit of activity. The vasodilatory capacity of the arterial beds in skeletal muscle increases, promoting greater delivery of oxygen and fuels to exercising muscle. Concurrently, the venous drainage capacity in muscle is enhanced, ensuring that lactic acid will not accumulate in contracting tissues. These adaptive changes in physiological responses are accompanied by increases in the number, size, and activity of skeletal muscle mitochondria along with the content of TCA cycle enzymes and components of the electron transport chain. These changes markedly enhance the oxidative capacity of exercising muscle.

**Ann R.** Ann R. is experiencing fatigue for several reasons. She has iron deficiency anemia, which affects both iron-containing hemoglobin in her red blood cells, iron in aconitase and succinic dehydrogenase, as well as iron in the heme proteins of the electron transport chain. She may also be

In skeletal muscle and other tissues, ATP is generated by anaerobic glycolysis when the rate of aerobic respiration is inadequate to meet the rate of ATP utilization. Under these circumstances, the rate of pyruvate production exceeds the cell's capacity to oxidize NADH in the electron transport chain, and hence, to oxidize pyruvate in the TCA cycle. The excess pyruvate is reduced to lactate. Because lactate is an acid, its accumulation affects the muscle and causes pain and swelling.

**Table 17.2    Diseases Discussed in Chapter 17**

| Disease or Disorder | Environmental or Genetic | Comments |
|---|---|---|
| Obesity | Both | Increased physical activity, without increasing caloric intake, will lead to weight loss and increased exercise capacity. One effect of increased aerobic exercise is increasing the number and size of mitochondria in the muscle cells. |
| Anorexia nervosa | Both | Patients who have been malnourished for some time may exhibit subclinical deficiencies in many vitamins, including riboflavin and niacin, factors required for energy generation. |
| Congestive heart failure linked to alcoholism | Both | Thiamine deficiency, brought about by chronic alcohol ingestion, leads to dilation of the blood vessels, inefficient energy production by the heart, and failure to adequately pump blood throughout the body. The vitamin $B_1$ deficiency reduces the activity of pyruvate dehydrogenase and the TCA cycle, severely restricting ATP generation. |
| Leigh disease (subacute necrotizing encephalopathy) | Genetic | Deficiencies of the pyruvate dehydrogenase complex (PDC), as well as of pyruvate carboxylase, are inherited disorders leading to lactic acidemia. In its most severe form, PDC deficiency presents with overwhelming lactic acidosis at birth, with death in the neonatal period. Even in less severe forms, neurological symptoms arise due to the brains' dependence on glucose metabolism for energy. The most common PDC deficiency is X-linked, in the α-subunit of the pyruvate decarboxylase ($E_1$) subunit. Pyruvate carboxylase deficiency also leads to mental retardation. |

TCA, tricarboxylic acid; ATP, adenosine triphosphate.

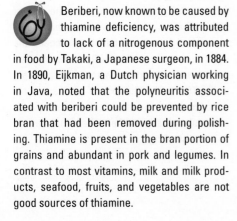

Riboflavin has a wide distribution in foods, and small amounts are present as coenzymes in most plant and animal tissues. Eggs, lean meats, milk, broccoli, and enriched breads and cereals are especially good sources. A portion of our niacin requirement can be met by synthesis from tryptophan. Meat (especially red meat), liver, legumes, milk, eggs, alfalfa, cereal grains, yeast, and fish are good sources of niacin and tryptophan.

Beriberi, now known to be caused by thiamine deficiency, was attributed to lack of a nitrogenous component in food by Takaki, a Japanese surgeon, in 1884. In 1890, Eijkman, a Dutch physician working in Java, noted that the polyneuritis associated with beriberi could be prevented by rice bran that had been removed during polishing. Thiamine is present in the bran portion of grains and abundant in pork and legumes. In contrast to most vitamins, milk and milk products, seafood, fruits, and vegetables are not good sources of thiamine.

experiencing the consequences of multiple vitamin deficiencies, including thiamine, riboflavin, and niacin (the vitamin precursor of $NAD^+$). It is less likely, but possible, that she also has subclinical deficiencies of pantothenate (the precursor of CoA) or biotin. As a result, Ann's muscles must use glycolysis as their primary source of energy, which results in sore muscles.

Riboflavin deficiency generally occurs in conjunction with other water-soluble vitamin deficiencies. The classic deficiency symptoms are cheilosis (inflammation of the corners of the mouth), glossitis (magenta tongue), and seborrheic ("greasy") dermatitis. It is also characterized by sore throat, edema of the pharyngeal and oral mucous membranes, and a normochromic, normocytic anemia. However, it is not known whether the glossitis and dermatitis are actually due to multiple vitamin deficiencies.

**Al M.** Al M. presents a second time with an alcohol-related high-output form of heart failure, sometimes referred to as wet beriberi or as the beriberi heart (see Chapter 7). The term "wet" refers to the fluid retention, which may eventually occur when left ventricular contractility is so compromised that cardiac output, although initially relatively "high," cannot meet the "demands" of the peripheral vascular beds, which have dilated in response to the thiamine deficiency.

The cardiomyopathy is due to the persistent high output required because of the dilated peripheral vasculature and also likely related to a reduction in the normal biochemical function of the vitamin thiamine in heart muscle. Inhibition of the α-keto acid dehydrogenase complexes causes accumulation of α-keto acids in heart muscle (and in blood), which may result in a chemically induced cardiomyopathy. Impairment of two other functions of thiamine may also contribute to the cardiomyopathy. TPP serves as the coenzyme for transketolase in the pentose phosphate pathway, and pentose phosphates accumulate in thiamine deficiency. In addition, thiamine triphosphate (a different coenzyme form) may function in $Na^+$ conductance channels.

Immediate treatment with large doses (50 to 100 mg) of intravenous thiamine may produce a measurable decrease in cardiac output and increase in peripheral vascular resistance as early as 30 minutes after the initial injection. Dietary supplementation of thiamine is not as effective because ethanol consumption interferes with thiamine absorption. Because ethanol also affects the absorption of most water-soluble vitamins or their conversion to the coenzyme form, **Al M.** was also given a bolus containing a multivitamin supplement.

## REVIEW QUESTIONS-CHAPTER 17

1. A patient diagnosed with thiamine deficiency exhibited fatigue and muscle cramps. The muscle cramps have been related to an accumulation of metabolic acids. Which one of the following metabolic acids is most likely to accumulate under these conditions?

   A. Isocitric acid
   B. Succinic acid
   C. Malic acid
   D. Oxaloacetic acid
   E. Pyruvic acid

2. During exercise, stimulation of the tricarboxylic acid cycle results principally from which one of the following?

   A. Allosteric activation of isocitrate dehydrogenase by increased NADH
   B. Stimulation of the flux through a number of enzymes by a decreased $NADH/NAD^+$ ratio
   C. Allosteric activation of fumarase by increased ADP
   D. A rapid decrease in the concentration of four-carbon intermediates
   E. Product inhibition of citrate synthase

3. $CO_2$ production by the tricarboxylic acid cycle would be increased to the greatest extent by a genetic abnormality that resulted in which one of the following?

   A. A 50% increase in the oxygen content of the cell
   B. A 50% decrease in the $V_{max}$ of α-ketoglutarate dehydrogenase

   C. A 50% increase in the $K_m$ of isocitrate dehydrogenase
   D. A 50% increase in the concentration of ADP in the mitochondrial matrix
   E. A 50% increase in $K_m$ of citrate synthase

4. The pyruvate dehydrogenase complex is directly activated by which one of the following?

   A. Dephosphorylation by pyruvate dehydrogenase phosphatase
   B. An increase of NADH
   C. An increase of acetyl CoA
   D. A decrease of $Ca^{2+}$
   E. An increase in the concentration of ATP

5. The TCA cycle is deemed "cyclic" because of the utilization and regeneration of which one of the following?

   A. Citrate
   B. Succinyl CoA
   C. Malate
   D. α-Ketoglutarate
   E. Oxaloacetate

# 18 Oxidative Phosphorylation, Mitochondrial Function, and Oxygen Radicals

## CHAPTER OUTLINE

# KEY POINTS

- The reduced cofactors generated during fuel oxidation donate their electrons to the mitochondrial electron transport chain.
- The electron transport chain transfers the electrons to $O_2$, which is reduced to water.
- As electrons travel through the electron transport chain, protons are transferred from the mitochondrial matrix to the cytosolic side of the inner mitochondrial membrane.
- The asymmetric distribution of protons across the inner mitochondrial membrane generates an electrochemical gradient across the membrane.
- The electrochemical gradient consists of a change in pH ($\Delta$pH) across the membrane and a difference in charge ($\Delta\varphi$) across the membrane.
- Proton entry into the mitochondrial matrix is energetically favorable and drives the synthesis of ATP via the ATP synthase.
- Respiration (oxygen consumption) is normally coupled to ATP synthesis; if one process is inhibited, the other is also inhibited.
- Uncouplers allow respiration to continue in the absence of ATP synthesis, as the energy inherent in the proton gradient is released as heat.
- Through a number of enzymatic and nonenzymatic processes, oxygen can accept a single electron to form reactive oxygen species.
- The major reactive oxygen species are the radicals superoxide and hydroxyl radical and the nonradical hydrogen peroxide.
- Reactive oxygen species cause damage to lipids, proteins, and DNA within cells.
- NO reacts with oxygen or superoxide to form a family of reactive nitrogen-oxygen species.
- Cellular defense mechanisms against radical damage include defense enzymes, antioxidants, and compartmentalization of free radicals.
- Cellular defense enzymes include superoxide dismutase, catalase, and glutathione peroxidase.
- Antioxidants include vitamins E and C and plant flavonoids.

# THE WAITING ROOM

**Cora N.** was recovering uneventfully from her heart attack 1 month earlier when she won the Georgia state lottery. When she heard her number announced over television, she experienced crushing chest pain, grew short of breath, and passed out. She regained consciousness as she was being rushed to the hospital emergency room.

On initial examination, her blood pressure was extremely high and her heart rhythm irregular. **Cora N.** is experiencing yet another myocardial infarction. Her blood levels of creatine kinase-MB (CK-MB) and troponin I (TnI) were elevated. An electrocardiogram showed unequivocal evidence of severe lack of $O_2$ (ischemia) in the muscles of the anterior and lateral walls of her heart. Life support measures including nasal $O_2$ were initiated. An intravenous drip of nitroglycerin, a vasodilating agent, was started in an effort to reduce her hypertension (it will also help to decrease her "preload" by vasodilating the vessels going to the heart). She was also given a β-blocker, which will also help decrease her blood pressure as well as decrease the work of her heart by slowing her heart rate. After her blood pressure was well controlled and because the hospital did not have a cardiac catheterization laboratory, a decision was made to administer intravenous tissue plasminogen activator (TPA) in

**Cora N.** is experiencing a second myocardial infarction (see Chapter 16). Ischemia (low blood flow) has caused hypoxia (low levels of $O_2$) in the threatened area of her heart muscle, resulting in inadequate generation of ATP for the maintenance of low intracellular $Na^+$ and $Ca^{2+}$ levels. As a consequence, the myocardial cells in that specific location have become swollen and the cytosolic proteins creatine kinase (MB isoform) and troponin (heart isoform) have leaked into the blood (see Ann J., Chapters 4 and 5).

an attempt to break up any intracoronary artery blood clots in vessels supplying the ischemic myocardium (thrombolytic therapy).

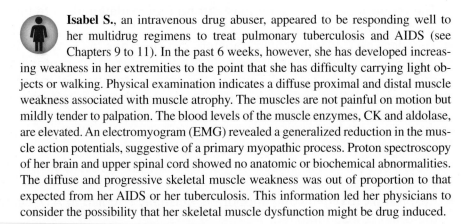

**Isabel S.**, an intravenous drug abuser, appeared to be responding well to her multidrug regimens to treat pulmonary tuberculosis and AIDS (see Chapters 9 to 11). In the past 6 weeks, however, she has developed increasing weakness in her extremities to the point that she has difficulty carrying light objects or walking. Physical examination indicates a diffuse proximal and distal muscle weakness associated with muscle atrophy. The muscles are not painful on motion but mildly tender to palpation. The blood levels of the muscle enzymes, CK and aldolase, are elevated. An electromyogram (EMG) revealed a generalized reduction in the muscle action potentials, suggestive of a primary myopathic process. Proton spectroscopy of her brain and upper spinal cord showed no anatomic or biochemical abnormalities. The diffuse and progressive skeletal muscle weakness was out of proportion to that expected from her AIDS or her tuberculosis. This information led her physicians to consider the possibility that her skeletal muscle dysfunction might be drug induced.

## I. OXIDATIVE PHOSPHORYLATION

Generation of ATP from **oxidative phosphorylation** requires an electron donor (NADH or FAD[2H]), an electron acceptor ($O_2$), an intact inner mitochondrial membrane that is impermeable to protons, all the components of the electron transport chain, and ATP synthase. It is regulated by the rate of ATP utilization.

### A. Overview of Oxidative Phosphorylation

Our understanding of oxidative phosphorylation is based on the **chemiosmotic hypothesis**, which proposes that the energy for ATP synthesis is provided by an electrochemical gradient across the inner mitochondrial membrane. This electrochemical gradient is generated by the components of the electron transport chain, which pump protons across the inner mitochondrial membrane as they sequentially accept and donate electrons (Fig. 18.1). The final acceptor is $O_2$, which is reduced to $H_2O$.

### 1. ELECTRON TRANSFER FROM NADH TO $O_2$

In the **electron transport chain**, electrons donated by NADH or FAD(2H) are passed sequentially through a series of electron carriers embedded in the inner mitochondrial membrane. Each of the components of the electron transfer chain is reduced as it accepts an electron and then oxidized as it passes the electrons to the next member

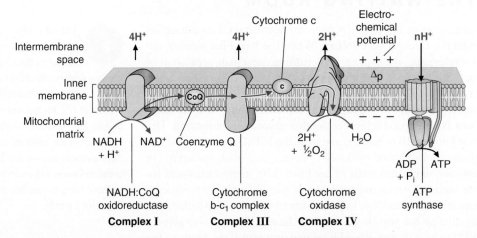

**FIG. 18.1.** Oxidative phosphorylation. *Red arrows* show the path of electron transport from NADH to $O_2$. As electrons pass through the chain, protons are pumped from the mitochondrial matrix to the intermembrane space, thereby establishing an electrochemical potential gradient, $\Delta p$, across the inner mitochondrial membrane. The positive and negative charges on the membrane denote the membrane potential ($\Delta \varphi$). $\Delta p$ drives protons into the matrix through a pore in ATP synthase, which uses the energy to form ATP from ADP and $P_i$.

of the chain. From NADH, electrons are transferred sequentially through **NADH dehydrogenase (complex I)**, **coenzyme Q (CoQ)**, **the cytochrome b-$c_1$ complex (complex III)**, **cytochrome c**, and finally **cytochrome c oxidase (complex IV)**. NADH dehydrogenase, the cytochrome b-$c_1$ complex, and cytochrome c oxidase are multisubunit protein complexes that span the inner mitochondrial membrane. CoQ is a lipid-soluble quinone that is not protein bound and is free to diffuse in the lipid membrane. It transports electrons from complex I to complex III and is an intrinsic part of the proton pumps for each of these complexes. Cytochrome c is a small protein in the intermembrane space that transfers electrons from the b-$c_1$ complex to cytochrome oxidase. The terminal complex, cytochrome c oxidase, contains the binding site for $O_2$. As $O_2$ accepts electrons from the chain, it is reduced to $H_2O$.

## 2.  THE ELECTROCHEMICAL POTENTIAL GRADIENT

At each of the three large membrane-spanning complexes in the chain, electron transfer is accompanied by proton pumping across the membrane. There is an energy drop of approximately 16 kcal in reduction potential as electrons pass through each of these complexes, which provides the energy required to move protons against a concentration gradient. The membrane is impermeable to protons, so they cannot diffuse through the lipid bilayer back into the matrix. Thus, in actively respiring mitochondria, the intermembrane space and cytosol may be approximately 0.75 pH units lower than the matrix.

The transmembrane movement of protons generates an electrochemical gradient with two components: the membrane potential (the external face of the membrane has a positive charge relative to the matrix side) and the proton gradient (the intermembrane space has a higher proton concentration and is, therefore, more acidic than the matrix) (see Fig. 18.1). The electrochemical gradient is sometimes called the **proton motive force** because it is the energy that pushes the protons to reenter the matrix to equilibrate on both sides of the membrane. The protons are attracted to the more negatively charged matrix side of the membrane, where the pH is more alkaline.

## 3.  ATP SYNTHASE

**ATP synthase** ($F_0F_1$ATPase), the enzyme that generates ATP, is a multisubunit enzyme containing an inner membrane portion ($F_0$) and a stalk and headpiece ($F_1$) that project into the matrix (Fig. 18.2). The 12 **c** subunits in the membrane form a rotor

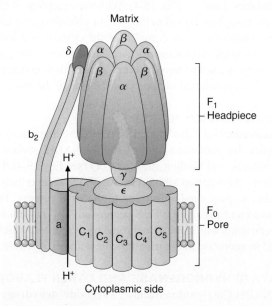

***FIG. 18.2.*** ATP synthase ($F_0F_1$ATPase). Note that the matrix side of the mitochondrial inner membrane is at the **top** of the figure.

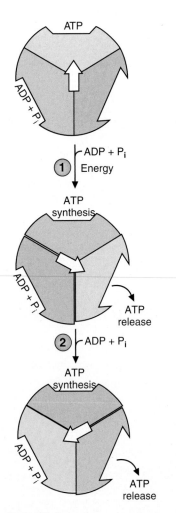

**FIG. 18.3.** Binding change mechanism for ATP synthesis. The three αβ-subunit pairs of the ATP synthase headpiece have binding sites that can exist in three different conformations, depending on the position of the γ-stalk subunit. *(1)* When ADP + P_i bind to an open site and the proton influx rotates the γ-spindle *(white arrow)*, the conformation of the subunits change and ATP is released from one site. (ATP dissociation is thus the energy-requiring step). Bound ADP and P_i combine to form ATP at another site. *(2)* As the ADP + P_i bind to the new open site and the γ-shaft rotates, the conformations of the sites change again and ATP is released. ADP and P_i combine to form another ATP.

that is attached to a central asymmetric shaft composed of ε- and γ-subunits. The headpiece is composed of three αβ-subunit pairs. Each β-subunit contains a catalytic site for ATP synthesis. The headpiece is held stationary by a δ-subunit attached to a long b subunit connected to the a subunit in the membrane.

The influx of protons through the proton channel turns the rotor. The proton channel is formed by the **c** subunit on one side and the **a** subunit on the other side (see Fig. 18.2). Although the channel is continuous, it has two offset portions: one portion opens directly to the intermembrane space and one portion opens directly to the matrix. In the current model, each c subunit contains a glutamyl carboxyl group that extends into the proton channel. Because this carboxyl group accepts a proton from the intermembrane space, the c subunit rotates into the hydrophobic lipid membrane. The rotation exposes a different proton-containing c subunit to the portion of the channel that is open directly to the matrix side. Because the matrix has a lower proton concentration, the glutamyl carboxylic acid group releases a proton into the matrix portion of the channel. Rotation is completed by an attraction between the negatively charged glutamyl residue and a positively charged arginine group on the a subunit.

According to the binding change mechanism, as the asymmetric shaft rotates to a new position, it forms different binding associations with the αβ-subunits. The new position of the shaft alters the conformation of one β-subunit so that it releases a molecule of ATP and another subunit spontaneously catalyzes synthesis of ATP from inorganic phosphate (P_i), one proton, and adenosine diphosphate (ADP) (Fig. 18.3). Thus, energy from the electrochemical gradient is used to change the conformation of the ATP synthase subunits so that the newly synthesized ATP is released. Twelve c subunits are hypothesized and it takes 12 protons to complete one turn of the rotor and synthesize three molecules of ATP.

## B. Oxidation–Reduction Components of the Electron Transport Chain

Electron transport to $O_2$ occurs via a series of oxidation–reduction steps in which each successive component of the chain is reduced as it accepts electrons and oxidized as it passes electrons to the next component of the chain. The oxidation–reduction components of the chain include flavin mononucleotide (FMN), iron-sulfur (Fe-S) centers, CoQ, and Fe in the cytochromes b, $c_1$, c, a, and $a_3$. Copper is also a component of cytochromes a and $a_3$ (Fig. 18.4). With the exception of CoQ, all of these electron acceptors are tightly bound to the protein subunits of the carriers.

The reduction potential of each complex of the chain is at a lower energy level than the previous complex, so that energy is released as electrons pass through each complex. This energy is used to move protons against their concentration gradient, so that they become concentrated on the cytosolic side of the inner membrane.

### 1. NADH:COQ OXIDOREDUCTASE

NADH:CoQ oxidoreductase (also named NADH dehydrogenase) is an enormous 42-subunit complex that contains a binding site for NADH, several FMN and Fe-S center binding proteins, and binding sites for CoQ (see Fig. 18.4). FMN, like FAD, is synthesized from the vitamin riboflavin. An FMN accepts two electrons from NADH and is able to pass single electrons to the Fe-S centers. The Fe-S centers transfer electrons to and from CoQ. Fe-S centers are also present in other enzyme systems, such as proteins within the cytochrome $b$-$c_1$ complex, which transfers electrons to CoQ and in aconitase in the tricarboxylic acid (TCA) cycle.

### 2. SUCCINATE DEHYDROGENASE AND OTHER FLAVOPROTEINS

In addition to NADH:CoQ oxidoreductase, **succinate dehydrogenase** and other flavoproteins in the inner mitochondrial membrane also pass electrons to CoQ (see Fig. 18.4). Succinate dehydrogenase is part of the TCA cycle and also a component

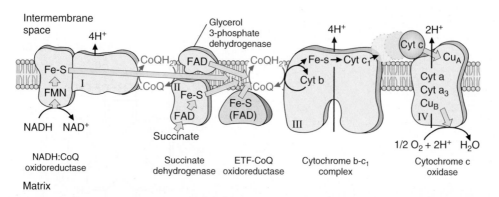

**FIG. 18.4.** Components of the electron transfer chain. NADH:CoQ oxidoreductase (complex I) spans the membrane and has a proton pumping mechanism involving CoQ. The electrons go from CoQ to the cytochrome b–$c_1$ complex (complex III); electron transfer does not involve complex II. Succinate dehydrogenase (complex II), glycerol-3-phosphate dehydrogenase, and ETF:Q oxidoreductase all transfer electrons to CoQ, but they do not span the membrane and do not have a proton pumping mechanism. As CoQ accepts protons from the matrix side, it is converted to $CoQH_2$. Electrons are transferred from complex III to complex IV (cytochrome c oxidase) by cytochrome c, a small cytochrome in the intermembrane space that has reversible binding sites on the b–$c_1$ complex and cytochrome c oxidase.

of complex II of the electron transport chain. ETF-CoQ oxidoreductase accepts electrons from ETF (**e**lectron-**t**ransferring **f**lavoprotein), which acquires them from fatty acid oxidation and other pathways. Glycerol-3-phosphate dehydrogenase is a flavoprotein that is part of a shuttle for reoxidizing cytosolic NADH.

The free energy drop in electron transfer between NADH and CoQ of approximately $-13$ to $-14$ kcal is able to support movement of four protons. However, the FAD in succinate dehydrogenase (as well as ETF-CoQ oxidoreductase and glycerol-3-phosphate dehydrogenase) is at roughly the same redox potential as CoQ and no energy is released as they transfer electrons to CoQ. These proteins do not span the membrane and consequently do not have a proton pumping mechanism.

### 3. COENZYME Q

CoQ is the only component of the electron transport chain that is not protein bound. CoQ is very hydrophobic (Fig. 18.5), which enables it to freely diffuse amongst the lipids of the inner mitochondrial membrane. When the oxidized quinone form accepts a single electron (to form the semiquinone), it forms a free radical (a compound with a single electron in an orbital). The transfer of single electrons makes it the major site for generation of toxic oxygen free radicals in the body (see Section IV).

The semiquinone can accept a second electron and two protons from the matrix side of the membrane to form the fully reduced quinone. The mobility of CoQ in the membrane, its ability to accept one or two electrons, and its ability to accept and donate protons enable it to participate in the proton pumps for both complexes I and III as it shuttles electrons between them. CoQ is also called **ubiquinone** because quinones with similar structures are found in all plants and animals.

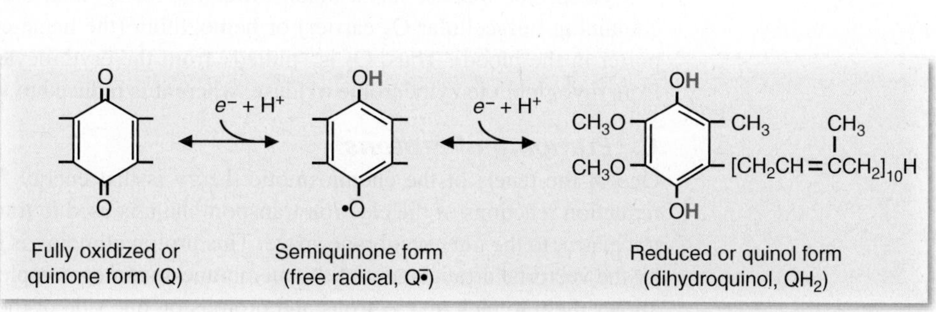

**FIG. 18.5.** Structure of CoQ. CoQ contains a quinone with a long lipophilic side chain comprising 10 isoprenoid units (thus, it is sometimes called $CoQ_{10}$.) CoQ can accept one electron ($e^-$) to become the half-reduced form or $2\ e^-$ to become fully reduced.

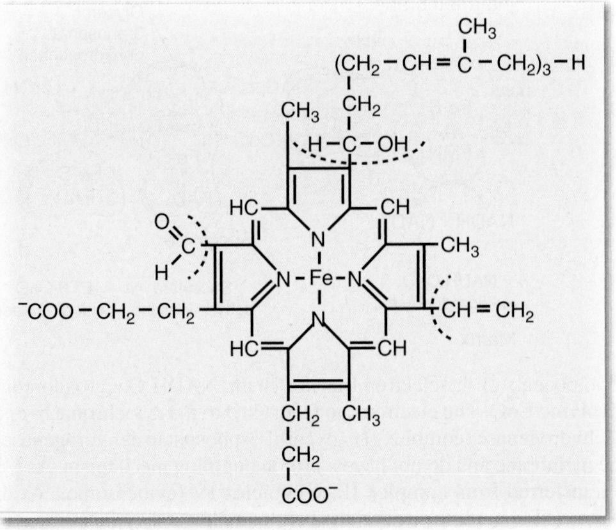

*FIG. 18.6.* Heme A. Heme A is found in cytochromes a and $a_3$. Cytochromes are proteins containing a heme chelated with an iron atom. Hemes are derivatives of protoporphyrin IX. Each cytochrome has a heme with different modifications of the side chains (indicated with *dashed lines*), resulting in a slightly different reduction potential and, consequently, a different position in the sequence of electron transfer.

Although iron deficiency anemia is characterized by decreased levels of hemoglobin and other iron-containing proteins in the blood, the iron-containing cytochromes and Fe-S centers of the electron transport chain in tissues such as skeletal muscle are affected as rapidly. Fatigue in iron deficiency anemia, in patients such as **Ann R.** (see Chapter 13), results in part from the reduction of electron transport for ATP production.

### 4. CYTOCHROMES

The remaining components in the electron transport chain are cytochromes (see Fig. 18.4). Each cytochrome is a protein that contains a bound heme (i.e., an Fe atom bound to a porphyrin nucleus similar in structure to the heme in hemoglobin) (Fig. 18.6).

Because of differences in the protein component of the cytochromes and small differences in the heme structure, each heme has a different reduction potential. The cytochromes of the b-$c_1$ complex have a higher energy level than those of cytochrome oxidase (a and $a_3$). Thus, energy is released by electron transfer between complexes III and IV. The iron atoms in the cytochromes are in the $Fe^{3+}$ state. As they accept an electron, they are reduced to $Fe^{2+}$. As they are reoxidized to $Fe^{3+}$, the electrons pass to the next component of the electron transport chain.

### 5. COPPER AND THE REDUCTION OF OXYGEN

The last cytochrome complex is cytochrome oxidase, which passes electrons from cytochrome c to $O_2$ (see Fig. 18.4). It contains cytochromes a and $a_3$ and the $O_2$ binding site. A whole oxygen molecule, $O_2$, must accept four electrons to be reduced to two $H_2O$ molecules. Bound copper ($Cu^+$) ions in the cytochrome oxidase complex facilitate the collection of the four electrons and the reduction of $O_2$.

Cytochrome oxidase has a much lower $K_m$ for $O_2$ than myoglobin (the heme-containing intracellular $O_2$ carrier) or hemoglobin (the heme-containing $O_2$ transporter in the blood). Thus, $O_2$ is "pulled" from the erythrocyte to myoglobin and from myoglobin to cytochrome oxidase, where it is reduced to water.

### C. Pumping of Protons

One of the tenets of the chemiosmotic theory is that energy from the oxidation–reduction reactions of the electron transport chain is used to transport protons from the matrix to the intermembrane space. This proton pumping is generally facilitated by the vectorial arrangement of the membrane-spanning complexes. Their structure allows them to pick up electrons and protons on one side of the membrane and release protons on the other side of the membrane as they transfer an electron to the next component of the chain.

The significance of the direct link between the electron transfer and proton movement is that one cannot occur without the other (the processes are said to be "coupled"). Thus, when protons are not being used for ATP synthesis, the proton gradient and the membrane potential build up. This "proton back pressure" controls the rate of proton pumping, which controls electron transport and $O_2$ consumption.

## D. Energy Yield from the Electron Transport Chain

The overall free energy release from oxidation of NADH by $O_2$ is approximately $-53$ kcal, and from FAD(2H), it is approximately $-41$ kcal. This $\Delta G^0$ is so negative that the chain is never reversible; we never synthesize $O_2$ from $H_2O$. The negative $\Delta G^0$ also drives NADH and FAD(2H) formation from the pathways of fuel oxidation, such as the TCA cycle and glycolysis, to completion.

Overall, each NADH donates two electrons, equivalent to the reduction of one-half of an $O_2$ molecule. A generally (but not universally) accepted estimate of the stoichiometry of ATP synthesis is that four protons are pumped at complex I, four protons at complex III, and two at complex IV. With four protons translocated for each ATP synthesized, an estimated 2.5 ATPs are formed for each NADH oxidized and 1.5 ATPs for each of the other FAD(2H)-containing flavoproteins that donate electrons to CoQ. (This calculation neglects proton requirements for the transport of phosphate and substrates from the cytosol as well as the basal proton leak.) Thus, only approximately 30% of the energy available from NADH and FAD(2H) oxidation by $O_2$ is used for ATP synthesis. Some of the remaining energy in the electrochemical potential is used for the transport of anions and $Ca^{2+}$ into the mitochondrion. The remainder of the energy is released as heat. Consequently, the electron transport chain is also our major source of heat.

## E. Respiratory Chain Inhibition and Sequential Transfer

In the cell, electron flow in the electron transport chain must be sequential from NADH or a flavoprotein all the way to $O_2$ to generate ATP (see Fig. 18.4). In the absence of $O_2$ (**anoxia**), there is no ATP generated from oxidative phosphorylation because electrons back up in the chain. Even complex I cannot pump protons to generate the electrochemical gradient, because every molecule of CoQ already has electrons that it cannot pass down the chain without an $O_2$ to accept them at the end. The action of the respiratory chain inhibitor **cyanide**, which binds to cytochrome oxidase, is similar to that of anoxia; it prevents proton pumping by all three complexes. Complete inhibition of the b-$c_1$ complex prevents pumping at cytochrome oxidase because there is no donor of electrons; it prevents pumping at complex I because there is no electron acceptor. Although complete inhibition of any one complex inhibits proton pumping at all of the complexes, partial inhibition of proton pumping can occur when only a fraction of the molecules of a complex contain bound inhibitor. The partial inhibition results in a partial decrease of the maximal rate of ATP synthesis. Table 18.1 lists chemical inhibitors of oxidative phosphorylation and indicates the steps within either electron transport or ATP synthesis at which they act.

**Table 18.1  Inhibitors of Oxidative Phosphorylation**

| Inhibitor | Site of Inhibition |
|---|---|
| Rotenone, Amytal | Transfer of electrons from complex I to coenzyme Q |
| Antimycin C | Transfer of electrons from complex III to cytochrome c |
| Carbon monoxide (CO) | Transfer of electrons from complex IV to oxygen |
| Cyanide (CN) | Transfer of electrons through complex IV to oxygen |
| Atractyloside | Inhibits the adenine nucleotide translocase (ANT) |
| Oligomycin | Inhibits proton flow through the $F_0$ component of the ATP synthase |
| Dinitrophenol | An uncoupler; facilitates proton transfer across the inner mitochondrial membrane |
| Valinomycin | A potassium ionophore; facilitates potassium ion transfer across the inner mitochondrial membrane |

ATP, adenosine triphosphate.

**Cora N.** has a lack of $O_2$ in the anterior and lateral walls of her heart caused by severe ischemia (lack of blood flow), resulting from clots within certain coronary arteries at the site of ruptured atherosclerotic plaques. The limited availability of $O_2$ to act as an electron acceptor will decrease proton pumping and generation of an electrochemical potential gradient across the inner mitochondrial membrane of ischemic cells. As a consequence, the rate of ATP generation in these specific areas of her heart will decrease, thereby triggering events that lead to irreversible cell injury.

Intravenous nitroprusside rapidly lowers elevated blood pressure through its direct vasodilating action. Fortunately, it was required in **Cora N.**'s case only for several hours. During prolonged infusions of 24 to 48 hours or more, nitroprusside slowly breaks down to produce cyanide, an inhibitor of the cytochrome c oxidase complex. Because small amounts of cyanide are detoxified in the liver by conversion to thiocyanate, which is excreted in the urine, the conversion of nitroprusside to cyanide can be monitored by following blood thiocyanate levels.

Cyanide binds to the $Fe^{3+}$ in the heme of the cytochrome $aa_3$ component of cytochrome c oxidase and prevents electron transport to $O_2$. Mitochondrial respiration and energy production cease, and cell death rapidly occurs. The central nervous system is the primary target for cyanide toxicity. Acute inhalation of high concentrations of cyanide (e.g., smoke inhalation during a fire) provokes a brief central nervous system stimulation rapidly followed by convulsion, coma, and death. Acute exposure to lower amounts can cause lightheadedness, breathlessness, dizziness, numbness, and headaches.

**Q:** Decreased activity of the electron transport chain can result from inhibitors as well as from mutations in mtDNA and nuclear DNA. Why does an impairment of the electron transport chain result in lactic acidosis?

## II. OXPHOS DISEASES

Clinical diseases involving components of oxidative phosphorylation (referred to as **OXPHOS diseases**) are among the most commonly encountered class of degenerative diseases. The clinical pathology may be caused by gene mutations in either mitochondrial DNA (mtDNA) or nuclear DNA (nDNA) that encode proteins required for normal oxidative phosphorylation.

### A. Mitochondrial DNA and OXPHOS Diseases

The mtDNA is a small, double-stranded circular DNA with 16,569 nucleotide pairs. It encodes 13 subunits of the complexes involved in oxidative phosphorylation. In addition, mtDNA encodes the necessary components for translation of its mRNA: a large and small ribosomal RNA (rRNA) and 22 transfer RNAs (tRNAs). Mutations in mtDNA have been identified as deletions, duplications, or point mutations. Disorders associated with these mutations are outlined in Table 18.2.

Mitochondrial disorders display maternal inheritance. The egg contains approximately 300,000 molecules of mtDNA packaged into mitochondria. These are

**Table 18.2   Examples of OXPHOS Diseases Arising from mtDNA Mutations**

| Syndrome | Characteristic Symptoms | mtDNA Mutation |
|---|---|---|
| **I. mtDNA rearrangements in which genes are deleted or duplicated** | | |
| Kearns-Sayre syndrome | Onset before 20 years of age, characterized by ophthalmoplegia, atypical retinitis pigmentosa, mitochondrial myopathy, and one of the following: cardiac conduction defect, cerebellar syndrome, or elevated CSF proteins | Deletion of contiguous segments of tRNA and OXPHOS polypeptides, or duplication mutations consisting of tandemly arranged normal mtDNA and an mtDNA with a deletion mutation |
| Pearson syndrome | Systemic disorder of oxidative phosphorylation that predominantly affects bone marrow | Deletion of contiguous segments of tRNA and OXPHOS polypeptides, or duplication mutations consisting of tandemly arranged normal mtDNA and a mtDNA with a deletion mutation |
| **II. mtDNA point mutations in tRNA or ribosomal RNA genes** | | |
| MERRF (**m**yoclonic **e**pilepsy and **r**agged **r**ed **f**iber disease) | Progressive myoclonic epilepsy, a mitochondrial myopathy with ragged red fibers, and a slowly progressive dementia. Onset of symptoms: late childhood to adult | $tRNA^{Lys}$ |
| MELAS (mitochondrial **m**yopathy, **e**ncephalomyopathy, **l**actic **a**cidosis, and **s**trokelike episodes) | Progressive neurodegenerative disease characterized by strokelike episodes first occurring between 5 and 15 years of age and a mitochondrial myopathy | 80%–90% mutations in $tRNA^{Leu}$ |
| **III. mtDNA missense mutations in OXPHOS polypeptides** | | |
| Leigh disease (subacute necrotizing encephalopathy) | Mean age of onset, 1.5–5 years; clinical manifestations include optic atrophy, ophthalmoplegia, nystagmus, respiratory abnormalities, ataxia, hypotonia, spasticity, and developmental delay or regression | 7%–20% of cases have mutations in $F_0$ subunits of $F_0F_1ATPase$. |
| LHON (**L**eber **h**ereditary **o**ptic **n**europathy) | Late onset, acute optic atrophy | 90% of European and Asian cases result from mutation in NADH dehydrogenase |

mtDNA, mitochondrial DNA; CSF, cerebrospinal fluid; tRNA, transfer RNA; OXPHOS, oxidative phosphorylation.

retained during fertilization, whereas those of the sperm do not enter the egg or are lost. As cells divide during mitosis and meiosis, mitochondria replicate by fission but various amounts of mitochondria with mutant and wild-type DNA are distributed to each daughter cell. Thus, any cell can have a mixture of mitochondria, each with mutant or wild-type mtDNAs (termed heteroplasmy). The mitotic and meiotic segregation of the heteroplasmic mtDNA mutation results in variable oxidative phosphorylation deficiencies between patients with the same mutation and even among a patient's own tissues.

The disease pathology usually becomes worse with age because a small amount of normal mitochondria might confer normal function and exercise capacity while the patient is young. As the patient ages, somatic (spontaneous) mutations in mtDNA accumulate from the generation of free radicals within the mitochondria. These mutations frequently become permanent, partly because mtDNA does not have access to the same repair mechanisms available for nDNA. Even in normal individuals, somatic mutations result in a decline of oxidative phosphorylation capacity with age. At some stage, the ATP-generating capacity of a tissue falls below the tissue-specific threshold for normal function. In general, symptoms of these defects appear in one or more of the tissues with the highest ATP demands: nervous tissue, heart, skeletal muscle, and kidney.

### B. Other Genetic Disorders of Oxidative Phosphorylation

Genetic mutations also have been reported for mitochondrial proteins that are encoded by nDNA. Most of the estimated 1,000 proteins required for oxidative phosphorylation are encoded by nDNA, whereas mtDNA encodes only 13 subunits of the oxidative phosphorylation complexes (including ATP synthase). Coordinate regulation of expression of nuclear and mtDNA, import of proteins into the mitochondria, assembly of the complexes, and regulation of mitochondrial fission are nuclear encoded.

nDNA mutations differ from mtDNA mutations in several important respects. These mutations do not show a pattern of maternal inheritance but are usually autosomal recessive. The mutations are uniformly distributed to daughter cells and therefore are expressed in all tissues containing the allele for a particular tissue-specific isoform. However, phenotypic expression still will be most apparent in tissues with high ATP requirements.

### III. COUPLING OF ELECTRON TRANSPORT AND ATP SYNTHESIS

The electrochemical gradient couples the rate of the electron transport chain to the rate of ATP synthesis. Because electron flow requires proton pumping, electron flow cannot occur faster than protons are used for ATP synthesis (coupled oxidative phosphorylation) or returned to the matrix by a mechanism that short circuits the ATP synthase pore (uncoupling).

### A. Regulation through Coupling

As ATP chemical bond energy is used by energy-requiring reactions, ADP and $P_i$ concentrations increase. The more ADP present to bind to the ATP synthase, the greater will be the proton flow through the ATP synthase pore from the intermembrane space to the matrix. Thus, as ADP levels rise, proton influx increases and the electrochemical gradient decreases (Fig. 18.7). The proton pumps of the electron transport chain respond with increased proton pumping and electron flow to maintain the electrochemical gradient. The result is increased $O_2$ consumption. The increased oxidation of NADH in the electron transport chain and the increased concentration of ADP stimulate the pathways of fuel oxidation, such as the TCA cycle, to supply more NADH and FAD(2H) to the electron transport chain. For example,

 The effect of inhibition of electron transport is an impaired oxidation of pyruvate, fatty acids, and other fuels. In many cases, the inhibition of mitochondrial electron transport results in higher than normal levels of lactate and pyruvate in the blood and an increased lactate/pyruvate ratio. NADH oxidation requires the completed transfer of electrons from NADH to $O_2$, and a defect anywhere along the chain will result in the accumulation of NADH and a decrease of $NAD^+$. The increase in NADH/$NAD^+$ inhibits pyruvate dehydrogenase and causes the accumulation of pyruvate. It also increases the conversion of pyruvate to lactate (anaerobic glycolysis), and elevated levels of lactate appear in the blood. A large number of genetic defects of the proteins in respiratory chain complexes have, therefore, been classified together as congenital lactic acidosis.

 A patient experienced spontaneous muscle jerking (myoclonus) in her mid-teens and her condition progressed over 10 years to include debilitating myoclonus, neurosensory hearing loss, dementia, hypoventilation, and mild cardiomyopathy. Energy metabolism was affected in the central nervous system, heart, and skeletal muscle, resulting in lactic acidosis. A history indicated that the patient's mother, her grandmother, and two maternal aunts had symptoms involving either nervous or muscular tissue (clearly a case of maternal inheritance). However, no other relative had identical symptoms. The symptoms and history of the patient are those of myoclonic epileptic ragged red fiber disease (MERRF). The affected tissues (central nervous system and muscle) are two of the tissues with the highest ATP requirements. Most cases of MERRF are caused by a point mutation in mitochondrial tRNA$^{Lys}$ (mtRNA$^{Lys}$). The mitochondria, obtained by muscle biopsy, are enlarged and show abnormal patterns of cristae. The muscle tissue also shows ragged red fibers.

 How does shivering generate heat?

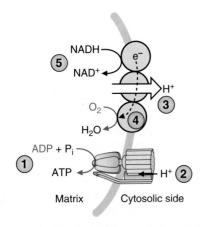

**FIG. 18.7.** Control of $O_2$ consumption by ADP. The concentration of ADP (or the phosphate potential [ATP]/[ADP][$P_i$]) controls the rate of $O_2$ consumption. *(1)* ADP is phosphorylated to ATP by ATP synthase. *(2)* The release of the ATP requires proton flow through ATP synthase into the matrix. *(3)* The use of protons from the intermembrane space for ATP synthesis decreases the proton gradient. *(4)* As a result, the electron transport chain pumps more protons, and $O_2$ is reduced to $H_2O$. *(5)* As NADH donates electrons to the electron transport chain, $NAD^+$ is regenerated and returns to the TCA cycle or other NADH-producing pathways.

A skeletal muscle biopsy performed on **Isabel S.** indicated proliferation of subsarcolemmal mitochondria with degeneration of muscle fibers (ragged red fibers) in approximately 55% of the total fibers observed. An analysis of mtDNA indicated no genetic mutations but did show a moderate quantitative depletion of mtDNA.

Isabel's AIDS was being treated with zidovudine (azidotyhymidine, AZT), which also can act as an inhibitor of the mtDNA polymerase (polymerase γ). A review of the drug's potential adverse effects showed that, rarely, it may cause varying degrees of mtDNA depletion in different tissues, including skeletal muscle. The depletion may cause a severe mitochondrial myopathy, including ragged red fiber accumulation within the skeletal muscle cells associated with ultrastructural abnormalities in their mitochondria.

**A:** Shivering results from muscular contraction, which increases the rate of ATP hydrolysis. As a consequence of proton entry for ATP synthesis, the electron transport chain is stimulated. Oxygen consumption increases, as does the amount of energy lost as heat by the electron transport chain.

during exercise, we use more ATP for muscle contraction, consume more $O_2$, oxidize more fuel (which means burn more calories), and generate more heat from the electron transport chain. If we rest, the rate of ATP utilization decreases, proton influx decreases, the electrochemical gradient increases, and proton back pressure decreases the rate of the electron transport chain. NADH and FAD(2H) cannot be oxidized as rapidly in the electron transport chain and, consequently, their buildup inhibits the enzymes that generate them.

The system is poised to maintain very high levels of ATP at all times. In most tissues, the rate of ATP utilization is nearly constant over time. However, in skeletal muscles, the rates of ATP hydrolysis change dramatically as the muscle goes from rest to rapid contraction. Even under these circumstances, ATP concentration decreases by only approximately 20% because it is so rapidly regenerated. In the heart, $Ca^{2+}$ activation of TCA cycle enzymes provides an extra push to NADH generation so that neither ATP nor NADH levels fall as ATP demand is increased. The electron transport chain has a very high capacity and can respond very rapidly to any increase in ATP utilization.

## B. Uncoupling ATP Synthesis from Electron Transport

When protons leak back into the matrix without going through the ATP synthase pore, they dissipate the electrochemical gradient across the membrane without generating ATP. This phenomenon is called "uncoupling" oxidative phosphorylation. It occurs with chemical compounds, known as uncouplers, and it occurs physiologically with uncoupling proteins (UCPs) that form proton conductance channels through the membrane. Uncoupling of oxidative phosphorylation results in increased $O_2$ consumption and heat production as electron flow and proton pumping attempt to maintain the electrochemical gradient.

### 1. CHEMICAL UNCOUPLERS OF OXIDATIVE PHOSPHORYLATION

**Chemical uncouplers,** also known as **proton ionophores,** are lipid-soluble compounds that rapidly transport protons from the cytosolic to the matrix side of the inner mitochondrial membrane (Fig. 18.8). Because the proton concentration is higher in the intermembrane space than in the matrix, uncouplers pick up protons from the intermembrane space. Their lipid solubility enables them to diffuse through the inner mitochondrial membrane while carrying protons and release these protons on the matrix side. The rapid influx of protons dissipates the electrochemical potential gradient; therefore, the mitochondria are unable to synthesize ATP. Eventually, mitochondrial integrity and function are lost.

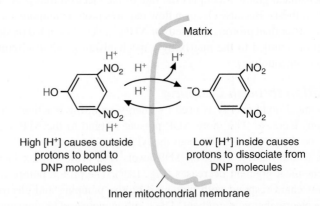

**FIG. 18.8.** Action of uncouplers. Dinitrophenol (DNP) is lipid soluble and can therefore diffuse across the membrane. It has a dissociable proton with a $pK_a$ near 7.2. Thus, in the intermembrane space where [$H^+$] is high (pH low), DNP picks up a proton, which it carries across the membrane. At the lower proton concentration of the matrix, the $H^+$ dissociates. As a consequence, cells cannot maintain their electrochemical gradient or synthesize ATP.

## 2. UNCOUPLING PROTEINS AND THERMOGENESIS

**UCPs** form channels through the inner mitochondrial membrane that are able to conduct protons from the intermembrane space to the matrix, thereby short-circuiting ATP synthase.

The UCPs exist as a family of proteins: UCP1 (thermogenin) is expressed in brown adipose tissue, UCP2 is found in most cells, UCP3 is found principally in skeletal muscle, and UCP4 and UCP5 are found in the nervous system. These are highly regulated proteins that, when activated, increase the amount of energy from fuel oxidation that is being released as heat. However, recent data indicates that this may not be the primary role of UCP2 and UCP3. It has been hypothesized that UCP3 acts as a transport protein to remove fatty acid anions and lipid peroxides from the mitochondria, thereby reducing the risk of forming $O_2$ free radicals and thus decreasing the occurrence of mitochondrial and cell injury.

UCP1 (thermogenin) is associated with heat production in **brown adipose tissue**. The major function of brown adipose tissue is nonshivering thermogenesis, whereas the major function of white adipose tissue is the storage of triacylglycerols in white lipid droplets. The brown color arises from the large number of mitochondria that participate. Human infants, who have little voluntary control over their environment and may kick their blankets off at night, have brown fat deposits along the neck, the breastplate, between the scapulae, and around the kidneys to protect them from cold. However, there is very little brown fat in most adults.

In response to cold, sympathetic nerve endings release norepinephrine, which activates a lipase in brown adipose tissue that releases fatty acids from triacylglycerols. Fatty acids serve as a fuel for the tissue (i.e., are oxidized to generate the electrochemical potential gradient and ATP) and participate directly in the proton conductance channel by activating UCP1 along with reduced CoQ. When UCP1 is activated by fatty acids, it transports protons from the cytosolic side of the inner mitochondrial membrane back into the mitochondrial matrix without ATP generation. Thus, it partially uncouples oxidative phosphorylation and generates additional heat.

## 3. PROTON LEAK AND RESTING METABOLIC RATE

A low level of proton leak across the inner mitochondrial membrane occurs in our mitochondria all of the time, and our mitochondria, thus, are normally partially uncoupled. It has been estimated that more than 20% of our resting metabolic rate (see Chapter 1) is the energy expended to maintain the electrochemical gradient dissipated by our basal proton leak (also referred to as global proton leak). Some of the proton leak results from permeability of the membrane associated with proteins embedded in the lipid bilayer. An unknown amount may result from UCPs.

## IV. *O₂ AND THE GENERATION OF REACTIVE OXYGEN SPECIES*

The generation of **reactive oxygen species** (**ROS**) from $O_2$ in our cells is a natural everyday occurrence. The electrons that contribute to their formation are usually derived from reduced electron carriers of the electron transport chain. ROS are formed as accidental products of nonenzymatic and enzymatic reactions. Occasionally, they are deliberately synthesized in enzyme-catalyzed reactions. Ultraviolet radiation and pollutants in the air can increase formation of toxic $O_2$-containing compounds.

### A. *The Radical Nature of O₂*

A **radical**, by definition, is a molecule that has a single unpaired electron in an orbital. A **free radical** is a radical capable of independent existence. (Radicals formed in an enzyme-active site during a reaction, for example, are not considered free radicals unless they can dissociate from the protein to interact with other molecules.) Radicals are highly reactive and initiate chain reactions by extracting an electron from a neighboring molecule to complete their own orbitals. Although the transition metals (e.g., Fe, Cu, and Mo) have single electrons in orbitals, they are not

 Salicylate, which is a degradation product of aspirin in humans, is lipid soluble and has a dissociable proton. In high concentrations, as in salicylate poisoning, salicylate is able to partially uncouple mitochondria. The decline of ATP concentration in the cell and consequent increase of AMP in the cytosol stimulates glycolysis. The overstimulation of the glycolytic pathway (see Chapter 19) results in increased levels of lactic acid in the blood and a metabolic acidosis. Fortunately, **Dennis V.** did not develop this consequence of aspirin poisoning (see Chapter 2).

The two unpaired electrons in $O_2$ have the same (parallel) spin and are called antibonding electrons. In contrast, C—C and C—H bonds each contain two electrons, which have antiparallel spins and form a thermodynamically stable pair. As a consequence, $O_2$ cannot readily oxidize a co-valent bond because one of its electrons would have to flip its spin around to make new pairs. The difficulty in changing spins is called the *spin restriction*. Without spin restriction, organic life forms could not have developed in the $O_2$ atmosphere on earth because they would be spontaneously oxidized by $O_2$. Instead, $O_2$ is confined to slower one-electron reactions catalyzed by metals (or metalloenzymes).

To decrease occurrence of nonenzymatic radical formation, accessibility to transition metals, such as $Fe^{2+}$ and $Cu^+$, are highly restricted in cells or in the body as a whole. Events that release iron from cellular storage sites, such as a crushing injury, are associated with increased free radical injury.

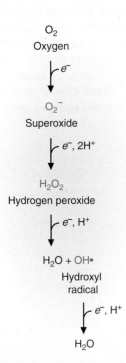

**FIG. 18.9.** Reduction of $O_2$ by four one-electron steps. The four one-electron reduction steps for $O_2$ progressively generate superoxide, $H_2O_2$, and the hydroxyl radical plus water. Superoxide is sometimes written $O_2^-$ to better illustrate its single unpaired electron. $H_2O_2$, the half-reduced form of $O_2$, has accepted two electrons and is therefore not an $O_2$ radical.

usually considered free radicals because they are relatively stable, do not initiate chain reactions, and are bound to proteins in the cell.

The oxygen atom is a **biradical**, which means it has two single electrons in different orbitals. These electrons cannot both travel in the same orbital because they have parallel spins (spin in the same direction). Although $O_2$ is very reactive from a thermodynamic standpoint, its single electrons cannot react rapidly with the paired electrons found in the covalent bonds of organic molecules. As a consequence, $O_2$ reacts slowly through the acceptance of single electrons in reactions that require a catalyst (such as a metal-containing enzyme).

$O_2$ is capable of accepting a total of four electrons, which reduces it to $H_2O$ (Fig. 18.9). When $O_2$ accepts one electron, **superoxide** is formed. Superoxide is still a radical because it has one unpaired electron remaining. This reaction is not thermodynamically favorable and requires a moderately strong reducing agent that can donate single electrons (e.g., the radical form of CoQ in the electron transport chain). When superoxide accepts an electron, it is reduced to **hydrogen peroxide ($H_2O_2$)**, which is not a radical. The **hydroxyl radical** is formed in the next one-electron reduction step in the reduction sequence. Finally, acceptance of the last electron reduces the hydroxyl radical to $H_2O$.

### B. Characteristics of Reactive Oxygen Species

Reactive free radicals extract electrons (usually as hydrogen atoms) from other compounds to complete their own orbitals, thereby initiating free radical chain reactions. The hydroxyl radical is probably the most potent of the ROS. It initiates chain reactions that form lipid peroxides and organic radicals and adds directly to compounds. The superoxide anion is also highly reactive but has limited lipid solubility and cannot diffuse far. However, it can generate the more reactive hydroxyl and hydroperoxy radicals by reacting nonenzymatically with $H_2O_2$.

$H_2O_2$, although not actually a radical, is a weak oxidizing agent that is classified as an ROS because it can generate the hydroxyl radical (OH•). Transition metals, such as $Fe^{2+}$ or $Cu^+$, catalyze formation of the hydroxyl radical from $H_2O_2$ in nonenzymatic reactions. Because $H_2O_2$ is lipid soluble, it can diffuse through membranes and generate OH• at localized $Fe^{2+}$- or $Cu^+$-containing sites, such as the components of the electron transport chain within the mitochondria.

Organic radicals are generated when superoxide or the hydroxyl radical indiscriminately extract electrons from other molecules. Organic peroxy radicals are intermediates of chain reactions, such as lipid peroxidation.

An additional group of oxygen-containing radicals, termed reactive nitrogen-oxygen species (RNOS), contains nitrogen as well as $O_2$ (see Section VI). These radicals are derived principally from the free radical nitric oxide (NO), which is produced endogenously by the enzyme NO synthase. NO combines with $O_2$ or superoxide to produce additional RNOS.

### C. Major Sources of Primary Reactive Oxygen Species in the Cell

ROS are constantly being formed in the cell; approximately 3% to 5% of the $O_2$ we consume is converted to oxygen free radicals. Some are produced as accidental byproducts of normal enzymatic reactions that escape from the active site of metal-containing enzymes during oxidation reactions. Others, such as $H_2O_2$, are physiological products of oxidases in peroxisomes. Deliberate production of toxic free radicals occurs in the inflammatory response. Drugs, natural radiation, air pollutants, and other chemicals also can increase formation of free radicals in cells.

### 1. GENERATION OF SUPEROXIDE

One of the major sites of superoxide generation is CoQ in the mitochondrial electron transport chain (Fig. 18.10). The one-electron reduced form of CoQ (CoQH•) is free within the membrane and can accidentally transfer an electron to dissolved $O_2$, thereby forming superoxide. In contrast, when $O_2$ binds to cytochrome oxidase and accepts electrons, none of the $O_2$ radical intermediates are released from the enzyme and no ROS are generated.

## 2.  OXIDASES, OXYGENASES, AND PEROXIDASES

Most of the oxidases, peroxidases, and oxygenases in the cell bind $O_2$ and transfer single electrons to it via a metal. Free radical intermediates of these reactions may be accidentally released before the reduction is complete.

Cytochrome P450 enzymes are a major source of free radicals "leaked" from reactions. Because these enzymes catalyze reactions in which single electrons are transferred to $O_2$ and an organic substrate, the possibility of accidentally generating and releasing free radical intermediates is high. Induction of P450 enzymes by alcohol, drugs, or chemical toxicants leads to increased cellular injury. When substrates for cytochrome P450 enzymes are not present, its potential for destructive damage is diminished by repression of gene transcription.

$H_2O_2$ and lipid peroxides are generated enzymatically as major reaction products by a number of oxidases present in peroxisomes, mitochondria, and the endoplasmic reticulum. For example, peroxisomal fatty acid oxidation generates $H_2O_2$ rather than FAD(2H) during the oxidation of very long chain fatty acids (see Chapter 20).

## 3.  IONIZING RADIATION

Cosmic rays that continuously bombard the earth, radioactive chemicals, and x-rays are forms of **ionizing radiation**. Ionizing radiation has a high enough energy level that it can split water into hydroxyl and hydrogen radicals, thus leading to radiation damage to the skin, mutations, cancer, and cell death. It also may generate organic radicals through direct collision with organic cellular components.

## V.  OXYGEN RADICAL REACTIONS WITH CELLULAR COMPONENTS

Oxygen radicals produce cellular dysfunction by reacting with lipids, proteins, carbohydrates, and DNA to extract electrons (summarized in Fig. 18.11). Evidence of free radical damage has been described in greater than 100 disease states. In some

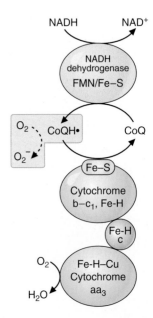

**FIG.  18.10.** Generation of superoxide by CoQ in the electron transport chain. In the process of transporting electrons to $O_2$, some of the electrons escape when CoQH• accidentally interacts with $O_2$ to form superoxide. Fe-H represents the Fe-heme center of the cytochromes.

 During **Cora N.'s** ischemia (decreased blood flow), the ability of her heart to generate ATP from oxidative phosphorylation was compromised. The damage appeared to accelerate when $O_2$ was first reintroduced (reperfused) into the tissue. During ischemia, CoQ and the other single-electron components of the electron transport chain become saturated with electrons. When $O_2$ is reintroduced (reperfusion), electron donation to $O_2$ to form superoxide is increased. The increase of superoxide results in enhanced formation of hydrogen peroxide and the hydroxyl radical. Macrophages in the area clean up cell debris from ischemic injury and produce nitric oxide, which may further damage mitochondria by generating RNOS that attack Fe-S centers and cytochromes in the electron transport chain. Thus, these radicals, which increase in concentration when $O_2$ is introduced into the system, may actually amplify the damage done by the original ischemic event and increase the infarct size.

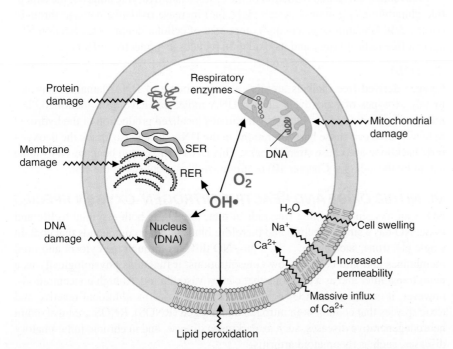

**FIG. 18.11.** Free radical–mediated cellular injury. Superoxide and the hydroxyl radical initiate lipid peroxidation in the cellular, mitochondrial, nuclear, and endoplasmic reticulum membranes. The increase in cellular permeability results in an influx of $Ca^{2+}$, which causes further mitochondrial damage. The cysteine sulfhydryl groups and other amino acid residues on proteins are oxidized and degraded. nDNA and mtDNA can be oxidized, resulting in strand breaks and other types of damage. RNOS (NO, $NO_2$, and peroxynitrites) have similar effects.

of these diseases, free radical damage is the primary cause of the disease; in others, it enhances complications of the disease.

### A. Membrane Attack: Formation of Lipid and Lipid Peroxy Radicals

Chain reactions that form lipid-free radicals and lipid peroxides in membranes make a major contribution to ROS-induced injury. An initiator (such as a hydroxyl radical produced locally in a nonenzymatic reaction) begins the chain reaction. It extracts a hydrogen atom, preferably from the double bond of a polyunsaturated fatty acid in a membrane lipid. The chain reaction is propagated when $O_2$ adds to form lipid peroxyl radicals and lipid peroxides. Eventually, lipid degradation occurs, forming such products as malondialdehyde (from fatty acids with three or more double bonds) and ethane and pentane (from the ω-terminal carbons of three- and six-carbon fatty acids, respectively). Malondialdehyde appears in the blood and urine and is used as an indicator of free radical damage.

Peroxidation of lipid molecules invariably changes or damages lipid molecular structure. In addition to the self-destructive nature of membrane lipid peroxidation, the aldehydes that are formed can cross-link proteins. When the damaged lipids are the constituents of biological membranes, the cohesive lipid bilayer arrangement and stable structural organization is disrupted (see Fig. 18.11). Disruption of mitochondrial membrane integrity may result in further free radical production.

### B. Proteins and Peptides

In proteins, the amino acids proline, histidine, arginine, cysteine, and methionine are particularly susceptible to hydroxyl radical attack and oxidative damage. As a consequence of oxidative damage, the protein may fragment or residues cross-link with other residues. Free radical attack on protein cysteine residues can result in cross-linking and formation of aggregates that prevents their degradation. However, oxidative damage increases the susceptibility of other proteins to proteolytic digestion.

Free radical attack and oxidation of the cysteine sulfhydryl residues of the tripeptide glutathione (γ-glutamyl cysteinylglycine) increase oxidative damage throughout the cell. Glutathione is a major component of cellular defense (see Section VII) against free radical injury and its oxidation reduces its protective effects.

### C. DNA

Oxygen-derived free radicals are also a major source of DNA damage. Approximately 20 types of oxidatively altered DNA molecules have been identified. The nonspecific binding of $Fe^{2+}$ to DNA facilitates localized production of the hydroxyl radical, which can cause base alterations in the DNA. It can also attack the deoxyribose backbone and cause strand breaks. This DNA damage can be repaired to some extent by the cell (see Chapter 10) or minimized by apoptosis of the cell.

## VI. NITRIC OXIDE AND REACTIVE NITROGEN–OXYGEN SPECIES

NO is an oxygen-containing free radical that, like $O_2$, is both essential to life and toxic. NO has a single electron and therefore binds to other compounds that contain single electrons, such as $Fe^{3+}$. As a gas, NO diffuses through the cytosol and lipid membranes and into cells. At low concentrations, it functions physiologically as a neurotransmitter and as a hormone that causes vasodilation. At high concentrations, however, it combines with $O_2$ or with superoxide to form additional reactive and toxic species that contain both nitrogen and oxygen (RNOS). RNOS are involved in neurodegenerative diseases, such as Parkinson disease, and in chronic inflammatory diseases, such as rheumatoid arthritis.

When NO is present in very high concentrations (e.g., during inflammation), it combines nonenzymatically with superoxide to form peroxynitrite ($ONOO^-$) or with $O_2$ to form dinitrogen trioxide ($N_2O_3$) (Fig. 18.12). Peroxynitrite, although it is not a free radical, is a strong oxidizing agent that is stable and directly toxic. It can

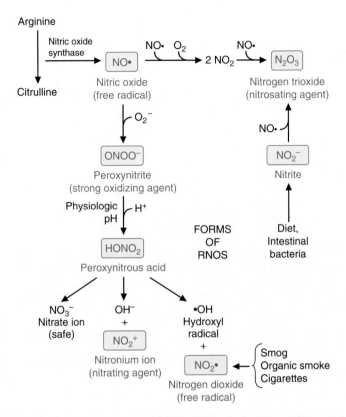

**FIG. 18.12.** Formation of RNOS from NO. RNOS are shown in *red*. The type of damage caused by each RNOS is shown in parentheses. Of all the nitrogen–oxygen-containing compounds shown, only nitrate is relatively nontoxic. $NO_2$ is one of the toxic agents present in smog, automobile exhaust, gas ranges, pilot lights, cigarette smoke, and smoke from forest fires or burning buildings.

diffuse through the cell and lipid membranes to interact with a wide range of targets, including the methionine side chain in proteins and $-SH$ groups (e.g., Fe-S centers in the electron transport chain). It also breaks down to form additional RNOS, including the free radical nitrogen dioxide ($NO_2$), which is an effective initiator of lipid peroxidation. Peroxynitrite products also react (nitration) with aromatic rings, forming compounds such as nitrotyrosine or nitroguanosine. $N_2O_3$, which can be derived from either $NO_2$ or nitrite, is the agent of nitrosative stress, and it nitrosylates sulfhydryl and similarly reactive groups in the cell. Nitrosylation usually interferes with the proper functioning of the protein or lipid that has been modified. Thus, RNOS can do as much oxidative and free-radical damage as non–nitrogen-containing ROS as well as nitrating and nitrosylating compounds. The result is widespread and includes inhibition of a large number of enzymes, mitochondrial lipid peroxidation, inhibition of the electron transport chain and energy depletion, single-stranded or double-stranded breaks in DNA, and modification of bases in DNA.

## VII. CELLULAR DEFENSES AGAINST OXYGEN TOXICITY

Our defenses against $O_2$ toxicity fall into the categories of antioxidant defense enzymes, dietary and endogenous antioxidants (free radical scavengers), cellular compartmentation, metal sequestration, and repair of damaged cellular components. The antioxidant defense enzymes react with ROS and cellular products of free radical chain reactions to convert them to nontoxic products.

Dietary antioxidants, such as vitamin E and flavonoids, and endogenous antioxidants, such as urate, can terminate free radical chain reactions. Defense through compartmentation refers to separation of species and sites involved in ROS

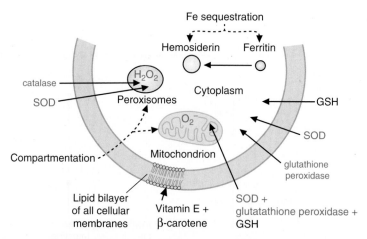

**FIG. 18.13.** Compartmentation of free radical defenses. Various defenses against ROS are found in the different subcellular compartments of the cell. The location of free radical defense enzymes (shown in *red*) matches the type and amount of ROS generated in each subcellular compartment. The highest activities of these enzymes are found in the liver, adrenal gland, and kidney where mitochondrial and peroxisomal contents are high, and cytochrome P450 enzymes are found in abundance in the smooth endoplasmic reticulum. The enzymes SOD and glutathione peroxidase are present as isozymes in the different compartments. Another form of compartmentation involves the sequestration of Fe, which is stored as mobilizable Fe in ferritin. Excess Fe is stored in nonmobilizable hemosiderin deposits. Glutathione (GSH) is a nonenzymatic antioxidant.

The intracellular form of the $Cu^+$–$Zn^{2+}$ SOD is encoded by the *SOD1* gene. To date, 58 mutations in this gene have been discovered in individuals affected by familial amyotrophic lateral sclerosis (ALS or Lou Gehrig disease). How a mutation in this gene leads to the symptoms of this disease has yet to be understood. It is important to note that only 5% to 10% of the total cases of diagnosed ALS are caused by the familial form. Recent work has indicated that mutations in enzymes involved in RNA processing also lead to familial and sporadic ALS.

generation from the rest of the cell (Fig. 18.13). For example, many of the enzymes that produce $H_2O_2$ are sequestered in peroxisomes with a high content of antioxidant enzymes. Repair mechanisms for DNA and for removal of oxidized fatty acids from membrane lipids are available to the cell. Oxidized amino acids on proteins are continuously repaired through protein degradation and resynthesis of new proteins.

## A. Antioxidant Scavenging Enzymes

The enzymatic defense against ROS includes superoxide dismutase, catalase, and glutathione peroxidase.

### 1. SUPEROXIDE DISMUTASE

Conversion of superoxide anion to $H_2O_2$ and $O_2$ (dismutation) by superoxide dismutase (SOD) is often called the primary defense against oxidative stress because superoxide is such a strong initiator of chain reactions (Fig. 18.14A). SOD exists as three isoenzyme forms, a $Cu^+$–$Zn^{2+}$ form present in the cytosol, a $Mn^{2+}$ form present in mitochondria, and a $Cu^+$–$Zn^{2+}$ form found extracellularly. The activity of $Cu^+$–$Zn^{2+}$ SOD is increased by chemicals or conditions (such as hyperbaric oxygen) that increase the production of superoxide.

### 2. CATALASE

$H_2O_2$, once formed, must be reduced to water to prevent it from forming the hydroxyl radical. One of the enzymes that is capable of reducing $H_2O_2$ is catalase (see Fig. 18.14B). Catalase is found principally in peroxisomes and, to a lesser extent, in the cytosol and microsomal fraction of the cell. The highest activities are found in tissues with a high peroxisomal content (kidney and liver). In cells of the immune system, catalase serves to protect the cell against its own respiratory burst.

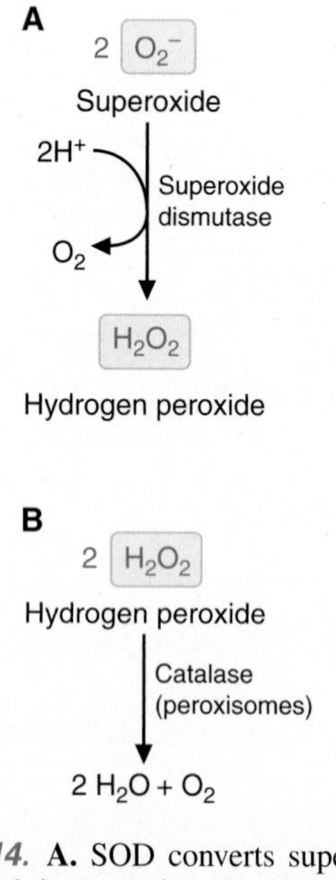

### 3. GLUTATHIONE PEROXIDASE AND GLUTATHIONE REDUCTASE

Glutathione (γ-glutamyl cysteinylglycine) is one of the body's principal means of protecting against oxidative damage (see also Chapter 24). Glutathione is a tripeptide composed of glutamate, cysteine, and glycine, with the amino group of cysteine

**A**

2 $O_2^-$

Superoxide

2H$^+$

Superoxide dismutase

$O_2$

$H_2O_2$

Hydrogen peroxide

**B**

2 $H_2O_2$

Hydrogen peroxide

Catalase (peroxisomes)

2 $H_2O$ + $O_2$

**FIG. 18.14. A.** SOD converts superoxide to $H_2O_2$, which is nontoxic unless it is converted to other ROS. **B.** Catalase reduces $H_2O_2$. (ROS is shown in a *yellow box*.)

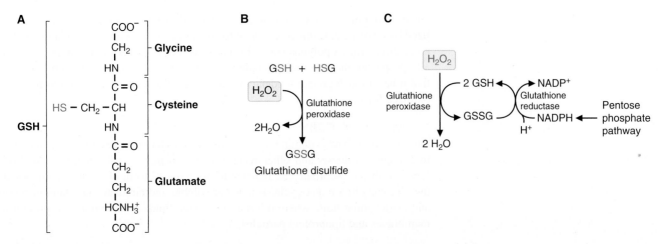

**FIG. 18.15.** Glutathione peroxidase reduces $H_2O_2$ to water. **A.** The structure of glutathione. The sulfhydryl group of glutathione, which is oxidized to a disulfide, is shown in *red*. **B.** Glutathione peroxidase transfers electrons from glutathione (GSH) to $H_2O_2$. **C.** Glutathione redox cycle. Glutathione reductase regenerates reduced glutathione. (ROS is shown in the *yellow box*.)

joined in peptide linkage to the γ-carboxyl group of glutamate (Fig. 18.15). In reactions that are catalyzed by glutathione peroxidases, the reactive sulfhydryl groups reduce $H_2O_2$ to water and lipid peroxides to nontoxic alcohols. In these reactions, two glutathione molecules are oxidized to form a single-molecule glutathione disulfide. The sulfhydryl groups are also oxidized in nonenzymatic chain-terminating reactions with organic radicals.

Glutathione peroxidases exist as a family of selenium enzymes with somewhat different properties and tissue locations. Within cells, they are found principally in the cytosol and mitochondria and are the major means for removing $H_2O_2$ produced outside of peroxisomes. They contribute to our dietary requirement for selenium and account for the protective effect of selenium in the prevention of free radical injury.

Once oxidized, glutathione (GSSG) is formed, it must be reduced back to the sulfhydryl form by glutathione reductase in a redox cycle (see Fig. 18.15C). Glutathione reductase contains a FAD and catalyzes transfer of electrons from NADPH to the disulfide bond of GSSG. NADPH is thus essential for protection against free radical injury. The major source of NADPH for this reaction is the pentose phosphate pathway (see Chapter 24).

### B. Nonenzymatic Antioxidants (Free Radical Scavengers)

Free radical scavengers convert free radicals to a nonradical, nontoxic form in nonenzymatic reactions. Most free radical scavengers are antioxidants, compounds that neutralize free radicals by donating a hydrogen atom (with its one electron) to the radical. Antioxidants, therefore, reduce free radicals and are themselves oxidized in the reaction. Dietary free radical scavengers (e.g., vitamin E, ascorbic acid, carotenoids, and flavonoids) as well as endogenously produced free radical scavengers (e.g., urate and melatonin) have a common structural feature: a conjugated double-bond system that may be an aromatic ring.

### 1. VITAMIN E

Vitamin E (α-tocopherol), the most widely distributed antioxidant in nature, is a lipid-soluble antioxidant vitamin that functions principally to protect against lipid peroxidation in membranes (see Fig. 18.13). Vitamin E comprises a number of tocopherols that differ in their methylation pattern. Among these, α-tocopherol is the most potent antioxidant and is present in the largest amounts in our diet.

Vitamin E is an efficient antioxidant and nonenzymatic terminator of free radical chain reactions, and it has little pro-oxidant activity. When vitamin E donates an electron to a lipid peroxy radical, it is converted to a free radical form that is stabilized by resonance. If this free radical form were to act as a pro-oxidant and abstract an electron from a polyunsaturated lipid, it would be oxidizing that lipid and actually propagate the free radical chain reaction. The chemistry of vitamin E is such that it has a much greater tendency to donate a second electron and go to the fully oxidized form.

## 2. ASCORBIC ACID

Although ascorbate (vitamin C) is an oxidation–reduction coenzyme that functions in collagen synthesis and other reactions, it also plays a role in free radical defense. Reduced ascorbate can regenerate the reduced form of vitamin E by donating electrons in a redox cycle. It is water soluble and circulates unbound in blood and extracellular fluid, where it has access to the lipid-soluble vitamin E present in membranes and lipoprotein particles.

## 3. CAROTENOIDS

Carotenoids is a term applied to β-carotene (the precursor of vitamin A) and similar compounds with functional oxygen-containing substituents on the rings, such as zeaxanthin and lutein. These compounds can exert antioxidant effects as well as quench singlet oxygen. (Singlet oxygen is a highly reactive oxygen species in which there are no unpaired electrons in the outer orbitals, but there is one orbital that is completely empty.) Epidemiologic studies have shown a correlation between diets that are high in fruits and vegetables and health benefits, leading to the hypothesis that carotenoids might slow the progression of cancer, atherosclerosis, and other degenerative diseases by acting as chain-breaking antioxidants. However, in clinical trials, β-carotene supplements had either no effect or an undesirable effect. Its ineffectiveness may be due to the pro-oxidant activity of the free radical form.

In contrast, epidemiologic studies relating the intake of lutein and zeaxanthin with decreased incidence of age-related macular degeneration have received progressive support. These two carotenoids are concentrated in the macula (the central portion of the retina) and are called the **macular carotenoids**.

## 4. OTHER DIETARY ANTIOXIDANTS

Flavonoids are a group of structurally similar compounds that contain two spatially separate aromatic rings and are found in red wine, green tea, chocolate, and other plant-derived foods. Flavonoids have been hypothesized to contribute to our free radical defenses in a number of ways. Some flavonoids inhibit enzymes responsible for superoxide anion production, such as xanthine oxidase. Others efficiently chelate iron and copper, making it impossible for these metals to participate in free radical reactions. They also may act as free radical scavengers by donating electrons to superoxide or lipid peroxy radicals or stabilize free radicals by complexing with them.

## 5. ENDOGENOUS ANTIOXIDANTS

A number of compounds that are synthesized endogenously for other functions, or as urinary excretion products, also function nonenzymatically as free radical antioxidants. Uric acid is formed from the degradation of purines and is released into extracellular fluids, including blood, saliva, and lung lining fluid. Together with protein thiols, it accounts for the major free radical–trapping capacity of plasma. It is particularly important in the upper airways, where there are few other antioxidants. It can directly scavenge hydroxyl radicals, oxyheme oxidants formed between the reaction of hemoglobin and peroxy radicals, and peroxyl radicals themselves. Having acted as a scavenger, uric acid produces a range of oxidation products that are subsequently excreted.

Melatonin, which is a secretory product of the pineal gland, is a neurohormone that functions in regulation of our circadian rhythm, light–dark signal transduction, and sleep induction. In addition to these receptor-mediated functions, it functions as a nonenzymatic free radical scavenger that donates an electron (as hydrogen) to

Age-related macular degeneration (AMD) is the leading cause of blindness in the United States among persons older than 50 years of age, and it affects 1.7 million people worldwide. In AMD, visual loss is related to oxidative damage to the retinal pigment epithelium (RPE) and the choriocapillaris epithelium. The photoreceptor/retinal pigment complex is exposed to sunlight, it is bathed in near-arterial levels of $O_2$, and the membranes contain high concentrations of polyunsaturated fatty acids, all of which are conducive to oxidative damage. Lipofuscin granules, which accumulate in the RPE throughout life, may serve as photosensitizers, initiating damage by absorbing blue light and generating singlet oxygen (an energetically excited form of oxygen) that forms other radicals. Dark sunglasses are protective. Epidemiologic studies showed that the intake of lutein and zeaxanthin in dark green leafy vegetables (e.g., spinach and collard greens) also may be protective. Lutein and zeaxanthin accumulate in the macula and protect against free radical damage by absorbing blue light and quenching singlet oxygen.

"neutralize" free radicals. It also can react with ROS and RNOS to form addition products, thereby undergoing suicidal transformations. Its effectiveness is related to both its lack of pro-oxidant activity and its joint hydrophilic/hydrophobic nature, which allows it to pass through membranes and the blood–brain barrier.

## VIII. TRANSPORT THROUGH INNER AND OUTER MITOCHONDRIAL MEMBRANES

Most of the newly synthesized ATP that is released into the mitochondrial matrix must be transported out of the mitochondria, where it is used for energy-requiring processes such as active ion transport, muscle contraction, or biosynthetic reactions. Likewise, ADP, phosphate, pyruvate, and other metabolites must be transported into the matrix. This requires transport of compounds through both the inner and outer mitochondrial membranes.

### A.  Transport through the Inner Mitochondrial Membrane

The inner mitochondrial membrane forms a tight permeability barrier to all polar molecules, including ATP, ADP, $P_i$; anions such as pyruvate; and cations such as $Ca^{2+}$, $H^+$, and $K^+$. Yet, the process of oxidative phosphorylation depends on rapid and continuous transport of many of these molecules across the inner mitochondrial membrane (Fig. 18.16). Ions and other polar molecules are transported across the inner mitochondrial membrane by specific protein translocases that nearly balance charge during the transport process. Most of the exchange transport is a form of active transport that generally uses energy from the electrochemical potential gradient, either the membrane potential or the proton gradient.

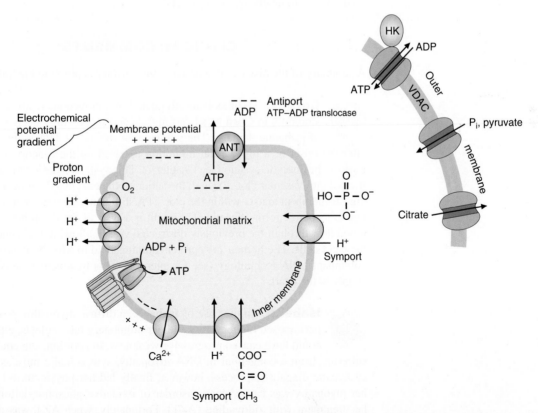

**FIG. 18.16.** Transport of compounds across the inner and outer mitochondrial membranes. The electrochemical potential gradient drives the transport of ions across the inner mitochondrial membrane on specific translocases. Each translocase is composed of specific membrane-spanning helices that bind only specific compounds (adenine nucleotide translocase [ANT]). In contrast, the outer membrane contains relatively large unspecific pores called VDAC through which a wide range of ions diffuse. These bind cytosolic proteins such as hexokinase (HK), which enables HK to have access to newly exported ATP.

ATP-ADP translocase (also called ANT for **a**denine **n**ucleotide **t**ranslocase) transports ATP formed in the mitochondrial matrix to the intermembrane space in a specific 1:1 exchange for ADP produced from energy-requiring reactions outside of the mitochondria (see Fig. 18.16). Because ATP contains four negative charges and ADP contains only three, the exchange is promoted by the electrochemical potential gradient because the net effect is the transport of one negative charge from the matrix to the cytosol. Similar antiports exist for most metabolic anions. In contrast, $P_i$ and pyruvate are transported into the mitochondrial matrix on specific transporters called **symports** together with a proton. A specific transport protein for $Ca^{2+}$ uptake, called the $Ca^{2+}$ uniporter, is driven by the electrochemical potential gradient, which is negatively charged on the matrix side of the membrane relative to the cytosolic side. Other transporters include the dicarboxylate transporter (malate-phosphate exchange), the tricarboxylate transporter (citrate-malate exchange), the aspartate-glutamate transporter, and the malate-$\alpha$-ketoglutarate transporter.

### B. Transport through the Outer Mitochondrial Membrane

Whereas the inner mitochondrial membrane is highly impermeable, the outer mitochondrial membrane is permeable to compounds with a molecular weight up to approximately 6,000 daltons because it contains large nonspecific pores called voltage-dependent anion channels (VDACs) that are formed by mitochondrial porins (see Fig. 18.16). These channels are "open" at low transmembrane potential, with a preference for anions such as phosphate, chloride, pyruvate, citrate, and adenine nucleotides. VDACs thus facilitate translocation of these anions between the intermembrane space and the cytosol. Several cytosolic kinases, such as the hexokinase that initiates glycolysis, bind to the cytosolic side of the channel, where they have ready access to newly synthesized ATP.

## CLINICAL COMMENTS

A summary of the diseases discussed in this chapter is presented in Table 18.3.

**Cora N.** Thrombolysis stimulated by intravenous recombinant TPA restored $O_2$ to **Cora N.'s** heart muscle and successfully decreased the extent of ischemic damage. The rationale for the use of TPA within 4 to 6 hours after the onset of a myocardial infarction is based on the function of the normal intrinsic fibrinolytic system (see Chapter 7). This system is designed to dissolve unwanted intravascular clots through the action of the enzyme plasmin, a protease that digests the fibrin matrix within the clot. TPA stimulates the conversion of plasminogen to its active form, plasmin. The result is a lysis of the thrombus and improved blood flow through the previously obstructed vessel, allowing fuels and $O_2$ to reach the heart cells. The human TPA protein administered to Mrs. N. is produced by recombinant DNA technology (see Chapter 14). This treatment rapidly restored $O_2$ supply to the heart.

**Isabel S.** In the case of **Isabel S.**, a diffuse myopathic process was superimposed on her AIDS and her pulmonary tuberculosis, either of which could have caused progressive weakness. In addition, she could have been suffering from a congenital mtDNA myopathy, symptomatic only as she ages. A systematic diagnostic process, however, finally led her physician to conclude that her myopathy was caused by a disorder of oxidative phosphorylation induced by her treatment with zidovudine (AZT). Fortunately, when AZT was discontinued, Ivy's myopathic symptoms gradually subsided. A repeat skeletal muscle biopsy performed 4 months later showed that her skeletal muscle cell mtDNA had been restored to normal and that she had experienced a reversible drug-induced disorder of oxidative phosphorylation.

**Table 18.3    Diseases Discussed in Chapter 18**

| Disease or Disorder | Environmental or Genetic | Comments |
|---|---|---|
| Myocardial infarction | Both | The lack of oxygen in the anterior and lateral walls of the heart is caused by severe ischemia due to clots formed within certain coronary arteries at the site of ruptured atherosclerotic plaques. The limited availability of oxygen to act as an electron acceptor decreases the proton motive force across the inner mitochondrial membrane of ischemic cells. This leads to reduced ATP generation, triggering events that lead to irreversible cell injury. Further damage to the heart muscle can occur due to free radical generation after oxygen is reintroduced to the cells that were temporarily ischemic, a process known as ischemic reperfusion injury. |
| AIDS treatment complication | Environmental | AZT, a component of AIDS treatment cocktails, can act as an inhibitor of mitochondrial DNA polymerase. Under rare conditions, it can lead to a depletion of mitochondrial DNA in cells, leading to a severe mitochondrial myopathy. |
| Iron deficiency anemia | Environmental | Lack of iron for heme synthesis, leading to reduced oxygen delivery to cells, and reduced iron in the electron transfer chain, leading to muscle weakness. |
| Cyanide poisoning | Environmental | Cyanide binds to the $Fe^{3+}$ in the heme of cytochrome $aa_3$, a component of cytochrome oxidase. Mitochondrial respiration and energy production cease, and cell death rapidly occurs. |
| Mitochondrial disorders | Genetic | Many types of mutations, leading to altered mitochondrial function and reduced energy production, due to mutations in the mitochondrial DNA. See Table 18.2 for a partial listing of these disorders. |
| Free radical disease | Both | Damage caused to proteins and lipids due to free radical generation may lead to cellular dysfunction. |
| Amyotrophic lateral sclerosis (ALS) | Both | The genetic form of ALS is due to mutations in superoxide dismutase, leading to difficulty in disposing of superoxide radicals, leading to cell damage due to excessive ROS. |
| Age-related macular degeneration | Both | Oxidative damage occurs in the retinal pigment epithelium, leading to first, reduced vision, and second, to blindness. |

ATP, adenosine triphosphate; AZT, azidothymidine; ROS, reactive oxygen species.

## REVIEW QUESTIONS-CHAPTER 18

1. Consider the following experiment. Carefully isolated liver mitochondria are incubated in the presence of a limiting amount of malate. Three minutes after adding the substrate, cyanide is added and the reaction allowed to proceed for another 7 minutes. At this point in time, which one of the following components of the electron transfer chain will be in an oxidized state?

   A. Complex I
   B. Complex II
   C. Complex III
   D. Coenzyme Q
   E. Cytochrome c

2. Consider the following experiment. Carefully isolated liver mitochondria are placed in a weakly buffered solution. Malate is added as an energy source, and an increase in oxygen consumption confirms that the electron transfer chain is functioning properly within these organelles. Valinomycin and potassium are then added to the mitochondrial suspension. Valinomycin is a drug that allows potassium ions to freely cross the inner mitochondrial membrane. What is the effect of valinomycin on the proton-motive force that had been generated by the oxidation of malate?

   A. The proton-motive force will be decreased but to a value greater than zero.
   B. The proton-motive force will be reduced to a value of zero.

C. There will be no change in the proton-motive force.

D. The proton-motive force will be increased.

E. The proton-motive force will be decreased to a value less than zero.

3. A 25-year-old female presents with chronic fatigue. A series of blood tests are ordered, and the results suggest that her red blood cell count is low due to iron deficiency anemia. Such a deficiency may play a part in leading to fatigue due to which one of the following?

A. She is not producing as much $H_2O$ in the electron transport chain, leading to dehydration, which has resulted in fatigue.

B. Iron forms a chelate with NADH and FAD(2H) that is necessary for them to donate their electrons to the electron transport chain.

C. Iron acts as a cofactor for α-ketoglutarate DH in the TCA cycle, a reaction required for the flow of electrons through the electron transport chain.

D. Iron accompanies the protons that are pumped from the mitochondrial matrix to the cytosolic side of the inner mitochondrial membrane. Without iron, the proton gradient cannot be maintained to produce adequate ATP.

E. Her decrease in Fe-S centers is impairing the transfer of electrons in the electron transport chain.

4. Rotenone, an inhibitor of NADH dehydrogenase, was originally used for fishing. When it was sprinkled on a lake, fish would absorb it through their gills and die. Until recently, it was used in the United States as an organic pesticide and was recommended for tomato plants. It was considered nontoxic to mammals and birds, which cannot readily absorb it. What effect would rotenone have on ATP production by heart mitochondria, if it could be absorbed?

A. There would be a 10% reduction in ATP production.

B. There would be a 50% reduction in ATP production.

C. There would be a 95% reduction in ATP production.

D. There would be no reduction in ATP production.

5. The level of oxidative damage to mitochondrial DNA is 10 times greater than that to nuclear DNA. This could be due, in part, to which one of the following?

A. Superoxide dismutase is present in the mitochondria.

B. The nucleus lacks glutathione.

C. The nuclear membrane presents a barrier to reactive oxygen species.

D. Mitochondrial DNA lacks histones.

E. The mitochondrial membrane is permeable to reactive oxygen species.

# 19  Generation of ATP from Glucose: Glycolysis

## CHAPTER OUTLINE

## KEY POINTS

- Glycolysis is the pathway in which glucose is oxidized and cleaved to form pyruvate.
- The enzymes of glycolysis are in the cytosol.
- Glucose is the major sugar in our diet; all cells can utilize glucose for energy.
- Glycolysis generates two molecules of ATP through substrate-level phosphorylation and two molecules of NADH.
- The cytosolic NADH generated via glycolysis transfers its reducing equivalents to mitochondrial $NAD^+$ via shuttle systems across the inner mitochondrial membrane.
- The pyruvate generated during glycolysis can enter the mitochondria and be oxidized completely to $CO_2$ by pyruvate dehydrogenase and the TCA cycle.
- Anaerobic glycolysis will generate energy in cells with a limited supply of oxygen or few mitochondria.
- Under anaerobic conditions, pyruvate is reduced to lactate by NADH, thereby regenerating the $NAD^+$ required for glycolysis to continue.
- Glycolysis is regulated to ensure that ATP homeostasis is maintained.

# THE WAITING ROOM

**Otto S.,** a 26-year-old medical student, had gained weight during his first sedentary year in medical school. During his second year, he began watching his diet, jogging for an hour four times each week, and playing tennis twice a week. He has decided to compete in a 5-km race. To prepare for the race, he begins training with wind sprints, bouts of alternately running and walking.

**Ivan A.** is a 56-year-old morbidly obese accountant (see Chapters 1 and 2). He decided to see his dentist because he felt excruciating pain in his teeth when he ate ice cream. He really likes sweets and keeps hard candy in his pocket. The dentist noted from Mr. A.'s history that he had numerous cavities as a child in his baby teeth. At this visit, the dentist found cavities in two of Mr. A.'s teeth.

## I. GLYCOLYSIS

**Glycolysis** is one of the principle pathways for generating ATP in cells and is present in all cell types. The central role of glycolysis in fuel metabolism is related to its ability to generate ATP with and without oxygen ($O_2$). The oxidation of glucose to pyruvate generates ATP from **substrate-level phosphorylation** (the transfer of phosphate from high-energy intermediates of the pathway to ADP) and NADH. Subsequently, the pyruvate may be oxidized to carbon dioxide ($CO_2$) in the TCA cycle and ATP generated from electron transfer to $O_2$ in **oxidative phosphorylation**. However, if the pyruvate and NADH from glycolysis are converted to lactate (**anaerobic glycolysis**), ATP can be generated in the absence of $O_2$ via substrate-level phosphorylation.

Glucose is readily available from our diet, internal glycogen stores, and the blood. Carbohydrate provides 50% or more of the calories in most diets, and glucose is the major carbohydrate. Other dietary sugars, such as fructose and galactose, are oxidized by conversion to intermediates of glycolysis. Glucose is stored in cells as glycogen, which can provide an internal source of fuel for glycolysis in emergency situations (e.g., decreased supply of fuels and $O_2$ during ischemia due to a reduced blood flow). Insulin and other hormones maintain blood glucose at a constant level (glucose homeostasis), thereby ensuring that glucose is always available to cells that depend on glycolysis for generation of ATP.

In addition to serving as an anaerobic and aerobic source of ATP, glycolysis is an anabolic pathway that provides biosynthetic precursors. For example, in liver and adipose tissue, this pathway generates pyruvate as a precursor for fatty acid biosynthesis. Glycolysis also provides precursors for the synthesis of amino acids and of nucleotides. The integration of glycolysis with other anabolic pathways is discussed in Chapter 30.

### A. The Reactions of Glycolysis

The glycolytic pathway, which cleaves 1 mole of glucose to 2 moles of the three-carbon compound pyruvate, consists of a preparative phase and an ATP-generating phase:

1. In the initial **preparative phase** of glycolysis, glucose is phosphorylated twice by ATP and cleaved into two triose phosphates (Fig. 19.1).
2. In the **ATP-generating phase**, glyceraldehyde 3-phosphate (glyceraldehyde 3P) (a triose phosphate) is oxidized by $NAD^+$ and phosphorylated using inorganic phosphate. The high-energy phosphate bond generated in this step is transferred to ADP to form ATP. The remaining phosphate is also rearranged to form another

After a high-carbohydrate meal, glucose is the major fuel for almost all tissues. Exceptions include intestinal mucosal cells, which transport glucose from the gut into the blood, and cells in the proximal convoluted tubule of the kidney, which return glucose from the renal filtrate to the blood. During fasting, the brain continues to oxidize glucose because it has a limited capacity for the oxidation of fatty acids or other fuels. Cells also continue to use glucose for the portion of their ATP generation that must be met by anaerobic glycolysis because of either a limited oxygen supply or a limited capacity for oxidative phosphorylation (e.g., the red blood cell).

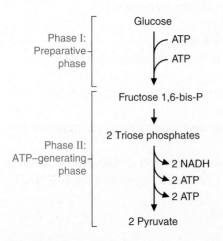

**FIG. 19.1.** Phases of the glycolytic pathway.

high-energy phosphate bond that is transferred to ADP. Because there were 2 moles of triose phosphate formed, the yield from the ATP-generating phase is 4 moles of ATP and 2 moles of NADH. The result is a net yield of 2 moles of ATP, 2 moles of NADH, and 2 moles of pyruvate per mole of glucose.

## 1. CONVERSION OF GLUCOSE TO GLUCOSE-6-PHOSPHATE

Glucose metabolism begins with transfer of a phosphate from ATP to glucose to form glucose-6-phosphate (G6P) (Fig. 19.2). Phosphorylation of glucose commits it to metabolism within the cell because G6P cannot be transported back across the plasma membrane.

The enzymes that catalyze the phosphorylation of glucose are named **hexokinases**, a family of tissue-specific isoenzymes that differ in their kinetic properties. The isoenzyme found in liver and β-cells of the pancreas has a much higher $K_m$ than other hexokinases and is called **glucokinase**.

## 2. CONVERSION OF GLUCOSE-6-PHOSPHATE TO THE TRIOSE PHOSPHATES

In the remainder of the preparative phase of glycolysis, G6P is isomerized to fructose 6-phosphate (F6P), again phosphorylated, and subsequently cleaved into two three-carbon fragments (Fig. 19.3).

The next step of glycolysis is the phosphorylation of F6P to fructose 1,6-bisphosphate (F1,6-bisP) by phosphofructokinase-1 (PFK-1). This phosphorylation requires ATP and is thermodynamically and kinetically irreversible. Therefore, PFK-1, a highly regulated enzyme in cells, irrevocably commits glucose to the glycolytic pathway. Like hexokinase, PFK-1 exists as tissue-specific isoenzymes whose regulatory properties match variations in the role of glycolysis in different tissues.

F1,6-bisP is cleaved into two phosphorylated three-carbon compounds (triose phosphates) by aldolase (see Fig. 19.3). Aldolase exists as tissue-specific isozymes, which all catalyze the cleavage of F1,6-bisP but differ in their specificites for fructose 1-phosphate. Dihydroxyacetone phosphate (DHAP) is isomerized to glyceraldehyde 3P, which is a triose phosphate. Thus, for every mole of glucose entering glycolysis, 2 moles of glyceraldehyde 3P continue through the pathway.

## 3. OXIDATION AND SUBSTRATE-LEVEL PHOSPHORYLATION

In the next part of the glycolytic pathway, glyceraldehyde 3P is oxidized and phosphorylated so that subsequent intermediates of glycolysis can donate phosphate to ADP to generate ATP. The first reaction in this sequence, catalyzed by glyceraldehyde 3P dehydrogenase, is really the key to the pathway (see Fig. 19.3). This enzyme oxidizes the aldehyde group of glyceraldehyde 3P to a high-energy acyl phosphate, generating 1,3-bisphosphoglycerate, and transfers the electrons to $NAD^+$ to form NADH. The formation of this high-energy phosphate bond is the start of **substrate-level phosphorylation** (the formation of a high-energy phosphate bond in the absence of $O_2$).

In the next reaction, the high-energy phosphate bond of 1,3-bisphosphoglycerate is transferred to ADP to form ATP by 3-phosphoglycerate kinase. The energy of the acyl phosphate bond is high enough ($\sim$10 kcal/mole) so that transfer to ADP is an energetically favorable process, although it is a reversible reaction. 3-Phosphoglycerate is the other product of this reaction.

To transfer the remaining low-energy phosphoester on 3-phosphoglycerate to ADP, it must be converted into a high-energy bond. This conversion is accomplished by moving the phosphate to the second carbon (forming 2-phosphoglycerate via phosphoglycerate mutase) and then removing water to form phosphoenolpyruvate (PEP) via enolase. The enol phosphate bond is a high-energy bond (its hydrolysis releases approximately 14 kcal/mole of energy), so the transfer of phosphate to ADP by pyruvate kinase is energetically favorable (see Fig. 19.3) and not reversible. This final reaction converts PEP to pyruvate.

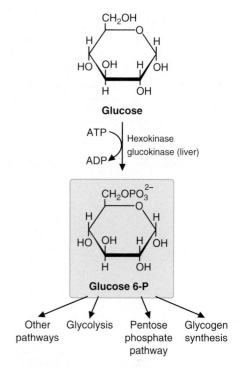

*FIG. 19.2.* G6P metabolism.

G6P is a branch point in carbohydrate metabolism. It is a precursor for almost every pathway that uses glucose, including glycolysis, the pentose phosphate pathway, and glycogen synthesis. From the opposite point of view, it can also be generated from other pathways of carbohydrate metabolism, such as glycogenolysis (breakdown of glycogen), the pentose phosphate pathway, and gluconeogenesis (the synthesis of glucose from noncarbohydrate sources).

Arsenic poisoning is caused by the presence of a large number of different arsenious compounds that are effective metabolic inhibitors. Acute accidental or intentional arsenic poisoning requires high doses and involves arsenate ($AsO_4^{3-}$) and arsenite ($AsO_3^{2-}$). Arsenite, which is 10 times more toxic than arsenate, binds to neighboring sulfhydryl groups, such as those in dihydrolipoate and in nearby cysteine pairs (vicinal) found in α-keto acid dehydrogenase complexes and in succinate dehydrogenase. Arsenate weakly inhibits enzymatic reactions involving phosphate, including the glyceraldehyde-3-P dehydrogenase step in glycolysis. Thus, both aerobic and anaerobic ATP production can be inhibited. The low doses of arsenic compounds in water supplies are a major public health concern but are associated with increased risk of cancer rather than direct toxicity.

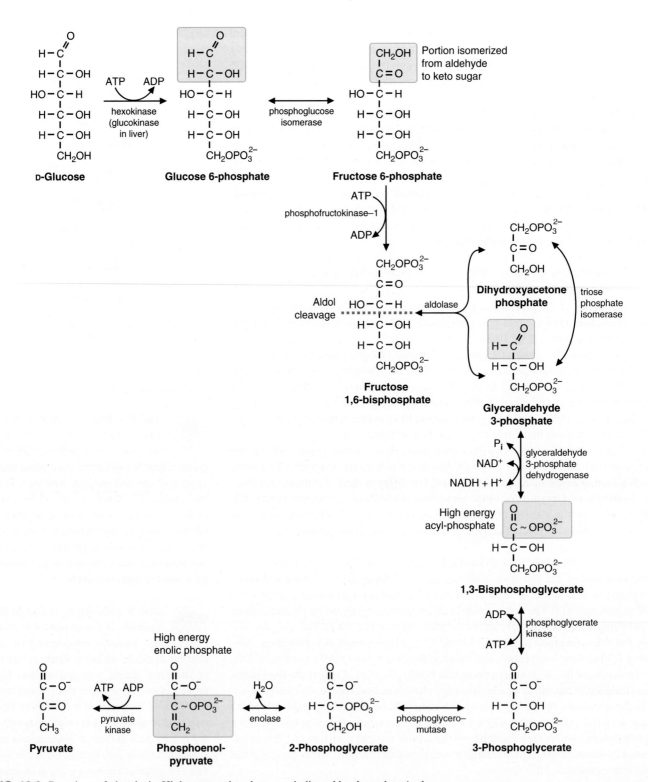

**FIG. 19.3.** Reactions of glycolysis. High-energy phosphates are indicated by the *red squiggles*.

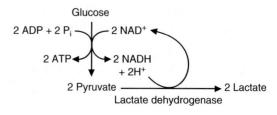

**A. Aerobic glycolysis**

**B. Anaerobic glycolysis**

**FIG. 19.4.** Alternate fates of pyruvate. **A.** The pyruvate produced by glycolysis enters mitochondria and is oxidized to $CO_2$ and $H_2O$. The reducing equivalents in NADH enter mitochondria via a shuttle system. **B.** Pyruvate is reduced to lactate in the cytosol, thereby using the reducing equivalents in NADH.

## 4.  SUMMARY OF THE GLYCOLYTIC PATHWAY

The overall net reaction in the glycolytic pathway is

$$\text{Glucose} + 2NAD^+ + 2P_i + 2ADP \rightarrow 2Pyruvate + 2NADH + 4H^+ + 2ATP + 2H_2O$$

The pathway occurs with an overall negative $\Delta G^{0'}$ of approximately $-22$ kcal/mole. Therefore, it cannot be reversed without the expenditure of energy.

## B.  Oxidative Fates of Pyruvate and NADH

The NADH produced from glycolysis must be continuously reoxidized back to $NAD^+$ to provide an electron acceptor for the glyceraldehyde 3P dehydrogenase reaction and prevent product inhibition. Without oxidation of this NADH, glycolysis cannot continue. There are two alternate routes for oxidation of cytosolic NADH (Fig. 19.4):

1. An aerobic route that involves pathways (known as shuttles) that transfer reducing equivalents across the mitochondrial membrane and ultimately to the electron transport chain and $O_2$ (see Fig. 19.4A).
2. An anaerobic route in which NADH is reoxidized in the cytosol by lactate dehydrogenase (LDH), which reduces pyruvate to lactate (see Fig. 19.4B).

Shuttles are required for the oxidation of cytosolic NADH by the electron transport chain because the inner mitochondrial membrane is impermeable to NADH, and no transport protein exists that can directly translocate NADH across this membrane. Consequently, NADH is reoxidized to $NAD^+$ in the cytosol by a reaction that transfers the electrons to DHAP in the glycerol 3-phosphate (glycerol 3P) shuttle and oxaloacetate in the malate–aspartate shuttle. The $NAD^+$ that is formed in the cytosol returns to glycolysis while glycerol 3P or malate carry the reducing equivalents that are ultimately transferred across the inner mitochondrial membrane. Thus, these shuttles transfer electrons and not NADH per se.

## 1.  GLYCEROL 3-PHOSPHATE SHUTTLE

The **glycerol 3P shuttle** is the major shuttle in most tissues. In this shuttle, cytosolic $NAD^+$ is regenerated by cytoplasmic glycerol 3P dehydrogenase, which transfers electrons from NADH to DHAP to form glycerol 3P (Fig. 19.5). Glycerol 3P then diffuses through the outer mitochondrial membrane to the inner mitochondrial membrane, where the electrons are donated to a membrane-bound flavin adenine

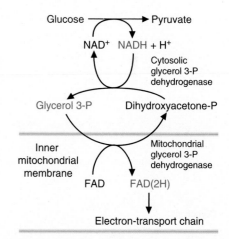

**FIG. 19.5.** Glycerol 3P shuttle. Because $NAD^+$ and NADH cannot cross the mitochondrial membrane, shuttles transfer the reducing equivalents into mitochondria. DHAP is reduced to glycerol 3P by cytosolic glycerol 3P dehydrogenase using cytosolic NADH produced in glycolysis. Glycerol 3P then reacts in the inner mitochondrial membrane with mitochondrial glycerol 3P dehydrogenase, which transfers the electrons to FAD and regenerates DHAP, which returns to the cytosol. The electron transport chain transfers the electrons to $O_2$, which generates approximately 1.5 ATP for each FAD(2H) that is oxidized.

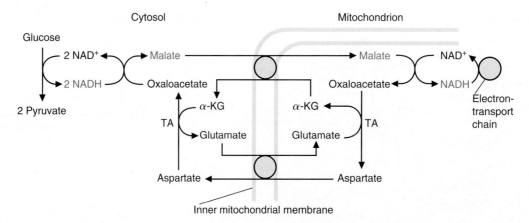

**FIG. 19.6.** Malate–aspartate shuttle. NADH produced by glycolysis reduces oxaloacetate (OAA) to malate, which crosses the mitochondrial membrane and is reoxidized to OAA. The mitochondrial NADH donates electrons to the electron transport chain, with 2.5 moles of ATP generated for each mole of NADH. To complete the shuttle, OAA must return to the cytosol, although it cannot be directly transported on a translocase. Instead, it is transaminated to aspartate, which is then transported out to the cytosol, where it is transaminated back to OAA. The translocators exchange compounds in such a way that the shuttle is completely balanced. *TA*, transamination reaction; α-*KG*, α-ketoglutarate.

dinucleotide (FAD)-containing glycerophosphate dehydrogenase. This enzyme, like succinate dehydrogenase, ultimately donates electrons to coenzyme Q (CoQ), resulting in an energy yield of approximately 1.5 ATP from oxidative phosphorylation. DHAP returns to the cytosol to continue the shuttle. The sum of the reactions in this shuttle system is simply

$$NADH_{cytosol} + H^+ + FAD_{mitochondria} \rightarrow NAD^+ +\ _{cytosol} + FAD(2H)_{mitochondria}$$

### 2. MALATE–ASPARTATE SHUTTLE

Many tissues contain both the glycerol 3P shuttle and the malate–aspartate shuttle. In the **malate–aspartate shuttle** (Fig. 19.6), cytosolic $NAD^+$ is regenerated by cytosolic malate dehydrogenase, which transfers electrons from NADH to cytosolic oxaloacetate to form malate.

Malate is transported across the inner mitochondrial membrane by a specific translocase, which exchanges malate for α-ketoglutarate. In the matrix, malate is oxidized back to oxaloacetate by mitochondrial malate dehydrogenase, and NADH is generated. This NADH can donate electrons to the electron transport chain with generation of approximately 2.5 moles of ATP per mole of NADH. The newly formed oxaloacetate cannot pass back through the inner mitochondrial membrane under physiological conditions, so aspartate is used to return the oxaloacetate carbon skeleton to the cytosol. In the matrix, transamination reactions transfer an amino group to oxaloacetate to form aspartate, which is transported out to the cytosol (using an aspartate-glutamate exchange translocase) and converted back to oxaloacetate through another transamination reaction. The sum of all the reactions of this shuttle system is simply

$$NADH_{cytosol} + NAD^+\ _{matrix} \rightarrow NAD^+\ _{cytosol} + NADH_{matrix}$$

## C. Anaerobic Glycolysis

When the oxidative capacity of a cell is limited (e.g., such as in the red blood cell, which has no mitochondria), the pyruvate and NADH produced from glycolysis cannot be oxidized aerobically. The NADH is therefore oxidized to $NAD^+$ in the cytosol by reduction of pyruvate to lactate. This reaction is catalyzed by LDH (Fig. 19.7). The net reaction for anaerobic glycolysis is

$$Glucose + 2\ ADP + 2\ P_i \rightarrow 2\ Lactate + 2\ ATP + 2\ H_2O + 2\ H^+$$

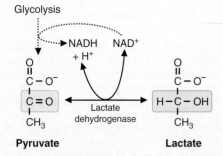

**FIG. 19.7.** LDH reaction. Pyruvate, which may be produced by glycolysis, is reduced to lactate. The reaction, which occurs in the cytosol, requires NADH and is catalyzed by LDH. This reaction is readily reversible.

## 1.  ENERGY YIELD OF AEROBIC VERSUS ANAEROBIC GLYCOLYSIS

In both aerobic and anaerobic glycolysis, each mole of glucose generates 2 moles of ATP, 2 moles of NADH, and 2 moles of pyruvate. The energy yield from anaerobic glycolysis (glucose to two lactate) is only 2 moles of ATP per mole of glucose, as the NADH is recycled to $NAD^+$ by reducing pyruvate to lactate. Neither the NADH nor pyruvate produced is thus used for further energy generation. However, when $O_2$ is available and cytosolic NADH can be oxidized via a shuttle system, pyruvate can also enter the mitochondria and be completely oxidized to $CO_2$ via pyruvate dehydrogenase (PDH) and the TCA cycle. The oxidation of pyruvate via this route generates roughly 12.5 moles of ATP per mole of pyruvate. If the cytosolic NADH is oxidized by the glycerol 3P shuttle, approximately 1.5 moles of ATP are produced per NADH. If, instead, the NADH is oxidized by the malate–aspartate shuttle, approximately 2.5 moles are produced. Thus, the two NADH molecules produced during glycolysis can lead to 3 to 5 molecules of ATP being produced, depending on which shuttle system is used to transfer the reducing equivalents. Because each mole of pyruvate produced can give rise to 12.5 moles of ATP, altogether, 30 to 32 moles of ATP can be produced from one mole of glucose oxidized to $CO_2$.

To produce the same amount of ATP per unit time from anaerobic glycolysis as from the complete aerobic oxidation of glucose to $CO_2$, anaerobic glycolysis must occur approximately 15 times faster and use approximately 15 times more glucose. Cells achieve this high rate of glycolysis by expressing high levels of glycolytic enzymes. In certain skeletal muscles and in most cells during hypoxic crises, high rates of glycolysis are associated with rapid degradation of internal glycogen stores to supply the required G6P.

**Q:** What are the energy-generating steps as pyruvate is completely oxidized to carbon dioxide to generate 12.5 moles of ATP per mole of pyruvate?

## 2.  ACID PRODUCTION IN ANAEROBIC GLYCOLYSIS

Anaerobic glycolysis results in acid production in the form of $H^+$. Glycolysis forms pyruvic acid, which is reduced to **lactic acid**. At an intracellular pH of 7.35, lactic acid dissociates to form the carboxylate anion, **lactate**, and $H^+$ (the pKa for lactic acid is 3.85). Lactate and the $H^+$ are both transported out of the cell into interstitial fluid by a transporter on the plasma membrane and eventually diffuse into the blood. If the amount of lactate generated exceeds the buffering capacity of the blood, the pH drops below the normal range, resulting in lactic acidosis (see Chapter 2).

## 3.  TISSUES DEPENDENT ON ANAEROBIC GLYCOLYSIS

Many tissues, including red and white blood cells, the kidney medulla, the tissues of the eye, and skeletal muscles, rely on anaerobic glycolysis for at least a portion of their ATP requirements. Tissues (or cells) that are heavily dependent on anaerobic glycolysis usually have a low ATP demand, high levels of glycolytic enzymes, and few capillaries, such that $O_2$ must diffuse over a greater distance to reach target cells. The lack of mitochondria, or the increased rate of glycolysis, is often related to some aspect of cell function. For example, the mature red blood cell has no mitochondria because oxidative metabolism might interfere with its function in transporting $O_2$ bound to hemoglobin. Some of the lactic acid generated by anaerobic glycolysis in skin is secreted in sweat, where it acts as an antibacterial agent. Many large tumors use anaerobic glycolysis for ATP production and lack capillaries in their core.

In tissues with some mitochondria, both aerobic and anaerobic glycolysis occur simultaneously. The relative proportion of the two pathways depends on the mitochondrial oxidative capacity of the tissue and its $O_2$ supply and may vary among cell types within the same tissue because of cell distance from the capillaries. When a cell's energy demand exceeds the capacity of the rate of the electron transport chain and oxidative phosphorylation to produce ATP, glycolysis is activated, and the increased $NADH/NAD^+$ ratio will direct excess pyruvate into lactate. Because under these conditions PDH, the TCA cycle, and the electron transport chain are operating as fast as they can, anaerobic glycolysis is meeting the need for additional ATP.

The dental caries in **Ivan A.'s** mouth were caused principally by the low pH generated from lactic acid production by oral bacteria. Below a pH of 5.5, decalcification of tooth enamel and dentine occurs. Mr. A.'s dentist explained that bacteria in his dental plaque could convert all the sugar in his candy into acid in less than 20 minutes. The acid is buffered by bicarbonate and other buffers in saliva, but saliva production decreases in the evening. Thus, the acid could dissolve the hydroxyapatite in his tooth enamel during the night.

In the complete oxidation of pyruvate to carbon dioxide, four steps generate NADH (pyruvate dehydrogenase, isocitrate dehydrogenase, α-ketoglutarate dehydrogenase, and malate dehydrogenase). One step generates FAD(2H) (succinate dehydrogenase) and one substrate-level phosphorylation (succinate thiokinase). Thus, because each mole of NADH generates 2.5 moles of ATP, the overall contribution by NADH is 10 moles of ATP. The FAD(2H) generates an additional 1.5 moles of ATP, and the substrate-level phosphorylation provides one more. Therefore, 10 + 1.5 + 1 = 12.5 moles of ATP.

## 4. FATE OF LACTATE

Lactate released from cells undergoing anaerobic glycolysis is taken up by other tissues (primarily the liver, heart, and skeletal muscle) and oxidized back to pyruvate. In the liver, the pyruvate is used to synthesize glucose (gluconeogenesis), which is returned to the blood. The cycling of lactate and glucose between peripheral tissues and liver is called the **Cori cycle**.

In many other tissues, lactate is oxidized to pyruvate, which is then oxidized to $CO_2$ in the TCA cycle. Although the equilibrium of the LDH reaction favors lactate production, flux occurs in the opposite direction if NADH is being rapidly oxidized in the electron transport chain (or being used for gluconeogenesis):

$$Lactate + NAD^+ \rightarrow Pyruvate + NADH + H^+$$

The heart, with its huge mitochondrial content and oxidative capacity, is able to use lactate released from other tissues as a fuel. During an exercise such as bicycle riding, lactate released into the blood from skeletal muscles in the leg might be used by resting skeletal muscles in the arm. In the brain, glial cells and astrocytes produce lactate, which is used by neurons or released into the blood.

## II.  OTHER FUNCTIONS OF GLYCOLYSIS

Glycolysis, in addition to providing ATP, generates precursors for biosynthetic pathways (Fig. 19.8). Intermediates of the pathway can be converted to ribose 5-phosphate, the sugar incorporated into nucleotides such as ATP. Other sugars, such as UDP-glucose, mannose, and sialic acid, are also formed from intermediates of glycolysis. Serine is synthesized from 3-phosphoglycerate and alanine from pyruvate. The backbone of triacylglycerols, glycerol 3P, is derived from DHAP in the glycolytic pathway.

The liver is the major site of biosynthetic reactions in the body. In addition to those pathways mentioned previously, the liver synthesizes fatty acids from the

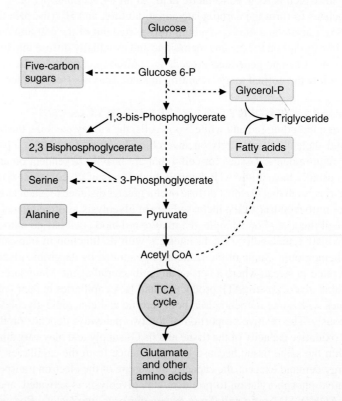

**FIG. 19.8.** Biosynthetic functions of glycolysis. Compounds formed from intermediates of glycolysis are shown in the *boxes*. These pathways are discussed in later chapters. *Dotted lines* indicate that more than one step is required for the conversion shown in the figure.

pyruvate generated by glycolysis. It also synthesizes glucose from lactate, glycerol 3P, and amino acids in the gluconeogenic pathway, which is principally a reversal of glycolysis. Consequently, in liver, many of the glycolytic enzymes exist as isoenzymes with properties suited for these functions.

## III. REGULATION OF GLYCOLYSIS BY THE NEED FOR ATP

One of the major functions of glycolysis is the generation of ATP so the pathway is regulated to maintain ATP homeostasis in all cells. PFK-1 and PDH, which links glycolysis and the TCA cycle, are both major regulatory sites that respond to feedback indicators of the rate of ATP utilization (Fig. 19.9). The supply of G6P for glycolysis is tissue-dependent and can be regulated at the steps of glucose transport into cells, glycogenolysis (the degradation of glycogen to form glucose), or the rate of glucose phosphorylation by hexokinase isoenzymes. Other regulatory mechanisms integrate the ATP-generating role of glycolysis with its anabolic roles.

The bisphosphoglycerate shunt is a "side reaction" of the glycolytic pathway in which 1,3-bisphosphoglycerate is converted to 2,3-bisphosphoglycerate (2,3-BPG). Red blood cells form 2,3-BPG to serve as an allosteric inhibitor of $O_2$ binding to heme (see Chapter 5). 2,3-BPG reenters the glycolytic pathway via dephosphorylation to 3-phosphoglycerate. It also functions as a coenzyme in the conversion of 3-phosphoglycerate to 2-phosphoglycerate by the glycolytic enzyme phosphoglyceromutase. Because 2,3-BPG is not depleted by its role in this catalytic process, most cells need only very small amounts.

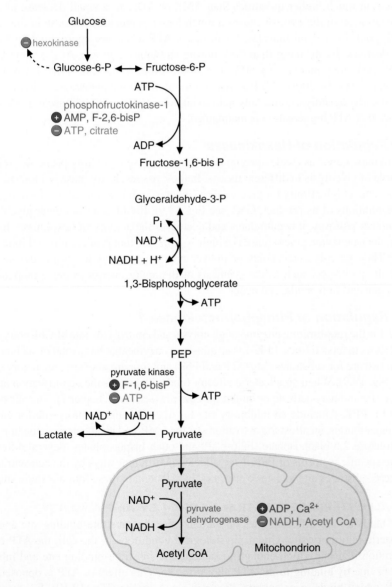

**FIG. 19.9.** Major sites of regulation in the glycolytic pathway. Hexokinase and PFK-1 are the major regulatory enzymes in skeletal muscle. The activity of PDH in the mitochondrion determines whether pyruvate is converted to lactate or to acetyl CoA. The regulation shown for pyruvate kinase only occurs for the liver (L) isoenzyme.

**Otto S.** has started high-intensity exercise that will increase the production of lactate in his exercising skeletal muscles. In skeletal muscles, the amount of aerobic versus anaerobic glycolysis that occurs varies with intensity of the exercise, with duration of the exercise, with the type of skeletal muscle fiber involved, and with the level of training. Human skeletal muscles are usually combinations of type I fibers (called fast glycolytic fibers or white muscle fibers) and type IIb fibers (called slow oxidative fibers or red muscle fibers). The designation "fast" or "slow" refers to the fibers rate of shortening, which is determined by the isoenzyme of myosin ATPase present. Compared with glycolytic fibers, oxidative fibers have a higher content of mitochondria and myoglobin, which gives them a red color. The gastrocnemius, a muscle in the leg used for running, has a high content of type IIb fibers. However, these fibers will still produce lactate during sprints when the ATP demand exceeds their oxidative capacity.

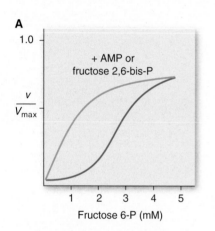

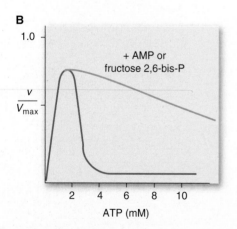

*FIG. 19.10.* Regulation of PFK-1 by AMP, ATP, and F2,6-bisP. **A.** AMP and F2,6-bisP activate PFK-1. **B.** ATP, as a substrate, increases the rate of the reaction at low concentrations but allosterically inhibits the enzyme at high concentrations.

All of the regulatory enzymes of glycolysis exist as tissue-specific isoenzymes, which alter the regulation of the pathway to match variations in conditions and needs in different tissues. For example, in the liver, an isoenzyme of pyruvate kinase introduces an additional regulatory site in glycolysis that contributes to the inhibition of glycolysis when the reverse pathway, gluconeogenesis, is activated.

## A. Relationship between ATP, ADP, and AMP Concentrations

The AMP levels within the cytosol provide a better indicator of the rate of ATP utilization than the ATP concentration itself. The concentration of AMP in the cytosol is determined by the equilibrium position of the adenylate kinase reaction.

$$\text{Adenylate kinase}$$
$$2\ \text{ADP} \leftrightarrow \text{AMP} + \text{ATP}$$

The equilibrium is such that hydrolysis of ATP to ADP in energy-requiring reactions increases both the ADP and AMP contents of the cytosol. However, ATP is present in much higher quantities than AMP or ADP, so a small decrease of ATP concentration in the cytosol causes a much larger percentage increase in the small AMP pool. In skeletal muscles, for instance, ATP levels are approximately 5 mM and decrease by no more than 20% during strenuous exercise. At the same time, ADP levels may increase by 50%, and AMP levels, which are in the micromolar range, increase by 300%. AMP activates several metabolic pathways, including glycolysis, glycogenolysis, and fatty acid oxidation (particularly in muscle tissues), to ensure that ATP homeostasis is maintained.

## B. Regulation of Hexokinases

Hexokinases exist as tissue-specific isoenzymes whose regulatory properties reflect the role of glycolysis in different tissues. In most tissues, hexokinase is a low-$K_m$ enzyme with a high affinity for glucose (see Chapter 7). It is inhibited by physiological concentrations of its product, G6P (see Fig. 19.9). If G6P does not enter glycolysis or another pathway, it accumulates and decreases the activity of hexokinase. In the liver, the isoenzyme glucokinase is a high-$K_m$ enzyme that is not readily inhibited by G6P. Thus, glycolysis can continue in liver even when energy levels are high so that anabolic pathways, such as the synthesis of the major energy storage compounds, glycogen and fatty acids, can occur.

## C. Regulation of Phosphofructokinase-1

PFK-1 is the rate-limiting enzyme of glycolysis and controls the rate of G6P entry into glycolysis in most tissues. PFK-1 is an allosteric enzyme that has a total of six binding sites: two are for substrates (Mg-ATP and F6P) and four are allosteric regulatory sites (see Fig. 19.9). When an allosteric effector binds, it changes the conformation at the active site and may activate or inhibit the enzyme (see also Chapter 7). The allosteric sites for PFK-1 include an inhibitory site for Mg-ATP, an inhibitory site for citrate and other anions, an allosteric activation site for AMP, and an allosteric activation site for fructose 2,6-bisphosphate (F2,6-bisP) and other bisphosphates. Several different tissue-specific isoforms of PFK-1 are affected in different ways by the concentration of these substrates and allosteric effectors, but all contain these four allosteric sites.

### 1. ALLOSTERIC REGULATION OF PFK-1 BY AMP AND ATP

ATP binds to two different sites on the enzyme: the substrate-binding site and an allosteric inhibitory site. Under physiological conditions in the cell, the ATP concentration is usually high enough to saturate the substrate-binding site and inhibit the enzyme by binding to the ATP allosteric site. This effect of ATP is opposed by AMP, which binds to a separate allosteric activator site (Fig. 19.10). For most of the PFK-1 isoenzymes, the binding of AMP increases the affinity of the enzyme for F6P (e.g., shifts the kinetic curve to the left). Thus, increases in AMP concentration can greatly increase the rate of the enzyme (see Fig. 19.10), particularly when F6P concentrations are low.

## 2. REGULATION OF PFK-1 BY FRUCTOSE 2,6-BISPHOSPHATE

F2,6-bisP is also an allosteric activator of PFK-1 that opposes ATP inhibition. Its effect on the rate of activity of PFK-1 is qualitatively similar to that of AMP, but it has a separate binding site. F2,6-bisP is not an intermediate of glycolysis but is synthesized by an enzyme that phosphorylates F6P at the 2-position. The enzyme is therefore named phosphofructokinase-2 (PFK-2); it is a bifunctional enzyme with two separate domains: a kinase domain and a phosphatase domain. At the kinase domain, F6P is phosphorylated to F2,6-bisP and at the phosphatase domain, F2,6-bisP is hydrolyzed back to F6P. PFK-2 is regulated through changes in the ratio of activity of the two domains. For example, in skeletal muscles, high concentrations of F6P activate the kinase and inhibit the phosphatase, thereby increasing the concentration of F2,6-bisP and activating glycolysis.

PFK-2 can also be regulated through phosphorylation by serine-threonine protein kinases. The liver isoenzyme contains a phosphorylation site near the amino terminal that decreases the activity of the kinase and increases the phosphatase activity. This site is phosphorylated by the cAMP-dependent protein kinase (protein kinase A) and is responsible for decreased levels of liver F2,6-bisP during fasting conditions (as modulated by circulating glucagon levels, which is discussed in detail in Chapters 21 and 26). The cardiac isoenzyme contains a phosphorylation site near the carboxy terminal that can be phosphorylated in response to adrenergic activators of contraction (such as norepinephrine) and by increased AMP levels. Phosphorylation at this site increases the kinase activity and increases F2,6-bisP levels, thereby contributing to the activation of glycolysis.

## 3. ALLOSTERIC INHIBITION OF PFK-1 AT THE CITRATE SITE

The function of the citrate-anion allosteric site is to integrate glycolysis with other pathways. For example, the inhibition of PFK-1 by citrate may play a role in decreasing glycolytic flux in the heart during the oxidation of fatty acids.

### D.  Regulation of Pyruvate Kinase

Pyruvate kinase exists as tissue-specific isoenzymes, designated as R (red blood cells), L (liver), and M1/M2 (muscle and other tissues). The M form present in brain, heart, and muscle contains no allosteric sites, and pyruvate kinase does not contribute to the regulation of glycolysis in these tissues. However, the liver isoenzyme can be inhibited through phosphorylation by the cAMP-dependent protein kinase and by several allosteric effectors that contribute to the inhibition of glycolysis during fasting conditions. These allosteric effectors include activation by F1,6-bisP, which ties the rate of pyruvate kinase to that of PFK-1, and inhibition by ATP, which signifies high energy levels.

### E.  Pyruvate Dehydrogenase Regulation and Glycolysis

PDH is also regulated principally by the rate of ATP utilization (see Chapter 17) through rapid phosphorylation to an inactive form. Thus, in a normal respiring cell, with an adequate supply of $O_2$, glycolysis and the TCA cycle are activated together, and glucose can be completely oxidized to $CO_2$. However, when tissues do not have an adequate supply of $O_2$ to meet their ATP demands, the increased NADH/NAD$^+$ ratio inhibits PDH, but AMP activates glycolysis. A proportion of the pyruvate is then reduced to lactate to allow glycolysis to continue.

## IV. LACTIC ACIDEMIA

Lactate production is a normal part of metabolism. In the absence of disease, elevated lactate levels in the blood are associated with anaerobic glycolysis during exercise. In lactic acidosis, lactic acid accumulates in blood to levels that significantly affect the pH (lactate levels greater than 5 mM and a decrease of blood pH below 7.2).

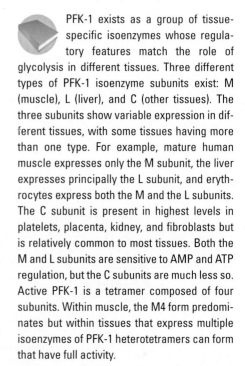

PFK-1 exists as a group of tissue-specific isoenzymes whose regulatory features match the role of glycolysis in different tissues. Three different types of PFK-1 isoenzyme subunits exist: M (muscle), L (liver), and C (other tissues). The three subunits show variable expression in different tissues, with some tissues having more than one type. For example, mature human muscle expresses only the M subunit, the liver expresses principally the L subunit, and erythrocytes express both the M and the L subunits. The C subunit is present in highest levels in platelets, placenta, kidney, and fibroblasts but is relatively common to most tissues. Both the M and L subunits are sensitive to AMP and ATP regulation, but the C subunits are much less so. Active PFK-1 is a tetramer composed of four subunits. Within muscle, the M4 form predominates but within tissues that express multiple isoenzymes of PFK-1 heterotetramers can form that have full activity.

Under ischemic conditions, AMP levels within the heart increase rapidly because of the lack of ATP production via oxidative phosphorylation. The increase in AMP levels activates the AMP-activated protein kinase, which phosphorylates the heart isoenzyme of PFK-2 to activate its kinase activity. This results in increased levels of F2,6-bisP, which activates PFK-1 along with AMP such that the rate of glycolysis can increase to compensate for the lack of ATP production via aerobic means.

During **Cora N.'s** myocardial infarction, the ischemic area in her heart had a limited supply of $O_2$ and blood-borne fuels. The absence of oxygen for oxidative phosphorylation would decrease the levels of ATP and increase those of AMP, an activator of PFK-1 and the AMP-activated protein kinase, resulting in a compensatory increase of anaerobic glycolysis and lactate production. However, obstruction of a vessel leading to her heart would decrease lactate removal, resulting in a decrease of intracellular pH. Under these conditions, at very low pH levels, glycolysis is inhibited and unable to compensate for the lack of oxidative phosphorylation.

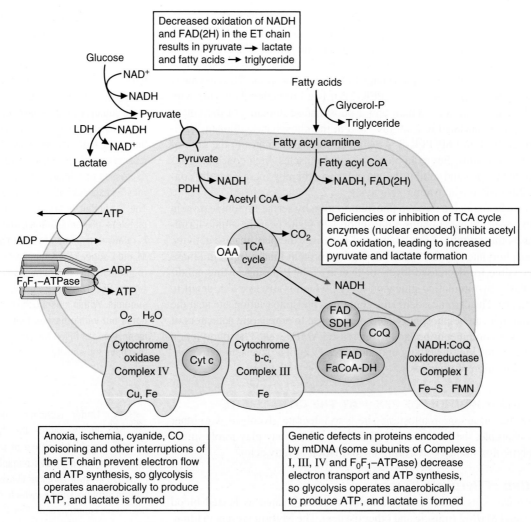

Decreased oxidation of NADH and FAD(2H) in the ET chain results in pyruvate → lactate and fatty acids → triglyceride

Deficiencies or inhibition of TCA cycle enzymes (nuclear encoded) inhibit acetyl CoA oxidation, leading to increased pyruvate and lactate formation

Anoxia, ischemia, cyanide, CO poisoning and other interruptions of the ET chain prevent electron flow and ATP synthesis, so glycolysis operates anaerobically to produce ATP, and lactate is formed

Genetic defects in proteins encoded by mtDNA (some subunits of Complexes I, III, IV and $F_0F_1$–ATPase) decrease electron transport and ATP synthesis, so glycolysis operates anaerobically to produce ATP, and lactate is formed

*FIG. 19.11.* Pathways leading to lactic acidemia.

Lactic acidosis generally results from a greatly increased $NADH/NAD^+$ ratio in tissues (Fig. 19.11). The increased NADH concentration prevents pyruvate oxidation in the TCA cycle and directs pyruvate to lactate. To compensate for the decreased ATP production from oxidative metabolism, PFK-1, and therefore, the entire glycolytic pathway is activated. For example, consumption of high amounts of alcohol, which is rapidly oxidized in the liver and increases NADH levels, can result in lactic acidosis. Hypoxia in any tissue increases lactate production as cells attempt to compensate for a lack of $O_2$ for oxidative phosphorylation.

Several other problems that interfere either with the electron transport chain or pyruvate oxidation in the TCA cycle result in lactic acidemia (see Fig. 19.11). For example, oxidative phosphorylation diseases increase the $NADH/NAD^+$ ratio and inhibit PDH (see Chapter 18). Pyruvate accumulates and is converted to lactate to allow glycolytic ATP production to proceed. Similarly, impaired PDH activity from an inherited deficiency of $E_1$ (the decarboxylase subunit of the complex), or from severe thiamine deficiency, increases blood lactate levels (see Chapter 17). Pyruvate carboxylase deficiency also can result in lactic acidosis (see Chapter 16) because of an accumulation of pyruvate.

Lactic acidosis can also result from inhibition of lactate utilization in gluconeogenesis (e.g., hereditary fructose intolerance, which is due to a defective aldolase gene). If other pathways that use G6P are blocked, G6P can be shunted into glycolysis and lactate production (e.g., glucose-6-phosphatase deficiency).

## CLINICAL COMMENTS

Diseases discussed in this chapter are summarized in Table 19.1.

**Otto S.** In skeletal muscles, lactate production occurs when the need for ATP exceeds the capacity of the mitochondria for oxidative phosphorylation. Thus, increased lactate production accompanies an increased rate of the TCA cycle. The extent to which skeletal muscles use aerobic versus anaerobic glycolysis to supply ATP varies with the intensity of exercise. During low-intensity exercise, the rate of ATP use is lower, and fibers can generate this ATP from oxidative phosphorylation, with the complete oxidation of glucose to $CO_2$. However, when **Otto S.** sprints, a high-intensity exercise, the ATP demand exceeds the rate at which the electron transport chain and TCA cycle can generate ATP from oxidative phosphorylation. The increased AMP level signals the need for additional ATP and stimulates PFK-1. The $NADH/NAD^+$ ratio directs the increase in pyruvate production toward lactate. The fall in pH causes muscle fatigue and pain. As Otto trains, the amounts of mitochondria and myoglobin in his skeletal muscle fibers increase, and these fibers rely less on anaerobic glycolysis.

**Ivan A.** Ivan A. had two sites of dental caries: one on a smooth surface and one in a fissure. The decreased pH resulting from lactic acid production by lactobacilli, which grow anaerobically within the fissure, is a major cause of fissure caries. *Streptococcus mutans* (*S. mutans*) plays a major role in smooth surface caries because it secretes dextran, an insoluble polysaccharide, which forms the base for plaque. *S. mutans* contains dextransucrase, a glucosyltransferase that transfers glucosyl units from dietary sucrose (the glucose-fructose disaccharide in sugar and sweets) to form the α(1→6) and α(1→3) linkages between the glucosyl units in dextran. Dextransucrase is specific for sucrose and does not catalyze the polymerization of free glucose or glucose from other disaccharides or polysaccharides. Thus, sucrose is responsible for the cariogenic potential of candy. The sticky water-insoluble dextran mediates the attachment of *S. mutans* and other bacteria to the tooth surface. This also keeps the acids produced from these bacteria close to the enamel surface. Fructose from sucrose is converted to intermediates of glycolysis and is rapidly metabolized to lactic acid. Other bacteria present in the plaque produce different acids from anaerobic metabolism, such as acetic acid and formic acid. The decrease in pH that results initiates demineralization of the hydroxyapatite of the tooth enamel. **Ivan A.'s** caries in his baby teeth could have been caused by sucking on bottles containing fruit juice. The sugar in fruit juice is also sucrose. Babies who fall asleep with a bottle of fruit juice or milk (milk can also decrease the pH) in their mouth may develop caries. Rapid decay of these baby teeth can harm the development of their permanent teeth.

**Table 19.1   Diseases Discussed in Chapter 19**

| Disease or Disorder | Environmental or Genetic | Comments |
| --- | --- | --- |
| Obesity | Both | Lactate production via anaerobic glycolysis in the muscle occurs during vigorous exercise for weight loss and causes muscle pain and fatigue. |
| Dental caries | Environmental | Effects of carbohydrate metabolism on oral flora and acid production |
| Lactic acidemia | Both | Elevated lactic acid due to mutations in a variety of enzymes involved in carbohydrate and energy metabolism |

1.  Starting with glyceraldehyde 3-phosphate and synthesizing one molecule of pyruvate, the net yield of ATP and NADH would be which one of the following?

    A.  Two ATP and one NADH
    B.  Two ATP and two NADH
    C.  One ATP and two NADH
    D.  One ATP and one NADH
    E.  Three ATP and two NADH

2.  Which one of the following statements correctly describes an aspect of glycolysis?

    A.  ATP is formed by oxidative phosphorylation.
    B.  Pyruvate kinase is the rate-limiting enzyme.
    C.  The reactions take place in the matrix of the mitochondria.
    D.  One pyruvate and three $CO_2$ are formed from the oxidation of one glucose molecule.
    E.  Two ATP are used in the beginning of the pathway.

3.  A person who is exercising at a high-intensity level will exhibit which one of the following biochemical changes in the muscle?

    A.  A high $NAD^+$:NADH ratio when compared to a person at rest

    B.  An increased velocity of the lactate dehydrogenase reaction
    C.  A high ratio of ATP:ADP when compared to a person at rest
    D.  Decreased $O_2$ consumption
    E.  A decreased velocity of the NADH dehydrogenase reaction

4.  The role of fructose 2,6-bisphosphate in glycolysis is which one of the following?

    A.  It is an intermediate of glycolysis.
    B.  It antagonizes phosphofructokinase-1.
    C.  It synthesizes phosphofructokinase-1.
    D.  It allosterically activates phosphofructokinase-1.
    E.  It catalyzes a reaction that produces NADH.

5.  Which one of the following statements best describes the activity of phosphofructokinase-1 in the presence of AMP, as compared to the absence of AMP?

    A.  The $K_m$ is increased, with a decreased $V_{max}$.
    B.  The $K_m$ is increased, with an increased $V_{max}$.
    C.  The $K_m$ is decreased, with no change in the $V_{max}$.
    D.  The $K_m$ is decreased, with a decreased $V_{max}$.
    E.  The $K_m$ is increased, with no change in the $V_{max}$.

# 20 Oxidation of Fatty Acids and Ketone Bodies

## CHAPTER OUTLINE

**I. FATTY ACIDS AS FUELS**
A. Characteristics of fatty acids used as fuels
B. Transport and activation of long-chain fatty acids
   1. Cellular uptake of long-chain fatty acids
   2. Activation of long-chain fatty acids
   3. Fates of fatty acyl coenzyme A's
   4. Transport of long-chain fatty acids into mitochondria
C. β-Oxidation of long-chain fatty acids
   1. The β-oxidation spiral
   2. Energy yield of β-oxidation
   3. Chain length specificity in β-oxidation
   4. Oxidation of unsaturated fatty acids
   5. Odd-chain-length fatty acids
D. Oxidation of medium-chain-length fatty acids
E. Regulation of β-oxidation

**II. ALTERNATIVE ROUTES OF FATTY ACID OXIDATION**
A. Peroxisomal oxidation of fatty acids
   1. Very long chain fatty acids
   2. Long-chain branched-chain fatty acids
B. ω-Oxidation of fatty acids

**III. METABOLISM OF KETONE BODIES**
A. Synthesis of ketone bodies
B. Oxidation of ketone bodies as fuels

**IV. THE ROLE OF FATTY ACIDS AND KETONE BODIES IN FUEL HOMEOSTASIS**
A. Preferential utilization of fatty acids
B. Tissues that use ketone bodies
C. Regulation of ketone body synthesis

## KEY POINTS

- Fatty acids are a major fuel for humans.
- During overnight fasting, fatty acids become the major fuel for cardiac muscle, skeletal muscle, and liver.
- The nervous system has a limited ability to use fatty acids as fuel. The liver converts fatty acids to ketone bodies, which can be used by the nervous system as a fuel during prolonged periods of fasting.
- Fatty acids are released from adipose tissue triacylglycerols under appropriate hormonal stimulation.
- In cells, fatty acids are activated to fatty acyl CoA derivatives by acyl CoA synthetases.
- Acyl CoAs are transported into the mitochondria for oxidation via carnitine.
- ATP is generated from fatty acids by the pathway of β-oxidation.
- In β-oxidation, the fatty acyl group is sequentially oxidized to yield FAD(2H), NADH, and acetyl CoA.
- Unsaturated and odd-chain-length fatty acids require additional reactions for their metabolism.
- β-Oxidation is regulated by the levels of FAD(2H), NADH, and acetyl CoA.
- The entry of fatty acids into mitochondria is regulated by malonyl CoA levels.
- Alternate pathways for very long chain and branched-chain fatty acid oxidation occur within peroxisomes.

# THE WAITING ROOM

**Otto S.** was disappointed that he did not place in his 5-km race and has decided that short-distance running is probably not right for him. After careful consideration, he decides to train for a marathon by running 12 miles three times per week. He is now 13 lb over his ideal weight, and he plans on losing this weight while studying for his pharmacology finals. He considers a variety of dietary supplements to increase his endurance and selects one that contains carnitine, Coenzyme Q (CoQ), pantothenate, riboflavin, and creatine.

**Lola B.** is a 16-year-old girl. Since age 14 months, she has experienced recurrent episodes of profound fatigue associated with vomiting and increased perspiration, which required hospitalization. These episodes occurred only if she fasted for more than 8 hours. Because her mother gave her food late at night and woke her early in the morning for breakfast, Lola's physical and mental development had progressed normally.

On the day of admission for this episode, Lola had missed breakfast, and by noon, she was extremely fatigued, nauseated, sweaty, and limp. She was unable to hold any food in her stomach and was rushed to the hospital, where an infusion of glucose was started intravenously. Her symptoms responded dramatically to this therapy.

Her initial serum glucose level was low at 38 mg/dL (reference range for fasting serum glucose levels = 70 to 100 mg/dL). Her blood urea nitrogen (BUN) level was slightly elevated at 26 mg/dL (reference range = 8 to 25 mg/dL) because of vomiting, which led to a degree of dehydration. Her blood levels of liver transaminases were slightly elevated, although her liver was not palpably enlarged. Despite elevated levels of free fatty acids (4.3 mM) in the blood, blood ketone bodies were below normal.

**Dianne A.**, a 27-year-old female with type 1 diabetes mellitus, had been admitted to the hospital in a ketoacidotic coma a year ago (see Chapter 2). She had been feeling drowsy and had been vomiting for 24 hours before that admission. At the time of admission, she was clinically dehydrated, her blood pressure was low, and her breathing was deep and rapid (Kussmaul breathing). Her pulse was rapid, and her breath had the odor of acetone. Her arterial blood pH was 7.08 (reference range = 7.36 to 7.44), and her blood ketone body levels were 15 mM (normal is approximately 0.2 mM for a person on a normal diet).

## I.  FATTY ACIDS AS FUELS

The **fatty acids** oxidized as fuels are principally **long-chain fatty acids** released from adipose tissue triacylglycerol stores between meals, during overnight fasting, and during periods of increased fuel demand (e.g., during exercise). Adipose tissue triacylglycerols are derived from two sources: dietary lipids and triacylglycerols synthesized in the liver. The major fatty acids oxidized are the long-chain fatty acids, palmitate, oleate, and stearate because they are highest in concentration in dietary lipids and are also synthesized in the human.

Between meals, a decreased insulin level and increased levels of insulin counterregulatory hormones (e.g., glucagon) activate lipolysis and free fatty acids are transported to tissues bound to serum albumin. Within tissues, energy is derived from oxidation of fatty acids to acetyl CoA in the pathway of **β-oxidation**. Most of the enzymes involved in fatty acid oxidation are present as two or three isoenzymes,

The liver transaminases measured in the blood are aspartate aminotransferase (AST), which was formerly called serum glutamate-oxaloacetate transaminase (SGOT), and alanine aminotransferase (ALT), which was formerly called serum glutamate pyruvate transaminase (SGPT). Elevation of liver enzymes reflects damage to the liver plasma membrane.

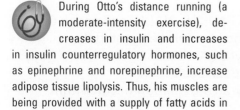

During Otto's distance running (a moderate-intensity exercise), decreases in insulin and increases in insulin counterregulatory hormones, such as epinephrine and norepinephrine, increase adipose tissue lipolysis. Thus, his muscles are being provided with a supply of fatty acids in the blood that they can use as a fuel.

which have different but overlapping specificities for the chain length of the fatty acid. Metabolism of **unsaturated fatty acids**, **odd-chain-length fatty acids**, and **medium-chain-length fatty acids** requires variations of this basic pattern. The **acetyl CoA** produced from fatty acid oxidation is principally oxidized in the tricarboxylic acid (TCA) cycle or converted to **ketone bodies** in the liver.

## A. Characteristics of Fatty Acids Used as Fuels

Fat constitutes approximately 38% of the calories in the average North American diet. Of this, more than 95% of the calories are present as **triacylglycerols** (three fatty acids esterified to a glycerol backbone). During ingestion and absorption, dietary triacylglycerols are broken down into their constituents and then reassembled for transport to adipose tissue in chylomicrons (see Chapter 1). Thus, the fatty acid composition of adipose triacylglycerols varies with the type of food consumed.

The most common dietary fatty acids are the saturated long-chain fatty acids palmitate (C16) and stearate (C18), the monounsaturated fatty acid oleate (C18:1), and the polyunsaturated essential fatty acid, linoleate (C18:2). (To review fatty acid nomenclature, consult Chapter 3.) Animal fat contains principally saturated and monounsaturated long-chain fatty acids, whereas vegetable oils contain linoleate and some longer chain and polyunsaturated fatty acids. They also contain smaller amounts of branched-chain and odd-chain-length fatty acids. Medium-chain-length fatty acids are present principally in dairy fat (e.g., milk, butter), maternal milk, and vegetable oils.

Adipose tissue triacylglycerols also contain fatty acids synthesized in the liver, principally from excess calories ingested as glucose. The pathway of fatty acid synthesis generates palmitate, which can be elongated to form stearate, and unsaturated to form oleate. These fatty acids are assembled into triacylglycerols and transported to adipose tissues as the lipoprotein very low density lipoprotein (VLDL).

## B. Transport and Activation of Long-Chain Fatty Acids

Long-chain fatty acids are hydrophobic and, therefore, water insoluble. In addition, they are toxic to cells because they can disrupt the hydrophobic bonding between amino acid side chains in proteins. Consequently, they are transported in the blood and in cells bound to proteins.

### 1. CELLULAR UPTAKE OF LONG-CHAIN FATTY ACIDS

During fasting and other conditions of metabolic need, long-chain fatty acids are released from adipose tissue triacylglycerols by lipases. They travel in the blood bound in the hydrophobic binding pocket of albumin, the major serum protein.

Fatty acids enter cells both by a saturable transport process and by diffusion through the lipid plasma membrane. A fatty acid–binding protein in the plasma membrane facilitates transport. An additional fatty acid–binding protein binds the fatty acid intracellularly and may facilitate its transport to the mitochondrion. The free fatty acid concentration in cells is, therefore, extremely low.

### 2. ACTIVATION OF LONG-CHAIN FATTY ACIDS

Fatty acids must be activated to acyl CoA derivatives before they can participate in β-oxidation and other metabolic pathways (Fig. 20.1). The process of activation involves an acyl CoA synthetase (also called a thiokinase) that uses ATP energy to form the fatty acyl CoA thioester bond. In this reaction, the β-bond of ATP is cleaved to form a fatty acyl adenosine monophosphate (AMP) intermediate and pyrophosphate (PPi). Subsequent cleavage of PPi helps to drive the reaction.

The acyl CoA synthetase that activates long-chain fatty acids, 12 to 20 carbons in length, is present in three locations in the cell: the endoplasmic reticulum, outer mitochondrial membranes, and peroxisomal membranes (Table 20.1). This enzyme has no activity toward C22 or longer fatty acids and little activity below C12. In contrast, the synthetase for activation of very long chain fatty acids is present in

**Lola B.** developed symptoms during fasting, when adipose tissue lipolysis was elevated. Under these circumstances, muscle tissue, liver, and many other tissues are oxidizing fatty acids as a fuel. After overnight fasting, approximately 60% to 70% of our energy supply is derived from the oxidation of fatty acids.

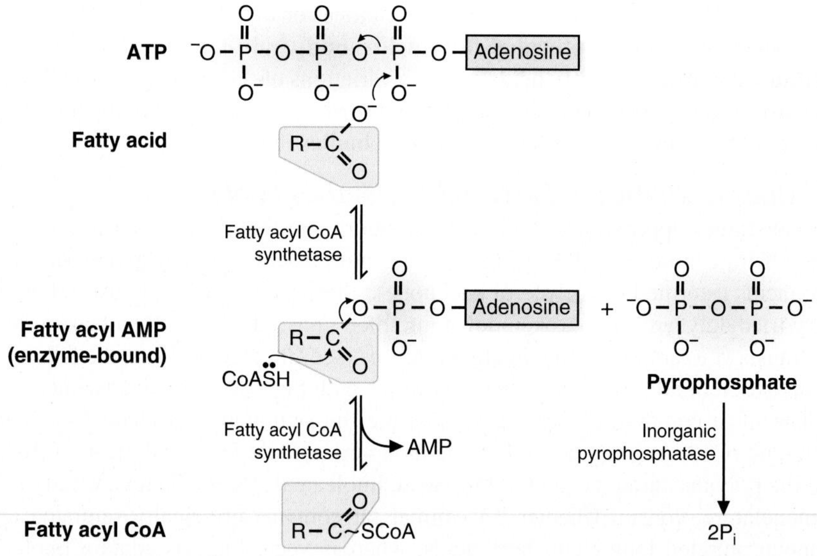

**FIG. 20.1.** Activation of a fatty acid by a fatty acyl CoA synthetase. The fatty acid is activated by reacting with ATP to form a high-energy fatty acyl AMP and PPi. The AMP is then exchanged for CoA. PPi is cleaved by a pyrophosphatase.

**Table 20.1   Chain Length Specificity of Fatty Acid Activation and Oxidation Enzymes**

| Enzyme | Chain Length | Comments |
|---|---|---|
| *Acyl CoA synthetases* | | |
| Very long chain | 14–26 | Found only in peroxisomes |
| Long chain | 12–20 | Enzyme present in membranes of endoplasmic reticulum, mitochondria, and peroxisomes to facilitate different metabolic routes of acyl CoAs. |
| Medium chain | 6–12 | Exists as many variants, present only in mitochondrial matrix of kidney and liver. Also involved in xenobiotic metabolism. |
| Acetyl | 2–4 | Present in cytoplasm and possibly mitochondrial matrix. |
| *Acyltransferases* | | |
| CPTI | 12–16 | Although maximum activity is for fatty acids 12–16 carbons long, it also acts on many smaller acyl CoA derivatives. |
| Medium chain (octanoyl-carnitine transferase) | 6–12 | Substrate is medium-chain acyl CoA derivatives generated during peroxisomal oxidation. |
| Carnitine acetyltransferase | 2 | High level in skeletal muscle and heart to facilitate use of acetate as a fuel. |
| *Acyl CoA dehydrogenases* | | |
| VLCAD | 14–20 | Present in inner mitochondrial membrane. |
| LCAD | 12–18 | Members of same enzyme family, which also includes acyl CoA dehydrogenases for carbon skeleton of branched-chain amino acids. |
| MCAD | 4–12 | — |
| SCAD | 4–6 | — |
| *Other enzymes* | | |
| Enoyl CoA hydratase, short chain | >4 | Also called crotonase. Activity decreases with increasing chain length. |
| L-3-Hydroxyacyl CoA dehydrogenase, short chain | 4–16 | Activity decreases with increasing chain length |
| Acetoacetyl CoA thiolase | 4 | Specific for acetoacetyl CoA |
| Trifunctional protein | 12–16 | Complex of long-chain enoyl hydratase, acyl CoA dehydrogenase and a thiolase with broad specificity. Most active with longer chains. |

CPTI, carnitine palmitoyl transferase I; VLCAD, very long chain acyl CoA dehydrogenase; LCAD, long-chain acyl CoA dehydrogenase; MCAD, medium-chain acyl CoA dehydrogenase; SCAD, short-chain acyl CoA dehydrogenase.

peroxisomes, and the medium-chain-length fatty acid–activating enzyme is present only in the mitochondrial matrix of liver and kidney cells.

## 3. FATES OF FATTY ACYL COENZYME A'S

Fatty acyl CoA formation, like the phosphorylation of glucose, is a prerequisite to metabolism of the fatty acid in the cell. The multiple locations of the long-chain acyl CoA synthetase reflect the location of different metabolic routes taken by fatty acyl CoA derivatives in the cell (e.g., triacylglycerol and phospholipid synthesis in the endoplasmic reticulum, oxidation and plasmalogen synthesis in the peroxisome, and β-oxidation in mitochondria). In the liver and some other tissues, fatty acids that are not being used for energy generation are reincorporated (reesterified) into triacylglycerols.

## 4. TRANSPORT OF LONG-CHAIN FATTY ACIDS INTO MITOCHONDRIA

**Carnitine** serves as the carrier that transports activated long-chain fatty acyl groups across the inner mitochondrial membrane (Fig. 20.2). Carnitine acyltransferases are able to reversibly transfer an activated fatty acyl group from CoA to the hydroxyl group of carnitine to form an acylcarnitine ester. The reaction is reversible, so that the fatty acyl CoA derivative can be regenerated from the carnitine ester.

Carnitine palmitoyltransferase I (CPTI; also called carnitine acyltransferase I, CATI), the enzyme that transfers long-chain fatty acyl groups from CoA to carnitine, is located on the outer mitochondrial membrane (Fig. 20.3). Fatty acylcarnitine crosses the inner mitochondrial membrane with the aid of a translocase. The fatty acyl group is transferred back to CoA by a second enzyme, carnitine palmitoyl transferase II (CPTII or CATII). The carnitine released in this reaction returns to the cytosolic side of the mitochondrial membrane by the same translocase that brings

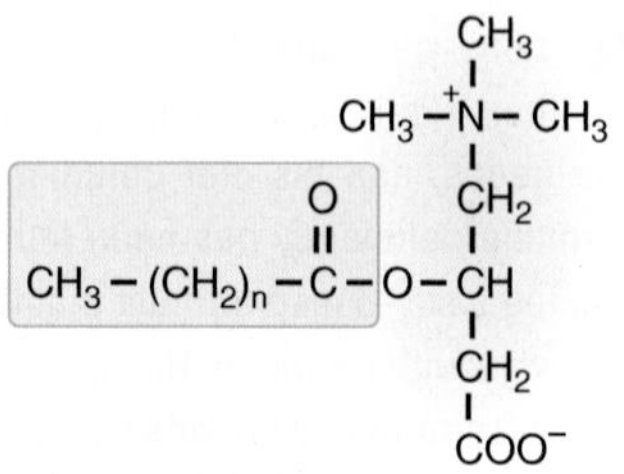

**Fatty acylcarnitine**

**FIG. 20.2.** Structure of fatty acylcarnitine. Carnitine palmitoyltransferases catalyze the reversible transfer of a long-chain fatty acyl group from the fatty acyl CoA to the hydroxyl group of carnitine. The atoms in the *green box* originate from the fatty acyl CoA.

Several inherited diseases in the metabolism of carnitine or acylcarnitines have been described. These include defects in the following enzymes or systems: the transporter for carnitine uptake into muscle, CPTI, carnitine-acylcarnitine translocase, and CPTII. Classical CPTII deficiency, the most common of these diseases, is characterized by adolescent to adult onset of recurrent episodes of acute myoglobinuria precipitated by prolonged exercise or fasting. During these episodes, the patient is weak and may be somewhat hypoglycemic with diminished ketosis (hypoketosis), but metabolic decompensation is not severe. Lipid deposits are found in skeletal muscles. Both creatine phosphokinase (CPK) and long-chain acylcarnitines are elevated in the blood. The activity of CPTII in fibroblasts is approximately 25% of normal. The residual CPTII activity probably accounts for the mild effect on liver metabolism. In contrast, when CPTII deficiency presents in infants, CPTII levels are less than 10% of normal, the hypoglycemia and hypoketosis are severe, hepatomegaly occurs from the triacylglycerol deposits, and cardiomyopathy is also present.

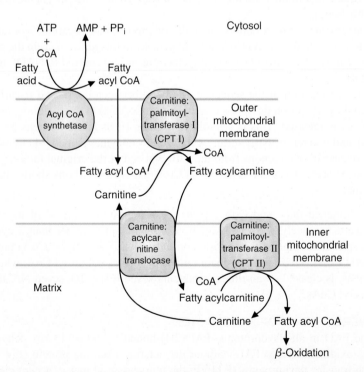

**FIG. 20.3.** Transport of long-chain fatty acids into mitochondria. The fatty acyl CoA crosses the outer mitochondrial membrane. CPTI in the outer mitochondrial membrane transfers the fatty acyl group to carnitine and releases CoASH. The fatty acyl carnitine is translocated into the mitochondrial matrix as carnitine moves out. CPTII on the inner mitochondrial membrane transfers the fatty acyl group back to CoASH to form fatty acyl CoA in the matrix.

**Otto S.'s** power supplement contains carnitine. However, his body can synthesize enough carnitine to meet his needs, and his diet contains carnitine. Carnitine deficiency has been found only in infants fed a soy-based formula that was not supplemented with carnitine. His other supplements likewise probably provide no benefit but are designed to facilitate fatty acid oxidation during exercise. Riboflavin is the vitamin precursor of FAD, which is required for acyl CoA dehydrogenases and ETFs. CoQ is synthesized in the body, but it is the recipient in the electron transport chain for electrons passed from complexes I and II and the ETFs. Some reports suggest that supplementation with pantothenate, the precursor of CoA, improves performance.

fatty acylcarnitine to the matrix side. Long-chain fatty acyl CoA, now located within the mitochondrial matrix, is a substrate for β-oxidation.

Carnitine is obtained from the diet or synthesized from the side chain of lysine by a pathway that begins in skeletal muscle and is completed in the liver. The reactions use S-adenosylmethionine to donate methyl groups, and vitamin C (ascorbic acid) is also required for these reactions. Skeletal muscles have a high-affinity uptake system for carnitine, and most of the carnitine in the body is stored in skeletal muscle.

### C. β-Oxidation of Long-Chain Fatty Acids

The oxidation of fatty acids to acetyl CoA in the β-oxidation spiral conserves energy as FAD(2H) and NADH. FAD(2H) and NADH are oxidized in the electron transport chain, generating ATP from oxidative phosphorylation. Acetyl CoA is oxidized in the TCA cycle or converted to ketone bodies.

#### 1. THE β-OXIDATION SPIRAL

The fatty acid β-oxidation pathway sequentially cleaves the fatty acyl group into two-carbon acetyl CoA units, beginning with the carboxyl end attached to CoA. Before cleavage, the β-carbon is oxidized to a keto group in two reactions that generate NADH and FAD(2H); thus, the pathway is called β-oxidation. As each acetyl group is released, the cycle of β-oxidation and cleavage begins again, but each time the fatty acyl group is two carbons shorter.

The β-oxidation pathway consists of four separate steps or reactions (Fig. 20.4):

1. In the first step, a double bond is formed between the β- and α-carbons by an acyl CoA dehydrogenase that transfers electrons to FAD. The double bond is in the *trans* configuration (a $\Delta^2$-*trans* double bond).
2. In the next step, an –OH from water is added to the β-carbon, and an –H from water is added to the α-carbon. The enzyme for this reaction is called an **enoyl hydratase** (hydratases add the elements of water, and "-ene" in a name denotes a double bond).
3. In the third step of β-oxidation, the hydroxyl group on the β-carbon is oxidized to a ketone by a hydroxyacyl CoA dehydrogenase. In this reaction, as in the conversion of most alcohols to ketones, the electrons are transferred to $NAD^+$ to form NADH.
4. In the last reaction of the sequence, the bond between the β- and α-carbons is cleaved by a reaction that links Coenzyme A (CoASH) to the β-carbon, and acetyl CoA is released. This is a thiolytic reaction (lysis refers to breakage of the bond, and thio refers to the sulfur), catalyzed by enzymes named β-ketothiolases. The release of two carbons from the carboxyl end of the original fatty acyl CoA produces acetyl CoA and a fatty acyl CoA that is two carbons shorter than the original.

The β-oxidation spiral uses the same reactions that occur in the TCA cycle when succinate is converted to oxaloacetate; only the enzymes of the reactions are different.

The shortened fatty acyl CoA repeats these four steps until all of its carbons are converted to acetyl CoA. β-Oxidation is thus a spiral rather than a cycle. In the last spiral, cleavage of the four-carbon fatty acyl CoA (butyryl CoA) produces two acetyl CoAs. Thus, an even-chain fatty acid such as palmitoyl CoA, which has 16 carbons, is cleaved seven times, producing seven FAD(2H), seven NADH, and eight acetyl CoAs.

#### 2. ENERGY YIELD OF β-OXIDATION

Like the FAD in all flavoproteins, FAD(2H) bound to the acyl CoA dehydrogenases is oxidized back to FAD without dissociating from the protein (Fig. 20.5). Electron-transfer flavoproteins (ETF) in the mitochondrial matrix accept electrons from the enzyme-bound FAD(2H) and transfer these electrons to the electron transfer flavoprotein–CoQ oxidoreductase (ETF-QO) in the inner mitochondrial membrane. ETF-QO, also a flavoprotein, transfers the electrons to CoQ in the electron transport

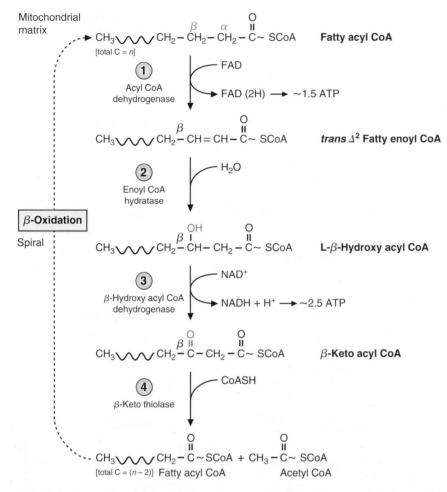

*FIG. 20.4.* Steps of β-oxidation. The four steps are repeated until an even-chain fatty acid is completely converted to acetyl CoA. The FAD(2H) and NADH are reoxidized by the electron transport chain, producing ATP.

*FIG. 20.5.* Transfer of electrons from acyl CoA dehydrogenase to the electron transport chain. An FAD is tightly bound to each protein in these three-electron transfer reactions. *ETF,* electron-transferring flavoprotein; *ETF-QO,* electron-transferring flavoprotein–Coenzyme Q oxidoreductase.

chain. Oxidative phosphorylation thus generates approximately 1.5 ATP for each FAD(2H) produced in the β-oxidation spiral.

The total energy yield from the oxidation of 1 mole of palmityl CoA to 8 moles of acetyl CoA is therefore 28 moles of ATP: 1.5 for each of the 7 FAD(2H), and 2.5 for each of the 7 NADH. To calculate the energy yield from oxidation of 1 mole of palmitate, 2 ATP need to be subtracted from the total because 2 high-energy phosphate bonds are cleaved when palmitate is activated to palmityl CoA.

### 3. CHAIN LENGTH SPECIFICITY IN β-OXIDATION

The four reactions of β-oxidation are catalyzed by sets of enzymes that are each specific for fatty acids with different chain lengths (see Table 20.1). The acyl CoA dehydrogenases, which catalyze the first step of the pathway, are part of an enzyme family that has four different ranges of specificity. The subsequent steps of the spiral use enzymes specific for long- or short-chain enoyl CoAs. Although these enzymes are structurally distinct, their specificities overlap to some extent. As the fatty acyl chains are shortened by consecutive cleavage of two acetyl units, they are transferred from enzymes that act on longer chains to those that act on shorter chains. Medium- or short-chain fatty acyl CoA that may be formed from dietary fatty acids or transferred from peroxisomes enters the spiral at the enzyme most active for fatty acids of its chain length.

**Q:** What is the total ATP yield for the oxidation of 1 mole of palmitic acid to carbon dioxide and water?

**A:** Palmitic acid is 16-carbons long with no double bonds, so it requires seven oxidation spirals to be completely converted to acetyl CoA. After 7 spirals, there are 7 FAD(2H)s, 7 NADHs, and 8 acetyl CoAs. Each NADH yields 2.5 ATP, each FAD(2H) yields 1.5 ATP, and each acetyl CoA yields 10 ATP as it is processed around the TCA cycle. This then yields 17.5 + 10.5 + 80.5 = 108 ATP. However, activation of palmitic acid to palmityl CoA requires two high-energy bonds, so the net yield is 108 − 2 or 106 moles of ATP per mole of palmitate oxidized completely to carbon dioxide and water.

After reviewing **Lola B.'s** previous hospital records, a specialist suspected that Lola's medical problems were caused by a disorder in fatty acid metabolism. A battery of tests showed that Lola's blood contained elevated levels of several partially oxidized medium-chain fatty acids, such as octanoic acid (8:0) and 4-decenoic acid (10:1, $\Delta^4$). A urine specimen showed an increase in organic acid metabolites of medium-chain fatty acids containing 6 to 10 carbons, including medium-chain acylcarnitine derivatives. The profile of acylcarnitine species in the urine was characteristic of a genetically determined MCAD deficiency. In this disease, long-chain fatty acids are metabolized by β-oxidation to a medium-chain-length acyl CoA such as octanoyl CoA. Because further oxidation of this compound is blocked in MCAD deficiency, the medium-chain acyl group is transferred back to carnitine. These acylcarnitines are water soluble and appear in blood and urine. The specific enzyme deficiency was demonstrated in cultured fibroblasts from Lola's skin as well as in her circulating monocytic leukocytes.

In LCAD deficiency, fatty acylcarnitines accumulate in the blood. Those containing 14 carbons predominate. However, these do not appear in the urine.

Linoleate is obtained from the diet and cannot be synthesized by the human; thus, it is considered an essential fatty acid (along with linolenic acid, *cis* $\Delta^{9,12,15}$ C18:3). Therefore, only that portion of linoleate that is not needed for other processes will undergo β-oxidation.

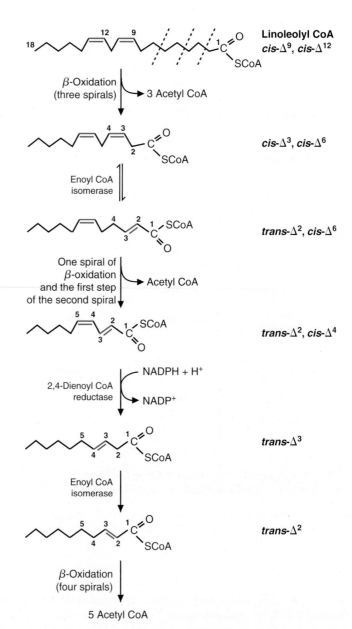

**FIG. 20.6.** Oxidation of linoleate. After three spirals of β-oxidation *(dashed lines)*, there is now a 3,4-*cis* double bond and a 6,7-*cis* double bond. The 3,4-*cis* double bond is isomerized to a 2,3-*trans* double bond, which is in the proper configuration for the normal enzymes to act. One spiral of β-oxidation occurs, plus the first step of a second spiral. A reductase that uses NADPH now converts these two double bonds (between carbons 2 and 3 and carbons 4 and 5) to one double bond between carbons 3 and 4 in a *trans* configuration. The isomerase (which can act on double bonds that are in either the *cis* or the *trans* configuration) moves this double bond to the 2,3-*trans* position, and β-oxidation can resume.

## 4. OXIDATION OF UNSATURATED FATTY ACIDS

Approximately one-half of the fatty acids in the human diet are unsaturated, containing *cis* double bonds, with oleate (C18:1,$\Delta^9$) and linoleate (18:2,$\Delta^{9,12}$) being the most common. In β-oxidation of saturated fatty acids, a *trans* double bond is created between the second and third ($\alpha$ and $\beta$) carbons. For unsaturated fatty acids to undergo the β-oxidation spiral, their *cis* double bonds must be isomerized to *trans* double bonds that will end up between the second and third carbons during β-oxidation, or the double bond must be reduced. The process is illustrated for the polyunsaturated fatty acid linoleate in Figure 20.6. Linoleate undergoes β-oxidation until one double bond is between carbons 3 and 4 near the carboxyl end of the fatty acyl chain, and the other is between carbons 6 and 7. An isomerase moves the double bond from the 3,4 position so that it is *trans* and in the 2,3 position and β-oxidation continues. When a conjugated pair of double bonds is formed (two double bonds separated by one single bond) at positions 2 and 4, an NADPH-dependent reductase reduces the pair to one *trans* double bond at position 3. Then, isomerization and β-oxidation resume.

In oleate (C18:1,$\Delta^9$), there is only one double bond between carbons 9 and 10. It is handled by an isomerization reaction similar to that shown for the double bond at position 9 of linoleate.

## 5. ODD-CHAIN-LENGTH FATTY ACIDS

Fatty acids containing an odd number of carbon atoms undergo β-oxidation, producing acetyl CoA, until the last spiral, when five carbons remain in the fatty acyl CoA. In this case, cleavage by thiolase produces acetyl CoA and a three-carbon fatty acyl CoA, propionyl CoA. Carboxylation of propionyl CoA yields methylmalonyl CoA, which is ultimately converted to succinyl CoA in a vitamin $B_{12}$–dependent reaction (Fig. 20.7). Propionyl CoA also arises from the oxidation of branched-chain amino acids.

The propionyl CoA to succinyl CoA pathway is a major anaplerotic route for the TCA cycle and is used in the degradation of valine, isoleucine, and several other compounds. In the liver, this route provides precursors of oxaloacetate, which is converted to glucose. Thus, this small proportion of the odd-carbon-number fatty acid chain can be converted to glucose. In contrast, the acetyl CoA formed from β-oxidation of even-chain-number fatty acids in the liver either enters the TCA cycle, where it is principally oxidized to $CO_2$ or is converted to ketone bodies.

## D. Oxidation of Medium-Chain-Length Fatty Acids

Dietary medium-chain-length fatty acids are more water soluble than long-chain fatty acids and are not stored in adipose triacylglycerol. After a meal, they enter the blood and pass into the portal vein to the liver. In the liver, they enter the mitochondrial matrix by the monocarboxylate transporter and are activated to acyl CoA derivatives in the mitochondrial matrix. Medium-chain-length acyl CoAs, such as long-chain acyl CoAs, are oxidized to acetyl CoA via the β-oxidation spiral. Medium-chain acyl CoAs also can arise from the peroxisomal oxidation pathway.

## E. Regulation of β-Oxidation

Fatty acids are used as fuels principally when they are released from adipose tissue triacylglycerols in response to hormones that signal fasting or increased demand. Many tissues, such as muscle and kidney, oxidize fatty acids completely to $CO_2$ and $H_2O$. In these tissues, the acetyl CoA produced by β-oxidation enters the TCA cycle. The FAD(2H) and the NADH from β-oxidation and the TCA cycle are reoxidized by the electron transport chain, and ATP is generated. The process of β-oxidation is regulated by the cells' requirements for energy (i.e., by the levels of ATP and NADH) because fatty acids cannot be oxidized any faster than NADH and FAD(2H) are reoxidized in the electron transport chain.

Fatty acid oxidation may also be restricted by the mitochondrial CoASH pool size. Acetyl CoASH units must enter the TCA cycle or another metabolic pathway to regenerate CoASH required for formation of the fatty acyl CoA derivative from fatty acylcarnitine.

An additional type of regulation occurs at CPTI. CPTI is inhibited by malonyl CoA, which is synthesized in the cytosol of many tissues by acetyl CoA carboxylase (Fig. 20.8). Acetyl CoA carboxylase is regulated by several different mechanisms, some of which are tissue dependent. In skeletal muscles and liver, it is inhibited when phosphorylated by the AMP-activated protein kinase (AMP-PK). Thus, during

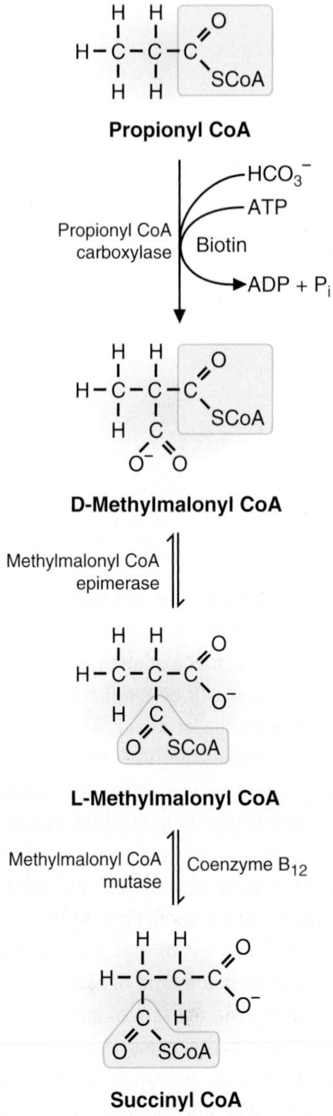

**Propionyl CoA**

Propionyl CoA carboxylase   HCO$_3^-$   ATP   Biotin   ADP + P$_i$

**D-Methylmalonyl CoA**

Methylmalonyl CoA epimerase

**L-Methylmalonyl CoA**

Methylmalonyl CoA mutase   Coenzyme B$_{12}$

**Succinyl CoA**

**FIG. 20.7.** Conversion of propionyl CoA to succinyl CoA. Succinyl CoA, an intermediate of the TCA cycle, can form malate, which can be converted to glucose in the liver through the process of gluconeogenesis. Certain amino acids also form glucose by this route (see Chapter 32).

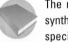

The medium-chain-length acyl CoA synthetase has a broad range of specificity and will activate to a CoA derivative a variety of metabolites. Once a metabolite CoA is formed, the carboxyl group is frequently conjugated with glycine to form a urinary excretion product. With certain disorders of fatty acid oxidation, medium- and short-chain fatty acylglycines may appear in the urine together with acylcarnitine or dicarboxylic acids. Octanoylglycine, for example, will appear in the urine of a patient with MCAD deficiency.

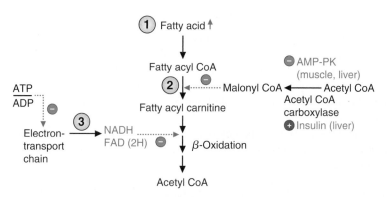

*FIG. 20.8.* Regulation of β-oxidation. *(1)* Hormones control the supply of fatty acids in the blood. *(2)* CPTI is inhibited by malonyl CoA, which is synthesized by acetyl CoA carboxylase (ACC). AMP-PK is the AMP-activated protein kinase. *(3)* The rate of ATP use controls the rate of the electron transport chain, which regulates the oxidative enzymes of β-oxidation and the TCA cycle.

As **Otto S.** runs, his skeletal muscles increase their use of ATP and their rate of fuel oxidation. Fatty acid oxidation is accelerated by the increased rate of the electron transport chain. As ATP is used and AMP increases, an AMP-PK acts to facilitate fuel utilization and maintain ATP homeostasis. Phosphorylation of acetyl CoA carboxylase results in a decreased level of malonyl CoA and increased activity of carnitine palmitoyl CoA transferase I. At the same time, AMP-PK facilitates the recruitment of glucose transporters into the plasma membrane of skeletal muscle, thereby increasing the rate of glucose uptake. AMP and hormonal signals also increase the supply of glucose 6-P from glycogenolysis. Thus, his muscles are supplied with more fuel, and all the oxidative pathways are accelerated.

exercise, when AMP levels increase, AMP-PK is activated and phosphorylates acetyl CoA carboxylase, which becomes inactive. Consequently, malonyl CoA levels decrease, CPTI is activated, and the β-oxidation of fatty acids is able to restore ATP homeostasis and decrease AMP levels. In liver, in addition to the regulation by the AMP-PK, acetyl CoA carboxylase is activated by insulin-dependent mechanisms leading to elevated citrate, an allosteric activator, which promotes the conversion of malonyl CoA to palmitate in the fatty acid synthesis pathway. Thus, in the liver, malonyl CoA inhibition of CPTI prevents newly synthesized fatty acids from being oxidized.

β-Oxidation is strictly an aerobic pathway, dependent on oxygen, a good blood supply, and adequate levels of mitochondria. Tissues that lack mitochondria, such as red blood cells, cannot oxidize fatty acids by β-oxidation. Fatty acids also do not serve as a significant fuel for the brain. They are not used by adipocytes, whose function is to store triacylglycerols to provide a fuel for other tissues. Those tissues that do not use fatty acids as a fuel, or use them only to a limited extent, use ketone bodies instead.

## II. ALTERNATIVE ROUTES OF FATTY ACID OXIDATION

Fatty acids that are not readily oxidized by the enzymes of β-oxidation enter alternative pathways of oxidation, including peroxisomal β- and α-oxidation and microsomal ω-oxidation. The function of these pathways is to convert as much as possible of the unusual fatty acids to compounds that can be used as fuels or biosynthetic precursors and to convert the remainder to compounds that can be excreted in bile or urine. During prolonged fasting, fatty acids released from adipose triacylglycerols may enter the ω-oxidation or peroxisomal β-oxidation pathway, even though they have a normal composition. These pathways not only use fatty acids, they act on xenobiotic (a term used to cover all organic compounds that are foreign to an organism) carboxylic acids that are large hydrophobic molecules resembling fatty acids.

### A. Peroxisomal Oxidation of Fatty Acids

A small proportion of our diet consists of very long chain fatty acids (20 or more carbons) or branched-chain fatty acids arising from degradative products of chlorophyll. Very long chain fatty acid synthesis also occurs within the body, especially in cells of the brain and nervous system, which incorporate them into the sphingolipids of myelin. These fatty acids are oxidized by **peroxisomal β- and α-oxidation pathways**, which are essentially chain-shortening pathways.

## 1. VERY LONG CHAIN FATTY ACIDS

Very long chain fatty acids of 24 to 26 carbons are oxidized exclusively in peroxisomes by a sequence of reactions similar to mitochondrial β-oxidation in that they generate acetyl CoA and NADH. However, the peroxisomal oxidation of straight-chain fatty acids stops when the chain reaches four to six carbons in length. Some of the long-chain fatty acids also may be oxidized by this route.

The long-chain fatty acyl CoA synthetase is present in the peroxisomal membrane, and the acyl CoA derivatives enter the peroxisome by a transporter that does not require carnitine. The first enzyme of peroxisomal β-oxidation is an oxidase, which donates electrons directly to molecular oxygen and produces hydrogen peroxide ($H_2O_2$) (Fig. 20.9). (In contrast, the first enzyme of mitochondrial β-oxidation is a dehydrogenase that contains FAD and transfers the electrons to the electron transport chain via ETF.) Thus, the first enzyme of peroxisomal oxidation is not linked to energy production. The three remaining steps of β-oxidation are catalyzed by enoyl CoA hydratase, hydroxyacyl CoA dehydrogenase, and thiolase, enzymes with activities similar to those found in mitochondrial β-oxidation but encoded by different genes. Thus, one NADH and one acetyl CoA are generated for each turn of the spiral. The peroxisomal β-oxidation spiral continues generating acetyl CoA until a medium-chain acyl CoA, which may be as short as butyryl CoA, is produced.

Within the peroxisome, the acetyl groups can be transferred from CoA to carnitine by an acetylcarnitine transferase, or they can enter the cytosol. A similar reaction converts medium-chain-length acyl CoAs and the short-chain butyryl CoA to acylcarnitine derivatives. These acylcarnitines diffuse from the peroxisome to the mitochondria, pass through the outer mitochondrial membrane, and are transported through the inner mitochondrial membrane via the carnitine translocase system. They are converted back to acyl CoAs by carnitine acyltransferases appropriate for their chain length and enter the normal pathways for β-oxidation and acetyl CoA metabolism. The electrons from NADH and acetyl CoA can also pass from the peroxisome to the cytosol. The export of NADH-containing electrons occurs through use of a shuttle system similar to those described for NADH electron transfer into the mitochondria.

## 2. LONG-CHAIN BRANCHED-CHAIN FATTY ACIDS

Two of the most common branched-chain fatty acids in the diet are phytanic acid and pristanic acid, which are degradation products of chlorophyll and thus are consumed in green vegetables (Fig. 20.10). Animals do not synthesize branched-chain fatty acids. These two multimethylated fatty acids are oxidized in peroxisomes to the level of a branched C8 fatty acid, which is then transferred to mitochondria. The pathway is therefore similar to that for the oxidation of straight very long chain fatty acids.

Phytanic acid, a multimethylated C20 fatty acid, is first oxidized to pristanic acid using the α-oxidation pathway (see Fig. 20.10). Phytanic acid hydroxylase introduces a hydroxyl group on the α-carbon, which is then oxidized to a carboxyl group with release of the original carboxyl group as $CO_2$. By shortening the fatty acid by one carbon, the methyl groups will appear on the α-carbon rather than the β-carbon during the β-oxidation spiral and can no longer interfere with oxidation of the β-carbon. Peroxisomal β-oxidation thus can proceed normally, releasing propionyl CoA and acetyl CoA with alternate turns of the spiral. When a medium-chain-length of approximately eight carbons is reached, the fatty acid is transferred to the mitochondrion as a carnitine derivative, and β-oxidation is resumed.

## B. ω-Oxidation of Fatty Acids

Fatty acids may also be oxidized at the ω-carbon of the chain (the terminal methyl group) by enzymes in the endoplasmic reticulum (Fig. 20.11). The ω-methyl group is first oxidized to an alcohol by an enzyme that uses cytochrome P450, molecular

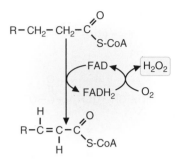

**FIG. 20.9.** Oxidation of fatty acids in peroxisomes. The first step of β-oxidation is catalyzed by an FAD-containing oxidase. The electrons are transferred from FAD(2H) to $O_2$, which is reduced to $H_2O_2$.

 Several inherited deficiencies of peroxisomal enzymes have been described. Zellweger syndrome, which results from defective peroxisomal biogenesis, leads to complex developmental and metabolic phenotypes that affect, principally, the liver and the brain. One of the metabolic characteristics of these diseases is an elevation of C26:0 and C26:1 fatty acid levels in plasma. Refsum disease is caused by a deficiency in a single peroxisomal enzyme, the phytanoyl CoA hydroxylase that carries out α-oxidation of phytanic acid. Symptoms include retinitis pigmentosa, cerebellar ataxia, and chronic polyneuropathy. Because phytanic acid is obtained solely from the diet, placing patients on a low-phytanic acid diet has resulted in marked improvement.

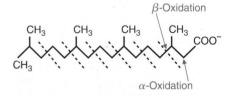

**FIG. 20.10.** Oxidation of phytanic acid. A peroxisomal α-hydroxylase oxidizes the α-carbon, and its subsequent oxidation to a carboxyl group releases the carboxyl carbon as $CO_2$. Subsequent spirals of peroxisomal β-oxidation alternately release propionyl and acetyl CoA. At a chain length of approximately eight carbons, the remaining branched fatty acid is transferred to mitochondria as a medium-chain carnitine derivative.

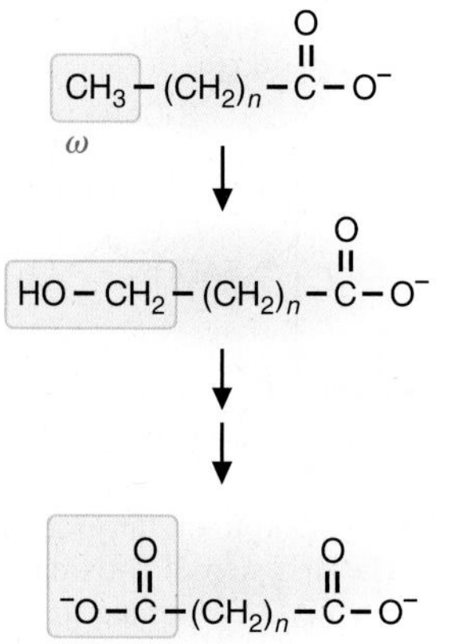

FIG. 20.11. ω-Oxidation of fatty acids converts them to dicarboxylic acids.

Normally, ω-oxidation is a minor process. However, in conditions that interfere with β-oxidation (such as carnitine deficiency or deficiency in an enzyme of β-oxidation), ω-oxidation produces dicarboxylic acids in increased amounts. These dicarboxylic acids are excreted in the urine.

**Lola B.** was excreting dicarboxylic acids in her urine, particularly, adipic acid (which has six carbons) and suberic acid (which has eight carbons).

$$—OOC—CH_2—CH_2—CH_2—CH_2—COO—$$
Adipic acid

$$—OOC—CH_2—CH_2—CH_2—CH_2—CH_2—CH_2—COO—$$
Suberic acid

Octanoylglycine was also found in the urine.

oxygen, and NADPH. Dehydrogenases convert the alcohol group to a carboxylic acid. The dicarboxylic acids produced by ω-oxidation can undergo β-oxidation, forming compounds with 6 to 10 carbons that are water soluble. Such compounds may then enter blood, be oxidized as medium-chain fatty acids, or be excreted in urine as medium-chain dicarboxylic acids.

The pathways of peroxisomal α- and β-oxidation and microsomal ω-oxidation are not feedback regulated. These pathways function to decrease levels of water-insoluble fatty acids or of xenobiotic compounds with a fatty acid–like structure that would become toxic to cells at high concentrations. Thus, their rate is regulated by the availability of substrate.

## III. METABOLISM OF KETONE BODIES

Overall, fatty acids released from adipose triacylglycerols serve as the major fuel for the body during fasting. These fatty acids are completely oxidized to $CO_2$ and $H_2O$ by some tissues. In the liver, much of the acetyl CoA generated from β-oxidation of fatty acids is used for synthesis of the ketone bodies acetoacetate and β-hydroxybutyrate, which enter the blood. In skeletal muscles and other tissues, these ketone bodies are converted back to acetyl CoA, which is oxidized in the TCA cycle with generation of ATP. An alternate fate of acetoacetate in tissues is the formation of cytosolic acetyl CoA.

### A. Synthesis of Ketone Bodies

In the liver, ketone bodies are synthesized in the mitochondrial matrix from acetyl CoA generated from fatty acid oxidation (Fig. 20.12). The thiolase reaction of fatty acid oxidation, which converts acetoacetyl CoA to two molecules of acetyl CoA, is a reversible reaction, although formation of acetoacetyl CoA is not the favored direction. Therefore, when acetyl CoA levels are high, this reaction can generate acetoacetyl CoA for ketone body synthesis. The acetoacetyl CoA will react with acetyl CoA to produce 3-hydroxy-3-methylglutaryl CoA (HMG-CoA). The enzyme that catalyzes this reaction is HMG-CoA synthase. In the next reaction of the pathway, HMG-CoA lyase catalyzes the cleavage of HMG-CoA to form acetyl CoA and acetoacetate.

Acetoacetate can enter the blood directly or it can be reduced by β-hydroxybutyrate dehydrogenase to β-hydroxybutyrate, which enters the blood (see Fig. 20.12). This dehydrogenase reaction is readily reversible and interconverts these two ketone bodies, which exist in an equilibrium ratio determined by the $NADH/NAD^+$ ratio of the mitochondrial matrix. Under normal conditions, the ratio of β-hydroxybutyrate to acetoacetate in the blood is approximately 1:1.

An alternatative fate of acetoacetate is spontaneous decarboxylation, a nonenzymatic reaction that cleaves acetoacetate into $CO_2$ and acetone (see Fig. 20.12). Because acetone is volatile, it is expired by the lungs. A small amount of acetone may be further metabolized in the body.

### B. Oxidation of Ketone Bodies as Fuels

Acetoacetate and β-hydroxybutyrate can be oxidized as fuels in most tissues, including skeletal muscle, brain, certain cells of the kidney, and cells of the intestinal mucosa. Cells transport both acetoacetate and β-hydroxybutyrate from the circulating blood into the cytosol and into the mitochondrial matrix. Here, β-hydroxybutyrate is oxidized back to acetoacetate by β-hydroxybutyrate dehydrogenase. This reaction produces NADH. Subsequent steps convert acetoacetate to acetyl CoA (Fig. 20.13).

In mitochondria, acetoacetate is activated to acetoacetyl CoA by succinyl CoA acetoacetate CoA transferase. As the name suggests, CoA is transferred from succinyl CoA, a TCA cycle intermediate, to acetoacetate. Although the liver produces ketone bodies, it does not use them because this thiotransferase enzyme is not present in sufficient quantity.

One molecule of acetoacetyl CoA is cleaved to two molecules of acetyl CoA by acetoacetyl CoA thiolase, the same enzyme involved in β-oxidation. The principal fate of this acetyl CoA is oxidation in the TCA cycle.

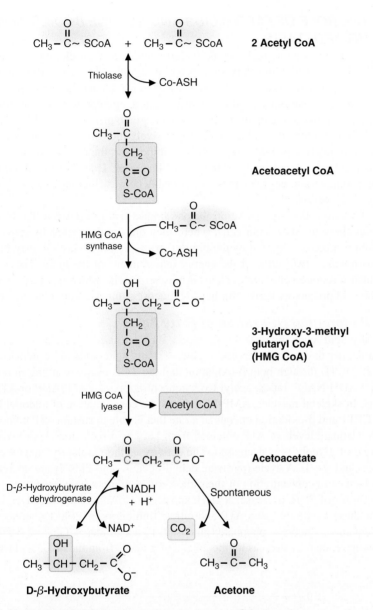

FIG. 20.12. Synthesis of the ketone bodies acetoacetate, β-hydroxybutyrate, and acetone. The portion of HMG-CoA shown in the tinted box is released as acetyl CoA, and the remainder of the molecule forms acetoacetate. Acetoacetate is reduced to β-hydroxybutyrate or decarboxylated to acetone. Note that the dehydrogenase that interconverts acetoacetate and β-hydroxybutyrate is specific for the D-isomer. Thus, it differs from the dehydrogenases of β-oxidation, which act on 3-hydroxy acyl CoA derivatives and is specific for the L-isomer.

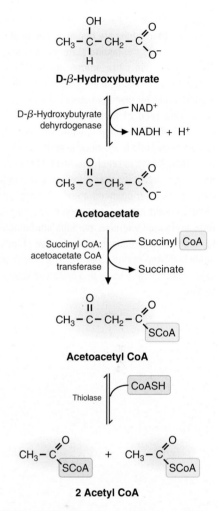

FIG. 20.13. Oxidation of ketone bodies. β-Hydroxybutyrate is oxidized to acetoacetate, which is activated by accepting a CoA group from succinyl CoA. Acetoacetyl CoA is cleaved to two acetyl CoA, which enter the TCA cycle and are oxidized.

The energy yield from oxidation of acetoacetate is equivalent to the yield for oxidation of two molecules of acetyl CoA in the TCA cycle (20 ATP) minus the energy for activation of acetoacetate (1 ATP). The energy of activation is calculated at one high-energy phosphate bond because succinyl CoA is normally converted to succinate in the TCA cycle, with generation of one molecule of GTP (the energy equivalent of ATP). However, when the high-energy thioester bond of succinyl CoA is transferred to acetoacetate, succinate is produced without the generation of this GTP. Oxidation of β-hydroxybutyrate generates one additional NADH. Therefore, the net energy yield from one molecule of β-hydroxybutyrate is approximately 21.5 molecules of ATP.

 Ketogenic diets, which are high-fat diets with a 3:1 ratio of lipid to carbohydrate, are being used to reduce the frequency of epileptic seizures in children. The reason for its effectiveness in the treatment of epilepsy is not known. Ketogenic diets are also used to treat children with pyruvate dehydrogenase deficiency. Ketone bodies can be used as a fuel by the brain in the absence of pyruvate dehydrogenase. They also can provide a source of cytosolic acetyl CoA for acetylcholine synthesis. They often contain medium-chain triglycerides, which induce ketosis more effectively than long-chain triglycerides.

Children are more prone to ketosis than adults are because their bodies enter the fasting state more rapidly. Their bodies use more energy per unit mass (because their muscle to adipose tissue ratio is higher), and liver glycogen stores are depleted faster (the ratio of their brain mass to liver mass is higher). In children, blood ketone body levels reach 2 mM in 24 hours; in adults, it takes more than 3 days to reach this level. Mild pediatric infections that cause anorexia and vomiting are the most common cause of ketosis in children. Mild ketosis is observed in children after prolonged exercise, perhaps attributable to an abrupt decrease in muscular use of fatty acids liberated during exercise. The liver then oxidizes these fatty acids and produces ketone bodies.

## IV. THE ROLE OF FATTY ACIDS AND KETONE BODIES IN FUEL HOMEOSTASIS

Fatty acids are used as fuels whenever fatty acid levels are elevated in the blood, that is, during fasting and starvation; because of a high-fat, low-carbohydrate diet; or during long-term, low- to mild-intensity exercise. Under these conditions, a decrease in insulin and increased levels of glucagon, epinephrine, or other hormones stimulate adipose tissue lipolysis. Fatty acids begin to increase in the blood approximately 3 to 4 hours after a meal and progressively increase with time of fasting up to approximately 2 to 3 days (Fig. 20.14). In the liver, the rate of ketone body synthesis increases as the supply of fatty acids increases. However, the blood level of ketone bodies continues to increase, presumably because their utilization by skeletal muscles decreases.

After 2 to 3 days of starvation, ketone bodies rise to a level in the blood that enables them to enter brain cells, where they are oxidized, thereby reducing the amount of glucose required by the brain. During prolonged fasting, they may supply as much as two-thirds of the energy requirements of the brain. The reduction in glucose requirements spares skeletal muscle protein, which is a major source of amino acid precursors needed for hepatic glucose synthesis from gluconeogenesis.

### A. Preferential Utilization of Fatty Acids

As fatty acid levels increase in the blood, they are used by skeletal muscles and certain other tissues in preference to glucose. Fatty acid oxidation generates NADH and FAD(2H) through both β-oxidation and the TCA cycle, resulting in relatively high NADH/NAD$^+$ ratios, acetyl CoA concentration, and ATP/ADP or ATP/AMP levels. In skeletal muscles, AMP-PK adjusts the concentration of malonyl CoA so that CPT1 and β-oxidation operate at a rate that is able to sustain ATP homeostasis. With adequate levels of ATP obtained from fatty acid (or ketone body) oxidation, the rate of glycolysis is decreased. The activity of the regulatory enzymes in glycolysis and the TCA cycle (pyruvate dehydrogenase and PFK-1) are decreased by the changes in concentration of their allosteric regulators (concentrations of ADP, an activator of PDH, decrease; NADH, and acetyl CoA, inhibitors of PDH, increase under these conditions; and ATP and citrate, inhibitors of PFK-1, increase). As a consequence, glucose-6-phophate (glucose 6-P) accumulates. Glucose 6-P inhibits hexokinase, thereby decreasing the uptake of glucose from the blood and its rate of

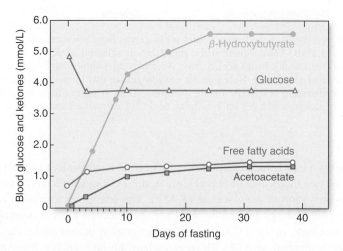

**FIG. 20.14.** Levels of ketone bodies in the blood at various times during fasting. Glucose levels remain relatively constant, as do levels of fatty acids. Ketone body levels, however, increase markedly, rising to levels at which they can be used by the brain and other nervous tissue. (From Cahill GF Jr, Aoki TT. How metabolism affects clinical problems. *Med Times.* 1970;98:106.)

entry into glycolysis. In skeletal muscles, this pattern of fuel metabolism is facilitated by the decrease in insulin concentration. Preferential utilization of fatty acids does not, however, restrict the ability of glycolysis to respond to an increase in AMP or ADP levels, such as might occur during exercise or oxygen limitation.

## B. Tissues that Use Ketone Bodies

Skeletal muscles, the heart, the liver, and many other tissues use fatty acids as their major fuel during fasting and other conditions that increase fatty acids in the blood. However, several other tissues (or cell types), such as the brain, use ketone bodies to a greater extent. For example, cells of the intestinal muscosa, which transport fatty acids from the intestine to the blood, use ketone bodies and amino acids during starvation rather than fatty acids. Adipocytes, which store fatty acids in triacylglycerols, do not use fatty acids as a fuel during fasting but can use ketone bodies. Ketone bodies cross the placenta and can be used by the fetus. Almost all tissues and cell types, with the exception of liver and red blood cells, are able to use ketone bodies as fuels.

## C. Regulation of Ketone Body Synthesis

Several events, in addition to the increased supply of fatty acids from adipose triacylglycerols, promote hepatic ketone body synthesis during fasting. The decreased insulin/glucagon ratio results in inhibition of acetyl CoA carboxylase and decreased malonyl CoA levels, which activates CPTI, thereby allowing fatty acyl CoA to enter the pathway of β-oxidation (Fig. 20.15). When oxidation of fatty acyl CoA to acetyl CoA generates enough NADH and FAD(2H) to supply the ATP needs of the liver, acetyl CoA is diverted from the TCA cycle into ketogenesis and oxaloacetate in the TCA cycle is diverted toward malate and into glucose synthesis (gluconeogenesis). This pattern is regulated by the NADH/NAD$^+$ ratio, which

The level of total ketone bodies in **Dianne A.'s** blood greatly exceeds normal fasting levels and the mild ketosis produced during exercise. In a person on a normal mealtime schedule, total blood ketone bodies rarely exceed 0.2 mM. During prolonged fasting, they may rise to 4 to 5 mM. Levels above 7 mM are considered evidence of ketoacidosis because the acid produced must reach this level to exceed the bicarbonate buffer system in the blood and compensatory respiration (Kussmaul breathing) (see Chapter 2).

Why can red blood cells not use ketone bodies for energy?

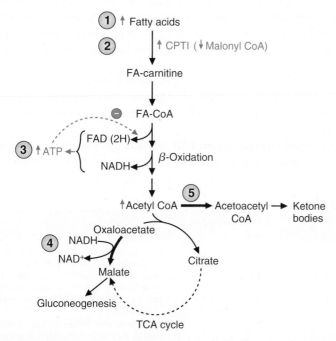

**FIG. 20.15.** Regulation of ketone body synthesis. *(1)* The supply of fatty acids is increased. *(2)* The malonyl CoA inhibition of CPTI is lifted by inactivation of acetyl CoA carboxylase. *(3)* β-Oxidation supplies NADH and FAD(2H), which are used by the electron transport chain for oxidative phosphorylation. As ATP levels increase, less NADH is oxidized, and the NADH/NAD$^+$ ratio is increased. *(4)* Oxaloacetate is converted into malate because of the high NADH levels, and the malate enters the cytoplasm for gluconeogenesis. *(5)* Acetyl CoA is diverted from the TCA cycle into ketogenesis, in part because of low oxaloacetate levels, which reduces the rate of the citrate synthase reaction.

Red blood cells lack mitochondria, which is the site of ketone body utilization.

is relatively high during β-oxidation. As the length of time of fasting continues, increased transcription of the gene for mitochondrial HMG-CoA synthase facilitates high rates of ketone body production. Although the liver has been described as "altruistic" because it provides ketone bodies for other tissues, it is simply getting rid of fuel that it does not need.

## CLINICAL COMMENTS

Diseases discussed in this chapter are summarized in Table 20.2.

**Otto S.** As **Otto S.** runs, he increases the rate at which his muscles oxidize all fuels. The increased rate of ATP utilization stimulates the electron transport chain, which oxidizes NADH and FAD(2H) much faster, thereby increasing the rate at which fatty acids are oxidized. During exercise, he also uses muscle glycogen stores, which contribute glucose to glycolysis. In some of the fibers, the glucose is used anaerobically, thereby producing lactate. Some of the lactate will be used by his heart and some will be taken up by the liver to be converted to glucose. As he trains, he increases his mitochondrial capacity, as well as his oxygen delivery, resulting in an increased ability to oxidize fatty acids and ketone bodies. As he runs, he increases fatty acid release from adipose tissue triacylglycerols. In the liver, fatty acids are being converted to ketone bodies, providing his muscles with another fuel. As a consequence, he experiences mild ketosis after his 12-mile run.

**Lola B.** Recently, medium-chain acyl CoA dehydrogenase (MCAD) deficiency, the cause of **Lola B.'s** problems, has emerged as one of the most common of the inborn errors of metabolism, with a carrier frequency ranging from 1 in 40 in northern European populations to less than 1 in 100 in Asians. Overall, the predicted disease frequency for MCAD deficiency is 1 in 15,000 persons. More than 25 enzymes and specific transport proteins participate in mitochondrial fatty acid metabolism. At least 15 of these have been implicated in inherited diseases in the human.

MCAD deficiency is an autosomal recessive disorder caused by the substitution of a T for an A at position 985 of the MCAD gene. This mutation causes a lysine to replace a glutamate residue in the protein, resulting in the production of an unstable dehydrogenase.

The most frequent manifestation of MCAD deficiency is intermittent hypoketotic hypoglycemia during fasting (low levels of ketone bodies and low levels of glucose

**Table 20.2   Diseases Discussed in Chapter 20**

| Disease or Disorder | Environmental or Genetic | Comments |
| --- | --- | --- |
| Obesity | Both | The contribution of fatty acids to overall energy metabolism and energy storage. |
| MCAD deficiency | Genetic | Lack of medium-chain acyl CoA dehydrogenase activity, leading to hypoglycemia and reduced ketone body formation under fasting conditions. |
| Type 1 diabetes | Both | Ketoacidosis; overproduction of ketone bodies due to lack of insulin and metabolic dysregulation in the liver. |
| Zellweger syndrome | Genetic | A defect in peroxisome biogenesis, leading to a lack of peroxisomes, inability to synthesize plasmalogens, or oxidize very long chain fatty acids. |
| LCAD deficiency | Genetic | A lack of long-chain acyl CoA dehydrogenase activity, leading to hypoglycemia. |

MCAD, medium-chain acyl CoA dehydrogenase; LCAD, long-chain acyl CoA dehydrogenase.

in the blood). Fatty acids normally would be oxidized to $CO_2$ and $H_2O$ under these conditions. In MCAD deficiency, however, fatty acids are oxidized only until they reach medium-chain length. As a result, the body must rely to a greater extent on oxidation of blood glucose to meet its energy needs.

However, hepatic gluconeogenesis appears to be impaired in MCAD. Inhibition of gluconeogenesis may be caused by the lack of hepatic fatty acid oxidation to supply the energy required for gluconeogenesis or by the accumulation of unoxidized fatty acid metabolites that inhibit gluconeogenic enzymes. As a consequence, liver glycogen stores are depleted more rapidly and hypoglycemia results. The decrease in hepatic fatty acid oxidation results in less acetyl CoA for ketone body synthesis and, consequently, a hypoketotic hypoglycemia develops.

Some of the symptoms once ascribed to hypoglycemia are now believed to be caused by the accumulation of toxic fatty acid intermediates, especially in those patients with only mild reductions in blood glucose levels. **Lola B.'s** mild elevation in the blood of liver transaminases may reflect an infiltration of her liver cells with unoxidized medium-chain fatty acids.

The management of MCAD-deficient patients includes the intake of a relatively high-carbohydrate diet and the avoidance of fasting for more than 2 to 6 hours during infancy and then no more than 12 hours later in life.

 **Dianne A.** Dianne A., a 26-year-old woman with type 1 diabetes mellitus, was admitted to the hospital in diabetic ketoacidosis. In this complication of diabetes mellitus, an acute deficiency of insulin, coupled with a relative excess of glucagon, results in a rapid mobilization of fuel stores from muscle (amino acids) and adipose tissue (fatty acids). Some of the amino acids are converted to glucose and fatty acids are converted to ketones (acetoacetate, β-hydroxybutyrate, and acetone). The high glucagon/insulin ratio promotes the hepatic production of ketones. In response to the metabolic "stress," the levels of insulin-antagonistic hormones, such as catecholamines, glucocorticoids, and growth hormone, are increased in the blood. The insulin deficiency further reduces the peripheral utilization of glucose and ketones. Because of this interrelated dysmetabolism, plasma glucose levels can reach 500 mg/dL (27.8 mmol/L) or more (normal fasting levels are 70 to 100 mg/dL, or 3.9 to 5.5 mmol/L), and plasma ketones can rise to levels of 8 to 15 mmol/L or more (normal is in the range of 0.2 to 2 mmol/L, depending on the fed state of the individual).

The increased glucose presented to the renal glomeruli induces an osmotic diuresis, which further depletes intravascular volume, further reducing the renal excretion of hydrogen ions and glucose. As a result, the metabolic acidosis worsens, and the hyperosmolarity of the blood increases, at times exceeding 330 mOsm/kg (normal is in the range of 285 to 295 mOsm/kg). The severity of the hyperosmolar state correlates closely with the degree of central nervous system dysfunction and may end in coma and even death if left untreated.

## REVIEW QUESTIONS-CHAPTER 20

1. A lack of the enzyme ETF:CoQ oxidoreductase leads to death. This is due to which one of the following?

   A. The energy yield from glucose utilization is dramatically reduced.

   B. The energy yield from alcohol utilization is dramatically reduced.

   C. The energy yield from fatty acid utilization is dramatically reduced.

   D. The energy yield from ketone body utilization is dramatically reduced.

   E. The energy yield from glycogen degradation is dramatically reduced.

2.  The ATP yield from the complete oxidation of one mole of a C18:0 fatty acid to carbon dioxide and water would be closest to which **ONE** of the following?

    A.  105
    B.  115
    C.  120
    D.  125
    E.  130

3.  An individual with a deficiency of an enzyme in the pathway for carnitine synthesis is not obtaining adequate amounts of carnitine in the diet. Which one of the following would you expect to be increased during fasting in this individual as compared to an individual with an adequate intake and synthesis of carnitine?

    A.  Fatty acid oxidation
    B.  Ketone body synthesis
    C.  Blood glucose levels
    D.  The levels of very long chain fatty acids in the blood
    E.  The levels of dicarboxylic acids in the blood

4.  If your patient has classic carnitine:palmitoyl transferase II deficiency, which one of the following laboratory test results would you expect to observe?

    A.  Elevated ketone body levels in the blood
    B.  Elevated blood acylcarnitine levels

C.  Elevated blood glucose levels
D.  Reduced blood creatine phosphokinase levels
E.  Reduced blood fatty acid levels

5.  A 6-month-old infant is brought to your office due to frequent crying episodes, lethargy, and poor eating. These symptoms were especially noticeable after the child had an ear infection, at which time he did not eat well. The parents stated that this has happened before, but they found if they fed the child frequently the lethargic episodes could be reduced in number. The results of blood work indicated that the child was hypoglycemic and hypoketotic. Six to eight carbon chain dicarboxylic acids and acylcarnitine derivatives were found in the urine of the child as well. Based on your understanding of fatty acid metabolism, which enzyme would you expect to be defective in this child?

    A.  CPT-1
    B.  CPT-II
    C.  LCAD
    D.  MCAD
    E.  Carnitine: acylcarnitine translocase

# 21 Basic Concepts in the Regulation of Fuel Metabolism by Insulin, Glucagon, and Other Hormones

## CHAPTER OUTLINE

I. METABOLIC HOMEOSTASIS

II. MAJOR HORMONES OF METABOLIC HOMEOSTASIS

III. SYNTHESIS AND RELEASE OF INSULIN AND GLUCAGON
   A. Endocrine pancreas
   B. Synthesis and secretion of insulin
   C. Stimulation and inhibition of insulin release
   D. Synthesis and secretion of glucagon

IV. MECHANISMS OF HORMONE ACTION
   A. Signal transduction by hormones that bind to plasma membrane receptors
      1. Signal transduction by insulin
      2. Signal transduction by glucagon
   B. Signal transduction by cortisol and other hormones that interact with intracellular receptors
   C. Signal transduction by epinephrine and norepinephrine

## KEY POINTS

- Insulin and glucagon are the two major hormones that regulate fuel mobilization and storage.
- Insulin and glucagon maintain blood glucose levels near 80 to 100 mg/dL despite varying carbohydrate intake during the day.
- Glucose homeostasis is the maintenance of constant blood glucose levels.
- If dietary intake of all fuels is in excess of immediate need, it is stored as either glycogen or fat.
- Appropriately stored fuels are mobilized when demand requires.
- Insulin is released in response to carbohydrate ingestion and promotes glucose utilization as a fuel and glucose storage as fat and glycogen.
- Glucagon is decreased in response to a carbohydrate meal and elevated during fasting.
- Glucagon promotes glucose production via glycogenolysis (glycogen degradation) and gluconeogenesis (glucose synthesis from amino acids and other noncarbohydrate precursors).
- Increased levels of glucagon relative to insulin also stimulate the release of fatty acids from adipose tissue.
- Insulin secretion is regulated principally by blood glucose levels.
- Glucagon release is regulated principally through suppression by glucose and by insulin.
- Glucagon acts by binding to a receptor on the cell surface, which stimulates the synthesis of the intracellular second messenger, cAMP.
- cAMP activates protein kinase A, which phosphorylates key regulatory enzymes, activating some and inhibiting others.
- Insulin acts via a receptor tyrosine kinase and leads to the dephosphorylation of the key enzymes phosphorylated in response to glucagon.

# THE WAITING ROOM

**Deborah S.** returned to her physician for her monthly office visit. She has been seeing her physician for over a year because of obesity and elevated blood glucose levels. She still weighed 198 lb, despite trying to adhere to her diet. Her blood glucose level at the time of the visit, 2 hours after lunch, was 221 mg/dL (reference range = 80 to 140). Deborah suffers from type 2 diabetes, an impaired response to insulin. Understanding the actions of insulin and glucagon are critical for understanding this disorder.

**Connie C.** is a 46-year-old woman who 6 months earlier began noting episodes of fatigue and confusion as she finished her daily prebreakfast jog. These episodes were occasionally accompanied by blurred vision and an unusually urgent sense of hunger. The ingestion of food relieved all of her symptoms within 25 to 30 minutes. In the last month, these attacks have occurred more frequently throughout the day and she has learned to diminish their occurrence by eating between meals. As a result, she has recently gained 8 lb.

A random serum glucose level done at 4:30 PM during her first office visit was subnormal at 67 mg/dL. Her physician, suspecting she was having episodes of hypoglycemia, ordered a series of fasting serum glucose, insulin, and c-peptide levels. In addition, he asked Connie to keep a careful daily diary of all of the symptoms that she experienced when her attacks were most severe.

Fatty acids provide an example of the influence that the level of a compound in the blood has on its own rate of metabolism. The concentration of fatty acids in the blood is the major factor determining whether skeletal muscles will use fatty acids or glucose as a fuel (see Chapter 24). In contrast, hormones are (by definition) carriers of messages between their sites of synthesis and their target tissues. Insulin and glucagon, for example, are two hormonal messengers that participate in the regulation of fuel metabolism by carrying messages that reflect the timing and composition of our dietary intake of fuels. Epinephrine, however, is a fight-or-flight hormone that signals an immediate need for increased fuel availability. Its level is regulated principally through the activation of the sympathetic nervous system.

## I. METABOLIC HOMEOSTASIS

Living cells require a constant source of fuels from which to derive adenosine triphosphate (ATP) for the maintenance of normal cell function and growth. Therefore, a balance must be achieved between carbohydrate, fat, and protein intake; their rates of oxidation; and their rates of storage when they are present in excess of immediate need. Alternatively, when the demand for these substrates increases, the rate of mobilization from storage sites and the rate of their de novo synthesis also require balanced regulation. The control of the balance between substrate need and substrate availability is referred to as metabolic homeostasis. The intertissue integration required for metabolic homeostasis is achieved in three principal ways:

- The concentration of nutrients or metabolites in the blood affects the rate at which they are used or stored in different tissues.
- Hormones carry messages to individual tissues about the physiological state of the body and nutrient supply or demand.
- The central nervous system uses neural signals to control tissue metabolism, either directly or through the release of hormones.

Insulin and glucagon are the two major hormones that regulate fuel storage and mobilization (Fig. 21.1). Insulin is the major anabolic hormone of the body. It promotes the storage of fuels and the utilization of fuels for growth. Glucagon is the major hormone of fuel mobilization. Other hormones, such as epinephrine, are released as a response of the central nervous system to hypoglycemia, exercise, or other types of physiologic stress. Epinephrine and other stress hormones also increase the availability of fuels (Fig. 21.2).

Glucose has a special role in metabolic homeostasis. Many tissues (e.g., the brain, red blood cells, kidney medulla, exercising skeletal muscle) depend on glycolysis for all or a part of their energy needs. As a consequence, these tissues

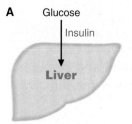

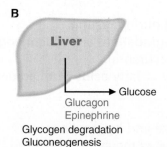

*FIG. 21.1.* Insulin and the insulin counter-regulatory hormones. **A.** Insulin promotes glucose storage as triglyceride (TG) or glycogen. **B.** Glucagon and epinephrine promote glucose release from the liver, activating glycogenolysis and gluconeogenesis. Cortisol will stimulate both glycogen synthesis and gluconeogenesis.

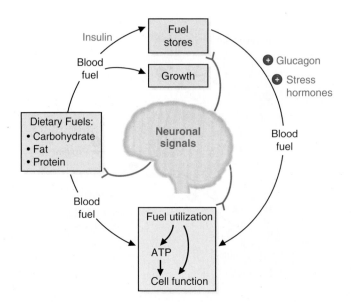

**FIG. 21.2.** Signals that regulate metabolic homeostasis. The major stress hormones are epinephrine and cortisol.

require uninterrupted access to glucose to meet their rapid rate of ATP use. In the adult, a minimum of 190 g glucose is required per day, approximately 150 g for the brain and 40 g for other tissues. Significant decreases of blood glucose below 60 mg/dL limit glucose metabolism in the brain and elicit hypoglycemic symptoms (as experienced by **Connie C.**), presumably because the overall process of glucose flux through the blood–brain barrier, into the interstitial fluid, and subsequently into the neuronal cells is slow at low blood glucose levels because of the $K_m$ values of the glucose transporters required for this to occur (see Chapter 22).

The continuous efflux of fuels from storage depots, during exercise, for example, is necessitated by the high amounts of fuel required each day to meet the need for ATP under these conditions. Disastrous results would occur if even a day's supply of glucose, amino acids, and fatty acids could not enter cells normally and were instead left circulating in the blood. Glucose and amino acids would be at such high concentrations in the circulation that the hyperosmolar effect would cause progressively severe neurologic deficits and even coma. The concentration of glucose and amino acids would rise above the renal tubular threshold for these substances (the maximal concentration in the blood at which the kidney can completely resorb metabolites), and some of these compounds would be wasted as they spilled over into the urine. Nonenzymatic glycosylation of proteins would increase at higher blood glucose levels altering the function of tissues in which these proteins reside. Triacylglycerols, present primarily in chylomicrons and very low density lipoproteins (VLDL) would rise in the blood, increasing the likelihood of atherosclerotic vascular disease. These potential metabolic derangements emphasize the need to maintain a normal balance between fuel storage and fuel use.

## II.  MAJOR HORMONES OF METABOLIC HOMEOSTASIS

The hormones that contribute to metabolic homeostasis respond to changes in the circulating levels of fuels that, in part, are determined by the timing and composition of our diet. Insulin and glucagon are considered the major hormones of metabolic homeostasis because they continuously fluctuate in response to our daily eating pattern. They provide good examples of the basic concepts of hormonal regulation. Certain features of the release and action of other insulin counterregulatory

Hyperglycemia may cause a constellation of symptoms such as polyuria and subsequent polydipsia (increased thirst). The inability to move glucose into cells necessitates the oxidation of lipids as an alternative fuel. As a result, adipose stores are used, and the patient with poorly controlled diabetes mellitus loses weight in spite of a good appetite. Extremely high levels of serum glucose can cause a hyperosmolar hyperglycemic state in patients with type 2 diabetes mellitus. Such patients usually have sufficient insulin responsiveness to block fatty acid release and ketone body formation, but they are unable to significantly stimulate glucose entry into peripheral tissues. The severely elevated levels of glucose in the blood compared with those inside the cell leads to an osmotic effect that causes water to leave the cells and enter the blood. Because of the osmotic diuretic effect of hyperglycemia, the kidney produces more urine, leading to dehydration, which, in turn, may lead to even higher levels of blood glucose. If dehydration becomes severe, further cerebral dysfunction occurs and the patient may become comatose. Chronic hyperglycemia also produces pathological effects through the nonenzymatic glycosylation of a variety of proteins. Hemoglobin A (HbA), one of the proteins that becomes glycosylated, forms $HbA_{1c}$ (see Chapter 7). **Deborah S.'s** high levels of $HbA_{1c}$ (12% of the total HbA, compared with the reference range of 4.7% to 6.4%) indicate that her blood glucose has been significantly elevated over the last 12 to 14 weeks, the half-life of hemoglobin in the bloodstream.

All membrane and serum proteins exposed to high levels of glucose in the blood or interstitial fluid are candidates for nonenzymatic glycosylation. This process distorts protein structure and slows protein degradation, which leads to an accumulation of these products in various organs, thereby adversely affecting organ function. These events contribute to the long-term microvascular and macrovascular complications of diabetes mellitus, which include diabetic retinopathy, nephropathy, and neuropathy (microvascular), in addition to coronary artery, cerebral artery, peripheral artery disease, and atherosclerosis (macrovascular).

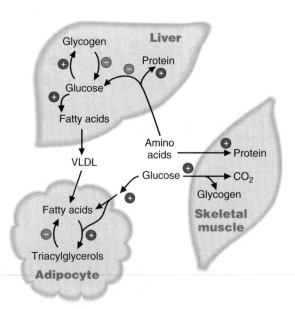

**FIG. 21.3.** Major sites of insulin action in fuel metabolism. *VLDL*, very low density lipoprotein; ⊕, stimulated by insulin; ⊖, inhibited by insulin.

**Connie C.'s** studies confirmed that her fasting serum glucose levels were below normal with an inappropriately high insulin level. She continued to experience the fatigue, confusion, and blurred vision she had described on her first office visit. These symptoms are referred to as the neuroglycopenic manifestations of severe hypoglycemia (neurologic symptoms resulting from an inadequate supply of glucose to the brain for the generation of ATP).

Connie also noted the symptoms that are part of the adrenergic response to hypoglycemic stress. Stimulation of the sympathetic nervous system (because of the low levels of glucose reaching the brain) results in the release of epinephrine, a stress hormone, from the adrenal medulla. Elevated epinephrine levels cause tachycardia (rapid heart rate), palpitations, anxiety, tremulousness, pallor, and sweating.

In addition to the symptoms described by **Connie C.**, individuals may experience confusion, light-headedness, headache, aberrant behavior, blurred vision, loss of consciousness, or seizures. When severe or prolonged, death may occur.

hormones, such as epinephrine, norepinephrine, and cortisol, will be described and compared with insulin and glucagon.

Insulin is the major anabolic hormone that promotes the storage of nutrients: glucose storage as glycogen in liver and muscle, conversion of glucose to triacylglycerols in liver and their storage in adipose tissue, and amino acid uptake and protein synthesis in skeletal muscle (Fig. 21.3). It also increases the synthesis of albumin and other proteins by the liver. Insulin promotes the use of glucose as a fuel by facilitating its transport into muscle and adipose tissue. At the same time, insulin acts to inhibit fuel mobilization.

Glucagon acts to maintain fuel availability in the absence of dietary glucose by stimulating the release of glucose from liver glycogen (see Chapter 23); by stimulating gluconeogenesis from lactate, glycerol, and amino acids (see Chapter 26); and, in conjunction with decreased insulin, by mobilizing fatty acids from adipose triacylglycerols to provide an alternate source of fuel (see Chapter 20 and Fig. 21.4). Its sites of action are principally the liver and adipose tissue; it has no influence on skeletal muscle metabolism because muscle cells lack glucagon receptors. The message carried by glucagon is that "Glucose is gone"; that is, the current supply of glucose is inadequate to meet the immediate fuel requirements of the body.

The release of insulin from the β-cells of the pancreas is dictated primarily by the level of glucose bathing the β-cells in the islets of Langerhans. The highest levels of insulin occur approximately 30 to 45 minutes after a high-carbohydrate meal (Fig. 21.5). They return to basal levels as the blood glucose concentration falls, approximately 120 minutes after the meal. The release of glucagon from the α-cells of the pancreas, conversely, is controlled principally through a reduction of glucose and/or a rise in the concentration of insulin in blood, bathing the α-cells in the pancreas. Therefore, the lowest levels of glucagon occur after a high-carbohydrate meal. Because all of the effects of glucagon are opposed by insulin, the simultaneous stimulation of insulin release and suppression of glucagon secretion by a high-carbohydrate meal provides integrated control of carbohydrate, fat, and protein metabolism.

Insulin and glucagon are not the only regulators of fuel metabolism. The intertissue balance between the use and storage of glucose, fat, and protein is also accom-

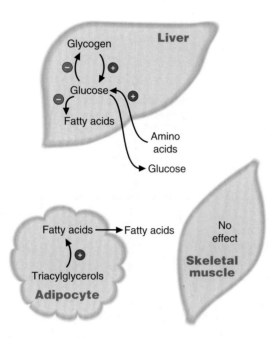

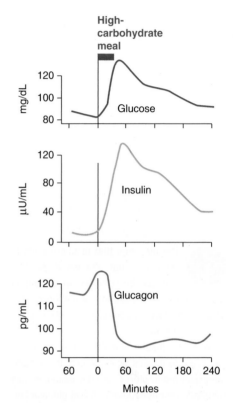

**FIG. 21.4.** Major sites of glucagon action in fuel metabolism. ⊕, pathways stimulated by glucagon; ⊖, pathways inhibited by glucagon.

**FIG. 21.5.** Blood glucose, insulin, and glucagon levels after a high-carbohydrate meal.

plished by the circulating levels of metabolites in the blood, by neuronal signals, and by the other hormones of metabolic homeostasis (epinephrine, norepinephrine, cortisol, and others) (Table 21.1). These hormones oppose the actions of insulin by mobilizing fuels. Like glucagon, they are insulin counterregulatory hormones (Fig. 21.6). Of all these hormones, only insulin and glucagon are synthesized and released in direct response to changing levels of fuels in the blood. The release of cortisol, epinephrine, and norepinephrine is mediated by neuronal signals. Rising levels of the insulin counterregulatory hormones in the blood reflect, for the most part, a current increase in the demand for fuel.

**Table 21.1    Physiological Actions of Insulin and Insulin Counterregulatory Hormones**

| Hormone | Function | Major Metabolic Pathways Affected |
|---|---|---|
| Insulin | • Promotes fuel storage after a meal<br>• Promotes growth | • Stimulates glucose storage as glycogen (muscle and liver)<br>• Stimulates fatty acid synthesis and storage after a high-carbohydrate meal<br>• Stimulates amino acid uptake and protein synthesis |
| Glucagon | • Mobilizes fuels<br><br>• Maintains blood glucose levels during fasting | • Activates gluconeogenesis and glycogenolysis (liver) during fasting<br>• Activates fatty acid release from adipose tissue |
| Epinephrine | • Mobilizes fuels during acute stress | • Stimulates glucose production from glycogen (muscle and liver)<br>• Stimulates fatty acid release from adipose issue |
| Cortisol | • Provides for changing requirements during stress | • Stimulates amino acid mobilization from muscle protein<br>• Stimulates gluconeogenesis to produce glucose for liver glycogen synthesis<br>• Stimulates fatty acid release from adipose tissue |

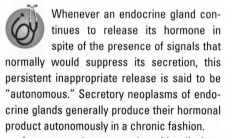

FIG. 21.6. Major insulin counterregulatory hormones. The stress of a low blood glucose level mediates the release of the major insulin counterregulatory hormones through neuronal signals. Hypoglycemia is one of the stress signals that stimulates the release of cortisol, epinephrine, and norepinephrine. Adrenocorticotropic hormone *(ACTH)* is released from the pituitary and stimulates the release of cortisol (a glucocorticoid) from the adrenal cortex. Neuronal signals stimulate the release of epinephrine from the adrenal medulla and norepinephrine from nerve endings. Neuronal signals also play a minor role in the release of glucagon. Although norepinephrine has counterregulatory actions, it is not a major counterregulatory hormone.

The message that insulin carries to tissues is that glucose is plentiful and can be used as an immediate fuel or can be converted to storage forms such as triacylglycerol in adipocytes or glycogen in liver and muscle.

Because insulin stimulates the uptake of glucose into tissues where it may be immediately oxidized or stored for later oxidation, this regulatory hormone lowers blood glucose levels. Therefore, one of the possible causes of **Connie C.'s** hypoglycemia is an insulinoma, a tumor that produces excessive insulin.

Whenever an endocrine gland continues to release its hormone in spite of the presence of signals that normally would suppress its secretion, this persistent inappropriate release is said to be "autonomous." Secretory neoplasms of endocrine glands generally produce their hormonal product autonomously in a chronic fashion.

Autonomous hypersecretion of insulin from a suspected pancreatic β-cell tumor (an insulinoma) can be demonstrated in several ways. The simplest test is to simultaneously draw blood for the measurement of both glucose and insulin at a time when the patient is spontaneously experiencing the characteristic adrenergic or neuroglycopenic symptoms of hypoglycemia. During such a test, **Connie C.'s** glucose levels fell to 45 mg/dL (normal = 80 to 100 mg/dL), and her ratio of insulin to glucose was far higher than normal. The elevated insulin levels markedly increased glucose uptake by the peripheral tissues, resulting in a dramatic lowering of blood glucose levels. In normal individuals, as blood glucose levels drop, insulin levels also drop.

## III. SYNTHESIS AND RELEASE OF INSULIN AND GLUCAGON

### A. Endocrine Pancreas

Insulin and glucagon are synthesized in different cell types of the endocrine pancreas, which consists of microscopic clusters of small glands, the islets of Langerhans, scattered among the cells of the exocrine pancreas. The α-cells secrete glucagon, and the β-cells secrete insulin into the hepatic portal vein via the pancreatic veins.

### B. Synthesis and Secretion of Insulin

Insulin is a polypeptide hormone. The active form of insulin is composed of two polypeptide chains (the A chain and the B chain) linked by two interchain disulfide bonds. The A chain has an additional intrachain disulfide bond (Fig. 21.7).

Insulin, like many other polypeptide hormones, is synthesized as a preprohormone that is converted in the rough endoplasmic reticulum (RER) to proinsulin. The "pre-" sequence, a short hydrophobic signal sequence at the N-terminal end, is cleaved as it enters the lumen of the RER. Proinsulin folds into the proper conformation and disulfide bonds are formed between the cysteine residues. It is then transported in microvesicles to the Golgi complex. It leaves the Golgi complex in storage vesicles, where a protease removes the biologically inactive "connecting peptide" (C-peptide) and a few small remnants, resulting in the formation of biologically active insulin (see Fig. 21.7). Zinc ions are also transported in these storage vesicles. Cleavage of the C-peptide decreases the solubility of the resulting insulin, which then coprecipitates with zinc. Exocytosis of the insulin storage vesicles from the cytosol of the β-cell into the blood is stimulated by rising levels of glucose in the blood bathing the β-cells.

Glucose enters the β-cell via specific glucose transporter proteins known as GLUT2 (see Chapter 22). Glucose is phosphorylated through the action of glucokinase to form glucose-6-phosphate, which is metabolized through glycolysis, the tricarboxylic acid

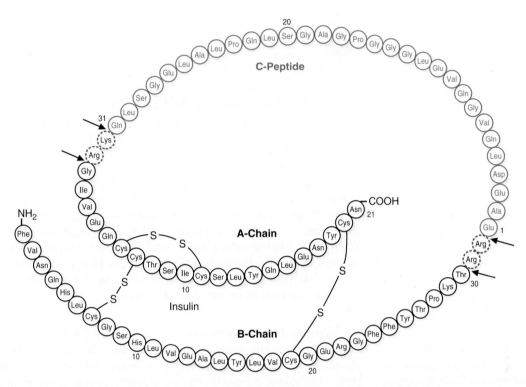

**FIG. 21.7.** Cleavage of proinsulin to insulin. Proinsulin is converted to insulin by proteolytic cleavage, which removes the C-peptide and a few additional amino acid residues. Cleavage occurs at the *arrows*. (From Murray RK, et al. Harper's Biochemistry, 23rd Ed. Stanford, CT: Appleton & Lange, 1993:560.)

(TCA) cycle, and oxidative phosphorylation. These reactions result in an increase in ATP levels within the β-cell (*circle 1* in Fig. 21.8). As the β-cell [ATP]/[ADP] ratio increases, the activity of a membrane-bound, ATP-dependent $K^+$ channel ($K^+_{ATP}$) is inhibited (i.e., the channel is closed) (*circle 2* in Fig. 21.8). The closing of this channel leads to a membrane depolarization (as the membrane is normally hyperpolarized, see *circle 3*, Fig. 21.8), which activates a voltage-gated $Ca^{2+}$ channel that allows $Ca^{2+}$ to enter the β-cell such that intracellular $Ca^{2+}$ levels increase significantly (*circle 4*, Fig. 21.8). The increase in intracellular $Ca^{2+}$ stimulates the fusion of insulin containing exocytotic vesicles with the plasma membrane, resulting in insulin secretion (*circle 5*, Fig. 21.8). Thus, an increase in glucose levels within the β-cells initiates insulin release.

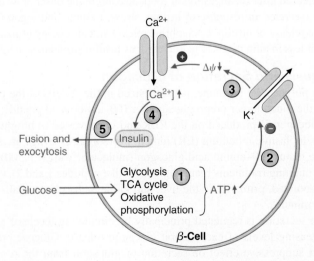

**FIG. 21.8.** Release of insulin by the β-cells. Details are provided in the text.

A rare form of diabetes known as maturity-onset diabetes of the young (MODY) results from mutations in either pancreatic glucokinase or specific nuclear transcription factors. MODY type 2 is caused by a glucokinase mutation that results in an enzyme with reduced activity because of either an elevated $K_m$ for glucose or a reduced $V_{max}$ for the reaction. Because insulin release depends on normal glucose metabolism within the β-cell that yields a critical [ATP]/[ADP] ratio in the β-cell, individuals with this glucokinase mutation cannot significantly metabolize glucose unless glucose levels are higher than normal. Thus, although these patients can release insulin, they do so at higher than normal glucose levels and are, therefore, almost always in a hyperglycemic state. Interestingly, however, these patients are somewhat resistant to the long-term complications of chronic hyperglycemia. The mechanism for this seeming resistance is not well understood.

Neonatal diabetes is an inherited disorder in which newborns develop diabetes within the first 3 months of life. The diabetes may be permanent, requiring lifelong insulin treatment, or transient. The most common mutation leading to permanent neonatal diabetes is in the *KCNJ11* gene, which encodes a subunit of the $K^+_{ATP}$ channel in various tissues including the pancreas. This is an activating mutation, which keeps the $K^+_{ATP}$ channel open and less susceptible to ATP inhibition. If the $K^+_{ATP}$ channel cannot be closed, activation of the $Ca^{2+}$ channel will not occur and insulin secretion will be impaired.

### C.  Stimulation and Inhibition of Insulin Release

The release of insulin occurs within minutes after the pancreas is exposed to a high glucose concentration. The threshold for insulin release is approximately 80 mg glucose/dL. Above 80 mg/dL, the rate of insulin release is not an all-or-nothing response but is proportional to the glucose concentration up to approximately 300 mg/dL glucose. As insulin is secreted, the synthesis of new insulin molecules is stimulated, so that secretion is maintained until blood glucose levels fall. Insulin is rapidly removed from the circulation and degraded by the liver (and, to a lesser extent, by kidney and skeletal muscle), so that blood insulin levels decrease rapidly once the rate of secretion slows.

Several factors other than the blood glucose concentration can modulate insulin release. The pancreatic islets are innervated by the autonomic nervous system, including a branch of the vagus nerve. These neural signals help to coordinate insulin release with the secretory signals initiated by the ingestion of fuels. However, signals from the central nervous system are not required for insulin secretion. Certain amino acids also can stimulate insulin secretion, although the amount of insulin released during a high-protein meal is very much lower than that released by a high-carbohydrate meal. Gastric inhibitory polypeptide (GIP) and glucagonlike peptide 1 (GLP-1), gut hormones released after the ingestion of food, also aid in the onset of insulin release. Epinephrine, secreted in response to fasting, stress, trauma, and vigorous exercise, decreases the release of insulin. Epinephrine release signals energy utilization, which indicates that less insulin needs to be secreted, as insulin stimulates energy storage.

### D.  Synthesis and Secretion of Glucagon

Glucagon, a polypeptide hormone, is synthesized in the α-cells of the pancreas by cleavage of the much larger preproglucagon, a 160–amino acid peptide. Like insulin, preproglucagon is produced on the RER and is converted to proglucagon as it enters the endoplasmic reticulum (ER) lumen. Proteolytic cleavage at various sites produces the mature 29–amino acid glucagon (molecular weight 3,500) and larger glucagon-containing fragments (named glucagonlike peptides 1 and 2). Glucagon is rapidly metabolized, primarily in the liver and kidneys. Its plasma half-life is only about 3 to 5 minutes.

Glucagon secretion is regulated principally by circulating levels of glucose and insulin. Increasing levels of each inhibit glucagon release. Glucose probably has both a direct suppressive effect on secretion of glucagon from the α-cell as well as an indirect effect, the latter being mediated by its ability to stimulate the release

**Deborah S.** is taking a sulfonylurea compound known as glipizide to treat her diabetes. The sulfonylureas act on the $K^+_{ATP}$ channels on the surface of the pancreatic β-cells. The $K^+_{ATP}$ channels contain pore-forming subunits (encoded by the *KCNJ11* gene) and regulatory subunits (the subunit to which sulfonylurea compounds bind encoded by the *SUR1* gene). The binding of the drug to the sulfonylurea receptor closes $K^+$ channels (as do elevated ATP levels), which, in turn, increases $Ca^{2+}$ movement into the interior of the β-cell. This influx of calcium modulates the interaction of the insulin storage vesicles with the plasma membrane of the β-cell, resulting in the release of insulin into the circulation.

Measurements of proinsulin and the connecting peptide between the α- and β-chains of insulin (C-peptide) in **Connie C.'s** blood during her hospital fast provided confirmation that she had an insulinoma. Insulin and C-peptide are secreted in approximately equal proportions from the β-cell, but C-peptide is not cleared from the blood as rapidly as insulin. Therefore, it provides a reasonably accurate estimate of the rate of insulin secretion. Plasma C-peptide measurements could also be potentially useful in treating patients with diabetes mellitus because they provide a way to estimate the degree of endogenous insulin secretion in patients who are receiving exogenous insulin, which lacks the C-peptide.

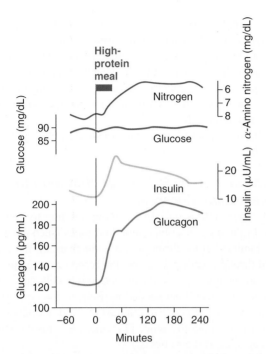

**FIG. 21.9.** Release of insulin and glucagon in response to a high-protein meal. This figure shows the increase in the release of insulin and glucagon into the blood after an overnight fast followed by the ingestion of 100 g protein (equivalent to a slice of roast beef). Insulin levels do not increase nearly as much as they do after a high-carbohydrate meal (see Fig. 21.5). The levels of glucagon, however, significantly increase above those present in the fasting state.

of insulin. The direction of blood flow in the islets of the pancreas carries insulin from the β-cells in the center of the islets to the peripheral α-cells, where it suppresses glucagon secretion.

Conversely, certain hormones stimulate glucagon secretion. Among these are the catecholamines (including epinephrine) and cortisol.

Many amino acids also stimulate glucagon release (Fig. 21.9). Thus, the high levels of glucagon that would be expected in the fasting state do not decrease after a high-protein meal. In fact, glucagon levels may increase, stimulating gluconeogenesis in the absence of dietary glucose. The relative amounts of insulin and glucagon in the blood after a mixed meal depend on the composition of the meal, because glucose stimulates insulin release and amino acids stimulate glucagon release. However, amino acids also induce insulin secretion but not to the same extent that glucose does. Although this may seem paradoxical, it actually makes good sense. Insulin release stimulates amino acid uptake by tissues and enhances protein synthesis. However, because glucagon levels also increase in response to a protein meal and the critical factor is the insulin to glucagon ratio, sufficient glucagon is released that gluconeogenesis is enhanced (at the expense of protein synthesis), and the amino acids that are taken up by the tissues serve as a substrate for gluconeogenesis. The synthesis of glycogen and triglycerides is also reduced when glucagon levels rise in the blood.

## IV. MECHANISMS OF HORMONE ACTION

For a hormone to affect the flux of substrates through a metabolic pathway, it must be able to change the rate at which that pathway proceeds by increasing or decreasing the rate of the slowest step(s). Either directly or indirectly, hormones affect the activity of specific enzymes or transport proteins that regulate the flux through a pathway. Thus, ultimately, the hormone must either cause the amount of the substrate for the enzyme to increase (if substrate supply is a rate-limiting factor), change the conformation at the active site by phosphorylating the enzyme, change the concentration of

 Patients with type 1 diabetes mellitus, such as **Dianne A.**, have almost undetectable levels of insulin in their blood. Patients with type 2 diabetes mellitus, such as **Deborah S.**, conversely, have normal or even elevated levels of insulin in their blood; however, the level of insulin in their blood is inappropriately low relative to their elevated blood glucose concentration. In type 2 diabetes mellitus, skeletal muscle, liver, and other tissues exhibit a resistance to the actions of insulin. As a result, insulin has a smaller than normal effect on glucose and fat metabolism in such patients. Levels of insulin in the blood must be higher than normal to maintain normal blood glucose levels. In the early stages of type 2 diabetes mellitus, these compensatory adjustments in insulin release may keep the blood glucose levels near the normal range. Over time, as the β-cells' capacity to secrete high levels of insulin declines, blood glucose levels increase, and exogenous insulin becomes necessary.

During the "stress" of hypoglycemia, the autonomic nervous system stimulates the pancreas to secrete glucagon, which tends to restore the serum glucose level to normal. The increased activity of the adrenergic nervous system (through epinephrine) also alerts a patient, such as **Connie C.**, to the presence of increasingly severe hypoglycemia. Hopefully, this will induce the patient to ingest simple sugars or other carbohydrates, which, in turn, will also increase glucose levels in the blood. **Connie C.** gained 8 lb before resection of her pancreatic insulin-secreting adenoma through this mechanism.

an allosteric effector of the enzyme, or change the amount of the protein by inducing or repressing its synthesis or by changing its turnover rate or location. Insulin, glucagon, and other hormones use all of these regulatory mechanisms to regulate the rate of flux in metabolic pathways. The effects mediated by phosphorylation or changes in the kinetic properties of an enzyme occur rapidly within minutes. In contrast, it may take hours for induction or repression of enzyme synthesis to change the amount of an enzyme in the cell.

The details of hormone action were previously described in Chapter 8 and are only summarized here.

### A. Signal Transduction by Hormones that Bind to Plasma Membrane Receptors

Hormones initiate their actions on target cells by binding to specific receptors or binding proteins. In the case of polypeptide hormones (such as insulin and glucagon) and catecholamines (epinephrine and norepinephrine), the action of the hormone is mediated through binding to a specific receptor on the plasma membrane. The first message of the hormone is transmitted to intracellular enzymes by the activated receptor and an intracellular second messenger; the hormone does not need to enter the cell to exert its effects. (In contrast, steroid hormones such as cortisol and the thyroid hormone triiodothyronine [$T_3$] enter the cytosol and eventually move into the cell nucleus to exert their effects.)

The mechanism by which the message carried by the hormone ultimately affects the rate of the regulatory enzyme in the target cell is called **signal transduction**. The three basic types of signal transduction for hormones binding to receptors on the plasma membrane are (a) receptor coupling to adenylate cyclase which produces cyclic adenosine monophosphate (cAMP), (b) receptor kinase activity, and (c) receptor coupling to hydrolysis of phosphatidylinositol bisphosphate (PIP$_2$). The hormones of metabolic homeostasis each use one of these mechanisms to carry out their physiological effect. In addition, some hormones and neurotransmitters act through receptor coupling to gated ion channels (previously described in Chapter 8).

### 1. SIGNAL TRANSDUCTION BY INSULIN

Insulin initiates its action by binding to a receptor on the plasma membrane of insulin's many target cells (see Fig. 8.12). The insulin receptor has two types of subunits: the α-subunits to which insulin binds, and the β-subunits, which span the membrane and protrude into the cytosol. The cytosolic portion of the β-subunit has tyrosine kinase activity. On binding of insulin, the tyrosine kinase phosphorylates tyrosine residues on the β-subunit (autophosphorylation) as well as on several other enzymes within the cytosol. A principal substrate for phosphorylation by the receptor, insulin receptor substrate 1 (IRS-1), then recognizes and binds to various signal transduction proteins in regions referred to as SH$_2$ domains. IRS-1 is involved in many of the physiological responses to insulin through complex mechanisms that are the subject of intensive investigation. The basic tissue-specific cellular responses to insulin, however, can be grouped into five major categories: (a) insulin reverses glucagon-stimulated phosphorylation, (b) insulin works through a phosphorylation cascade that stimulates the phosphorylation of several enzymes, (c) insulin induces and represses the synthesis of specific enzymes, (d) insulin acts as a growth factor and has a general stimulatory effect on protein synthesis, and (e) insulin stimulates glucose and amino acid transport into cells (Fig. 21.10).

Several mechanisms have been proposed for the action of insulin in reversing glucagon-stimulated phosphorylation of the enzymes of carbohydrate metabolism. From the student's point of view, the ability of insulin to reverse glucagon-stimulated phosphorylation occurs as if it were lowering cAMP and stimulating phosphatases that could remove those phosphates added by protein kinase A. In reality, the mechanism is more complex and still not fully understood.

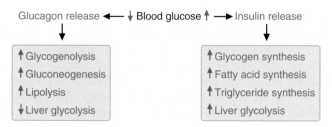

*FIG. 21.10.* Pathways regulated by the release of glucagon (in response to a lowering of blood glucose levels) and insulin (released in response to an elevation of blood glucose levels). Tissue-specific differences occur in the response to these hormones, as detailed in subsequent chapters of this text.

## 2.  SIGNAL TRANSDUCTION BY GLUCAGON

The pathway for signal transduction by glucagon is one that is common to several hormones; the glucagon receptor is coupled to adenylate cyclase and cAMP production (see Fig. 8.13). Glucagon, through G proteins, activates the membrane-bound adenylate cyclase, increasing the synthesis of the intracellular second messenger 3′,5′-cyclic AMP (cAMP) (see Fig. 7.9A). cAMP activates protein kinase A (cAMP-dependent protein kinase), which changes the activity of enzymes by phosphorylating them at specific serine residues. Phosphorylation activates some enzymes and inhibits others.

The G proteins, which couple the glucagon receptor to adenylate cyclase, are proteins in the plasma membrane that bind guanosine triphosphate (GTP) and have dissociable subunits that interact with both the receptor and adenylate cyclase. In the absence of glucagon, the stimulatory $G_s$ protein complex binds guanosine diphosphate (GDP) but cannot bind to the unoccupied receptor or adenylate cyclase (see Fig. 8.14). Once glucagon binds to the receptor, the receptor also binds the $G_s$ complex, which then releases GDP and binds GTP. The α-subunit then dissociates from the βγ-subunits and binds to adenylate cyclase, thereby activating it. As the GTP on the α-subunit is hydrolyzed to GDP, the subunit dissociates and recomplexes with the β- and γ-subunits. Only continued occupancy of the glucagon receptor can keep adenylate cyclase active.

Although glucagon works by activating adenylate cyclase, a few hormones inhibit adenylate cyclase. In this case, the inhibitory G protein complex is called a **$G_i$ complex**.

cAMP is very rapidly degraded to AMP by a membrane-bound phosphodiesterase. The concentration of cAMP is thus very low in the cell so changes in its concentration can occur rapidly in response to changes in the rate of synthesis. The amount of cAMP present at any time is a direct reflection of hormone binding and the activity of adenylate cyclase. It is not affected by ATP, ADP, or AMP levels in the cell.

cAMP transmits the hormone signal to the cell by activating protein kinase A (cAMP-dependent protein kinase). As cAMP binds to the regulatory subunits of protein kinase A, these subunits dissociate from the catalytic subunits, which are thereby activated. Activated protein kinase A phosphorylates serine residues of key regulatory enzymes in the pathways of carbohydrate and fat metabolism. Some enzymes are activated and others are inhibited by this change in phosphorylation state. The message of the hormone is terminated by the action of semispecific protein phosphatases that remove phosphate groups from the enzymes. The activity of the protein phosphatases is also controlled through hormonal regulation.

Changes in the phosphorylation state of proteins that bind to cAMP response elements (CREs) in the promoter region of genes contribute to the regulation of gene transcription by several cAMP-coupled hormones (see Chapter 13). For instance, cAMP response element binding protein (CREB) is directly phosphorylated by protein kinase A, a step essential for the initiation of transcription. Phosphorylation at other sites on CREB, by a variety of kinases, may also play a role in regulating transcription.

cAMP is the intracellular second messenger for a number of hormones that regulate fuel metabolism. The specificity of the physiological response to each hormone results from the presence of specific receptors for that hormone in target tissues. For example, glucagon activates glucose production from glycogen in liver but not in skeletal muscle because glucagon receptors are present in liver but absent in skeletal muscle. However, skeletal muscle has adenylate cyclase, cAMP, and protein kinase A, which can be activated by epinephrine binding to the $β_2$-receptors in the membrane of muscle cells. Liver cells also have epinephrine receptors.

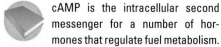 Phosphodiesterase is inhibited by methylxanthines, a class of compounds that includes caffeine. Would the effect of a methylxanthine on fuel metabolism be similar to fasting or to a high-carbohydrate meal?

**A:** Inhibition of phosphodiesterase by methylxanthine would increase cAMP and have the same effects on fuel metabolism as would an increase of glucagon and epinephrine, as in the fasted state. Increased fuel mobilization would occur through glycogenolysis (the release of glucose from glycogen) and through lipolysis (the release of fatty acids from triacylglycerols).

The mechanism for signal transduction by glucagon illustrates some of the important principles of hormonal signaling mechanisms. The first principle is that specificity of action in tissues is conferred by the receptor on a target cell for glucagon. In general, the major actions of glucagon occur in liver, adipose tissue, and certain cells of the kidney that contain glucagon receptors. The second principle is that signal transduction involves amplification of the first message. Glucagon and other hormones are present in the blood in very low concentrations. However, these minute concentrations of hormone are adequate to initiate a cellular response because the binding of one molecule of glucagon to one receptor ultimately activates many protein kinase A molecules, each of which phosphorylates hundreds of downstream enzymes. The third principle involves integration of metabolic responses. For instance, the glucagon-stimulated phosphorylation of enzymes simultaneously activates glycogen degradation, inhibits glycogen synthesis, and inhibits glycolysis in the liver (see Fig. 21.10). The fourth principle involves augmentation and antagonism of signals. An example of augmentation involves the actions of glucagon and epinephrine (which is released during exercise). Although these hormones bind to different receptors, each can increase cAMP and stimulate glycogen degradation. A fifth principle is that of rapid signal termination. In the case of glucagon, both the termination of the $G_s$ protein activation and the rapid degradation of cAMP contribute to signal termination.

## B. Signal Transduction by Cortisol and Other Hormones that Interact with Intracellular Receptors

Signal transduction by the glucocorticoid cortisol and other steroids that have glucocorticoid activity and by thyroid hormone involves hormone binding to intracellular (cytosolic) receptors or binding proteins, after which this hormone-binding protein complex, if not already in the nucleus, moves into the nucleus, where it interacts with chromatin. This interaction changes the rate of gene transcription in the target cells (see Chapter 13). The cellular responses to these hormones continue as long as the target cell is exposed to the specific hormones. Thus, disorders that cause a chronic excess in their secretion will result in an equally persistent influence on fuel metabolism. For example, chronic stress such as that seen in prolonged sepsis may lead to varying degrees of glucose intolerance if high levels of epinephrine and cortisol persist.

The effects of cortisol on gene transcription are usually synergistic to those of certain other hormones. For instance, the rates of gene transcription for some of the enzymes in the pathway for glucose synthesis from amino acids (gluconeogenesis) are induced by glucagon as well as by cortisol.

## C. Signal Transduction by Epinephrine and Norepinephrine

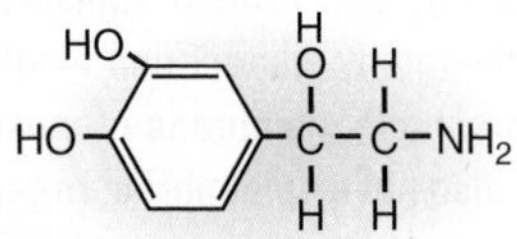

Epinephrine and norepinephrine are catecholamines (Fig. 21.11). They can act as neurotransmitters or as hormones. A neurotransmitter allows a neural signal to be transmitted across the juncture or synapse between the nerve terminal of a proximal nerve axon and the cell body of a distal neuron. A hormone, conversely, is released into the blood and travels in the circulation to interact with specific receptors on the plasma membrane or cytosol of the target organ. The general effect of these catecholamines is to prepare us for fight or flight. Under these acutely stressful circumstances, these "stress" hormones increase fuel mobilization, cardiac output, blood flow, and so on, which enable us to meet these stresses. The catecholamines bind to adrenergic receptors (the term *adrenergic* refers to nerve cells or fibers that are part of the involuntary or autonomic nervous system, a system that employs norepinephrine as a neurotransmitter).

There are nine different types of adrenergic receptors: $\alpha_{1A}$, $\alpha_{1B}$, $\alpha_{1D}$, $\alpha_{2A}$, $\alpha_{2B}$, $\alpha_{2C}$, $\beta_1$, $\beta_2$, and $\beta_3$. Only the three $\beta$- and $\alpha_1$- receptors are discussed here. The three $\beta$-receptors work through the adenylate cyclase–cAMP system, activating a $G_s$ protein, which activates adenylate cyclase, and eventually protein kinase A. The $\beta_1$-receptor is the major adrenergic receptor in the human heart and is primarily stimulated by norepinephrine. On activation, the $\beta_1$-receptor increases the rate of muscle contraction.

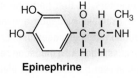

**FIG. 21.11.** Structure of epinephrine and norepinephrine. Epinephrine and norepinephrine are synthesized from tyrosine and act as both hormones and neurotransmitters. They are catecholamines, the term catechol referring to a ring structure containing two hydroxyl groups.

The $\beta_2$-receptor is present in liver, skeletal muscle, and other tissues and is involved in the mobilization of fuels (such as the release of glucose through glycogenolysis). It also mediates vascular, bronchial, and uterine smooth muscle contraction. Epinephrine is a much more potent agonist for this receptor than norepinephrine, whose major action is neurotransmission. The $\beta_3$-receptor is found predominantly in adipose tissue and to a lesser extent in skeletal muscle. Activation of this receptor stimulates fatty acid oxidation and thermogenesis, and agonists for this receptor may prove to be beneficial weight loss agents. The $\alpha_1$-receptors, which are postsynaptic receptors, mediate vascular and smooth muscle contraction as well as glycogenolysis in liver. The $\alpha_1$-receptors work through the $PIP_2$ system via activation of a $G_q$ protein and phospholipase C-$\beta$.

## CLINICAL COMMENTS

Diseases discussed in this chapter are summarized in Table 21.2.

**Deborah S.** Deborah S. has type 2 diabetes mellitus (formerly called non–insulin-dependent diabetes mellitus), whereas **Dianne A.** has type 1 diabetes mellitus (formally designated insulin-dependent diabetes mellitus). Although the pathogenesis differs for these major forms of diabetes mellitus, both cause varying degrees of hyperglycemia. In type 1 diabetes mellitus, the pancreatic $\beta$-cells are gradually destroyed by antibodies directed at a variety of proteins within the $\beta$-cells. As insulin secretory capacity by the $\beta$-cells gradually diminishes below a critical level, the symptoms of chronic hyperglycemia develop rapidly. In type 2 diabetes mellitus, these symptoms develop more subtly and gradually over the course of months or years. Eighty-five percent or more of type 2 patients are obese and, like **Ivan A.**, have a high waist-hip ratio with regard to adipose tissue disposition. This abnormal distribution of fat in the visceral (peri-intestinal) adipocytes is associated with reduced sensitivity of fat cells, muscle cells, and liver cells to the actions of insulin outlined previously. This insulin resistance can be diminished through weight loss, specifically in the visceral depots.

**Connie C.** Connie C. underwent an ultrasonographic (ultrasound) study of her upper abdomen, which showed a 2.6-cm mass in the midportion of her pancreas. With this finding, her physicians decided that further noninvasive studies would not be necessary before surgery and removal of the mass. At the time of surgery, a yellow-white 2.8-cm mass consisting primarily of insulin-rich $\beta$-cells was resected from her pancreas. No cytologic changes of malignancy were seen on cytologic examination of the surgical specimen, and no evidence of malignant behavior by the tumor (such as local metastases) was found. Connie had an uneventful postoperative recovery and no longer experienced the signs and symptoms of insulin-induced hypoglycemia.

**Deborah S.**, a patient with type 2 diabetes mellitus, is experiencing insulin resistance. Her levels of circulating insulin are normal to high, although inappropriately low for her elevated level of blood glucose. However, her insulin target cells, such as muscle and fat, do not respond as those of a nondiabetic subject would to this level of insulin. For most type 2 patients, the site of insulin resistance is subsequent to binding of insulin to its receptor; that is, the number of receptors and their affinity for insulin is near normal. However, the binding of insulin at these receptors does not elicit most of the normal intracellular effects of insulin discussed previously. Consequently, there is little stimulation of glucose metabolism and storage after a high-carbohydrate meal and little inhibition of hepatic gluconeogenesis.

**Table 21.2   Diseases Discussed in Chapter 21**

| Disease or Disorder | Environmental or Genetic | Comments |
|---|---|---|
| Type 2 diabetes | Both | Emergence of insulin resistance due to a wide variety of causes; tissues do not respond to insulin as they normally would. |
| Insulinoma | Both | Periodic release of insulin from a tumor of the $\beta$-cells, leading to hypoglycemic symptoms, which are accompanied by excessive appetite and weight gain. |
| Hyperglycemia | Both | Constantly elevated levels of glucose in the circulation due to a wide variety of causes. Hyperglycemia leads to protein glycation and potential loss of protein function in a variety of tissues. |
| Type 1 diabetes | Both | No production of insulin by the $\beta$-cells due to an autoimmune destruction of the $\beta$-cells. Hyperglycemia and ketoacidosis may result from the lack of insulin. |
| Maturity onset diabetes of the young | Genetic | Form of diabetes caused by specific mutations, such as a mutation in pancreatic glucokinase, which alters the set point for insulin release from the $\beta$-cells. |
| Neonatal diabetes | Genetic | One cause of neonatal diabetes is a mutation in a subunit of the potassium channel in various tissues. Such a mutation in the pancreas leads to permanent opening of the potassium channel, keeping intracellular calcium levels low and difficulty in releasing insulin from the $\beta$-cells. |

1. A patient with type I diabetes mellitus takes an insulin injection before eating dinner but then gets distracted and does not eat. About 3 hours later, the patient becomes shaky, sweaty, and confused. These symptoms have occurred due to which one of the following?

   A. Low blood glucose levels
   B. Increased glucagon release from the pancreas
   C. Decreased glucagon release from the pancreas
   D. High blood glucose levels
   E. Elevated blood ketone levels

2. Caffeine is a potent inhibitor of the enzyme cAMP phosphodiesterase. Which one of the following consequences would you expect to occur in the liver after drinking two cups of strong expresso coffee?

   A. An inhibition of protein kinase A
   B. An enhancement of glycolytic activity
   C. A reduced rate of glucose export to the circulation
   D. A prolonged response to insulin
   E. A prolonged response to glucagon

3. Assume that a rise in blood glucose concentration from 5 to 10 mM would result in insulin release by the pancreas. A mutation in pancreatic glucokinase can lead to MODY due to which one of the following within the pancreatic β-cell?

   A. An inability to raise cAMP levels
   B. An inability to raise ATP levels

   C. An inability to stimulate gene transcription
   D. An inability to activate glycogen degradation
   E. An inability to raise intracellular lactate levels

4. A patient is rushed to the emergency room after a fainting episode. Blood glucose levels were extremely low; insulin levels were normal, but there was no detectable C-peptide. The cause of the fainting episode may be due to which one of the following?

   A. An insulin-producing tumor
   B. A glucagon-producing tumor
   C. An overdose of glucagon
   D. An overdose of insulin
   E. An overdose of epinephrine

5. Assume that an individual had a glucagon-secreting pancreatic tumor (glucagonoma). Which one of the following is most likely to result from hyperglucagonemia?

   A. Hypoglycemia
   B. Weight loss
   C. Increased muscle protein synthesis
   D. Decreased lipolysis
   E. Increased liver glycolytic rate

# 22 Digestion, Absorption, and Transport of Carbohydrates

## CHAPTER OUTLINE

## KEY POINTS

- The major carbohydrates in the American diet are starch, lactose, and sucrose.
- Starch is a polysaccharide composed of many glucose units linked together through α-1,4- and α-1,6-glycosidic bonds (see Fig. 3.11).
- Lactose is a disaccharide composed of glucose and galactose.
- Sucrose is a disaccharide composed of glucose and fructose.
- Digestion converts all dietary carbohydrates to their respective monosaccharides.
- Amylase digests starch; it is found in the saliva and pancreas, which releases it into the small intestine.
- Intestinal epithelial cells contain disaccharidases, which cleave lactose, sucrose, and digestion products of starch into monosaccharides.
- Dietary fiber is composed of polysaccharides that cannot be digested by human enzymes.
- Monosaccharides are transported into the absorptive intestinal epithelial cells via active transport systems.
- Monosaccharides released into the blood via the intestinal epithelial cells are recovered by tissues that utilize facilitative transporters.

# THE WAITING ROOM

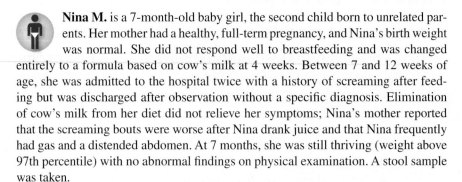

**Deborah S.'s** fasting and postprandial blood glucose levels are frequently above the normal range in spite of good compliance with insulin therapy. Her physician has referred her to a dietician skilled in training diabetic patients in the successful application of an appropriate American Diabetes Association diet. As part of the program, Ms. S. is asked to incorporate foods containing fiber into her diet, such as whole grains (e.g., wheat, oats, corn), legumes (e.g., peas, beans, lentils), tubers (e.g., potatoes, peanuts), and fruits.

**Nina M.** is a 7-month-old baby girl, the second child born to unrelated parents. Her mother had a healthy, full-term pregnancy, and Nina's birth weight was normal. She did not respond well to breastfeeding and was changed entirely to a formula based on cow's milk at 4 weeks. Between 7 and 12 weeks of age, she was admitted to the hospital twice with a history of screaming after feeding but was discharged after observation without a specific diagnosis. Elimination of cow's milk from her diet did not relieve her symptoms; Nina's mother reported that the screaming bouts were worse after Nina drank juice and that Nina frequently had gas and a distended abdomen. At 7 months, she was still thriving (weight above 97th percentile) with no abnormal findings on physical examination. A stool sample was taken.

The dietary sugar in fruit juice and other sweets is sucrose, a disaccharide composed of glucose and fructose joined through their anomeric carbons. **Nina M.'s** symptoms of pain and abdominal distension are caused by an inability to digest sucrose or absorb fructose, which are converted to gas by colonic bacteria. Nina's stool sample had a pH of 5 and gave a positive test for sugar. The possibility of carbohydrate malabsorption was considered, and a hydrogen breath test was recommended.

## I.  DIETARY CARBOHYDRATES

Carbohydrates are the largest source of calories in the average American diet and usually constitute 40% to 45% of our caloric intake. The plant **starches amylopectin** and **amylose**, which are present in grains, tubers, and vegetables, constitute approximately 50% to 60% of the carbohydrate calories consumed. These starches are polysaccharides, containing 10,000 to 1 million glucosyl units. In amylose, the glucosyl residues form a straight chain linked via α-1,4-glycosidic bonds; in amylopectin, the α-1,4-chains contain branches connected via α-1,6-glycosidic bonds (Fig. 22.1). The other major sugar found in fruits and vegetables is **sucrose**, a disaccharide of glucose and fructose (see Fig. 22.1). Sucrose and small amounts of the monosaccharides **glucose** and **fructose** are the major natural sweeteners found in fruit, honey, and vegetables. **Dietary fiber**, the part of the diet that cannot be digested by human enzymes of the intestinal tract, is also composed principally of plant polysaccharides and a polymer called **lignin**.

Many foods derived from animals, such as meat or fish, contain very little carbohydrate except for small amounts of glycogen (which has a structure similar to amylopectin) and glycolipids. The major dietary carbohydrate of animal origin is **lactose**, a disaccharide composed of glucose and galactose that is found exclusively in milk and milk products (see Fig. 22.1).

Although all cells require glucose for metabolic functions, neither glucose nor other sugars are specifically required in the diet. Glucose can be synthesized from many amino acids found in dietary protein. Fructose, galactose, xylulose, and all the other sugars required for metabolic processes in the human can be synthesized from glucose.

## II.  DIGESTION OF DIETARY CARBOHYDRATES

In the digestive tract, dietary polysaccharides and disaccharides are converted to monosaccharides by **glycosidases**, enzymes that hydrolyze the glycosidic bonds between the sugars. All of these enzymes exhibit some specificity for the sugar, the

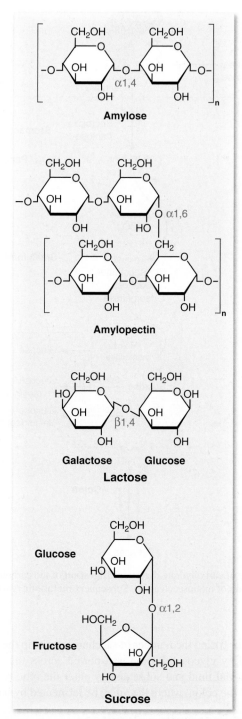

***FIG. 22.1.*** The structures of common dietary carbohydrates. For disaccharides and higher, the sugars are linked through glycosidic bonds between the anomeric carbon of one sugar and a hydroxyl group on another sugar. The glycosidic bond may be either α or β, depending on its position above or below the plane of the sugar containing the anomeric carbon (see Chapter 3, Section II.A, to review terms used in the description of sugars). The starch amylose is a polysaccharide of glucose residues linked with α-1,4-glycosidic bonds. Amylopectin is amylose with the addition of α-1,6-glycosidic branch points. Dietary sugars may be monosaccharides (single sugar residues), disaccharides (two sugar residues), oligosaccharides (several sugar residues), or polysaccharides (hundreds of sugar residues). For clarity, the hydrogen atoms are not shown in the figure.

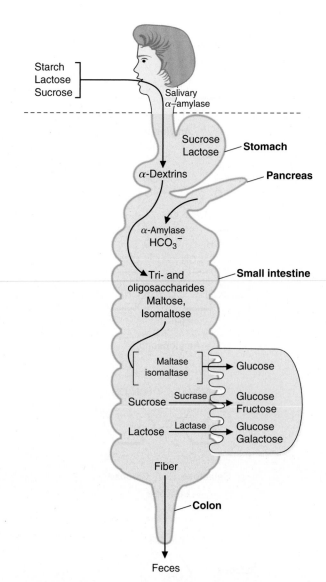

**FIG. 22.2.** Overview of carbohydrate digestion. **Digestion** of the carbohydrates occurs first, followed by **absorption** of monosaccharides. Subsequent **metabolic** reactions occur after the sugars are absorbed.

glycosidic bond ($\alpha$ or $\beta$) and the number of saccharide units in the chain. The monosaccharides formed by glycosidases are transported across the intestinal mucosal cells into the interstitial fluid and subsequently enter the bloodstream. Undigested carbohydrates enter the colon, where they may be fermented by bacteria (Fig. 22.2).

## A. Salivary and Pancreatic $\alpha$-Amylase

The digestion of starch (amylopectin and amylose) begins in the mouth, where chewing mixes the food with saliva. The salivary glands secrete approximately 1 L of liquid per day into the mouth, containing **salivary $\alpha$-amylase** and other components. $\alpha$-Amylase is an **endoglucosidase**, which means that it hydrolyzes internal $\alpha$-1,4 bonds between glucosyl residues at random intervals in the polysaccharide chains (Fig. 22.3). The shortened polysaccharide chains that are formed are called **$\alpha$-dextrins**. Salivary $\alpha$-amylase is largely inactivated by the acidity of the stomach contents, which contain HCl secreted by the parietal cells.

The acidic gastric juice enters the duodenum, the upper part of the small intestine, where digestion continues. Secretions from the exocrine pancreas (approximately

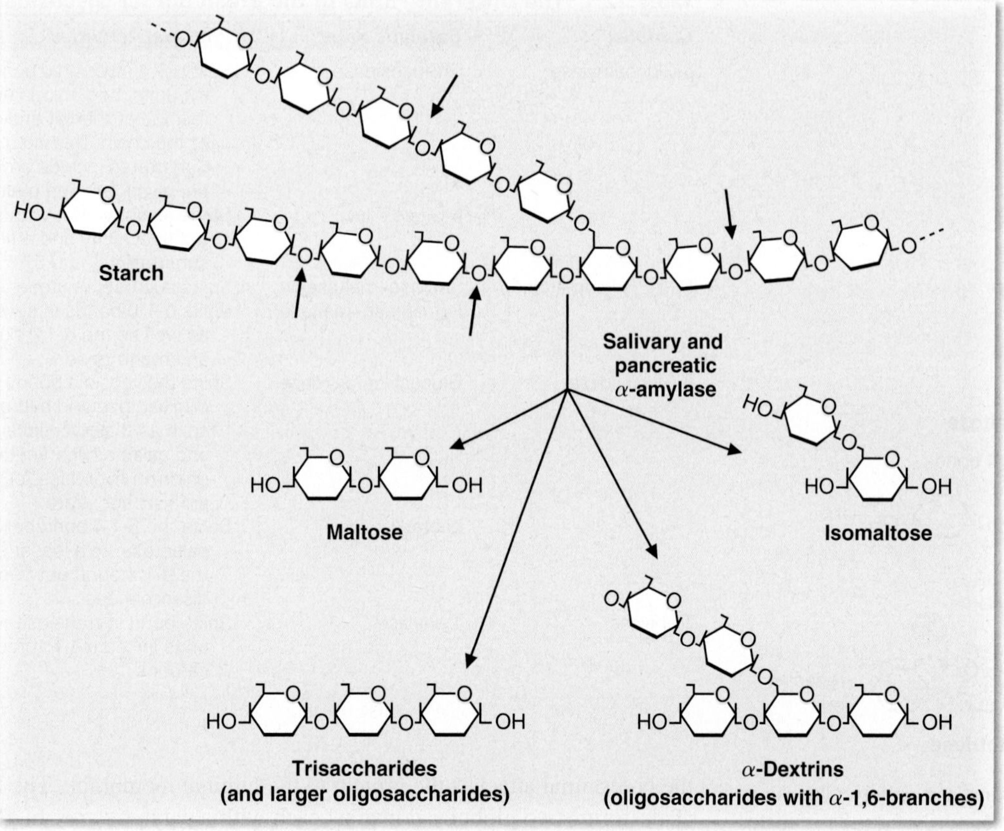

**Starch**

**Salivary and pancreatic α-amylase**

**Maltose**

**Isomaltose**

**Trisaccharides**
**(and larger oligosaccharides)**

**α-Dextrins**
**(oligosaccharides with α-1,6-branches)**

*FIG. 22.3.* Action of salivary and pancreatic α-amylase.

1.5 L/day) flow down the pancreatic duct and also enter the duodenum. These secretions contain bicarbonate ($HCO_3^-$), which neutralizes the acidic pH of stomach contents, and digestive enzymes, including pancreatic α-amylase.

Pancreatic α-amylase continues to hydrolyze the starches and glycogen, forming the disaccharide maltose, the trisaccharide maltotriose, and oligosaccharides. These oligosaccharides, called **limit dextrins**, are usually four to nine glucosyl units long and contain one or more α-1,6 branches. The two glucosyl residues that contain the α-1,6-glycosidic bond eventually become the disaccharide isomaltose, but α-amylase does not cleave these branched oligosaccharides all the way down to isomaltose.

α-Amylase has no activity toward sugar-containing polymers other than glucose linked by α-1,4 bonds. α-Amylase displays no activity toward the α-1,6 bond at branch points and has little activity for the α-1,4 bond at the nonreducing end of a chain.

### B. Disaccharidases of the Intestinal Brush Border Membrane

The dietary disaccharides lactose and sucrose, as well as the products of starch digestion, are converted to monosaccharides by glycosidases attached to the membrane in the brush border of absorptive cells. The different glycosidase activities are found in four glycoproteins: glucoamylase, the sucrase–maltase complex, the smaller glycoprotein trehalase, and lactase-glucosylceramidase (Table 22.1). These glycosidases are collectively called the **small intestinal disaccharidases**, although glucoamylase is really an oligosaccharidase.

### 1. GLUCOAMYLASE

Glucoamylase and the sucrase–isomaltase complex have similar structures and exhibit a great deal of sequence homogeneity. A membrane-spanning domain near

Amylase activity in the gut is abundant and is not normally rate limiting for the process of digestion. Alcohol-induced pancreatitis or surgical removal of part of the pancreas can decrease pancreatic secretion. Pancreatic exocrine secretion into the intestine can also be decreased due to cystic fibrosis in which mucus blocks the pancreatic duct, which eventually degenerates. However, pancreatic exocrine secretion can be decreased to 10% of normal and still not affect the rate of starch digestion, because amylases are secreted in the saliva and pancreatic fluid in excessive amounts. In contrast, protein and fat digestion are more strongly affected in cystic fibrosis.

**Table 22.1  The Different Forms of the Brush Border Glycosidases**

| Complex | Catalytic Sites | Principal Activities |
|---|---|---|
| β-Glucoamylase | α-Glucosidase | Split α-1,4-glycosidic bonds between glucosyl units, beginning sequentially with the residue at the tail end (nonreducing end) of the chain. This is an exoglycosidase. Substrates include amylase, amylopectin, glycogen, and maltose. |
| | β-Glucosidase | Same as above but with slightly different specificity and affinities for the substrates. |
| Sucrase–isomaltase | Sucrase–maltase | Splits sucrose, maltose, and maltotriose |
| | Isomaltase–maltase | Splits α-1,6 bonds in several limit dextrins, as well as the α-1,4 bonds in maltose and maltotriose |
| β-Glycosidase | Glucosylceramidase | Splits β-glycosidic bonds between glucose or galactose and hydrophobic residues, such as the glycolipids glucosylceramide and galactosylceramide. Also known as phlorizin hydrolase for its activity on an artificial substrate. |
| | Lactase | Splits the β-1,4 bond between glucose and galactose. To a lesser extent also splits the β-1,4 bond between some cellulose disaccharides. |
| Trehalase | Trehalase | Splits bond in trehalose, which is 2 glucosyl units linked α-1,1 through their anomeric carbons. |

**Maltose**

α-1,4 bond

**Maltotriose**

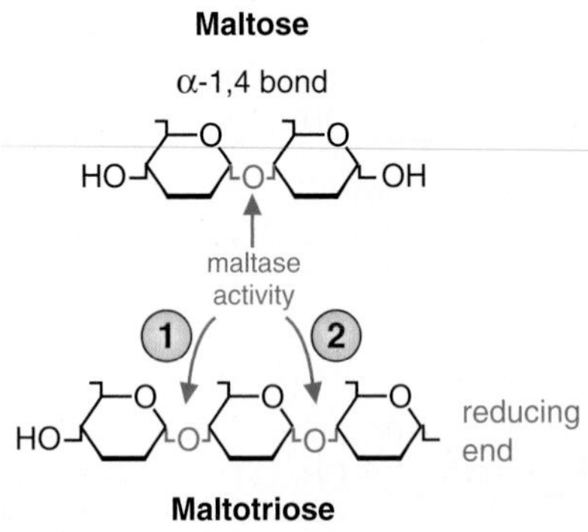

**FIG. 22.4.** Glucoamylase activity. Glucoamylase is an α-1,4-exoglycosidase that initiates cleavage at the nonreducing end of the sugar. Thus, for maltotriose, the bond labeled *1* is hydrolyzed first, which then allows the bond at position *2* to be the next one hydrolyzed.

Individuals with genetic deficiencies of the sucrase–isomaltase complex show symptoms of sucrose intolerance but are able to digest normal amounts of starch in a meal without problems. The maltase activity in the glucoamylase complex and residual activity in the sucrase–isomaltase complex (which is normally present in excess of need) is apparently sufficient to digest normal amounts of dietary starch.

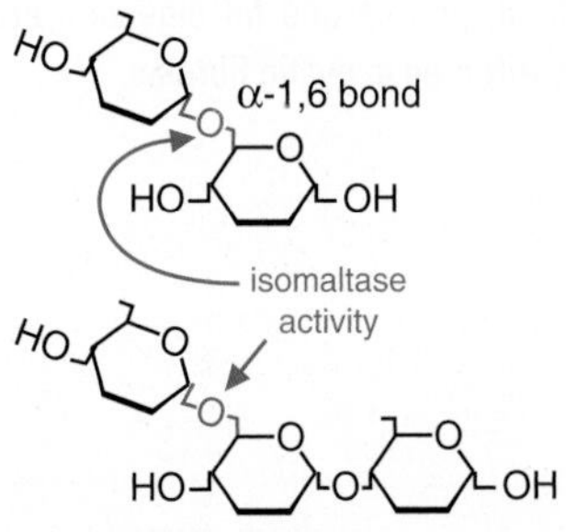

**FIG. 22.5.** Isomaltase activity. *Arrows* indicate the α-1,6 bonds that are cleaved.

the N-terminal attaches the protein to the luminal membrane. The long polypeptide chain forms two globular domains, each with a catalytic site. In glucoamylase, the two catalytic sites have similar activities, with only small differences in substrate specificity. The protein is heavily glycosylated with oligosaccharides that protect it from digestive proteases.

Glucoamylase is an **exoglucosidase** that is specific for the α-1,4 bonds between glucosyl residues (Fig. 22.4). It begins at the nonreducing end of a polysaccharide or limit dextrin and sequentially hydrolyzes the bonds to release glucose monosaccharides. It will digest a limit dextrin down to isomaltose, the glucosyl disaccharide with an α-1,6-branch, that is subsequently hydrolyzed principally by the isomaltase activity in the sucrase–isomaltase complex.

### 2. SUCRASE–ISOMALTASE COMPLEX

The structure of the sucrase–isomaltase complex is similar to that of glucoamylase, and these two proteins have a high degree of sequence homology. However, after the single polypeptide chain of sucrase–isomaltase is inserted through the membrane and the protein protrudes into the intestinal lumen, an intestinal protease clips it into two separate subunits that remain attached to each other. Each subunit has a catalytic site that differs in substrate specificity from the other through noncovalent interactions. The sucrase–maltase site accounts for approximately 100% of the intestine's ability to hydrolyze sucrose in addition to maltase activity; the isomaltase–maltase site accounts for almost all of the intestine's ability to hydrolyze α-1,6 bonds (Fig. 22.5), in addition to maltase activity. Together, these sites account for approximately 80% of the maltase activity of the small intestine. The remainder of the maltase activity is found in the glucoamylase complex.

### 3. TREHALASE

Trehalase is only half as long as the other disaccharidases and has only one catalytic site. It hydrolyzes the glycosidic bond in trehalose, a disaccharide composed of two glucosyl units linked by an α-bond between their anomeric carbons (Fig. 22.6).

Trehalose, which is found in insects, algae, mushrooms, and other fungi, is not currently a major dietary component in the United States. However, unwitting consumption of trehalose can cause nausea, vomiting, and other symptoms of severe gastrointestinal distress if consumed by an individual deficient in the enzyme. Trehalase deficiency was discovered when a woman became very sick after eating mushrooms and was initially thought to have α-amanitin poisoning.

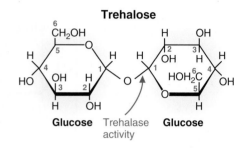

**Trehalose**

**Glucose**    Trehalase activity    **Glucose**

*FIG. 22.6.* Trehalose. This disaccharide contains two glucose moieties linked by an unusual bond that joins their anomeric carbons. It is cleaved by trehalase.

### 4. β-GLYCOSIDASE COMPLEX (LACTASE-GLUCOSYLCERAMIDASE)

The β-glycosidase complex is another large glycoprotein found in the brush border that has two catalytic sites extending in the lumen of the intestine. However, its primary structure is very different from the other enzymes. The lactase catalytic site hydrolyzes the β-bond connecting glucose and galactose in lactose (a β-galactosidase activity; Fig. 22.7). The major activity of the other catalytic site in humans is the β-bond between glucose or galactose and ceramide in glycolipids (this catalytic site is sometimes called **phlorizin hydrolase**, named for its ability to hydrolyze an artificial substrate).

### 5. LOCATION WITHIN THE INTESTINE

The production of maltose, maltotriose, and limit dextrins by pancreatic α-amylase occurs in the duodenum, the most proximal portion of the small intestine. Sucrase–isomaltase activity is highest in the jejunum, where the enzymes can hydrolyze sucrose and the products of starch digestion. β-Glycosidase activity is also highest in the jejunum. Glucoamylase activity increases progressively along the length of the small intestine and its activity is highest in the ileum. Thus, it presents a final opportunity for digestion of starch oligomers that have escaped amylase and disaccharidase activities at the more proximal regions of the intestine.

## C. Metabolism of Sugars by Colonic Bacteria

Not all of the starch ingested as part of foods is normally digested in the small intestine (Fig. 22.8). Starches that are high in amylose or are less well hydrated (e.g., starch in dried beans) are resistant to digestion and enter the colon. Dietary fiber and undigested sugars also enter the colon. Here, colonic bacteria rapidly metabolize the saccharides, forming gases, short-chain fatty acids, and lactate. The major short-chain fatty acids formed are acetic acid (two carbons), propionic acid (three carbons), and butyric acid (four carbons). The short-chain fatty acids are absorbed by the colonic mucosal cells and can provide a substantial source of energy for these cells. The major gases formed are hydrogen ($H_2$) gas, carbon dioxide ($CO_2$), and methane ($CH_4$). These gases are released through the colon, resulting in flatulence, or in the breath. Incomplete products of digestion in the intestines increase the retention of water in the colon, resulting in diarrhea.

## D. Lactose Intolerance

**Lactose intolerance** refers to a condition of pain, nausea, and flatulence after the ingestion of foods containing lactose, most notably dairy products. Although it is often caused by low levels of lactase, it also can be caused by intestinal injury (defined in the following text). The lactose that is not absorbed is converted by colonic bacteria to lactic acid, $CH_4$ gas, and $H_2$ gas (Fig. 22.9). The osmotic effect of the lactose and lactic acid in the bowel lumen is responsible for the diarrhea often seen as part of this syndrome. Similar symptoms can result from sensitivity to milk proteins (milk intolerance) or from the malabsorption of other dietary sugars.

### 1. NONPERSISTENT AND PERSISTENT LACTASE

Lactase activity increases in the human from about 6 to 8 weeks of gestation, and it rises during the late gestational period (27 to 32 weeks) through full term. It remains high for about 1 month after birth and then begins to decline. For most of

**Nina M.** was given a hydrogen breath test, a test measuring the amount of hydrogen gas released after consuming a test dose of sugar. The association of **Nina M.'s** symptoms with her ingestion of fruit juices suggests that she might have a problem resulting from low sucrase activity or an inability to absorb fructose. Her ability to thrive and her adequate weight gain suggest that any deficiencies of the sucrase–isomaltase complex must be partial and do not result in a functionally important reduction in maltase activity. (Maltase activity is also present in the glucoamylase complex). Her urine tested negative for sugar, suggesting the problem is in digestion or absorption, because only sugars that are absorbed and enter the blood can be found in urine. The basis of the hydrogen breath test is that if a sugar is not absorbed, it is metabolized in the intestinal lumen by bacteria that produce various gases, including hydrogen. The test is often accompanied by measurements of the amount of sugar that appear in the blood or feces and acidity of the feces.

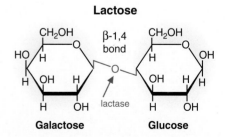

**Lactose**

β-1,4 bond

lactase

**Galactose**    **Glucose**

*FIG. 22.7.* Lactase activity. Lactase is a β-galactosidase. It cleaves the β-galactoside lactose, the major sugar in milk, forming galactose and glucose.

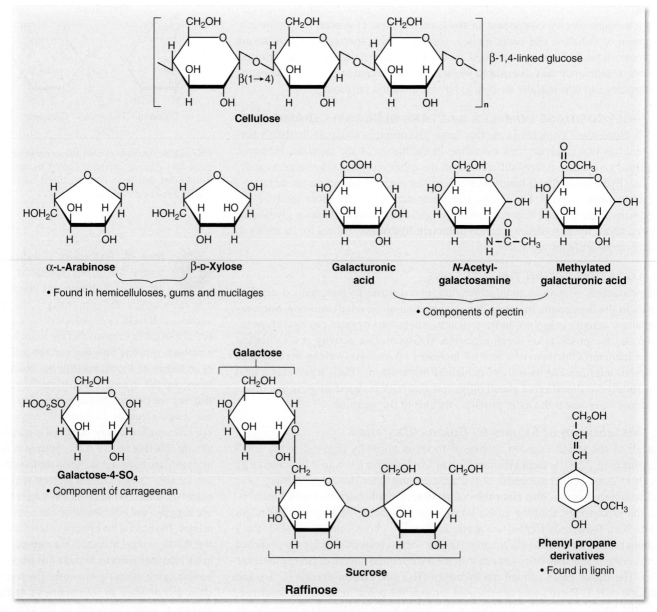

**FIG. 22.8.** Some indigestible carbohydrates. These compounds are components of dietary fiber.

the world's population, lactase activity decreases to adult levels at approximately 5 to 7 years of age. Adult levels are less than 10% of that present in infants. These populations have adult hypolactasia (formerly called adult lactase deficiency) and exhibit the lactase nonpersistence phenotype. In people who are derived mainly from western Northern Europeans and milk-dependent Nomadic tribes of Saharan Africa, the levels of lactase remain at or only slightly below infant levels throughout adulthood (lactase persistence phenotype). Thus, adult hypolactasia is the normal condition for most of the world's population.

In contrast, congenital lactase deficiency is a severe autosomal recessive inherited disease in which lactase activity is significantly reduced or totally absent. The disorder presents as soon as the newborn is fed breast milk or lactose-containing formula, resulting in watery diarrhea, weight loss, and dehydration. Treatment consists of removal of lactose from the diet, which allows for normal growth and development to occur.

## 2. INTESTINAL INJURY

Intestinal diseases that injure the absorptive cells of the intestinal villi diminish lactase activity along the intestine, producing a condition known as secondary lactase deficiency. Kwashiorkor (protein malnutrition), colitis, gastroenteritis, tropical and nontropical sprue, and excessive alcohol consumption fall into this category. These diseases also affect other disaccharidases, but sucrase, maltase, isomaltase, and glucoamylase activities are usually present at such excessive levels that there are no pathological effects. Lactase is usually the first activity lost and the last to recover.

## III. DIETARY FIBER

Dietary fiber is the portion of the diet resistant to digestion by human digestive enzymes. It consists principally of plant materials that are polysaccharide derivatives and lignin (see Fig. 22.8). The components of fiber are often divided into the categories of soluble and insoluble fiber, according to their ability to dissolve in water. Insoluble fiber consists of three major categories: cellulose, hemicellulose, and lignins. Soluble fiber categories include pectins, mucilages, and gums (see the online Table A22.1 @ ). Although human enzymes cannot digest fiber, the bacterial flora in the normal human gut may metabolize the more soluble dietary fibers to gases and short-chain fatty acids, much as they do undigested starch and sugars. Some of these fatty acids may be absorbed and used by the colonic epithelial cells of the gut, and some may travel to the liver through the hepatic portal vein. We may obtain as much as 10% of our total calories from compounds produced by bacterial digestion of substances in our digestive tract.

In 2005, the Committee on Dietary Reference Intakes issued new guidelines for fiber ingestion; anywhere from 25 to 38 g/day, depending on age and sex of the individual. It was also recommended that 14 g of fiber should accompany every 1,000 calories ingested. No distinction was made between soluble and insoluble fibers. Adult males between the ages of 14 and 49 years require 38 g of fiber per day; males aged 50 years or more are recommended to consume 30 g of fiber per day. Females from ages 4 to 8 years require 25 g/day; from ages 9 to 16 years, 26 g/day; and from ages 19 to 50 years, 25 g/day. Women older than 50 years of age are recommended to consume 21 g of fiber per day. These numbers are increased during pregnancy and lactation. One beneficial effect of fiber is seen in diverticular disease in which sacs or pouches may develop in the colon because of a weakening of the muscle and submucosal structures. Fiber is thought to "soften" the stool, thereby reducing pressure on the colonic wall and enhancing expulsion of feces.

## IV. ABSORPTION OF SUGARS

Once the carbohydrates have been split into monosaccharides, the sugars are transported across the intestinal epithelial cells and into the blood for distribution to all tissues. Not all complex carbohydrates are digested at the same rate within the intestine, and some carbohydrate sources lead to a near-immediate rise in blood glucose levels after ingestion, whereas others slowly raise blood glucose levels over an extended period after ingestion. The **glycemic index** of a food is an indication of how rapidly blood glucose levels rise after consumption. Glucose and maltose have the highest glycemic indices (142, with white bread defined as an index of 100). Online Table A22.2 @ indicates the glycemic index for a variety of food types. It is of interest to note that cornflakes and potatoes have high glycemic indices, whereas yogurt and skim milk have particularly low glycemic indices.

### A. Absorption by the Intestinal Epithelium

Glucose is transported through the absorptive cells of the intestine by facilitated diffusion and by $Na^+$-dependent facilitated transport. (See Chapter 8 for a description of transport mechanisms.) Glucose, therefore, enters the absorptive cells by binding

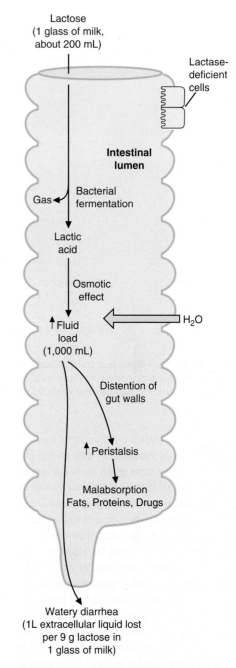

**FIG. 22.9.** Summary of the metabolic fate of lactose in lactase-deficient individuals. The bacteria in the intestine metabolize the lactose to gases and lactic acid, which generates an osmotic imbalance between the intestinal lumen and the cells lining the lumen. Water leaves the cells lining the intestinal lumen to correct this osmotic imbalance, which leads to a watery diarrhea.

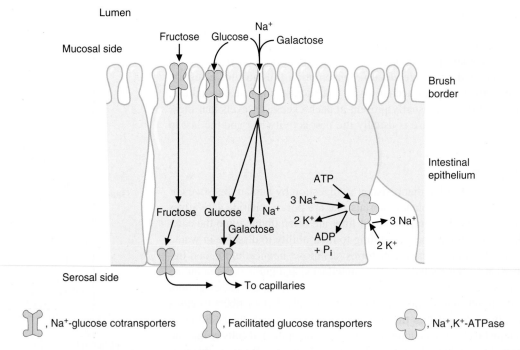

**FIG. 22.10.** $Na^+$-dependent and facilitative transporters in the intestinal epithelial cells. Both glucose and fructose are transported by the facilitated glucose transporters on the luminal and serosal sides of the absorptive cells. Glucose and galactose are transported by the $Na^+$-glucose cotransporters on the luminal (mucosal) side of the absorptive cells.

The glycemic response to ingested foods depends not only on the glycemic index of the foods but also on the fiber and fat content of the food as well as its method of preparation. Highly glycemic carbohydrates can be consumed before and after exercise because their metabolism results in a rapid entry of glucose into the blood, where it is then immediately available for muscle use. Low-glycemic carbohydrates enter the circulation slowly and can be used to best advantage if consumed before exercise such that as exercise progresses, glucose is slowly being absorbed from the intestine into the circulation in which it can be used to maintain blood glucose levels during the exercise period.

to transport proteins, membrane-spanning proteins that bind the glucose molecule on one side of the membrane and release it on the opposite side. This is necessary because the glucose molecule is extremely polar and cannot diffuse through the hydrophobic phospholipid bilayer of the cell membrane. Each hydroxyl group of the glucose molecule forms at least two hydrogen bonds with water molecules, and random movement would require energy to dislodge the polar hydroxyl groups from their hydrogen bonds and to disrupt the Van der Waals forces between the hydrocarbon tails of the fatty acids in the membrane phospholipid. Two types of glucose transport proteins are present in the intestinal absorptive cells: the $Na^+$-dependent glucose transporters and the facilitative glucose transporters (Fig. 22.10).

### 1. NA$^+$-DEPENDENT TRANSPORTERS

$Na^+$-dependent glucose transporters, which are located on the luminal side of the absorptive cells, enable these cells to concentrate glucose from the intestinal lumen.

The dietician explained to **Deborah S.** the rationale for a person with diabetes to take an American Diabetes Association diet plan. It is important for Deborah to add a variety of fibers to her diet. The gel-forming, water-retaining pectins and gums delay gastric emptying and retard the rate of absorption of disaccharides and monosaccharides, thus reducing the rate at which blood glucose levels rise. The glycemic index of foods also needs to be considered for appropriate maintenance of blood glucose levels in persons with diabetes. Consumption of a low glycemic index diet results in a lower rise in blood glucose levels after eating, which can be more easily controlled by exogenous insulin. For example, **Deborah S.** is advised to eat pasta and rice (glycemic indices of 67 and 65, respectively) instead of potatoes (glycemic index of 80 to 120, depending on the method of preparation) and to incorporate breakfast cereals composed of wheat bran, barley, and oats into her morning routine.

A low intracellular $Na^+$ concentration is maintained by a $Na^+,K^+$-ATPase on the serosal (blood) side of the cell that uses the energy from adenosine triphosphate (ATP) cleavage to pump $Na^+$ out of the cell into the blood. Thus, the transport of glucose from a low concentration in the lumen to a high concentration in the cell is promoted by the cotransport of $Na^+$ from a high concentration in the lumen to a low concentration in the cell (secondary active transport). Similar transporters are found in the epithelial cells of the kidney, which are thus able to transport glucose against its concentration gradient.

## 2. FACILITATIVE GLUCOSE TRANSPORTERS

Facilitative glucose transporters, which do not bind $Na^+$, are located on the serosal side of the cells. Glucose moves via the facilitative transporters from the high concentration inside the cell to the lower concentration in the blood without the expenditure of energy. In addition to the $Na^+$-dependent glucose transporters, facilitative transporters for glucose also exist on the luminal side of the absorptive cells. The various types of facilitative glucose transporters found in the plasma membranes of cells (referred to as GLUT 1 to GLUT 5) are described in Table 22.2. One common structural theme to these proteins is that they all contain 12 membrane-spanning domains. Note that the sodium-linked transporter on the luminal side of the intestinal epithelial cell is not a member of the GLUT family.

## 3. GALACTOSE AND FRUCTOSE ABSORPTION THROUGH GLUCOSE TRANSPORTERS

Galactose is absorbed through the same mechanisms as glucose. It enters the absorptive cells on the luminal side via the $Na^+$-dependent glucose transporters and facilitative glucose transporters and is transported through the serosal side on the facilitative glucose transporters.

Fructose both enters and leaves absorptive epithelial cells by facilitated diffusion, apparently via transport proteins that are part of the GLUT family. The transporter on the luminal side has been identified as GLUT 5. Although this transporter can transport glucose, it has a much higher activity with fructose (see Fig. 22.10). Other fructose transport proteins may also be present. For reasons as yet unknown, fructose is absorbed at a much more rapid rate when it is ingested as sucrose than when it is ingested as a monosaccharide.

**Table 22.2  Properties of the GLUT 1 to GLUT 5 Isoforms of the Glucose Transport Proteins**

| Transporter | Tissue Distribution | Comments |
|---|---|---|
| GLUT 1 | Human erythrocyte<br>Blood–brain barrier<br>Blood–retinal barrier<br>Blood–placental barrier<br>Blood–testis barrier | Expressed in cell types with barrier functions; a high-affinity glucose transport system. |
| GLUT 2 | Liver<br>Kidney<br>Pancreatic β-cell<br>Serosal surface of intestinal mucosa cells | A high-capacity, low-affinity transporter<br>May be used as the glucose sensor in the pancreas |
| GLUT 3 | Brain (neurons) | Major transporter in the central nervous system; a high-affinity system |
| GLUT 4 | Adipose tissue<br>Skeletal muscle<br>Heart muscle | Insulin-sensitive transporter. In the presence of insulin, the number of GLUT 4 transporters increases on the cell surface; a high-affinity system. |
| GLUT 5 | Intestinal epithelium<br>Spermatozoa | This is actually a fructose transporter. |

Genetic techniques have identified additional GLUT transporters (GLUT 6 to 12), but the role of these transporters has not yet been fully described.

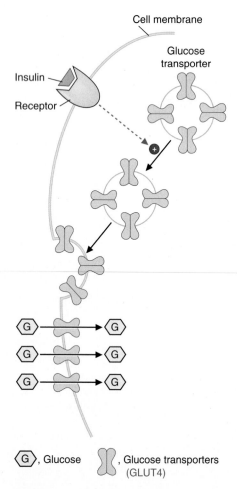

*Cell membrane*

*Glucose transporter*

*Insulin*

*Receptor*

$+$

G → G

G → G

G → G

G , Glucose          , Glucose transporters (GLUT4)

**FIG. 22.11.** Stimulation by insulin of glucose transport into muscle and adipose cells. Binding of insulin to its cell membrane receptor causes vesicles containing glucose transport proteins to move from inside the cell to the cell membrane.

### B. Transport of Monosaccharides into Tissues

The properties of the GLUT transport proteins differ among tissues, reflecting the function of glucose metabolism in each tissue. In most cell types, the rate of glucose transport across the cell membrane is not rate limiting for glucose metabolism. This is because the isoform of transporter present in these cell types has a relatively low $K_m$ for glucose (i.e., a low concentration of glucose will result in half the maximal rate of glucose transport) or is present in relatively high concentration in the cell membrane so that the intracellular glucose concentration reflects that in the blood. Because the hexokinase isozyme present in these cells has an even lower $K_m$ for glucose (0.05 to 0.10 mM), variations in blood glucose levels do not affect the intracellular rate of glucose phosphorylation. However, in several tissues, the rate of transport becomes rate limiting when the serum level of glucose is low or when low levels of insulin signal the absence of dietary glucose.

The erythrocyte (red blood cell) is an example of a tissue in which glucose transport is not rate limiting. Although the glucose transporter (GLUT 1) has a $K_m$ of 1 to 7 mM, it is present in extremely high concentrations, constituting approximately 5% of all membrane proteins. Consequently, as the blood glucose levels fall from a postprandial level of 140 mg/dL (7.5 mM) to the normal fasting level of 80 mg/dL (4.5 mM) or even the hypoglycemic level of 40 mg/dL (2.2 mM), the supply of glucose is still adequate for the rates at which glycolysis and the pentose phosphate pathway operate.

In the liver, the $K_m$ for the glucose transporter (GLUT 2) is relatively high compared with that of other tissues, probably 15 mM or above. This is in keeping with the liver's role as the organ that maintains blood glucose levels. Thus, the liver will only convert glucose into other energy storage molecules only when blood glucose levels are high, such as the time immediately after ingesting a meal. In muscle and adipose tissue, the transport of glucose is greatly stimulated by insulin. The mechanism involves the recruitment of glucose transporters (specifically, GLUT 4) from intracellular vesicles into the plasma membrane (Fig. 22.11). In adipose tissue, the stimulation of glucose transport across the plasma membrane by insulin increases its availability for the synthesis of fatty acids and glycerol from the glycolytic pathway. In skeletal muscle, the stimulation of glucose transport by insulin increases its availability for glycolysis and glycogen synthesis.

## V.  GLUCOSE TRANSPORT THROUGH THE BLOOD–BRAIN BARRIER AND INTO NEURONS

A hypoglycemic response is elicited by a decrease of blood glucose concentration to some point between 18 and 54 mg/dL (1 and 3 mM). The hypoglycemic response is a result of a decreased supply of glucose to the brain and starts with lightheadedness and dizziness and may progress to coma. The slow rate of transport of glucose through the blood–brain barrier (from the blood into the cerebrospinal fluid) at low levels of glucose is thought to be responsible for this neuroglycopenic response. Glucose transport from the cerebrospinal fluid across the plasma membranes of neurons is rapid and is not rate limiting for ATP generation from glycolysis.

In the brain, the endothelial cells of the capillaries have extremely tight junctions, and glucose must pass from the blood into the extracellular cerebrospinal fluid by GLUT 1 transporters in the endothelial cell membranes (Fig. 22.12) and then through the basement membrane. Measurements of the overall process of glucose transport from the blood into the brain (mediated by GLUT 3 on neural cells) show a $K_{m,app}$ of 7 to 11 mM and a maximal velocity not much greater than the rate of glucose utilization by the brain. Thus, decreases of blood glucose below the fasting level of 80 to 90 mg/dL (approximately 5 mM) are likely to significantly affect the rate of glucose metabolism in the brain, because of reduced glucose transport into the brain.

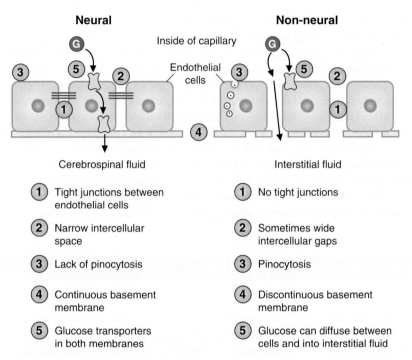

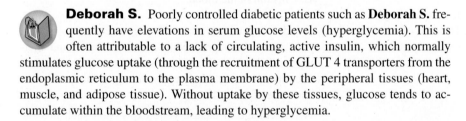

*FIG. 22.12.* Glucose transport through the capillary endothelium in neural and nonneural tissues. Characteristics of transport in each type of tissue are listed by numbers that refer to the numbers in the drawing. *G*, glucose.

## CLINICAL COMMENTS

Diseases discussed in this chapter are summarized in Table 22.3.

 **Deborah S.** Poorly controlled diabetic patients such as **Deborah S.** frequently have elevations in serum glucose levels (hyperglycemia). This is often attributable to a lack of circulating, active insulin, which normally stimulates glucose uptake (through the recruitment of GLUT 4 transporters from the endoplasmic reticulum to the plasma membrane) by the peripheral tissues (heart, muscle, and adipose tissue). Without uptake by these tissues, glucose tends to accumulate within the bloodstream, leading to hyperglycemia.

**Nina M.** The large amount of $H_2$ produced on fructose ingestion suggested that **Nina M.'s** problem was one of a deficiency in fructose transport into the absorptive cells of the intestinal villi. If fructose were being

**Table 22.3   Diseases Discussed in Chapter 22**

| Disease or Disorder | Environmental or Genetic | Comments |
|---|---|---|
| Lactose intolerance | Both | Reduced levels of lactase on the intestinal epithelial cell surface lead to reduced lactose digestion in the intestinal lumen, providing substrate for flora in the large intestine. Metabolism of the lactose by these bacteria leads to the generation of organic acids and gases. |
| Type 2 diabetes | Both | Diets consisting of low glycemic index carbohydrates will be beneficial in controlling the rise in blood glucose levels after eating. |
| Fructose malabsorption | Genetic | Inability to absorb fructose in the small intestine, leading to colonic bacteria metabolism of fructose and the generation of organic acids and gases. |

absorbed properly, the fructose would not have traveled to the colonic bacteria, which metabolized the fructose to generate the hydrogen gas. To confirm the diagnosis, a jejunal biopsy was taken; lactase, sucrase, maltase, and trehalase activities were normal in the jejunal cells. The tissue was also tested for the enzymes of fructose metabolism; these were in the normal range as well. Although Nina had no sugar in her urine, malabsorption of disaccharides can result in their appearance in the urine if damage to the intestinal mucosal cells allows their passage into the interstitial fluid. When Nina was placed on a diet free of fruit juices and other foods containing fructose, she did well and could tolerate small amounts of pure sucrose.

More than 50% of the adult population is estimated to be unable to absorb fructose in high doses (50 g), and more than 10% cannot completely absorb 25 g fructose. These individuals, like those with other disorders of fructose metabolism, must avoid fruits and other foods containing high concentrations of fructose.

## REVIEW QUESTIONS-CHAPTER 22

1.  An alcoholic patient developed a pancreatitis that affected his exocrine pancreatic function. He exhibited discomfort after eating a high-carbohydrate meal. The patient most likely had a reduced ability to digest which one of the following?

    A.  Lactose
    B.  Fiber
    C.  Starch
    D.  Sucrose
    E.  Maltose

2.  A patient with type 1 diabetes neglects to take his insulin injections while on a weekend vacation. The cells of which one of the following tissues would be most greatly affected by this mistake?

    A.  Muscle
    B.  Brain
    C.  Liver
    D.  Red blood cells
    E.  Pancreas

3.  After digestion of a piece of cake that contains flour, milk, and sucrose as its primary ingredients, the major carbohydrate products entering the blood are which one of the following?

    A.  Glucose
    B.  Fructose and galactose
    C.  Galactose and glucose
    D.  Glucose, galactose, and fructose
    E.  Fructose and glucose

4.  A patient has a genetic defect that causes intestinal epithelial cells to produce disaccharidases of much lower activity than normal. Compared with a normal person, after eating a bowl of milk and oatmeal sweetened with table sugar, this patient will exhibit higher levels of which one of the following?

    A.  Starch in the stool
    B.  Maltose, sucrose, and lactose in the stool
    C.  Galactose and fructose in the blood
    D.  Glycogen in the muscle
    E.  Insulin in the blood

5.  An individual who is recovering from colitis notes that, upon eating dairy products, severe flatulence and diarrhea result. This problem had never been evident before the colitis. The most likely explanation for this problem is which one of the following?

    A.  A change in lactase gene expression such that the gene is turned off
    B.  A mutation in the lactase gene that produces an inactive enzyme
    C.  An inhibitor of RNA polymerase that results in no transcription of the lactase gene
    D.  Physical damage to the intestinal epithelial cells such that lactase is lost from the membrane
    E.  Physical damage to the pancreas, such that bicarbonate cannot enter the intestine

# 23  Formation and Degradation of Glycogen

## CHAPTER OUTLINE

I. STRUCTURE OF GLYCOGEN

II. FUNCTION OF GLYCOGEN IN SKELETAL MUSCLE AND LIVER

III. SYNTHESIS AND DEGRADATION OF GLYCOGEN
   A. Glycogen synthesis
   B. Glycogen degradation

IV. DISORDERS OF GLYCOGEN METABOLISM

V. REGULATION OF GLYCOGEN SYNTHESIS AND DEGRADATION
   A. Regulation of glycogen metabolism in liver
      1. Nomenclature of enzymes metabolizing glycogen
      2. Regulation of liver glycogen metabolism by insulin and glucagon

   3. Activation of a phosphorylation cascade by glucagon
   4. Inhibition of glycogen synthase by glucagon-directed phosphorylation
   5. Regulation of protein phosphatases
   6. Insulin in liver glycogen metabolism
   7. Blood glucose levels and glycogen synthesis and degradation
   8. Epinephrine and calcium in the regulation of liver glycogen levels
      a. Epinephrine acting at β-receptors
      b. Epinephrine acting at α-receptors
   B. Regulation of glycogen synthesis and degradation in skeletal muscle

## KEY POINTS

- Glycogen is the storage form of glucose, composed of glucosyl units linked by α-1,4-glycosidic bonds with α-1,6 branches occurring about every 8 to 10 glucosyl units.
- Glycogen synthesis requires energy.
- Glycogen synthase transfers a glucosyl residue from the activated intermediate UDP-glucose to the ends of existing glycogen chains during glycogen synthesis. The branching enzyme creates α-1,6 linkages in the glycogen chain.
- Glycogenolysis is the degradation of glycogen. Glycogen phosphorylase catalyzes a phosphorolysis reaction, utilizing exogenous inorganic phosphate to break α-1,4 linkages at the ends of glycogen chains, releasing glucose-1-phosphate. The debranching enzyme hydrolyzes the α-1,6 linkages in glycogen, releasing free glucose.
- Liver glycogen supplies blood glucose.
- Glycogen synthesis and degradation are regulated in the liver by hormonal changes, which signify the need for or excess of blood glucose.
- Lack of dietary glucose, signaled by a decrease of the insulin/glucagon ratio, activates liver glycogenolysis and inhibits glycogen synthesis. Epinephrine also activates liver glycogenolysis.

continued

- Glucagon and epinephrine release lead to phosphorylation of glycogen synthase (inactivating it) and glycogen phosphorylase (activating it).
- Glycogenolysis in muscle supplies glucose-6-phosphate for adenosine triphosphate synthesis in the glycolytic pathway.
- Muscle glycogen phosphorylase is allosterically activated by adenosine monophosphate as well as by phosphorylation.
- Increases in sarcoplasmic $Ca^{2+}$ stimulates phosphorylation of muscle glycogen phosphorylase.

# THE WAITING ROOM

A newborn baby girl, **Gretchen C.**, was born after a 38-week gestation. Her mother, a 36-year-old woman, had developed a significant viral infection that resulted in a prolonged, severe loss of appetite with nausea in the month preceding delivery, leading to minimal food intake. Fetal bradycardia (slower than normal fetal heart rate) was detected with each uterine contraction of labor, a sign of possible fetal distress and the baby was delivered emergently.

At birth, Gretchen was cyanotic (a bluish discoloration caused by a lack of adequate oxygenation of tissues) and limp. She responded to several minutes of assisted ventilation. Her Apgar score of 3 was low at 1 minute after birth but improved to a score of 7 at 5 minutes.

The Apgar score is an objective estimate of the overall condition of the newborn, determined at both 1 and 5 minutes after birth. The best score is 10 (normal in all respects).

Physical examination in the nursery at 10 minutes showed a thin, malnourished female newborn. Her body temperature was slightly low, her heart rate was rapid, and her respiratory rate of 55 breaths per minute was elevated. Gretchen's birth weight was only 2,100 g, compared with a normal value of 3,300 g. Her length was 47 cm, and her head circumference was 33 cm (low normal). The laboratory reported that Gretchen's serum glucose level when she was unresponsive was 14 mg/dL. A glucose value below 40 mg/dL (2.5 mM) is considered to be abnormal in newborn infants.

At 5 hours of age, she was apneic (not breathing) and unresponsive. Ventilatory resuscitation was initiated and a cannula placed in the umbilical vein. Blood for a glucose level was drawn through this cannula, and 5 mL of a 20% glucose solution was injected. Gretchen slowly responded to this therapy.

**Jim B.'s** treadmill exercise and most other types of moderate exercise involving whole body movement (running, skiing, dancing, tennis) increase the use of blood glucose and other fuels by skeletal muscles. The blood glucose is normally supplied by the stimulation of liver glycogenolysis and gluconeogenesis.

**Jim B.**, a 19-year-old body builder, was rushed to the hospital emergency room in a coma. One-half hour earlier, his mother had heard a loud crashing sound in the basement where Jim had been lifting weights and completing his daily workout on the treadmill. She found her son on the floor having severe jerking movements of all muscles (a grand mal seizure).

In the emergency room, the doctors learned that despite the objections of his family and friends, Jim regularly used androgens and other anabolic steroids in an effort to bulk up his muscle mass.

On initial physical examination, he was comatose with occasional involuntary jerking movements of his extremities. Foamy saliva dripped from his mouth. He had bitten his tongue and had lost bowel and bladder control at the height of the seizure.

The laboratory reported a serum glucose level of 18 mg/dL (extremely low). The intravenous infusion of 5% glucose (5 g of glucose per 100 mL of solution), which had been started earlier, was increased to 10%. In addition, 50 g glucose was given over 30 seconds through the intravenous tubing.

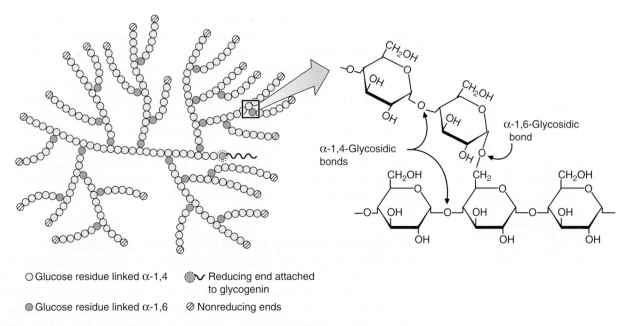

**FIG. 23.1.** Glycogen structure. Glycogen is composed of glucosyl units linked by α-1,4-glycosidic bonds and α-1,6-glycosidic bonds. The branches occur more frequently in the center of the molecule and less frequently in the periphery. The anomeric carbon that is not attached to another glucosyl residue (the reducing end) is attached to the protein glycogenin by a glycosidic bond. The hydrogen atoms have been omitted from this figure for clarity.

## I.  STRUCTURE OF GLYCOGEN

**Glycogen**, the storage form of glucose, is a branched glucose polysaccharide composed of chains of glucosyl units linked by α-1,4 bonds with α-1,6 branches every 8 to 10 residues (Fig. 23.1). In a molecule of this highly branched structure, only one glucosyl residue has an anomeric carbon that is not linked to another glucose residue. This anomeric carbon at the beginning of the chain is attached to the protein glycogenin. The other ends of the chains are called **nonreducing ends** because they cannot form a carbonyl group when converted to straight chain form (see Chapter 3). The branched structure permits rapid degradation and rapid synthesis of glycogen because enzymes can work on several chains simultaneously from the multiple nonreducing ends.

Glycogen is present in tissues as polymers of very high molecular weight ($10^7$ to $10^8$ Da) collected together in glycogen particles. The enzymes involved in glycogen synthesis and degradation and some of the regulatory enzymes are bound to the surface of the glycogen particles.

## II.  FUNCTION OF GLYCOGEN IN SKELETAL MUSCLE AND LIVER

Glycogen is found in most cell types, where it serves as a reservoir of glucosyl units for adenosine triphosphate (ATP) generation from glycolysis.

Glycogen is degraded mainly to **glucose-1-phosphate**, which is converted to **glucose-6-phosphate (G6P)** in a process called **glycogenolysis**. In skeletal muscle and other cell types, G6P enters the glycolytic pathway (Fig. 23.2). Glycogen is an extremely important fuel source for skeletal muscle when ATP demands are high and when G6P is used rapidly in anaerobic glycolysis. In many other cell types, the small glycogen reservoir serves a similar purpose; it is an emergency fuel source that supplies glucose for the generation of ATP in the absence of oxygen or during restricted blood flow. In general, glycogenolysis and glycolysis are activated together in these cells.

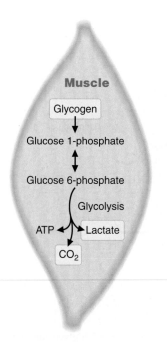

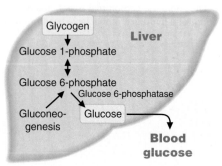

**FIG. 23.2.** Glycogenolysis in skeletal muscle and liver. Glycogen stores serve different functions in muscle cells and liver. In the muscle and most other cell types, glycogen stores serve as a fuel source for the generation of ATP. In the liver, glycogen stores serve as a source of blood glucose.

Regulation of glycogen synthesis serves to prevent futile cycling and waste of ATP. Futile cycling (also called substrate cycling) refers to a situation in which a substrate is converted to a product through one pathway, and the product converted back to the substrate through another pathway. Because the biosynthetic pathway is energy-requiring, futile cycling results in a waste of high-energy phosphate bonds. Thus, glycogen synthesis is activated when glycogen degradation is inhibited and vice versa.

Glycogen serves a very different purpose in liver than in skeletal muscle and other tissues (see Fig. 23.2). Liver glycogen is the first and immediate source of glucose for the maintenance of blood glucose levels. In the liver, the G6P that is generated from glycogen degradation is hydrolyzed to glucose by glucose-6-phosphatase, an enzyme present only in the liver and kidneys. Glycogen degradation thus provides a readily mobilized source of blood glucose as dietary glucose decreases or as exercise increases the use of blood glucose by muscles.

The pathways of glycogenolysis and gluconeogenesis in the liver both supply blood glucose, and consequently, these two pathways are activated together by glucagon. Gluconeogenesis, the synthesis of glucose from amino acids and other gluconeogenic precursors (discussed in detail in Chapter 26), also forms G6P so that glucose-6-phosphatase serves as a "gateway" to the blood for both pathways (see Fig. 23.2).

## III. SYNTHESIS AND DEGRADATION OF GLYCOGEN

Glycogen synthesis, like almost all the pathways of glucose metabolism, begins with the phosphorylation of glucose to G6P by hexokinase or, in the liver, glucokinase (Fig. 23.3). G6P is the precursor of glycolysis, the pentose phosphate pathway, and of pathways for the synthesis of other sugars. In the pathway for glycogen synthesis, G6P is converted to glucose-1-phosphate by phosphoglucomutase, a reversible reaction.

Glycogen is both formed from and degraded to glucose-1-phosphate, but the biosynthetic and degradative pathways are separate and involve different enzymes (see Fig. 23.3). The biosynthetic pathway is an energy-requiring pathway; high-energy

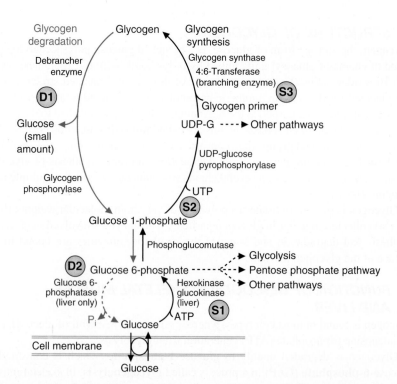

**FIG. 23.3.** Scheme of glycogen synthesis and degradation. (*S1*) G6P is formed from glucose by hexokinase in most cells, and glucokinase in the liver. It is a metabolic branch point for the pathways of glycolysis, the pentose phosphate pathway, and glycogen synthesis. (*S2*) UDP-G is synthesized from glucose-1-phosphate. UDP-G is the branch point for glycogen synthesis and other pathways requiring the addition of carbohydrate units. (*S3*) Glycogen synthesis is catalyzed by glycogen synthase and the branching enzyme. (*D1*) Glycogen degradation is catalyzed by glycogen phosphorylase and a debrancher enzyme. (*D2*) Glucose-6-phosphatase in the liver (and, to a small extent, the kidney) generates free glucose from G6P.

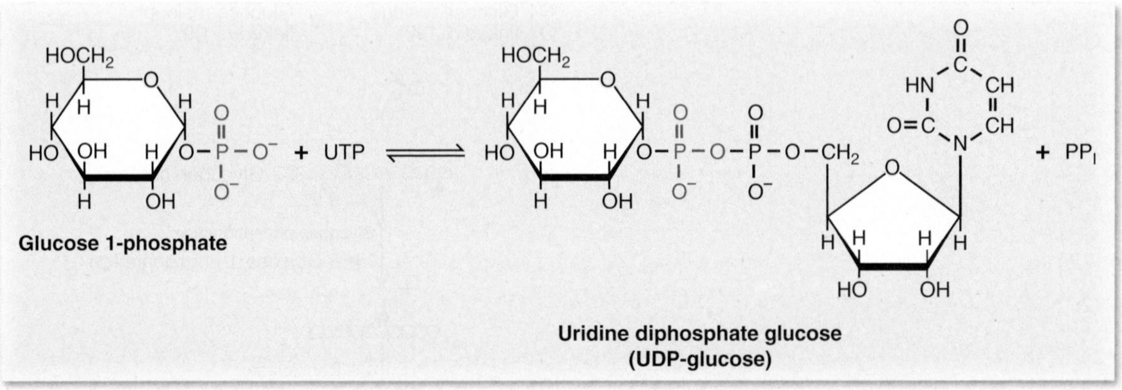

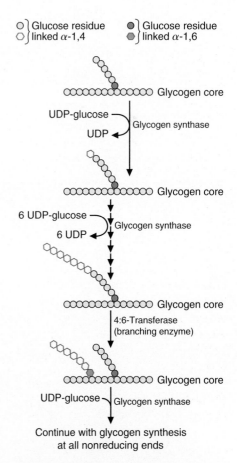

FIG. 23.4. Formation of UDP-G. The high-energy phosphate bond of *UTP* provides the energy for the formation of a high-energy bond in UDP-G. Pyrophosphate *(PPi)*, released by the reaction, is cleaved to two inorganic phosphate (P$_i$).

phosphate from uridine triphosphate (UTP) is used to activate the glucosyl residues to uridine diphosphate glucose (UDP-G) (Fig. 23.4). In the degradative pathway, the glycosidic bonds between the glucosyl residues in glycogen are simply cleaved by the addition of phosphate to produce glucose-1-phosphate (or water to produce free glucose), and UDP-G is not resynthesized. The existence of separate pathways for the formation and degradation of important compounds is a common theme in metabolism. Because the synthesis and degradation pathways use different enzymes, one can be activated while the other is inhibited.

## A. Glycogen Synthesis

Glycogen synthesis requires the formation of α-1,4-glycosidic bonds to link glucosyl residues in long chains and the formation of an α-1,6 branch every 8 to 10 residues (Fig. 23.5). Most of glycogen synthesis occurs through the lengthening of the polysaccharide chains of a preexisting glycogen molecule (a glycogen primer) in which the reducing end of the glycogen is attached to the protein glycogenin. To lengthen the glycogen chains, glucosyl residues are added from UDP-G to the nonreducing ends of the chain by glycogen synthase. The anomeric carbon of each glucosyl residue is attached in an α-1,4-glycosidic bond to the hydroxyl of carbon 4 of the terminal glucosyl residue. When the chain reaches approximately 11 residues in length, a 6- to 8-residue piece is cleaved by amylo-4,6-transferase (an activity of the branching enzyme) and reattached to a glucosyl unit by an α-1,6 bond. Both chains continue to lengthen until they are long enough to produce two new branches. This process continues, producing highly branched molecules. Branching of glycogen serves two major roles: increased sites for synthesis and degradation and enhancing the solubility of the molecule. **Glycogen synthase**, the enzyme that attaches the glucosyl residues in 1,4 bonds, is the regulated step in the pathway.

The synthesis of new glycogen primer molecules also occurs. Glycogenin, the protein to which glycogen is attached, glycosylates itself (autoglycosylation) by attaching the glucosyl residue of UDP-G to the hydroxyl side chain of a serine residue in the protein. The protein then extends the carbohydrate chain (using UDP-G as the substrate) until the glucosyl chain is long enough to serve as a substrate for glycogen synthase.

## B. Glycogen Degradation

Glycogen is degraded by two enzymes: **glycogen phosphorylase** and the **debrancher enzyme** (Fig. 23.6). Glycogen degradation is a phosphorolysis reaction (breaking of a bond using a phosphate ion as a nucleophile). Enzymes that catalyze

FIG. 23.5. Glycogen synthesis. See text for details.

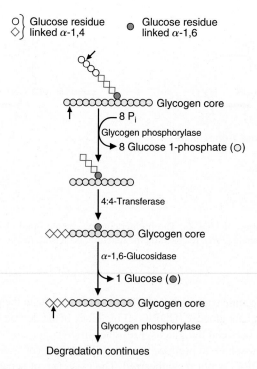

*FIG. 23.6.* Glycogen degradation. See text for details.

phosphorolysis reactions are named phosphorylases. Because more than one type of phosphorylase exists, the substrate usually is included in the name of the enzyme, such as glycogen phosphorylase or purine nucleoside phosphorylase.

The enzyme glycogen phosphorylase starts at the nonreducing end of a chain and successively cleaves glucosyl residues by adding phosphate to the anomeric carbon of the terminal glycosidic bond, thereby releasing glucose-1-phosphate and producing a free 4'-hydroxyl group on the glucose residue now at the end of the glycogen chain. However, glycogen phosphorylase cannot act on the glycosidic bonds of the four glucosyl residues closest to a branch point because the branching chain sterically hinders a proper fit into the catalytic site of the enzyme. The debrancher enzyme, which catalyzes the removal of the four residues closest to the branch point, has two catalytic activities: it acts as a transferase and as an α-1,6-glucosidase. As a transferase, the debrancher first removes a unit containing three glucose residues and adds it to the end of a longer chain by an α-1,4-glycosidic bond. The one glucosyl residue remaining at the α-1,6 branch is hydrolyzed by the amylo-1,6-glucosidase activity of the debrancher, resulting in the release of free glucose. Thus, one glucose and approximately 7 to 9 glucose-1-phosphate residues are released for every branch point.

Some degradation of glycogen also occurs within lysosomes when glycogen particles become surrounded by membranes that then fuse with the lysosomal membranes. A lysosomal glucosidase hydrolyzes this glycogen to glucose.

## IV. DISORDERS OF GLYCOGEN METABOLISM

A series of inborn errors of metabolism, the glycogen storage diseases, result from deficiencies in the enzymes of glycogen metabolism (Table 23.1). The diseases are labeled I through XI and O. Several disorders have different subtypes, as indicated in the legend of Table 23.1. Glycogen phosphorylase, the key regulatory enzyme of glycogen degradation, is encoded by different genes in the muscle and liver (tissue-specific isozymes), and thus, a person may have a defect in one and not the other.

**Table 23.1   Glycogen Storage Diseases**

| Type | Enzyme Affected | Primary Organ Involved | Manifestations[a] |
|------|-----------------|------------------------|-------------------|
| O | Glycogen synthase | Liver | Hypoglycemia, hyperketonemia, failure to thrive, early death |
| I[b] | Glucose-6-phosphatase (Von Gierke disease) | Liver | Enlarged liver and kidney, growth failure, severe fasting hypoglycemia, acidosis, lipemia, thrombocyte dysfunction |
| II | Lysosomal α-glucosidase (Pompe disease): may see clinical symptoms in childhood, juvenile, or adult life stages, depending on the nature of the mutation | All organs with lysosomes | Infantile form: early-onset progressive muscle hypotonia, cardiac failure, death before age 2 years. Juvenile form: later onset myopathy with variable cardiac involvement. Adult form: limb girdle, muscular dystrophy–like features. Glycogen deposits accumulate in lysosomes. |
| III | Amylo-1,6-glucosidase (debrancher): form IIIa is the liver and muscle enzymes, form IIIb is a liver-specific form, and IIIc a muscle-specific form. | Liver, skeletal muscle, heart | Fasting hypoglycemia; hepatomegaly in infancy in some myopathic features. Glycogen deposits have short outer branches. |
| IV | Amylo-4,6-glucosidase (branching enzyme) (Andersen disease) | Liver | Hepatosplenomegaly; symptoms may arise from a hepatic reaction to the presence of a foreign body (glycogen with long outer branches). Usually fatal. |
| V | Muscle glycogen phosphorylase (McArdle disease) (expressed as either adult or infantile form) | Skeletal muscle | Exercise-induced muscular pain, cramps, and progressive weakness, sometimes with myoglobinuria. |
| VI[c] | Liver glycogen phosphorylase (Hers disease) and its activating system (includes mutations in liver phosphorylase kinase and liver protein kinase A) | Liver | Hepatomegaly, mild hypoglycemia; good prognosis. |
| VII | Phosphofructokinase-I (Tarui syndrome) | Muscle, red blood cells | As in type V; in addition, enzymopathic hemolysis |
| XI | GLUT2 (glucose/galactose transporter); Fanconi-Bickel syndrome | Intestine, pancreas, kidney, liver | Glycogen accumulation in liver and kidney; rickets, growth retardation, glucosuria |

[a]All of these diseases except type O are characterized by increased glycogen deposits.
[b]Glucose-6-phosphatase is composed of several subunits that also transport glucose, glucose-6-phosphate (G6P), phosphate, and pyrophosphate across the endoplasmic reticulum membranes. Therefore, there are several subtypes of this disease corresponding to defects in the different subunits. Type Ia is a lack of glucose-6-phosphatase activity; type Ib is a lack of G6P translocase activity; type Ic is a lack of phosphotranslocase activity; type Id is a lack of glucose translocase activity.
[c]Glycogen storage diseases IX (hepatic phosphorylase kinase) and X (hepatic protein kinase A) have been reclassified to VI, which now refers to the hepatic glycogen phosphorylase activating system.
(*Sources:* Parker PH, Ballew M, Greene HL. Nutritional management of glycogen storage disease. *Annu Rev Nutr.* 1993;13:83–109. Copyright © 1993 by Annual Reviews, Inc; Shin YS. Glycogen storage disease: clinical, biochemical and molecular heterogeneity. *Semin Ped Neurol.* 2006;13:115–120; Ozen H. Glycogen storage diseases: new perspectives. *World J Gastroenterol.* 2007;13:2541–2553.)

## V.  REGULATION OF GLYCOGEN SYNTHESIS AND DEGRADATION

The regulation of glycogen synthesis in different tissues matches the function of glycogen in each tissue. Liver glycogen serves principally for the support of blood glucose during fasting or during extreme need (e.g., exercise) and the degradative and biosynthetic pathways are regulated principally by changes in the insulin/glucagon ratio and by blood glucose levels, which reflect the availability of dietary glucose

Maternal blood glucose readily crosses the placenta to enter the fetal circulation. During the last 9 or 10 weeks of gestation, glycogen formed from maternal glucose is deposited in the fetal liver under the influence of the insulin-dominated hormonal milieu of that period. At birth, maternal glucose supplies cease, causing a temporary physiological drop in glucose levels in the newborn's blood, even in normal healthy infants. This drop serves as one of the signals for glucagon release from the newborn's pancreas, which, in turn, stimulates glycogenolysis. As a result, the glucose levels in the newborn return to normal.

Healthy, full-term babies have adequate stores of liver glycogen to survive short (12 hours) periods of caloric deprivation provided other aspects of fuel metabolism are normal. Because **Gretchen C.'s** mother was markedly anorexic during the critical period when the fetal liver is normally synthesizing glycogen from glucose supplied in the maternal blood, Gretchen's liver glycogen stores were below normal. Thus, because fetal glycogen is the major source of fuel for the newborn in the early hours of life, Gretchen became profoundly hypoglycemic within 5 hours of birth because of her low levels of stored carbohydrate.

**Q:** A patient was diagnosed as an infant with type III glycogen storage disease, a deficiency of debrancher enzyme (see Table 23.1). The patient had hepatomegaly (an enlarged liver) and experienced bouts of mild hypoglycemia. To diagnose the disease, glycogen was obtained from the patient's liver by biopsy after the patient had fasted overnight and compared with normal glycogen. The glycogen samples were treated with a preparation of commercial glycogen phosphorylase and commercial debrancher enzyme. The amounts of glucose-1-phosphate and glucose produced in the assay were then measured. The ratio of glucose-1-phosphate to glucose for the normal glycogen sample was 9:1, and the ratio for the patient was 3:1. Can you explain these results?

**Table 23.2   Regulation of Liver and Muscle Glycogen Stores**

| State | Regulators | Response of Tissue |
|---|---|---|
| *Liver* | | |
| Fasting | Blood: glucagon ↑<br>Insulin ↓<br>Tissue: cAMP ↑ | Glycogen degradation ↑<br>Glycogen synthesis ↓ |
| Carbohydrate meal | Blood: glucagon ↓<br>Insulin ↑<br>Glucose ↑<br>Tissue: cAMP ↓<br>Glucose ↑ | Glycogen degradation ↓<br>Glycogen synthesis ↑ |
| Exercise and stress | Blood: epinephrine ↑<br>Tissue: cAMP ↑<br>$Ca^{2+}$-calmodulin ↑ | Glycogen degradation ↑<br>Glycogen synthesis ↓ |
| *Muscle* | | |
| Fasting (rest) | Blood: insulin ↓ | Glycogen synthesis ↓<br>Glucose transport ↓ |
| Carbohydrate meal (rest) | Blood: insulin ↑ | Glycogen synthesis ↑<br>Glucose transport ↑ |
| Exercise | Blood: epinephrine ↑<br>Tissue: AMP ↑<br>$Ca^{2+}$-calmodulin ↑<br>cAMP ↑ | Glycogen synthesis ↓<br>Glycogen degradation ↑<br>Glycolysis ↑ |

↑, increased compared with other physiological states; ↓, decreased compared with other physiological states.

(Table 23.2). Degradation of liver glycogen is also activated by epinephrine, which is released in response to exercise, hypoglycemia, or other stress situations in which there is an immediate demand for blood glucose. In contrast, in skeletal muscles, glycogen is a reservoir of glucosyl units for the generation of ATP from glycolysis and glucose oxidation. As a consequence, muscle glycogenolysis is regulated principally by adenosine monophosphate (AMP), which signals a lack of ATP, and by $Ca^{2+}$ released during contraction. Epinephrine, which is released in response to exercise and other stress situations, also activates skeletal muscle glycogenolysis. The glycogen stores of resting muscle decrease very little during fasting.

## A.  Regulation of Glycogen Metabolism in Liver

Liver glycogen is synthesized after a carbohydrate meal, when blood glucose levels are elevated and degraded as blood glucose levels decrease. When an individual eats a carbohydrate-containing meal, blood glucose levels immediately increase, insulin levels increase, and glucagon levels decrease (see Fig. 21.5). The increase of blood glucose levels and the rise of the insulin/glucagon ratio inhibit glycogen degradation and stimulate glycogen synthesis. The immediate increased transport of glucose into peripheral tissues and storage of blood glucose as glycogen helps to bring circulating blood glucose levels back to the normal 80- to 100-mg/dL range of the fasted state. As the length of time after a carbohydrate-containing meal increases, insulin levels decrease and glucagon levels increase. The fall of the insulin/glucagon ratio results in inhibition of the biosynthetic pathway and activation of the degradative pathway. As a result, liver glycogen is rapidly degraded to glucose, which is released into the blood.

Although glycogenolysis and gluconeogenesis are activated together by the same regulatory mechanisms, glycogenolysis responds more rapidly with a greater outpouring of glucose. A substantial proportion of liver glycogen is degraded early within a fast (30% after 4 hours). The rate of glycogenolysis is fairly constant for the first 23 hours; but in a prolonged fast, the rate decreases significantly as the liver glycogen supplies dwindle. Liver glycogen stores are therefore a rapidly rebuilt and degraded store of glucose, ever responsive to small and rapid changes of blood glucose levels.

## 1.  NOMENCLATURE OF ENZYMES METABOLIZING GLYCOGEN

Both glycogen phosphorylase and glycogen synthase are covalently modified to regulate their activity. When activated by covalent modification, glycogen phosphorylase is referred to as **glycogen phosphorylase *a*** (remember **a** for active); when the covalent modification is removed, and the enzyme is inactive, it is referred to as **glycogen phosphorylase *b***. Glycogen synthase, when it is not covalently modified, is active and can be designated **glycogen synthase *a*** or **glycogen synthase I** (the I stands for *independent* of modifiers for activity). When glycogen synthase is covalently modified, it is inactive, in the form of **glycogen synthase *b*** or **glycogen synthase D** (for *dependent* on a modifier for activity).

## 2. REGULATION OF LIVER GLYCOGEN METABOLISM BY INSULIN AND GLUCAGON

Insulin and glucagon regulate liver glycogen metabolism by changing the phosphorylation state of glycogen phosphorylase in the degradative pathway and glycogen synthase in the biosynthetic pathway. An increase of glucagon and decrease of insulin during the fasting state initiates a cyclic adenosine monophosphate (cAMP)-directed phosphorylation cascade, which results in the phosphorylation of glycogen phosphorylase to an active enzyme, and the phosphorylation of glycogen synthase to an inactive enzyme (Fig. 23.7). As a consequence, glycogen degradation is stimulated, and glycogen synthesis is inhibited.

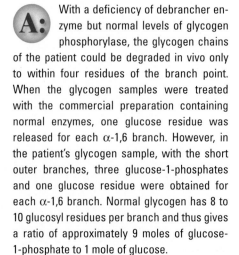

With a deficiency of debrancher enzyme but normal levels of glycogen phosphorylase, the glycogen chains of the patient could be degraded in vivo only to within four residues of the branch point. When the glycogen samples were treated with the commercial preparation containing normal enzymes, one glucose residue was released for each α-1,6 branch. However, in the patient's glycogen sample, with the short outer branches, three glucose-1-phosphates and one glucose residue were obtained for each α-1,6 branch. Normal glycogen has 8 to 10 glucosyl residues per branch and thus gives a ratio of approximately 9 moles of glucose-1-phosphate to 1 mole of glucose.

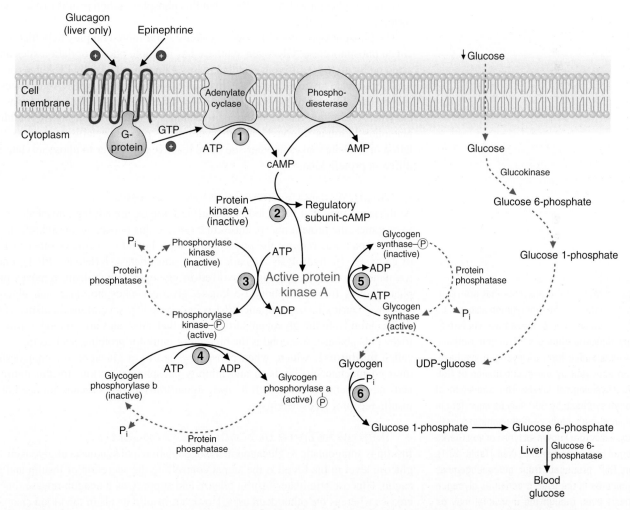

***FIG. 23.7.*** Regulation of glycogen synthesis and degradation in the liver. *(1)* Glucagon binding to the serpentine glucagon receptor or epinephrine binding to a serpentine β-receptor in the liver activates adenylate cyclase via G proteins, which synthesizes cAMP from ATP. *(2)* cAMP binds to PKA (cAMP-dependent protein kinase), thereby activating the catalytic subunits. *(3)* PKA activates phosphorylase kinase by phosphorylation. *(4)* Phosphorylase kinase adds a phosphate to specific serine residues on glycogen phosphorylase *b*, thereby converting it to the active glycogen phosphorylase *a*. *(5)* PKA also phosphorylates glycogen synthase, thereby decreasing its activity. *(6)* Because of the inhibition of glycogen synthase and the activation of glycogen phosphorylase, glycogen is degraded to glucose-1-phosphate. The *red dashed lines* denote reactions that are decreased in the livers of fasting individuals.

### 3. ACTIVATION OF A PHOSPHORYLATION CASCADE BY GLUCAGON

Glucagon regulates glycogen metabolism through its intracellular second messenger cAMP and protein kinase A (PKA) (see Chapter 21). Glucagon, by binding to its cell membrane receptor, transmits a signal through G proteins that activates adenylate cyclase, causing cAMP levels to increase (see Fig. 23.7). cAMP binds to the regulatory subunits of PKA, which dissociate from the catalytic subunits. The catalytic subunits of PKA are activated by the dissociation and phosphorylate the enzyme phosphorylase kinase, activating it. Phosphorylase kinase is the protein kinase that converts the inactive liver glycogen phosphorylase *b* conformer to the active glycogen phosphorylase *a* conformer by transferring a phosphate from ATP to a specific serine residue on the phosphorylase subunits. Because of the activation of glycogen phosphorylase, glycogenolysis is stimulated.

### 4. INHIBITION OF GLYCOGEN SYNTHASE BY GLUCAGON-DIRECTED PHOSPHORYLATION

When glycogen degradation is activated by the cAMP-stimulated phosphorylation cascade, glycogen synthesis is simultaneously inhibited. The enzyme glycogen synthase is also phosphorylated by PKA, but this phosphorylation results in a less active form, glycogen synthase *b*.

The phosphorylation of glycogen synthase is far more complex than that of glycogen phosphorylase. Glycogen synthase has multiple phosphorylation sites and is acted on by up to 10 different protein kinases. Phosphorylation by PKA does not, by itself, inactivate glycogen synthase. Instead, phosphorylation by PKA facilitates the subsequent addition of phosphate groups by other kinases, and these inactivate the enzyme. A term that has been applied to changes of activity resulting from multiple phosphorylation is "hierarchical" or "synergistic" phosphorylation; the phosphorylation of one site makes another site more reactive and easier to phosphorylate by a different protein kinase.

### 5. REGULATION OF PROTEIN PHOSPHATASES

At the same time that PKA and phosphorylase kinase are adding phosphate groups to enzymes, the protein phosphatases that remove this phosphate are inhibited. Protein phosphatases remove the phosphate groups, bound to serine or other residues of enzymes, by hydrolysis. Hepatic protein phosphatase-1 (hepatic PP-1), one of the major protein phosphatases involved in glycogen metabolism, removes phosphate groups from phosphorylase kinase, glycogen phosphorylase, and glycogen synthase. During fasting, hepatic PP-1 is inactivated by several mechanisms. One is dissociation from the glycogen particle, such that substrates are no longer available to the phosphatase. A second is the binding of inhibitor proteins, such as the protein called **inhibitor-1**, which, when phosphorylated by a glucagon (or epinephrine)-directed mechanism, binds to and inhibits phosphatase action. Insulin indirectly activates hepatic PP-1 through its own signal transduction cascade initiated at the insulin receptor tyrosine kinase.

### 6. INSULIN IN LIVER GLYCOGEN METABOLISM

Insulin is antagonistic to glucagon in the degradation and synthesis of glycogen. The glucose level in the blood is the signal controlling the secretion of insulin and glucagon. Glucose stimulates insulin release and suppresses glucagon release; one increases whereas the other decreases. However, insulin levels in the blood change to a greater degree with the fasting-feeding cycle than do the glucagon levels, and thus, insulin is considered the principal regulator of glycogen synthesis and degradation. The role of insulin in glycogen metabolism is often overlooked because the mechanism by which insulin reverses all of the effects of glucagon on individual metabolic enzymes is still under investigation. In addition to the activation of hepatic

Most of the enzymes that are regulated by phosphorylation also can be converted to the active conformation by allosteric effectors. Glycogen synthase *b*, the less active form of glycogen synthase, can be activated by the accumulation of G6P above physiological levels. The activation of glycogen synthase by G6P may be important in individuals with glucose-6-phosphatase deficiency, a disorder known as type I or von Gierke glycogen storage disease (see Table 23.1). When G6P produced from gluconeogenesis accumulates in the liver, it activates glycogen synthesis even though the individual may be hypoglycemic and have low insulin levels. G6P is also elevated, resulting in the inhibition of glycogen phosphorylase. As a consequence, large glycogen deposits accumulate and hepatomegaly occurs.

PP-1 through the insulin-receptor tyrosine kinase phosphorylation cascade, insulin may activate the phosphodiesterase that converts cAMP to AMP, thereby decreasing cAMP levels and inactivating PKA. Regardless of the mechanisms involved, insulin is able to reverse all of the effects of glucagon and is the most important hormonal regulator of blood glucose levels.

## 7. BLOOD GLUCOSE LEVELS AND GLYCOGEN SYNTHESIS AND DEGRADATION

When an individual eats a high-carbohydrate meal, glycogen degradation immediately stops. Although the changes in insulin and glucagon levels are relatively rapid (10 to 15 minutes), the direct inhibitory effect of rising glucose levels on glycogen degradation is even more rapid. Glucose, as an allosteric effector, inhibits liver glycogen phosphorylase *a* by stimulating dephosphorylation of this enzyme. As insulin levels rise and glucagon levels fall, cAMP levels decrease and PKA reassociates with its inhibitory subunits and becomes inactive. The protein phosphatases are activated, and phosphorylase *a* and glycogen synthase *b* are dephosphorylated. The collective result of these effects is rapid inhibition of glycogen degradation and rapid activation of glycogen synthesis.

## 8. EPINEPHRINE AND CALCIUM IN THE REGULATION OF LIVER GLYCOGEN LEVELS

Epinephrine, the fight-or-flight hormone, is released from the adrenal medulla in response to neural signals reflecting an increased demand for glucose. To flee from a dangerous situation, skeletal muscles use increased amounts of blood glucose to generate ATP. As a result, liver glycogenolysis must be stimulated. In the liver, epinephrine stimulates glycogenolysis through two different types of receptors, the α- and β-agonist receptors.

### a. Epinephrine Acting at β-Receptors

Epinephrine, acting at the β-receptors, transmits a signal through G proteins to adenylate cyclase, which increases cAMP and activates PKA. Hence, regulation of glycogen degradation and synthesis in liver by epinephrine and glucagon are similar (see Fig. 23.7).

### b. Epinephrine Acting at α-Receptors

Epinephrine also binds to α-receptors in the hepatocyte. This binding activates glycogenolysis and inhibits glycogen synthesis principally by increasing the $Ca^{2+}$ levels in the liver. The effects of epinephrine at the α-agonist receptor are mediated by the phosphatidylinositol bisphosphate ($PIP_2$)-$Ca^{2+}$ signal transduction system, one of the principal intracellular second messenger systems employed by many hormones (Fig. 23.8) (also see Chapter 8).

In the $PIP_2$-$Ca^{2+}$ signal transduction system, the signal is transferred from the epinephrine receptor to membrane-bound phospholipase C by G proteins. Phospholipase C hydrolyzes $PIP_2$ to form diacylglycerol (DAG) and inositol trisphosphate ($IP_3$). $IP_3$ stimulates the release of $Ca^{2+}$ from the endoplasmic reticulum. $Ca^{2+}$ and DAG activate protein kinase C. The amount of calcium bound to one of the calcium-binding proteins, calmodulin, is also increased.

Calcium/calmodulin associates as a subunit with a number of enzymes and modifies their activities. It binds to inactive phosphorylase kinase, thereby partially activating this enzyme. (The fully activated enzyme is both bound to the calcium-calmodulin subunit and phosphorylated.) Phosphorylase kinase then phosphorylates glycogen phosphorylase *b*, thereby activating glycogen degradation. Calcium/calmodulin is also a modifier protein that activates one of the glycogen synthase kinases (calcium-calmodulin synthase kinase). Protein kinase C, calcium-calmodulin synthase kinase, and phosphorylase kinase all phosphorylate glycogen synthase at

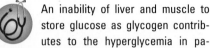

An inability of liver and muscle to store glucose as glycogen contributes to the hyperglycemia in patients, such as **Dianne A.**, with type 1 diabetes mellitus and in patients, such as **Deborah S.**, with type 2 diabetes mellitus. The absence of insulin in type 1 diabetes mellitus patients and the high levels of glucagon result in decreased activity of glycogen synthase. Glycogen synthesis in skeletal muscles of type 1 patients is also limited by the lack of insulin-stimulated glucose transport. Insulin resistance in type 2 patients has the same effect.

An injection of insulin suppresses glucagon release and alters the insulin/glucagon ratio. The result is rapid uptake of glucose into skeletal muscle and rapid conversion of glucose to glycogen in skeletal muscle and liver.

In the neonate, the release of epinephrine during labor and birth normally contributes to restoring blood glucose levels. Unfortunately, **Gretchen C.** did not have adequate liver glycogen stores to support a rise in her blood glucose levels.

**Q:** A series of inborn errors of metabolism, the glycogen storage diseases, result from deficiencies in the enzymes of glycogenolysis (see Table 23.1). Muscle glycogen phosphorylase, the key regulatory enzyme of glycogen degradation, is genetically different from liver glycogen phosphorylase, and thus, a person may have a defect in one and not the other. Why do you think that a genetic deficiency in muscle glycogen phosphorylase (McArdle disease) is a mere inconvenience, whereas a deficiency of liver glycogen phosphorylase (Hers disease) can be lethal?

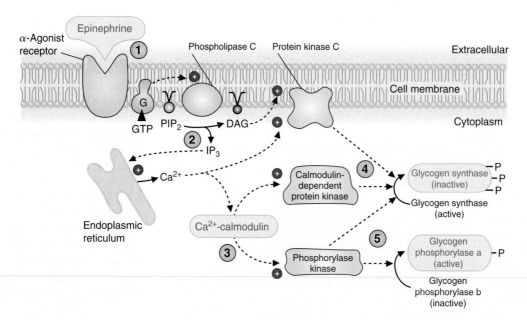

**FIG. 23.8.** Regulation of glycogen synthesis and degradation by epinephrine and $Ca^{2+}$. *(1)* The effect of epinephrine binding to α-agonist receptors in liver transmits a signal via G proteins to phospholipase C, which hydrolyzes $PIP_2$ to DAG and $IP_3$. *(2)* $IP_3$ stimulates the release of $Ca^{2+}$ from the endoplasmic reticulum. *(3)* $Ca^{2+}$ binds to the modifier protein calmodulin, which activates calmodulin-dependent protein kinase and phosphorylase kinase. Both $Ca^{2+}$ and DAG activate protein kinase C. *(4)* These three kinases phosphorylate glycogen synthase at different sites and decrease its activity. *(5)* Phosphorylase kinase phosphorylates glycogen phosphorylase *b* to the active form. It therefore activates glycogenolysis as well as inhibiting glycogen synthesis.

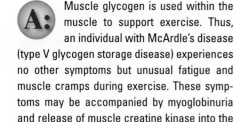 Muscle glycogen is used within the muscle to support exercise. Thus, an individual with McArdle's disease (type V glycogen storage disease) experiences no other symptoms but unusual fatigue and muscle cramps during exercise. These symptoms may be accompanied by myoglobinuria and release of muscle creatine kinase into the blood.

Liver glycogen is the first reservoir for the support of blood glucose levels, and a deficiency in glycogen phosphorylase or any of the other enzymes of liver glycogen degradation can result in fasting hypoglycemia. The hypoglycemia is usually mild because patients can still synthesize glucose from gluconeogenesis (see Table 23.1).

different serine residues on the enzyme, thereby inhibiting glycogen synthase and thus glycogen synthesis.

The effect of epinephrine in the liver, therefore, enhances or is synergistic with the effects of glucagon. Epinephrine release during bouts of hypoglycemia or during exercise can stimulate hepatic glycogenolysis and inhibit glycogen synthesis very rapidly.

### B. Regulation of Glycogen Synthesis and Degradation in Skeletal Muscle

The regulation of glycogenolysis in skeletal muscle is related to the availability of ATP for muscular contraction. Skeletal muscle glycogen produces glucose-1-phosphate and a small amount of free glucose. Glucose-1-phosphate is converted to G6P, which is committed to the glycolytic pathway; the absence of glucose-6-phosphatase in skeletal muscle prevents conversion of the glucosyl units from glycogen to blood glucose. Skeletal muscle glycogen is therefore degraded only when the demand for ATP generation from glycolysis is high. The highest demands occur during anaerobic glycolysis, which requires more moles of glucose for each ATP produced than oxidation of glucose to $CO_2$ (see Chapter 19). Anaerobic glycolysis occurs in tissues that have fewer mitochondria, a higher content of glycolytic enzymes, and higher levels of glycogen or fast-twitch glycolytic fibers. It occurs most frequently at the onset of exercise—before vasodilation occurs to bring in blood-borne fuels. The regulation of skeletal muscle glycogen degradation therefore must respond very rapidly to the need for ATP, indicated by the increase in AMP.

The regulation of skeletal muscle glycogen synthesis and degradation differs from that in liver in several important respects:

1. Glucagon has no effect on muscle, and thus glycogen levels in muscle do not vary with the fasting or feeding state.

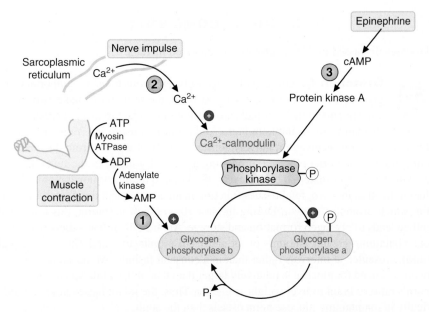

 **Jim B.** gradually regained consciousness with continued infusions of high-concentration glucose titrated to keep his serum glucose level between 120 and 160 mg/dL. Although he remained somnolent and moderately confused over the next 12 hours, he was eventually able to tell his physicians that he had self-injected approximately 25 units of regular (short-acting) insulin every 6 hours while eating a high-carbohydrate diet for the last 2 days preceding his seizure. Normal subjects under basal conditions secrete an average of 40 units of insulin daily. He had last injected insulin just before exercising. An article in a body-building magazine that he had recently read cited the anabolic effects of insulin on increasing muscle mass. He had purchased the insulin and necessary syringes from the same underground drug source from whom he regularly bought his anabolic steroids.

Normally, muscle glycogenolysis supplies the glucose required for the kinds of high-intensity exercise that require anaerobic glycolysis, such as weight-lifting. Jim's treadmill exercise also uses blood glucose, which is supplied by liver glycogenolysis. The high serum insulin levels, resulting from the injection he gave himself just before his workout, activated both glucose transport into skeletal muscle and glycogen synthesis while inhibiting glycogen degradation. His exercise, which would continue to use blood glucose, could normally be supported by breakdown of liver glycogen. However, glycogen synthesis in his liver was activated, and glycogen degradation was inhibited by the insulin injection.

**FIG. 23.9.** Activation of muscle glycogen phosphorylase during exercise. Glycogenolysis in skeletal muscle is initiated by muscle contraction, neural impulses, and epinephrine. *(1)* AMP produced from the degradation of ATP during muscular contraction allosterically activates glycogen phosphorylase *b*. *(2)* The neural impulses that initiate contraction release $Ca^{2+}$ from the sarcoplasmic reticulum. The $Ca^{2+}$ binds to calmodulin, which is a modifier protein that activates phosphorylase kinase. *(3)* Phosphorylase kinase is also activated through phosphorylation by PKA. The formation of cAMP and the resultant activation of PKA are initiated by the binding of epinephrine to plasma membrane receptors.

2. AMP is an allosteric activator of the muscle isozyme of glycogen phosphorylase but not liver glycogen phosphorylase (Fig. 23.9).
3. The effects of $Ca^{2+}$ in muscle result principally from the release of $Ca^{2+}$ from the sarcoplasmic reticulum after neural stimulation and not from epinephrine-stimulated uptake.
4. Glucose is not a physiological inhibitor of glycogen phosphorylase *a* in muscle.
5. Glycogen is a stronger feedback inhibitor of muscle glycogen synthase than of liver glycogen synthase, resulting in a smaller amount of stored glycogen per gram weight of muscle tissue.

However, the effects of epinephrine-stimulated phosphorylation by PKA on skeletal muscle glycogen degradation and glycogen synthesis are similar to those occurring in liver (see Fig. 23.7).

Muscle glycogen phosphorylase is a genetically distinct isoenzyme of liver glycogen phosphorylase and contains an amino acid sequence that has a purine nucleotide-binding site. When AMP binds to this site, it changes the conformation at the catalytic site to a structure very similar to that in the phosphorylated enzyme. Thus, hydrolysis of ATP to adenosine diphosphate (ADP) and the consequent increase of AMP generated by adenylate kinase during muscular contraction can directly stimulate glycogenolysis to provide fuel for the glycolytic pathway. AMP also stimulates glycolysis by activating phosphofructokinase-1, so this one effector activates both glycogenolysis and glycolysis. The activation of the calcium-calmodulin subunit of phosphorylase kinase by the $Ca^{2+}$ released from the sarcoplasmic reticulum during muscle contraction also provides a direct and rapid means of stimulating glycogen degradation.

## CLINICAL COMMENTS

Diseases discussed in this chapter are summarized in Table 23.3.

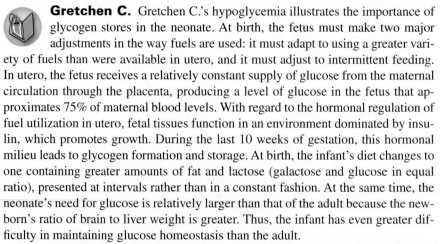

**Gretchen C.** Gretchen C.'s hypoglycemia illustrates the importance of glycogen stores in the neonate. At birth, the fetus must make two major adjustments in the way fuels are used: it must adapt to using a greater variety of fuels than were available in utero, and it must adjust to intermittent feeding. In utero, the fetus receives a relatively constant supply of glucose from the maternal circulation through the placenta, producing a level of glucose in the fetus that approximates 75% of maternal blood levels. With regard to the hormonal regulation of fuel utilization in utero, fetal tissues function in an environment dominated by insulin, which promotes growth. During the last 10 weeks of gestation, this hormonal milieu leads to glycogen formation and storage. At birth, the infant's diet changes to one containing greater amounts of fat and lactose (galactose and glucose in equal ratio), presented at intervals rather than in a constant fashion. At the same time, the neonate's need for glucose is relatively larger than that of the adult because the newborn's ratio of brain to liver weight is greater. Thus, the infant has even greater difficulty in maintaining glucose homeostasis than the adult.

At the moment that the umbilical cord is clamped, the normal neonate is faced with a metabolic problem: the high insulin levels of late fetal existence must be quickly reversed to prevent hypoglycemia. This reversal is accomplished through the secretion of the counterregulatory hormones epinephrine and glucagon. Glucagon release is triggered by the normal decline of blood glucose after birth. The neural response that stimulates the release of both glucagon and epinephrine is activated by the anoxia, cord clamping, and tactile stimulation that are part of a normal delivery. These responses have been referred to as the "normal sensor function" of the neonate.

Within 3 to 4 hours of birth, these counterregulatory hormones reestablish normal serum glucose levels in the newborn's blood through their glycogenolytic and gluconeogenic actions. The failure of Gretchen's normal "sensor function" was partly the result of maternal malnutrition, which resulted in an inadequate deposition of glycogen in Gretchen's liver before birth. The consequence was a serious degree of postnatal hypoglycemia.

The ability to maintain glucose homeostasis during the first few days of life also depends on the activation of gluconeogenesis and the mobilization of fatty acids. Fatty acid oxidation in the liver not only promotes gluconeogenesis (see Chapter 26) but also generates ketone bodies. The neonatal brain has an enhanced capacity to use ketone bodies relative to that of infants (4-fold) and adults (40-fold). This ability is consistent with the relatively high fat content of breast milk.

**Table 23.3   Diseases Discussed in Chapter 23**

| Disease or Disorder | Environmental or Genetic | Comments |
| --- | --- | --- |
| Newborn hypoglycemia | Environmental | Poor maternal nutrition may lead to inadequate glycogen levels in the newborn, resulting in hypoglycemia during the early fasting period after birth. |
| Insulin overdose | Environmental | Insulin taken without carbohydrate ingestion will lead to severe hypoglycemia, due to stimulation of glucose uptake by peripheral tissues, leading to insufficient glucose in the circulation for proper functioning of the nervous system. |
| Glycogen storage diseases | Genetic | These have been summarized in Table 23.1. Affect storage and use of glycogen, with different levels of severity, from mild to fatal. |

**Jim B.**  Jim B. attempted to build up his muscle mass with androgens and with insulin. The anabolic (nitrogen-retaining) effects of androgens on skeletal muscle cells enhance muscle mass by increasing amino acid flux into muscle and by stimulating protein synthesis. Exogenous insulin has the potential to increase muscle mass by similar actions and also by increasing the content of muscle glycogen.

The most serious side effect of exogenous insulin administration is the development of severe hypoglycemia, such as what occurred in **Jim B.'s** case. The immediate adverse effect relates to an inadequate flow of fuel (glucose) to the metabolizing brain. When hypoglycemia is extreme, the patient may suffer a seizure and, if the hypoglycemia worsens, irreversible brain damage may occur. If prolonged, the patient will lapse into a coma and may die.

## REVIEW QUESTIONS-CHAPTER 23

1. A patient has large deposits of liver glycogen, which, after an overnight fast, had shorter than normal branches. This abnormality could be caused by a defective from of which one of the following proteins or activities?

    A. Glycogen phosphorylase
    B. Amylo-1,6-glucosidase
    C. Glucagon receptor
    D. Glycogenin
    E. Amylo-4,6-transferase

2. An adolescent patient with a deficiency of muscle phosphorylase was examined while exercising her forearm by squeezing a rubber ball. Compared with a normal person performing the same exercise, this patient would exhibit which one of the following?

    A. Exercise for a longer time without fatigue
    B. Have increased glucose levels in blood drawn from her forearm
    C. Have lower levels of glycogen in biopsies of her forearm muscle
    D. Hyperglycemia
    E. Have decreased lactate levels in blood drawn from her forearm

3. In a glucose tolerance test, an individual in the basal metabolic state ingests a large amount of glucose. If the individual expresses no metabolic disorder, this ingestion should result in which one of the following?

    A. An enhanced glycogen synthase activity in the liver
    B. An increased ratio of glycogen phosphorylase *a* to glycogen phosphorylase *b* in the liver

    C. An increased rate of lactate formation by red blood cells
    D. An inhibition of protein phosphatase I activity in the liver
    E. An increase of cAMP levels in the liver

4. An individual is exhibiting fasting hypoglycemia. A liver biopsy has indicated elevated levels of glycogen with normal structure. A glucagon challenge to the patient only raises blood glucose levels 10% that expected from a normal individual. A likely defect in this patient is in which one of the following enzymes?

    A. Glycogen phosphorylase
    B. Glycogen synthase
    C. Protein kinase A
    D. Glucose-6-phosphatase
    E. UDP-glucose pyrophosphorylase

5. Allosteric activation of glycogen phosphorylase *b* in the muscle is due to which one of the following?

    A. AMP
    B. Glucose
    C. Glucose-6-phosphate
    D. ADP
    E. ATP

# 24 Pathways of Sugar and Alcohol Metabolism: Fructose, Galactose, Pentose Phosphate Pathway, and Ethanol Metabolism

## CHAPTER OUTLINE

## KEY POINTS

- Fructose is ingested principally as the monosaccharide or as part of sucrose. Fructose metabolism generates fructose 1-phosphate, which is then converted to intermediates of the glycolytic pathway.
- Galactose is ingested principally as lactose, which is converted to glucose and galactose in the intestine. Galactose metabolism generates first galactose 1-phosphate, which is converted to UDP-galactose. The end product is glucose-1-phosphate, which is isomerized to glucose-6-phosphate, which then enters glycolysis.
- The energy yield through glycolysis for both fructose and galactose is the same as for glucose metabolism.
- The pentose phosphate pathway consists of both oxidative and nonoxidative reactions.
- The oxidative steps of the pentose phosphate pathway generate NADPH and ribulose 5-phosphate from glucose-6-phosphate.
  - Ribulose 5-phosphate is converted to ribose 5-phosphate for nucleotide biosynthesis.
  - NADPH is utilized as reducing power for biosynthetic pathways.
- The nonoxidative steps of the pentose phosphate pathway reversibly convert five-carbon sugars to fructose 6-phosphate and glyceraldehyde 3-phosphate.
- Ethanol is metabolized to acetate primarily in the liver, generating NADH.

continued

■ The enzymes involved in ethanol metabolism are alcohol and aldehyde dehydrogenases.

■ Under conditions of high or chronic ethanol ingestion, a microsomal ethanol oxidizing system (MEOS) is induced, composed of cytochrome P450 enzymes in the endoplasmic reticulum.

■ Acute effects of ethanol ingestion arise principally from the generation of NADH, which increases the $NADH/NAD^+$ ratio of the liver. This leads to the following:
  ■ Inhibition of fatty acid oxidation
  ■ Inhibition of ketogenesis
  ■ Lactic acidosis
  ■ Hypoglycemia

■ Long-term effects of ethanol are due to acetaldehyde and free radical production, which leads to fatty liver, hepatitis, and liver cirrhosis.

## THE WAITING ROOM

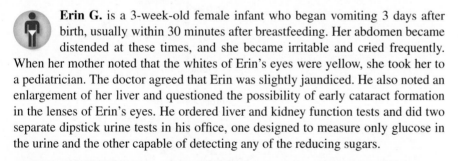

**Candice S.** is an 18-year-old girl who presented to her physician for a precollege physical examination. While taking her medical history, the doctor learned that she carefully avoided eating all fruits and any foods that contained table sugar. She related that from a very early age, she had learned that these foods caused severe weakness and symptoms suggestive of low blood sugar, such as tremulousness and sweating. Her medical history also indicated that her mother told her that once she started drinking and eating more than breast milk, she became a more irritable baby who often cried incessantly, especially after meals, and vomited frequently. At these times, Candice's abdomen had become distended, and she became drowsy and apathetic. Her mother had intuitively eliminated certain foods from Candice's diet, after which the severity and frequency of these symptoms diminished.

**Erin G.** is a 3-week-old female infant who began vomiting 3 days after birth, usually within 30 minutes after breastfeeding. Her abdomen became distended at these times, and she became irritable and cried frequently. When her mother noted that the whites of Erin's eyes were yellow, she took her to a pediatrician. The doctor agreed that Erin was slightly jaundiced. He also noted an enlargement of her liver and questioned the possibility of early cataract formation in the lenses of Erin's eyes. He ordered liver and kidney function tests and did two separate dipstick urine tests in his office, one designed to measure only glucose in the urine and the other capable of detecting any of the reducing sugars.

**Al M.** was found lying semiconscious at the bottom of the stairs by his landlady when she returned from an overnight visit with friends. His face had multiple bruises and his right forearm was grotesquely angulated. Non-bloody dried vomitus stained his clothing. Mr. M. was rushed by ambulance to the emergency room at the nearest hospital. In addition to multiple bruises and the compound fracture of his right forearm, he had deep and rapid (Kussmaul) breathing and was moderately dehydrated.

Initial laboratory studies showed a relatively large anion gap of 34 mmol/L (reference range = 9 to15 mmol/L). An arterial blood gas analysis (which measures pH in addition to the levels of dissolved $O_2$ and $CO_2$) confirmed the presence of a metabolic acidosis. Mr. M.'s blood alcohol level was only slightly elevated. His serum glucose was 68 mg/dL (low normal).

The anion gap is calculated by subtracting the sum of the value for serum chloride and for the serum HCO$_3^-$ content from the serum sodium concentration. If the gap is greater than normal (8 to 16 mEq/L), it suggests that acids such as the ketone bodies acetoacetate and β-hydroxybutyrate are present in the blood in increased amounts.

Jaundice is a yellow discoloration involving the sclerae (the "whites" of the eyes) and skin. It is caused by the deposition of bilirubin, a yellow degradation product of heme. Bilirubin accumulates in the blood under conditions of liver injury, bile duct obstruction, and excessive degradation of heme.

Mr. M. developed a fever of 101.5°F on the second day of his hospitalization for acute alcoholism. One of his physicians noticed that one of the lacerations on his arm was swollen with some pus drainage. The pus was cultured and gram-positive cocci were found and identified as *Staphlococcus aureus*. Because his landlady stated that he had an allergy to penicillin and the concern over methicillin-resistant *S. aureus*, Mr. M. was started on a course of the antibiotic combination of trimethoprim and sulfamethoxazole (TMP/sulfa). To his landlady's knowledge, he had never been treated with a sulfa drug previously.

On the third day of therapy with TMP/sulfa for his infection, Mr. M. was slightly jaundiced. His hemoglobin level had fallen by 3.5 g/dL from its value at admission, and his urine was red-brown because of the presence of free hemoglobin. Mr. M. had apparently suffered acute hemolysis (lysis or destruction of some of his red blood cells) induced by his infection and exposure to the sulfa drug.

## I.  FRUCTOSE

**Fructose** is found in the diet as a component of sucrose in fruit, as a free sugar in honey, and in high-fructose corn syrup. Fructose enters epithelial cells and other types of cells by facilitated diffusion on the GLUT 5 transporter. It is metabolized to intermediates of glycolysis. Problems with fructose absorption and metabolism are relatively more common than with other sugars.

### A.  Fructose Metabolism

Fructose is metabolized by conversion to glyceraldehyde 3-phosphate (glyceraldehyde 3-P) and dihydroxyacetone phosphate, which are intermediates of glycolysis (Fig. 24.1). The steps parallel those of glycolysis. The first step in the metabolism of fructose, as with glucose, is phosphorylation. Fructokinase, the major kinase involved, is found primarily in the liver, intestine, and kidney, and phosphorylates fructose in the 1-position. Fructokinase has a high $V_{max}$ and rapidly

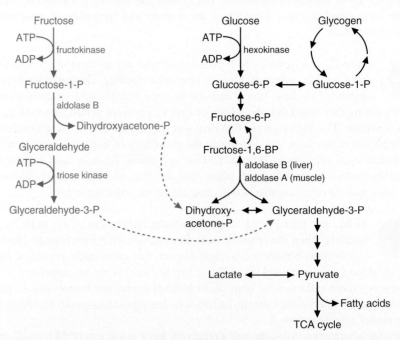

**FIG. 24.1.** Fructose metabolism. The pathway for the conversion of fructose to dihydroxyacetone phosphate and glyceraldehyde 3-P is shown in *red*. These two compounds are intermediates of glycolysis and are converted in the liver principally to glucose, glycogen, or fatty acids. In the liver, aldolase B cleaves both fructose 1-P in the pathway for fructose metabolism and fructose 1,6-bisphosphate in the pathway for glycolysis.

When individuals with defects of aldolase B ingest fructose, the extremely high levels of fructose 1-P that accumulate in the liver and kidney cause several adverse effects. Hypoglycemia results from inhibition of glycogenolysis and gluconeogenesis. Glycogen phosphorylase (and possibly phosphoglucomutase and other enzymes of glycogen metabolism) are inhibited by the accumulated fructose 1-P. Aldolase B is required for glucose synthesis from glyceraldehyde 3-P and dihydroxyacetone phosphate, and its low activity in aldolase B–deficient individuals is further decreased by the accumulated fructose 1-P. The inhibition of gluconeogenesis results in lactic acidosis.

The accumulation of fructose 1-P also substantially depletes the phosphate pools. The fructokinase reaction uses ATP at a rapid rate such that the mitochondria regenerate ATP rapidly, which leads to a drop in free phosphate levels. The low levels of phosphate release inhibition of AMP deaminase, which converts AMP to inosine monophosphate (IMP). The nitrogenous base of IMP (hypoxanthine) is degraded to uric acid. The lack of phosphate and depletion of adenine nucleotides lead to a loss of ATP, further contributing to the inhibition of biosynthetic pathways, including gluconeogenesis.

phosphorylates fructose as it enters the cell. The fructose 1-phosphate (fructose 1-P) formed is not an intermediate of glycolysis but rather is cleaved by aldolase B to dihydroxyacetone phosphate (an intermediate of glycolysis) and glyceraldehyde. Glyceraldehyde is then phosphorylated to glyceraldehyde 3-P by triose kinase. Dihydroxyacetone phosphate and glyceraldehyde 3-P are intermediates of the glycolytic pathway and can proceed through it to pyruvate, the tricarboxylic acid (TCA) cycle, and fatty acid synthesis. Alternately, these intermediates can also be converted to glucose by gluconeogenesis. In other words, the fate of fructose parallels that of glucose.

The metabolism of fructose occurs principally in the liver and, to a lesser extent, in the small intestinal mucosa and proximal epithelium of the renal tubule because these tissues express both fructokinase and aldolase B. Aldolase exists as several isoforms: aldolases A, B, C, and fetal aldolase. Although all of these aldolase isoforms can cleave fructose 1,6-bisphosphate, the intermediate of glycolysis, only aldolase B can also cleave fructose 1-P. Aldolase A, present in muscle and most other tissues, and aldolase C, present in brain, have almost no ability to cleave fructose 1-P. Fetal aldolase, present in the liver before birth, is similar to aldolase C.

Aldolase B is the rate-limiting enzyme of fructose metabolism, although it is not a rate-limiting enzyme of glycolysis. It has a much lower affinity for fructose 1-P than fructose 1,6-bisphosphate and is very slow at physiological levels of fructose 1-P. As a consequence, after ingesting a high dose of fructose, normal individuals accumulate fructose 1-P in the liver while it is slowly converted to glycolytic intermediates. Individuals with hereditary fructose intolerance (a deficiency of aldolase B) accumulate much higher amounts of fructose 1-P in their livers.

Other tissues also have the capacity to metabolize fructose but do so much more slowly. The hexokinase isoforms present in muscle, adipose tissue, and other tissues can convert fructose to fructose 6-phosphate (fructose 6-P) but react so much more efficiently with glucose. As a result, fructose phosphorylation is very slow in the presence of physiological levels of intracellular glucose and glucose-6-phosphate (glucose 6-P).

## B. Synthesis of Fructose in the Polyol Pathway

Fructose can be synthesized from glucose in the **polyol pathway**. The polyol pathway is named for the first step of the pathway in which sugars are reduced to the sugar alcohol by the enzyme aldose reductase (Fig. 24.2). Glucose is reduced to the sugar alcohol sorbitol, and sorbitol is then oxidized to fructose. This pathway is present in seminal vesicles, which synthesize fructose for the seminal fluid. Spermatozoa use fructose as a major fuel source while in the seminal fluid and then switch to glucose

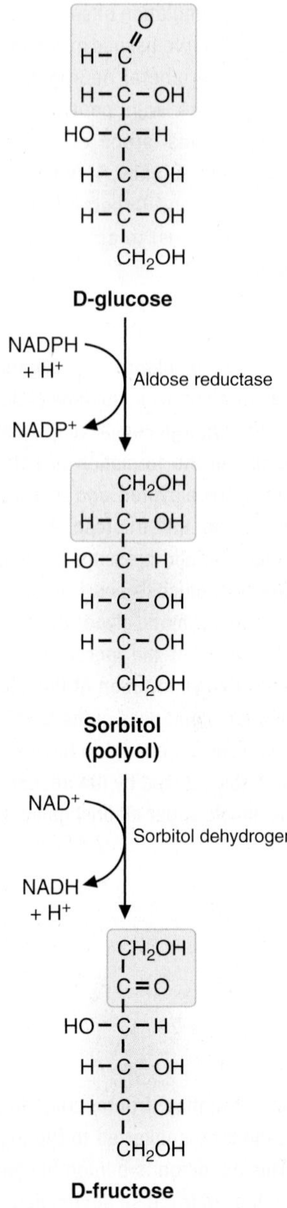

**FIG. 24.2.** The polyol pathway converts glucose to fructose.

**Q:** Essential fructosuria is a rare and benign genetic disorder caused by a deficiency of the enzyme fructokinase. Why is this disease benign, when a deficiency of aldolase B (hereditary fructose intolerance) can be fatal?

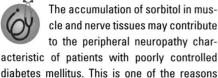 The accumulation of sorbitol in muscle and nerve tissues may contribute to the peripheral neuropathy characteristic of patients with poorly controlled diabetes mellitus. This is one of the reasons it is so important for **Dianne A.** (who has type 1 diabetes mellitus) and **Deborah S.** (who has type 2 diabetes mellitus) to achieve good glycemic control.

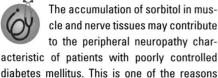 The accumulation of sugars and sugar alcohols in the lens of patients with hyperglycemia (e.g., diabetes mellitus) results in the formation of cataracts. Glucose levels are elevated and increase the synthesis of sorbitol and fructose. As a consequence, a high osmotic pressure is created in the lens. The high glucose and fructose levels also result in nonenzymatic glycosylation of lens proteins. The result of the increased osmotic pressure and the glycosylation of the lens protein is an opaque cloudiness of the lens known as a cataract. **Erin G.** seemed to have an early cataract, probably caused by the accumulation of galactose and its sugar alcohol galactitol.

**A:** In essential fructosuria, fructose cannot be converted to fructose 1-P. This condition is benign because no toxic metabolites of fructose accumulate in the liver, and the patient remains nearly asymptomatic. Some of the ingested fructose is slowly phosphorylated by hexokinase in nonhepatic tissues and metabolized by glycolysis and some appears in the urine. There is no renal threshold for fructose; the appearance of fructose in the urine (fructosuria) does not require a high fructose concentration in the blood.

Hereditary fructose intolerance, conversely, results in the accumulation of fructose 1-P and fructose. By inhibiting glycogenolysis and gluconeogenesis, the high levels of fructose 1-P caused the hypoglycemia that **Candice S.** experienced as an infant when she became apathetic and drowsy and as an adult when she experienced sweating and tremulousness.

once in the female reproductive tract. Utilization of fructose is thought to prevent acrosomal breakdown of the plasma membrane (and consequent activation) while the spermatozoa are still in the seminal fluid.

The polyol pathway is present in many tissues, but its function in all tissues is not understood. Aldose reductase is relatively nonspecific, and its major function may be the metabolism of an aldehyde sugar other than glucose. The activity of this enzyme can lead to major problems in the lens of the eye where it is responsible for the production of sorbitol from glucose and galactitol from galactose. When the concentration of glucose or galactose is elevated in the blood, their respective sugar alcohols are synthesized in the lens more rapidly than they are removed, resulting in increased osmotic pressure within the lens.

## II.  GALACTOSE METABOLISM: METABOLISM TO GLUCOSE-1-PHOSPHATE

Dietary **galactose** is metabolized principally by phosphorylation to galactose 1-phosphate (galactose 1-P) and then conversion to uridine diphosphate-galactose (UDP-galactose) and glucose-1-phosphate (glucose 1-P) (Fig. 24.3). The phosphorylation of galactose, again an important first step in the pathway, is carried out by a specific kinase, galactokinase. The formation of UDP-galactose is accomplished by attack of the phosphate oxygen on galactose 1-P on the α phosphate of UDP-glucose, releasing glucose 1-P while forming UDP-galactose. The enzyme that catalyzes this reaction is galactose 1-P uridylyltransferase. The UDP-galactose is then converted to UDP-glucose by the reversible UDP-glucose epimerase (the configuration of the hydroxyl group on carbon 4 is reversed in this reaction). The net result of this sequence of reactions is that galactose is converted to glucose 1-P at the expense of one high-energy bond of adenosine triphosphate (ATP). The sum of these reactions is indicated in the equations that follow:

1. Galactose + ATP $\xrightarrow{\text{Galactokinase}}$ Galactose 1-P + ADP

2. Galactose 1-P + UDP-glucose $\xrightarrow[\text{uridylyltransferase}]{\text{Galactose 1-P}}$ UDP-galactose + glucose 1-P

3. UDP-galactose $\xrightarrow{\text{UDP-glucose epimerase}}$ UDP-glucose

*Net Equation: Galactose + ATP → Glucose 1-P + ADP*

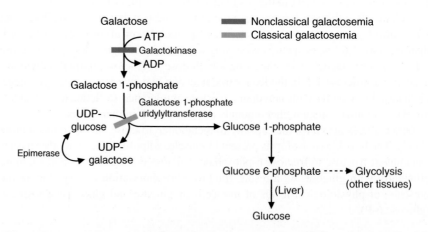

**FIG. 24.3.** Metabolism of galactose. Galactose is phosphorylated to galactose 1-P by galactokinase. Galactose 1-P reacts with UDP-glucose to release glucose 1-P. Galactose, thus, can be converted to blood glucose, enter glycolysis, or enter any of the metabolic routes of glucose. In classical galactosemia, a deficiency of galactose 1-P uridylyltransferase (shown in *green*) results in the accumulation of galactose 1-P in tissues and the appearance of galactose in the blood and urine. In nonclassical galactosemia, a deficiency of galactokinase (shown in *red*) results in the accumulation of galactose.

**Erin G.'s** urine was negative for glucose when measured with the glucose oxidase strip but was positive for the presence of a reducing sugar. The reducing sugar was identified as galactose. Her liver function tests showed an increase in serum bilirubin and in several liver enzymes. Albumin was present in her urine. These findings and the clinical history increased her physician's suspicion that Erin had classical galactosemia.

Classical galactosemia is caused by a deficiency of galactose 1-P uridylyltransferase. In this disease, galactose 1-P accumulates in tissues, and galactose is elevated in the blood and urine. This condition differs from the rarer deficiency of galactokinase (nonclassical galactosemia) in which galactosemia and galactosuria occur but galactose 1-P is not formed. Both enzyme defects result in cataracts from galactitol formation by aldose reductase in the polyol pathway. Aldose reductase has a relatively high $K_m$ for galactose, approximately 12 to 20 mM, so that galactitol is formed only in galactosemic patients who have eaten galactose. Galactitol is not further metabolized and diffuses out of the lens very slowly. Thus, hypergalactosemia is even more likely to cause cataracts than hyperglycemia. **Erin G.**, although she is only 3 weeks old, appeared to have early cataracts forming in the lens of her eyes.

One of the most serious problems of classical galactosemia is an irreversible mental retardation. Realizing this problem, **Erin G.'s** physician wanted to begin immediate dietary therapy. A test that measures galactose 1-P uridylyltransferase activity in erythrocytes was ordered. The enzyme activity was virtually absent, confirming the diagnosis of classical galactosemia.

---

The enzymes for galactose conversion to glucose 1-P are present in many tissues, including the adult erythrocyte, fibroblasts, and fetal tissues. The liver has high activity of these enzymes and can convert dietary galactose to blood glucose and glycogen. The fate of dietary galactose, like that of fructose, therefore, parallels that of glucose. The ability to metabolize galactose is even higher in infants than in adults. Newborn infants ingest up to 1 g galactose per kilogram per feeding (as lactose). Yet, the rate of metabolism is so high that the blood level in the systemic circulation is less than 3 mg/dL, and none of the galactose is lost in the urine.

## III. THE PENTOSE PHOSPHATE PATHWAY

The **pentose phosphate pathway** is essentially a scenic bypass route around the first stage of glycolysis that generates NADPH and ribose 5-phosphate (ribose-5-P) (as well as other pentose sugars). Glucose 6-P is the common precursor for both pathways. The oxidative first stage of the pentose phosphate pathway generates two moles of NADPH per glucose 6-P oxidized. The second stage of the pentose phosphate pathway (the nonoxidative phase) generates ribose 5-P and converts unused intermediates to fructose 6-P and glyceraldehyde 3-P in the glycolytic pathway. All cells require NADPH for reductive detoxification, and most cells require ribose 5-P for nucleotide synthesis. Consequently, the pathway is present in all cells. The enzymes reside in the cytosol, as do the enzymes of glycolysis.

### A. Oxidative Phase of the Pentose Phosphate Pathway

In the oxidative first phase of the pentose phosphate pathway, glucose 6-P undergoes an oxidation and decarboxylation to a pentose sugar, ribulose 5-phosphate (ribulose 5-P) (Fig. 24.4). The first enzyme of this pathway, glucose 6-P dehydrogenase, oxidizes the aldehyde at carbon 1 and reduces $NADP^+$ to NADPH. The gluconolactone that is formed is rapidly hydrolyzed to 6-phosphogluconate, a sugar acid with a carboxylic acid group at carbon 1. The next oxidation step releases this carboxyl group as $CO_2$, with the electrons being transferred to $NADP^+$. This reaction is mechanistically very similar to the one catalyzed by isocitrate dehydrogenase in the TCA cycle. Thus, 2 moles of NADPH per mole of glucose 6-P are formed from this portion of the pathway.

NADPH rather than NADH is generally used in the cell for pathways that require the input of electrons for reductive reactions because the ratio of $NADPH/NADP^+$ is much greater than the $NADH/NAD^+$ ratio. The NADH generated from fuel oxidation is rapidly oxidized back to $NAD^+$ by NADH dehydrogenase in the electron transport chain, so the level of NADH is very low in the cell.

NADPH can be generated from a number of reactions in the liver and other tissues but not in red blood cells. For example, in tissues with mitochondria, an energy-requiring transhydrogenase located near the complexes of the electron transport chain can transfer reducing equivalents from NADH to $NADP^+$ to generate NADPH.

NADPH, however, cannot be directly oxidized by the electron transport chain, and the ratio of NADPH to $NADP^+$ in cells is greater than one. The reduction potential of NADPH, therefore, can contribute to the energy needed for biosynthetic processes and provide a constant source of reducing power for detoxification reactions.

Doctors suspected that the underlying factor in the destruction of **Al M.'s** red blood cells was an X-linked defect in the gene that codes for glucose 6-P dehydrogenase. The red blood cell is dependent on this enzyme for a source of NADPH to maintain reduced levels of glutathione, one of its major defenses against oxidative stress (see Chapter 18). Glucose 6-P dehydrogenase deficiency is the most common known enzymopathy, affecting approximately 7% of the world's population and about 2% of the U.S. population. Most glucose 6-P dehydrogenase–deficient individuals are asymptomatic but can undergo an episode of hemolytic anemia if exposed to certain drugs, to certain types of infections, or if they ingest fava beans. When questioned, Al M. replied that he did not know what a fava bean was and had no idea whether he was sensitive to them.

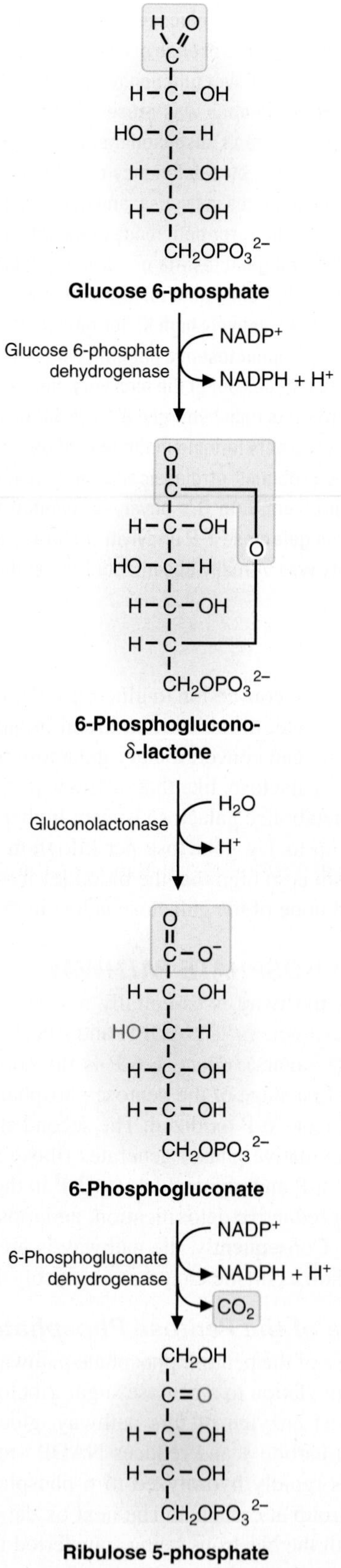

**Glucose 6-phosphate**

Glucose 6-phosphate dehydrogenase

NADP+

NADPH + H+

**6-Phosphoglucono-δ-lactone**

Gluconolactonase

$H_2O$

H+

**6-Phosphogluconate**

6-Phosphogluconate dehydrogenase

NADP+

NADPH + H+

$CO_2$

**Ribulose 5-phosphate**

**FIG. 24.4.** Oxidative portion of the pentose phosphate pathway. Carbon 1 of glucose 6-P is oxidized to an acid and then released as $CO_2$ in an oxidation followed by a decarboxylation reaction. Each of the oxidation steps generates an NADPH.

The ribulose 5-P formed from the action of the two oxidative steps is isomerized to produce ribose 5-P (a ketose-to-aldose conversion, similar to fructose 6-P being isomerized to glucose 6-P). The ribose 5-P can then enter the pathway for nucleotide synthesis, if needed, or can be converted to glycolytic intermediates, as described in the following text for the nonoxidative phase of the pentose phosphate pathway. The pathway through which the ribose 5-P travels is determined by the needs of the cell at the time of its synthesis.

## B. Nonoxidative Phase of the Pentose Phosphate Pathway

The nonoxidative reactions of this pathway are *reversible reactions* that allow intermediates of glycolysis (specifically glyceraldehyde 3-P and fructose 6-P) to be converted to five-carbon sugars (such as ribose 5-P) and vice versa. The needs of the cell determine which direction this pathway proceeds. If the cell has produced ribose 5-P but does not need to synthesize nucleotides, then the ribose 5-P is converted back to glycolytic intermediates. If the cells still requires NADPH, the ribose 5-P is converted back into glucose 6-P using nonoxidative reactions. And finally, if the cell already has a high level of NADPH but needs to produce nucleotides, the oxidative reactions of the pentose phosphate pathway are inhibited, and the glycolytic intermediates fructose 6-P and glyceraldehyde 3-P are used to produce the five-carbon sugars using exclusively the nonoxidative phase of the pentose phosphate pathway. The nonoxidative portion of the pentose phosphate pathway consists of a series of rearrangement and transfer reactions that first convert ribulose 5-P to ribose 5-P and xylulose 5-phosphate (xylulose 5-P) (Fig. 24.5), and then, the ribose 5-P and xylulose 5-P are converted to intermediates of the glycolytic pathway. The enzymes involved are an isomerase, epimerase, transketolase, and transaldolase.

The epimerase and isomerase convert ribulose 5-P to two other five-carbon sugars (see Fig. 24.5). The isomerase converts ribulose 5-P to ribose 5-P. The epimerase changes the stereochemical position of one hydroxyl group (at carbon 3), converting ribose 5-P to xylulose 5-P.

Transketolase transfers two-carbon fragments of keto sugars (sugars with a keto group at carbon 2) to other sugars. Transketolase picks up a two-carbon fragment from xylulose 5-P by cleaving the carbon–carbon bond between the keto group and the adjacent carbon, thereby releasing glyceraldehyde 3-P (Fig. 24.6). Two reactions in the pentose phosphate pathway use transketolase; in the first, the two-carbon keto fragment from xylulose 5-P is transferred to ribose 5-P to form sedoheptulose 7-phosphate, and in the other, a two-carbon keto fragment (usually derived from xylulose 5-P) is transferred to erythrose 4-phosphate to form fructose 6-P.

Transaldolase transfers a three-carbon keto fragment from sedoheptulose 7-phosphate to glyceraldehyde 3-P to form erythrose 4-phosphate and fructose 6-P (Fig. 24.7). This reaction is similar to the aldolase reaction in glycolysis, and the enzyme uses an active site amino group from the side chain of lysine to catalyze the reaction.

The net result of the metabolism of 3 moles of ribulose 5-P in the pentose phosphate pathway is the formation of 2 moles of fructose 6-P and 1 mole of glyceraldehyde 3-P, which then continue through the glycolytic pathway with the production of NADH, ATP, and pyruvate. Because the pentose phosphate pathway begins with glucose 6-P and feeds back into the glycolytic pathway, it is sometimes called the **hexose monophosphate shunt** (a shunt or a pathway for glucose 6-P). The reaction sequence starting from glucose 6-P and involving both the oxidative and nonoxidative phases of the pathway is shown in Figure 24.8.

The reactions catalyzed by the epimerase, isomerase, transketolase, and transaldolase are all reversible reactions under physiological conditions. Thus, ribose 5-P required for purine and pyrimidine synthesis can be generated from intermediates of

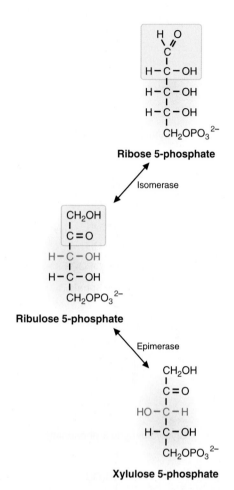

**FIG. 24.5.** Ribulose 5-P can be epimerized (to xylulose 5-P) at carbon 3 (shown in *red*) or isomerized (to ribose 5-P) as shown in the *yellow box.*

The transketolase activity of red blood cells is used to measure thiamine nutritional status and diagnose the presence of thiamine deficiency. The activity of transketolase is measured in the presence and absence of added thiamine pyrophosphate. If the thiamine intake of a patient is adequate, the addition of thiamine pyrophosphate does not increase the activity of transketolase because it already contains bound thiamine pyrophosphate. If the patient is thiamine deficient, transketolase activity will be low, and adding thiamine pyrophosphate will greatly stimulate the reaction. **Al M.** was diagnosed previously as having beriberi heart disease resulting from thiamine deficiency. The diagnosis was based on laboratory tests confirming the thiamine deficiency.

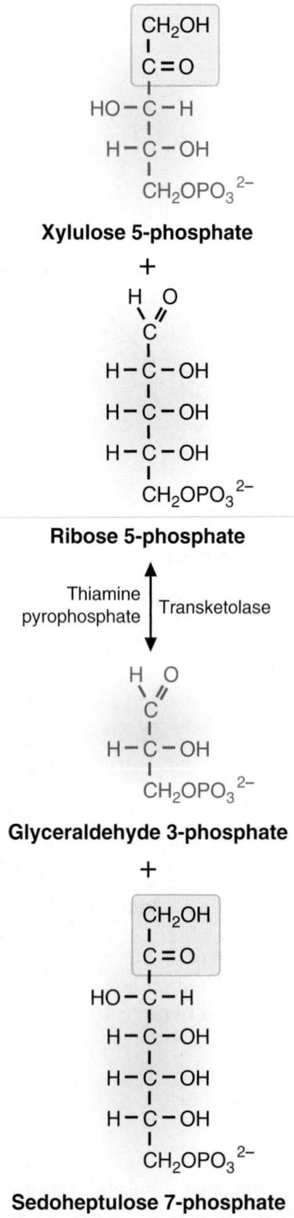

**FIG. 24.6.** Two-carbon unit transferred by transketolase. Transketolase cleaves the bond next to the keto group and transfers the two-carbon keto fragment to an aldehyde. Thiamine pyrophosphate carries the two-carbon fragment, forming a covalent bond with the carbon of the keto group.

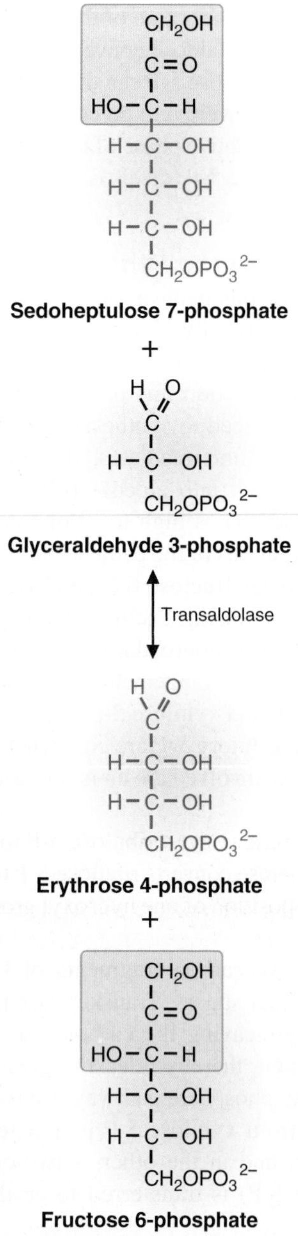

**FIG. 24.7.** Transaldolase transfers a three-carbon fragment that contains an alcohol group next to a keto group.

the glycolytic pathway, as well as from the oxidative phase of the pentose phosphate pathway. The sequence of reactions that generate ribose 5-P from intermediates of glycolysis is indicated as follows:

1. Fructose 6-P + Glyceraldehyde 3-P $\xleftrightarrow{\text{\textit{Transketolase}}}$ Erythrose 4-P + Xylulose 5-P

2. Erythrose 4-P + Fructose 6-P $\xrightarrow{\text{\textit{Transaldolase}}}$ Sedoheptulose 7-P + Glyceraldehyde 3-P

3. Sedoheptulose 7-P + Glyceraldehyde 3-P $\xleftrightarrow{\text{\textit{Transketolase}}}$ Ribose 5-P + Xylulose 5-P

4. 2 Xyulose 5-P $\xleftrightarrow{\text{\textit{Epimerase}}}$ 2 Ribulose 5-P

5. 2 Ribulose 5-P $\xleftrightarrow{\text{\textit{Isomerase}}}$ 2 Ribose 5-P

*Net Equation: 2 Fructose 6-P + Glyceraldehyde 3-P $\leftrightarrow$ 3 Ribose 5-P*

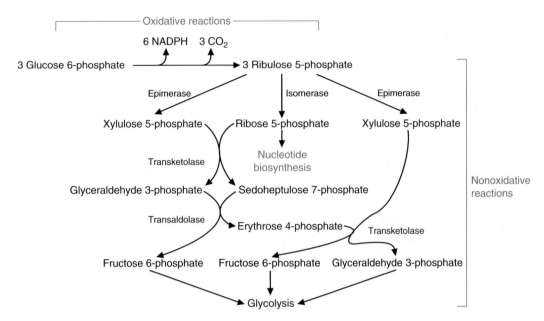

***FIG. 24.8.*** A balanced sequence of reactions in the pentose phosphate pathway. The interconversion of sugars in the pentose phosphate pathway results in conversion of three glucose 6-P to 6 NADPH, three $CO_2$, two fructose 6-P, and one glyceraldehyde 3-P.

## C. Role of the Pentose Phosphate Pathway in Generation of NADPH

In general, the oxidative phase of the pentose phosphate pathway is the major source of NADPH in cells. The glutathione-mediated defense against oxidative stress is common to all cell types (including red blood cell), and the requirement for NADPH to maintain levels of reduced glutathione probably accounts for the universal distribution of the pentose phosphate pathway among different types of cells. Figure 24.9 illustrates the importance of this pathway in maintaining the membrane integrity of the red blood cells. NADPH is also used for anabolic pathways, such as fatty acid synthesis, cholesterol synthesis, and fatty acid chain elongation. It is the source of reducing equivalents for cytochrome P450 hydroxylation of aromatic compounds, steroids, alcohols, and drugs. The highest concentrations of glucose 6-P dehydrogenase are found in phagocytic cells where NADPH oxidase uses NADPH to form superoxide from molecular oxygen. The superoxide then generates hydrogen peroxide, which kills the microorganisms taken up by the phagocytic cells (see Chapter 18).

The entry of glucose 6-P into the pentose phosphate pathway is controlled by the cellular concentration of NADPH. NADPH is a strong product inhibitor of glucose 6-P dehydrogenase, the first enzyme of the pathway. As NADPH is oxidized in other pathways, the product inhibition of glucose 6-P dehydrogenase is relieved, and the rate of the enzyme is accelerated to produce more NADPH.

In the liver, the synthesis of fatty acids from glucose is a major route of NADPH reoxidation. The synthesis of liver glucose 6-P dehydrogenase, like the key enzymes of glycolysis and fatty acid synthesis, is induced by the increased insulin:glucagon ratio after a high-carbohydrate meal. A summary of the possible routes glucose 6-P may follow using the pentose phosphate pathway is presented in Table 24.1.

## IV. ETHANOL METABOLISM

**Ethanol** is a small molecule that is both lipid and water soluble. It is therefore readily absorbed from the intestine by passive diffusion. A small percentage of ingested ethanol (0% to 5%) enters the gastric mucosal cells of the upper gastrointestinal (GI) tract (tongue, mouth, esophagus, and stomach), where it is metabolized. The remainder enters the blood. Of this, 85% to 98% is metabolized in the liver, and only

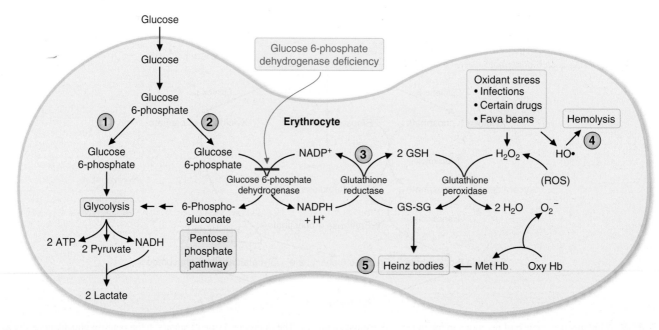

**FIG. 24.9.** Hemolysis caused by reactive oxygen species (ROS). *(1)* Maintenance of the integrity of the erythrocyte membrane depends on its ability to generate ATP and NADH from glycolysis. *(2)* NADPH is generated by the pentose phosphate pathway. *(3)* NADPH is used for the reduction of oxidized glutathione (GSSG) to reduced glutathione (GSH). Glutathione is necessary for the removal of $H_2O_2$ and lipid peroxides generated by ROS. *(4)* In the erythrocytes of healthy individuals, the continuous generation of superoxide ion from the nonenzymatic oxidation of hemoglobin provides a source of ROS. The glutathione defense system is compromised by glucose 6-P dehydrogenase deficiency, infections, certain drugs, and the purine glycosides of fava beans. *(5)* As a consequence, Heinz bodies, aggregates of cross-linked hemoglobin, form on the cell membranes and subject the cell to mechanical stress as it tries to go through small capillaries. The action of the ROS on the cell membrane as well as mechanical stress from the lack of deformability result in hemolysis.

Individual variations in the quantity of the isoenzymes which metabolize ethanol and acetaldehyde influence several factors, such as the rate of ethanol clearance from the blood, the degree of inebriation exhibited by an individual, and differences in individual susceptibility to the development of alcohol-induced liver disease.

2% to 10% is excreted through the lungs or kidneys. The major enzymes involved in metabolizing ethanol are alcohol dehydrogenase, acetaldehyde dehydrogenase, and the microsomal ethanol oxidizing system (MEOS).

## A. Alcohol Dehydrogenase

The major route of ethanol metabolism in the liver is through liver **alcohol dehydrogenase (ADH)**, a cytosolic enzyme that oxidizes ethanol to acetaldehyde with reduction of $NAD^+$ to NADH (Fig. 24.10). If it is not removed by metabolism, acetaldehyde exerts toxic actions in the liver and can enter the blood and exert toxic effects in other tissues.

ADH exists as a family of isoenzymes with varying specificity for chain length of the alcohol substrate (see Table A24.1 of the online supplement @ ). Ethanol is a small molecule that does not exhibit much in the way of unique structural

**Table 24.1   Cellular Needs Dictate the Direction of the Pentose Phosphate Pathway Reactions**

| Cellular Need | Direction of Pathway |
|---|---|
| NADPH only | Oxidative reactions produce NADPH; nonoxidative reactions convert ribulose 5-P to glucose 6-P to produce more NADPH |
| NADPH + ribose 5-P | Oxidative reactions produce NADPH and ribulose 5-P; the isomerase converts ribulose 5-P to ribose 5-P. |
| Ribose 5-P only | Only the nonoxidative reactions. High NADPH inhibits glucose 6-P dehydrogenase, so transketolase and transaldolase will be used to convert fructose 6-P and glyceraldehyde 3-P to ribose 5-P. |
| NADPH and pyruvate | Both the oxidative and nonoxidative reactions are used. The oxidative reactions generate NADPH and ribulose 5-P. The nonoxidative reactions convert the ribulose 5-P to fructose 6-P and glyceraldehyde 3-P, and glycolysis will convert these intermediates to pyruvate. |

characteristics and, at high concentrations, is nonspecifically metabolized by many members of the ADH family. The ADHs that exhibit the highest specificity for ethanol are members of the ADH1 family. Humans have three genes for this family of ADHs, each of which exists as allelic variants (polymorphisms).

The ADH1 family members are present in high quantities in the liver, representing approximately 3% of all soluble protein. These ADHs, commonly referred to collectively as liver alcohol dehydrogenase, have a low $K_m$ for ethanol between 0.02 and 5 mM (high affinities). Thus, the liver is the major site of ethanol metabolism and the major site at which the toxic metabolite acetaldehyde is generated.

Although the ADH4 and ADH2 enzymes make minor contributions to ethanol metabolism, they may contribute to its toxic effects. Ethanol concentrations can be quite high in the upper GI tract (e.g., beer is approximately 0.8 M ethanol), and acetaldehyde generated here by ADH4 enzymes (gastric ADH) might contribute to the risk for cancer associated with heavy drinking. ADH2 genes are expressed primarily in the liver and at lower levels in the lower GI tract.

### B. Acetaldehyde Dehydrogenases

Acetaldehyde is oxidized to acetate with the generation of NADH by acetaldehyde dehydrogenases (ALDH) (see Fig. 24.10). More than 80% of acetaldehyde oxidation in the human liver is normally catalyzed by mitochondrial acetaldehyde dehydrogenase (ALDH2), which has a high affinity for acetaldehyde ($K_m$ of 0.2 μM) and is highly specific. However, individuals with a common allelic variant of ALDH2 (designated as ALDH2*2) have a greatly decreased capacity for acetaldehyde metabolism due to an increased $K_m$ (46 μM) and a decreased $V_{max}$ (0.017 unit/mg vs. 0.60 units/mg).

Most of the remainder of acetaldehyde oxidation occurs through a cytosolic acetaldehyde dehydrogenase (ALDH1). Additional ALDHs act on a variety of organic alcohols, toxins, and pollutants.

### C. Fate of Acetate

Acetate, which has no toxic effects, may be activated to acetyl CoA in the liver (where it can enter either the TCA cycle or the pathway for fatty acid synthesis). However, most of the acetate that is generated enters the blood and is activated to acetyl CoA in skeletal muscles and other tissues. Acetate is generally considered nontoxic and is a normal constituent of the diet.

The activation of acetate to acetyl CoA is catalyzed by acetyl CoA synthetase in a reaction similar to the reaction catalyzed by fatty acyl CoA synthetases. In the liver, the principle isoform of acetyl CoA synthetase (ACS I) is a cytosolic enzyme that generates acetyl CoA for the cytosolic pathways of cholesterol and fatty acid synthesis. Acetate entry into these pathways is under regulatory control by mechanisms involving cholesterol or insulin. Thus, most of the acetate generated enters the blood.

Acetate is taken up and oxidized by other tissues, notably heart and skeletal muscle, which have a high concentration of the mitochondrial acetyl CoA synthetase isoform (ACS II). This enzyme is present in the mitochondrial matrix. It therefore generates acetyl CoA that can directly enter the TCA cycle and be oxidized to $CO_2$.

### D. Microsomal Ethanol Oxidizing System

The other principal route of ethanol oxidation in the liver is the **MEOS**, which also oxidizes ethanol to acetaldehyde (Fig. 24.11). The principal microsomal enzyme involved is a cytochrome P450 mixed-function oxidase isozyme (CYP2E1), which uses NADPH as an additional electron donor and $O_2$ as an electron acceptor. This route accounts for only a small percentage of ethanol oxidation in a moderate drinker (Fig. 24.12). The cytochrome P450 enzymes all have two major catalytic protein components: an electron-donating reductase system that transfers electrons from NADPH (cytochrome P450 reductase) and a cytochrome P450. The cytochrome

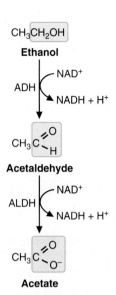

**FIG. 24.10.** The pathway of ethanol metabolism. *ADH*, alcohol dehydrogenase; *ALDH*, acetaldehyde dehydrogenase.

 The accumulation of acetaldehyde causes nausea and vomiting, and, therefore, inactive ALDHs are associated with a distaste for alcoholic beverages and protection against alcoholism. In one of the common allelic variants of ALDH2 (ALDH2*2), a single amino acid substitution increases the $K_m$ for acetaldehyde 23-fold (lowers the affinity) and decreases the $V_{max}$ 35-fold, resulting in a very inactive enzyme. Homozygosity for the ALDH2*2 allele affords absolute protection against alcoholism; no individual with this genotype has been found among alcoholics. Alcoholics are frequently treated with ALDH inhibitors (e.g., disulfiram) to help them abstain from alcohol intake. Unfortunately, alcoholics who continue to drink while taking this drug are exposed to the toxic effects of elevated acetaldehyde levels.

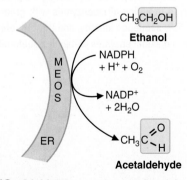

**FIG. 24.11.** The reaction catalyzed by the MEOS (which includes CYP2E1) in the endoplasmic reticulum *(ER)*.

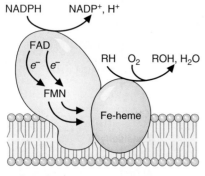

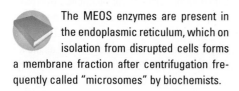

FIG. 24.12. General structure of cytochrome P450 enzymes. $O_2$ binds to the P450 Fe heme in the active site and is activated to a reactive form by accepting electrons. The electrons are donated by the cytochrome P450 reductase, which contains a flavin adenine dinucleotide (FAD) plus a flavin mononucleotide (FMN) or Fe—S center to facilitate the transfer of single electrons from NADPH to $O_2$. The P450 enzymes involved in steroidogenesis have a somewhat different structure. For CYP2E1, *RH* is ethanol ($CH_3CH_2OH$) and *ROH* is acetaldehyde ($CH_3COH$).

The MEOS enzymes are present in the endoplasmic reticulum, which on isolation from disrupted cells forms a membrane fraction after centrifugation frequently called "microsomes" by biochemists.

CYP represents **cy**tochrome **P**450. P450 is an Fe heme similar to that found in the cytochromes of the electron transport chain ("P" denotes the heme **p**igment, and 450 is the wavelength of visible light absorbed by the pigment). In CYP2E1, the "2" refers to the gene family, which comprises isoenzymes with greater than 40% amino acid sequence identity. The "E" refers to the subfamily, a grouping of isoenzymes with greater than 55% sequence identity, and the "1" refers to the individual enzymes within this subfamily.

P450 protein contains the binding sites for $O_2$ and the substrate (e.g., ethanol) and carries out the reaction.

### 1. CYP2E1

The MEOS is part of the superfamily of cytochrome P450 enzymes, all of which catalyze similar oxidative reactions. Within the superfamily, at least 10 distinct gene families are found in mammals. More than 100 different cytochrome P450 isozymes exist within these 10 gene families. Each isoenzyme has a distinct classification according to its structural relationship with other isoenzymes. The isoenzyme that has the highest activity toward ethanol is called **CYP2E1**. A great deal of overlapping specificity exists among the various P450 isoenzymes, and ethanol is also oxidized by several other P450 isoenzymes. MEOS refers to the combined ethanol-oxidizing activity of all the P450 enzymes.

CYP2E1 has a much higher $K_m$ for ethanol than the ADH1 family members (11 mM [51 mg/dL] compared with 0.02 to 5 mM [0.09 to 22.5 mg/dL]). Thus, a greater proportion of ingested ethanol is metabolized through CYP2E1 at high levels of ethanol consumption than at low levels.

### 2. INDUCTION OF P450 ENZYMES

The P450 enzymes are inducible both by their most specific substrate and by substrates for some of the other cytochrome P450 enzymes. Chronic consumption of ethanol increases hepatic CYP2E1 levels approximately 5-fold to 10-fold. However, it also causes a 2-fold to 4-fold increase in some of the other P450s from the same subfamily, from different subfamilies, and even from different gene families. The endoplasmic reticulum undergoes proliferation, with a general increase in the content of microsomal enzymes, including those that are not directly involved in ethanol metabolism.

The increase in CYP2E1 with ethanol consumption occurs through transcriptional, posttranscriptional, and posttranslational regulation. Increased levels of mRNA resulting from induction of gene transcription or stabilization of message are found in actively drinking patients. The protein is also stabilized against degradation. In general, the mechanism for induction of P450 enzymes by their substrates occurs through the binding of the substrate (or related compound) to an intracellular receptor protein followed by binding of the activated receptor to a response element in the target gene. Ethanol induction of CYP2E1 appears to act via stabilization of the protein and protection against degradation (an increased half-life for the synthesized protein).

Although induction of CYP2E1 increases ethanol clearance from the blood, it has negative consequences. Acetaldehyde may be produced faster than it can be metabolized by ALDHs, thereby increasing the risk of hepatic injury. An increased amount of acetaldehyde can enter the blood and can damage other tissues. In addition, cytochrome P450 enzymes are capable of generating free radicals, which may also lead to increased hepatic injury and cirrhosis.

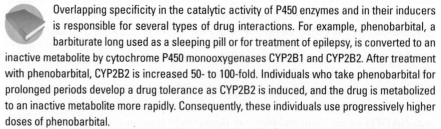

Overlapping specificity in the catalytic activity of P450 enzymes and in their inducers is responsible for several types of drug interactions. For example, phenobarbital, a barbiturate long used as a sleeping pill or for treatment of epilepsy, is converted to an inactive metabolite by cytochrome P450 monooxygenases CYP2B1 and CYP2B2. After treatment with phenobarbital, CYP2B2 is increased 50- to 100-fold. Individuals who take phenobarbital for prolonged periods develop a drug tolerance as CYP2B2 is induced, and the drug is metabolized to an inactive metabolite more rapidly. Consequently, these individuals use progressively higher doses of phenobarbital.

Ethanol is an inhibitor of the phenobarbital-oxidizing P450 system. When large amounts of ethanol are consumed, the inactivation of phenobarbital is directly or indirectly inhibited. Therefore, when high doses of phenobarbital and ethanol are consumed at the same time, toxic levels of the barbiturate can accumulate in the blood.

### E. Energy Yield of Ethanol Oxidation

The ATP yield from ethanol oxidation to acetate varies with the route of ethanol metabolism. If ethanol is oxidized by the major route of cytosolic ADH and mitochondrial ALDH, one cytosolic and one mitochondrial NADH are generated with a maximum yield of 5 ATP. Oxidation of acetyl CoA in the TCA cycle and electron transport chain leads to the generation of 10 high-energy phosphate bonds. However, activation of acetate to acetyl CoA requires two high-energy phosphate bonds (one in the cleavage of ATP to adenosine monophosphate [AMP] and pyrophosphate and one in the cleavage of pyrophosphate to phosphate), which must be subtracted. Thus, the maximum total energy yield is 13 moles of ATP per mole of ethanol.

In contrast, oxidation of ethanol to acetaldehyde by CYP2E1 consumes energy in the form of NADPH, which is equivalent to 2.5 ATP. Thus, for every mole of ethanol metabolized by this route, only a maximum of 8.0 moles of ATP can be generated (10 ATP from acetyl CoA oxidation through the TCA cycle, minus 2 for acetate activation; the NADH generated by aldehyde dehydrogenase is balanced by the loss of NADPH in the MEOS step).

## V. TOXIC EFFECTS OF ETHANOL METABOLISM

Alcohol-induced liver disease, a common and sometimes fatal consequence of chronic ethanol abuse, may manifest itself in three forms: fatty liver, alcohol-induced hepatitis, and cirrhosis. Each may occur alone, or they may be present in any combination in a given individual. Alcohol-induced cirrhosis is discovered in up to 9% of all autopsies performed in the United States, with a peak incidence in patients 40 to 55 years of age.

However, ethanol ingestion also has acute effects on liver metabolism including inhibition of fatty acid oxidation and stimulation of triacylglycerol synthesis, leading to a fatty liver. It also can result in ketoacidosis or lactic acidosis and cause hypoglycemia or hyperglycemia, depending on the dietary state. These effects are considered reversible.

In contrast, acetaldehyde and free radicals generated from ethanol metabolism can result in alcohol-induced hepatitis, a condition in which the liver is inflamed and cells become necrotic and die. Diffuse damage to hepatocytes results in cirrhosis, characterized by fibrosis (scarring), disturbance of the normal architecture and blood flow, loss of liver function, and ultimately, hepatic failure.

### A. Acute Effects of Ethanol Arising from the Increased NADH/NAD⁺ Ratio

Many of the acute effects of ethanol ingestion arise from the increased $NADH/NAD^+$ ratio in the liver (Fig. 24.13). At lower levels of ethanol intake, the rate of ethanol oxidation is regulated by the supply of ethanol (usually determined by how much ethanol we consume) and the rate at which NADH is reoxidized in the electron transport chain. NADH is not a very effective product inhibitor of ADH or ALDH, and there is no other feedback regulation by ATP, ADP, or AMP. As a consequence, NADH generated in the cytosol and mitochondria tends to accumulate, increasing the $NADH/NAD^+$ ratio to high levels (see Fig. 24.13, *circle 1*). The increase is even greater as the mitochondria become damaged from acetaldehyde or free radical injury.

#### 1. CHANGES IN FATTY ACID METABOLISM

The high $NADH/NAD^+$ ratio generated from ethanol oxidation inhibits the oxidation of fatty acids, which accumulate in the liver (see Fig. 24.13, *circles 2* and *3*). These fatty acids are reesterified into triacylglycerols by combining with glycerol 3-phosphate (glycerol 3-P). The increased $NADH/NAD^+$ ratio increases the availability of glycerol 3-P by promoting its synthesis from intermediates of glycolysis. The triacylglycerols are incorporated into very low density lipoproteins (VLDL), which accumulate in the liver and enter the blood, resulting in an ethanol-induced hyperlipidemia.

As blood ethanol concentration rises above 18 mM (the legal intoxication limit is now defined as 0.08% in most states of the United States, which is approximately 18 mM), the brain and central nervous system are affected. Induction of CYP2E1 increases the rate of ethanol clearance from the blood, thereby contributing to increased alcohol tolerance. However, the apparent ability of a chronic alcoholic to drink without appearing inebriated is partly a learned behavior.

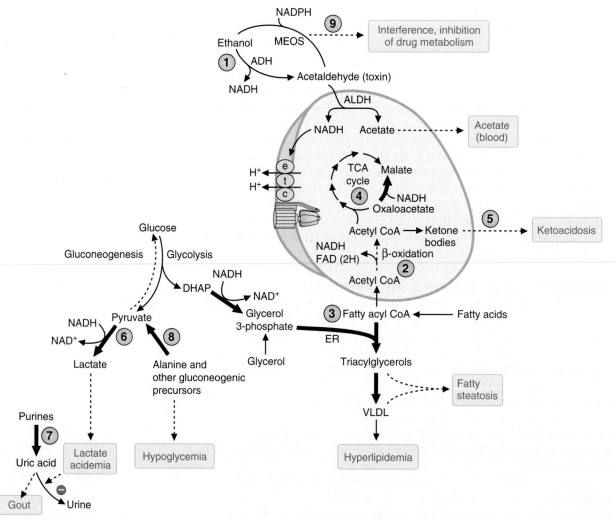

**FIG. 24.13.** Acute effects of ethanol metabolism on lipid metabolism in the liver. *(1)* Metabolism of ethanol generates a high NADH/NAD$^+$ ratio. *(2)* The high NADH/NAD$^+$ ratio inhibits fatty acid oxidation and the TCA cycle, resulting in accumulation of fatty acids. *(3)* Fatty acids are reesterified to glycerol 3-P by acyltransferases in the endoplasmic reticulum. Glycerol 3-P levels are increased because a high NADH/NAD$^+$ ratio favors its formation from dihydroxyacetone phosphate (an intermediate of glycolysis). Ethanol-stimulated increases of endoplasmic reticulum enzymes also favors triacylglycerol formation. *(4)* NADH generated from ethanol oxidation can meet the requirements of the cell for ATP generation from oxidative phosphorylation. Thus, acetyl CoA oxidation in the TCA cycle is inhibited. *(5)* The high NADH/NAD$^+$ ratio shifts OAA toward malate, and acetyl CoA is directed into ketone body synthesis. Options *(6)* through *(8)* are discussed in the text.

Although just a few drinks may result in hepatic fat accumulation, chronic consumption of alcohol greatly enhances the development of a fatty liver. Reesterification of fatty acids into triacylglycerols by fatty acyl CoA transferases in the endoplasmic reticulum is enhanced (see Fig. 24.13). Because the transferases are microsomal enzymes, they are induced by ethanol consumption just as MEOS is induced. The result is a fatty liver (hepatic steatosis).

The source of the fatty acids can be dietary fat, fatty acids synthesized in the liver, or fatty acids released from adipose tissue stores. Adipose tissue lipolysis increases after ethanol consumption, possibly because of a release of epinephrine.

## 2.   ALCOHOL-INDUCED KETOACIDOSIS

Fatty acids that are oxidized are converted to acetyl CoA and subsequently to ketone bodies (acetoacetate and β-hydroxybutyrate). Enough NADH is generated from oxidation of ethanol and fatty acids that there is no need to oxidize acetyl CoA in the TCA cycle. The very high NADH/NAD$^+$ ratio shifts all of the oxaloacetate (OAA) in the TCA cycle to malate, leaving the OAA levels too low for citrate synthase to synthesize citrate (see Fig. 24.13, *circle 4*). The acetyl CoA enters the pathway for ketone body synthesis instead of the TCA cycle.

Although ketone bodies are being produced at a high rate, their metabolism in other tissues is restricted by the supply of acetate, which is the preferred fuel. Thus, the blood concentration of ketone bodies may be much higher than found under normal fasting conditions.

### 3.  LACTIC ACIDOSIS, HYPERURICEMIA, AND HYPOGLYCEMIA

Another consequence of the very high NADH/NAD$^+$ ratio is that the balance in the lactate dehydrogenase reaction is shifted toward lactate, resulting in a lactic acidosis (see Fig. 24.13, *circle 6*). The elevation of blood lactate may decrease excretion of uric acid (see Fig. 24.13, *circle 7*) by the kidney. Consequently, patients with gout (which results from precipitated uric acid crystals in the joints) are advised not to drink excessive amounts of ethanol. Increased degradation of purines also may contribute to hyperuricemia.

The increased NADH/NAD$^+$ ratio also can cause hypoglycemia in a fasting individual who has been drinking and is dependent on gluconeogenesis to maintain blood glucose levels (see Fig. 24.13, *circles 6* and *8*). Alanine and lactate are major gluconeogenic precursors that enter gluconeogenesis as pyruvate. The high NADH/NAD$^+$ ratio shifts the lactate dehydrogenase equilibrium to lactate, so that pyruvate formed from alanine is converted to lactate and cannot enter gluconeogenesis. The high NADH/NAD$^+$ ratio also prevents other major gluconeogenic precursors, such as OAA and glycerol, from entering the gluconeogenic pathway.

In contrast, ethanol consumption with a meal may result in a transient hyperglycemia, possibly because the high NADH/NAD$^+$ ratio inhibits glycolysis at the glyceraldehyde 3-P dehydrogenase step.

### B.  Acetaldehyde Toxicity

Many of the toxic effects of chronic ethanol consumption result from accumulation of acetaldehyde, which is produced from ethanol by both ADHs and MEOS. Acetaldehyde accumulates in the liver and is released into the blood after heavy doses of ethanol. It is highly reactive and binds covalently to amino groups, sulfhydryl groups, nucleotides, and phospholipids to form "adducts." These adducts will lead to a decrease in hepatic protein synthesis, increased free radical formation and damage, and leads to liver cirrhosis and loss of liver function.

**Al M.**'s admitting physician suspected an alcohol-induced ketoacidosis superimposed on a starvation ketoacidosis. Tests showed that his plasma-free fatty acid level was elevated, and his plasma β-hydroxybutyrate level was 40 times the upper limit of normal. The increased NADH/NAD$^+$ ratio from ethanol consumption inhibited the TCA cycle and shifted acetyl CoA from fatty acid oxidation into the pathway of ketone body synthesis.

---

### CLINICAL COMMENTS

Diseases discussed in this chapter are summarized in Table 24.2.

**Candice S.** Hereditary fructose intolerance (HFI) is caused by a low level of fructose 1-P aldolase activity in aldolase B. Aldolase B is an isozyme of fructose 1,6-bisphosphate aldolase that is also capable of cleaving fructose 1-P. In persons of European descent, the most common defect is a single missense mutation in exon 5 (G → C), resulting in an amino acid substitution (Ala → Pro). As a result of this substitution, a catalytically impaired aldolase B is synthesized in abundance. The exact prevalence of HFI in the United States is not established but is approximately 1 per 15,000 to 25,000 population. The disease is transmitted by an autosomal recessive inheritance pattern.

**Table 24.2   Diseases Discussed in Chapter 24**

| Disease or Disorder | Environmental or Genetic | Comments |
|---|---|---|
| Obesity | Both | Ethanol is a nutrient, and its caloric content can contribute to obesity. |
| Alcoholism | Both | Alcohol addiction (alcoholism) may occur, leading to damage of internal organs by acetaldehyde production. |
| Jaundice | Environmental | Altered liver function leads to a reduced ability to conjugate and solubilize bilirubin, which leads to bilirubin deposition in the eyes and skin, giving them a yellow pallor. Jaundice is an indication of liver disease. |
| Liver fibrosis | Environmental | Excessive damage to liver due to alcohol metabolism, particularly acetaldehyde accumulation, leading to extensive collagen secretion and loss of liver function. |
| Hereditary fructose intolerance | Genetic | Lack of aldolase B, leading to an accumulation of fructose 1-phosphate (fructose 1-P) after fructose ingestion. The increased levels of fructose 1-P interfere with glycogen metabolism and can lead to hypoglycemia. |
| Galactosemia | Genetic | Mutations in either galactokinase or galactose 1-phosphate uridylyltransferase, leading to elevated galactose and/or galactose 1-phosphate levels. This can lead to cataract formation (high galactose) and mental retardation (elevated galactose 1-phosphate levels) if not treated early in life. |
| Glucose-6-phosphate dehydrogenase deficiency | Genetic, X-linked | Lack of glucose-6-phosphate dehydrogenase activity leads to hemolytic anemia in the presence of strong oxidizing agents. |

When affected patients such as **Candice S.** ingest fructose, fructose is converted to fructose 1-P. Because of the deficiency of aldolase B, fructose 1-P cannot be further metabolized to dihydroxyacetone phosphate and glyceraldehyde and accumulates in those tissues that have fructokinase (liver, kidney, and small intestine). Fructose is detected in the urine with the reducing sugar test (see Chapter 5). A DNA screening test (based on the generation of a new restriction site by the mutation) now provides a safe method to confirm a diagnosis of HFI.

In infants and small children, the major symptoms include poor feeding, vomiting, intestinal discomfort, and failure to thrive. The greater the ingestion of dietary fructose, the more severe is the clinical reaction. The result of prolonged ingestion of fructose is ultrastructural changes in the liver and kidney that result in hepatic and renal failure. HFI is usually a disease of infancy because adults with fructose intolerance who have survived avoid the ingestion of fruits, table sugar, and other sweets.

 **Erin G.** Erin G. has galactosemia, which is caused by a deficiency of galactose 1-P uridylyltransferase; it is one of the most common genetic diseases. Galactosemia is an autosomal recessive disorder of galactose metabolism that occurs in about 1 in 60,000 newborns. All of the states in the United States screen newborns for this disease because failure to begin immediate treatment results in mental retardation. Failure to thrive is the most common initial clinical symptom. Vomiting or diarrhea occurs in most patients, usually starting within a few days of milk ingestion. Signs of deranged liver function, jaundice or hepatomegaly, are present almost as frequently after the first week of life. The jaundice of intrinsic liver disease may be accentuated by the severe hemolysis in some patients. Cataracts have been observed within a few days of birth.

Management of patients requires eliminating galactose from the diet. Failure to eliminate this sugar results in progressive liver failure and death. In infants, artificial milk made from casein or soybean hydrolysate is used.

**Al M.**  Al M.'s pus culture sent on the second day of his admission for acute alcoholism grew out *S. aureus*. This organism has become resistant to a variety of antibiotics, so TMP/Sulfa treatment was initiated. Unfortunately, it appeared that Mr. M. had suffered an acute hemolysis (lysis or destruction of some of his red blood cells), probably induced by exposure to the sulfa drug and his infection with *S. aureus*. The hemoglobin that escaped from the lysed red blood cells was filtered by his kidneys and appeared in his urine.

By mechanisms that are not fully delineated, certain drugs (such as sulfa drugs and antimalarials), a variety of infectious agents, and exposure to fava beans can cause red blood cell destruction in individuals with a genetic deficiency of glucose 6-P dehydrogenase. Presumably, these patients cannot generate enough reduced NADPH to defend against the reactive oxygen species (ROS). Although erythrocytes lack most of the other enzymatic sources of NADPH for the glutathione antioxidant system, they do have the defense mechanisms provided by the antioxidant vitamins E and C and catalase. Thus, individuals who are not totally deficient in glucose 6-P dehydrogenase remain asymptomatic unless an additional oxidative stress, such as an infection, generates additional oxygen radicals.

Some drugs, such as the antimalarial primaquine and the sulfonamide that **Al M.** is taking, affect the ability of red blood cells to defend against oxidative stress. Fava beans, which look like fat string beans and are sometimes called **broad beans**, contain the purine glycosides vicine and isouramil. These compounds react with glutathione. It has been suggested that cellular levels of reduced glutathione (GSH) decrease to such an extent that critical sulfhydryl groups in some key proteins cannot be maintained in reduced form.

The highest prevalence rates for glucose 6-P dehydrogenase deficiency are found in tropical Africa and Asia, in some areas of the Middle East and the Mediterranean, and in Papua New Guinea. The geographic distribution of this deficiency is similar to that of sickle cell trait and is probably also related to the relative resistance it confers against the malaria parasite.

Because the individuals with this deficiency are asymptomatic unless they are exposed to an "oxidant challenge," the clinical course of the hemolytic anemia is usually self-limited if the causative agent is removed. However, genetic polymorphism accounts for a substantial variability in the severity of the disease. Severely affected patients may have a chronic hemolytic anemia and other sequelae even without known exposure to drugs, infection, and other causative factors. In such patients, neonatal jaundice is also common and can be severe enough to cause death.

**Al M.** was also suffering from acute effects of high ethanol ingestion in the absence of food intake. Both heavy ethanol consumption and low caloric intake increase adipose tissue lipolysis and elevate blood fatty acids. As a consequence of his elevated hepatic NADH/NAD$^+$ ratio, acetyl CoA produced from fatty acid oxidation was diverted from the TCA cycle into the pathway of ketone body synthesis. Because his skeletal muscles were using acetate as a fuel, ketone body utilization was diminished, resulting in ketoacidosis. **Al M.'s** moderately low blood glucose level also suggests that his high hepatic NADH level prevented pyruvate and glycerol from entering the gluconeogenic pathway. Pyruvate is diverted to lactate, which may have contributed to his metabolic acidosis and anion gap.

Rehydration with intravenous fluids containing glucose and potassium was initiated. Al's initial potassium was low, possibly secondary to vomiting. An orthopedic surgeon was consulted regarding the compound fracture of his right forearm.

1. An alcoholic is brought to the emergency room due to a hypoglycemic coma. In addition to treating the patient with an intravenous glucose infusion, the patient was also tested for the level of transketolase activity in blood cells in order to determine if which one of the following vitamins was deficient?

   A. Niacin
   B. Riboflavin
   C. Pantothenic acid
   D. Thiamine
   E. Biotin

2. Intravenous fructose feeding can lead to lactic acidosis due to which one of the following?

   A. Bypassing the regulated pyruvate kinase step
   B. Bypassing the regulated PFK-1 step
   C. Allosterically activating aldolase B
   D. Allosterically activating lactate dehydrogenase
   E. Increasing the [ATP]/[ADP] ratio in the liver

3. A man of Mediterranean descent was prescribed a drug which was a strong oxidizing agent. The man rapidly developed hemolytic anemia, a problem he had never experienced before. This individual would have difficulty with which one of the following reactions?

   A. Glucose to glucose-6-phosphate in the liver
   B. Glucose-1-phosphate to UDP-glucose in the liver

   C. Glucose-6-phosphate to 6-phosphogluconate in all cells
   D. Glucose-6-phosphate to fructose 6-phosphate in all cells
   E. 6-phosphogluconate to ribulose 5-phosphate in all cells

4. A patient was found to have elevated levels of galactose and galactitol in the blood but low cellular levels of galactose 1-phosphate. Which one of the following enzymes is most likely defective in this patient?

   A. Galactokinase
   B. Hexokinase
   C. UDP-glucose epimerase
   D. Phosphoglucomutase
   E. Galactose 1-phosphate uridylyl transferase

5. The enzymes that metabolize ethanol exist as a variety of isozymes in the general population. A slow activity isozyme of which one of the following enzymes is most likely responsible for reducing the tolerance an individual might have to drinking alcohol?

   A. Alcohol dehydrogenase
   B. Acetyl CoA synthetase
   C. Microsome ethanol oxidizing system
   D. Acetyl CoA carboxylase
   E. Aldehyde dehydrogenase

## 25 Synthesis of Glycosides, Lactose, Glycoproteins, Glycolipids, and Proteoglycans

## CHAPTER OUTLINE

## KEY POINTS

- Reactions between sugars or the formation of sugar derivatives utilize sugars activated by attachment to nucleotides (a nucleotide sugar).
- UDP-glucose and UDP-galactose are substrates for many glycosyltransferase reactions.
- Lactose is formed from UDP-galactose and glucose.
- UDP-glucose is oxidized to UDP-glucuronate, which forms glucuronide derivatives of various hydrophobic compounds, making them more readily excreted in urine or bile than the parent compound.
- Glycoproteins and glycolipids contain various types of carbohydrate residues.
- The carbohydrates in glycoproteins can be either *O*-linked or *N*-linked and are synthesized in the endoplasmic reticulum and Golgi apparatus.
- For *O*-linked carbohydrates, the carbohydrates are added sequentially (via nucleotide sugar precursors), beginning with a sugar linked to the hydroxyl group of the amino acid side chains of serine or threonine.
- For *N*-linked carbohydrates, the branched carbohydrate chain is first synthesized on dolichol phosphate and then transferred to the amide nitrogen of an asparagine residue of the protein.
- Glycolipids belong to the class of sphingolipids, synthesized from nucleotide sugars that add carbohydrate groups to the base ceramide.
- Defects in the degradation of glycosphingolipids leads to a class of lysosomal diseases known as the sphingolipidoses.

continued

■ Proteoglycans consist of a core protein covalently attached to many long, linear chains of glycosaminoglycans, which contain repeating disaccharide units. Proteoglycans are synthesized in the endoplasmic reticulum and Golgi complex.

■ The major carbohydrates in glycosaminoglycans are a hexosamine and uronic acid, along with sulfated carbohydrates.

■ Failure to appropriately degrade proteoglycans within the lysosome leads to a set of disorders known as the mucopolysaccharidoses.

# THE WAITING ROOM

To help support herself through medical school, **Edna R.** works evenings in a hospital blood bank. She is responsible for ensuring that compatible donor blood is available to patients who need blood transfusions. As part of her training, Edna has learned that the external surfaces of all blood cells contain large numbers of antigenic determinants. These determinants are often glycoproteins or glycolipids that differ from one individual to another. As a result, all blood transfusions expose the recipient to many foreign immunogens. Most of these, fortunately, do not induce antibodies, or they induce antibodies that elicit little or no immunological response. For routine blood transfusions, therefore, tests are performed only for the presence of antigens that determine whether the patient's blood type is A, B, AB, or O, and Rh(D)-positive or -negative.

**Jay S.'s** psychomotor development has become progressively more abnormal (see Chapter 12). At 2 years of age, he is obviously mentally retarded and nearly blind. His muscle weakness has progressed to the point that he cannot sit up or even crawl. As the result of a weak cough reflex, he is unable to clear his normal respiratory secretions and has had recurrent respiratory infections.

**Sarah L.** (first introduced in Chapter 11) noted a moderate reduction in pain and swelling in the joints of her fingers while she was taking her immunosuppressant medication. At her next checkup, her rheumatologist described to Sarah the underlying inflammatory tissue changes that her systemic lupus erythematosus (SLE) was causing in the joint tissues.

## I. INTERCONVERSIONS INVOLVING NUCLEOTIDE SUGARS

Activated sugars attached to nucleotides are converted to other sugars, oxidized to sugar acids, and joined to proteins, lipids, or other sugars through **glycosidic bonds**.

### A. Reactions of UDP-glucose

**Uridine diphosphate (UDP)-glucose** is an activated sugar nucleotide (see Fig. 23.4) that is a precursor of glycogen and lactose; UDP-glucuronate and glucuronides; and the carbohydrate chains in proteoglycans, glycoproteins, and glycolipids. In the synthesis of many of the carbohydrate portions of these compounds, a sugar is transferred from the nucleotide sugar to an alcohol or other nucleophilic group to form a glycosidic bond (Fig. 25.1). The use of UDP as a leaving group in the reaction provides the energy for formation of the new bond. The enzymes that form glycosidic bonds are sugar transferases (e.g., glycogen synthase is a glucosyltransferase). Transferases are also involved in the formation of the glycosidic bonds in bilirubin glucuronides, proteoglycans, and lactose.

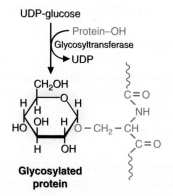

**FIG. 25.1.** Glycosyltransferases. These enzymes transfer sugars from nucleotide sugars to nucleophilic amino acid residues on proteins, such as the hydroxyl group of serine or the amide group of asparagine. Other transferases transfer specific sugars from a nucleotide sugar to a hydroxyl group of other sugars. The bond formed between the anomeric carbon of the sugar and the nucleophilic group of another compound is a glycosidic bond.

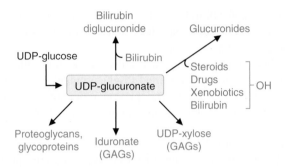

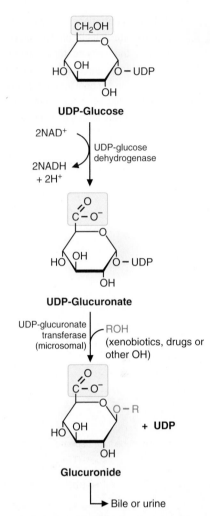

**FIG. 25.2.** Metabolic routes of UDP-glucuronate. UDP-glucuronate is formed from UDP-glucose (shown in *black*). Glucuronate from UDP-glucuronate is incorporated into GAGs where certain of the glucuronate residues are converted to iduronate. UDP-glucuronate is a precursor of UDP-xylose, another sugar residue incorporated into GAGs. Glucuronate is also transferred to the carboxyl groups of bilirubin or the alcohol groups of steroids, drugs, and xenobiotics to form glucuronides. The "-ide" in the name glucuronide denotes that these compounds are glycosides. Xenobiotics are pharmacologically, endocrinologically, or toxicologically active substances not produced endogenously and, therefore, are foreign to an organism. Drugs are an example of xenobiotics.

## B. Formation of UDP-glucuronate

One of the major routes of UDP-glucose metabolism is the formation of **UDP-glucuronate**, which serves as a precursor of other sugars and of glucuronides (Fig. 25.2). Glucuronate is formed by the oxidation of the alcohol on carbon 6 of glucose to an acid (through two oxidation states) by a $NAD^+$-dependent dehydrogenase (Fig. 25.3). Glucuronate is also present in the diet and can be formed from the degradation of inositol (the sugar alcohol that forms inositol trisphosphate [$IP_3$]), an intracellular second messenger for many hormones.

## C. Glucuronides: A Source of Negative Charges

The function of glucuronate in the excretion of bilirubin, drugs, xenobiotics, and other compounds containing a hydroxyl group is to add negative charges and increase their solubility. Bilirubin is a degradation product of heme that is formed in the reticuloendothelial system and is only slightly soluble in plasma. It is transported to the liver bound to albumin. In the liver, glucuronate residues are transferred from UDP-glucuronate to two carboxyl groups on bilirubin, sequentially forming bilirubin monoglucuronide and bilirubin diglucuronide, the "conjugated" forms of

**FIG. 25.3.** Formation of glucuronate and glucuronides. A glycosidic bond is formed between the anomeric hydroxyl of glucuronate (at carbon 1) and the hydroxyl group of a nonpolar compound. The negatively charged carboxyl group of the glucuronate increases the water solubility and allows otherwise nonpolar compounds to be excreted in the urine or bile. The hydrogen atoms have been omitted from the figure for clarity.

A failure of the liver to transport, store, or conjugate bilirubin results in the accumulation of unconjugated bilirubin in the blood. Jaundice (or icterus), the yellowish tinge to the skin and the whites of the eyes (sclerae) experienced by **Erin G.** (see Chapter 24), occurs when plasma becomes supersaturated with bilirubin (>2 to 2.5 mg/dL) and the excess diffuses into tissues. When bilirubin levels are measured in the blood, one can measure either indirect bilirubin (this is the nonconjugated form of bilirubin, which is bound to albumin), direct bilirubin (the conjugated, water-soluble form), or total bilirubin (the sum of the direct and indirect levels). If total bilirubin levels are high, then a determination of direct and indirect bilirubin is needed to appropriately determine a cause for the elevation of total bilirubin.

Many full-term newborns develop jaundice, termed neonatal jaundice. It is usually caused by an increased destruction of red blood cells after birth (the fetus has an unusually large number of red blood cells) and an immature bilirubin conjugating system in the liver. This leads to elevated levels of nonconjugated bilirubin, which is deposited in hydrophobic (fat) environments. If bilirubin levels reach a certain threshold at the age of 48 hours, the newborn is a candidate for phototherapy, in which the child is placed under lamps that emit light between the wavelengths of 425 and 475 nm. Bilirubin absorbs this light, undergoes chemical changes, and becomes more water soluble. Usually, within a week of birth, the newborn's liver can handle the load generated from red blood cell turnover.

**Q:** High concentrations of galactose 1-phosphate inhibit phosphoglucomutase, the enzyme that converts glucose-6-phosphate to glucose-1-phosphate. How can this inhibition account for the hypoglycemia and jaundice that accompany galactose 1-phosphate uridylyltransferase deficiency?

bilirubin. The more soluble bilirubin diglucuronide (as compared with unconjugated bilirubin, as two negative charges have been added to the molecule) is then actively transported into the bile for excretion.

Many xenobiotics, drugs, steroids, and other compounds with hydroxyl groups and low solubility in water are converted to glucuronides in a similar fashion by glucuronyltransferases present in the endoplasmic reticulum (ER) and cytoplasm of the liver and kidney. This is one of the major conjugation pathways for excretion of these compounds.

Glucuronate, once formed, can reenter the pathways of glucose metabolism through reactions that eventually convert it to D-xylulose 5-phosphate, an intermediate of the pentose phosphate pathway. In most mammals other than humans, an intermediate of this pathway is the precursor of ascorbic acid (vitamin C). Humans, however, are deficient in this pathway and cannot synthesize vitamin C.

### D. Synthesis of UDP-Galactose and Lactose from Glucose

**Lactose** is synthesized from UDP-galactose and glucose (Fig. 25.4). However, galactose is not required in the diet for lactose synthesis because galactose can be synthesized from glucose.

#### 1. CONVERSION OF GLUCOSE TO GALACTOSE

Galactose and glucose are **epimers**; they differ only in the stereochemical position of one hydroxyl group at carbon 4. Thus, the formation of UDP-galactose from UDP-glucose is an **epimerization** (see Fig. 24.3). The epimerase does not actually transfer the hydroxyl group; it oxidizes the hydroxyl to a ketone by transferring electrons to $NAD^+$ and then donates electrons back to re-form the alcohol group on the other side of the carbon.

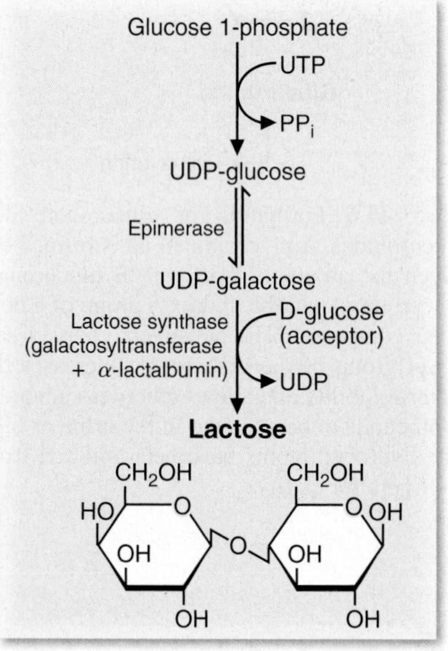

#### 2. LACTOSE SYNTHESIS

Lactose is unique in that it is synthesized only in the mammary gland of the female adult for short periods during lactation. Lactose synthase, an enzyme present in the ER of the lactating mammary gland, catalyzes the last step in lactose biosynthesis, the transfer of galactose from UDP-galactose to glucose (see Fig. 25.4). Lactose synthase has two protein subunits, a galactosyltransferase and an α-lactalbumin. α-Lactalbumin is a modifier protein synthesized after parturition (childbirth) in response to the hormone prolactin. This enzyme subunit lowers the $K_m$ of the galactosyltransferase for glucose from 1,200 to 1 mM, thereby increasing the rate of lactose synthesis. In the absence of α-lactalbumin, galactosyltransferase transfers galactosyl units to glycoproteins.

### E. Formation of Sugars for Glycolipid and Glycoprotein Synthesis

The transferases that produce the oligosaccharide and polysaccharide side chains of glycolipids and attach sugar residues to proteins are specific for the sugar moiety and for the donating nucleotide (e.g., UDP, cytidine monophosphate [CMP], or guanosine diphosphate [GDP]). Some of the sugar nucleotides used for **glycoprotein**, **proteoglycan**, and **glycolipid** formation (see Chapters 3 and 8 for a description of these compounds) include the derivatives of glucose and galactose that we have already discussed as well as acetylated amino sugars and derivatives of mannose. The reason for the large variety of sugars attached to proteins and lipids is that they have relatively specific and different functions, such as targeting a protein toward a membrane; providing recognition sites on the cell surface for other cells, hormones, or viruses; or acting as lubricants or molecular sieves. A more complete list is available in Table A25.1 of the online supplement @.

The pathways for utilization and formation of many of these sugars are summarized in Figure A25.1 of the online supplement @. Many of the steps are reversible,

**FIG. 25.4.** Lactose synthesis. Lactose is a disaccharide composed of galactose and glucose. UDP-galactose for the synthesis of lactose in the mammary gland is usually formed from the epimerization of UDP-glucose. Lactose synthase catalyzes the attack of the C4 alcohol group of glucose on the anomeric carbon of the galactose, releasing UDP and forming a glycosidic bond. Lactose synthase is composed of a galactosyltransferase and α-lactalbumin, which is a regulatory subunit.

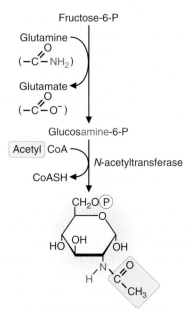

**N-Acetylglucosamine-6-P**

*FIG. 25.5.* The formation of *N*-acetylglucosamine 6-phosphate. The amino sugar is formed by a transfer of the amino group from the amide of glutamine to a carbon of the sugar. The amino group is acetylated by the transfer of an acetyl group from acetyl CoA. The hydrogen atoms from the sugar have been omitted for clarity.

**A:** The inhibition of phosphoglucomutase by galactose 1-phosphate results in hypoglycemia by interfering with both the formation of UDP-glucose (the glycogen precursor) and the degradation of glycogen back to glucose-6-phosphate. Ninety percent of glycogen degradation leads to glucose-1-phosphate, which can only be converted to glucose-6-phosphate by phosphoglucomutase. When phosphoglucomutase activity is inhibited, less glucose-6-phosphate production occurs, and hence, less glucose is available for export. Thus, the stored glycogen is only approximately 10% efficient in raising blood glucose levels, and hypoglycemia results. UDP-glucose levels are reduced because glucose-1-phosphate is required to synthesize UDP-glucose, and in the absence of phosphoglucomutase activity, glucose-6-phosphate cannot be converted to glucose-1-phosphate. This prevents the formation of UDP-glucuronate, which is necessary to convert bilirubin to the diglucuronide form for transport into the bile. Bilirubin accumulates in tissues, giving them a yellow color (jaundice).

so that glucose and other dietary sugars enter a common pool from which the diverse sugars can be formed. Mannose, like galactose, is an epimer of glucose, and mannose and glucose are interconverted by epimerization reactions at carbon 2. *N*-acetylmannosamine is the precursor of *N*-acetylneuraminic acid (NANA, a sialic acid), which is found in many glycoproteins. The negative charge on sialic acid is obtained by the addition of a three-carbon carboxyl moiety from phosphoenolpyruvate. GDP-mannose is the precursor of GDP-fucose, another sugar found in many glycoproteins.

Of particular note is that the amino sugars are all derived from glucosamine 6-phosphate. To synthesize glucosamine 6-phosphate, an amino group is transferred from the amide of glutamine to fructose 6-phosphate (Fig. 25.5). Amino sugars, such as glucosamine, can then be *N*-acetylated by an acetyltransferase. *N*-Acetyltransferases are present in the ER and cytosol and provide another means of chemically modifying sugars, metabolites, drugs, and xenobiotic compounds. Individuals may vary greatly in their capacity for acetylation reactions.

## II.   GLYCOPROTEINS

### A.   Structure and Function

Glycoproteins contain short carbohydrate chains covalently linked to either serine/threonine or asparagine residues in the protein. These oligosaccharide chains are often branched, and they do not contain repeating disaccharides (Fig. 25.6). Most proteins in the blood are glycoproteins. They serve as hormones, antibodies, enzymes (including those of the blood clotting cascade), and as structural components of the extracellular matrix. Collagen contains galactosyl units and disaccharides composed of galactosyl-glucose attached to hydroxylysine residues (see Chapter 5). The secretions of mucus-producing cells, such as salivary mucin, are glycoproteins.

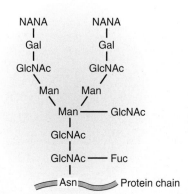

*FIG. 25.6.* An example of a branched glycoprotein. *NANA*, *N*-acetylneuraminic acid; *Gal*, galactose; *Glc-NAc*, N-acetylglucosamine; *Man*, mannose; *Fuc*, fucose.

Although most glycoproteins are secreted from cells, some are segregated in lysosomes, where they serve as the lysosomal enzymes that degrade various types of cellular and extracellular material. Other glycoproteins are produced like secretory proteins, but hydrophobic regions of the protein remain attached to the cell membrane, and the carbohydrate portion extends into the extracellular space. These glycoproteins serve as receptors for compounds such as hormones, as transport proteins, and as cell attachment and cell–cell recognition sites. Bacteria and viruses also bind to these sites.

### B. Synthesis

The protein portion of glycoproteins is synthesized on ribosomes attached to the ER. The carbohydrate chains are attached to the protein in the lumen of the ER and the Golgi complex. In some cases, the initial sugar is added to a serine or a threonine residue in the protein, and the carbohydrate chain is extended by the sequential addition of sugar residues to the nonreducing end. UDP sugars are the precursors for the addition of four of the seven sugars that are usually found in glycoproteins—glucose, galactose, *N*-acetylglucosamine, and *N*-acetylgalactosamine. GDP sugars are the precursors for the addition of mannose and L-fucose, and CMP-NANA is the precursor for NANA. Dolichol phosphate (a long-chain hydrocarbon synthesized from isoprene units) is involved in transferring branched sugar chains to the amide nitrogen of asparagine residues. Sugars are removed and added as the glycoprotein moves from the ER through the Golgi complex (Fig. 25.7). As discussed in Chapter 12, the carbohydrate chain is used as a targeting marker for lysosomal enzymes.

## III. GLYCOLIPIDS

### A. Structure and Function

Glycolipids are derivatives of the lipid sphingosine. These **sphingolipids** include the **cerebrosides** and the **gangliosides** (Fig. 25.8; see also Fig. 3.15). They contain ceramide, with carbohydrate moieties attached to its hydroxymethyl group.

Glycolipids are involved in intercellular communication. Oligosaccharides of identical composition are present in both the glycolipids and glycoproteins associated with the cell membrane, where they serve as cell recognition factors. For example, carbohydrate residues in these oligosaccharides are the antigens of the ABO blood group substances (Fig. 25.9).

By identifying the nature of antigenic determinants on the surface of the donor's red blood cells, **Edna R.** is able to classify the donor's blood as belonging to certain specific blood groups. These antigenic determinants are located in the oligosaccharides of the glycoproteins and glycolipids of the cell membranes. The most important blood group in humans is the ABO group, which comprises two antigens, A and B. Individuals with the A antigen on their cells belong to blood group A. Those with B belong to group B, and those with both A and B belong to group AB. The absence of both the A and the B antigen results in blood type O (see Fig. 25.9).

The blood group substances are oligosaccharide components of glycolipids and glycoproteins found in most cell membranes. Those located on red blood cells have been studied extensively. A single genetic locus with two alleles determines an individual's blood type. These genes encode glycosyltransferases involved in the synthesis of the oligosaccharides of the blood group substances.

Most individuals can synthesize the H substance, an oligosaccharide that contains a fucose linked to a galactose at the nonreducing end of the blood group substance (see Fig. 25.9). Type A individuals produce an *N*-acetylgalactosamine transferase (encoded by the A gene) that attaches *N*-acetylgalactosamine to the galactose residue of the H substance. Type B individuals produce a galactosyltransferase (encoded by the B gene) that links galactose to the galactose residue of the H substance. Type AB individuals have both alleles and produce both transferases. Thus, some of the oligosaccharides of their blood group substances contain *N*-acetylgalactosamine and some contain galactose. Type O individuals produce a defective transferase, and therefore, they do not attach either *N*-acetylgalactosamine or galactose to the H substance. Thus, individuals of blood type O have only the H substance.

**A**

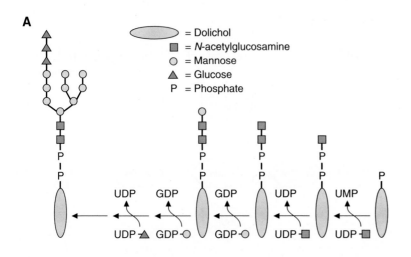

**B**

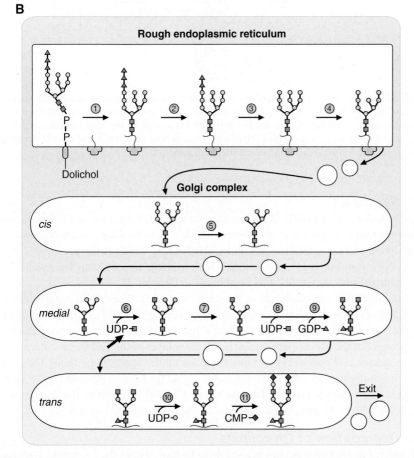

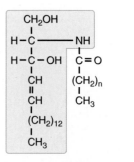

**Galactocerebroside**

**Ganglioside**

**Ceramide**

**FIG. 25.8.** Structures of cerebrosides and gangliosides. In these glycolipids, sugars are attached to ceramide (shown below the glycolipids). The *boxed portion* of ceramide is sphingosine, from which the name *sphingolipids* is derived.

**FIG. 25.7.** Action of dolichol phosphate in synthesizing the high-mannose form of oligosaccharides (**A**) and processing of these carbohydrate groups (**B**). Transfer of the branched oligosaccharide from dolichol phosphate to a protein in the lumen of the rough endoplasmic reticulum (RER) (*step 1*) and processing of the oligosaccharide (*steps 2–11*). *Steps 1* through *4* occur in the RER. The glycoprotein is transferred in vesicles to the Golgi complex where further modifications of the oligosaccharides occur (steps *5–11*). (**B** modified with permission from Kornfeld R, Kornfeld S. Annu Rev Biochem 1985;54:640. Copyright 1985 by Annual Reviews, Inc.)

**Blood Type**

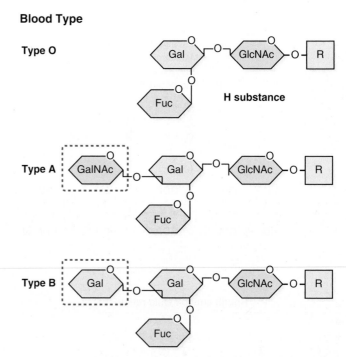

**FIG. 25.9.** Structures of the blood group substances. Note that these structures are the same except that type A has *N*-acetylgalactosamine *(GalNAc)* at the nonreducing end, type B has galactose *(Gal)*, and type O has neither. *R* is either a protein or the lipid ceramide. Each antigenic determinant is boxed. Type AB blood contains both the type A and type B structures. *Fuc,* fucose; *GlcNAc,* *N*-acetylglucosamine; *Gal,* galactose.

**Q:** **Edna R.** determined that a patient's blood type was AB. The new surgical resident was eager to give this patient a blood transfusion and, because AB blood is rare and an adequate amount was not available in the blood bank, he requested type A blood. Should Edna give him type A blood for his patient?

**Jay S.** has Tay-Sachs disease, which belongs to a group of gangliosidoses that include Fabry and Gaucher diseases. They mainly affect the brain, the skin, and the reticuloendothelial system (e.g., liver and spleen). In these diseases, complex lipids accumulate. Each of these lipids contains a ceramide as part of its structure (see Table 25.1). The rate at which the lipid is synthesized is normal. However, the lysosomal enzyme required to degrade it is not very active, either because it is made in deficient quantities because of a mutation in a gene that specifically codes for the enzyme or because a critical protein required to activate the enzyme is deficient. Because the lipid cannot be degraded, it accumulates and causes degeneration of the affected tissues with progressive malfunction, such as the psychomotor deficits that occur as a result of the central nervous system involvement seen in most of these storage diseases.

## B. Synthesis

Cerebrosides are synthesized from ceramide and UDP-glucose or UDP-galactose. They contain a single sugar (a monosaccharide). Gangliosides contain oligosaccharides produced from UDP sugars and CMP-NANA, which is the precursor for the *N*-acetylneuraminic acid residues that branch from the linear chain. The synthesis of the sphingolipids is described in more detail in Chapter 28.

Sphingolipids are produced in the Golgi complex. Their lipid component becomes part of the membrane of the secretory vesicle that buds from the *trans* face of the Golgi. After the vesicle membrane fuses with the cell membrane, the lipid component of the glycolipid remains in the outer layer of the cell membrane, and the carbohydrate component extends into the extracellular space. Sometimes, the carbohydrate component is used as a recognition signal for foreign proteins; for example, cholera toxin (which affected **Dennis V.,** see Chapter 8) binds to the carbohydrate portion of the GM1 ganglioside to allow its catalytic subunit to enter the cell.

## C. Degradation of Glycolipids

Glycolipid degradation occurs in a stepwise fashion within the lysosome, with each step catalyzed by a different enzyme. Defects in the degradation of the gangliosides (and other sphingolipids) lead to a set of diseases known as the sphingolipidoses (gangliosidoses) (Table 25.1). A defect in virtually any step in the degradative pathway will lead to a disease.

## IV. PROTEOGLYCANS

A major component of a cell's **extracellular matrix (ECM)** are proteoglycans. The proteoglycans act to form a gel that embeds structural proteins, such as collagen, within the ECM. They are found in interstitial connective tissues, such as the synovial fluid of the joints, the vitreous humor of the eye, arterial walls, bone, cartilage, and cornea. Proteoglycans consist of polysaccharides called **glycosaminoglycans**

**Table 25.1   Defective Enzymes in the Gangliosidoses**

| Disease | Enzyme Deficiency | Accumulated Lipid |
|---|---|---|
| Fucosidosis | α-Fucosidase | Cer–Glc–Gal–GalNAc–Gal:Fuc H-isoantigen |
| Generalized gangliosidosis | $G_{M1}$-β-galactosidase | Cer–Glc–Gal(NeuAc)–GalNAc:Gal $G_{M1}$ ganglioside |
| Tay-Sachs disease | Hexosaminidase A | Cer–Glc–Gal(NeuAc):GalNAc $G_{M2}$ ganglioside |
| Tay-Sachs variant or Sandhoff disease | Hexosaminidase A and B | Cer–Glc–Gal–Gal:GalNAc Globoside plus $G_{M2}$ ganglioside |
| Fabry disease | α-Galactosidase | Cer–Glc–Gal:Gal globotriaosylceramide |
| Ceramide lactoside lipidosis | Ceramide lactosidase (β-galactosidase) | Cer–Glc:Gal ceramide lactoside |
| Metachromatic leukodystrophy | Arylsulfatase A | Cer–Gal:$OSO_3^{-3}$ sulfogalactosylceramide |
| Krabbe disease | β-Galactosidase | Cer:Gal galactosylceramide |
| Gaucher disease | β-Glucosidase | Cer:Glc glucosylceramide |
| Niemann-Pick disease | Sphingomyelinase | Cer:P–choline Sphingomyelin |
| Farber disease | Ceramidase | Acyl:sphingosine ceramide |

NeuAc, N-acetylneuraminic acid; Cer, ceramide; Glc, glucose; Gal, galactose; Fuc, fucose. The colon indicates the bond which cannot be broken due to the enzyme deficiency associated with the disease.

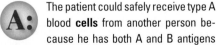

**A:** The patient could safely receive type A blood **cells** from another person because he has both A and B antigens on his own cells and does not have antibodies in his serum to either type A or B cells. However, he should not be given type A serum (or type A whole blood) because type A serum contains antibodies to type B antigens, which are present on his cells.

(GAGs) linked to a core protein. The overall charge on the GAGs is negative, which allow the proteoglycan to bind positively charged ions and form hydrogen bonds with trapped water molecules, thereby creating a hydrated gel. The gel provides a flexible mechanical support to the ECM. The gel also acts as a filter that allows the diffusion of ions (e.g., $Ca^{+2}$), $H_2O$, and other small molecules, but slows diffusion of proteins and movement of cells. The gel also acts as a lubricant. Some specific functions of proteoglycans and GAGs are outlined in Table A25.2 of the online supplement @.

## A.  Structure and Function

The major components of the proteoglycans are the GAGs (formerly called mucopolysaccharides). GAGs are long, unbranched polysaccharides composed of repeating disaccharide units (Fig. 25.10). The repeating disaccharides usually contain an iduronic or uronic acid and a hexosamine and are frequently sulfated. Consequently, they carry a negative charge, are hydrated, and act as lubricants. After synthesis, proteoglycans are secreted from cells; thus, they function extracellularly. Because the long, negatively charged GAG chains repel each other, the proteoglycans occupy a very large space and act as "molecular sieves," determining which substances enter or leave cells. Their properties also give resilience and a degree of flexibility to substances such as cartilage, permitting compression and reexpansion of the molecule to occur.

At least seven types of GAGs exist, which differ in the monosaccharides present in their repeating disaccharide units—chondroitin sulfate, dermatan sulfate, heparin, heparin sulfate, hyaluronic acid, and keratan sulfates I and II. Except for hyaluronic acid (which is a single, long polysaccharide with no sulfate groups), the GAGs are linked to proteins, usually attached covalently to serine or threonine residues (Fig. 25.11). Keratan sulfate I is attached to asparagine.

## B.  Synthesis

The protein component of the proteoglycans is synthesized on ribosomes attached to the ER. It enters the lumen of this organelle, where the initial glycosylations occur. UDP sugars serve as the precursors that add sugar units one at a time, first to the protein and then to the nonreducing end of the growing carbohydrate chain (Fig. 25.12). Glycosylation occurs initially in the lumen of the ER and subsequently in the Golgi complex. Glycosyltransferases, the enzymes that add sugars to the chain, are specific for the sugar being added, the type of linkage that is formed, and the sugars already

The principal components of the matrix of cartilage are collagen and proteoglycans, both of which are produced and degraded by the chondrocytes that are embedded in this matrix. An autoimmune attack on articular proteins alters the balance between cartilage degradation and formation. The resulting loss of cartilage organization accompanied by an inflammatory response is responsible for the symptoms experienced by **Sarah L.**

The collagen component forms a network of fine fibrils that give shape to the cartilage. The proteoglycans embedded in the cartilage are responsible for its compressibility and its deformability.

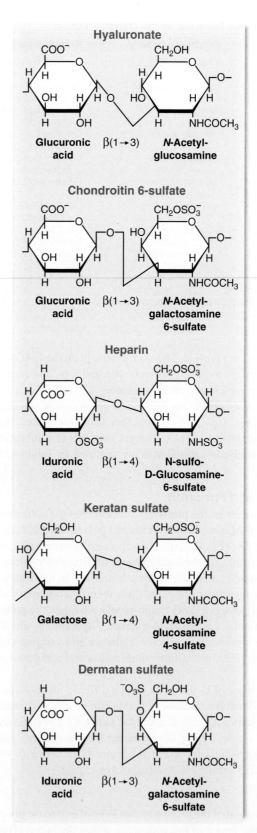

***FIG. 25.10.*** Repeating disaccharides of some GAGs. These repeating disaccharides usually contain an *N*-acetylated sugar and a uronic acid, which usually is glucuronic acid or iduronic acid. Sulfate groups are often present but are not included in the sugar names in this figure. Iduronic acid and glucuronic acid are epimers at position 5 of the sugar.

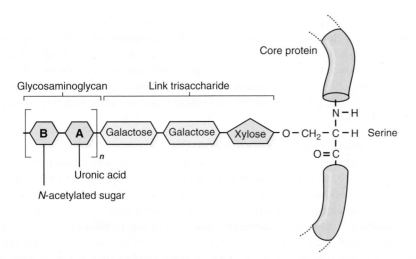

**FIG. 25.11.** Attachment of GAGs to proteins. The sugars are linked to a serine or threonine residue of the protein. *A* and *B* represent the sugars of the repeating disaccharide.

present in the chain. Once the initial sugars are attached to the protein, the alternating action of two glycosyltransferases adds the sugars of the repeating disaccharide to the growing GAG chain. Sulfation occurs after addition of the sugar. 3′-Phosphoadenosine 5′-phosphosulfate (PAPS), also called **active sulfate**, provides the sulfate groups. An epimerase converts glucuronic acid residues to iduronic acid residues.

The long polysaccharide side chains of the proteoglycans in cartilage contain many anionic groups. This high concentration of negative charges attracts cations that create a high osmotic pressure within cartilage, drawing water into this specialized connective tissue and placing the collagen network under tension. At equilibrium, the resulting tension balances the swelling pressure caused by the proteoglycans. The complementary roles of this macromolecular organization give cartilage its resilience. Cartilage can thus withstand the compressive load of weight bearing and then reexpand to its previous dimensions when that load is relieved.

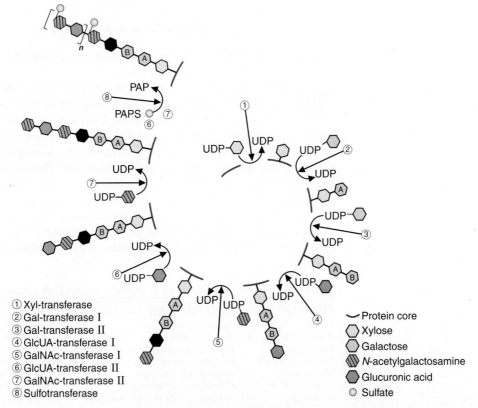

① Xyl-transferase
② Gal-transferase I
③ Gal-transferase II
④ GlcUA-transferase I
⑤ GalNAc-transferase I
⑥ GlcUA-transferase II
⑦ GalNAc-transferase II
⑧ Sulfotransferase

⌒ Protein core
⬡ Xylose
⬡ Galactose
⬡ *N*-acetylgalactosamine
⬡ Glucuronic acid
○ Sulfate

**FIG. 25.12.** Synthesis of chondroitin sulfate. Sugars are added to the protein one at a time, with UDP sugars serving as the precursors. Initially a xylose residue is added to a serine in the protein. Then two galactose residues are added, followed by a glucuronic acid (GlcUA) and an *N*-acetylglucosamine (GalNAc). Subsequent additions occur by the alternating action of two enzymes that produce the repeating disaccharide units. One enzyme *(6)* adds GlcUA residues, and the other *(7)* adds *GalNAc*. As the chain grows, sulfate groups are added by phosphoadenosine phosphosulfate (PAPS). (Modified from Roden L. In: Fishman WH, ed. Metabolic Conjugation and Metabolic Hydrolysis, vol II. Orlando, FL: Academic Press, 1970:401.)

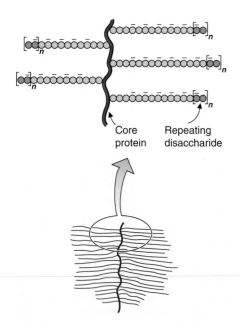

*FIG. 25.13.* "Bottlebrush" structure of a proteoglycan with a magnified segment.

After synthesis, the proteoglycan is secreted from the cell. Its structure resembles a bottlebrush with many glycosaminoglycan chains extending from the core protein (Fig. 25.13). The proteoglycans may form large aggregates, noncovalently attached by a "link" protein to hyaluronic acid. The proteoglycans interact with the adhesion protein, fibronectin, which is attached to an integrin (protein) embedded within the plasma membrane. Cross-linked fibers of collagen also associate with this complex, forming the ECM.

## C.  Degradation of Proteoglycans

Lysosomal enzymes degrade proteoglycans, glycoproteins, and glycolipids, which are brought into the cell by the process of endocytosis. Lysosomes fuse with the endocytic vesicles, and lysosomal proteases digest the protein component. The carbohydrate component is degraded by lysosomal glycosidases.

Lysosomes contain both **endoglycosidases** and **exoglycosidases**. The endoglycosidases cleave the chains into shorter oligosaccharides. Then exoglycosidases, specific for each type of linkage, remove the sugar residues, one at a time, from the nonreducing ends.

Deficiencies of lysosomal glycosidases cause partially degraded carbohydrates from proteoglycans, glycoproteins, and glycolipids to accumulate within membrane-enclosed vesicles inside cells. These "residual bodies" can cause marked enlargement of the organ with impairment of its function.

In the clinical disorders known as the mucopolysaccharidoses (caused by accumulation of partially degraded GAGs), deformities of the skeleton may occur, along with cardiac changes, eye problems, and cognitive dysfunction, depending on the type of mucopolysaccharidosis disorder (Table 25.2).

## CLINICAL COMMENTS

Diseases discussed in this chapter are summarized in Table 25.3.

 **Edna R.**  During her stint in the hospital blood bank, **Edna R.** learned that the importance of the ABO blood group system in transfusion therapy is based on two principles (Table 25.4): (a) Antibodies to A and to B antigens occur naturally in the blood serum of persons whose red blood cell surfaces lack the corresponding antigen (i.e., individuals with A antigens on their red blood cells have B antibodies in their serum and vice versa). These antibodies may arise as a result of previous exposure to cross-reacting antigens in bacteria and foods or to blood transfusions. (b) Antibodies to A and B are usually present in high titers and are capable of activating the entire complement system. As a result, these antibodies may cause intravascular destruction of a large number of incompatible red blood cells given inadvertently during a blood transfusion. Individuals with type AB blood

**Table 25.2    Defective Enzymes in the Mucopolysaccharidoses**

| Disease | Enzyme Deficiency | Accumulated Products |
|---|---|---|
| Hunter | Iduronate sulfatase | Heparan sulfate, dermatan sulfate |
| Hurler + Scheie | α-L-Iduronidase | Heparan sulfate, dermatan sulfate |
| Maroteaux-Lamy | *N*-Acetylgalactosamine sulfatase | Dermatan sulfate |
| Mucolipidosis VII | β-Glucuronidase | Heparan sulfate, dermatan sulfate |
| Sanfilippo A | Heparan sulfamidase | Heparan sulfate |
| Sanfilippo B | *N*-Acetylglucosaminidase | Heparan sulfate |
| Sanfilippo D | *N*-Acetylglucosamine 6-sulfatase | Heparin sulfate |

These disorders share many clinical features, although there are significant variations between disorders, and even within a single disorder, based on the amount of residual activity remaining. In most cases, multiple organ systems are affected (with bone and cartilage being a primary target). For some disorders, there is significant neuronal involvement, leading to mental retardation.

**Table 25.3    Diseases Discussed in Chapter 25**

| Disease or Disorder | Environmental or Genetic | Comments |
|---|---|---|
| Blood transfusions | Environmental/ genetic | Blood typing is dependent on antigens on the cell surface, particularly the carbohydrate content of the antigen. |
| Tay-Sachs disease | Genetic | Lack of hexosaminidase A activity, leading to an accumulation of $G_{M2}$ in the lysosomes |
| Jaundice | Both | Lack of ability to conjugate bilirubin with glucuronic acid in the liver |
| Sphingolipidoses | Genetic | Defects in ganglioside and sphingolipid degradation, as summarized in Table 25.1 |
| Lupus | Environmental | Alterations in cell matrix components due to an autoimmune induced trigger |
| Mucopolysaccharidoses | Genetic | Defects in the breakdown of mucopolysaccharides, found primarily in the extracellular matrix. See Table 25.2 for more details on these diseases. |

have both A and B antigens and do not produce antibodies to either. Hence, they are "universal" recipients. They can safely receive red blood cells from individuals of A, B, AB, or O blood type. (However, they cannot safely receive serum from these individuals because it contains antibodies to A or B antigens.) Those with type O blood do not have either antigen. They are "universal" donors; that is, their red cells can safely be infused into type A, B, O, or AB individuals. (However, their serum contains antibodies to both A and B antigens and cannot safely be used.)

The second important red blood cell group is the Rh group. It is important because one of its antigenic determinants, the D antigen, is a very potent immunogen, stimulating the production of a large number of antibodies. The unique carbohydrate composition of the glycoproteins that constitute the antigenic determinants on red blood cells in part contributes to the relative immunogenicity of the A, B, and Rh (D) red blood cell groups in human blood.

**Jay S.** Tay-Sachs disease, the problem afflicting **Jay S.**, is an autosomal recessive disorder that is rare in the general population (1 in 300,000 births), but its prevalence in Jews of Eastern European (Ashkenazi) extraction (who make up 90% of the Jewish population in the United States) is much higher (1 in 3,600 births). One in 28 Ashkenazi Jews carries this defective gene. Its presence can be discovered by measuring the tissue level of the protein produced by the gene (hexosaminidase A) or by recombinant DNA techniques. Skin fibroblasts of concerned couples planning a family are frequently used for these tests.

Carriers of the affected gene have a reduced but functional level of this enzyme that normally hydrolyzes a specific bond between an N-acetyl-D-galactosamine and a D-galactose residue in the polar head of the ganglioside.

No effective therapy is available. Enzyme replacement has met with little success because of the difficulties in getting the enzyme across the blood–brain barrier.

**Sarah L.** Articular cartilage is a living tissue with a turnover time determined by a balance between the rate of its synthesis and that of its degradation. The chondrocytes that are embedded in the matrix of intra-articular

**Table 25.4    Characteristics of the ABO Blood Groups**

| Red cell type | O | A | B | AB |
|---|---|---|---|---|
| Possible genotypes | OO | AA or AO | BB or BO | AB |
| Antibodies in serum | Anti-A and -B | Anti-B | Anti-A | None |
| Frequency (in Caucasians) | 45% | 40% | 10% | 5% |
| Can accept blood types | O | A, O | B, O | A, B, AB, O |

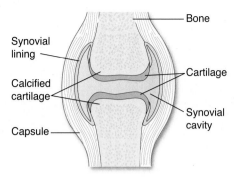

**FIG. 25.14.** A simplified view of a joint, indicating the location of the cartilage covering the ends of the long bones.

cartilage participate in both its synthesis and its enzymatic degradation. The latter occurs as a result of cleavage of proteoglycan aggregates by enzymes produced and secreted by the chondrocytes.

In SLE, the condition that affects **Sarah L.**, this delicate balance is disrupted in favor of enzymatic degradation, leading to dissolution of articular cartilage and, with it, the loss of its critical cushioning functions. The functional properties of a normal joint depend, in part, on the presence of a soft, well-lubricated, deformable, and compressible layer of cartilaginous tissue covering the long bones that constitute the joint (Fig. 25.14). The underlying mechanisms responsible for this process in SLE involve an autoimmune-induced inflammation. In this sense, SLE is an "autoimmune" disease because antibodies are produced by the host that attack "self" proteins. This process excites the local release of cytokines such as interleukin-1 (IL-1), which increases the proteolytic activity of the chondrocytes, causing further loss of articular proteins such as the proteoglycans. The associated inflammatory cascade is responsible for **Sarah L.'s** joint pain.

 **REVIEW QUESTIONS–CHAPTER 25**

1.  Which one of the following statements best describes a mother with classical galactosemia?

    A.  She can convert galactose to UDP-galactose for lactose synthesis during lactation.
    B.  She can utilize galactose as a precursor to glucose production.
    C.  She can utilize galactose to produce glycogen.
    D.  She will have lower than normal serum galactose levels after drinking milk.
    E.  She can form galactose 1-phosphate from galactose.

2.  A newborn is diagnosed with neonatal jaundice. In this patient, a significant amount of the bilirubin produced lacks which one of the following carbohydrates?

    A.  Glucose
    B.  Gluconate
    C.  Galactose
    D.  Glucuronate
    E.  Galactitol

3.  A woman, shortly after giving birth to her first child, was discovered to be unable to synthesize lactose. Analysis of various glycoproteins in her serum indicated that there was no defect in the carbohydrate chains nor was the carbohydrate content of her cell surface glycolipids altered. This woman may have a mutation in which one of the following proteins or class of proteins?

    A.  A glucosyltransferase
    B.  α-Lactalbumin

    C.  A galactosyltransferase
    D.  Lactase
    E.  A lactosyltransferase

4.  The only blood available in the blood bank is type A. Which one of the following answers best describes which blood type(s) can receive type A cells without a severe immune reaction?

    A.  Types A and AB
    B.  Type A only
    C.  Types A and B
    D.  Types A, B, and AB
    E.  Types A, B, AB, and O
    F.  Types A, B, and O

5.  The underlying mechanism via which glycosaminoglycans allow for the formation of a gel-like substance in the extracellular matrix is which one of the following?

    A.  Charge attraction between glycosaminoglycan chains
    B.  Charge repulsion between glycosaminoglycan chains
    C.  Hydrogen bonding between glycosaminoglycan chains
    D.  Covalent cross-linking between glycosaminoglycan chains
    E.  Hydroxylation of adjacent glycosaminoglycan chains

# 26 Gluconeogenesis and Maintenance of Blood Glucose Levels

## CHAPTER OUTLINE

## KEY POINTS

- The process of glucose production is termed gluconeogenesis. Gluconeogenesis occurs primarily in the liver.
- The major precursors for glucose production are lactate, glycerol, and amino acids.
- The gluconeogenic pathway utilizes the reversible reactions of glycolysis, plus additional reactions to bypass the irreversible steps.
  - Pyruvate carboxylase (pyruvate to oxaloacetate) and phosphoenolpyruvate carboxykinase (PEPCK; oxaloacetate to phosphoenolpyruvate [PEP]) bypass the pyruvate kinase step.
  - Fructose 1,6-bisphosphatase (fructose 1,6-bisphosphate to fructose 6-phosphate) bypasses the phosphofructokinase-1 step.
  - Glucose-6-phosphatase (glucose-6-phosphate to glucose) bypasses the glucokinase step.
- Gluconeogenesis and glycogenolysis are carefully regulated such that blood glucose levels can be maintained at a constant level during fasting. The regulation of triglyceride metabolism is also linked to the regulation of blood glucose levels.

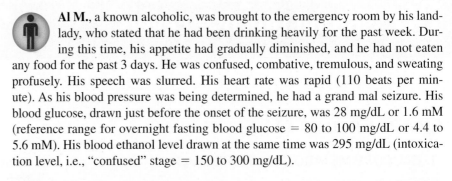

# THE WAITING ROOM

**Q:** What clinical signs and symptoms help to distinguish a coma caused by an excess of blood glucose and ketone bodies due to a deficiency of insulin (diabetic ketoacidosis [DKA]) from a coma caused by a sudden lowering of blood glucose (hypoglycemic coma) induced by the inadvertent injection of excessive insulin, the current problem experienced by **Dianne A.**?

**Al M.**, a known alcoholic, was brought to the emergency room by his landlady, who stated that he had been drinking heavily for the past week. During this time, his appetite had gradually diminished, and he had not eaten any food for the past 3 days. He was confused, combative, tremulous, and sweating profusely. His speech was slurred. His heart rate was rapid (110 beats per minute). As his blood pressure was being determined, he had a grand mal seizure. His blood glucose, drawn just before the onset of the seizure, was 28 mg/dL or 1.6 mM (reference range for overnight fasting blood glucose = 80 to 100 mg/dL or 4.4 to 5.6 mM). His blood ethanol level drawn at the same time was 295 mg/dL (intoxication level, i.e., "confused" stage = 150 to 300 mg/dL).

**Dianne A.** could not remember whether she had taken her 6:00 PM insulin dose, when in fact, she had done so. Unfortunately, she decided to give herself the evening dose (for the second time). When she did not respond to her alarm clock at 6:00 AM the following morning, her roommate tried unsuccessfully to awaken her. The roommate called an ambulance, and Dianne was rushed to the hospital emergency room in a coma. Her pulse and blood pressure at admission were normal. Her skin was flushed and slightly moist. Her respirations were slightly slow.

Diabetes mellitus (DM) should be suspected if a venous plasma glucose level drawn regardless of when food was last eaten (a "random" sample of blood glucose) is "unequivocally elevated" (i.e., ≥200 mg/dL), particularly in a patient who manifests the classic signs and symptoms of chronic hyperglycemia (polydipsia, polyuria, blurred vision, headaches, rapid weight loss, sometimes accompanied by nausea and vomiting). To confirm the diagnosis, the patient should fast overnight (10 to16 hours), and the blood glucose measurement should be repeated. Values of less than 100 mg/dL are considered normal. Values greater than or equal to 126 mg/dL are indicative of DM. Glycosylated hemoglobin (HbA$_{1c}$) can also be measured to make the diagnosis and, if greater than 6.5%, is diagnostic for DM. Values of fasting blood glucose between 101 and 125 mg/dL are designated impaired fasting glucose (IFG or prediabetes), and these individuals are at increased risk to eventually develop overt DM. The determination that fasting blood glucose levels of 126 mg/dL or a percentage of HbA$_{1c}$ of greater than 6.5% is diagnostic for DM is based on data indicating that at those levels of glucose or HbA$_{1c}$, patients begin to develop complications of DM, specifically retinopathy.

The renal tubular transport maximum in the average healthy subject is such that glucose will not appear in the urine until the blood glucose level exceeds 180 mg/dL. As a result, reagent tapes (Tes-Tape or Dextrostix) designed to detect the presence of glucose in the urine are not sensitive enough to establish a diagnosis of early DM.

## I. GLUCOSE METABOLISM IN THE LIVER

Glucose serves as a fuel for most tissues of the body. It is the major fuel for certain tissues such as the brain and red blood cells. After a meal, food is the source of blood glucose. The liver oxidizes glucose and stores the excess as glycogen. The liver also uses the pathway of glycolysis to convert glucose to pyruvate, which provides carbon for the synthesis of fatty acids. Glycerol-3-phosphate, produced from glycolytic intermediates, combines with fatty acids to form triacylglycerols, which are secreted into the blood in very low density lipoproteins (VLDL; further explained in Chapter 27). During fasting, the liver releases glucose into the blood, so that glucose-dependent tissues do not suffer from a lack of energy. Two mechanisms are involved in this process: glycogenolysis and gluconeogenesis. Hormones, particularly insulin and glucagon, dictate whether glucose flows through glycolysis or whether the reactions are reversed and glucose is produced via gluconeogenesis.

## II. GLUCONEOGENESIS

**Gluconeogenesis**, the process by which glucose is synthesized from noncarbohydrate precursors, occurs mainly in the liver under fasting conditions. Under the more extreme conditions of starvation, the kidney cortex also may produce glucose. For the most part, the glucose produced by the kidney cortex is used by the kidney medulla but some may enter the bloodstream.

Starting with pyruvate, most of the steps of gluconeogenesis are simply reversals of those of glycolysis (Fig. 26.1). In fact, these pathways differ at only three points. Enzymes involved in catalyzing these steps are regulated so that either glycolysis or gluconeogenesis predominates, depending on physiological conditions.

Most of the steps of gluconeogenesis use the same enzymes that catalyze the process of glycolysis. The flow of carbon, however, is in the reverse direction. Three reaction sequences of gluconeogenesis differ from the corresponding steps of glycolysis. They involve the conversion of pyruvate to phosphoenolpyruvate (PEP)

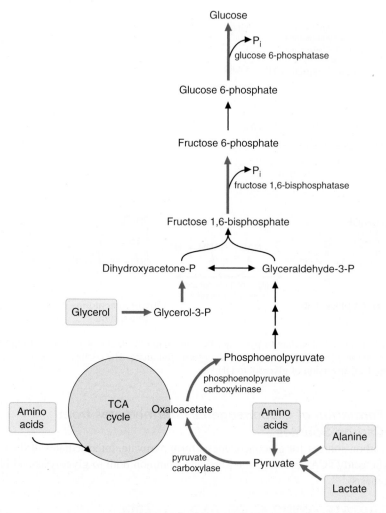

**FIG. 26.1.** Key reactions of gluconeogenesis. The precursors are amino acids (particularly alanine), lactate, and glycerol. *Heavy red arrows* indicate steps that differ from those of glycolysis.

 Comatose patients in diabetic keto-acidosis have the smell of acetone (a derivative of the ketone body acetoacetate) on their breath. In addition, DKA patients have deep, relatively rapid respirations typical of acidotic patients (Kussmaul breathing). These respirations result from an acidosis-induced stimulation of the respiratory center in the brain. More $CO_2$ is exhaled in an attempt to reduce the amount of acid in the body: $H^+ + HCO_3 \rightarrow H_2CO_3 \rightarrow H_2O + CO_2$ (exhaled). These signs are not observed in a hypoglycemic coma.

The severe hyperglycemia of DKA also causes an osmotic diuresis (i.e., glucose entering the urine carries water with it), which, in turn, causes a contraction of blood volume. Volume depletion may be aggravated by vomiting, which is common in patients with DKA. DKA may cause dehydration (dry skin), a low blood pressure, and a rapid heartbeat. These respiratory and hemodynamic alterations are not seen in patients with hypoglycemic coma. The flushed, wet skin of hypoglycemic coma is in contrast to the dry skin observed in DKA.

and the reactions that remove phosphate from fructose 1,6-bisphosphate to form fructose 6-phosphate and glucose-6-phosphate to form glucose (see Fig. 26.1). The conversion of pyruvate to PEP is catalyzed during gluconeogenesis by a series of enzymes instead of the single enzyme used for glycolysis. The reactions that remove phosphate from fructose 1,6-bisphosphate and from glucose-6-phosphate each use single enzymes that differ from the corresponding enzymes of glycolysis. Although phosphate is added during glycolysis by kinases, which use adenosine triphosphate (ATP), it is removed during gluconeogenesis by phosphatases that release inorganic phosphate ($P_i$) via hydrolysis reactions.

## A. Precursors for Gluconeogenesis

The three major carbon sources for gluconeogenesis in humans are lactate, glycerol, and amino acids, particularly alanine. Lactate is produced by anaerobic glycolysis in tissues such as exercising muscle or red blood cells as well as by adipocytes during the fed state. Glycerol is released from adipose stores of triacylglycerol, and amino acids come mainly from amino acid pools in muscle, where they may be obtained by degradation of muscle protein. Alanine, the major gluconeogenic amino acid, is produced in the muscle from other amino acids and from glucose (see Chapter 32). Because ethanol metabolism only gives rise to acetyl coenzyme A (acetyl CoA), the carbons of ethanol cannot be used for gluconeogenesis.

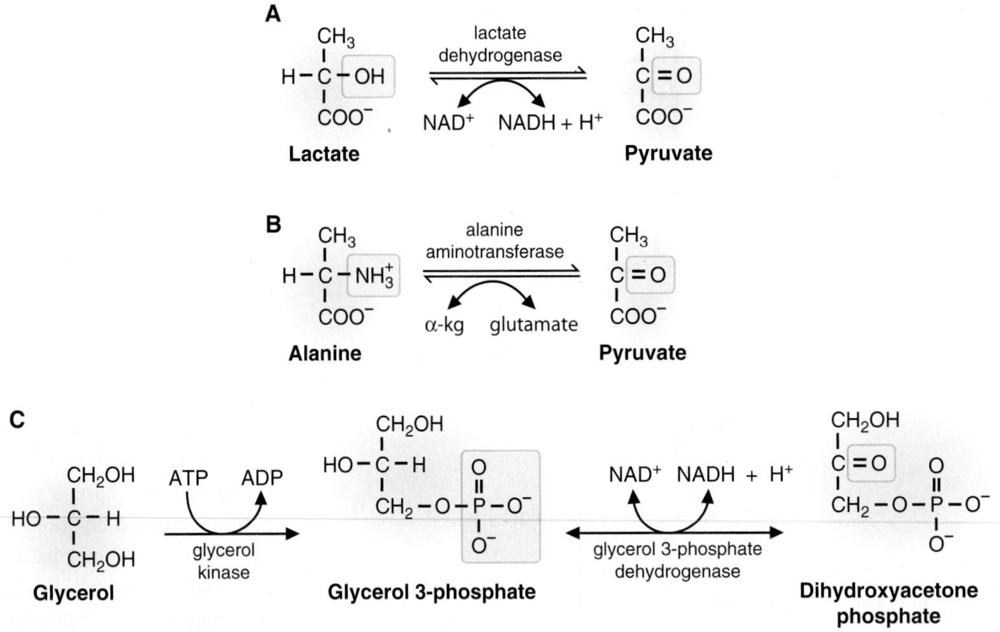

**FIG. 26.2.** Metabolism of gluconeogenic precursors. **A.** Conversion of lactate to pyruvate. **B.** Conversion of alanine to pyruvate. In this reaction, alanine aminotransferase transfers the amino group of alanine to α-ketoglutarate (α-kg) to form glutamate. The coenzyme for this reaction, pyridoxal phosphate, accepts and donates the amino group. **C.** Conversion of glycerol to DHAP.

### B. Formation of Gluconeogenic Intermediates from Carbon Sources

The carbon sources for gluconeogenesis form pyruvate, intermediates of the tricarboxylic acid (TCA) cycle, or intermediates common both to glycolysis and gluconeogenesis.

#### 1. LACTATE, AMINO ACIDS, AND GLYCEROL

Pyruvate is produced in the liver from the gluconeogenic precursors lactate and alanine. Lactate dehydrogenase oxidizes lactate to pyruvate, generating NADH (Fig. 26.2A), and alanine aminotransferase converts alanine to pyruvate (see Fig. 26.2B).

Although alanine is the major gluconeogenic amino acid, other amino acids, such as serine, serve as carbon sources for the synthesis of glucose because they also form pyruvate, the substrate for the initial step in the process. Some amino acids form intermediates of the TCA cycle (see Chapter 21), which can enter the gluconeogenic pathway.

The carbons of glycerol are gluconeogenic because they form dihydroxyacetone phosphate (DHAP), a glycolytic intermediate (see Fig. 26.2C).

#### 2. PROPIONATE

Fatty acids with an odd number of carbon atoms, which are obtained mainly from vegetables in the diet, produce propionyl CoA from the three carbons at the ω-end of the chain (see Chapter 20). These carbons are relatively minor precursors of glucose in humans. Propionyl CoA is converted to methylmalonyl CoA, which is rearranged to form succinyl CoA, a four-carbon intermediate of the TCA cycle that can be used for gluconeogenesis. The remaining carbons of an odd-chain fatty acid form acetyl CoA, from which no net synthesis of glucose occurs.

### C. Pathway of Gluconeogenesis

Gluconeogenesis occurs by a pathway that reverses many, but not all, of the steps of glycolysis.

Excessive ethanol metabolism blocks the production of gluconeogenic precursors. Cells have limited amounts of NAD, which exist either as NAD$^+$ or as NADH. As the levels of NADH rise, those of NAD$^+$ fall and the ratio of the concentrations of NADH and NAD$^+$ ([NADH]/[NAD$^+$]) increases. In the presence of ethanol, which is very rapidly oxidized in the liver, the [NADH]/[NAD$^+$] ratio is much higher than it is in the normal fasting liver (see Fig. 24.10). High levels of NADH drive the lactate dehydrogenase reaction toward lactate. Therefore, lactate cannot enter the gluconeogenic pathway, and pyruvate that is generated from alanine is converted to lactate. Because glycerol is oxidized by NAD$^+$ during its conversion to DHAP, the conversion of glycerol to glucose is also inhibited when NADH levels are elevated. Consequently, the major precursors lactate, alanine, and glycerol are not used as efficiently for gluconeogenesis under conditions in which alcohol metabolism is high.

## 1. CONVERSION OF PYRUVATE TO PHOSPHOENOLPYRUVATE

In glycolysis, PEP is converted to pyruvate by pyruvate kinase. In gluconeogenesis, a series of steps are required to accomplish the reversal of this reaction (Fig. 26.3). Pyruvate is carboxylated by pyruvate carboxylase to form oxaloacetate. This enzyme, which requires biotin, is the catalyst of an anaplerotic (refilling) reaction of the TCA cycle (see Chapter 17). In gluconeogenesis, this reaction replenishes the oxaloacetate that is used for the synthesis of glucose (see Fig. 17.13).

The $CO_2$ that was added to pyruvate to form oxaloacetate is released in the reaction catalyzed by phosphoenolpyruvate carboxykinase (PEPCK), which generates PEP (Fig. 26.4). For this reaction, guanosine triphosphate (GTP) provides a source of energy as well as the phosphate group of PEP. Pyruvate carboxylase is found in mitochondria. In various species, PEPCK is located either in the cytosol or in mitochondria, or it is distributed between these two compartments. In humans, the enzyme is distributed about equally in each compartment.

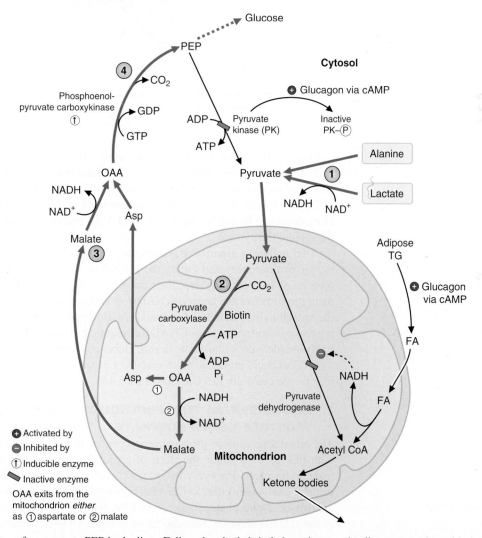

**FIG. 26.3.** Conversion of pyruvate to PEP in the liver. Follow the *shaded* circled numbers on the diagram, starting with the precursors, alanine and lactate. The first step is the conversion of alanine and lactate to pyruvate. Pyruvate then enters the mitochondria and is converted to oxaloacetate (OAA) *(circle 2)* by pyruvate carboxylase. Pyruvate dehydrogenase has been inactivated by both the NADH and acetyl CoA generated from fatty acid oxidation, which allows OAA production for gluconeogenesis. The OAA formed in the mitochondria is converted to either malate or aspartate to enter the cytoplasm via the malate–aspartate shuttle. In the cytoplasm, the malate or aspartate is converted back into OAA *(circle 3)*, and PEPCK will convert it to PEP *(circle 4)*. The PEP formed is not converted to pyruvate because pyruvate kinase has been inactivated by phosphorylation by the cAMP-dependent protein kinase under these conditions. The *white* circled numbers are alternate routes for exit of carbon from the mitochondrion using the malate–aspartate shuttle. *FA*, fatty acid; *TG*, triacylglycerol.

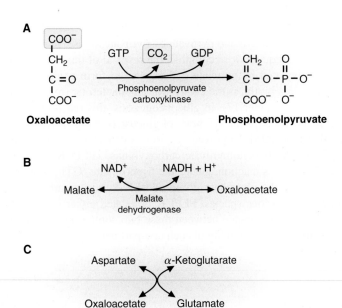

**FIG. 26.4.** Generation of PEP from gluconeogenic precursors. **A.** Conversion of oxaloacetate to PEP using PEPCK. **B.** Interconversion of oxaloacetate and malate. **C.** Transamination of aspartate to form oxaloacetate. Note that the cytosolic reaction is the reverse of the mitochondrial reaction shown in Figure 26.3.

Oxaloacetate, generated from pyruvate by pyruvate carboxylase or from amino acids that form intermediates of the TCA cycle, does not readily cross the mitochondrial membrane. It is either decarboxylated to form PEP by the mitochondrial PEPCK or it is converted to malate or aspartate (see Fig. 26.4B,C). The conversion of oxaloacetate to malate requires NADH. PEP, malate, and aspartate can be transported into the cytosol.

After malate or aspartate traverses the mitochondrial membrane (acting as a carrier of oxaloacetate) and enters the cytosol, it is reconverted to oxaloacetate by reversal of the reactions described earlier (see Figs. 26.4B,C). The conversion of malate to oxaloacetate generates NADH. Whether oxaloacetate is transported across the mitochondrial membrane as malate or aspartate depends on the need for reducing equivalents in the cytosol. NADH is required to reduce 1,3-bisphosphoglycerate to glyceraldehyde 3-phosphate during gluconeogenesis.

Oxaloacetate, produced from malate or aspartate in the cytosol, is converted to PEP by the cytosolic PEPCK (see Fig. 26.4A).

## 2. CONVERSION OF PHOSPHOENOLPYRUVATE TO FRUCTOSE 1,6-BISPHOSPHATE

The remaining steps of gluconeogenesis occur in the cytosol (Fig. 26.5). Starting with PEP as a substrate, the steps of glycolysis are reversed to form glyceraldehyde 3-phosphate. For every two molecules of glyceraldehyde 3-phosphate that are formed, one is converted to DHAP. These two triose phosphates, DHAP and glyceraldehyde 3-phosphate, condense to form fructose 1,6-bisphosphate by a reversal of the aldolase reaction. Because glycerol forms DHAP, it enters the gluconeogenic pathway at this level.

## 3. CONVERSION OF FRUCTOSE 1,6-BISPHOSPHATE TO FRUCTOSE 6-PHOSPHATE

The enzyme fructose 1,6-bisphosphatase releases $P_i$ from fructose 1,6-bisphosphate to form fructose 6-phosphate. This is not a reversal of the phosphofructokinase-1 (PFK-1) reaction; ATP is not produced when the phosphate is removed from the 1-position of fructose 1,6-bisphosphate because that is a low-energy phosphate

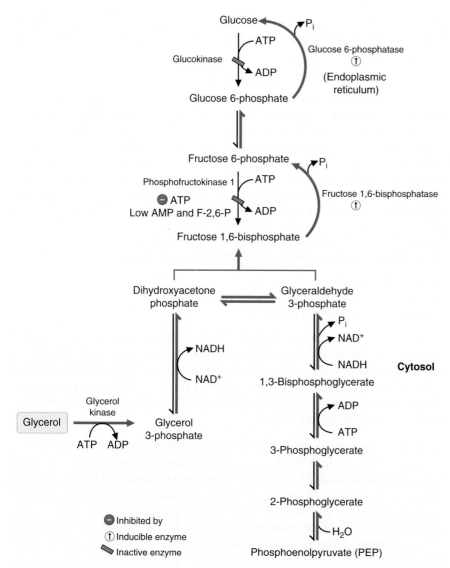

***FIG. 26.5.*** Conversion of phosphoenolpyruvate and glycerol to glucose. Gluconeogenic reactions are indicated by the *red arrows*. Glucokinase is inactive because of the low levels of glucose in the cell (below the $K_m$ for glucokinase), whereas PFK-1 is inactive because of the low concentration of the allosteric activators AMP and fructose 2,6-bisphosphate, coupled with high concentrations of ATP, an allosteric inhibitor.

bond. Rather, $P_i$ is released in this hydrolysis reaction. In the next reaction of gluconeogenesis, fructose 6-phosphate is converted to glucose-6-phosphate by the same isomerase used in glycolysis (phosphoglucose isomerase).

## 4.  CONVERSION OF GLUCOSE-6-PHOSPHATE TO GLUCOSE

Glucose-6-phosphatase hydrolyzes $P_i$ from glucose-6-phosphate, and free glucose is released into the blood. As with fructose 1,6-bisphosphatase, this is not a reversal of the glucokinase reaction because the phosphate bond in glucose-6-phosphate is a low-energy bond and ATP is not generated at this step.

Glucose-6-phosphatase is located in the membrane of the endoplasmic reticulum. It is used not only in gluconeogenesis but also to produce blood glucose from the breakdown of liver glycogen.

## D.  Regulation of Gluconeogenesis

Although gluconeogenesis occurs during fasting, it is also stimulated during prolonged exercise, by a high-protein diet, and under conditions of stress. The factors

**Al M.** had not eaten for 3 days, so he had no dietary source of glucose, and his liver glycogen stores were essentially depleted. He was solely dependent on gluconeogenesis to maintain his blood glucose levels. One of the consequences of ethanol ingestion and the subsequent rise in NADH levels is that the major carbon sources for gluconeogenesis cannot readily be converted to glucose (the high [NADH/NAD$^+$] ratio favors lactate formation from pyruvate, malate formation from oxaloacetate, and glycerol-3-phosphate formation from DHAP). During his alcoholic binges, Mr. M. became hypoglycemic. His blood glucose level was 28 mg/dL.

Amino acids that form intermediates of the TCA cycle are converted to malate, which enters the cytosol and is converted to oxaloacetate, which proceeds through gluconeogenesis to form glucose. When excessive amounts of ethanol are ingested, elevated NADH levels inhibit the conversion of malate to oxaloacetate in the cytosol. Therefore, carbons from amino acids that form intermediates of the TCA cycle cannot be converted to glucose as readily.

that promote the overall flow of carbon from pyruvate to glucose include the availability of substrate and changes in the activity or amount of certain key enzymes of glycolysis and gluconeogenesis.

## 1. AVAILABILITY OF SUBSTRATE

Gluconeogenesis is stimulated by the flow of its major substrates (glycerol, lactate, and amino acids) from peripheral tissues to the liver. Glycerol is released from adipose tissue whenever the levels of insulin are low and the levels of glucagon or the "stress" hormones, epinephrine and cortisol (a glucocorticoid), are elevated in the blood (see Chapter 21). Lactate is produced by muscle during exercise and by red blood cells. Amino acids are released from muscle whenever insulin is low or when cortisol is elevated. Amino acids are also available for gluconeogenesis when the dietary intake of protein is high and intake of carbohydrate is low.

## 2. ACTIVITY OR AMOUNT OF KEY ENZYMES

Three sequences in the pathway of gluconeogenesis are regulated:

1. Pyruvate → PEP
2. Fructose 1,6-bisphosphate → fructose 6-phosphate
3. Glucose-6-phosphate → glucose

These steps correspond to those in glycolysis that are catalyzed by regulatory enzymes. The enzymes involved in these steps of gluconeogenesis differ from those that catalyze the reverse reactions in glycolysis. The net flow of carbon, whether from glucose to pyruvate (glycolysis) or from pyruvate to glucose (gluconeogenesis), depends on the relative activity or amount of these glycolytic or gluconeogenic enzymes (Fig. 26.6 and Table 26.1).

## 3. CONVERSION OF PYRUVATE TO PHOSPHOENOLPYRUVATE

Pyruvate, a key substrate for gluconeogenesis, is derived from lactate and amino acids, particularly alanine. Pyruvate is not converted to acetyl CoA under conditions that favor gluconeogenesis because pyruvate dehydrogenase is relatively inactive. Instead, pyruvate is converted to oxaloacetate by pyruvate carboxylase. Subsequently, oxaloacetate is converted to PEP by PEPCK. The following is a description of activity states of enzymes under which PEP will be used to form glucose rather than pyruvate.

- **Pyruvate dehydrogenase is inactive.** Under conditions of fasting, insulin levels are low and glucagon levels are elevated. Consequently, fatty acids and glycerol are released from the triacylglycerol stores of adipose tissue. Fatty acids travel to the liver, where they undergo β-oxidation, producing acetyl CoA, NADH, and ATP. As a consequence, the concentration of adenosine diphosphate (ADP) decreases. These changes result in the phosphorylation of pyruvate dehydrogenase to the inactive form. Therefore, pyruvate is not converted to acetyl CoA (see Chapter 18).
- **Pyruvate carboxylase is active.** Acetyl CoA, which is produced by oxidation of fatty acids, activates pyruvate carboxylase. Therefore, pyruvate, derived from lactate or alanine, is converted to oxaloacetate.
- **PEPCK is induced.** Oxaloacetate produces PEP in a reaction catalyzed by PEPCK. Cytosolic PEPCK is an inducible enzyme, which means that the quantity of the enzyme in the cell increases because of increased transcription of its gene and increased translation of its mRNA. The major inducer is cyclic adenosine monophosphate (cAMP), which is increased by hormones that activate adenylate cyclase. Adenylate cyclase produces cAMP from ATP. Glucagon is the hormone that causes cAMP to rise during fasting, whereas epinephrine acts during exercise or stress. cAMP activates protein kinase A, which phosphorylates a set of specific transcription factors (cAMP response element binding protein [CREB]) that stimulate transcription of the PEPCK gene (see Chapter 13). Increased synthesis

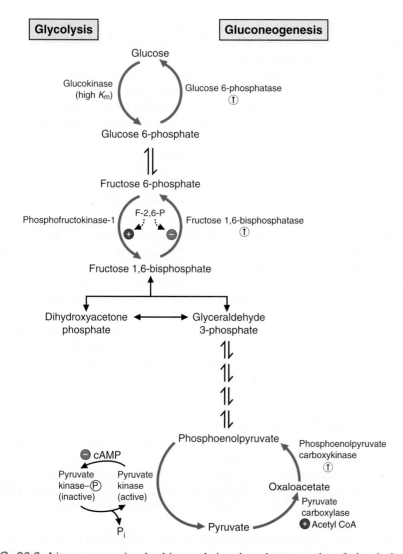

**FIG. 26.6.** Liver enzymes involved in regulating the substrate cycles of glycolysis and gluconeogenesis. *Heavy arrows* indicate the three substrate cycles. *F-2,6-P*, fructose 2,6-bisphosphate; ⊕, activated by; ⊖, inhibited by; ↑, inducible enzyme.

**Table 26.1   Regulation of Enzymes of Glycolysis and Gluconeogenesis in Liver**

| Enzyme | Mechanism |
| --- | --- |
| *A. Glycolytic enzymes* | |
| Pyruvate kinase | Activated by F1,6-BP |
| | Inhibited by ATP, alanine |
| | Inhibited by phosphorylation (glucagon and epinephrine lead to an increase in cAMP levels, which activates protein kinase A) |
| Phosphofructokinase-1 | Activated by F2,6-BP, AMP |
| | Inhibited by ATP, citrate |
| Glucokinase | High $K_m$ for glucose |
| | Induced by insulin |
| *B. Gluconeogenic enzymes* | |
| Pyruvate carboxylase | Activated by acetyl CoA |
| Phosphoenolpyruvate carboxykinase | Induced (increase in gene transcription) by glucagon, epinephrine, glucocorticoids |
| | Repressed by insulin |
| Glucose-6-phosphatase | Induced (increase in gene transcription) during fasting |
| Fructose 1,6-bisphosphatase | Inhibited by F2,6-BP, AMP |
| | Induced (increase in gene transcription) during fasting |

F1,6-BP, fructose 1,6-bisphosphate; ATP, adenosine triphosphate; cAMP, cyclic adenosine monophosphate; AMP, adenosine monophosphate; acetyl CoA, acetyl coenzyme A; F2,6-BP, fructose 2,6-bisphosphate.

of mRNA for PEPCK results in increased synthesis of the enzyme. Cortisol, the major human glucocorticoid, also induces PEPCK but through a different regulatory site on the PEPCK promoter.

- **Pyruvate kinase is inactive**. When glucagon is elevated, pyruvate kinase is phosphorylated and inactivated by a mechanism that involves cAMP and protein kinase A. Therefore, PEP is not reconverted to pyruvate. Rather, it continues along the pathway of gluconeogenesis. If PEP were reconverted to pyruvate, these substrates would simply cycle, causing a net loss of energy with no net generation of useful products. The inactivation of pyruvate kinase prevents such substrate cycling and promotes the net synthesis of glucose.

### 4. CONVERSION OF FRUCTOSE 1,6-BISPHOSPHATE TO FRUCTOSE 6-PHOSPHATE

The carbons of PEP reverse the steps of glycolysis, forming fructose 1,6-bisphosphate. Fructose 1,6-bisphosphatase acts on this bisphosphate to release $P_i$ and produce fructose 6-phosphate. A futile substrate cycle is prevented at this step because, under conditions that favor gluconeogenesis, the concentrations of the compounds that activate the glycolytic enzyme PFK-1 are low. These same compounds, fructose 2,6-bisphosphate (whose levels are regulated by insulin and glucagon) and adenosine monophosphate (AMP), are allosteric inhibitors of fructose 1,6-bisphosphatase. When the concentrations of these allosteric effectors are low, PFK-1 is less active, fructose 1,6-bisphosphatase is more active, and the net flow of carbon is toward fructose 6-phosphate and, thus, toward glucose. The synthesis of fructose 1,6-bisphosphatase is also induced during fasting.

### 5. CONVERSION OF GLUCOSE-6-PHOSPHATE TO GLUCOSE

Glucose-6-phosphatase catalyzes the conversion of glucose-6-phosphate to glucose, which is released from the liver cell. The glycolytic enzyme glucokinase, which catalyzes the reverse reaction, is relatively inactive during gluconeogenesis. Glucokinase, which has a high $S_{0.5}$ ($K_m$) for glucose, is not very active during fasting because the blood glucose level is lower (approximately 5 mM) than the $S_{0.5}$ of the enzyme.

Glucokinase is also an inducible enzyme. The concentration of the enzyme increases in the fed state, when blood glucose and insulin levels are elevated and decrease in the fasting state, when glucose and insulin are low.

### E. Energy is Required for the Synthesis of Glucose

During the gluconeogenic reactions, 6 moles of high-energy phosphate bonds are cleaved. Two moles of pyruvate are required for the synthesis of 1 mole of glucose. As 2 moles of pyruvate are carboxylated by pyruvate carboxylase, 2 moles of ATP are hydrolyzed. PEPCK requires 2 moles of GTP (the equivalent of 2 moles of ATP) to convert 2 moles of oxaloacetate to 2 moles of PEP. An additional 2 moles of ATP are used when 2 moles of 3-phosphoglycerate are phosphorylated, forming 2 moles of 1,3-bisphosphoglycerate. Energy in the form of reducing equivalents (NADH) is also required for the conversion of 1,3-bisphosphoglycerate to glyceraldehyde 3-phosphate. Under fasting conditions, the energy required for gluconeogenesis is obtained from β-oxidation of fatty acids. Defects in fatty acid oxidation can lead to hypoglycemia, in part, because of reduced fatty acid–derived energy production within the liver.

## III. CHANGES IN BLOOD GLUCOSE LEVELS AFTER A MEAL

After a high-carbohydrate meal, blood glucose rises from a fasting level of approximately 80 to 100 mg/dL (~5 mM) to a level of approximately 120 to 140 mg/dL (8 mM) within a period of 30 minutes to 1 hour. The concentration of glucose in the blood then begins to decrease, returning to the fasting range by approximately 2 hours after the meal (see also Chapter 22).

**Table 26.2   Blood Glucose Levels at Various Stages of Fasting**

| Stage of Fasting | Glucose (mg/dL) |
| --- | --- |
| Glucose, 700 g/d IV | 100 |
| Fasting, 12 h | 80 |
| Starvation, 3 d | 70 |
| Starvation, 5–6 wk | 65 |

IV, intravenous.
Source: Ruderman NB, Aoki TT, Cahill GF Jr. Gluconeogenesis and its disorders in man. In: Hanson RW, Mehlman MA, eds. *Gluconeogenesis: Its Regulation in Mammalian Species.* New York, NY: John Wiley & Sons; 1976:517.

Blood glucose levels increase as dietary glucose is digested and absorbed. The values go no higher than approximately 140 mg/dL in a normal, healthy person because tissues take up glucose from the blood, storing it for subsequent use and oxidizing it for energy. After the meal is digested and absorbed, blood glucose levels decline because cells continue to metabolize glucose.

If blood glucose levels continued to rise after a meal, the high concentration of glucose would cause the release of water from tissues as a result of the osmotic effect of glucose. Tissues would become dehydrated and their function would be affected. If hyperglycemia becomes severe, a hyperosmolar coma could result from dehydration of the brain.

Conversely, if blood glucose levels continued to drop after a meal, tissues that depend on glucose would suffer from a lack of energy. If blood glucose levels dropped abruptly, the brain would not be able to produce an adequate amount of ATP. Light-headedness and dizziness would result, followed by drowsiness and, eventually, coma. Red blood cells would not be able to produce enough ATP to maintain the integrity of their membranes. Hemolysis of these cells would decrease the transport of oxygen to the tissues of the body. Eventually, all tissues that rely on oxygen for energy production would fail to perform their normal functions. If the problem were severe enough, death could result.

Devastating consequences of glucose excess or insufficiency are normally avoided because the body is able to regulate its blood glucose levels. As the concentration of blood glucose approaches the normal fasting range of 80 to 100 mg/dL roughly 2 hours after a meal, the process of glycogenolysis is activated in the liver (see Chapter 23). Liver glycogen is the primary source of blood glucose during the first few hours of fasting. Subsequently, gluconeogenesis begins to play a role as an additional source of blood glucose. The carbon for gluconeogenesis, a pathway that occurs in the liver, is supplied by other tissues. Exercising muscle and red blood cells provide lactate through glycolysis, muscle also provides amino acids by degradation of protein, and glycerol is released from adipose tissue as triacylglycerol stores are mobilized.

Even during a prolonged fast, blood glucose levels do not decrease dramatically. After 5 to 6 weeks of starvation, blood glucose levels decrease to only approximately 65 mg/dL (Table 26.2).

## A. Blood Glucose Levels in the Fed State

The major factors involved in regulating blood glucose levels are the blood glucose concentration itself and hormones, particularly insulin and glucagon.

As blood glucose levels rise after a meal, the increased glucose concentration stimulates the β-cells of the pancreas to release insulin (Fig. 26.7). Certain amino acids, particularly arginine and leucine, also stimulate insulin release from the pancreas.

Blood levels of glucagon, which is secreted by the α-cells of the pancreas, may increase or decrease, depending on the content of the meal. Glucagon levels decrease in response to a high-carbohydrate meal, but they increase in response to a high-protein meal. After a typical mixed meal containing carbohydrate, protein, and fat, glucagon levels remain relatively constant, whereas insulin levels increase.

When **Dianne A.** inadvertently injected an excessive amount of insulin, she caused an acute reduction in her blood glucose levels 4 to 5 hours later while she was asleep. Had she been awake, she would have first experienced symptoms caused by a hypoglycemia-induced hyperactivity of her sympathetic nervous system (e.g., sweating, tremulousness, palpitations). Eventually, as her hypoglycemia became more profound, she would have experienced symptoms of "neuroglycopenia" (inadequate glucose supply to the brain), such as confusion, speech disturbances, emotional instability, possible seizure activity, and, finally, coma. While sleeping, she had reached this neuroglycopenic stage of hypoglycemia and could not be aroused at 6:00 AM.

**Ann R.**, who is recovering from anorexia nervosa (see Chapter 1) and whose intake of glucose and of glucose precursors has been severely restricted, has not developed any of these manifestations. Her lack of hypoglycemic symptoms can be explained by the very gradual reduction of her blood glucose levels as a consequence of near starvation and her ability to maintain blood glucose levels within an acceptable fasting range through hepatic gluconeogenesis. In addition, lipolysis of adipose triacylglycerols produces fatty acids, which are used as fuel and converted to ketone bodies by the liver. The oxidation of fatty acids and ketone bodies by the brain and muscle reduces the need for blood glucose.

In **Dianne's** case, the excessive dose of insulin inhibited lipolysis and ketone body synthesis, so these alternative fuels were not available to spare blood glucose. The rapidity with which hypoglycemia was induced could not be compensated for quickly enough by hepatic glycogenolysis and gluconeogenesis, which are inhibited by the insulin, and hypoglycemia ensued.

An immediate finger stick revealed that Dianne's capillary blood glucose level was less than 20 mg/dL. An intravenous infusion of a 50% solution of glucose was started, and her blood glucose level was determined frequently. When Dianne regained consciousness, the intravenous solution was eventually changed to 10% glucose. After 6 hours, her blood glucose levels stayed in the upper normal range, and she was able to tolerate oral feedings. She was transferred to the metabolic unit for overnight monitoring. By the next morning, her previous diabetes treatment regimen could be reestablished. The reasons that she had developed hypoglycemic coma were explained to Dianne, and she was discharged to the care of her family doctor.

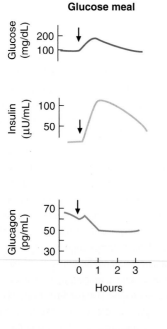

**Glucose meal**

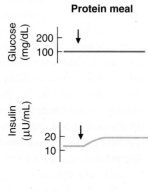

**Protein meal**

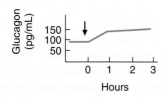

*FIG. 26.7.* Blood glucose, insulin, and gluca-gon levels after a high-carbohydrate meal and after a high-protein meal. The meals occurred at the time indicated by the *down arrows.*

## 1. FATE OF DIETARY GLUCOSE IN THE LIVER

After a meal, the liver oxidizes glucose to meet its immediate energy needs. Any excess glucose is converted to stored fuels. Glycogen is synthesized and stored in the liver, and glucose is converted to fatty acids and to the glycerol moiety that reacts with the fatty acids to produce triacylglycerols. These triacylglycerols are packaged in VLDL (see Chapter 1, Section IV.B.2) and transported to adipose tissue where the fatty acids are stored in adipose triacylglycerols. The VLDL can also deliver triglyc-eride (fatty acids) to the muscle for immediate oxidation, if required.

Regulatory mechanisms control the conversion of glucose to stored fuels. As the concentration of glucose increases in the hepatic portal vein, the concentration of glucose in the liver may increase from the fasting level of 80 to 100 mg/dL ($\sim$5 mM) to a concentration of 180 to 360 mg/dL (10 to 20 mM). Consequently, the velocity of the glucokinase reaction increases because this enzyme has a high $S_{0.5}$ ($K_m$) for glucose (see Fig. 7.4). Glucokinase is also induced by a high-carbohydrate diet; the quantity of the enzyme increases in response to elevated insulin levels.

Insulin promotes the storage of glucose as glycogen by countering the effects of glucagon-stimulated phosphorylation. The response to insulin activates the phos-phatases that dephosphorylate glycogen synthase (which leads to glycogen synthase activation) and glycogen phosphorylase (which leads to inhibition of the enzyme) (Fig. 26.8A). Insulin also promotes the synthesis of the triacylglycerols that are re-leased from the liver into the blood as VLDL. The regulatory mechanisms for this process are described in Chapter 28.

## 2. FATE OF DIETARY GLUCOSE IN PERIPHERAL TISSUES

Almost every cell in the body oxidizes glucose for energy. Certain critical tissues, particularly the brain, other nervous system tissues, and red blood cells depend es-pecially on glucose for their energy supply. The brain requires approximately 150 g of glucose per day. In addition, approximately 40 g of glucose per day is required by other glucose-dependent tissues. Furthermore, all tissues require glucose for the pentose phosphate pathway, and many tissues use glucose for synthesis of glycopro-teins and other carbohydrate-containing compounds.

Insulin stimulates the transport of glucose into adipose and muscle cells by pro-moting the recruitment of glucose transporters to the cell membrane (see Fig. 26.8C). Other tissues, such as the liver, brain, and red blood cells, have a different type of glucose transporter that is not as significantly affected by insulin.

In muscle, glycogen is synthesized after a meal by a mechanism similar to that in the liver (see Fig. 26.8B). Metabolic differences exist between these tissues (see Chapter 23), but in essence, insulin stimulates glycogen synthesis in resting muscle as it does in the liver. A key difference between muscle and liver is that insulin greatly stimulates the transport of glucose into muscle cells but only slightly stimu-lates its transport into liver cells.

## 3. RETURN OF BLOOD GLUCOSE TO FASTING LEVELS

After a meal has been digested and absorbed, blood glucose levels peak and then begin to decline. The uptake of dietary glucose by cells, particularly those in the liver, muscle, and adipose tissue, lowers blood glucose levels. By 2 hours after a meal, blood glucose levels return to the normal fasting level of less than 100 mg/dL.

### B. Blood Glucose Levels in the Fasting State

## 1. CHANGES IN INSULIN AND GLUCAGON LEVELS

During fasting, as blood glucose levels decrease, insulin levels decrease and gluca-gon levels rise. These hormonal changes cause the liver to degrade glycogen by the process of glycogenolysis and to produce glucose by the process of gluconeogenesis so that blood glucose levels are maintained.

## 2.  STIMULATION OF GLYCOGENOLYSIS

Within a few hours after a high-carbohydrate meal, glucagon levels begin to rise. Glucagon binds to cell surface receptors and activates adenylate cyclase, causing cAMP levels in liver cells to rise (see Fig. 23.7). cAMP activates protein kinase A, which phosphorylates and inactivates glycogen synthase. Therefore, glycogen synthesis decreases.

At the same time, protein kinase A stimulates glycogen degradation by a two-step mechanism. Protein kinase A phosphorylates and activates phosphorylase kinase. This enzyme, in turn, phosphorylates and activates glycogen phosphorylase.

Glycogen phosphorylase catalyzes the phosphorolysis of glycogen, producing glucose-1-phosphate, which is converted to glucose-6-phosphate. Dephosphorylation of glucose-6-phosphate by glucose-6-phosphatase produces free glucose, which then enters the blood.

## 3.  STIMULATION OF GLUCONEOGENESIS

By 4 hours after a meal, the liver is supplying glucose to the blood not only by the process of glycogenolysis but also by the process of gluconeogenesis. Hormonal changes cause peripheral tissues to release precursors that provide carbon for gluconeogenesis, specifically lactate, amino acids, and glycerol.

Regulatory mechanisms promote the conversion of gluconeogenic precursors to glucose (see Fig. 26.6). These mechanisms prevent the occurrence of potential futile (substrate) cycles, which would continuously convert substrates to products while consuming energy but producing no useful result. Such cycles are more currently referred to as substrate cycles, and they provide a means for rapid regulation of opposing metabolic pathways.

These regulatory mechanisms inactivate the glycolytic enzymes pyruvate kinase, PFK-1, and glucokinase during fasting and promote the flow of carbon to glucose via gluconeogenesis. These mechanisms operate at the three steps where glycolysis and gluconeogenesis differ (glucokinase vs. glucose-6-phosphatase, PFK-1 vs. fructose 1,6 bisphosphatase, pyruvate kinase vs. pyruvate carboxylase and PEPCK) as previously discussed in this chapter.

## 4.  STIMULATION OF LIPOLYSIS

The hormonal changes that occur during fasting stimulate the breakdown of adipose triacylglycerols. Consequently, fatty acids and glycerol are released into the blood (Fig. 26.9). Glycerol serves as a source of carbon for gluconeogenesis. Fatty acids become the major fuel of the body and are oxidized to $CO_2$ and $H_2O$ by various tissues, which enable these tissues to decrease their use of glucose. Fatty acids are also oxidized to acetyl CoA in the liver to provide energy for gluconeogenesis. In a prolonged fast, acetyl CoA is converted to ketone bodies, which enter the blood and serve as an additional fuel source for the muscle and the brain.

### C.  Blood Glucose Levels during Prolonged Fasting (Starvation)
During prolonged fasting, several changes occur in fuel use. These changes cause tissues to use less glucose than they use during a brief fast and to use predominantly

The pathophysiology leading to an elevation of blood glucose after a meal differs between patients with type 1 diabetes mellitus and those with type 2 diabetes mellitus. **Dianne A.**, who has type 1 disease, cannot secrete insulin adequately in response to a meal because of a defect in the β-cells of her pancreas. **Deborah S.**, however, has type 2 disease. In this form of the disorder, the cause of glucose intolerance is more complex, involving at least a delay in the release of relatively appropriate amounts of insulin after a meal combined with a degree of resistance to the actions of insulin in skeletal muscle and adipocytes. Excessive hepatic gluconeogenesis occurs even though blood glucose levels are elevated.

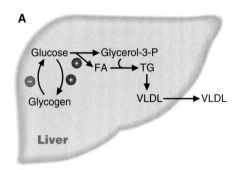

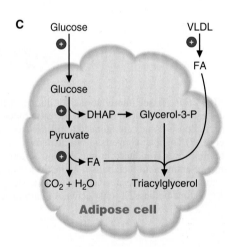

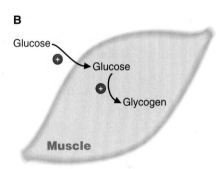

FIG. 26.8. Glucose metabolism in various tissues. **A.** Effect of insulin on glycogen synthesis and degradation and on VLDL synthesis in the liver. **B.** Glucose metabolism in resting muscle in the fed state. The transport of glucose into cells and the synthesis of glycogen are stimulated by insulin. **C.** Glucose metabolism in adipose tissue in the fed state. *DHAP*, dihydroxyacetone phosphate; *FA*, fatty acids; *TG*, triacylglycerols; ⊕, stimulated by insulin; ⊖, inhibited by insulin.

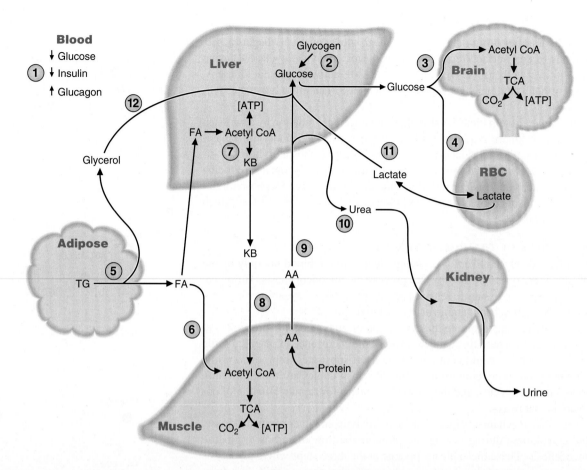

**FIG. 26.9.** Tissue interrelationships during fasting. *(1)* Blood glucose levels drop, decreasing insulin and raising blood glucagon levels. *(2)* Glycogenolysis is induced in the liver to raise blood glucose levels. *(3)* The brain uses the glucose released by the liver, as do the red blood cells *(4)*. *(5)* Adipose tissues are induced to release free fatty acids and glycerol from stored triglycerides. *(6)* The muscle and liver use fatty acids for energy. *(7)* The liver converts fatty acid derived–acetyl CoA to ketone bodies for export, which the muscles *(8)* and brain can use for energy. *(9)* Protein turnover is induced in muscle, and amino acids leave the muscle and travel to the liver for use as gluconeogenic precursors. *(10)* The high rate of amino acid metabolism in the liver generates urea, which travels to the kidney for excretion. *(11)* Red blood cells produce lactate, which returns to the liver as a substrate for gluconeogenesis. *(12)* The glycerol released from adipose tissue is used by the liver for gluconeogenesis. *KB*, ketone bodies; *FA*, fatty acids; *AA*, amino acids; *TG*, triacylglycerols.

fuels derived from adipose triacylglycerols (i.e., fatty acids and their derivatives, the ketone bodies). Therefore, blood glucose levels do not decrease drastically. In fact, even after 5 to 6 weeks of starvation, blood glucose levels are still in the range of 65 mg/dL (Fig. 26.10; see Table 26.2).

The major change that occurs in starvation is a dramatic elevation of blood ketone body levels after 3 to 5 days of fasting (see Chapter 20 and Fig. 26.10). At these levels, the brain and other nervous tissues begin to use ketone bodies and, consequently, they oxidize less glucose, requiring roughly one-third as much glucose (approximately 40 g/day) as under normal dietary conditions. As a result of reduced glucose utilization, the rate of gluconeogenesis in the liver decreases, as does the production of urea (see Fig. 26.10). Because in this stage of starvation, amino acids, obtained from the degradation of existing proteins, are the major gluconeogenic precursor; reducing glucose requirements in tissues reduces the rate of protein degradation and hence the rate of urea formation. Protein from muscle and other tissues is, therefore, spared because there is less need for amino acids for gluconeogenesis.

Body protein, particularly muscle protein, is not primarily a storage form of fuel in the same sense as glycogen or triacylglycerol; proteins have many functions beside fuel storage. For example, proteins function as enzymes, as structural proteins,

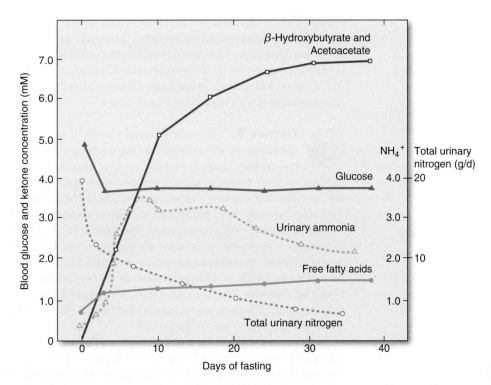

**FIG. 26.10.** Changes in blood fuels during fasting. The units for fatty acids, glucose, and ketone bodies are millimolar (on *left*) and for urinary nitrogen and ammonia are grams/day (on *right*). (Modified from Linder MC. *Nutritional Biochemistry and Metabolism with Clinical Applications.* 2nd ed. Norwalk, CT: Appleton & Lange; 1991:103. ©1991 Appleton & Lange.)

and in muscle contraction. If tissue protein is degraded to too great an extent, body function can be severely compromised. If starvation continues and no other problems such as infections occur, a starving individual usually dies because of severe protein loss that causes malfunction of major organs, such as the heart. Therefore, the increase in ketone body levels that results in the sparing of body protein allows individuals to survive for extended periods (weeks) without ingesting food.

### D. Blood Glucose Levels during Exercise

During exercise, mechanisms very similar to those that are used during fasting operate to maintain blood glucose levels. The liver maintains blood glucose levels through both glucagon- and epinephrine-induced glycogenolysis and gluconeogenesis. Recall that muscle glycogen is not used to maintain blood glucose levels; muscle cells lack glucose-6-phosphatase, so glucose cannot be produced from glucose-6-phosphate for export.

## CLINICAL COMMENTS

A summary of the diseases discussed in this chapter is presented in Table 26.3.

**Al M.** The chronic excessive ingestion of ethanol concurrent with a recent reduction in nutrient intake caused **Al M.'s** blood glucose level to decrease to 28 mg/dL. This degree of hypoglycemia caused the release of a number of "counterregulatory" hormones into the blood, including glucagon, growth hormone, cortisol, and epinephrine (adrenaline).

Some of the patient's signs and symptoms are primarily the result of an increase in adrenergic nervous system activity after a rapid decrease in blood glucose. The subsequent increase in epinephrine levels in the blood leads to tremulousness, excessive sweating, and rapid heart rate. Other manifestations arise when the brain has insufficient glucose, hence the term, "neuroglycopenic symptoms." Mr. M. was confused, combative, had slurred speech, and eventually had a grand mal seizure. If not treated quickly by intravenous glucose administration, Mr. M. may have lapsed into a coma. Permanent neurological deficits and even death may result if severe hypoglycemia is not corrected in 6 to 10 hours.

**Dianne A.** Chronically elevated levels of glucose in the blood may contribute to the development of the microvascular complications of diabetes mellitus, such as diabetic retinal damage, kidney damage, and nerve damage, as well as macrovascular complications such as cerebrovascular, peripheral vascular, and coronary vascular insufficiency. The precise mechanism by which long-term hyperglycemia induces these vascular changes is not fully established.

One postulated mechanism proposes that nonenzymatic glycation (glycosylation) of proteins in vascular tissue alters the structure and functions of these proteins. A protein that is exposed to chronically increased levels of glucose will covalently bind glucose, a process called **glycation** or **glycosylation**. This process is not regulated by enzymes. These nonenzymatically glycated proteins slowly form cross-linked protein adducts (often called advanced glycosylation end products) within the microvasculature and macrovasculature.

By cross-linking vascular matrix proteins and plasma proteins, chronic hyperglycemia may cause narrowing of the luminal diameter of the microvessels in the retina (causing diabetic retinopathy), the renal glomeruli (causing diabetic nephropathy), and the microvessels supplying peripheral and autonomic nerve fibers (causing diabetic neuropathy). The same process has been postulated to accelerate atherosclerotic change in the macrovasculature, particularly in the brain (causing strokes), the coronary arteries (causing heart attacks), and the peripheral arteries (causing peripheral arterial insufficiency and possibly gangrene). The abnormal lipid metabolism associated with poorly controlled diabetes mellitus also may contribute to the accelerated atherosclerosis associated with this metabolic disorder.

The publication of the Diabetes Control and Complications Trial followed by the United Kingdom Prospective Diabetes Study were the first big human studies to show that maintaining long-term controlled blood glucose levels in patients with diabetes, such as **Dianne A.** and **Deborah S.** (who has type 2 diabetes), favorably affects the course of microvascular complications. More recent studies have confirmed this, and although it is thought that controlling blood sugar decreases macrovascular complications, this has been harder to show in human studies.

**Table 26.3   Diseases Discussed in Chapter 26**

| Disease or Disorder | Environmental or Genetic | Comments |
|---|---|---|
| Ethanol-induced hypoglycemia | Environmental | Ethanol, combined with poor nutrition, leads to hypoglycemia due to excessive ethanol metabolism altering the NADH/NAD$^+$ ratio in the liver. |
| Insulin overdose | Environmental | Hypoglycemia as a result of insulin overdose due to insulin stimulation of glucose transport into muscle and fat cells. |
| Anorexia nervosa | Environmental | The use of ketone bodies as an alternative energy source during prolonged fasting preserves muscle protein as reduced levels of glucose are now required by the nervous system. |
| Weight loss | Environmental | Maintenance of blood glucose levels during dieting occurs due to glycogen release. |
| Diabetic keto-acidosis | Environmental | Excessive production of ketone bodies in a type 1 diabetic whose insulin levels are too low, coupled with hyperglycemia; rarely observed in type 2 diabetes. |

## REVIEW QUESTIONS-CHAPTER 26

1. A common intermediate in the conversion of glycerol and lactate to glucose is which one of the following?

   A. Glucose-6-phosphate
   B. Pyruvate
   C. Oxaloacetate
   D. Malate
   E. Phosphoenolpyruvate

2. A patient presented with a bacterial infection produced an endotoxin that inhibits phosphoenolpyruvate carboxykinase. In this patient, then, under these conditions, glucose production from which one of the following precursors would be inhibited?

   A. Glycerol
   B. Alanine
   C. Even-chain fatty acids
   D. Galactose
   E. Phosphoenolpyruvate

3. A patient arrives at the hospital via an ambulance. She is currently in a coma. Before lapsing into the coma, her symptoms included vomiting, dehydration, low blood pressure, and a rapid heartbeat. She also had relatively rapid respirations, resulting in more carbon dioxide exhaled. These symptoms are consistent with which one of the following conditions?

   A. The patient lacks a functional pancreas.
   B. Ketoalkalosis
   C. Diabetic ketoacidosis
   D. Hypoglycemic coma
   E. Insulin shock in a diabetic patient

4. Assume that an individual carries a mutation in muscle protein kinase A such that the protein is refractory to high levels of cAMP. Glycogen degradation in the muscle would occur, then, under conditions which lead to high intracellular levels of which one of the following?

   A. Glucose
   B. Glucose-6-phosphate
   C. Glucose-1-phosphate
   D. Intracellular calcium
   E. Intracellular magnesium

5. A 50-year-old overweight man visits his physician for a physical examination, and it is determined that his fasting blood glucose levels are elevated despite normal levels of insulin. An oral glucose tolerance test also demonstrates a normal rise in insulin levels after glucose is ingested but an abnormal, slow drop in circulating blood glucose levels. These findings can be best explained by which one of the following?

   A. Allosteric inhibition of glycolysis by the circulating glucose
   B. Impairment in the stimulation of glucose transport into the peripheral tissues
   C. Allosteric inhibition of glycogen synthesis by the circulating glucose
   D. A defect in muscle glucokinase
   E. A defect in pancreatic glucokinase

# 27   Digestion and Transport of Dietary Lipids

## CHAPTER OUTLINE

I. **DIGESTION OF TRIACYLGLYCEROLS**
   A. Action of bile salts
   B. Action of pancreatic lipase

II. **ABSORPTION OF DIETARY LIPIDS**

III. **SYNTHESIS OF CHYLOMICRONS**

IV. **TRANSPORT OF DIETARY LIPIDS IN THE BLOOD**

V. **FATE OF CHYLOMICRONS**

## KEY POINTS

- Triacylglycerols are the major fat source in the human diet.
- Lipases (lingual lipase in the saliva and gastric lipase in the stomach) perform limited digestion of triacylglycerol prior to entry into the intestine.
- As food enters the intestine, cholecystokinin is released, which signals the gallbladder to release bile acids and the exocrine pancreas to release digestive enzymes.
- Within the intestine, bile salts emulsify fats, which increase their accessibility to pancreatic lipase and colipase.
- Triacylglycerols are degraded to form free fatty acids and 2-monoacylgylcerol by pancreatic lipase and colipase.
- Dietary phospholipids are hydrolyzed by pancreatic phospholipase $A_2$ in the intestine.
- Dietary cholesterol esters (cholesterol esterified to a fatty acid) are hydrolyzed by pancreatic cholesterol esterase in the intestine.
- Micelles, consisting of bile acids and the products of fat digestion, form within the intestinal lumen and interact with the enterocyte membrane. Lipid-soluble components diffuse from the micelle into the cell.
- Bile salts are resorbed further down the intestinal tract and returned to the liver by the enterohepatic circulation.
- The intestinal epithelial cells resynthesize triacylglycerol and package them into nascent chylomicrons for release into the circulation.
- Once in circulation the nascent chylomicrons interact with high-density lipoprotein (HDL) particles and acquire two additional protein components: apolipoproteins C-II and E.
- ApoC-II activates lipoprotein lipase on capillary endothelium of muscle and adipose tissue, which digests the triglycerides in the chylomicron. The fatty acids released from the chylomicron enter the muscle for energy production or the fat cell for storage. The glycerol released is metabolized only in the liver.
- As the chylomicron loses triglyceride, its density increases and it becomes a chylomicron remnant. Chylomicron remnants are removed from circulation by the liver through specific binding of the remnant to apoE receptors on the liver membrane.
- Once in the liver the remnant is degraded, and the lipids are recycled.

# THE WAITING ROOM

**Will S.** had several episodes of mild back and lower extremity pain over the last year, probably caused by minor sickle cell crises. He then developed severe right upper abdominal pain radiating to his lower right chest and his right flank 36 hours before being admitted to the emergency department. He states that the pain is not like his usual crisis pain. Intractable vomiting began 12 hours after the onset of these new symptoms. He reports that his urine is the color of iced tea and his stool now has a light clay color.

On physical examination, his body temperature is slightly elevated and his heart rate is rapid. The whites of his eyes (the sclerae) are obviously jaundiced (or icteric, a yellow discoloration caused by the accumulation of bilirubin pigment). He is exquisitely tender to pressure over his right upper abdomen.

The emergency room physician suspects that Will is not in sickle cell crisis but instead has either acute cholecystitis (gallbladder inflammation) or a gallstone lodged in his common bile duct, causing cholestasis (the inability of the bile from the liver to reach his small intestine). His hemoglobin level was low at 7.6 mg/dL (reference range = 12 to 16 mg/dL) but unchanged from his baseline 3 months earlier. His serum total bilirubin level was 3.2 mg/dL (reference range = 0.2 to 1.0 mg/dL) and his direct (conjugated) bilirubin level was 0.9 mg/dL (reference range = 0 to 0.2 mg/dL).

Intravenous fluids were started; he was not allowed to take anything by mouth, a nasogastric tube was passed and placed on constant suction, and symptomatic therapy was started for pain and nausea. He was sent for an ultrasonographic (ultrasound) study of his upper abdomen.

**Al M.** has continued to abuse alcohol and to eat poorly. After a particularly heavy intake of vodka, a steady severe pain began in his upper mid abdomen. This pain spread to the left upper quadrant and eventually radiated to his mid back. He began vomiting nonbloody material and was brought to the hospital emergency room with fever, a rapid heartbeat, and a mild reduction in blood pressure. On physical examination, he was dehydrated and tender to pressure over the upper abdomen. His vomitus and stool were both negative for occult blood.

Blood samples were sent to the laboratory for a variety of hematological and chemical tests, including a measurement of serum amylase and lipase, digestive enzymes normally secreted from the exocrine pancreas through the pancreatic ducts into the lumen of the small intestine.

## I. DIGESTION OF TRIACYLGLYCEROLS

**Triacylglycerols** are the major fat in the human diet because they are the major storage lipid in the plants and animals that constitute our food supply. Triacylglycerols contain a glycerol backbone to which three fatty acids are esterified (see Fig. 3.13). The main route for digestion of triacylglycerols involves hydrolysis to fatty acids and 2-monoacylglycerol in the lumen of the intestine. However, the route depends to some extent on the chain length of the fatty acids. Lingual and gastric **lipases** are produced by cells at the back of the tongue and in the stomach, respectively. These lipases preferentially hydrolyze short- and medium-chain fatty acids (containing 12 or fewer carbon atoms) from dietary triacylglycerols. Therefore, they are most active in infants and young children who drink relatively large quantities of cow's milk, which contains triacylglycerols with a high percentage of short- and medium-chain fatty acids.

---

Currently, 38% of the calories (kcal) in the typical American diet come from fat. The content of fat in the diet increased from the early 1900s until the 1960s, and then decreased as we became aware of the unhealthy effects of a high-fat diet. According to current recommendations, fat should provide no more than 30% of the total calories of a healthy diet.

---

The mammary gland produces milk, which is the major source of nutrients for the breastfed human infant. The fatty acid composition of human milk varies, depending on the diet of the mother. However, long-chain fatty acids predominate, particularly palmitic, oleic, and linoleic acids. Although the amount of fat contained in human milk and cow's milk is similar, cow's milk contains more short- and medium-chain fatty acids and does not contain the long-chain polyunsaturated fatty acids found in human milk that are important in brain development.

Although the concentrations of pancreatic lipase and bile salts are low in the intestinal lumen of the newborn infant, the fat of human milk is still readily absorbed. This is true because lingual and gastric lipases produced by the infant partially compensate for the lower levels of pancreatic lipase. The human mammary gland also produces lipases that enter the milk. One of these lipases, which requires lower levels of bile salts than pancreatic lipase, is not inactivated by stomach acid and functions in the intestine for several hours.

## A. Action of Bile Salts

Dietary fat leaves the stomach and enters the small intestine, where it is **emulsified** (suspended in small particles in the aqueous environment) by bile salts (see Fig. 3.16). The bile salts are amphipathic compounds (containing both hydrophobic and hydrophilic components), synthesized in the liver (see Chapter 29 for the pathway) and secreted via the gallbladder into the intestinal lumen. The contraction of the gallbladder and secretion of pancreatic enzymes are stimulated by the gut hormone **cholecystokinin**, which is secreted by the intestinal cells when stomach contents enter the intestine. Bile salts act as detergents, binding to the globules of dietary fat as they are broken up by the peristaltic action of the intestinal muscle. This emulsified fat, which has an increased surface area as compared with unemulsified fat, is attacked by digestive enzymes from the pancreas (Fig. 27.1).

## B. Action of Pancreatic Lipase

The major enzyme that digests dietary triacylglycerols is a lipase produced in the pancreas. **Pancreatic lipase** is secreted along with another protein, **colipase**, in response to the release of cholecystokinin from the intestine. The peptide hormone secretin is also released by the small intestine in response to acidic conditions (such as the partially digested materials from the stomach, which contains HCl) entering the duodenum. Secretin signals the liver, pancreas, and certain intestinal cells to

In patients such as **Will S.** who have severe and recurrent episodes of increased red blood cell destruction (hemolytic anemia), greater than normal amounts of the red cell pigment heme must be processed by the liver and spleen. In these organs, heme (derived from hemoglobin) is degraded to bilirubin, which is excreted by the liver in the bile.

If large quantities of bilirubin are presented to the liver as a consequence of acute hemolysis, the capacity of the liver to conjugate it, that is, convert it to the water-soluble bilirubin diglucuronide, can be overwhelmed. As a result, a greater percentage of the bilirubin entering the hepatic biliary ducts in patients with hemolysis is in the less water-soluble forms. In the gallbladder, these relatively insoluble particles tend to precipitate as gallstones that are rich in calcium bilirubinate. In some patients, one or more stones may leave the gallbladder through the cystic duct and enter the common bile duct. Most pass harmlessly into the small intestine and are later excreted in the stool. Larger stones, however, may become entrapped in the lumen of the common bile duct, where they cause varying degrees of obstruction to bile flow (cholestasis) with associated ductal spasm, producing pain. If adequate amounts of bile salts do not enter the intestinal lumen, dietary fats cannot readily be emulsified and digested.

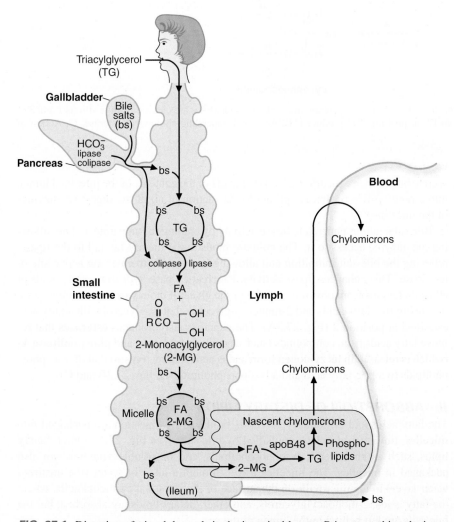

**FIG. 27.1.** Digestion of triacylglycerols in the intestinal lumen. Prior to reaching the intestine, lingual lipase (mouth) and gastric lipase (stomach) have begun digestion of the triacylglycerol. *FA*, fatty acid.

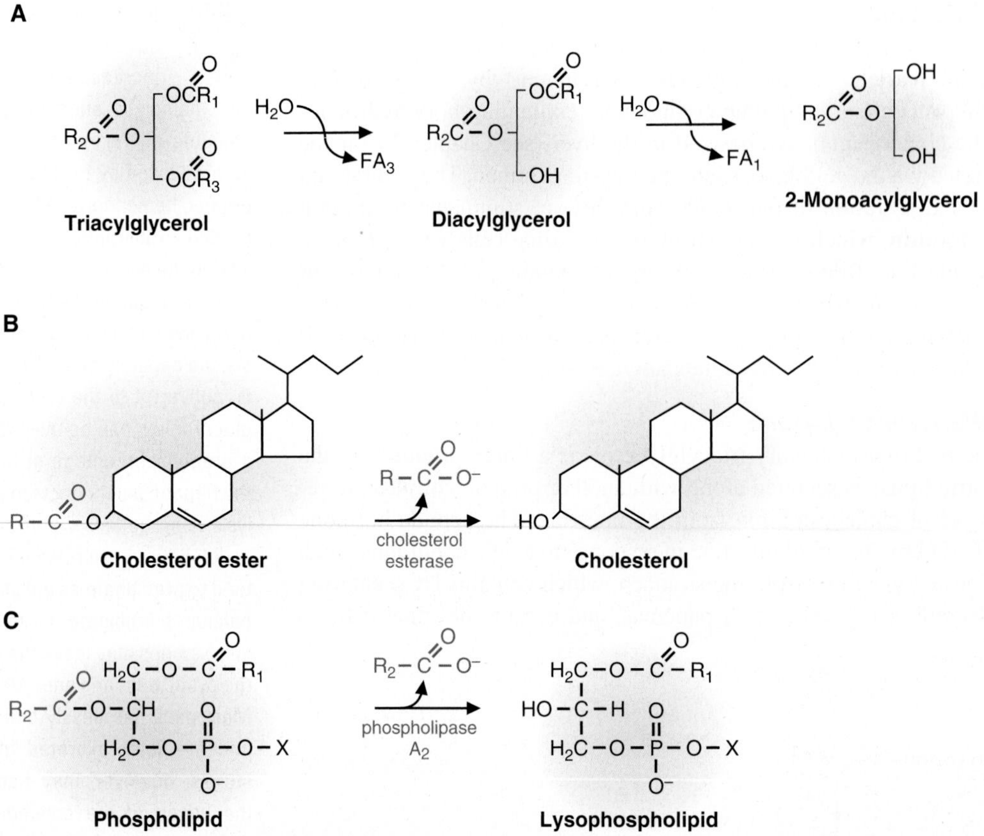

**A**

Triacylglycerol     Diacylglycerol     2-Monoacylglycerol

**B**

Cholesterol ester     Cholesterol

**C**

Phospholipid     Lysophospholipid

**FIG. 27.2.** Action of pancreatic enzymes on fat digestion. **A.** Action of pancreatic lipase. Fatty acids (FAs) are cleaved from positions 1 and 3 of the triacylglycerol, and a monoacylglycerol with an FA at position 2 is produced. **B.** Action of pancreatic cholesterol esterase. **C.** Action of phospholipase $A_2$.

**Al M.'s** serum levels of pancreatic amylase (which digests dietary starch) and pancreatic lipase were elevated, a finding consistent with a diagnosis of acute pancreatitis. The elevated levels of these enzymes in the blood are the result of their escape from the inflamed exocrine cells of the pancreas into the surrounding pancreatic veins. The cause of this inflammatory pancreatic process in this case was related to the toxic effect of acute and chronic excessive alcohol ingestion.

When he was finally able to tolerate a full diet, **Al M.'s** stools became bulky, glistening, yellow-brown, and foul smelling. They floated on the surface of the toilet water. What caused this problem?

secrete bicarbonate. Bicarbonate raises the pH of the contents of the intestinal lumen into a range (pH $\sim$6) that is optimal for the action of all of the digestive enzymes of the intestine.

Bile salts inhibit pancreatic lipase activity by coating the substrate and not allowing the enzyme access to it. The colipase binds to the dietary fat and to the lipase, relieving the bile salt inhibition and allowing triglyceride to enter the active site of the lipase. This enhances lipase activity. Pancreatic lipase hydrolyzes fatty acids of all chain lengths from positions 1 and 3 of the glycerol moiety of the triacylglycerol, producing free fatty acids and 2-monoacylglycerol, that is, glycerol with a fatty acid esterified at position 2 (Fig. 27.2A). The pancreas also produces **esterases** that remove fatty acids from compounds (such as cholesterol esters) and **phospholipase $A_2$** (which is released in its zymogen form and is activated by trypsin) that digests phospholipids to a free fatty acid and a lysophospholipid (see Fig. 27.2B and C).

## II. ABSORPTION OF DIETARY LIPIDS

The fatty acids and 2-monoacylglycerols produced by digestion are packaged into **micelles**, tiny microdroplets emulsified by bile salts (see Fig. 27.1). Other dietary lipids, such as cholesterol, lysophospholipids, and fat-soluble vitamins, are also packaged in micelles. The micelles travel through a layer of water (the unstirred water layer) to the microvilli on the surface of the intestinal epithelial cells, where the fatty acids, 2-monoacylglycerols, and other dietary lipids are absorbed, but the bile salts are left behind in the lumen of the gut.

The bile salts are extensively resorbed when they reach the ileum. Greater than 95% of the bile salts are recirculated, traveling through the enterohepatic circulation

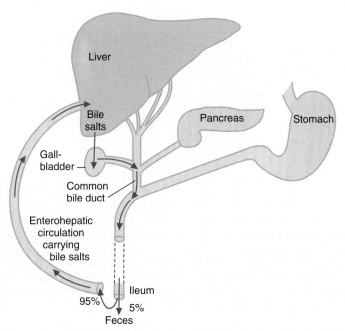

**FIG. 27.3.** Recycling of bile salts. Bile salts are synthesized in the liver, stored in the gallbladder, secreted into the small intestine, resorbed in the ileum, and returned to the liver via the enterohepatic circulation. Under normal circumstances, 5% or less of luminal bile acids are excreted in the stool.

to the liver, which secretes them into the bile for storage in the gallbladder and ejection into the intestinal lumen during another digestive cycle (Fig. 27.3).

Short- and medium-chain fatty acids (C4 to C12) do not require bile salts for their absorption. They are absorbed directly into intestinal epithelial cells. Because they do not need to be packaged to increase their solubility, they enter the portal blood (rather than the lymph) and are transported to the liver bound to serum albumin.

For bile salt micelles to form, the concentration of bile salts in the intestinal lumen must reach 5 to 15 μmol/mL. This critical micelle concentration (CMC) of bile salts is therefore required for optimal lipid absorption. Below the CMC, the bile salts are soluble; above the CMC, micelles will form.

## III. SYNTHESIS OF CHYLOMICRONS

Within the intestinal epithelial cells, the fatty acids and 2-monoacylglycerols are condensed by enzymatic reactions in the smooth endoplasmic reticulum to form triacylglycerols (Fig. 27.4). The reactions for triacylglycerol synthesis in intestinal

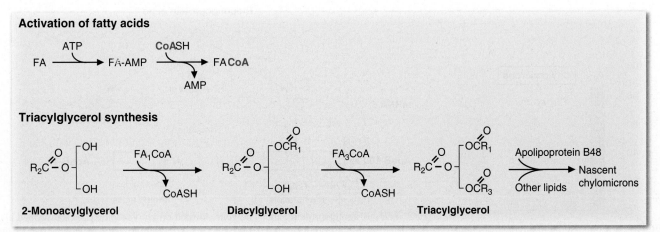

**FIG. 27.4.** Resynthesis of triacylglycerols in intestinal epithelial cells. Fatty acids (FA) produced by digestion are activated in intestinal epithelial cells and then esterified to the 2-monoacylglycerol produced by digestion. The triacylglycerols are packaged in chylomicrons and secreted into the lymph.

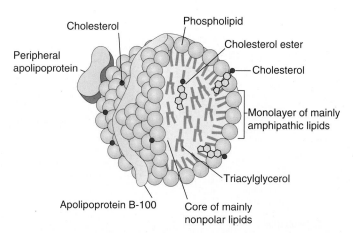

**FIG. 27.5.** Example of the structure of a blood lipoprotein. VLDL is depicted. Lipoproteins contain phospholipids and proteins on the surface, with their hydrophilic regions interacting with water. Hydrophobic molecules are in the interior of the lipoprotein. The hydroxyl group of cholesterol is near the surface. In cholesterol esters, the hydroxyl group is esterified to a fatty acid. Cholesterol esters are found in the interior of lipoproteins and are synthesized by reaction of cholesterol with an activated fatty acid (see Chapter 29).

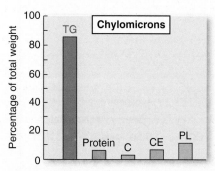

Because the fat-soluble vitamins (A, D, E, and K) are absorbed from micelles along with the long-chain fatty acids and 2-monoacylglycerols, prolonged obstruction of the duct that carries exocrine secretions from the pancreas and the gallbladder into the intestine (via the common duct) could lead to a deficiency of these metabolically important substances. If the obstruction of **Will S.'s** common duct continues, he will eventually suffer from a fat-soluble vitamin deficiency.

cells differ from those in liver and adipose cells in that 2-monoacylglycerol is an intermediate in triacylglycerol formation in intestinal cells, whereas phosphatidic acid is the necessary intermediate in other tissues.

Triacylglycerols, due to their insolubility in water, are packaged into lipoprotein particles (see Chapter 1). If triacylglycerols entered the blood directly, they would coalesce, impeding blood flow. Intestinal cells package triacylglycerols together with proteins and phospholipids in **chylomicrons**, which are lipoprotein particles that do not readily coalesce in aqueous solutions (Figs. 27.5 and 27.6). Chylomicrons also contain cholesterol and fat-soluble vitamins. The protein constituents of the lipoproteins are known as **apolipoproteins**.

The major apolipoprotein associated with chylomicrons as they leave the intestinal cells is B-48. The B-48 apolipoprotein is structurally and genetically related to the B-100 apolipoprotein synthesized in the liver that serves as a major protein of another lipid carrier, **very low density lipoprotein (VLDL)**. These two apolipoproteins are encoded by the same gene. In the intestine, the primary transcript of this gene undergoes RNA editing (Fig. 27.7). A stop codon is generated that causes a

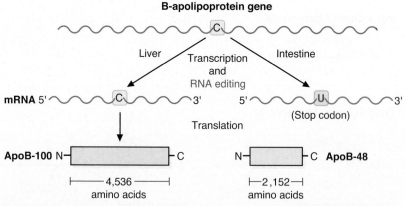

**FIG. 27.7.** B-apolipoprotein gene. The gene, located on chromosome 2, is transcribed and translated in liver to produce apoB-100, which is 4,536 amino acids in length (one of the longest single-polypeptide chains). In intestinal cells, RNA editing converts a cytosine (*C*) to a uracil (*U*) via deamination, producing a stop codon. Consequently, the B apolipoprotein of intestinal cells (apoB-48) contains only 2,152 amino acids. ApoB-48 is 48% of the size of apoB-100.

**FIG. 27.6.** Composition of a typical chylomicron. Although the composition varies to some extent, the major component is triacylglycerol (*TG*). *C*, cholesterol; *CE*, cholesterol ester; *PL*, phospholipid.

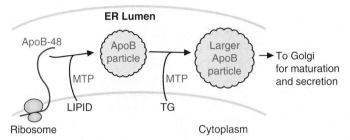

**FIG. 27.8.** A model of MTP action. MTP is required to transfer lipid to apoB-48 as it is synthesized and to transfer lipid from the cytoplasm to the ER lumen.

protein to be produced in the intestine that is 48% of the size of the protein produced in the liver; hence, the designations B-48 and B-100.

The protein component of the lipoproteins is synthesized on the rough endoplasmic reticulum (RER). Lipids, which are synthesized in the smooth endoplasmic reticulum, are complexed with the proteins to form the chylomicrons.

The assembly of chylomicrons within the endoplasmic reticulum (**ER**) of the intestinal epithelial cell (enterocyte) requires the activity of **microsomal triglyceride transfer protein** (**MTP**). The protein is a dimer of nonidentical subunits. MTP accelerates the transport of triglycerides, cholesterol esters, and phospholipids across membranes of subcellular organelles. It is required for both chylomicron assembly in the intestine and VLDL assembly in the liver. The lack of triglyceride transferase activity leads to the disease abetalipoproteinemia. This disorder affects both chylomicron assembly in the intestine and VLDL assembly in the liver. Both particles require a B apolipoprotein for their assembly (apoB-48 for chylomicrons, apoB-100 for VLDL), and MTP binds to the B apolipoproteins. For both chylomicron and VLDL assembly, a small apoB-containing particle is first produced within the lumen of the ER. The appropriate apoB is made on the RER and is inserted into the ER lumen during its synthesis (see Chapter 12). As the protein is being translated, lipid (a small amount of triglyceride) begins to associate with the protein, and the lipid association is catalyzed by MTP. This leads to the generation of small apoB-containing particles. These particles are not formed in patients with abetalipoproteinemia. The second stage of particle assembly is the fusion of the initial apoB particle with triacylglycerol droplets within the ER. The role of MTP in this second step is still under investigation; it may be required for the transfer of triacylglycerol from the cytoplasm to the lumen of the ER to form this lipid droplet. These steps are depicted in Figure 27.8.

## IV. TRANSPORT OF DIETARY LIPIDS IN THE BLOOD

By the process of exocytosis, nascent chylomicrons are secreted by the intestinal epithelial cells into the chyle of the lymphatic system and enter the blood through the thoracic duct. The lymph system is a network of vessels that surround interstitial cavities in the body. Cells secrete various compounds into the lymph, and the lymph vessels transport these fluids away from the interstitial spaces in the body tissues and into the bloodstream. In the case of the intestinal lymph system, the lymph enters the bloodstream via the thoracic duct. The design of these vessels prevents the contents of the blood from entering the lymphatic system. The lymph system is similar in composition to that of the blood but lacks the cells found in blood. Nascent chylomicrons begin to enter the blood within 1 to 2 hours after the start of a meal; as the meal is digested and absorbed, they continue to enter the blood for many hours. Initially, the particles are called nascent (newborn) chylomicrons. As they accept proteins from high-density lipoprotein (**HDL**) within the lymph and the blood, they become "mature" chylomicrons. HDL is the lipoprotein with the highest content of proteins, and lowest of triglyceride (see Chapter 29 for further discussion of HDL and other lipoproteins found in the body).

 The lack of triglyceride transfer activity leads to the disease **abetalipoproteinemia**. This disease affects both chylomicron assembly in the intestine and VLDL assembly in the liver. The complications of abetalipoproteinemia include lipid malabsorption, which causes steatorrhea and vomiting. This will also result in caloric deficiencies, weight loss, and clinical issues related to deficiencies in the lipid-soluble vitamins.

Because of their high triacylglycerol content, chylomicrons are the least dense of the blood lipoproteins. When blood is collected from patients with certain types of hyperlipoproteinemias (high concentrations of lipoproteins in the blood) in which chylomicron levels are elevated and the blood is allowed to stand in the refrigerator overnight, the chylomicrons float to the top of the liquid and coalesce, forming a creamy layer.

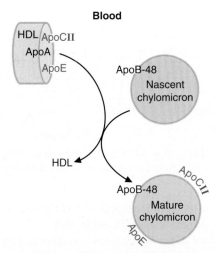

**FIG. 27.9.** Transfer of proteins from HDL to chylomicrons. Newly synthesized chylomicrons (nascent chylomicrons) mature as they receive apoC-II and apoE from HDL. HDL functions in the transfer of these apolipoproteins and also in transfer of cholesterol from peripheral tissues to the liver.

One manner in which individuals can lose weight is to inhibit the activity of pancreatic lipase. This would result in reduced fat digestion and absorption and a reduced caloric yield from the diet. The drug Orlistat is a chemically-synthesized derivative of lipstatin, a natural lipase inhibitor found in certain bacteria. The drug works in the intestinal lumen and forms a covalent bond with the active site serine residue of both gastric and pancreatic lipase, thereby inhibiting their activities. Nondigested triglycerides are not absorbed by the intestine and are eliminated in the feces. Under normal use of the drug, approximately 30% of dietary fat absorption is inhibited. Because excessive nondigested fat in the intestines can lead to gastrointestinal distress related to excessive intestinal gas formation, individuals who take this drug need to follow a diet with reduced daily intake of fat, which should be evenly distributed amongst the meals of the day.

HDL transfers proteins to the nascent chylomicrons, particularly apolipoprotein E (apoE) and apolipoprotein C-II (apoC-II) (Fig. 27.9). ApoE is recognized by membrane receptors, particularly those on the surface of liver cells, allowing apoE-bearing lipoproteins to enter these cells by endocytosis for subsequent digestion by lysosomes. ApoC-II acts as an activator of **lipoprotein lipase** (LPL), the enzyme on capillary endothelial cells, primarily within muscle and adipose tissue, that digests the triacylglycerols of the chylomicrons and VLDL in the blood.

## V. FATE OF CHYLOMICRONS

The triacylglycerols of the chylomicrons are digested by LPL attached to the proteoglycans in the basement membranes of endothelial cells that line the capillary walls (Fig. 27.10). LPL is produced by adipose cells, muscle cells (particularly cardiac

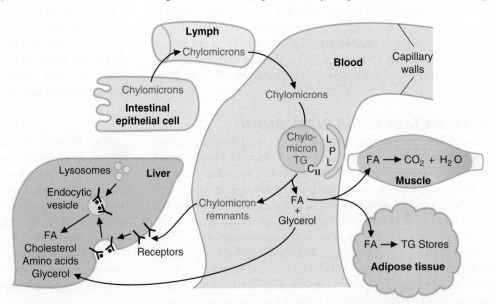

**FIG. 27.10.** Fate of chylomicrons. Chylomicrons are synthesized in intestinal epithelial cells, secreted into the lymph, pass into the blood, and become mature chylomicrons (see Fig. 27.9). On capillary walls in adipose tissue and muscle, *LPL* activated by apoC-II digests the triacylglycerols (*TG*) of chylomicrons to fatty acids and glycerol. Fatty acids (*FA*) are oxidized in muscle or stored in adipose cells as triacylglycerols. The remnants of the chylomicrons are taken up by the liver by receptor-mediated endocytosis (through recognition of apoE on the remnant). Lysosomal enzymes within the hepatocyte digest the remnants, releasing the products into the cytosol.

muscle), and cells of the lactating mammary gland. The isozyme synthesized in adipose cells has a higher $K_m$ than the isozyme synthesized in muscle cells. Therefore, adipose LPL is more active after a meal, when chylomicron levels are elevated in the blood. Insulin stimulates the synthesis and secretion of adipose LPL so that after a meal, when triglyceride levels increase in circulation, LPL has been upregulated (through insulin release) to facilitate the hydrolysis of fatty acids from the triglyceride.

The fatty acids released from triacylglycerols by LPL are not very soluble in water. They become soluble in blood by forming complexes with the protein albumin. The major fate of the fatty acids is storage as triacylglycerol in adipose tissue. However, these fatty acids also may be oxidized for energy in muscle and other tissues (see Fig. 27.10). The LPL in the capillaries of muscle cells has a lower $K_m$ than adipose LPL. Thus, muscle cells can obtain fatty acids from blood lipoproteins preferentially over adipose tissue whenever they are needed for energy, even if the concentration of the lipoproteins is low.

The glycerol released from chylomicron triacylglycerols by LPL may be used for triacylglycerol synthesis in the liver in the fed state.

The portion of a chylomicron that remains in the blood after LPL action is known as a **chylomicron remnant**. The remnant has lost many of the apoC molecules bound to the mature chylomicron, which exposes apoE. This remnant binds to receptors on hepatocytes (the major cells of the liver), which recognize apoE and is taken up by the process of endocytosis. Lysosomes fuse with the endocytic vesicles, and the chylomicron remnants are degraded by lysosomal enzymes. The products of lysosomal digestion (e.g., fatty acids, amino acids, glycerol, cholesterol, phosphate) can be reused by the cell.

 Heparin is a complex polysaccharide (a glycosaminoglycan) that is a component of proteoglycans (see Chapter 25). Isolated heparin is frequently used as an anticoagulant because it binds to antithrombin III (ATIII), and the activated ATIII then binds factors necessary for clotting and inhibits them from working. As LPL is bound to the capillary endothelium through binding to proteoglycans, heparin can also bind to LPL and dislodge it from the capillary wall. This leads to loss of LPL activity and an increase of triglyceride content in the blood.

## CLINICAL COMMENTS

A summary of the diseases discussed in this chapter is found in Table 27.1

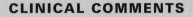 **Will S.** The upper abdominal ultrasound study showed a large gallstone lodged in **Will S.'s** common duct with dilation of this duct proximal to the stone. Will was scheduled for endoscopic retrograde cholangiopancreatography (ERCP). (An ERCP involves cannulation of the common bile duct—and, if necessary, the pancreatic duct—through a tube placed through the mouth and stomach and into the upper small intestine.) With this technique, a stone can be snared in the common duct and removed to relieve an obstruction.

If common duct obstruction is severe enough, bilirubin flows back into the venous blood draining from the liver. As a consequence, serum bilirubin levels, particularly

**Table 27.1   Diseases Discussed in Chapter 27**

| Disease or Disorder | Environmental or Genetic | Comments |
|---|---|---|
| Sickle cell disease | Genetic | Cholecystitis may result as a consequence of sickle cell disease due to increased red cell destruction in the spleen and an inability of the liver to conjugate all of the bilirubin resulting from heme degradation. |
| Alcoholism | Both | Pancreatitis may result from chronic alcohol abuse, leading to malabsorption problems within the intestine. |
| Abetalipoproteinemia | Genetic | Loss of MTP activity, leading to an inability to produce both chylomicrons and VLDL. Steatorrhea and fat-soluble vitamin deficiencies may result as well as a deficiency in required dietary fatty acids. |

MTP, microsomal triglyceride transfer protein; VLDL, very low density lipoprotein.

the indirect (unconjugated) fraction, increase. Tissues such as the sclerae of the eye take up this pigment, which causes them to become yellow (jaundiced, icteric). **Will S.'s** condition was severe enough to cause jaundice by this mechanism.

 **AI M.** Alcohol excess may produce proteinaceous plugs in the small pancreatic ducts, causing back pressure injury and autodigestion of the pancreatic acini drained by these obstructed channels. This process causes one form of acute pancreatitis. **Al M.** had an episode of acute alcohol-induced pancreatitis superimposed on a more chronic alcohol-related inflammatory process in the pancreas—in other words, a chronic pancreatitis. As a result of decreased secretion of pancreatic lipase through the pancreatic ducts and into the lumen of the small intestine, dietary fat was not absorbed at a normal rate, and steatorrhea (fat-rich stools) occurred. If abstinence from alcohol does not allow adequate recovery of the enzymatic secretory function of the pancreas, Mr. M. will have to take a commercial preparation of pancreatic enzymes with meals that contain even minimal amounts of fat.

## REVIEW QUESTIONS-CHAPTER 27

1. The most abundant component of chylomicrons is which one of the following?

    A. Phospholipid
    B. Cholesterol
    C. Cholesterol ester
    D. ApoB-48
    E. Triglyceride

2. The conversion of nascent chylomicrons to mature chylomicrons requires which one of the following?

    A. High-density lipoprotein (HDL)
    B. Bile salts
    C. 2-Monoacylglycerol
    D. Lipoprotein lipase (LPL)
    E. Lymphatic system

3. The apolipoproteins B-48 and B-100 are similar with respect to which one of the following?

    A. They are derived by alternative splicing of the same hnRNA.
    B. They are synthesized from the same gene.
    C. ApoB-48 is a proteolytic product of apoB-100.
    D. Both are found in mature chylomicrons.
    E. Both are found in very low density lipoproteins (VLDL).

4. Type III hyperlipidemia is due to a deficiency of apolipoprotein E. Analysis of the serum of patients with this disorder would exhibit which one of the following?

    A. An absence of chylomicrons after eating
    B. Above normal levels of VLDL immediately after eating
    C. Elevated triglyceride levels
    D. Normal triglyceride levels
    E. Below normal triglyceride levels

5. An obstruction of the pancreatic duct would lead to steatorrhea due to which one of the following?

    A. Lack of bile salts in the intestinal lumen
    B. Lack of phospholipase $A_2$ activity in the intestinal lumen
    C. Lack of cholesterol esterase activity in the intestinal lumen
    D. Lack of pancreatic lipase activity in the intestinal lumen
    E. Inability to salvage bile salts

# 28 Synthesis of Fatty Acids, Triacylglycerols, Eicosanoids, and the Major Membrane Lipids

## CHAPTER OUTLINE

## KEY POINTS

■ Fatty acids are synthesized mainly in the liver, primarily from glucose.

■ Glucose is converted to pyruvate via glycolysis, which enters the mitochondrion and forms both acetyl coenzyme A (CoA) and oxaloacetate, which then forms citrate.

■ The newly synthesized citrate is transported to the cytosol, where it is cleaved to form acetyl CoA, which is the source of carbons for fatty acid biosynthesis.

■ Two enzymes, acetyl CoA carboxylase (the key regulatory step) and fatty acid synthase, produce palmitic acid (16 carbons, no double bonds) from acetyl CoA. After activation to palmitoyl CoA, the fatty acid can be elongated or desaturated (adding double bonds) by enzymes in the endoplasmic reticulum.

■ The eicosanoids (prostaglandins, thromboxanes, and leukotrienes) are potent regulators of cellular function (such as the inflammatory response, smooth muscle contraction, blood pressure regulation,

continued

and bronchoconstriction and bronchodilation) and are derived from polyunsaturated fatty acids containing 20 carbon atoms.

■ The prostaglandins and thromboxanes require cyclooxygenase activity to be synthesized, whereas the leukotrienes require lipoxygenase activity.

■ Cyclooxygenase is the target of nonsteroidal anti-inflammatory drugs (NSAIDs), including aspirin, which covalently acetylates and inactivates the enzyme in platelets.

■ Fatty acids are used to produce triacylgylcerols (for energy storage) and glycerol phospholipids and sphingolipids (for structural components of cell membranes).

■ Liver-derived triacylglycerol is packaged with various apolipoproteins and secreted into the circulation as very low density lipoprotein (VLDL).

■ As with dietary chylomicrons, lipoprotein lipase in the capillaries of adipose tissue, muscle, and the lactating mammary gland digests the triacylglycerol of VLDL, forming fatty acids and glycerol.

■ Glycerophospholipids, synthesized from fatty acyl CoA and glycerol 3-phosphate, are all derived from phosphatidic acid. Various head groups are added to phosphatidic acid to form the mature glycerophospholipids.

■ Phospholipid degradation is catalyzed by phospholipases.

■ Sphingolipids are synthesized from sphingosine, which is derived from palmitoyl CoA and serine. Glycolipids, such as cerebrosides, globosides, and gangliosides, are sphingolipids.

■ The sole sphingosine-based phospholipid is sphingomyelin.

■ The adipocyte is an active endocrine organ, producing adipokines that help to regulate appetite and adipocyte size.

## THE WAITING ROOM

**Cora N.'s** hypertension and heart failure (see Chapter 16) have been well controlled on medication, and she has lost 10 lb since she had her recent heart attack. Her fasting serum lipid profile before discharge from the hospital indicated a significantly elevated serum low-density lipoprotein (LDL) cholesterol level of 175 mg/dL (recommended level for a patient with known coronary artery disease is 100 mg/dL or less), a serum triacylglycerol level of 280 mg/dL (reference range = 60 mg/dL to 150 mg/dL), and a serum high-density lipoprotein (HDL) cholesterol level of 34 mg/dL (reference range >50 mg/dL for healthy women). While she was still in the hospital, she was asked to obtain the most recent serum lipid profiles for her older brother and her younger sister, both of whom were experiencing chest pain. Her brother's profile showed normal triacylglycerols, moderately elevated LDL cholesterol, and significantly suppressed HDL cholesterol levels. Her sister's profile showed only hypertriglyceridemia (high blood triacylglycerols).

**Christy L.** was born 6 weeks prematurely. She appeared normal until about 30 minutes after delivery, when her respirations became rapid at 64 breaths per minute with audible respiratory grunting. The spaces between her ribs (intercostal spaces) retracted inward with each inspiration, and her lips and fingers became cyanotic from a lack of oxygen in her arterial blood. An arterial blood sample indicated a low partial pressure of oxygen ($Po_2$) and a slightly elevated partial pressure of carbon dioxide ($Pco_2$). The arterial pH was somewhat suppressed, in part, from an accumulation of lactic acid secondary to the hypoxemia (a low level of oxygen in her blood). A chest radiograph showed a fine reticular granularity of the lung tissue, especially in the left lower lobe area. From these clinical data, a diagnosis of respiratory distress syndrome (RDS), also known as hyaline membrane disease, was made.

Christy was immediately transferred to the neonatal intensive care unit, where, with intensive respiration therapy, she slowly improved.

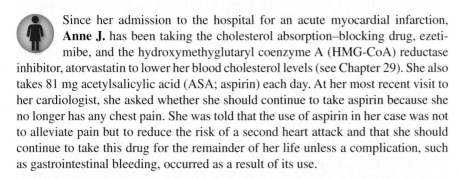

Since her admission to the hospital for an acute myocardial infarction, **Anne J.** has been taking the cholesterol absorption–blocking drug, ezetimibe, and the hydroxymethyglutaryl coenzyme A (HMG-CoA) reductase inhibitor, atorvastatin to lower her blood cholesterol levels (see Chapter 29). She also takes 81 mg acetylsalicylic acid (ASA; aspirin) each day. At her most recent visit to her cardiologist, she asked whether she should continue to take aspirin because she no longer has any chest pain. She was told that the use of aspirin in her case was not to alleviate pain but to reduce the risk of a second heart attack and that she should continue to take this drug for the remainder of her life unless a complication, such as gastrointestinal bleeding, occurred as a result of its use.

## I.  FATTY ACID SYNTHESIS

**Fatty acids** are synthesized whenever an excess of calories is ingested. The major source of carbon for the synthesis of fatty acids is dietary carbohydrate. An excess of dietary protein can also result in an increase in fatty acid synthesis. In this case, the carbon source is amino acids that can be converted to acetyl CoA or tricarboxylic acid (TCA) cycle intermediates (see Chapter 33). Fatty acid synthesis occurs primarily in the liver, although it can also occur, to a lesser extent, in adipose tissue.

When an excess of dietary carbohydrate is consumed, glucose is converted to acetyl CoA, which provides the two-carbon units that condense in a series of reactions on the fatty acid synthase complex, producing **palmitate**. Palmitate is then converted to other fatty acids. The fatty acid synthase complex is located in the cytosol and, therefore, it uses **cytosolic acetyl CoA**.

### A.  Conversion of Glucose to Cytosolic Acetyl Coenzyme A

The pathway for the synthesis of cytosolic acetyl CoA from glucose begins with glycolysis, which converts glucose to pyruvate in the cytosol (Fig. 28.1). Pyruvate enters mitochondria, where it is converted to acetyl CoA by pyruvate dehydrogenase and to oxaloacetate by pyruvate carboxylase. The pathway that pyruvate follows is dictated by the acetyl CoA levels in the mitochondria. When acetyl CoA levels are high, pyruvate dehydrogenase is inhibited, and pyruvate carboxylase activity is stimulated. As oxaloacetate levels increase because of the activity of pyruvate carboxylase, oxaloacetate condenses with acetyl CoA to form citrate. This condensation reduces

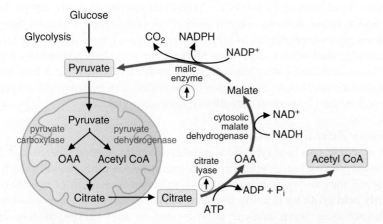

**FIG. 28.1.** Conversion of glucose to cytosolic acetyl CoA and the fate of citrate in the cytosol. Citrate lyase is also called citrate cleavage enzyme. *OAA*, oxaloacetate; ↑, inducible enzyme.

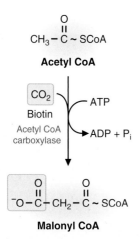

**FIG. 28.2.** Reaction catalyzed by acetyl CoA carboxylase. Initially, $CO_2$ is covalently attached to biotin, which is linked by an amide bond to the ε-amino group of a lysine residue of the enzyme. Hydrolysis of ATP is required for the attachment of $CO_2$ to biotin. Subsequently, the $CO_2$ is transferred to acetyl CoA.

AMP is a much more sensitive indicator of low energy levels than adenosine diphosphate (ADP) because of the adenylate kinase reaction. The [AMP]/[ATP] ratio is proportional to the square of the [ADP]/[ATP] ratio, so a 5-fold change in ADP levels corresponds to a 25-fold change in AMP levels.

the acetyl CoA levels, which leads to the activation of pyruvate dehydrogenase and inhibition of pyruvate carboxylase. Through such reciprocal regulation, citrate can be continuously synthesized and transported across the inner mitochondrial membrane. In the cytosol, citrate is cleaved by citrate lyase to re-form acetyl CoA and oxaloacetate. This circuitous route is required because pyruvate dehydrogenase, the enzyme that converts pyruvate to acetyl CoA, is found only in mitochondria and because acetyl CoA cannot directly cross the mitochondrial membrane.

Reduced nicotinamide-adenine dinucleotide phosphate (NADPH) is required for fatty acid synthesis and is generated by the pentose phosphate pathway (see Chapter 24) and from recycling of the oxaloacetate produced by citrate lyase (see Fig. 28.1). Oxaloacetate is converted back to pyruvate in two steps: the reduction of oxaloacetate to malate by oxidized nicotinamide adenine dinucleotide ($NAD^+$)-dependent malate dehydrogenase and the oxidation and decarboxylation of malate to pyruvate by a nicotinamide adenine dinucleotide phosphate ($NADP^+$)-dependent malate dehydrogenase (malic enzyme). The pyruvate formed by malic enzyme is reconverted to citrate. The NADPH that is generated by malic enzyme, along with the NADPH generated by glucose-6-phosphate dehydrogenase and gluconate 6-phosphate dehydrogenase in the pentose phosphate pathway, is used for the reduction reactions that occur on the fatty acid synthase complex as the fatty acid is synthesized.

The generation of cytosolic acetyl CoA from pyruvate is stimulated by elevation of the insulin/glucagon ratio after a carbohydrate meal. Insulin activates pyruvate dehydrogenase by stimulating the phosphatase that dephosphorylates the enzyme to an active form (see Chapter 16). The synthesis of malic enzyme, glucose-6-phosphate dehydrogenase, and citrate lyase is induced by the high insulin/glucagon ratio. The ability of citrate to accumulate and to leave the mitochondrial matrix for the synthesis of fatty acids is attributable to the allosteric inhibition of isocitrate dehydrogenase by high energy levels within the matrix under these conditions. The concerted regulation of glycolysis and fatty acid synthesis is described in Chapter 30.

### B. Conversion of Acetyl Coenzyme A to Malonyl Coenzyme A

Cytosolic acetyl CoA is converted to **malonyl CoA**, which serves as the immediate donor of the two carbon units that are added to the growing fatty acid chain on the fatty acid synthase complex. To synthesize malonyl CoA, **acetyl CoA carboxylase** adds a carboxyl group to acetyl CoA in a reaction that requires biotin and adenosine triphosphate (ATP) (Fig. 28.2).

Acetyl CoA carboxylase is the rate-limiting enzyme of fatty acid synthesis. Its activity is regulated by phosphorylation, allosteric modification, and induction/repression of its synthesis (Fig. 28.3). Citrate allosterically activates acetyl CoA carboxylase by causing the individual enzyme molecules (each composed of four subunits) to polymerize. Palmityl CoA, produced from palmitate (the end product of fatty acid synthase activity), inhibits acetyl CoA carboxylase. Phosphorylation by an adenosine monophosphate (AMP)-activated protein kinase inhibits the enzyme in the fasting state when energy levels are low. The enzyme is activated by dephosphorylation in the fed state when energy and insulin levels are high. A high insulin/glucagon ratio also results in induction of the synthesis of both acetyl CoA carboxylase and the next enzyme in the pathway, fatty acid synthase.

### C. Fatty Acid Synthase Complex

As an overview, fatty acid synthase sequentially adds two-carbon units from malonyl CoA to the growing fatty acyl chain to form palmitate. After the addition of each two-carbon unit, the growing chain undergoes two reduction reactions that require NADPH.

**Fatty acid synthase** is a very large enzyme composed of two identical subunits, which each have seven catalytic activities and an **acyl carrier protein (ACP)** segment in a continuous polypeptide chain. The ACP segment contains a phosphopantetheine residue that is derived from the cleavage of coenzyme A. The key feature

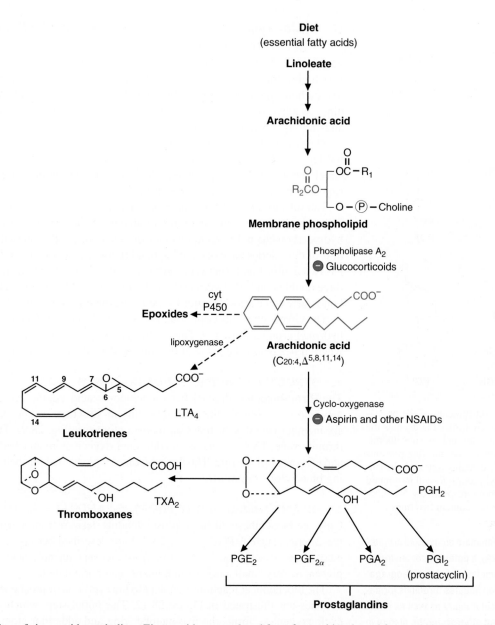

**FIG. 28.9.** Overview of eicosanoid metabolism. Eicosanoids are produced from fatty acids released from membrane phospholipids. In humans, arachidonic acid is the major precursor of the eicosanoids, which include the prostaglandins, leukotrienes, and thromboxanes. ⊖, "inhibits"; *cyt,* cytochrome; *NSAID,* nonsteroidal anti-inflammatory drug.

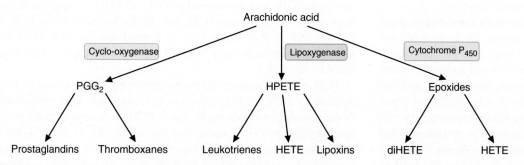

**FIG. 28.10.** Pathways for the metabolism of arachidonic acid.

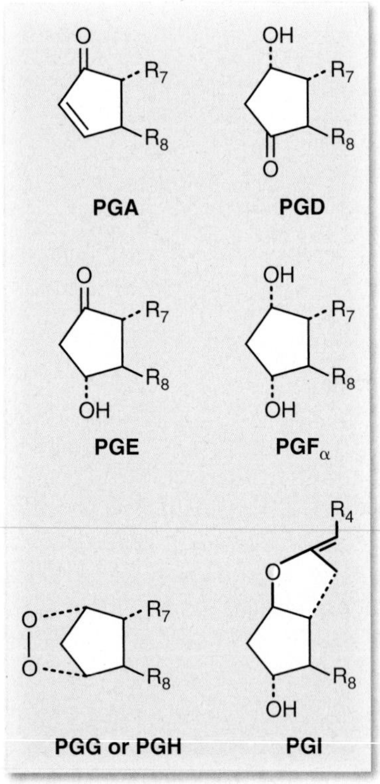

**FIG. 28.11.** Ring substituents of the prostaglandins (PG). The letter after PG denotes the configuration of the ring and its substituents. $R_4$, $R_7$, and $R_8$ represent the non-ring portions of the molecule. $R_4$ contains four carbons (including the carboxyl group). $R_7$ and $R_8$ contain seven and eight carbons, respectively. Note that the prostacyclins *(PGI)* contain two rings.

The predominant eicosanoid in platelets is TXA$_2$, a potent vasoconstrictor and a stimulator of platelet aggregation. The latter action initiates thrombus formation at sites of vascular injury as well as in the vicinity of a ruptured atherosclerotic plaque in the lumen of vessels such as the coronary arteries. Such thrombi may cause sudden total occlusion of the vascular lumen, causing acute ischemic damage to tissues distal to the block (i.e., acute myocardial infarction).

Aspirin, by covalently acetylating the active site of cyclooxygenase, blocks the production of TXA$_2$ from its major precursor, arachidonic acid. By causing this mild hemostatic defect, low-dose aspirin has been shown to be effective in prevention of acute myocardial infarction. For **Ivan A.** (who has symptoms of coronary heart disease), aspirin is used to prevent a first heart attack (primary prevention). For **Anne J.** and **Cora N.** (who already have had heart attacks), aspirin is used in hopes of preventing a second heart attack (secondary prevention).

## C. Cyclooxygenase Pathway: Synthesis of the Prostaglandins and Thromboxanes

### 1. STRUCTURES OF THE PROSTAGLANDINS

**Prostaglandins** are fatty acids containing 20 carbon atoms, including an internal five-carbon ring. In addition to this ring, each of the biologically active prostaglandins has a hydroxyl group at carbon 15, a double bond between carbons 13 and 14, and various substituents on the ring.

The nomenclature for the prostaglandins (PGs) involves the assignment of a capital letter (PGE), an Arabic numeral subscript (PGE$_1$), and for the PGF family, a Greek letter subscript (e.g., PGF$_{2\alpha}$). The capital letter, in this case "F," refers to the ring substituents shown in Figure 28.11.

The subscript that follows the capital letter (PGF$_1$) refers to the PG series 1, 2, or 3, determined by the number of unsaturated bonds present in the linear portion of the hydrocarbon chain. It does not include double bonds in the internal ring. Prostaglandins of the 1 series have one double bond (between carbons 13 and 14). The 2 series has two double bonds (between carbons 13 and 14 and 5 and 6), and the 3 series has three double bonds (between carbons 13 and 14, 5 and 6, and 17 and 18). The double bonds between carbons 13 and 14 are *trans*; the others are *cis*.

The Greek letter subscript, found only in the F series, refers to the position of the hydroxyl group at carbon 9. This hydroxyl group primarily exists in the α position, where it lies below the plane of the ring, as does the hydroxyl group at carbon 11.

### 2. STRUCTURE OF THE THROMBOXANES

The **thromboxanes**, derived from arachidonic acid via the cyclooxygenase pathway, closely resemble the prostaglandins in structure except that they contain a six-member ring that includes an oxygen atom (see Fig. 28.9). The most common thromboxane, TXA$_2$, contains an additional oxygen atom attached both to carbon 9 and carbon 11 of the ring. The thromboxanes were named for their action in producing blood clots (thrombi).

### 3. BIOSYNTHESIS OF THE PROSTAGLANDINS AND THROMBOXANES

Only the biosynthesis of those prostaglandins derived from arachidonic acid (e.g., the 2 series, such as PGE$_2$, PGI$_2$, TXA$_2$) are described because those derived from eicosatrienoic acid (the 1 series) or from eicosapentaenoic acid (the 3 series) are present in very small amounts in humans on a normal diet.

The biochemical reactions that lead to the synthesis of prostaglandins and thromboxanes are illustrated in Figure 28.12. The initial step, which is catalyzed by a cyclooxygenase, forms the five-member ring and adds four atoms of oxygen (two between carbons 9 and 11, and two at carbon 15) to form the unstable endoperoxide, PGG$_2$. The hydroperoxy group at carbon 15 is quickly reduced to a hydroxyl group by a peroxidase to form another endoperoxide, PGH$_2$.

The next step is tissue specific (see Fig. 28.12). Depending on the type of cell involved, PGH$_2$ may be reduced to PGE$_2$ or PGD$_2$ by specific enzymes (PGE synthase and PGD synthase). PGE$_2$ may be further reduced by PGE 9-ketoreductase to form PGF$_{2\alpha}$. PGF$_{2\alpha}$ also may be formed directly from PGH$_2$ by the action of an endoperoxide reductase. Some of the major functions of the prostaglandins are listed in Table 28.1.

PGH$_2$ may be converted to the thromboxane, TXA$_2$, a reaction catalyzed by TXA synthase (see Fig. 28.12). This enzyme is present in high concentration in platelets. In the vascular endothelium, however, PGH$_2$ is converted to the prostaglandin PGI$_2$ (prostacyclin) by PGI synthase (see Fig. 28.12). TXA$_2$ and PGI$_2$ have important antagonistic biological effects on vasomotor and smooth muscle tone and on platelet aggregation. Some of the known functions of the thromboxanes are listed in Table 28.2.

In the 1990s, the cyclooxygenase enzyme was found to exist as two distinct isoforms, designated COX-1 and COX-2. COX-1 is regarded as a constitutive form of

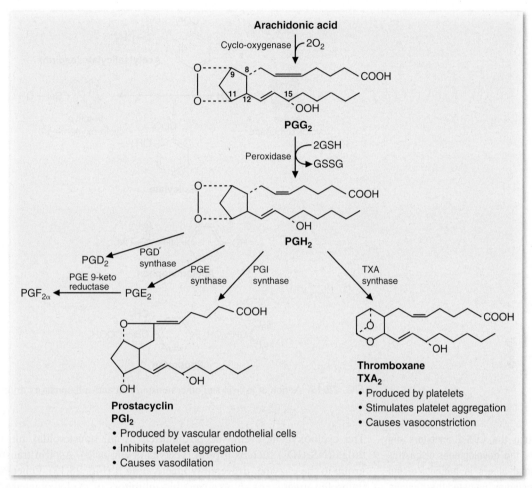

**FIG. 28.12.** Formation of prostaglandins (including the prostacyclin PGI$_2$) and thromboxane TXA$_2$ from arachidonic acid. The conversion of arachidonic acid to PGH$_2$ is catalyzed by a membrane-bound enzyme, prostaglandin endoperoxide synthase, which has cyclooxygenase and peroxidase activities. The reducing agent is glutathione *(GSH)*, which is oxidized to form a disulfide between the two glutathione molecules *(GSSG)*.

the enzyme, is widely expressed in almost all tissues, is the only form expressed in mature platelets, and is involved in the production of prostaglandins and thromboxanes for "normal" physiological functions. COX-2 is an inducible form of the enzyme regulated by a variety of cytokines and growth factors. COX-2 mRNA and protein levels are usually low in most healthy tissue but are expressed at high levels in inflamed tissue.

Because of the importance of prostaglandins in mediating the inflammatory response, drugs that block prostaglandin production should provide relief from pain.

Diets that include cold-water fish (e.g., salmon, mackerel, brook trout, herring), with a high content of polyunsaturated fatty acids, eicosapentaenoic acid (EPA) and docosahexaenoic acid (DHA), result in a high content of these fatty acids in membrane phospholipids. It has been suggested that such diets are effective in preventing heart disease, in part, because they lead to formation of more TXA$_3$ relative to TXA$_2$. TXA$_3$ is less effective in stimulating platelet aggregation than its counterpart in the 2 series, TXA$_2$.

**Table 28.1   Some Functions of the Prostaglandins**

| PGI$_2$, PGE$_2$, PGD$_2$ | PGF$_{2\alpha}$ |
|---|---|
| Increases | Increases |
| Vasodilation | Vasoconstriction |
| cAMP | Bronchoconstriction |
| Decreases | Smooth muscle contraction |
| Platelet aggregation | |
| Leukocyte aggregation | |
| IL-1[a] and IL-2 | |
| T-cell proliferation | |
| Lymphocyte migration | |

[a]IL, interleukin; a cytokine that augments the activity of many cells in the immune system.

**Table 28.2   Some Functions of Thromboxane A$_2$**

| Increases |
|---|
| Vasoconstriction |
| Platelet aggregation |
| Lymphocyte proliferation |
| Bronchoconstriction |

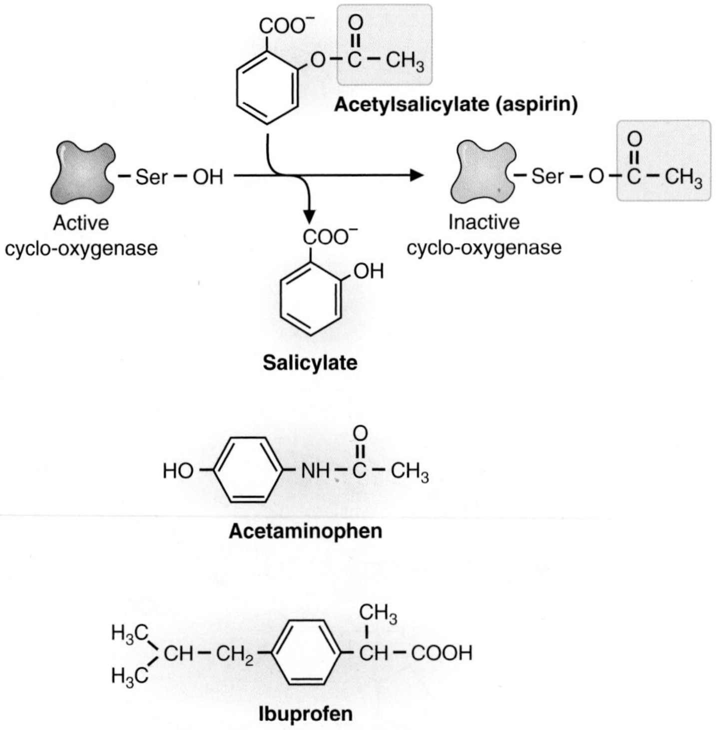

**FIG. 28.13.** Action of aspirin and other nonsteroidal anti-inflammatory drugs.

Although the COX-2 inhibitors did relieve the development of gastrointestinal ulcers in patients taking NSAIDs, further studies indicated that specific COX-2 inhibitors may have a negative effect on cardiovascular function. Vioxx was withdrawn from the market by its manufacturer because of these negative patient studies. It has been postulated that long-term use of COX-2 inhibitors alter the balance of prostacyclin (antithrombotic, $PGI_2$) and thromboxane (prothrombotic) because platelets, the major source of the thromboxanes, do not express COX-2 and thromboxane synthesis is not reduced with COX-2 inhibitors (see Fig. 28.12 and Table 28.3). This will tilt the balance of the eicosanoids synthesized toward a thrombotic pathway. The COX-2 inhibitors that remain on the market must be used with caution, as they are contraindicated in patients with ischemic heart disease or stroke.

The cyclooxygenase enzyme is inhibited by all nonsteroidal anti-inflammatory drugs (NSAIDs) such as aspirin (acetylsalicylic acid). Aspirin transfers an acetyl group to the enzyme, irreversibly inactivating it (Fig. 28.13). Other NSAIDs (e.g., ibuprofen, naproxen) act as reversible inhibitors of cyclooxygenase. Ibuprofen is the major ingredient in popular over-the-counter NSAIDs such as Motrin, Nuprin, and Advil (see Fig. 28.13). Although they have some relative selectivity for inhibiting either COX-1 or COX-2, NSAIDs block the activity of both isoforms. These findings provided the impetus for the development of selective COX-2 inhibitors, which are proposed to act as potent anti-inflammatory agents by inhibiting COX-2 activity, without the gastrointestinal (stomach ulcers) and antiplatelet side effects commonly associated with NSAID use. These adverse effects of NSAIDs are thought to be caused by COX-1 inhibition. An example of a selective COX-2 inhibitors is celecoxib (Celebrex). Some properties of COX-1 and COX-2 are indicated in Table 28.3.

**Table 28.3 Properties of COX-1 and COX-2**

| | COX-1 | COX-2 |
|---|---|---|
| Primary function | Platelet aggregation, stomach cytoprotection | Inflammation, hyperalgesia |
| Response to | | |
|   NSAIDs | Decreased activity | Decreased activity |
|   Steroids | No effect | Decreased synthesis and activity |
|   COX-2 inhibitor | No effect | Decreased activity |

Data adapted from Patrono and Baigent (see References [@]) indicate that low-dose aspirin (50 to 100 mg/day) reduces platelet $TXA_2$ levels by 97% with no effect on whole body $PGI_2$, thereby leading to cardioprotection. High-dose aspirin (650 to 1,300 mg/day), in addition to reducing $TXA_2$ levels, also reduced $PGI_2$ levels by 60% to 80%. COX-2 specific inhibitors, at high levels, had no effect on $TXA_2$ levels but reduced whole body $PGI_2$ levels by 60% to 80%, leading to an increased risk of myocardial infarction. NSAIDS, nonsteroidal anti-inflammatory drugs.

### 4. INACTIVATION OF THE PROSTAGLANDINS AND THROMBOXANES

Prostaglandins and thromboxanes are rapidly inactivated. Their half-lives ($t_{1/2}$) range from seconds to minutes. The prostaglandins are inactivated by oxidation of the 15-hydroxy group, critical for their activity, to a ketone. The double bond at carbon 13 is reduced. Subsequently, both β- and ω-oxidation of the nonring portions occur, producing dicarboxylic acids that are excreted in the urine. Active $TXA_2$ is rapidly metabolized to $TXB_2$ by cleavage of the oxygen bridge between carbons 9 and 11 to form two hydroxyl groups. $TXB_2$ has no biological activity.

## III. SYNTHESIS OF TRIACYLGLYCEROLS AND VERY LOW DENSITY LIPOPROTEIN PARTICLES

In liver and adipose tissue, **triacylglycerols** are produced by a pathway containing a phosphatidic acid intermediate (Fig. 28.14). Phosphatidic acid is also the precursor of the glycerolipids found in cell membranes and the blood lipoproteins.

The sources of glycerol 3-phosphate, which provides the glycerol moiety for triacylglycerol synthesis, differ in liver and adipose tissue. In liver, glycerol 3-phosphate is produced from the phosphorylation of glycerol by glycerol kinase or from the reduction of dihydroxyacetone phosphate (DHAP) derived from glycolysis. White adipose tissue lacks glycerol kinase and can produce glycerol 3-phosphate only from glucose via DHAP. Thus, adipose tissue can store fatty acids only when glycolysis is activated, that is, in the fed state.

In both adipose tissue and liver, triacylglycerols are produced by a pathway in which glycerol 3-phosphate reacts with fatty acyl CoA to form phosphatidic acid. Dephosphorylation of phosphatidic acid produces DAG. Another fatty acyl CoA reacts with the DAG to form a triacylglycerol (see Fig. 28.14).

The triacylglycerol, which is produced in the smooth endoplasmic reticulum of the liver, is packaged with cholesterol, phospholipids, and proteins (synthesized in the rough endoplasmic reticulum) to form VLDL (Fig. 28.15 and see Section III of Chapter 26). The microsomal triglyceride transfer protein (MTP), which is required for chylmicron assembly, is also required for VLDL assembly. The major protein of VLDL is apolipoprotein B-100 (apoB-100). There is one long apoB-100 molecule wound through the surface of each VLDL particle. ApoB-100 is encoded by the same gene as the apoB-48 of chylomicrons, but it is a larger protein. In intestinal cells, RNA editing produces a stop codon in the mRNA produced by the gene and a protein which is 48% of the size of apoB-100 (see Fig. 27.7).

VLDL is processed in the Golgi complex and secreted into the blood by the liver. The fatty acid residues of the triacylglycerols ultimately are stored in the triacylglycerols of adipose cells. Note that, in comparison to chylomicrons (see Chapter 27), VLDL particles are denser, as they contain a lower percentage of triglyceride (and hence more protein) than do the chylomicrons. Similar to chylomicrons, VLDL particles are first synthesized in a nascent form, and on entering the circulation, they acquire apolipoproteins C-II and E from HDL particles to become mature VLDL particles (see Chapter 27).

## IV. FATE OF VERY LOW DENSITY LIPOPROTEIN TRIACYLGLYCEROL

Lipoprotein lipase (LPL), which is attached to the basement membrane proteoglycans of capillary endothelial cells, cleaves the triacylglycerols in both VLDL and chylomicrons, forming fatty acids and glycerol. Apolipoprotein C-II, which these lipoproteins obtain from HDL, activates LPL. The fate of the VLDL particle after triglyceride has been removed by LPL is the generation of an intermediate-density lipoprotein (IDL) particle, which can further lose triglyceride to become an low-density lipoprotein (LDL) particle. The fate of the IDL and LDL particles is discussed in Chapter 29.

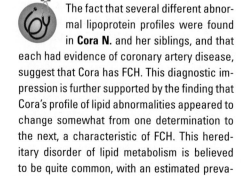

The fact that several different abnormal lipoprotein profiles were found in **Cora N.** and her siblings, and that each had evidence of coronary artery disease, suggest that Cora has FCH. This diagnostic impression is further supported by the finding that Cora's profile of lipid abnormalities appeared to change somewhat from one determination to the next, a characteristic of FCH. This hereditary disorder of lipid metabolism is believed to be quite common, with an estimated prevalence of about 1 per 100 in population.

The mechanisms for FCH are incompletely understood but may involve, in part, a genetically determined increase in the production of apoB-100. As a result, packaging of VLDL is increased, and blood VLDL levels may be elevated. Depending on the efficiency of lipolysis of VLDL by LPL, VLDL levels may be normal and LDL levels may be elevated, or both VLDL and LDL levels may be high. In addition, the phenotypic expression of FCH in any given family member may be determined by the degree of associated obesity, the diet, the use of specific drugs, or other factors that change over time. Additionally, FCH may be a multigenic trait, and even though the disease appears as an autosomal dominant trait in a pedigree analysis, no genes have yet been definitively linked to this condition.

**Q:** Why do some alcoholics have high VLDL levels?

The muscle LPL isozyme has a low $K_m$, which permits muscle to use the fatty acids of chylomicrons and VLDL as a source of fuel even when the blood concentration of these lipoproteins is very low. The LPL isozyme in adipose tissues has a high $K_m$ and is most active after a meal, when the blood levels of chylomicrons and VLDL are elevated.

Fatty acids for VLDL synthesis in the liver may be obtained from the blood or they may be synthesized from glucose. In a healthy individual, the major source of the fatty acids of VLDL triacylglycerol is excess dietary glucose. In individuals with diabetes mellitus, fatty acids mobilized from adipose triacylglycerols in excess of the oxidative capacity of tissues are a major source of the fatty acids reesterified in liver to VLDL triacylglycerol. These individuals frequently have elevated levels of blood triacylglycerols.

**A:** In alcoholism, NADH levels in the liver are elevated (see Chapter 24). High levels of NADH inhibit the oxidation of fatty acids. Therefore, fatty acids, mobilized from adipose tissue, are reesterified to glycerol 3-phosphate in the liver, forming triacylglycerols, which are packaged into VLDL and secreted into the blood. Elevated VLDL is frequently associated with chronic alcoholism. As alcohol-induced liver disease progresses, the ability to secrete the triacylglycerols is diminished, resulting in a fatty liver.

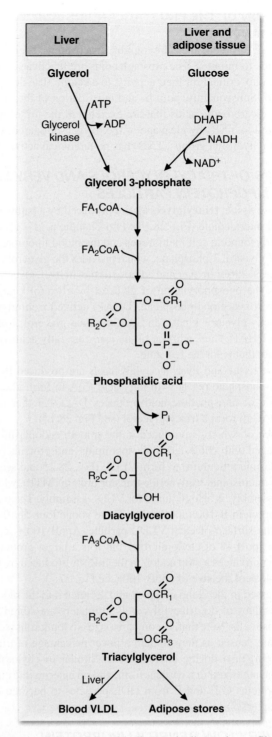

**FIG. 28.14.** Synthesis of triacylglycerol in liver and adipose tissue. Glycerol 3-phosphate is produced from glucose in both tissues. It is also produced from glycerol in liver but not in adipose tissue, which lacks glycerol kinase. The steps from glycerol 3-phosphate are the same in the two tissues. *FA*, fatty acyl group.

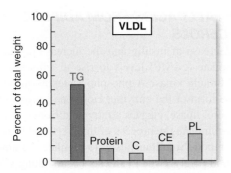

**FIG. 28.15.** Composition of a typical VLDL particle. The major component is triacylglycerol *(TG)*. *C*, cholesterol; *CE*, cholesterol ester; *PL*, phospholipid.

## V. STORAGE OF TRIACYLGLYCEROLS IN ADIPOSE TISSUE

After a meal, the triacylglycerol stores of adipose tissue increase (Fig. 28.16). Adipose cells synthesize LPL and secrete it into the capillaries of adipose tissue when the insulin/glucagon ratio is elevated. This enzyme digests the triacylglycerols of both chylomicrons and VLDL. The fatty acids enter adipose cells and are activated, forming fatty acyl CoA, which reacts with glycerol 3-phosphate to form triacylglycerol by the same pathway used in the liver (see Fig. 28.14). Because adipose tissue lacks glycerol kinase and cannot use the glycerol produced by LPL, the glycerol travels through the blood to the liver, which uses it for the synthesis of triacylglycerol. In adipose cells, under fed conditions, glycerol 3-phosphate is derived from glucose.

In addition to stimulating the synthesis and release of LPL, insulin stimulates glucose metabolism in adipose cells. Insulin leads to the activation of the glycolytic enzyme phosphofructokinase-1 (PFK-1) by an activation of the kinase activity of PFK-2, which increases fructose 2,6-bisphosphate levels. Insulin also stimulates the dephosphorylation of pyruvate dehydrogenase, so that the pyruvate produced by glycolysis can be oxidized in the TCA cycle. Furthermore, insulin stimulates the conversion of glucose to fatty acids in adipose cells, although the liver is the major site of fatty acid synthesis in humans.

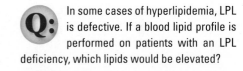 In some cases of hyperlipidemia, LPL is defective. If a blood lipid profile is performed on patients with an LPL deficiency, which lipids would be elevated?

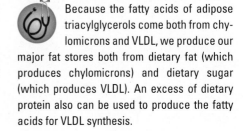 Because the fatty acids of adipose triacylglycerols come both from chylomicrons and VLDL, we produce our major fat stores both from dietary fat (which produces chylomicrons) and dietary sugar (which produces VLDL). An excess of dietary protein also can be used to produce the fatty acids for VLDL synthesis.

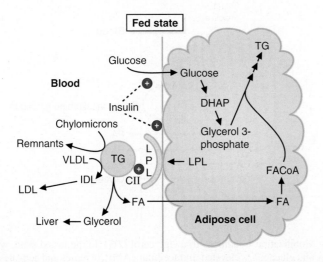

**FIG. 28.16.** Conversion of the fatty acid *(FA)* from the triacylglycerols *(TG)* of chylomicrons and VLDL to the *TG* stored in adipose cells. Note that insulin stimulates both the transport of glucose into adipose cells and the synthesis and secretion of LPL from the cells. Glucose provides the glycerol 3-phosphate for *TG* synthesis. Apolipoprotein C-II activates LPL.

Individuals with a defective LPL have high blood triacylglycerol levels. Their levels of chylomicrons and VLDL (which contain large amounts of triacylglycerols) are elevated because they are not digested at the normal rate by LPL. LPL can be dissociated from capillary walls by treatment with heparin (a glycosaminoglycan). Measurements can be made on blood after heparin treatment to determine whether LPL levels are abnormal.

## VI. RELEASE OF FATTY ACIDS FROM ADIPOSE TRIACYLGLYCEROLS

During fasting, the decrease of insulin and the increase of glucagon cause cyclic adenosine monophosphate (cAMP) levels to rise in adipose cells, stimulating lipolysis (Fig. 28.17). Protein kinase A phosphorylates hormone-sensitive lipase to produce a more active form of the enzyme. Hormone-sensitive lipase, also known as adipose triacylglycerol lipase, cleaves a fatty acid from a triacylglycerol. Subsequently, other lipases complete the process of lipolysis, and fatty acids and glycerol are released into the blood. Simultaneously, to regulate the amount of fatty acids released into circulation, triglyceride synthesis occurs along with the synthesis of glycerol 3-phosphate.

The fatty acids, which travel in the blood complexed with albumin, enter cells of muscle and other tissues, where they are oxidized to $CO_2$ and water to produce energy. During prolonged fasting, acetyl CoA produced by β-oxidation of fatty acids in the liver is converted to ketone bodies, which are released into the blood. The glycerol derived from lipolysis in adipose cells is used by the liver during fasting as a source of carbon for gluconeogenesis.

## VII. METABOLISM OF GLYCEROPHOSPHOLIPIDS AND SPHINGOLIPIDS

Fatty acids, obtained from the diet or synthesized from glucose, are the precursors of **glycerophospholipids** and **sphingolipids** (Fig. 28.18). These lipids are major components of cellular membranes. Glycerophospholipids are also components of blood lipoproteins, bile, and lung surfactant. They are the source of the polyunsaturated fatty acids, particularly arachidonic acid, that serve as precursors of the eicosanoids. **Ether glycerophospholipids** differ from other glycerophospholipids in that the alkyl or alkenyl chain (an alkyl chain with a double bond) is joined to carbon 1 of the glycerol moiety by an ether rather than an ester bond. Examples of ether lipids are the plasmalogens and platelet-activating factor (PAF). Sphingolipids are particularly important in signal transduction and in forming the myelin sheath surrounding nerves in the central nervous system.

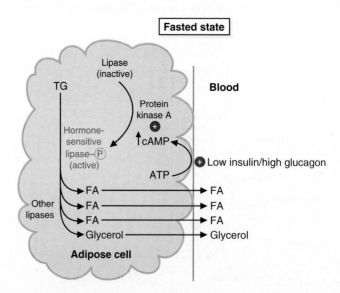

**FIG. 28.17.** Mobilization of adipose triacylglycerol *(TG)*. In the fasted state, when insulin levels are low and glucagon is elevated, intracellular cAMP increases and activates protein kinase A, which phosphorylates hormone-sensitive lipase (HSL). Phosphorylated HSL is active and initiates the breakdown of adipose *TG*. Re-esterification of fatty acids *(FA)* does occur, along with the synthesis of glycerol 3-phosphate, in the fasted state, to regulate the release of fatty acids from the adipocyte. HSL is also called triacylglycerol lipase.

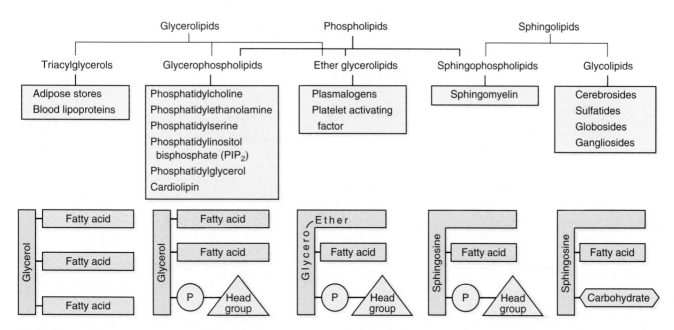

**FIG. 28.18.** Types of glycerolipids and sphingolipids. Glycerolipids contain glycerol and sphingolipids contain sphingosine. The category of phospholipids overlaps both glycerolipids and sphingolipids. The head groups include choline, ethanolamine, serine, inositol, glycerol, and phosphatidylglycerol. The carbohydrates are monosaccharides (which may be sulfated), oligosaccharides, and oligosaccharides with branches of NANA. *P*, phosphate.

In glycerolipids and ether glycerolipids, glycerol serves as the backbone to which fatty acids and other substituents are attached. Sphingosine, derived from serine, provides the backbone for sphingolipids.

## A.  Synthesis of Phospholipids Containing Glycerol

### 1.  GLYCEROPHOSPHOLIPIDS

The initial steps in the synthesis of glycerophospholipids are similar to those of triacylglycerol synthesis. Glycerol 3-phosphate reacts with two activated fatty acids to form phosphatidic acid. Two different mechanisms are then used to add a head group to the molecule. A head group is a chemical group, such as choline or serine, attached to the phosphate on carbon 3 of a glycerol moiety that contains hydrophobic groups, usually fatty acids, at positions 1 and 2. Head groups are hydrophilic, either charged or polar. The head groups all contain a free hydroxyl group, which is used to link to the phosphate on carbon 3 of the glycerol backbone.

In the first mechanism, phosphatidic acid is cleaved by a phosphatase to form DAG. DAG then reacts with an activated head group. In the synthesis of phosphatidylcholine, the head group choline is activated by combining with cytidine triphosphate (CTP) to form cytidine diphosphate (CDP)-choline (Fig. 28.19). Phosphocholine is then transferred to carbon 3 of DAG, and cytidine monophosphate (CMP) is released. Phosphatidylethanolamine is produced by a similar reaction involving CDP-ethanolamine.

Various types of interconversions occur among these phospholipids (see Fig. 28.19). Phosphatidylserine is produced by a reaction in which the ethanolamine moiety of phosphatidylethanolamine is exchanged for serine. Phosphatidylserine can be converted back to phosphatidylethanolamine by a decarboxylation reaction. Phosphatidylethanolamine can be methylated to form phosphatidylcholine (see Chapter 34).

In the second mechanism for the synthesis of glycerolipids, phosphatidic acid reacts with CTP to form CDP-DAG (Fig. 28.20). This compound can react with phosphatidylglycerol (which itself is formed from the condensation of CDP-DAG

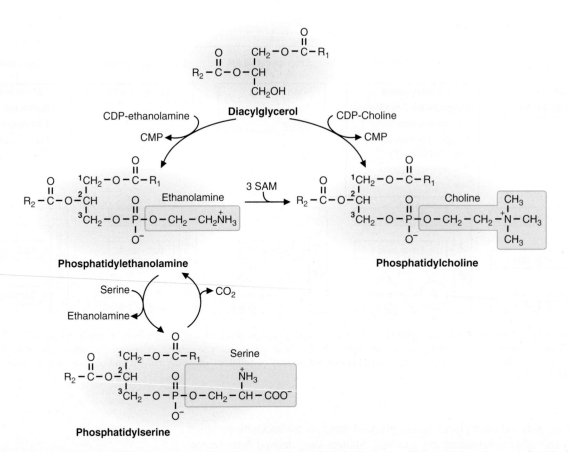

**FIG. 28.19.** Synthesis of phosphatidylcholine, phosphatidylethanolamine, and phosphatidylserine. The multiple pathways reflect the importance of phospholipids in membrane structure. For example, phosphatidylcholine (PC) can be synthesized from dietary choline when it is available. If choline is not available, PC can be made from dietary carbohydrate, although the amount synthesized is inadequate to prevent choline deficiency. *SAM*, is S-adenosylmethionine, a methyl group donor for many biochemical reactions (see Chapter 34).

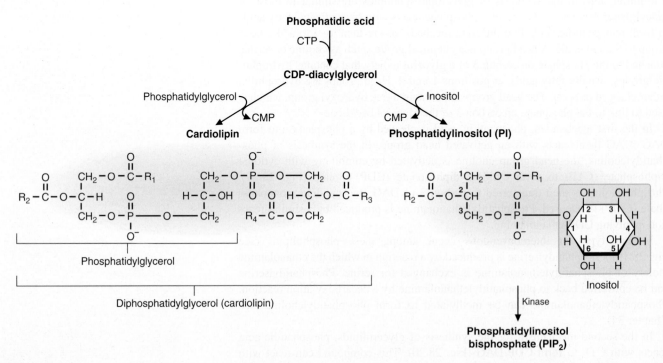

**FIG. 28.20.** Synthesis of cardiolipin and phosphatidylinositol.

and glycerol 3-phosphate) to produce cardiolipin or with inositol to produce phosphatidylinositol. Cardiolipin is a component of the inner mitochondrial membrane. Phosphatidylinositol can be phosphorylated to form phosphatidylinositol 4,5-bisphosphate ($PIP_2$), which is a component of cell membranes. In response to signals such as the binding of hormones to membrane receptors, $PIP_2$ can be cleaved to form the second messengers, DAG and inositol triphosphate ($IP_3$) (see Chapter 8).

### 2.  ETHER GLYCEROLIPIDS

The ether glycerolipids are synthesized from the glycolytic intermediate DHAP. A fatty acyl CoA reacts with carbon 1 of DHAP, forming an ester. This fatty acyl group is exchanged for a fatty alcohol, produced by reduction of a fatty acid. Thus, the ether linkage is formed. Then, the keto group on carbon 2 of the DHAP moiety is reduced and esterified to a fatty acid. Addition of the head group proceeds by a series of reactions analogous to those for synthesis of phosphatidylcholine. Formation of a double bond between carbons 1 and 2 of the alkyl group produces a plasmalogen. Ethanolamine plasmalogen is found in myelin and choline plasmalogen in heart muscle. PAF is similar to choline plasmalogen except that an acetyl group replaces the fatty acyl group at carbon 2 of the glycerol moiety, and the alkyl group on carbon 1 is saturated. PAF is released from phagocytic blood cells in response to various stimuli. It causes platelet aggregation, edema, and hypotension, and it is involved in the allergic response. Plasmalogen synthesis occurs within peroxisomes and, in individuals with Zellweger syndrome (a defect in peroxisome biogenesis), plasmalogen synthesis is compromised. If it is severe enough, this syndrome leads to death at a very early age.

### B.  Degradation of Glycerophospholipids

Phospholipases located in cell membranes or in lysosomes degrade glycerophospholipids. Phospholipase $A_1$ removes the fatty acyl group on carbon 1 of the glycerol moiety, and phospholipase $A_2$ removes the fatty acid on carbon 2 (Fig. 28.21). The C2 fatty acid in cell membrane phospholipids is usually an unsaturated fatty acid, which is frequently arachidonic acid. It is removed in response to signals for the synthesis of eicosanoids. The bond joining carbon 3 of the glycerol moiety to phosphate is cleaved by phospholipase C. Hormonal stimuli activate phospholipase C, which hydrolyzes $PIP_2$ to produce the second messengers, DAG and $IP_3$. The bond between the phosphate and the head group is cleaved by phospholipase D, producing phosphatidic acid and the free alcohol of the head group.

### C.  Sphingolipids

Sphingolipids serve in intercellular communication and as the antigenic determinants of the ABO blood groups. Some are used as receptors by viruses and bacterial toxins, although it is unlikely that this was the purpose for which they originally evolved.

 RDS of a premature infant such as **Christy L.** is, in part, related to a deficiency in the synthesis of a substance known as lung surfactant. The major constituents of surfactant are dipalmitoylphosphatidylcholine, phosphatidylglycerol, apolipoproteins (surfactant proteins: Sp-A,B,C), and cholesterol. These components of lung surfactant normally contribute to a reduction in the surface tension within the air spaces (alveoli) of the lung, preventing their collapse. The premature infant has not yet begun to produce adequate amounts of lung surfactant.

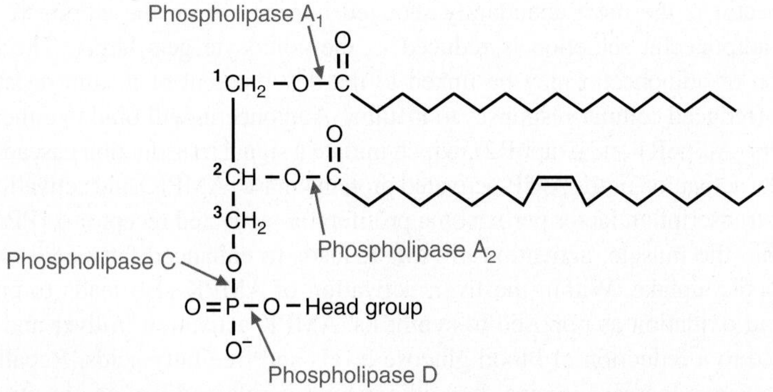

*FIG. 28.21.* Bonds cleaved by phospholipases.

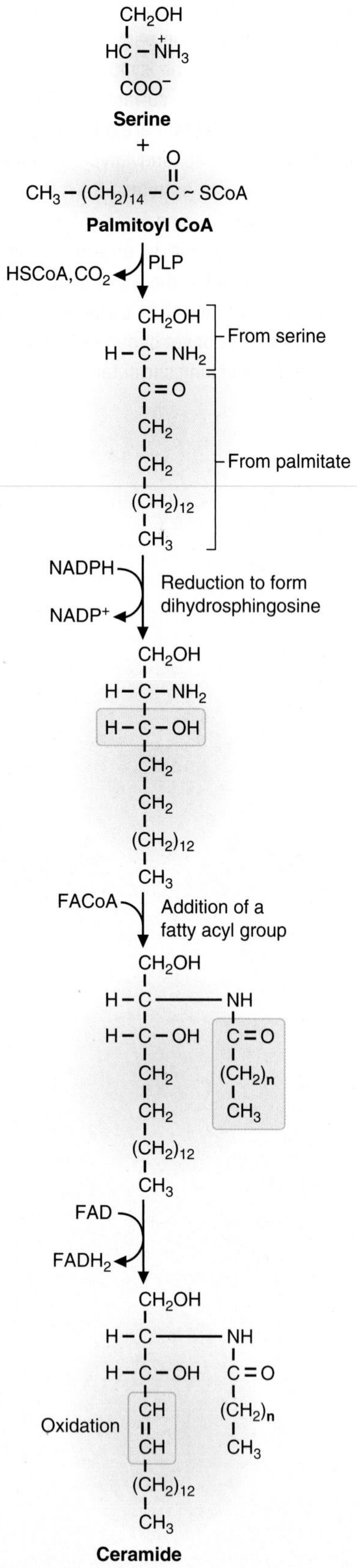

**FIG. 28.22.** Synthesis of ceramide. The changes that occur in each reaction are highlighted. *PLP*, pyridoxal phosphate.

The synthesis of sphingolipids begins with the formation of ceramide (Fig. 28.22). Serine and palmityl CoA condense to form a product that is reduced. A very long chain fatty acid (usually containing 22 carbons) forms an amide with the amino group, a double bond is generated, and ceramide is formed.

Ceramide reacts with phosphatidylcholine to form sphingomyelin, a component of the myelin sheath (Fig. 28.23), and the only sphingosine-based phospholipid. Ceramide also reacts with uridine diphosphate (UDP) sugars to form cerebrosides (which contain a single monosaccharide, usually galactose or glucose). Galactocerebroside may react with 3'-phosphoadenosine 5'-phosphosulfate (PAPS, an active sulfur donor) to form sulfatides, the major sulfolipids of the brain.

Additional sugars may be added to ceramide to form globosides, and gangliosides are produced by the addition of *N*-acetylneuraminic acid (NANA) as branches from the oligosaccharide chains (see Fig. 28.23).

Sphingolipids are degraded by lysosomal enzymes (see Table 25.1). Deficiencies of these enzymes result in a group of lysosomal storage diseases known as the sphingolipidoses.

## VIII. THE ADIPOCYTE AS AN ENDOCRINE ORGAN

It has become increasingly apparent in recent years that adipose tissue does more than just store triglyceride; it is also an active endocrine organ that secretes a variety of factors to regulate both glucose and fat metabolism. Two of the best characterized factors are leptin and adiponectin.

### A. Leptin

Leptin was initially discovered in an obese mouse model as a circulating factor that, when added to a genetically obese mouse (ob/ob), resulted in a loss of weight. Leptin binds to a receptor that is linked to janus kinase (JAK) (see Chapter 11), so leptin's signal is transmitted by variations in the activity of the signal transducer and activator of transcription (STAT) factors. Leptin is released from adipocytes as their triglyceride levels increase and binds to receptors in the hypothalamus, which leads to the release of neuropeptides that signal a cessation of eating (anorexigenic factors). Giving leptin to leptin-deficient patients will result in a weight loss, but administering leptin to obese patients does not have the same effect. It is believed that the lack of a leptin effect is due to the development of leptin resistance in many obese patients. Leptin resistance could result from the constant stimulation of the leptin receptors in obese individuals, leading to receptor desensitization. Another possibility is leptin-induced synthesis of factors that block leptin-induced signal transduction. As an example, leptin induces the synthesis of suppressor of cytokine signaling-3 (SOCS-3), a factor that antagonizes STAT activation. Long-term leptin stimulation may lead to constant expression of SOCS-3, which would result in a diminished cellular response to leptin.

### B. Adiponectin

Adiponectin is the most abundantly secreted hormone from the adipocyte. Unlike leptin, adiponectin secretion is reduced as the adipocyte gets larger. The reduced secretion of adiponectin may be linked to the development of insulin resistance in obesity (reduced cellular responses to insulin). Adiponectin will bind to either of two receptors (AdipoR1 and AdipoR2), which initiate a signal transduction cascade resulting in the activation of the AMP-activated protein kinase (AMPK) and activation of the nuclear transcription factor peroxisome proliferator–activated receptor α (PPARα).

Within the muscle, activation of AMPK leads to enhanced fatty acid oxidation and glucose uptake. Within the liver, activation of AMPK also leads to enhanced fatty acid oxidation as opposed to synthesis. AMPK activation in liver and muscle then lead to a reduction of blood glucose levels and free fatty acids. Recall that as the adipocytes increase in size, less adiponectin is released; so, as obesity occurs, it is more difficult for circulating fatty acids and glucose to be used by the tissues.

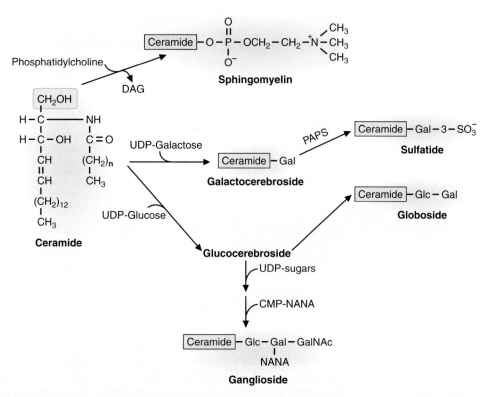

*FIG. 28.23.* Synthesis of sphingolipids from ceramide. Phosphocholine or sugars add to the hydroxymethyl group of ceramide (in *yellow box*) to form sphingomyelins, cerebrosides, sulfatides, globosides, and gangliosides. *Gal*, galactose; *Glc*, glucose; *GalNAc*, N-acetylgalactosamine; *NANA*, N-acetylneuraminic acid.

This contributes, in part, to the elevated glucose and fat levels seen in the circulation of obese patients (the insulin-resistance syndrome).

Activation of PPARα leads to enhanced fatty acid oxidation by the liver and muscle. PPARα is the target of the fibrate group of lipid-lowering drugs. PPARα activation leads to increased transcription of genes involved in fatty acid transport, energy uncoupling, and fatty acid oxidation.

The thiazolidinedione group of antidiabetic drugs (pioglitazone) can be used to control type 2 diabetes. These drugs bind to and activate PPARγ in adipose tissues, and lead, in part, to increased adiponectin synthesis and release, which aids in reducing circulating fat and glucose levels.

## CLINICAL COMMENTS

Diseases discussed in this chapter are summarized in Table 28.4.

**Cora N.** Because **Cora N.'s** lipid profile indicated an elevation in both serum triacylglycerols and LDL cholesterol, she was classified as having a combined hyperlipidemia. The dissimilarities in the lipid profiles of Cora and her two siblings, both of whom were experiencing anginal chest pain, are characteristic of the multigenic syndrome referred to as familial combined hyperlipidemia (FCH).

Approximately 1% of the North American population has FCH. It is the most common cause of coronary artery disease in the United States. In contrast to patients with familial hypercholesterolemia (FH), patients with FCH do not have fatty deposits within the skin or tendons (xanthomas) (see Chapter 29). In FCH, coronary artery disease usually appears by the fifth decade of life.

**Table 28.4    Diseases Discussed in Chapter 28**

| Disease or Disorder | Environmental or Genetic | Comments |
| --- | --- | --- |
| Obesity | Both | Weight gain will occur because of excessive calorie consumption; fat can be derived from carbohydrates, protein, and triglyceride in the diet. |
| Heart disease, familial combined hyperlipidemia (FCH) | Both | FCH, leading to elevated cholesterol and triglyceride levels in the serum. Levels of lipid in the blood, and symptoms displayed by patients, will vary from patient to patient. |
| Respiratory distress syndrome | Both | Inability of lungs to properly expand and contract due to lack of surfactant, a complex mixture of lipids and apolipoproteins. |
| Abetalipoproteinemia | Genetic | Lack of microsomal triglyceride transport protein, leading to reduced production of VLDL and chylomicrons within the liver and intestine, respectively. |
| Cardiac (protection against future myocardial infarctions) | Environmental | NSAIDs, such as aspirin, are used to block prostaglandin production via inhibition of cyclooxygenase. Low-dose aspirin provides potential protective effects for those with cardiovascular disease. |

VLDL, very low density lipoprotein; NSAIDS, nonsteroidal anti-inflammatory drugs.

Treatment of FCH includes restriction of dietary fat. Patients who do not respond adequately to dietary therapy are treated with antilipidemic drugs. Selection of the appropriate antilipidemic drugs depends on the specific phenotypic expression of the patient's multigenic disease as manifested by their particular serum lipid profile. In Cora's case, a decrease in both serum triacylglycerols and LDL cholesterol must be achieved. If possible, her serum HDL cholesterol level should also be raised to a level above 50 mg/dL.

To accomplish these therapeutic goals, her physician initially prescribed a statin (atorvastatin) and fast-release nicotinic acid (niacin), because these agents have the potential to lower serum triacylglycerol levels and cause a reciprocal rise in serum HDL cholesterol levels, as well as lowering serum total and LDL cholesterol levels. The mechanisms suggested for niacin's triacylglycerol-lowering action include enhancement of the action of LPL, inhibition of lipolysis in adipose tissue, and a decrease in esterification of triacylglycerols in the liver. The mechanism by which niacin lowers the serum total and LDL cholesterol levels is related to the decrease in hepatic production of VLDL. When the level of VLDL in the circulation decreases, the production of its daughter particles, IDL and LDL, also decreases. Cora found niacin's side effects of flushing and itching to be intolerable, and the drug was discontinued.

Statins, such as atorvastatin, inhibit cholesterol synthesis by inhibiting hydroxymethylglutaryl CoA (HMG-CoA) reductase, the rate-limiting enzyme in the pathway (see Chapter 29). After 3 months of therapy, atorvastatin decreased Cora's LDL cholesterol from a pretreatment level of 175 to 122 mg/dL (still higher than the recommended treatment goal of 100 mg/dL or less in a patient with established coronary artery disease). Her fasting serum triacylglycerol concentration was decreased from a pretreatment level of 280 to 178 mg/dL (a treatment goal for serum triacylglycerol when the pretreatment level is less than 500 mg/dL has not been established). In patients with diabetes, the goal is to bring the triacylglycerol level to 150 mg/dL or less.

Cora was also told to take 81 mg of aspirin every day. In the presence of aspirin, cyclooxygenase is irreversibly inactivated by acetylation. New cyclooxygenase molecules are not produced in platelets because platelets have no nuclei and, therefore, cannot synthesize new mRNA. Thus, the inhibition of cyclooxygenase by aspirin persists for the lifespan of the platelet (7 to 10 days). When aspirin is taken daily at doses between 81 and 325 mg, new platelets are affected as they are generated. Higher doses do not improve efficacy but do increase side effects, such as gastrointestinal bleeding and easy bruisability.

Patients with established or suspected atherosclerotic coronary disease, such as **Ann J., Cora N.,** and **Ivan A.,** benefit from the action of low-dose aspirin (approximately 81 mg/day), which produces a mild defect in hemostasis. This action of aspirin helps to prevent thrombus formation in the area of an atherosclerotic plaque at critical sites in the vascular tree.

 **Christy L. Christy L.** suffered from RDS, which is a major cause of death in the newborn. RDS is preventable if prematurity can be avoided by appropriate management of high-risk pregnancy and labor. Before delivery, the obstetrician must attempt to predict and possibly treat pulmonary prematurity in utero. For example, estimation of fetal head circumference by ultrasonography, monitoring for fetal arterial oxygen saturation, and determination of the ratio of the concentrations of phosphatidylcholine (lecithin) and that of sphingomyelin in the amniotic fluid may help to identify premature infants who are predisposed to RDS.

The administration of synthetic corticosteroids 48 to 72 hours before delivery of a fetus of less than 33 weeks of gestation in women who have toxemia of pregnancy, diabetes mellitus, or chronic renal disease may reduce the incidence or mortality of RDS by stimulating fetal synthesis of lung surfactant.

The administration of one dose of surfactant into the trachea of the premature infant immediately after birth, for babies with very poor respiratory function, can improve morbidity and mortality. In Christy's case, intensive therapy allowed her to survive this acute respiratory complication of prematurity.

## REVIEW QUESTIONS-CHAPTER 28

1. Which one of the following is involved in the synthesis of triacylglycerols in adipose tissue?

   A. Glycerol 3-phosphate derived from blood glycerol
   B. 2-monoacylgylcerol as an obligatory intermediate
   C. Lipoprotein lipase to catalyze the formation of ester bonds
   D. Acetoacetyl CoA as an obligatory intermediate
   E. Fatty acids obtained from chylomicrons and VLDL

2. A molecule of palmitic acid, attached to carbon 1 of the glycerol moiety of a triacylglycerol, is ingested and digested. It passes into the blood, is stored in a fat cell, and ultimately, is oxidized to carbon dioxide and water in a muscle cell. Choose the molecular complex in which the palmitate residue is carried from the lumen of the gut to the surface of the gut epithelial cell.

   A. Bile salt micelle
   B. VLDL
   C. Chylomicron
   D. Fatty acid–albumin complex
   E. LDL

3. A patient with hyperlipoproteinemia would be most likely to benefit from a low-carbohydrate diet if the lipoproteins that are elevated in blood are which one of the following?

   A. Chylomicrons
   B. VLDL
   C. LDL
   D. HDL
   E. IDL

4. Which one of the following drugs leads to the covalent modification, and inactivation, of both the COX-1 and COX-2 enzymes?

   A. Celebrex
   B. Tylenol
   C. Vioxx
   D. Aspirin
   E. Advil

5. Newly synthesized fatty acids are not immediately degraded due to which one of the following?

   A. Tissues that synthesize fatty acids do not contain the enzymes that degrade fatty acids.
   B. High NADPH levels inhibit β-oxidation.
   C. Transport of fatty acids into mitochondria is inhibited under conditions in which fatty acids are being synthesized.
   D. In the presence of insulin, the key fatty acid degrading enzyme is not induced.
   E. Newly synthesized fatty acids cannot be converted to their CoA derivatives.

# 29 Cholesterol Absorption, Synthesis, Metabolism, and Fate

## CHAPTER OUTLINE

## KEY POINTS

- Cholesterol regulates membrane fluidity and is a precursor of bile salts, steroid hormones (such as estrogen and testosterone), and vitamin D.
- Cholesterol, because of its hydrophobic nature, is transported in the blood as a component of lipoproteins.
- Within the lipoproteins, cholesterol can appear in its unesterified form in the outer shell of the particle or as cholesterol esters in the core of the particle.

continued

■ De novo cholesterol synthesis requires acetyl coenzyme A as a precursor, which is initially converted to hydroxymethylglutaryl coenzyme A (HMG-CoA). The cholesterol synthesized in this way is packaged, along with triglyceride, into very low density lipoprotein (VLDL) in the liver and then released into circulation.

  ■ The conversion of HMG-CoA to mevalonic acid, catalyzed by HMG-CoA reductase, is the regulated and rate-limiting step of cholesterol biosynthesis.

  ■ In the circulation, the triglycerides in VLDL are digested by lipoprotein lipase, which converts the particle to intermediate-density lipoprotein (IDL) and then to low-density lipoprotein (LDL).

  ■ IDL and LDL bind specifically to receptors on the liver cell, are internalized, and the particle components are recycled. LDL also binds to LDL receptors on peripheral tissue cells, delivering cholesterol to those cells.

  ■ A third lipoprotein particle, high-density lipoprotein (HDL), functions to transfer apolipoprotein E and apolipoprotein C-II to nascent chylomicrons and nascent VLDL.

  ■ HDL also participates in reverse cholesterol transport, the movement of cholesterol from cell membranes to the HDL particle, which returns the cholesterol to the liver.

  ■ Atherosclerotic plaques are associated with elevated levels of blood cholesterol levels. High levels of LDL are more strongly associated with the generation of atherosclerotic plaques, whereas high levels of HDL are protective because of their participation in reverse cholesterol transport.

  ■ Bile salts are recycled by the enterohepatic circulation, forming the secondary bile acids in the process.

  ■ The steroid hormones are derived from cholesterol, which is converted to pregnenolone, which is the precursor for the mineralocorticoids (such as aldosterone), the glucocorticoids (such as cortisol), and the sex steroids (such as testosterone and estrogen).

  ■ Lipid-lowering drugs act on a variety of targets within liver, intestine, and adipocytes.

## THE WAITING ROOM

At his next office visit, **Ivan A.'s** case was reviewed by his physician. Mr. A. has several of the major risk factors for coronary heart disease (CHD). These include a sedentary lifestyle, marked obesity, hypertension, hyperlipidemia, and early type 2 diabetes. Unfortunately, he has not followed his doctor's advice with regard to a diabetic diet designed to affect a significant loss of weight nor has he followed an aerobic exercise program. As a result, his weight has gone from 270 to 291 lb. After a 14-hour fast, his serum glucose is now 214 mg/dL (normal, <100 mg/dL), and his serum total cholesterol level is 314 mg/dL (desired level is 200 mg/dL or less). His serum triacylglycerol level is 295 mg/dL (desired level is 150 mg/dL or less), and his serum high-density lipoprotein (HDL) cholesterol is 24 mg/dL (desired level is ≥40 mg/dL for a man). His calculated serum low-density lipoprotein (LDL) cholesterol level is 231 mg/dL. According to recent guidelines, an LDL value of greater than 190 mg/dL merits starting medication to decrease risk for cardiovascular disease. Mr. A. exhibits sufficient criteria to be classified as having metabolic syndrome.

**Anne J.** was carefully followed by her physician after she survived her heart attack. Before she was discharged from the hospital, after a 14-hour fast, her serum triacylglycerol level was 158 mg/dL (slightly above the upper range of normal), and her HDL cholesterol level was low at 32 mg/dL (normal for women is ≥50 mg/dL). Her serum total cholesterol level was elevated at 420 mg/dL (reference range, ≤200 mg/dL for a female with known CHD). From these values, her LDL cholesterol level was calculated to be 356 mg/dL. Current guidelines recommend starting medications in her treatment because of her known cardiovascular disease.

Until recently, the concentration of LDL cholesterol could only be directly determined by sophisticated laboratory techniques not available for routine clinical use. As a consequence, the LDL cholesterol concentration in the blood was derived indirectly by using the Friedewald formula: the sum of the HDL cholesterol level and the triacylglycerol (TG) level divided by 5 (which gives an estimate of the VLDL cholesterol level) subtracted from the total cholesterol level.

LDL cholesterol = total cholesterol −
[HDL cholesterol + (TG/5)]

This equation yields inaccurate LDL cholesterol levels 15% to 20% of the time and fails completely when serum triacylglycerol levels exceed 400 mg/dL.

A recently developed test called LDL direct isolates LDL cholesterol by using a special immunoseparation reagent. Not only is this direct assay for LDL cholesterol more accurate than the indirect Friedewald calculation, it also is not affected by mildly to moderately elevated serum TG levels and can be used for a patient who has not fasted. It does not require the expense of determining serum total cholesterol, HDL cholesterol, and TG levels.

**Table 29.1   The Four Major Statin Benefit Groups**

| Patient Status | Statin Treatment |
|---|---|
| Patient exhibits clinical atherosclerotic cardiovascular disease (ASCVD)[a] | If age ≤75 years, a high-intensity statin[b]; if >75 years or not a candidate for a high-intensity statin, a moderate-intensity statin[c] |
| Patient with LDL cholesterol ≥190 mg/dL; no ASCVD | High-intensity statin (moderate-intensity statin if not a candidate for high-intensity statin) |
| Patients with type 1 or 2 diabetes aged 40–75 years old with LDL cholesterol between 70 and 189 mg/dL, without ASCVD | Moderate-intensity statin; if the calculated 10-year ASCVD risk is ≥7.5%, a high-intensity statin |
| No clinical ASCVD or diabetes with LDL cholesterol between 70 and 189 mg/dL and an estimated 10-year ASCVD risk of ≥7.5% | Moderate- to high-intensity statin |

[a]Clinical disease refers to acute coronary syndrome or a history of heart attacks, stable or unstable angina, coronary or other arterial revascularization, stroke, transient ischemic attacks (TIA), or peripheral arterial disease.
[b]A high-intensity statin is a daily dose of statin that lowers LDL cholesterol by approximately ≥50%.
[c]A moderate-intensity statin is a daily dose of statin that lowers LDL cholesterol by approximately 30% to 50%.
This table is derived from Stone NJ, Robinson J, Lichtenstein AH, et al. 2013 ACC/AHA guideline on the treatment of blood cholesterol to reduce atherosclerotic cardiovascular risk in adults: a report of the American College of Cardiology/American Heart Association task force on practice guidelines [published online ahead of print November 12, 2013]. *Circulation.* http://circ.ahajournals.org/content/early/2013/11/01/cir.0000437738.63853.7a.

Both of Ms. J.'s younger brothers had "very high" serum cholesterol levels and both had suffered heart attacks in their mid-40s. With this information, a tentative diagnosis of familial hypercholesterolemia type IIA was made, and the patient was started on a diet and medication as recommended by the American College of Cardiology and the American Heart Association Task Force. This panel recommends that decisions with regard to when dietary and drug therapy should be initiated are based on the serum LDL cholesterol level and cardiovascular risk, as detailed in Table 29.1.

Because a step I diet (Table 29.2) usually lowers serum total and LDL cholesterol levels by no more than 15%, Ms. J. was also started on a potent statin, atorvastatin, as she had already experienced a myocardial infarction.

Ezetimibe is a compound that, although structurally distinct from the sterols, lowers serum cholesterol levels by blocking cholesterol absorption by the enterocyte. The reduction of cholesterol absorption from the intestinal lumen has been shown to reduce blood levels of LDL cholesterol, particularly when used with a drug that also blocks endogenous cholesterol synthesis.

## I.   INTESTINAL ABSORPTION OF CHOLESTEROL

Cholesterol absorption by intestinal cells is a key regulatory point in human sterol metabolism because it ultimately determines what percentage of the 1,000 mg of biliary cholesterol produced by the liver each day and what percentage of the 300 mg of dietary cholesterol entering the gut per day is eventually absorbed into the blood. In normal subjects, approximately 55% of this intestinal pool enters the blood through the enterocyte each day. The details of diffusion-mediated cholesterol absorption from dietary sources was outlined in Chapter 27.

**Table 29.2   Dietary Therapy for Elevated Blood Cholesterol**

| Nutrient | Step I Diet | Step II Diet[a] |
|---|---|---|
| Cholesterol[b] | <300 mg/d | <200 mg/d |
| Total fat | ≤30%[b] | 30% |
| Saturated fat | 8%–10% | <7% |
| Polyunsaturated fat | ≤10% | ≤10% |
| Monounsaturated fat | ≤15% | ≤15% |
| Carbohydrates | ≥55% | ≥55% |
| Protein | ~15% | ~15% |
| Calories | To achieve and maintain desirable body weight | |

[a]The step II diet is applied if 3 months on the step I diet has failed to reduce blood cholesterol to the desired level (see Table 34.1).
[b]Except for the values given in milligrams per day, all values are percentage of total calories eaten daily.
Based on Summary of the second report of the National Cholesterol Education Program (NCEP) Expert Panel on Detection, Evaluation, and Treatment of High Blood Cholesterol in Adults (Adults Treatment Panel III). *JAMA.* 1993;269(23):3015–3023.

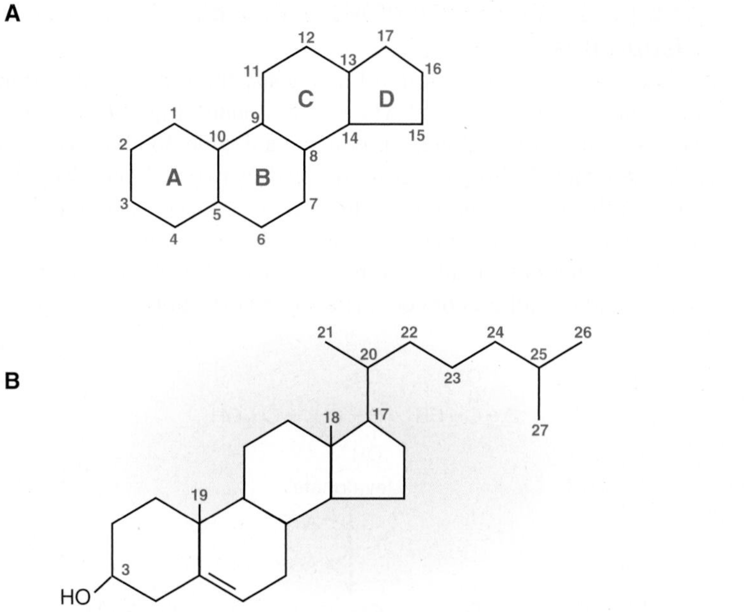

**A**

**B**

**FIG. 29.1.** The steroid ring nucleus and cholesterol. **A.** The basic ring structure of sterols; the perhydrocyclopentanophenanthrene nucleus. Each ring is labeled either *A*, *B*, *C*, or *D*. **B.** The structure of cholesterol.

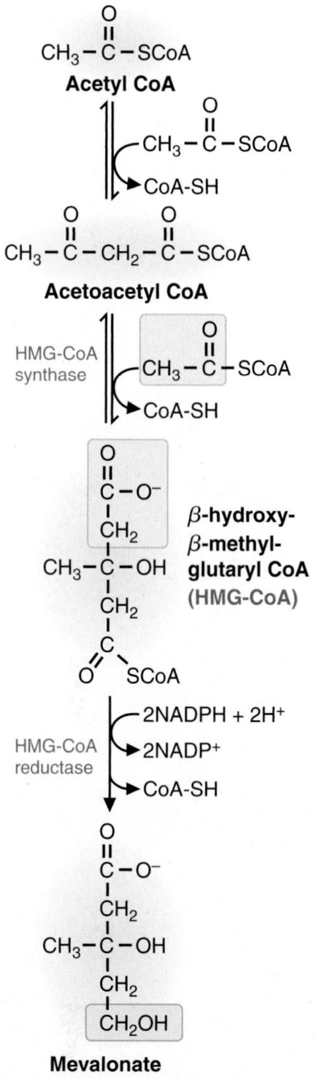

## II.  CHOLESTEROL SYNTHESIS

**Cholesterol** is an alicyclic compound whose basic structure contains four fused rings (Fig. 29.1A). In its free form, the cholesterol molecule contains a number of modifications to the basic ring structure (Fig. 29.1B). Of note is the hydroxyl group at C3. Approximately one-third of plasma cholesterol exists in the free (or unesterified) form. The remaining two-thirds exist as **cholesterol esters** in which a long-chain fatty acid (usually **linoleic acid**) is attached by ester linkage to this hydroxyl group. Esterified cholesterol is more hydrophobic than free cholesterol due to this modification.

All of the carbons of cholesterol are derived from one precursor, acetyl coenzyme A (CoA), which can be obtained from several sources, including the β-oxidation of fatty acids, the oxidation of ketogenic amino acids such as leucine and lysine (see Chapter 32), and the pyruvate dehydrogenase reaction.

The synthesis of cholesterol, like that of fatty acids, occurs in the cytoplasm and requires significant reducing power, which is supplied in the form of NADPH. Energy is also required, which is provided by the hydrolysis of high-energy thioester bonds of acetyl CoA and phosphoanhydride bonds of adenosine triphosphate (ATP). Cholesterol synthesis occurs in four stages.

## A.  Stage 1: Synthesis of Mevalonate from Acetyl CoA

The first stage of cholesterol synthesis leads to the production of the intermediate mevalonate (Fig. 29.2). The synthesis of mevalonate is the committed, rate-limiting step in cholesterol formation. In this cytoplasmic pathway, two molecules of acetyl CoA condense, forming acetoacetyl CoA, which then condenses with a third molecule of acetyl CoA to yield the six-carbon compound **3-hydroxy-3-methylglutaryl-CoA (HMG-CoA)**. *The committed step and major point of regulation of cholesterol synthesis in stage 1 involves reduction of HMG-CoA to mevalonate, a reaction catalyzed by* **HMG-CoA reductase**, *an enzyme embedded in the membrane of the endoplasmic reticulum.* The reducing equivalents for this reaction are donated by two molecules of NADPH. The regulation of the activity of HMG-CoA reductase is controlled in multiple ways and is discussed in Section II.E.

**FIG. 29.2.** The conversion of three molecules of acetyl CoA to mevalonic acid.

HMG-CoA is also an intermediate in ketone body synthesis (see Chapter 20); however, ketone body synthesis occurs in the mitochondria, whereas cholesterol synthesis occurs in the cytoplasm. Thus, there are different isozymes involved in synthesizing HMG-CoA (HMG-CoA synthase), depending on the cellular compartment.

### B. Stage 2: Conversion of Mevalonate to Two Activated Isoprenes

In the second stage of cholesterol synthesis, three phosphate groups are transferred from three molecules of ATP to mevalonate (Fig. 29.3). This allows for the decarboxylation of mevalonate, producing a double bond in the five-carbon product, $\Delta^3$-isopentenyl pyrophosphate, the first of two activated isoprenes necessary for the synthesis of cholesterol. The second activated isoprene is formed when $\Delta^3$-isopentenyl pyrophosphate is isomerized to dimethylallyl pyrophosphate (see Fig. 29.3). Isoprenes, in addition to being used for cholesterol biosynthesis, are also used in the synthesis of coenzyme Q and dolichol.

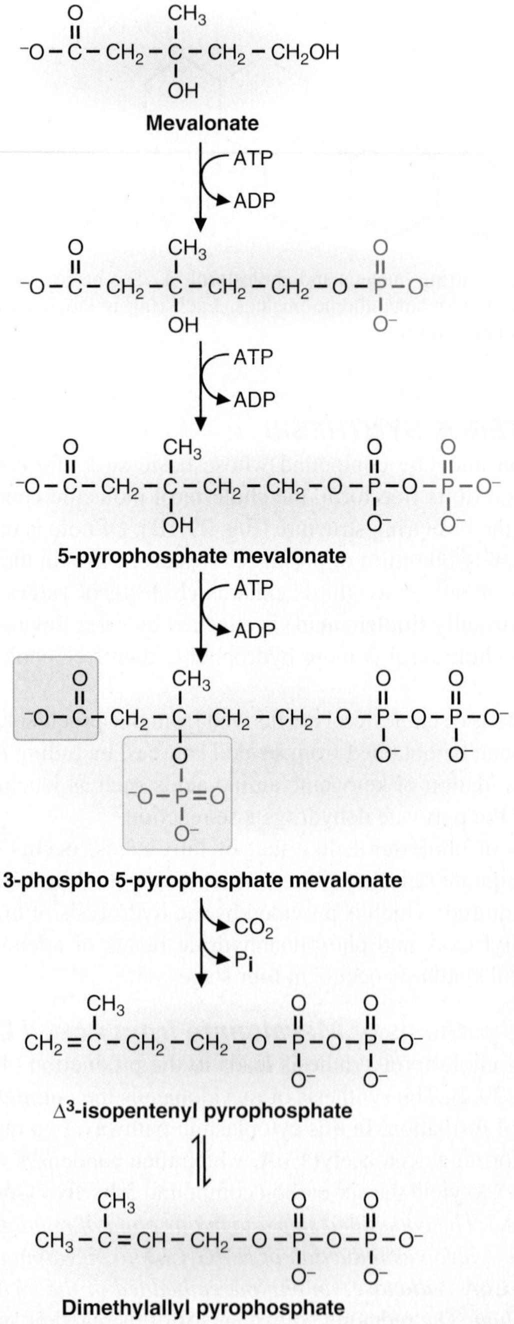

**FIG. 29.3.** The formation of activated isoprene units ($\Delta^3$-isopentenyl pyrophosphate and dimethylallyl pyrophosphate) from mevalonic acid. Note the large ATP requirement for these steps.

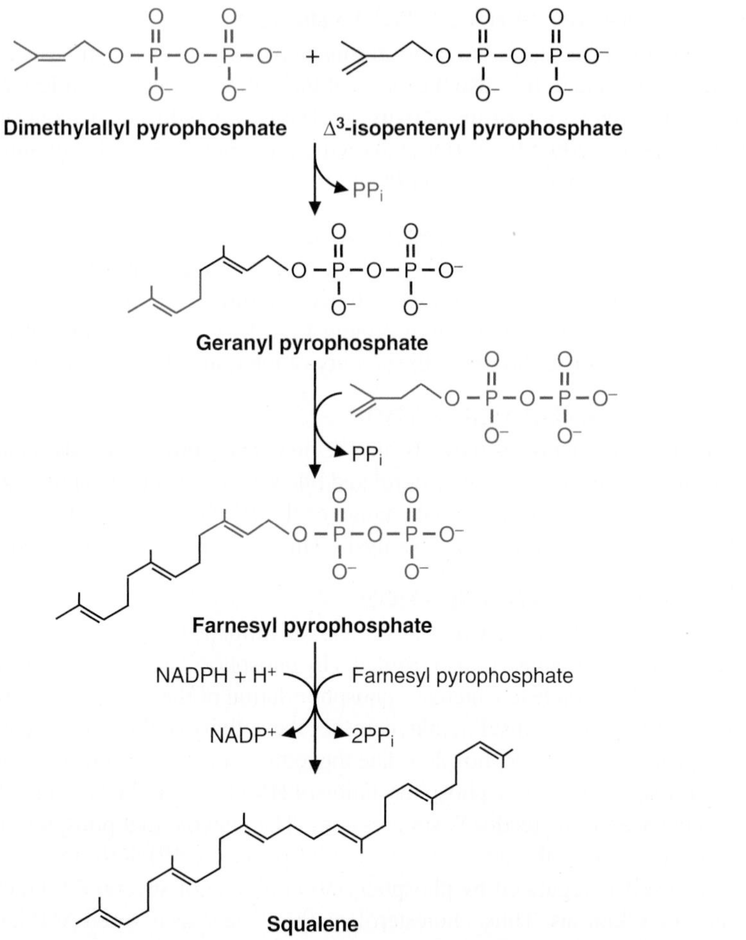

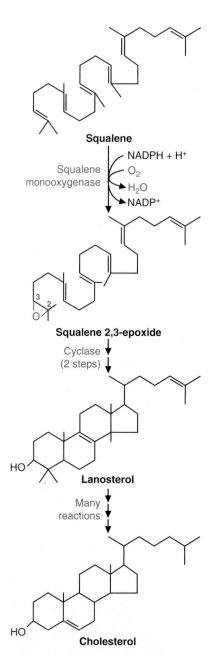

**FIG. 29.4.** The formation of squalene from six isoprene units. The activation of the isoprene units drives their condensation to form geranyl pyrophosphate, farnesyl pyrophosphate, and squalene.

## C. Stage 3: Condensation of Six Activated Five-Carbon Isoprenes to Squalene

The next stage in the biosynthesis of cholesterol involves the head-to-tail condensation of isopentenyl pyrophosphate and dimethylallyl pyrophosphate. The "head" in this case refers to the end of the molecule to which pyrophosphate is linked. In this reaction, the pyrophosphate group of dimethylallyl pyrophosphate is displaced and a 10-carbon chain, known as geranyl pyrophosphate, is generated (Fig. 29.4). Geranyl pyrophosphate then undergoes another head-to-tail condensation with isopentenyl pyrophosphate, resulting in the formation of the 15-carbon intermediate, farnesyl pyrophosphate. After this, two molecules of farnesyl pyrophosphate undergo a head-to-head fusion, and both pyrophosphate groups are removed to form squalene, a compound that was first isolated from the liver of sharks (genus *Squalus*). Squalene contains 30 carbons (24 in the main chain and 6 in the methyl group branches; see Fig. 29.4).

## D. Stage 4: Conversion of Squalene to the Steroid Nucleus

The enzyme squalene monooxygenase adds a single oxygen atom from $O_2$ to the end of the squalene molecule, forming an epoxide. NADPH then reduces the other oxygen atom of $O_2$ to $H_2O$. The unsaturated carbons of the squalene 2,3-epoxide are aligned in a way that allows conversion of the linear squalene epoxide into a cyclic structure. The cyclization leads to the formation of lanosterol, a sterol with the four-ring structure characteristic of the steroid nucleus. A series of complex reactions, containing many steps and elucidated in the late 1950s, leads to the formation of cholesterol (Fig. 29.5).

**FIG. 29.5.** The conversion of squalene to cholesterol. Squalene is shown in a different conformation than in Figure 29.4 to better indicate how the cyclization reaction occurs.

Farnesyl and geranyl groups can form covalent bonds with proteins, particularly the G proteins and certain protooncogene products involved in signal transduction. These hydrophobic groups anchor the proteins in the cell membrane.

### E.  Regulation of HMG-CoA Reductase

HMG-CoA reductase is the rate-limiting step of cholesterol synthesis and, as such, is highly regulated. It is also the target of the statins, which are cholesterol-lowering drugs. The regulation of the activity of HMG-CoA reductase is controlled in multiple ways, including transcriptional regulation, regulation of the amount of enzyme by proteolysis, and covalent modification.

#### 1.  TRANSCRIPTIONAL REGULATION

When intracellular sterol levels are low, transcription of the HMG-CoA reductase gene is enhanced due to increased activity of a transcription factor belonging to the sterol response element–binding protein (SREBP) family of transcription factors. As sterol levels rise, however, the activity of the transcription factor is reduced.

#### 2.  PROTEOLYTIC REGULATION

HMG-CoA reductase activity is also regulated by proteolytic degradation of the enzyme. Rising levels of cholesterol and bile salts in cells that synthesize these molecules lead to a conformational change of the HMG-CoA reductase, rendering the enzyme more susceptible to proteolysis. This, in turn, decreases its activity.

#### 3.  COVALENT MODIFICATION

In addition to the inductive and repressive influences previously mentioned, the activity of the reductase is also regulated by phosphorylation and dephosphorylation. Elevated glucagon levels increase phosphorylation of the enzyme, thereby inactivating it, whereas hyperinsulinemia increases the activity of the reductase by activating phosphatases, which dephosphorylate the reductase. Increased levels of intracellular sterols may also increase phosphorylation of HMG-CoA reductase, thereby reducing its activity as well (feedback suppression). The enzyme that phosphorylates HMG-CoA reductase is the adenosine monophosphate (AMP)-activated protein kinase, which itself is regulated by phosphorylation by one of several AMP-activated protein kinase kinases. Thus, cholesterol synthesis decreases when ATP levels are low and increases when ATP levels are high, similar to what occurs with fatty acid biosynthesis. As has been seen during the discussion of cholesterol biosynthesis, large amounts of ATP are required to synthesize cholesterol, so low energy levels will lead to inhibition of the pathway.

## III.  SEVERAL FATES OF CHOLESTEROL

Almost all mammalian cells are capable of producing cholesterol. Most of the biosynthesis of cholesterol, however, occurs within liver cells, although the gut, adrenal cortex, and gonads (as well as the placenta in pregnant women) also produce significant quantities of the sterol. A fraction of hepatic cholesterol is used for the synthesis of hepatic membranes, but the bulk of synthesized cholesterol is secreted from the hepatocyte as one of three moieties: cholesterol esters, biliary cholesterol (cholesterol found in the bile), or bile acids. Cholesterol ester production in the liver is catalyzed by acyl-CoA cholesterol acyltransferase (ACAT). ACAT catalyzes the transfer of a fatty acid from CoA to the hydroxyl group on carbon 3 of cholesterol (Fig. 29.6). The liver packages some of the very hydrophobic esterified cholesterol into the hollow core of lipoproteins, primarily very low density lipoprotein (VLDL). VLDL is secreted from the hepatocyte into the blood and transports the cholesterol esters (and triacylglycerols, phospholipids, apolipoproteins, etc.) to the tissues that require greater amounts of cholesterol than they can synthesize de novo. These tissues then use the cholesterol for the synthesis of membranes, for the formation of steroid hormones, and for the biosynthesis of vitamin D. The residual cholesterol esters not used in these ways are stored in the liver for later use.

The hepatic cholesterol pool also serves as a source of cholesterol for the synthesis of the relatively hydrophilic bile acids and their salts. These derivatives of cholesterol are very effective detergents because they contain both polar and nonpolar regions.

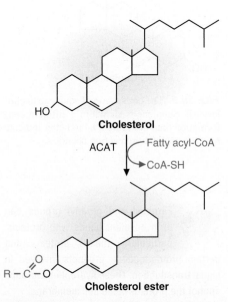

**FIG. 29.6.** The ACAT reaction, producing cholesterol esters. *ACAT*, acyl-CoA cholesterol acyltransferase.

They are introduced into the biliary ducts of the liver. They are stored and concentrated in the gallbladder and later discharged into the gut in response to the ingestion of food (see Chapter 27). They aid in the digestion of intraluminal lipids by forming micelles with them, which increases the surface area of lipids exposed to the digestive action of intraluminal lipases. On a low-cholesterol diet, the liver synthesizes approximately 800 mg of cholesterol per day to replace bile salts and cholesterol lost from the enterohepatic circulation into the feces. Conversely, a greater intake of dietary cholesterol suppresses the rate of hepatic cholesterol synthesis (feedback repression).

## IV. SYNTHESIS AND FATE OF BILE SALTS

**Bile salts** are synthesized in the liver from cholesterol by reactions that hydroxylate the steroid nucleus and cleave the side chain. In the first and rate-limiting reaction, an α-hydroxyl group is added to carbon 7 (on the α side of the B ring). The activity of the 7α-hydroxylase that catalyzes this step is decreased by an increase in bile salt concentration (Fig. 29.7). In subsequent steps, the double bond in the B ring is reduced and an additional hydroxylation may occur. Two different sets of compounds are produced. One set has α-hydroxyl groups at positions 3, 7, and 12 and produces the cholic acid series of bile salts. The other set has α-hydroxyl groups at positions 3 and 7 and produces the chenodeoxycholic acid series. Three carbons are

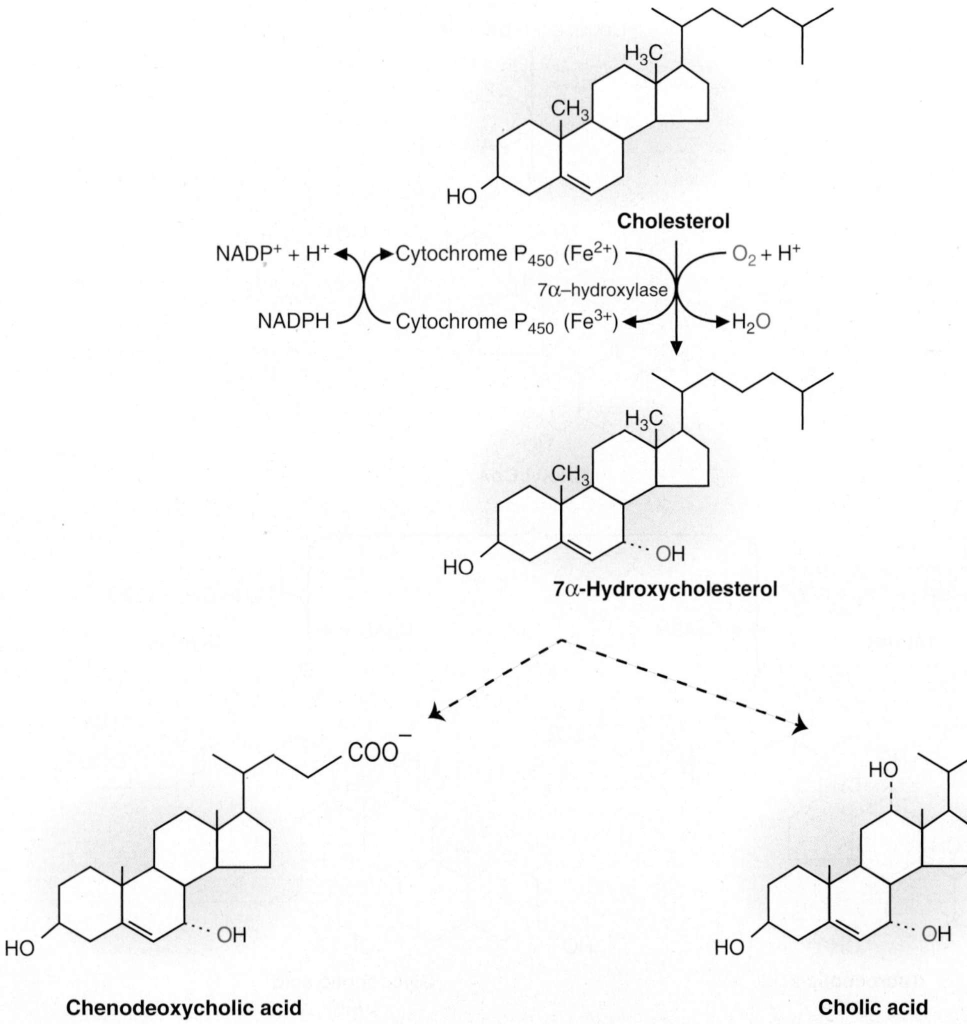

**FIG. 29.7.** Synthesis of bile salts. The rate-limiting step is the reaction catalyzed by 7α-hydroxylase. An α-hydroxyl group is formed at position 7 of cholesterol. This reaction is inhibited by bile salts. 7α-hydroxycholesterol then gives rise to cholic acid (which contains three hydroxyl groups) and chenodeoxycholic acid (which contains two hydroxyl groups).

removed from the side chain by an oxidation reaction. The remaining five-carbon fragment attached to the ring structure contains a carboxyl group.

The $pK_a$ of the bile acids is approximately 6. Therefore, in the contents of the intestinal lumen, which normally have a pH of 6, approximately 50% of the molecules are present in the protonated form, and 50% are ionized, which forms bile salts. (The terms *bile acids* and *bile salts* are often used interchangeably, but *bile salts* actually refer to the ionized form of the molecules.)

### A. Conjugation of Bile Salts

The carboxyl group at the end of the side chain of the bile salts is activated by a reaction that requires ATP and CoA. The CoA derivatives can react with either glycine or taurine (which is derived from cysteine), forming amides that are known as the conjugated bile salts. In glycocholic acid and glycochenodeoxycholic acid, the bile acids are conjugated with glycine. These compounds have a pK of approximately 4, so compared to their unconjugated forms, a higher percentage of the molecules is present in the ionized form at the pH of the intestine. The taurine conjugates, taurocholic and taurochenodeoxycholic acid, have a pK of approximately 2. Therefore, compared with the glycoconjugates, an even greater percentage of the molecules of these conjugates are ionized in the lumen of the gut (Fig. 29.8).

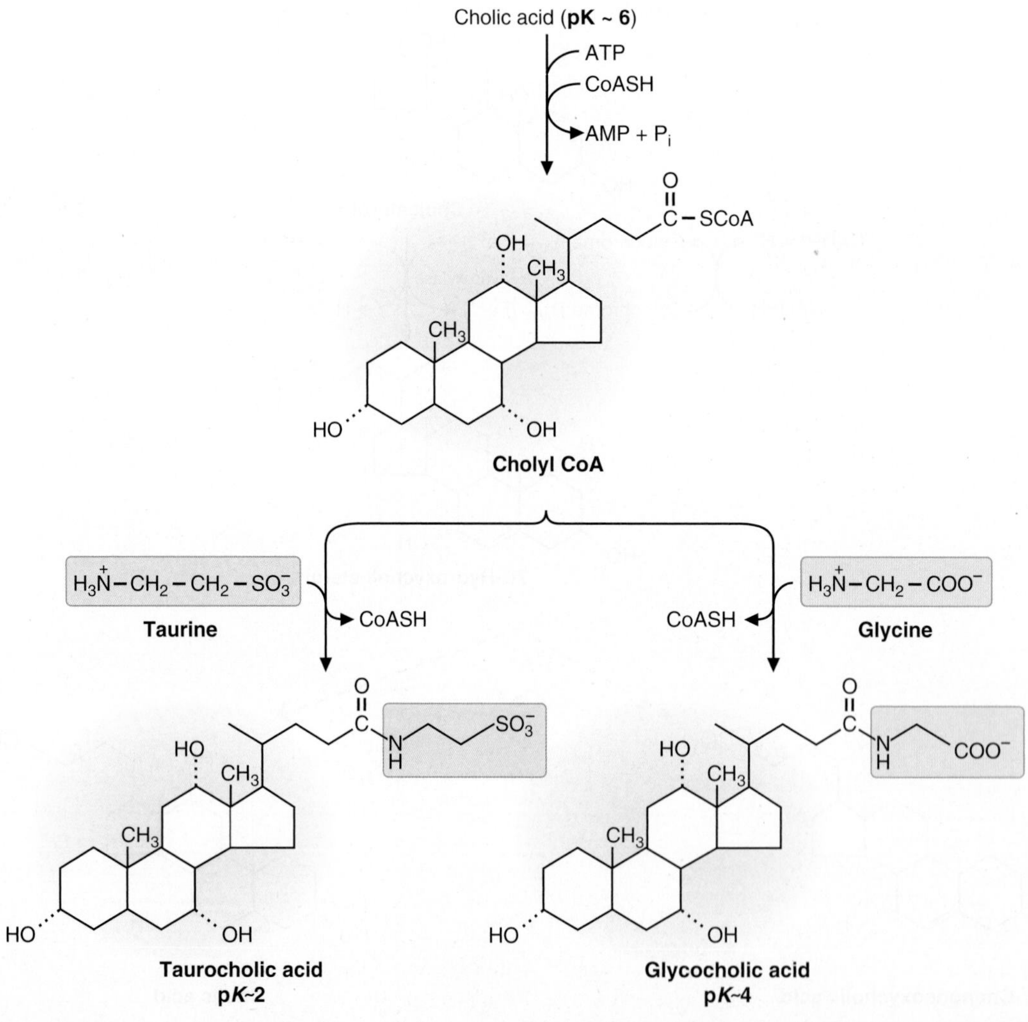

**FIG. 29.8.** Conjugation of bile salts. Conjugation lowers the pK of the bile salts, making them better detergents; that is, they are more ionized in the contents of the intestinal lumen (pH ≈ 6) than are the unconjugated bile salts (pK ≈ 6). The reactions are the same for the chenodeoxycholic acid series of bile salts.

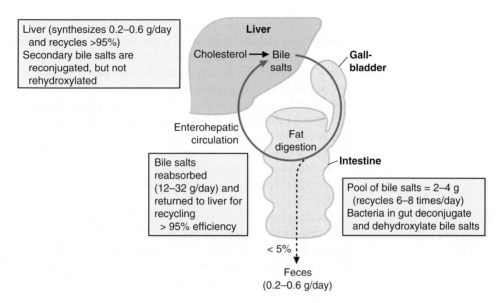

*FIG. 29.9.* Overview of bile salt metabolism.

## B. Fate of Bile Salts

Bile salts are produced in the liver and secreted into the bile (Fig. 29.9). They are stored in the gallbladder and released into the intestine during a meal, where they serve as detergents that aid in the digestion of dietary lipids (see Chapter 27).

Intestinal bacteria deconjugate and dehydroxylate the bile salts, removing the glycine and taurine residues and the hydroxyl group at position 7. The bile salts that lack a hydroxyl group at position 7 are called **secondary bile salts**. The deconjugated and dehydroxylated bile salts are less soluble and, therefore, are less readily resorbed from the intestinal lumen than the bile salts that have not been subjected to bacterial action (Fig. 29.10). Lithocholic acid, a secondary bile salt that has a hydroxyl group only at position 3, is the least soluble bile salt. Its major fate is excretion.

Greater than 95% of the bile salts are resorbed in the ileum and return to the liver via the enterohepatic circulation (via the portal vein; see Fig. 29.9). The secondary bile salts may be reconjugated in the liver, but they are not rehydroxylated. The bile salts are recycled by the liver, which secretes them into the bile. This enterohepatic recirculation of bile salts is extremely efficient. Less than 5% of the bile salts entering the gut are excreted in the feces each day. Because the steroid nucleus cannot be degraded in the body, the excretion of bile salts serves as a major route for removal of the steroid nucleus and, thus, of cholesterol from the body.

## V. TRANSPORT OF CHOLESTEROL BY THE BLOOD LIPOPROTEINS

Because they are hydrophobic and essentially insoluble in the water of the blood, cholesterol and cholesterol esters, like triacylglycerols and phospholipids, must be transported through the bloodstream packaged as **lipoproteins**. These macromolecules are water soluble. Each lipoprotein particle is composed of a core of hydrophobic lipids such as cholesterol esters and triacylglycerols surrounded by a shell of polar lipids (the phospholipids) and a variety of **apolipoproteins**, which allows a hydration shell to form around the lipoprotein (see Fig. 27.5). In addition, the shell contains a variety of apolipoproteins that also increase the water solubility of the lipoprotein. Free cholesterol molecules are dispersed throughout the lipoprotein shell to stabilize it in a way that allows it to maintain its spherical shape. The major carriers of lipids are **chylomicrons** (see Chapter 27), **VLDL**, and high-density lipoprotein (**HDL**). Metabolism of **VLDL** will lead to intermediate-density lipoprotein (**IDL**) and low-density lipoprotein (**LDL**). Metabolism of chylomicrons leads to formation of chylomicron remnants.

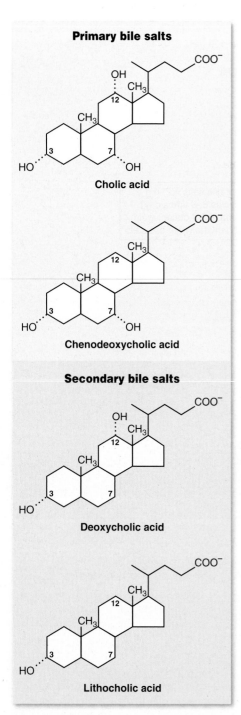

**Primary bile salts**

Cholic acid

Chenodeoxycholic acid

**Secondary bile salts**

Deoxycholic acid

Lithocholic acid

*FIG. 29.10.* Structures of the primary and secondary bile salts. Primary bile salts form conjugates with taurine or glycine in the liver. After secretion into the intestine, they may be deconjugated and dehydroxylated by the bacterial flora, forming secondary bile salts. Note that dehydroxylation occurs at position 7, forming the deoxy family of bile salts. Dehydroxylation at position 12 also leads to excretion of the bile salt.

Through this carrier mechanism, lipids leave their tissue of origin, enter the bloodstream, and are transported to the tissues, where their components are either used in synthetic or oxidative processes or stored for later use. The apolipoproteins ("apo-" describes the protein within the shell of the particle in its lipid-free form) not only add to the hydrophilicity and structural stability of the particle but they also have other functions as well: (a) They activate certain enzymes required for normal lipoprotein metabolism, and (b) they act as ligands on the surface of the lipoprotein that target specific receptors on peripheral tissues that require lipoprotein delivery for their innate cellular functions.

Ten principal apolipoproteins have been characterized. Their tissue source, molecular mass, distribution within lipoproteins, and metabolic functions are shown in Table 29.3.

The lipoproteins themselves are distributed among eight major classes. Some of their characteristics are summarized in Table 29.4. Each class of lipoprotein has a specific function determined by its apolipoprotein content, its tissue of origin, and the proportion of the macromolecule made up of triacylglycerols, cholesterol esters, free cholesterol, and phospholipids (see Tables 29.3 and 29.4).

### A. Chylomicrons

Chylomicrons (see Chapter 27 for a review of their metabolism) are the largest of the lipoproteins and the least dense because of their rich triacylglycerol content. They are synthesized from dietary lipids (the exogenous lipoprotein pathway) within the epithelial cells of the small intestine and then secreted into the lymphatic vessels draining the gut (see Chapter 27 and Fig. 27.10). They enter the bloodstream via the

**Table 29.3  Characteristics of the Major Apolipoproteins**

| Apolipoprotein | Primary Tissue Source | Molecular Mass (daltons) | Lipoprotein Distribution | Metabolic Function |
|---|---|---|---|---|
| ApoA-I | Intestine, liver | 28,016 | HDL (chylomicrons) | Activates LCAT; structural component of HDL |
| ApoA-II | Liver | 17,414 | HDL (chylomicrons) | Uncertain; may regulate transfer of apolipoproteins from HDL to other lipoprotein particles |
| ApoA-IV | Intestine | 46,465 | HDL (chylomicrons) | Uncertain; may be involved in assembly of HDL and chylomicrons |
| ApoB-48 | Intestine | 264,000 | Chylomicrons | Assembly and secretion of chylomicrons from small bowel |
| ApoB-100 | Liver | 540,000 | VLDL, IDL, LDL | VLDL assembly and secretion; structural protein of VLDL, IDL, and LDL; ligand for LDL receptor |
| ApoC-1 | Liver | 6,630 | Chylomicrons, VLDL, IDL, HDL | Unknown; may inhibit hepatic uptake of chylomicron and VLDL remnants |
| ApoC-II | Liver | 8,900 | Chylomicrons, VLDL, IDL, HDL | Cofactor activator of lipoprotein lipase (LPL) |
| ApoC-III | Liver | 8,800 | Chylomicrons, VLDL, IDL, HDL | Inhibitor of LPL; may inhibit hepatic uptake of chylomicrons and VLDL remnants |
| ApoE | Liver | 34,145 | Chylomicron remnants, VLDL, IDL, HDL | Ligand for binding of several lipoproteins to the LDL receptor, to the LDL receptor–related protein (LRP) and possibly to a separate apoE receptor |
| Apo(a) | Liver | | Lipoprotein "little" a (Lp[a]) | Unknown; consists of apoB-100 linked by a disulfide bond to apolipoprotein (a) |

HDL, high-density lipoprotein; LCAT, lecithin-cholesterol acyltransferase; VLDL, very low density lipoprotein; IDL, intermediate-density lipoprotein; LDL, low-density lipoprotein.

**Table 29.4 Characteristics of the Major Lipoproteins**

| Lipoprotein | Density Range (g/mL) | Particle Diameter Range (MM) | Electrophoretic Mobility | Lipid | | | Function |
| --- | --- | --- | --- | --- | --- | --- | --- |
| | | | | TG | Chol (%)[a] | PL | |
| Chylomicrons | 0.930 | 75–1,200 | Origin | 80–95 | 2–7 | 3–9 | Deliver dietary lipids |
| Chylomicron remnants | 0.930–1.006 | 30–80 | Slow pre-β | | | | Return dietary lipids to the liver |
| VLDL | 0.930–1.006 | 30–80 | Pre-β | 55–80 | 5–15 | 10–20 | Deliver endogenous lipids |
| IDL | 1.006–1.019 | 25–35 | Slow pre-β | 20–50 | 20–40 | 15–25 | Return endogenous lipids to the liver; precursor of LDL |
| LDL | 1.019–1.063 | 18–25 | β | 5–15 | 40–50 | 20–25 | Deliver cholesterol to cells |
| HDL$_2$ | 1.063–1.125 | 9–12 | α | 5–10 | 15–25 | 20–30 | Reverse cholesterol transport |
| HDL$_3$ | 1.125–1.210 | 5–9 | α | | | | Reverse cholesterol transport |
| Lip(a) | 1.050–1.120 | 25 | Pre-β | | | | |

[a]The remaining percent composition is composed of apolipoproteins.
TG, triacylglycerols; Chol, the sum of free and esterified cholesterol; PL, phospholipid; VLDL, very low density lipoprotein; IDL, intermediate-density lipoprotein; LDL, low-density lipoprotein; HDL, high-density lipoprotein.

left subclavian vein. The major apolipoproteins of chylomicrons are apolipoprotein B48 (apoB-48), apoC-II, and apoE (see Table 29.3). The apoC-II activates lipoprotein lipase (LPL), an enzyme that projects into the lumen of capillaries in adipose tissue, cardiac muscle, skeletal muscle, and the acinar cells of mammary tissue. This activation allows LPL to hydrolyze the triacylglycerol of the chylomicrons, leading to the release of fatty acids. The muscle cells then oxidize the fatty acids as fuel, whereas the adipocyte and mammary cells store them as triacylglycerols (fat) or, in the case of lactating breast, use them for milk formation. The partially hydrolyzed chylomicrons remaining in the bloodstream (the chylomicron remnants) have lost their apoC-II but still retain their apoE and apoB-48 proteins. Receptors in the plasma membranes of the liver cells bind to apoE on the surface of these remnants, allowing them to be taken up by the liver through a process of receptor-mediated endocytosis (see the following text).

## B. Very Low Density Lipoproteins

If dietary intake of carbohydrates exceeds the immediate fuel requirements of the liver, the excess carbohydrates are converted to triacylglycerols, which, along with free and esterified cholesterol, phospholipids, and the major apolipoprotein B100 (see Table 29.3), are packaged to form nascent VLDL (see Chapter 28). These particles are then secreted from the liver (the "endogenous" pathway of lipoprotein metabolism) into the bloodstream (Fig. 29.11), where they accept apoC-II and apoE from circulating HDL particles. This then forms the mature VLDL particle. VLDL are then transported from the hepatic veins to capillaries in skeletal and cardiac muscle and adipose tissue, as well as lactating mammary tissues, where LPL is activated by apoC-II in the VLDL particles. The activated enzyme facilitates the hydrolysis of the triglyceride in VLDL, causing the release of fatty acids and glycerol from a portion of core triacylglycerols. These fatty acids are oxidized as fuel by muscle cells, used in the resynthesis of triacylglycerols in fat cells, and used for milk production in the lactating breast. As the VLDL particles are depleted of triacylglycerol, **VLDL remnants** are formed. Approximately 50% of these remnants are taken up from the blood by liver cells through the binding of VLDL apoE to the hepatocyte plasma membrane apoE receptor followed by endocytic internalization of the VLDL remnant (similar to the fate of the chylomicron remnant).

## C. Intermediate-Density Lipoprotein and Low-Density Lipoproteins

Approximately half of the VLDL remnants are not taken up by the liver but, instead, have additional core triacylglycerols removed to form IDL, a specialized class of VLDL remnants. With the removal of additional triacylglycerols from IDL through the action of hepatic triglyceride lipase within hepatic sinusoids, LDL is generated from IDL. As can be seen in Table 29.4, the LDL particles are rich in cholesterol and

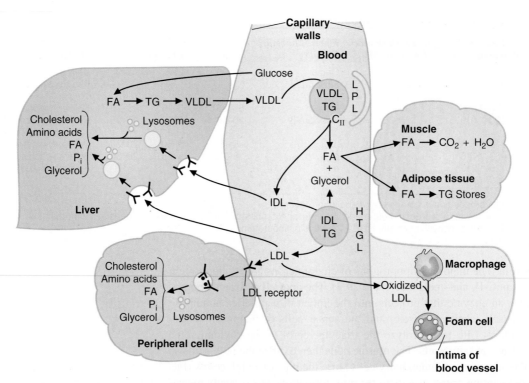

**FIG. 29.11.** Fate of VLDL. VLDL triacylglycerol (TG) is degraded by LPL, forming IDL. IDL can either be endocytosed by the liver through a receptor-mediated process or further digested, mainly by hepatic triacylglycerol lipase (HTGL), to form LDL. LDL may be endocytosed by receptor-mediated processes in the liver or in peripheral cells. LDL also may be oxidized and taken up by "scavenger" receptors on macrophages. The scavenger pathway plays a role in atherosclerosis. *FA*, fatty acids; *P*$_i$, inorganic phosphate.

cholesterol esters. Approximately 60% of the LDL is transported back to the liver, where its apoB-100 binds to specific apoB-100 receptors in the liver cell plasma membranes, allowing particles to be endocytosed into the hepatocyte. The remaining 40% of LDL particles is carried to extrahepatic tissues such as adrenocortical and gonadal cells that also have apoB-100 receptors, allowing them to internalize the LDL particles and use their cholesterol for the synthesis of steroid hormones. Some of the cholesterol of the internalized LDL is used for membrane synthesis and vitamin D synthesis as well. If an excess of LDL particles is present in the blood, this specific receptor-mediated uptake of LDL by hepatic and nonhepatic tissue becomes saturated. The "excess" LDL particles are now more readily available for nonspecific uptake of LDL by macrophages (scavenger cells) present near the endothelial cells of arteries. This exposure of vascular endothelial cells to high levels of LDL is believed to induce an inflammatory response by these cells, a process that has been suggested to initiate the complex cascade of atherosclerosis discussed in the following text.

### D. High-Density Lipoproteins

The fourth class of lipoproteins is HDL, which plays several roles in whole-body lipid metabolism.

#### 1. SYNTHESIS OF HIGH-DENSITY LIPOPROTEINS

HDL particles can be created by a number of mechanisms. The first is synthesis of nascent HDL by the liver and intestine as a relatively small molecule whose shell, like that of other lipoproteins, contains phospholipids, free cholesterol, and a variety of apolipoproteins, predominantly apoA-I, apoA-II, apoC-I, and apoC-II (see Table 29.3). Very low levels of triacylglycerols or cholesterol esters are found in the hollow core of this early, or nascent, version of HDL.

A second method for HDL generation is the budding of apolipoproteins from chylomicrons and VLDL particles as they are digested by LPL. The apolipoproteins (particularly apoA-I) and shells can then accumulate more lipid, as described in the following text.

A third method for HDL generation is free apoA-I, which may be shed from other circulating lipoproteins. The apoA-I acquires cholesterol and phospholipids from other lipoproteins and cell membranes to form nascent-like HDL particles within the circulation.

## 2. MATURATION OF NASCENT HIGH-DENSITY LIPOPROTEINS

In the process of maturation, the nascent HDL particles accumulate phospholipids and cholesterol from cells lining the blood vessels. As the central hollow core of nascent HDL progressively fills with cholesterol esters, HDL takes on a more globular shape to eventually form the mature HDL particle. The transfer of lipids to nascent HDL does not require enzymatic activity.

## 3. REVERSE CHOLESTEROL TRANSPORT

A major benefit of HDL particles derives from their ability to remove cholesterol from cholesterol-laden cells and to return the cholesterol to the liver, a process known as reverse cholesterol transport. This is particularly beneficial in vascular tissue; by reducing cellular cholesterol levels in the subintimal space, the likelihood that foam cells (lipid-laden macrophages that engulf oxidized LDL cholesterol and represent an early stage in the development of atherosclerotic plaque) will form within the blood vessel wall is reduced.

Reverse cholesterol transport requires a directional movement of cholesterol from the cell to the lipoprotein particle. Cells contain the protein ATP–binding casette 1 (ABC1) that uses ATP hydrolysis to move cholesterol from the inner leaflet of the membrane to the outer leaflet. Once the cholesterol has reached the outer membrane leaflet, the HDL particle can accept it, but if the cholesterol is not modified within the HDL particle, the cholesterol can leave the particle by the same route that it entered. To trap the cholesterol within the HDL core, the HDL particle acquires the enzyme lecithin cholesterol acyltransferase (LCAT) from the circulation. (LCAT is synthesized and secreted by the liver.) LCAT catalyzes the transfer of a fatty acid from the 2-position of lecithin (phosphatidylcholine) in the phospholipid shell of the particle to the 3-hydroxyl group of cholesterol, forming a cholesterol ester (Fig. 29.12). The cholesterol ester migrates to the core of the HDL particle and is no longer free to return to the cell.

Elevated levels of lipoprotein-associated cholesterol in the blood, particularly that associated with LDL and also the more triacylglycerol-rich lipoproteins, are associated with the formation of cholesterol-rich atheromatous plaques in the vessel walls, leading eventually to diffuse **atherosclerotic vascular disease** that can result in acute cardiovascular events, such as myocardial infarction, stroke, or symptomatic peripheral vascular insufficiency. High levels of HDL in the blood, therefore, are believed to be vasculoprotective because these high levels increase the rate of reverse cholesterol transport "away" from the blood vessels and "toward" the liver ("out of harm's way").

## 4. FATE OF HIGH-DENSITY LIPOPROTEIN CHOLESTEROL

Mature HDL particles can bind to specific receptors on hepatocytes (such as the apoE receptor), but the primary means of clearance of HDL from the blood is through its uptake by the scavenger receptor SR-B1. This receptor is present on many cell types. It does not carry out endocytosis per se, but once the HDL particle is bound to the receptor, its cholesterol and cholesterol esters are transferred into the cells. When depleted of cholesterol and its esters, the HDL particle dissociates from the SR-B1 receptor and reenters the circulation. SR-B1 receptors can be upregulated in certain cell types that require cholesterol for biosynthetic purposes, such as the

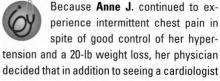

Two genetically determined disorders, familial HDL deficiency and Tangier disease, result from mutations in the ABC1 protein. Cholesterol-depleted HDL cannot transport free cholesterol from cells that lack the ability to express this protein. As a consequence, HDL is rapidly degraded. These disorders have established a role for ABC1 protein in the regulation of HDL levels in the blood.

Because **Anne J.** continued to experience intermittent chest pain in spite of good control of her hypertension and a 20-lb weight loss, her physician decided that in addition to seeing a cardiologist to further evaluate the chest pain, a second drug is needed to be added to her regimen to lower her blood LDL cholesterol level. Consequently, treatment with ezetimibe, a drug that blocks cholesterol absorption from the intestine, was added to complement the atorvastatin Anne was already taking.

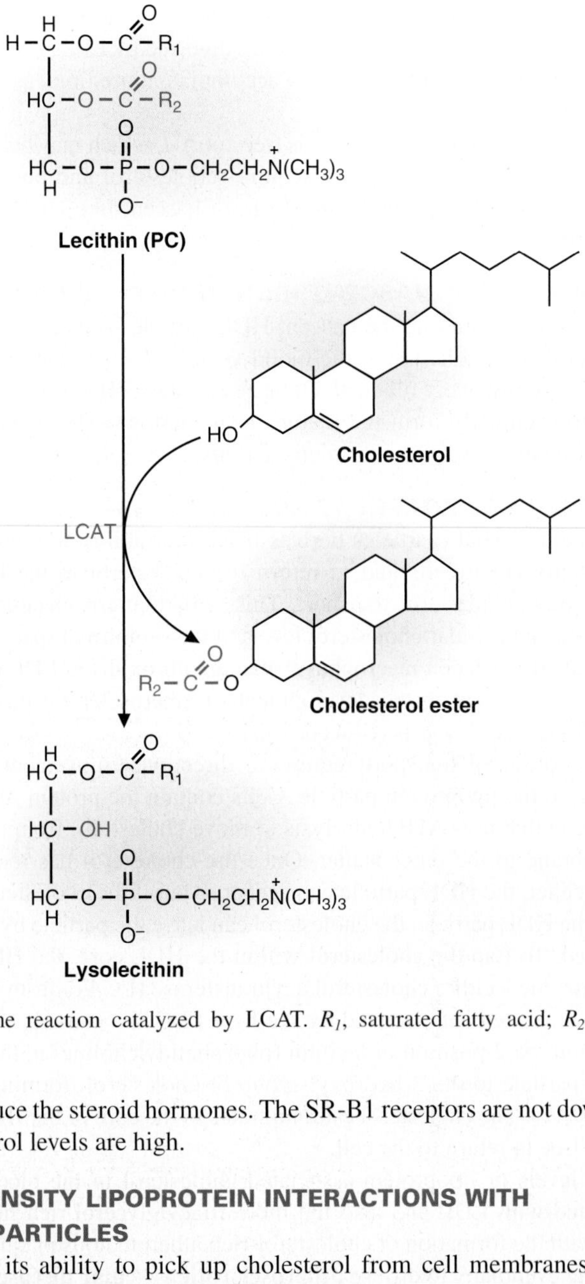

***FIG. 29.12.*** The reaction catalyzed by LCAT. $R_1$, saturated fatty acid; $R_2$, unsaturated fatty acid.

cells that produce the steroid hormones. The SR-B1 receptors are not downregulated when cholesterol levels are high.

## 5. HIGH-DENSITY LIPOPROTEIN INTERACTIONS WITH OTHER PARTICLES

In addition to its ability to pick up cholesterol from cell membranes, HDL also exchanges apolipoproteins and lipids with other lipoproteins in the blood. For example, HDL transfers apoE and apoC-II to chylomicrons and to VLDL. The apoC-II stimulates the degradation of the triacylglycerols of chylomicrons and VLDL by activating LPL (Fig. 29.13). After digestion of the chylomicrons and the VLDL triacylglycerols, apoE and apoC-II are transferred back to HDL. When HDL obtains free cholesterol from cell membranes, the free cholesterol is esterified at the third carbon of the A ring via the LCAT reaction (see Fig. 29.11). From this point, HDL either transports the free cholesterol and cholesterol esters directly to the liver, as described previously, or by cholesterol ester transfer protein (CETP) to circulating triacylglycerol-rich lipoproteins such as VLDL and VLDL remnants (see Fig. 29.13). In exchange, triacylglycerols from the latter lipoproteins are transferred to HDL. The greater the concentration of triacylglycerol-rich lipoproteins in the blood, the greater the rate of these exchanges.

The CETP exchange pathway may explain the observation that whenever triacylglycerol-rich lipoproteins are present in the blood in high concentrations, the

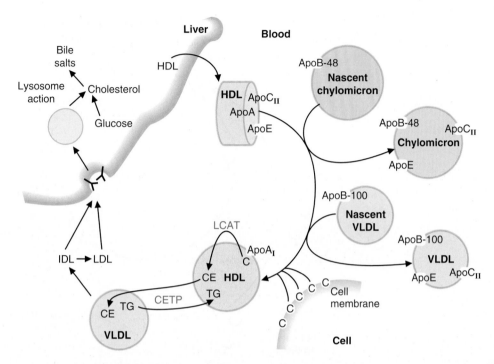

***FIG. 29.13.*** Functions and fate of HDL. Nascent HDL is synthesized in liver and intestinal cells. It exchanges proteins with chylomicrons and VLDL. HDL picks up cholesterol *(C)* from cell membranes. This cholesterol is converted to cholesterol ester *(CE)* by the LCAT reaction. HDL transfers *CE* to VLDL in exchange for triacylglycerol *(TG)*. The CETP mediates this exchange. *PL*, phospholipids.

amount of cholesterol reaching the liver via cholesterol-enriched VLDL and VLDL remnants increases, and a proportional reduction in the total amount of cholesterol and cholesterol esters that are directly transferred to the liver via HDL occurs. Mature HDL particles are designated as $HDL_3$; after reverse cholesterol transport and the accumulation of cholesterol esters, they become the atherogenic protective form, $HDL_2$. The CETP reaction then leads to the loss of cholesterol and gain of triacylglycerol such that the particles become larger and eventually regenerate $HDL_3$ particles (see Table 29.4). Hepatic lipase can then remove triacylglycerol from $HDL_3$ particles to regenerate $HDL_2$ particles.

## VI. RECEPTOR-MEDIATED ENDOCYTOSIS OF LIPOPROTEINS

As stated earlier, each lipoprotein particle contains specific apolipoproteins on its surface that act as ligands for specific plasma membrane receptors on target tissues such as the liver, the adrenal cortex, the gonads, and other cells that require one or more of the components of the lipoproteins. With the exception of the scavenger receptor SR-B1, the interaction of ligand and receptor initiates the process of endocytosis shown for LDL in Figure 29.14. The receptors for LDL, for example, are found in specific areas of the plasma membrane of the target cell for circulating lipoproteins. They are known as coated pits, and they contain a unique protein called **clathrin**. The plasma membrane in the vicinity of the receptor-LDL complex invaginates and fuses to form an endocytic vesicle. These vesicles then fuse with lysosomes, acidic subcellular vesicles that contain several degradative enzymes. The cholesterol esters of LDL are hydrolyzed to form free cholesterol, which is rapidly reesterified through the action of ACAT. This rapid reesterification is necessary to avoid the damaging effect of high levels of free cholesterol on cellular membranes.

As is true for the synthesis and activity of HMG-CoA reductase, the synthesis of the LDL receptor itself is subject to feedback inhibition by increasing levels of cholesterol within the cell. As cholesterol levels increase within the cell, synthesis of

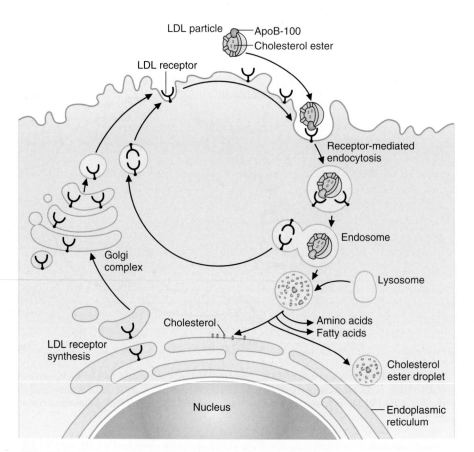

**FIG. 29.14.** Cholesterol uptake by receptor-mediated endocytosis.

the LDL receptor is inhibited. When the intracellular levels of cholesterol decrease, both synthesis of cholesterol from acetyl CoA and synthesis of LDL receptors are stimulated. An increased number of receptors (upregulation of receptor synthesis) results in an increased uptake of LDL cholesterol from the blood, with a subsequent reduction of circulating LDL cholesterol levels. At the same time, the cellular cholesterol pool is replenished. The upregulation of LDL receptors forms the basis of the mechanism of statin drugs lowering blood LDL levels.

## VII.  LIPOPROTEIN RECEPTORS

The best-characterized lipoprotein receptor, the LDL receptor, specifically recognizes apoB-100 and apoE. Therefore, this receptor binds VLDL, IDL, and chylomicron remnants in addition to LDL. The binding reaction is characterized by its saturability and occurs with high affinity and a narrow range of specificity. Other receptors, such as the LDL receptor–related proteins (LRP) and the macrophage scavenger receptor (notably types SR-A1 and SR-A2, which are located primarily near the endothelial surface of vascular endothelial cells), have broad specificity and bind many other ligands in addition to the blood lipoproteins.

### A.  The Low-Density Lipoprotein Receptor

The **LDL receptor** is essential for removing LDL from the circulation. Failure to do so can be detrimental to the cardiovascular system. The number of LDL receptors, the binding of LDL to its receptors, and the postreceptor binding process can be diminished for a variety of reasons, all of which may lead to an accumulation of LDL cholesterol in the blood and premature atherosclerosis. These abnormalities can result from mutations in one (heterozygous—seen in approximately 1 in 500 people) or both (homozygous—seen in about 1 in 1 million people) of the alleles for the LDL receptor (**familial hypercholesterolemia**). Heterozygotes produce approximately half of the normal complement of LDL receptors, whereas the homozygotes produce almost no LDL receptor protein (receptor-negative familial hypercholesterolemia).

The genetic mutations are mainly deletions, but insertions or duplications also occur as well as missense and nonsense mutations. Four classes of mutations have been identified. The first class involves "null" alleles that either direct the synthesis of no protein at all or a protein that cannot be precipitated by antibodies to the LDL receptor. In the second class, the alleles encode proteins, but they cannot be transported to the cell surface. The third class of mutant alleles encodes proteins that reach the cell surface but cannot bind LDL normally. Finally, the fourth class encodes proteins that reach the surface and bind LDL but fail to cluster and internalize the LDL particles. The result of each of these mutations is that blood levels of LDL are elevated because cells cannot take up these particles at a normal rate.

### B. Low-Density Lipoprotein Receptor–Related Protein

The **LRP** is structurally related to the LDL receptor but recognizes a broader spectrum of ligands. In addition to lipoproteins, it binds the blood proteins $\alpha_2$-macroglobulin (a protein that inhibits blood proteases) and tissue plasminogen activator (TPA) and its inhibitors. The LRP receptor recognizes the apoE of lipoproteins and binds remnants produced by the digestion of the triacylglycerols of chylomicrons and VLDL by LPL. Thus, one of its functions is believed to be the clearance of these remnants from the blood. The LRP receptor is abundant in the cell membranes of the liver, brain, and placenta. In contrast to the LDL receptor, synthesis of the LRP receptor is not significantly affected by an increase in the intracellular concentration of cholesterol. However, insulin causes the number of these receptors on the cell surface to increase, consistent with the need to remove chylomicron remnants that otherwise would accumulate after eating a meal.

### C. Macrophage Scavenger Receptors

Some cells, particularly the phagocytic macrophage, have nonspecific receptors known as **scavenger receptors** that bind various types of molecules, including oxidatively modified LDL particles. There are several different types of scavenger receptors. SR-B1 is used primarily for HDL binding, whereas the scavenger receptors expressed on macrophages are SR-A1 and SR-A2. Modification of LDL frequently involves oxidative damage, particularly of polyunsaturated fatty acyl groups (see Chapter 18). In contrast to the LDL receptors, the scavenger receptors are not subject to downregulation. The continued presence of scavenger receptors in the cell membrane allows the cells to take up oxidatively modified LDL long after intracellular cholesterol levels are elevated. When the macrophages become engorged with lipid, they are called **foam cells**. An accumulation of these foam cells in the subendothelial space of blood vessels form the earliest gross evidence of a developing atherosclerotic plaque known as a fatty streak.

The processes that cause oxidation of LDL involve superoxide radicals, nitric oxide, hydrogen peroxide, and other oxidants (see Chapter 18). Antioxidants, such as vitamin E, ascorbic acid (vitamin C), and carotenoids, may be involved in protecting LDL from oxidation.

### VIII. ANATOMIC AND BIOCHEMICAL ASPECTS OF ATHEROSCLEROSIS

The normal artery is composed of three distinct layers (Fig. 29.15). That which is closest to the lumen of the vessel, the **intima**, is lined by a monolayer of endothelial cells that are bathed by the circulating blood. Just beneath these specialized cells lies the **subintimal extracellular matrix** in which some vascular smooth muscle cells are embedded (the subintimal space). The middle layer, known as the **tunica media**, is separated from the intima by the **internal elastic lamina**. The

 **Anne J.'s** blood lipid levels (in milligrams per deciliter) were as follows:

| | |
|---|---|
| Triacylglycerol | 158 |
| Total cholesterol | 420 |
| HDL cholesterol | 32 |
| LDL cholesterol | 356 |

She was diagnosed as having familial hypercholesterolemia (FH) type IIA, which is caused by genetic defects in the gene that encodes the LDL receptor. As a result of the receptor defect, LDL cannot readily be taken up by cells, and its concentration in the blood is elevated.

LDL particles contain a high percentage, by weight, of cholesterol and cholesterol esters, more than other blood lipoproteins. However, LDL triacylglycerol levels are low because LDL is produced by digestion of the triacylglycerols of VLDL and IDL. Therefore, individuals with a type IIA hyperlipoproteinemia have very high blood cholesterol levels, but their levels of triacylglycerols may be in or near the normal range (see Table 29.4).

 **Ivan A.'s** blood lipid levels were as follows:

| | |
|---|---|
| Triacylglycerol | 295 |
| Total cholesterol | 314 |
| HDL cholesterol | 24 |
| LDL cholesterol | 231 |

The elevated serum levels of LDL cholesterol found in patients such as **Ivan A.** who have type 2 diabetes mellitus is multifactorial. One of the mechanisms responsible for this increase involves the presence of chronically elevated levels of glucose in the blood of poorly controlled diabetics. This prolonged hyperglycemia increases the rate of nonenzymatic attachment of glucose to various proteins in the body, a process referred to as glycation or glycosylation of proteins.

Glycation may adversely affect the structure or the function of the protein involved. For example, glycation of the LDL receptor and of proteins in the LDL particle may interfere with the normal "fit" of LDL particles with their specific receptors. As a result, less circulating LDL is internalized into cells by receptor-mediated endocytosis, and the serum LDL cholesterol level rises. Additionally, because Mr. A. is obese, he exhibits higher than normal levels of circulating free fatty acids, which the liver uses to increase the synthesis of VLDL, leading to hypertriglyceridemia.

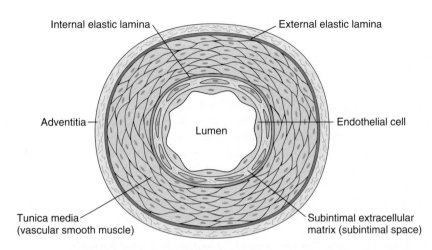

Internal elastic lamina

External elastic lamina

Adventitia

Endothelial cell

Lumen

Tunica media
(vascular smooth muscle)

Subintimal extracellular
matrix (subintimal space)

*FIG. 29.15.* The different layers of the arterial wall.

tunica media contains lamellae of smooth muscle cells surrounded by an elastin- and collagen-rich matrix. The external elastic lamina forms the border between the tunica media and the outermost layer, the **adventitia**. This layer contains nerve fibers and mast cells.

The initial step in the development of an atherosclerotic lesion within the wall of an artery is the formation of a **fatty streak**. A fatty streak is an accumulation of lipid-laden macrophages or foam cells in the subintimal space. These fatty streaks are visible as a yellow-white linear streak that bulges slightly into the lumen of the vessel. These streaks are initiated when one or more known vascular risk factors for atherosclerosis, all of which have the potential to injure the vascular endothelial cells, reach a critical threshold at the site of future lesions. Examples of such risk factors include elevated intra-arterial pressure (arterial hypertension); elevated circulating levels of various lipids such as LDL, chylomicron remnants, and VLDL remnants; low levels of circulating HDL; cigarette smoking; chronic elevations in blood glucose levels; high circulating levels of the vasoconstricting octapeptide angiotensin II; and others. The resulting insult to endothelial cells may trigger these cells to secrete adhesion molecules that bind to circulating monocytes and markedly slow their rate of movement past the endothelium. When these monocytic cells are slowed enough, they accumulate and have access to the physical spaces that exist between endothelial cells. This accumulation of monocytic cells resembles the classical inflammatory response to injury. These changes have led to the suggestion that atherosclerosis is, in fact, an inflammatory disorder and, therefore, is one that might be prevented or attenuated through the use of anti-inflammatory agents. Two such agents, acetylsalicylic acid (e.g., aspirin) and HMG-CoA reductase inhibitors (statins), have been shown to suppress the inflammatory cascade, whereas statins also inhibit the action of HMG-CoA reductase.

The monocytic cells are transformed into macrophages that migrate through the spaces between endothelial cells. They enter the subintimal space under the influence of chemoattractant cytokines secreted by vascular cells in response to exposure to oxidatively modified fatty acids within the lipoproteins.

These macrophages can replicate and exhibit augmented expression of receptors that recognize oxidatively modified lipoproteins. Unlike the classic LDL receptors on liver and many nonhepatic cells, these macrophage-bound receptors are high-capacity, low-specificity receptors (scavenger receptors). They bind to and internalize oxidatively modified fatty acids within LDLs to become subintimal foam cells as described previously. As these foam cells accumulate, they deform the overlying endothelium, causing microscopic separations between endothelial cells, exposing these foam cells and underlying extracellular matrix to the blood. These exposed

In addition to dietary therapy, aimed at reducing her blood cholesterol levels, **Anne J.** was treated with atorvastatin, an HMG-CoA reductase inhibitor. HMG-CoA reductase inhibitors decrease the rate of synthesis of cholesterol in cells. As cellular cholesterol levels decrease, the synthesis of LDL receptors increases. As the number of receptors increases on the cell surface, the uptake of LDL is accelerated. Consequently, the blood level of LDL cholesterol decreases. Anne was also treated with ezetimibe, which reduces cholesterol absorption from the intestinal lumen but has not been shown to decrease cardiovascular risk.

HDL is considered to be the "good cholesterol" because it accepts free cholesterol from peripheral tissues, such as cells in the walls of blood vessels. This cholesterol is converted to cholesterol ester, part of which is transferred to VLDL by CETP and returned to the liver by IDL and LDL. The remainder of the cholesterol is transferred directly as part of the HDL molecule to the liver. The liver reutilizes the cholesterol in the synthesis of VLDL, converts it to bile salts, or excretes it directly into the bile. HDL therefore tends to lower blood cholesterol levels. Lower blood cholesterol levels correlate with a lower rate of death caused by atherosclerosis.

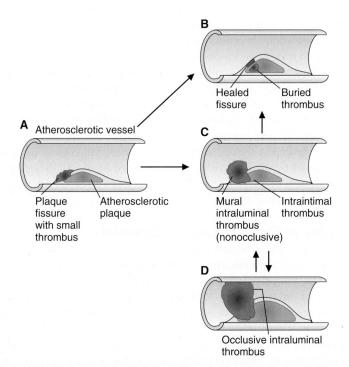

**FIG. 29.16.** Evolution of an atherosclerotic plaque. Plaque capsule eroded near the elbow of plaque, creating an early plaque fissure (**A**), which may heal as plaque increases in size (**B**) or may grow as thrombus expands, having an intraluminal portion and an intraintimal portion (**C**). If the fissure is not properly sealed, the thrombus may grow and completely occlude the vessel lumen (**D**), causing an acute infarction of tissues downstream of the vessel occlusion.

In patients such as **Anne J.** and **Ivan A.**, who have elevated levels of VLDL or LDL, HDL levels are often low. These patients are predisposed to atherosclerosis and suffer from a high incidence of heart attacks and strokes.

Exercise and estrogen administration both increase HDL levels. This is one of the reasons exercise is often recommended to aid in the prevention or treatment of heart disease. Prior to menopause, the incidence of heart attacks is relatively low in women, but it rises after menopause and increases to the level found in men by the age of 65 or 70 years. Moderate consumption of ethanol (alcohol) has also been correlated with increased HDL levels. Recent studies suggest that the beneficial amount of ethanol may be quite low, about two small glasses of wine a day, and that beneficial effects ascribed to ethanol may result from other components of wine and alcoholic beverages. In spite of the evidence that postmenopausal hormone replacement therapy (HRT) decreases circulating levels of LDL and increases HDL levels, data from controlled trials show that HRT may actually increase the rate of atherosclerotic vascular disease in these women. As a result, the accepted indications for estrogen administration are now limited to intolerable "hot flashes" or vaginal dryness.

areas serve as sites for platelet adhesion and aggregation. Activated platelets secrete cytokines that perpetuate this process and increase the potential for thrombus (clot) formation locally. As the evolving plaque matures, a **fibrous cap** forms over its expanding "roof," which now bulges into the vascular lumen, thereby partially occluding it. Vascular smooth muscle cells now migrate from the tunica media to the subintimal space and secrete additional plaque matrix material. The smooth muscle cells also secrete metalloproteinases that thin the fibrous cap near its "elbow" at the periphery of the plaque. This thinning progresses until the fibrous cap ruptures, allowing the plaque contents to physically contact the procoagulant elements present within the circulation. This leads to acute thrombus formation. If this thrombus completely occludes the remaining lumen of the vessel, an infarction of tissues distal to the occlusion (i.e., an acute myocardial infarction) may occur (Fig. 29.16). Most plaques that rupture also contain focal areas of calcification, which appears to result from the induction of the same cluster of genes as those that promote the formation of bone. The inducers for this process include oxidized sterols as well as transforming growth factor-β (TGF-β) derived from certain vascular cells.

Finally, high **intraluminal shear forces** develop in these thinning or eroded areas of the plaque's fibrous cap, inducing macrophages to secrete additional metalloproteinases that further degrade the arterial–fibrous cap matrix. This contributes further to plaque rupture and thrombus formation (see Fig. 29.16). The consequence is a macrovascular ischemic event, such as an acute myocardial infarction (AMI) or acute cerebrovascular accident (CVA).

## IX. STEROID HORMONES

Cholesterol is the precursor of all five classes of **steroid hormones**: glucocorticoids, mineralocorticoids, androgens, estrogens, and progestins. These hormones are synthesized in the adrenal cortex, ovaries, testes, and ovarian corpus luteum.

Steroid hormones are transported through the blood from their sites of synthesis to their target organs where, because of their hydrophobicity, they cross the cell membrane and bind to specific receptors in either the cytoplasm or nucleus. The bound receptors then bind to DNA to regulate gene transcription (see Chapter 14). Because of their hydrophobicity, steroid hormones must be complexed with a serum protein. Serum albumin can act as a nonspecific carrier for the steroid hormones, but there are specific carriers as well. The cholesterol used for steroid hormone synthesis is either synthesized in the tissues from acetyl CoA, extracted from intracellular cholesterol ester pools, or taken up by the cell in the form of cholesterol-containing lipoproteins (either internalized by the LDL receptor or absorbed by the SR-B1 receptor). The specific complement of enzymes present in the cells of an organ determines which hormones the organ can synthesize.

## A. Overview of Steroid Hormone Synthesis

The biosynthesis of glucocorticoids and mineralocorticoids (in the adrenal cortex) and that of sex steroids (in the adrenal cortex and gonads) requires several distinct cytochrome P450 enzymes (see Chapter 24). These monooxygenases are involved in the transfer of electrons from NADPH through electron transfer protein intermediates to molecular oxygen, which then oxidizes a variety of the ring carbons of cholesterol.

Cholesterol is converted to progesterone in the first two steps of synthesis of all steroid hormones. Cytochrome $P450_{SCC}$ side-chain cleavage enzyme (previously referred to as cholesterol desmolase and classified as CYP11A) is located in the mitochondrial inner membrane and removes six carbons from the side chain of cholesterol, forming pregnenolone, which has 21 carbons (Fig. 29.17). The next step, the conversion of pregnenolone to progesterone, is catalyzed by 3-β-hydroxysteroid dehydrogenase, an enzyme that is not a member of the cytochrome P450 family. Other steroid hormones are produced from progesterone by reactions that involve members of the P450 family. These include the mitochondrial enzyme cytochrome $P450_{C11}$ (CY11B1), which catalyzes β-hydroxylation at carbon 11 and two endoplasmic reticulum enzymes: $P450_{C17}$ (17-α-hydroxylase, CYP17) and $P450_{C21}$ (hydroxylation at carbon 21, CYP21). As the synthesis of the steroid hormones is discussed, notice how certain enzymes are used in more than one pathway. Defects in these enzymes lead to multiple abnormalities in steroid synthesis, which, in turn, results in a variety of abnormal phenotypes.

## B. Synthesis of Cortisol

The adrenocortical biosynthetic pathway that leads to **cortisol** synthesis occurs in the middle layer of the adrenal cortex known as the zona fasciculata. Free cholesterol is transported by an intracellular carrier protein to the inner mitochondrial membrane of cells, where the side chain is cleaved to form pregnenolone. Pregnenolone returns to the cytosol where it forms progesterone.

In the membranes of the endoplasmic reticulum, the enzyme $P450_{C17}$ (CYP17) catalyzes the hydroxylation of C17 of progesterone or pregnenolone and can also catalyze the cleavage of the two-carbon side chain of these compounds at C17 (a C17–C20 lyase activity), which forms androstenedione from 17-α-hydroxyprogesterone. These two separate functions of the same enzyme allow further steroid synthesis to proceed along two separate pathways: The 17-hydroxylated steroids that retain their side chains are precursors of cortisol (C21), whereas those from which the side chain was cleaved (C19 steroids) are precursors of androgens (male sex hormones) and estrogens (female sex hormones).

In the pathway of cortisol synthesis, the 17-hydroxylation of progesterone yields 17-α-hydroxyprogesterone, which, along with progesterone, is transported to the smooth endoplasmic reticulum. There, the membrane-bound $P450_{C21}$ (21-α-hydroxylase) enzyme catalyzes the hydroxylation of C21 of 17-α-hydroxyprogesterone

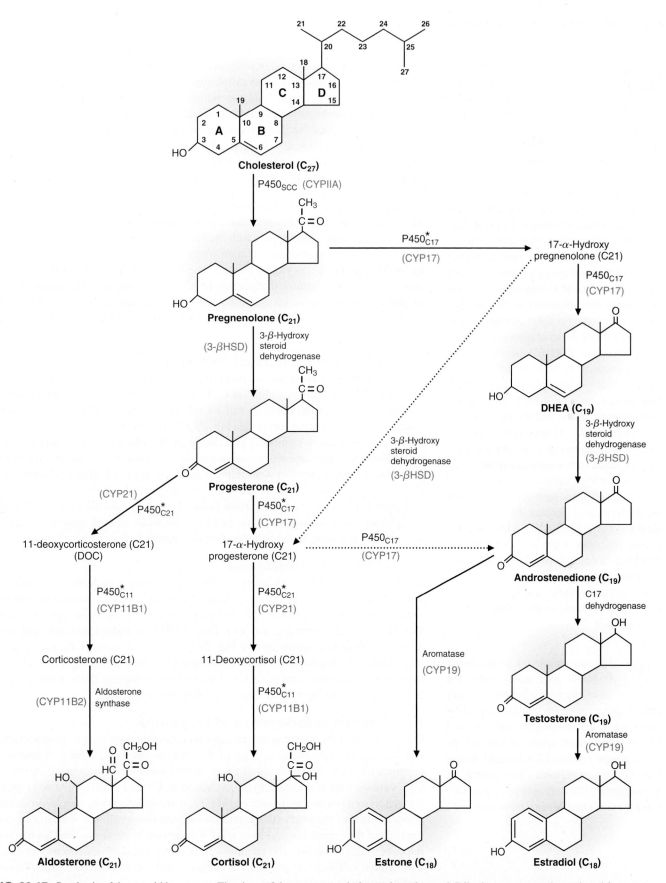

**FIG. 29.17.** Synthesis of the steroid hormones. The rings of the precursor, cholesterol, are lettered. Dihydrotestosterone is produced from testosterone by reduction of the carbon–carbon double bond in ring A. The *dashed lines* indicate alternative pathways to the major pathways indicated. The starred enzymes are those that may be defective in the condition congenital adrenal hyperplasia. CYP is a designation for a cytochrome P450–containing enzyme. *DHEA*, dehydroepiandrosterone.

Congenital adrenal hyperplasia (CAH) is a group of diseases caused by a genetically determined deficiency in a variety of enzymes required for cortisol synthesis. The most common deficiency is that of 21-α hydroxylase (CYP21), the activity of which is necessary to convert progesterone to 11-deoxycorticosterone and 17-α hydroxyprogesterone to 11-deoxycortisol. Thus, this deficiency reduces both aldosterone and cortisol production without affecting androgen production. If the enzyme deficiency is severe, the precursors for aldosterone and cortisol production are shunted to androgen synthesis, producing an overabundance of androgens, which leads to prenatal masculinization in females and postnatal virilization in males. Another enzyme deficiency in this group of diseases is that of 11-β hydroxylase (CYP11B1), which results in the accumulation of 11-deoxycorticosterone. An excess of this mineralocorticoid leads to hypertension (through binding of 11-deoxycorticosterone to the aldosterone receptor). In this form of CAH, 11-deoxycortisol also accumulates but its biological activity is minimal and no specific clinical signs and symptoms result. The androgen pathway is unaffected and the increased adrenocorticotropic hormone (ACTH) levels may increase the levels of adrenal androgens in the blood. A third possible enzyme deficiency is that of 17-α hydroxylase (CYP17). A defect in 17-α hydroxylase leads to aldosterone excess and hypertension; however, because adrenal androgen synthesis requires this enzyme, no virilization occurs in these patients.

Androstenedione can be purchased at health food stores under the name Andros. It is touted to improve athletic performance through its ability to be converted to testosterone. Its use has been banned by most major sports, although in 1998, it was a legal supplement in baseball. During that year, the drug received a lot of publicity, as the supplement had been used by a player who broke the major league home run record.

to form 11-deoxycortisol (and of progesterone to form deoxycorticosterone [DOC], a precursor of the mineralocorticoid aldosterone; see Fig. 29.17).

The final step in cortisol synthesis requires transport of 11-deoxycortisol back to the inner membrane of the mitochondria, where $P450_{C11}$ (11-β-hydroxylase, CYB11B1) catalyzes the β-hydroxylation of the substrate at carbon 21, in a reaction that requires molecular oxygen and electrons derived from NADPH, to form cortisol. The rate of biosynthesis of cortisol and other adrenal steroids depends on stimulation of the adrenal cortical cells by ACTH.

### C. Synthesis of Aldosterone

The synthesis of the potent mineralocorticoid **aldosterone** in the zona glomerulosa of the adrenal cortex also begins with the conversion of cholesterol to progesterone (see Fig. 29.17). Progesterone is then hydroxylated at C21, a reaction catalyzed by $P450_{C21}$ (CYP21), to yield 11-DOC. The $P450_{C11}$ (CYP11B1) enzyme system then catalyzes the reactions that convert DOC to corticosterone. The terminal steps in aldosterone synthesis, catalyzed by the P450 aldosterone system (CYP11B2), involve the oxidation of corticosterone to 18-hydroxycorticosterone, which is oxidized to aldosterone.

### D. Synthesis of the Adrenal Androgens

**Adrenal androgen** biosynthesis proceeds from cleavage of the two-carbon side chain of 17-hydroxypregnenolone at C17 to form the 19-carbon adrenal androgen dehydroepiandrosterone (DHEA) and its sulfate derivative (DHEAS) in the zona reticulosum of the adrenal cortex (see Fig. 29.17). These compounds, which are weak androgens, represent a significant percentage of the total steroid production by the normal adrenal cortex and are the major androgens synthesized in the adrenal gland.

Androstenedione, another weak adrenal androgen, is produced by oxidation of the β-hydroxy group to a carbonyl group by 3-β-hydroxysteroid dehydrogenase. This androgen is converted to **testosterone** primarily in extra-adrenal tissues. Although the adrenal cortex makes very little estrogen, the weak adrenal androgens may be converted to estrogens in the peripheral tissues, particularly in adipose tissue.

### E. Synthesis of Testosterone

In many ways, the pathways leading to androgen synthesis in the testicle are similar to those described for the adrenal cortex. In the human testicle, the predominant pathway leading to testosterone synthesis is through pregnenolone to 17-α-hydroxypregnenolone to DHEA (the $\Delta^5$ pathway), and then from DHEA to androstenedione, and from androstenedione to testosterone (see Fig. 29.17). As for all steroids, the rate-limiting step in testosterone production is the conversion of cholesterol to pregnenolone. In its target cells, the double bond in ring A of testosterone is reduced through the action of 5-α-reductase, forming the active hormone dihydrotestosterone.

### F. Synthesis of Estrogens and Progestins

Ovarian production of **estrogens**, **progestins** (compounds related to progesterone), and androgens requires the activity of the cytochrome P450 family of oxidative enzymes used for the synthesis of other steroid hormones. Ovarian estrogens are C18 steroids with a phenolic hydroxyl group at C3 and either a hydroxyl group (estradiol) or a ketone group (estrone) at C17. Although the major steroid-producing compartments of the ovary (the granulosa cell, the theca cell, the stromal cell, and the cells of the corpus luteum) have all of the enzyme systems required for the synthesis of multiple steroids, the granulosa cells secrete primarily estrogens, the thecal and stromal cells secrete primarily androgens, and the cells of the corpus luteum secrete primarily progesterone.

The ovarian granulosa cell, in response to stimulation by follicle-stimulating hormone (FSH) from the anterior pituitary gland and through the catalytic activity of P450 aromatase (CYP19), converts testosterone to estradiol, the predominant and most potent of the ovarian estrogens (see Fig. 29.17). Similarly, androstenedione is converted to estrone in the ovary, although the major site of estrone production from androstenedione occurs in extraovarian tissues, principally skeletal muscle and adipose tissue.

### G. Vitamin D Synthesis

**Vitamin D** is unique in that it can be either obtained from the diet (as vitamin $D_2$ or $D_3$) or synthesized from a cholesterol precursor, a process that requires reactions in the skin, liver, and intestine. The calciferols, including several forms of vitamin D, are a family of steroids that affect calcium homeostasis (Fig. 29.18). Cholecalciferol (vitamin $D_3$) requires ultraviolet light for its production from 7-dehydrocholesterol present in cutaneous tissues (skin) in animals and available from ergosterol in plants. This irradiation cleaves the carbon–carbon bond at C9–C10 to open the B ring to form cholecalciferol, an inactive precursor of 1,25-dihydroxy cholecalciferol (calcitriol). Calcitriol is the most potent biologically active form of vitamin D (see Fig. 29.18).

1,25-$(OH)_2D_3$ (calcitriol) is approximately 100 times more potent than 25-$(OH)$ $D_3$ in its actions, yet 25-$(OH)D_3$ is present in the blood in a concentration that may be 100 times greater, which suggests that it may play some role in calcium and phosphorus homeostasis.

The formation of calcitriol from cholecalciferol begins in the liver and ends in the kidney, where the pathway is regulated (see Fig. 29.18). The release of parathyroid hormone from the parathyroid gland results in activation of the last step of active hormone formation in the kidney, which is the hydroxylation of 25-hydroxycholecalciferol via a mixed function oxidase.

The biologically active forms of vitamin D are sterol hormones and, like other steroids, diffuse passively through the plasma membrane. In the intestine, bone, and kidney, the sterol then moves into the nucleus and binds to specific vitamin $D_3$ receptors. This complex activates genes that encode proteins mediating the action of active vitamin $D_3$. In the intestinal mucosal cell, for example, transcription of genes encoding calcium-transporting proteins is activated. These proteins are capable of carrying $Ca^{2+}$ (and phosphorus) absorbed from the gut lumen across the cell, making it available for eventual passage into the circulation.

## CLINICAL COMMENTS

Diseases discussed in this chapter are summarized in Table 29.5.

**Anne J.** Anne J. is typical of patients with essentially normal serum triacylglycerol levels and elevated serum total cholesterol levels that are repeatedly in the upper 1% of the general population (e.g., 325 to 500 mg/dL). When similar lipid abnormalities are present in other family members in a pattern of autosomal dominant inheritance and no secondary causes for these lipid alterations (e.g., hypothyroidism) are present, the entity referred to as familial hypercholesterolemia (FH) type IIA is the most likely cause of this hereditary dyslipidemia.

FH is a genetic disorder caused by an abnormality in one or more alleles responsible for the formation or the functional integrity of high-affinity LDL receptors on the plasma membrane of cells that normally initiate the internalization of circulating LDL and other blood lipoproteins.

Chronic hypercholesterolemia not only may cause the deposition of lipid within vascular tissues leading to atherosclerosis but also may cause the deposition of lipid within the skin and eye. When this occurs in the medial aspect of the upper and lower eyelids, it is referred to as xanthelasma. Similar deposits known as xanthomas may occur in the iris of the eye (arcus lipidalis) as well as the tendons of the hands ("knuckle pads") and Achilles tendons.

Rickets is a disorder of young children caused by a deficiency of vitamin D. Low levels of calcium and phosphorus in the blood are associated with skeletal deformities in these patients.

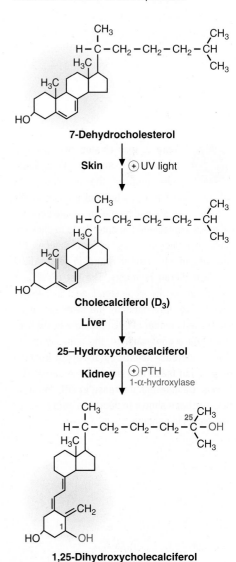

**FIG. 29.18.** Synthesis of active vitamin D. 1,25-$(OH)_2D_3$ is produced from 7-dehydrocholesterol, a precursor of cholesterol. In the skin, ultraviolet (UV) light produces cholecalciferol, which is hydroxylated at the 25-position in the liver and the 1-position in the kidney to form the active hormone. *PTH*, parathyroid hormone.

**Table 29.5    Diseases Discussed in Chapter 29**

| Disease or Disorder | Environmental or Genetic | Comments |
|---|---|---|
| Hypercholesterolemia | Both | Defined by elevated levels of cholesterol in the blood, often leading to coronary artery disease |
| Familial hypercholesterolemia, type II | Genetic | Defect in LDL receptor, leading to elevated cholesterol levels and premature death due to coronary artery disease |
| Virilization | Both | Excessive release of androgenic steroids due to a variety of causes. |
| Congenital adrenal hyperplasia (CAH) | Genetic | CAH is a constellation of disorders due to mutations in enzymes required for cortisol synthesis. One potential consequence is excessive androgen synthesis, which may lead to prenatal masculinization of females. The different symptoms observed between patients are due to different enzyme deficiencies in the patients. |
| Rickets | Environmental | Due to a lack of vitamin D, calcium metabolism is altered, leading to skeletal deformities. |

LDL, low-density lipoprotein.

**Anne J.** was treated with a statin (atorvastatin) and ezetimibe. Ezetimibe reduces the percentage of absorption of free cholesterol present in the lumen of the gut and hence the amount of cholesterol available to the enterocyte to package into chylomicrons. This, in turn, reduces the amount of cholesterol returning to the liver in chylomicron remnants. The net result is a reduction in the cholesterol pool in hepatocytes. The latter induces the synthesis of an increased number of LDL receptors by the liver cells. As a consequence, the capacity of the liver to increase hepatic uptake of LDL from the circulation leads to a decrease in serum LDL levels. Despite this decrease in LDL, the drug has not been shown to decrease cardiovascular events in patients.

Although therapy aimed at inserting competent LDL receptor genes into the cells of patients with homozygous FH is being designed for the future, the current approach in the heterozygote is to attempt to increase the rate of synthesis of LDL receptors in cells pharmacologically.

In addition to a HMG-CoA reductase inhibitor, **Anne J.** was treated with ezetimibe, a drug that blocks cholesterol absorption in the intestine, causing a portion of the dietary cholesterol to be carried into the feces rather than packaged into chylomicrons. This reduces the levels of chylomicron-based cholesterol and cholesterol delivered to the liver by chylomicron remnants.

HMG-CoA reductase inhibitors, such as atorvastatin, which Anne is also taking, stimulate the synthesis of additional LDL receptors by inhibiting HMG-CoA reductase, the rate-limiting enzyme for cholesterol synthesis. The subsequent decline in the intracellular free cholesterol pool stimulates the synthesis of additional LDL receptors. These additional receptors reduce circulating LDL cholesterol levels by increasing receptor-mediated endocytosis of LDL particles.

A combination of strict dietary and dual pharmacological therapy, aimed at decreasing the cholesterol levels of the body, is usually quite effective in correcting the lipid abnormality and hopefully, the associated risk of atherosclerotic cardiovascular disease in patients with heterozygous FH.

**Ivan A.** LDL cholesterol is the primary target of cholesterol-lowering therapy because both epidemiological and experimental evidence strongly suggest a benefit of lowering serum LDL cholesterol in the prevention of atherosclerotic cardiovascular disease. Similar evidence for raising subnormal levels of serum HDL cholesterol is less conclusive but adequate to support such efforts, particularly in high-risk patients, such as **Ivan A.**, who have multiple cardiovascular risk factors.

Despite diet, exercise, and an HMG-CoA reductase inhibitor, Mr. A.'s LDL cholesterol level is 231 mg/dL. According to Table 29.1, he is a candidate for more stringent dietary therapy and for drug treatment. He should be given a higher dose or more potent HMG-CoA reductase inhibitor. A low daily dose of aspirin (81 mg) could also be prescribed. It is important to gain early control of Mr. A.'s metabolic syndrome before the effect of insulin resistance can no longer be reversed. A variety of lipid-lowering agents are summarized in Table 29.6 .

**Table 29.6   Mechanism(s) of Action and Efficacy of Lipid-Lowering Agents**

| Agent | Mechanism of Action | Total Cholesterol | Percentage Change in Serum Lipid Level (Monotherapy) | | |
|---|---|---|---|---|---|
| | | | LDL Cholesterol | HDL Cholesterol | Triacylglycerols |
| Statins | Inhibit HMG-CoA reductase activity | ↓ 15–60 | ↓ 20–60 | ↑ 5–15 | ↓ 10–40 |
| Bile acid resins | Increase fecal excretion of bile salts | ↓ 15–20 | ↓ 10–25 | ↑ 3–5 | Variable, depending on pretreatment level of triacylglycerols (may increase) |
| Niacin | Activates LPL, reduces hepatic production of VLDL, reduces catabolism of HDL | ↓ 22–25 | ↓ 10–25 | ↑ 15–35 | ↓ 20–50 |
| Fibrates | Antagonize the transcription factor PPAR-α, causing an increase in LPL activity, a decrease in apoC-III production, and an increase in apoA-I production | ↓ 12–15 | Variable, depending on pretreatment levels of other lipids | ↑ 5–15 | ↓ 20–50 |
| Ezetimibe | Reduces intestinal absorption of free cholesterol from the gut lumen | ↓ 10–15 | ↓ 15–20 | ↑ 1–3 | ↓ 5–8 if triacylglycerols are high pretreatment |

LDL, low-density lipoprotein; HDL, high-density lipoprotein; HMG-CoA, β-hydroxy-β-methylglutaryl-CoA; LPL, lipoprotein lipase; VLDL, very low density lipoprotein; PPAR, peroxisome proliferator–activated receptor.
Adapted from Third report of the National Cholesterol Education Program (NCEP) expert panel on detection, evaluation, and treatment of high blood cholesterol in adults (Adult Treatment Panel III) final report. *Circulation.* 2002;106:3143–3457.

## REVIEW QUESTIONS-CHAPTER 29

1. Of the major risk factors for the development of atherosclerotic cardiovascular disease (ASCVD) such as sedentary lifestyle, obesity, cigarette smoking, diabetes mellitus, hypertension, and hyperlipidemia, which one, if present, is the only risk factor in a given patient without a history of having had a myocardial infarction that requires that the therapeutic goal for the serum LDL cholesterol level be less than 100 mg/dL?

   A. Obesity
   B. Cigarette smoking
   C. Diabetes mellitus
   D. Hypertension
   E. Sedentary lifestyle

2. If the intestinal pH decreases to 3.0 as a result of a deficiency of pancreatic exocrine secretion, which one of the following will be most negatively charged?

   A. Palmitate
   B. Cholic acid
   C. Cholesterol
   D. Glycocholic acid
   E. Taurocholic acid

3. A person with type IIA familial hypercholesterolemia had a blood cholesterol level of 360 mg/dL (recommended level <200 mg/dL) and blood triglyceride levels of 140 mg/dL (recommended level <150 mg/dL). The person most likely is expressing which one of the following?

   A. A decreased ability for receptor-mediated endocytosis of LDL
   B. A decreased ability to produce VLDL

   C. An increased ability to produce VLDL
   D. An elevation of HDL in the blood
   E. A decreased ability to convert VLDL to IDL

4. An article in the June 2002 issue of the Journal of Nutrition reported that S-allyl cysteine, which is found at high levels in garlic, increases the phosphorylation of HMG-CoA reductase. Which one of the effects listed below would be likely to result from ingesting large amounts of garlic?

   A. Increased cholesterol biosynthesis
   B. Decreased cholesterol biosynthesis
   C. Increased serum LDL levels
   D. Increased chylomicron levels
   E. Decreased frequency of vampire bites

5. Cholestyramine is used to reduce serum cholesterol because of its ability to interfere with the enterohepatic circulation of bile salts, resulting in increased amounts of bile salts in the feces. When this drug is given, the liver responds with increased synthesis of which one of the following?

   A. Vitamin K
   B. Lecithin
   C. Fatty acids
   D. Mevalonate
   E. Triglyceride

# 30 Integration of Carbohydrate and Lipid Metabolism

## CHAPTER OUTLINE

**I. REGULATION OF CARBOHYDRATE AND LIPID METABOLISM IN THE FED STATE**
  A. Mechanisms that affect glycogen and triacylglycerol synthesis in liver
    1. Glucokinase
    2. Glycogen synthase
    3. Phosphofructokinase-1 and pyruvate kinase
    4. Pyruvate dehydrogenase and pyruvate carboxylase
    5. Citrate lyase, malic enzyme, and glucose-6-phosphate dehydrogenase
    6. Acetyl CoA carboxylase
    7. Fatty acid synthase complex
  B. Mechanisms that affect the fate of chylomicrons and very low density lipoproteins
  C. Mechanisms that affect triacylglycerol storage in adipose tissue

**II. REGULATION OF CARBOHYDRATE AND LIPID METABOLISM DURING FASTING**
  A. Mechanisms in liver that serve to maintain blood glucose levels
  B. Mechanisms that affect lipolysis in adipose tissue
  C. Mechanisms that affect ketone body production by the liver
  D. Regulation of the use of glucose and fatty acids by muscle

**III. THE IMPORTANCE OF ADENOSINE MONOPHOSPHATE AND FRUCTOSE 2,6-BISPHOSPHATE**

**IV. THE ADENOSINE MONOPHOSPHATE–ACTIVATED PROTEIN KINASE**

**V. GENERAL SUMMARY**

## KEY POINTS

- Three key controlling elements determine whether a fuel is metabolized or stored: hormones, concentration of available fuels, and energy needs of the body.
- Key intracellular enzymes are generally regulated by allosteric activation and inhibition, by covalent modification, by transcriptional control, and by degradation.
- Regulation is complex in order to allow sensitivity and feedback to multiple stimuli so that an exact balance can be maintained between synthesis of a product and need for the product.
- The insulin/glucagon ratio is responsible for the hormonal regulation of carbohydrate and lipid metabolism.
- The key enzymes of glycolysis, fatty acid synthesis, glycogen synthesis, glycogenolysis, and gluconeogenesis are all regulated in a coordinated manner, allowing the appropriate pathways to be activated and inhibited without the creation of futile cycles.
- This chapter summarizes, in one package, all of the regulatory events discussed in the previous 14 chapters.

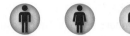

# THE WAITING ROOM

A few months after her last hospitalization, **Dianne A.** was once again brought to the hospital emergency room in diabetic ketoacidosis (DKA). Blood samples for glucose and electrolytes were drawn repeatedly during the first 24 hours. The hospital laboratory reported that the serum in each of these specimens appeared opalescent rather than having its normal clear or transparent appearance. This opalescence results from light scattering caused by the presence of elevated levels of triacylglycerol-rich lipoproteins in the blood.

When **Deborah S.** initially presented (see Chapter 21) with type 2 diabetes mellitus at age 39 years, she was approximately 30 lb higher than her ideal weight. Her high serum glucose levels were accompanied by abnormalities in her 14-hour fasting lipid profile. Her serum total cholesterol, low-density lipoprotein (LDL) cholesterol, and triacylglycerol levels were elevated, and her serum high-density lipoprotein (HDL) cholesterol level was lower than the normal range.

## I. REGULATION OF CARBOHYDRATE AND LIPID METABOLISM IN THE FED STATE

### A. Mechanisms That Affect Glycogen and Triacylglycerol Synthesis in Liver

After a meal, the liver synthesizes glycogen and triacylglycerol. The level of glycogen stored in the liver can increase from approximately 80 g after an overnight fast to a limit of approximately 200 to 300 g. Although the liver synthesizes triacylglycerol, it does not store this fuel but rather packages it in very low density lipoprotein (VLDL) and secretes it into the blood. The fatty acids of the VLDL triacylglycerols secreted from the liver are stored as adipose triacylglycerols. Adipose tissue has an almost infinite capacity to store fat, limited mainly by the ability of the heart to pump blood through the capillaries of the expanding adipose mass. Although we store fat throughout our bodies, it tends to accumulate in places where it does not interfere too much with our mobility: in the abdomen, hips, thighs, and buttocks.

Both the synthesis of liver glycogen and the conversion by the liver of dietary glucose to triacylglycerol (lipogenesis) are regulated by mechanisms involving key enzymes in these pathways.

#### 1. GLUCOKINASE

After a meal, glucose can be converted to glycogen or to triacylglycerol in the liver. For both processes, glucose is first converted to glucose-6-phosphate by glucokinase, a liver enzyme that has a high Michaelis constant ($K_m$) (low affinity) for glucose (Fig. 30.1). Because of the enzyme's low affinity for glucose, this enzyme is most active in the fed state, when the concentration of glucose is particularly high because the hepatic portal vein carries digestive products directly from the intestine to the liver. Synthesis of glucokinase is also induced by insulin (which is elevated after a meal) and repressed by glucagon (which is elevated during fasting). In keeping with the liver's function in maintaining blood glucose levels, this system is set up such that the liver can metabolize glucose only when sugar levels are high and not when sugar levels are low.

#### 2. GLYCOGEN SYNTHASE

In the conversion of glucose-6-phosphate to glycogen, the key regulatory enzyme is glycogen synthase. This enzyme is activated by dephosphorylation, which occurs when insulin is elevated and glucagon is decreased (Fig. 30.2) and by the increased level of glucose.

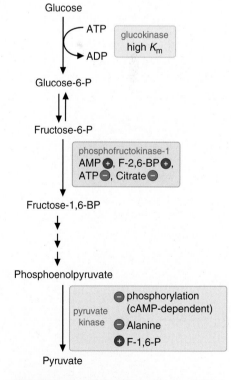

**FIG. 30.1.** Regulation of glucokinase, PFK-1, and pyruvate kinase in the liver. *Fructose-1,6-BP*, fructose 1,6-bisphosphate; *F-2,6-BP*, fructose 2,6-bisphosphate.

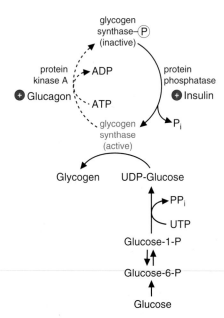

**FIG. 30.2.** Regulation of glycogen synthase. This enzyme is phosphorylated by a series of kinases, which are initiated by the cAMP-dependent protein kinase under fasting conditions. It is dephosphorylated and active after a meal, and glycogen is stored. *ADP*, adenosine diphosphate; *ATP*, adenosine triphosphate; *UDP*, uridine diphosphate; *UTP*, uridine triphosphate; ⓟ, phosphate; ⊕, activated by; ⊖, inhibited by.

### 3. PHOSPHOFRUCTOKINASE-1 AND PYRUVATE KINASE

For lipogenesis, glucose-6-phosphate is converted through glycolysis to pyruvate. Key enzymes that regulate this pathway in the liver are phosphofructokinase-1 (PFK-1) and pyruvate kinase. PFK-1 is allosterically activated in the fed state by fructose 2,6-bisphosphate and adenosine monophosphate (AMP) (see Fig. 30.1). PFK-2, the enzyme that produces the activator fructose 2,6-bisphosphate, is dephosphorylated and the kinase activity is active after a meal (see Chapter 19). Pyruvate kinase is also activated by dephosphorylation, which is stimulated by the increase of the insulin/glucagon ratio in the fed state (see Fig. 30.1).

### 4. PYRUVATE DEHYDROGENASE AND PYRUVATE CARBOXYLASE

The conversion of pyruvate to fatty acids requires a source of acetyl coenzyme A (CoA) in the cytosol. Pyruvate can only be converted to acetyl CoA in mitochondria, so it enters mitochondria and forms acetyl CoA through the pyruvate dehydrogenase (PDH) reaction. This enzyme is dephosphorylated and most active when its supply of substrates and adenosine diphosphate (ADP) is high, its products are used, and insulin is present (see Fig. 17.11).

Pyruvate is also converted to oxaloacetate. The enzyme that catalyzes this reaction, pyruvate carboxylase, is activated by acetyl CoA. Because acetyl CoA cannot cross the mitochondrial membrane directly to form fatty acids in the cytosol, it condenses with oxaloacetate, producing citrate. The citrate that is not required for tricarboxylic acid (TCA) cycle activity crosses the membrane and enters the cytosol.

As fatty acids are produced under conditions of high energy, the high NADH/NAD$^+$ ratio in the mitochondria inhibits isocitrate dehydrogenase, which leads to citrate accumulation within the mitochondrial matrix. As the citrate accumulates, it is transported out into the cytosol to donate carbons for fatty acid synthesis.

### 5. CITRATE LYASE, MALIC ENZYME, AND GLUCOSE-6-PHOSPHATE DEHYDROGENASE

In the cytosol, citrate is cleaved by citrate lyase, an inducible enzyme, to form oxaloacetate and acetyl CoA (Fig. 30.3). The acetyl CoA is used for fatty acid

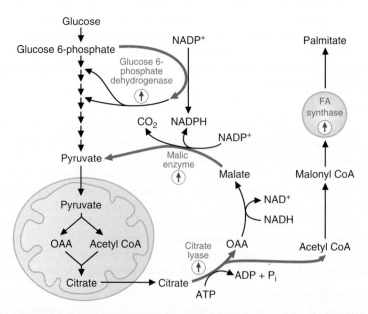

**FIG. 30.3.** Regulation of citrate lyase, malic enzyme, glucose-6-phosphate dehydrogenase, and fatty acid synthase. Citrate lyase, which provides acetyl CoA for fatty acid biosynthesis, the enzymes that provide NADPH (malic enzyme, glucose-6-phosphate dehydrogenase), as well as fatty acid synthase, are inducible (↑). *FA*, fatty acid.

biosynthesis and for cholesterol synthesis, pathways that are activated by insulin. Oxaloacetate is recycled to pyruvate via cytosolic malate dehydrogenase and malic enzyme, which is inducible. Malic enzyme generates NADPH for the reactions of the fatty acid synthase complex. NADPH is also produced by the two enzymes of the pentose phosphate pathway (see Chapter 24), glucose-6-phosphate dehydrogenase and 6-phosphogluconate dehydrogenase. Glucose-6-phosphate dehydrogenase is also induced by insulin.

## 6. ACETYL CoA CARBOXYLASE

Acetyl CoA is converted to malonyl CoA, which provides the two-carbon units for elongation of the growing fatty acyl chain on the fatty acid synthase complex. Acetyl CoA carboxylase, the enzyme that catalyzes the conversion of acetyl CoA to malonyl CoA, is controlled by three of the major mechanisms that regulate enzyme activity (Fig. 30.4). It is activated by citrate, which causes the enzyme to polymerize, and inhibited by long-chain fatty acyl CoA. A phosphatase stimulated by insulin activates the enzyme by dephosphorylation. The third means by which this enzyme is regulated is induction: The quantity of the enzyme increases in the fed state.

Malonyl CoA, the product of the acetyl CoA carboxylase reaction, provides the carbons for the synthesis of palmitate on the fatty acid synthase complex. Malonyl CoA also inhibits carnitine palmitoyltransferase I (CPTI, also known as carnitine acyltransferase I), the enzyme that prepares long-chain fatty acyl CoA for transport into mitochondria. In the fed state, when acetyl CoA carboxylase is active and malonyl CoA levels are elevated, newly synthesized fatty acids are converted to triacylglycerols for storage rather than being transported into mitochondria for oxidation and formation of ketone bodies.

## 7. FATTY ACID SYNTHASE COMPLEX

In a well-fed individual, the quantity of the fatty acid synthase complex is increased (see Fig. 30.3). The genes that produce this enzyme complex are induced by

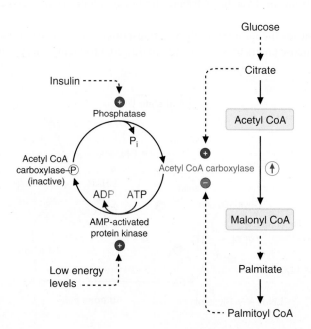

**FIG. 30.4.** Regulation of acetyl CoA carboxylase (ACC). ACC is regulated by activation and inhibition, by phosphorylation (mediated by the AMP-activated protein kinase) and dephosphorylation (via an insulin-stimulated phosphatase), and by induction and repression. It is active in the fed state.

increases in the insulin/glucagon ratio. The amount of the complex increases slowly after a few days of a high-carbohydrate diet.

Glucose-6-phosphate dehydrogenase, which generates NADPH in the pentose phosphate pathway, and malic enzyme, which produces NADPH, are also induced by the increase of insulin.

The palmitate produced by the synthase complex is converted to palmityl CoA and elongated and desaturated to form other fatty acyl CoA molecules, which are converted to triacylglycerols. These triacylglycerols are packaged and secreted into the blood as VLDL.

### B. Mechanisms That Affect the Fate of Chylomicrons and Very Low Density Lipoproteins

The lipoprotein triacylglycerols in chylomicrons and VLDL are hydrolyzed to fatty acids and glycerol by lipoprotein lipase (LPL), an enzyme attached to endothelial cells of capillaries in muscle and adipose tissue. The enzyme found in muscle, particularly heart muscle, has a low $K_m$ (high affinity) for these blood lipoproteins. Therefore, it acts even when these lipoproteins are present at very low concentrations in the blood. The fatty acids enter muscle cells and are oxidized for energy. The enzyme found in adipose tissue has a higher $K_m$ and is most active after a meal when blood lipoprotein levels are elevated.

### C. Mechanisms That Affect Triacylglycerol Storage in Adipose Tissue

Insulin stimulates adipose cells to synthesize and secrete LPL, which hydrolyzes the chylomicron and VLDL triacylglycerols. Apolipoprotein (apo) C-II, donated to chylomicrons and VLDL by HDL, activates LPL (Fig. 30.5).

Fatty acids released from chylomicrons and VLDL by LPL are stored as triacylglycerols in adipose cells. The glycerol released by LPL is not used by adipose cells because they lack glycerol kinase. Glycerol can be used by liver cells, however, because these cells do contain glycerol kinase. In the fed state, liver cells convert glycerol to the glycerol moiety of the triacylglycerols of VLDL, which is secreted from the liver to distribute the newly synthesized triglycerides to the tissues.

Insulin causes the number of glucose transporters in adipose cell membranes to increase. Glucose enters these cells and is oxidized, producing energy and providing

**Dianne A.** has type 1 diabetes mellitus, a disease associated with a severe deficiency or absence of insulin caused by destruction of the β cells of the pancreas. One of the effects of insulin is to stimulate production of LPL. Because of low insulin levels, Dianne tends to have low levels of this enzyme. Hydrolysis of the triacylglycerols in chylomicrons and in VLDL is decreased, and hypertriglyceridemia results.

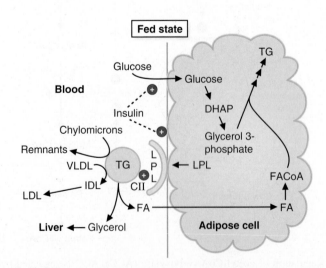

**FIG. 30.5.** Regulation of the storage of triacylglycerols (TG) in adipose tissue. Insulin stimulates the secretion of LPL from adipose cells and the transport of glucose into these cells. ApoC-II activates LPL. *FA*, fatty acids.

the glycerol 3-phosphate moiety for triacylglycerol synthesis (via the dihydroxy-acetone phosphate intermediate of glycolysis).

## II. REGULATION OF CARBOHYDRATE AND LIPID METABOLISM DURING FASTING

### A. Mechanisms in Liver That Serve to Maintain Blood Glucose Levels

During fasting, the insulin/glucagon ratio decreases. Liver glycogen is degraded to produce blood glucose because enzymes of glycogen degradation are activated by cyclic adenosine monophosphate (cAMP)-directed phosphorylation (see Fig. 23.7). Glucagon stimulates adenylate cyclase to produce cAMP, which activates protein kinase A. Protein kinase A phosphorylates phosphorylase kinase, which then phosphorylates and activates glycogen phosphorylase. Protein kinase A also phosphorylates but, in this case, *inactivates* glycogen synthase.

Gluconeogenesis is stimulated because the synthesis of phosphoenolpyruvate carboxykinase, fructose 1,6-bisphosphatase, and glucose-6-phosphatase is induced and because there is an increased availability of precursors. Fructose 1,6-bisphosphatase is also activated because the levels of its inhibitor, fructose 2,6-bisphosphate, are low (Fig. 30.6). During fasting, the activities of the corresponding enzymes of glycolysis are decreased.

Induction of enzyme synthesis requires activation of transcription factors. One of the factors that are activated is CREB, which stands for cAMP response element binding protein. CREB is phosphorylated and activated by the cAMP-dependent protein kinase A (PKA), which itself is activated upon glucagon or epinephrine stimulation. Other transcription factors are activated by cAMP, but the regulation of those factors by cAMP is not as well understood as it is for CREB.

### B. Mechanisms That Affect Lipolysis in Adipose Tissue

During fasting, as blood insulin levels fall and glucagon levels rise, the level of cAMP rises in adipose cells. Consequently, PKA is activated and causes phosphorylation of hormone-sensitive lipase (HSL). The phosphorylated form of this enzyme is active and cleaves fatty acids from triacylglycerols (Fig. 30.7). Other hormones (e.g., epinephrine, adrenocorticotropic hormone [ACTH], growth hormone) also activate this enzyme.

### C. Mechanisms That Affect Ketone Body Production by the Liver

As fatty acids are released from adipose tissue during fasting, they travel in the blood complexed with albumin. These fatty acids are oxidized by various tissues, particularly muscle. In the liver, fatty acids are transported into mitochondria because acetyl CoA carboxylase is inactive, malonyl CoA levels are low, and CPTI (carnitine acyltransferase I) is active. Acetyl CoA, produced by β-oxidation, is converted to ketone bodies. Ketone bodies are used as an energy source by many tissues (Table 30.1) to spare the use of glucose and the necessity of degrading muscle protein to provide the precursors for gluconeogenesis. The high levels of acetyl CoA in the liver (derived from fat oxidation) inhibit PDH (which prevents pyruvate from being converted to acetyl CoA) and activate pyruvate carboxylase, which produces oxaloacetate for gluconeogenesis. The oxaloacetate does not condense with acetyl CoA to form citrate for two reasons. The first is that under these conditions (a high rate of fat oxidation in the liver mitochondria), energy levels in the mitochondrial matrix are high; that is, there are high levels of NADH and ATP present. The high NADH level inhibits isocitrate dehydrogenase. As a result, citrate accumulates and inhibits citrate synthase from producing more citrate. The second reason that citrate synthesis is depressed is that

Dianne A. suffers from hyperglycemia because her insulin levels tend to be low and her glucagon levels tend to be high. Her muscle and adipose cells do not take glucose up at a normal rate, and she produces glucose by glycogenolysis and gluconeogenesis. As a result, her blood glucose levels are elevated. Deborah S. is in a similar metabolic state. However, in this case, she produces insulin, but her tissues are resistant to its actions.

Insulin normally inhibits lipolysis by decreasing the lipolytic activity of HSL in the adipocyte. Individuals such as Dianne A., who have a deficiency of insulin, have increased lipolysis and a subsequent increase in the concentration of free fatty acids in the blood. The liver, in turn, uses some of these fatty acids to synthesize triacylglycerols, which then are used in the hepatic production of VLDL. VLDL is not stored in the liver but is secreted into the blood, raising its serum concentration. Dianne also has low levels of LPL because of decreased insulin levels. Her hypertriglyceridemia is the result, therefore, of both overproduction of VLDL by the liver and decreased breakdown of VLDL triacylglycerol for storage in adipose cells.

The serum begins to appear cloudy when the triacylglycerol level reaches 200 mg/dL. As the triacylglycerol level increases still further, the degree of serum opalescence increases proportionately.

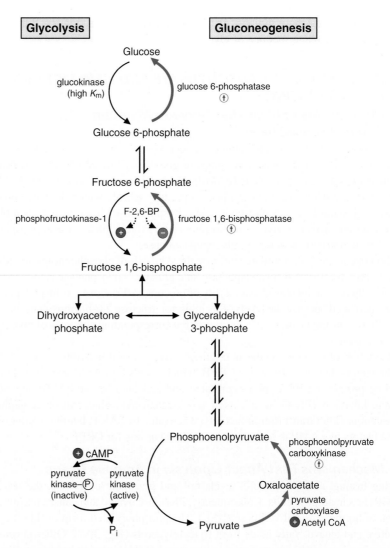

**FIG. 30.6.** Regulation of gluconeogenesis *(red arrows)* and glycolysis *(black arrows)* during fasting. The gluconeogenic enzymes phosphoenolpyruvate carboxykinase, fructose 1,6-bisphosphatase, and glucose-6-phosphatase are induced (↑). Fructose 1,6-bisphosphatase is also active because during fasting, the level of its inhibitor, fructose 2,6-bisphosphate, is low. The corresponding enzymes of glycolysis are not very active during fasting. The rate of glucokinase is low because it has a high $K_m$ for glucose and the glucose concentration is low. PFK-1 is not very active because the concentration of its activator fructose 2,6-bisphosphate is low. Pyruvate kinase is inactivated by cAMP-mediated phosphorylation. *F-2,6-BP,* fructose 2,6 bisphosphate.

the high NADH/NAD$^+$ ratio also diverts oxaloacetate into malate, such that the malate can exit the mitochondria (via the malate–aspartate shuttle) for use in gluconeogenesis.

### D. Regulation of the Use of Glucose and Fatty Acids by Muscle

During exercise, the fuel that is used initially by muscle cells is muscle glycogen. As exercise continues and the blood supply to the tissue increases, glucose is taken up from the blood and oxidized. Liver glycogenolysis and gluconeogenesis replenish the blood glucose supply. However, because insulin levels drop, the concentration of the GLUT4 glucose transporters in the membrane is reduced, thereby reducing glucose entry from the circulation into the muscle. However, muscle

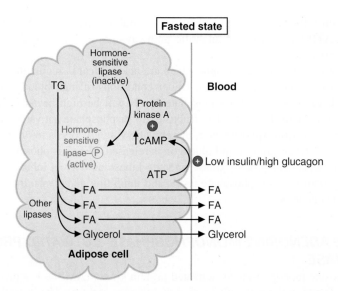

***FIG. 30.7.*** Regulation of HSL in adipose tissue. During fasting, the glucagon/insulin ratio rises, causing cAMP levels to be elevated. PKA is activated and phosphorylates HSL, activating this enzyme. HSL-P initiates the mobilization of adipose triacylglycerol by removing a fatty acid *(FA)*. Other lipases then act, producing fatty acids and glycerol. Insulin stimulates the phosphatase that inactivates HSL in the fed state.

GLUT4 transporters are also induced by high AMP levels, through the actions of the AMP-activated protein kinase. Thus, if energy levels are low and the concentration of AMP increases, glucose can still be transported from the circulation into the muscle to provide energy. This will most frequently be the case during periods of exercise.

However, as fatty acids become available because of increased lipolysis of adipose triacylglycerols, the exercising muscle begins to oxidize fatty acids. β-Oxidation produces NADH and acetyl CoA, which slow the flow of carbon from glucose through the reaction catalyzed by PDH. Thus, the oxidation of fatty acids provides a major portion of the increased demand for ATP generation and spares blood glucose.

## III.  THE IMPORTANCE OF ADENOSINE MONOPHOSPHATE AND FRUCTOSE 2,6-BISPHOSPHATE

The switch between catabolic and anabolic pathways is often regulated by the levels of AMP and fructose 2,6-bisphosphate in cells, particularly the liver. It is logical for AMP to be a critical regulator. Because a cell uses ATP in energy-requiring pathways, the levels of AMP accumulate more rapidly than that of ADP because of the adenylate kinase reaction (2 ADP → ATP and AMP). The rise in AMP levels then signals that more energy is required (usually through allosteric binding sites on enzymes and the activation of the AMP-activated protein kinase),

**Table 30.1   Fuel Utilization by Various Tissues during Starvation (Fasting)**

| *Tissue* | *Glucose* | *Fatty Acids* | *Ketone Bodies* |
|---|---|---|---|
| Nervous system | ++ | − | ++ |
| Skeletal muscle | − | ++ | ++ |
| Heart muscle | − | ++ | ++ |
| Liver | − | ++ | − |
| Intestinal epithelial cells | − | − | ++ |
| Kidney | − | + | + |

and the cell will switch to the activation of catabolic pathways. As AMP levels drop and ATP levels rise, the anabolic pathways are now activated to store the excess energy.

The levels of fructose 2,6-bisphosphate are also critical in regulating glycolysis versus gluconeogenesis in the liver. Under conditions of high blood glucose and insulin release, fructose 2,6-bisphosphate levels will be high because the PFK-2 kinase is in its activated state. The fructose 2,6-bisphosphate activates PFK-1 and inhibits fructose 1,6-bisphosphatase, thereby allowing glycolysis to proceed. When blood glucose levels are low and glucagon is released, PFK-2 is phosphorylated by the cAMP-dependent protein kinase and the kinase activity is inhibited, thereby lowering fructose 2,6-bisphosphate levels and inhibiting glycolysis, thereby favoring gluconeogenesis.

## IV. THE ADENOSINE MONOPHOSPHATE–ACTIVATED PROTEIN KINASE

The adenosine monophosphate–activated protein kinase (AMPK) is a pivotal regulatory molecule in the metabolism of carbohydrates and fats. The overall effect of AMPK activation in the liver is reduced fatty acid, cholesterol and triglyceride synthesis, and reduced protein synthesis. There is a concomitant increase in fatty acid oxidation to raise ATP levels. The overall effect is to reduce the activity of energy-requiring pathways and activate energy-generating pathways.

The AMPK can be activated in a number of ways, all of which depend on increased AMP levels within the cell. As the concentration of AMP increases, AMPK is activated by allosteric means, or by phosphorylation by the protein kinase LKB1, or by phosphorylation by a calmodulin kinase kinase. AMPK is inactivated by dephosphorylation by protein phosphatases or a decrease in AMP levels. Small changes in intracellular AMP levels can have profound effects on AMPK activity because of these multiple regulatory pathways.

AMPK is a heterotrimeric complex that consists of a catalytic subunit ($\alpha$) and two regulatory subunits ($\beta$ and $\gamma$). The allosteric activation of AMPK occurs via AMP binding to the $\alpha$-subunit; the phosphorylation activation of AMPK occurs via threonine phosphorylation on the $\alpha$-subunit. Different tissues express different isoforms of the $\alpha$-, $\beta$-, and $\gamma$-subunits, giving rise to a wide variety of isozymes of AMPK in the different tissues.

## V. GENERAL SUMMARY

All of the material in this chapter was presented previously. However, because this information is so critical for understanding biochemistry in a way that will allow it to be used in interpreting clinical situations, it was summarized in this chapter. In addition, the information presented previously under carbohydrate metabolism has been integrated with lipid metabolism. We have, for the most part, left out the role of allosteric modifiers and other regulatory mechanisms that finely coordinate these processes to an exquisite level. Because such details may be important for specific clinical situations, we hope this summary will serve as a framework to which the details can be fitted as students advance in their clinical studies.

Figure 30.8 is a comprehensive figure, and Tables 30.2 and 30.3 provide a list of the major regulatory enzymes of carbohydrate and lipid metabolism in the liver, an order of the events that occur and the mechanisms by which they are controlled. This figure and tables should help students to integrate this mass of material.

Now that many of the details of the pathways have been presented, it would be worthwhile to reread the first chapter of this book. A student who understands biochemistry within the context of fuel metabolism is in a very good position to solve clinical problems that involve metabolic derangements.

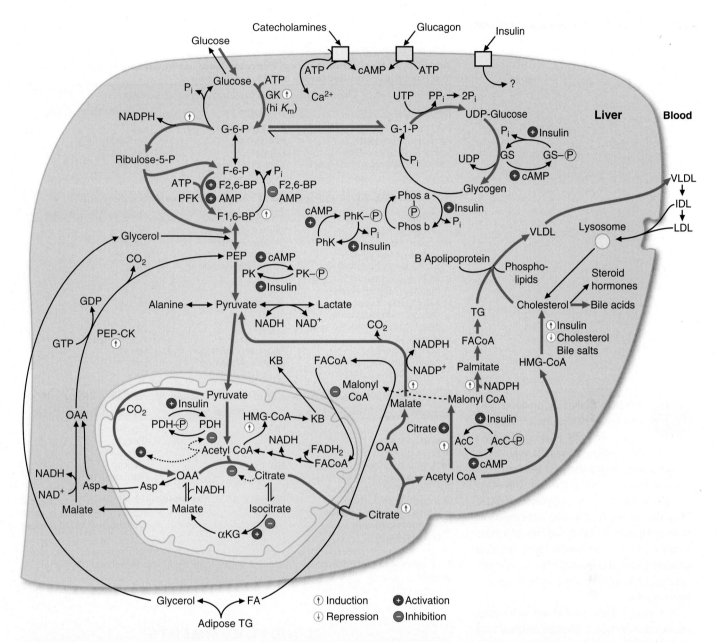

**FIG. 30.8.** Regulation of carbohydrate and lipid metabolism in the liver. *Solid red arrows* indicate the flow of metabolites in the fed state. *Solid black arrows* indicate the flow during fasting. *ACC*, acetyl CoA carboxylase; *αKG*, α-ketoglutarate; *F1,6-BP*, fructose 1,6-bisphosphate; *F2,6-BP*, fructose 2,6-bisphosphate; *F-6-P*, fructose 6-phosphate; *G-6-P*, glucose-6-phosphate; *FA*, fatty acid or fatty acyl group; *GK*, glucokinase; *GS*, glycogen synthase; *OAA*, oxaloacetate; *circled P*, phosphate group; *PEP*, phosphoenolpyruvate; *PFK*, phosphofructokinase-1; *Phos*, glycogen phosphorylase; *PhK*, phosphorylase kinase; *PK*, pyruvate kinase; *TG*, triacylglycerol.

**Table 30.2   Flowchart of Changes in Liver Metabolism**

| *When Blood Sugar Increases* | *When Blood Sugar Decreases* |
|---|---|
| Insulin is released, which leads to the **dephosphorylation** of | Glucagon is released, which leads to the **phosphorylation** of |
| • PFK-2 (kinase activity now active) | • PFK-2 (phosphatase activity now active) |
| • Pyruvate kinase (now active) | • Pyruvate kinase (now inactive) |
| • Glycogen synthase (now active) | • Glycogen synthase (now inactive) |
| • Phosphorylase kinase (now inactive) | • Phosphorylase kinase (now active) |
| • Glycogen phosphorylase (now inactive) | • Glycogen phosphorylase (now active) |
| • Pyruvate dehydrogenase (now active) | • Pyruvate dehydrogenase (now inactive) |
| • Acetyl CoA carboxylase (now active) | • Acetyl CoA carboxylase (now inactive) |
| Which leads to **active** | Which leads to **active** |
| • Glycolysis | • Glycogenolysis |
| • Fatty acid synthesis | • Fatty acid oxidation |
| • Glycogen synthesis | • Gluconeogenesis |

PFK-2, phosphofructokinase-2; CoA, coenzyme A.

**Table 30.3   Regulation of Liver Enzymes Involved in Glycogen, Blood Glucose, and Triacylglycerol Synthesis and Degradation**

| Liver Enzymes Regulated by Activation/Inhibition | | |
| --- | --- | --- |
| **Enzyme** | **Activated by** | **State in Which Active** |
| PFK-1 | Fructose 2,6-bisP, AMP | Fed |
| Pyruvate carboxylase | Acetyl CoA | Fed and fasting |
| Acetyl CoA carboxylase | Citrate | Fed |
| Carnitine palmitoyltransferase I | Loss of inhibitor (malonyl CoA) | Fasting |

| Liver Enzymes Regulated by Phosphorylation/Dephosphorylation | | |
| --- | --- | --- |
| **Enzyme** | **Active Form** | **State in Which Active** |
| Glycogen synthase | Dephosphorylated | Fed |
| Phosphorylase kinase | Phosphorylated | Fasting |
| Glycogen phosphorylase | Phosphorylated | Fasting |
| PFK-2/F2,6-bisphosphatase (acts as a kinase, increasing fructose 2,6-bisP levels) | Dephosphorylated | Fed |
| PFK-2/F2,6-bisphosphatase (acts as a phosphatase, decreasing fructose 2,6-bisP levels) | Phosphorylated | Fasting |
| Pyruvate kinase | Dephosphorylated | Fed |
| Pyruvate dehydrogenase | Dephosphorylated | Fed |
| Acetyl CoA carboxylase | Dephosphorylated | Fed |

| Liver Enzymes Regulated by Induction/Repression | | |
| --- | --- | --- |
| **Enzyme** | **State in Which Induced** | **Process Affected** |
| Glucokinase | Fed | Glucose → TG |
| Citrate lyase | Fed | Glucose → TG |
| Acetyl CoA carboxylase | Fed | Glucose → TG |
| Fatty acid synthase | Fed | Glucose → TG |
| Malic enzyme | Fed | Production of NADPH |
| Glucose-6-P dehydrogenase | Fed | Production of NADPH |
| Glucose-6-phosphatase | Fasted | Production of blood glucose |
| Fructose 1,6-bisphosphatase | Fasted | Production of blood glucose |
| Phosphoenolpyruvate carboxykinase | Fasted | Production of blood glucose |

AMP, adenosine monophosphate; fructose 2,6-bisP, fructose 2,6-bisphosphate; TG, triacylglycerol.

Because **Dianne A.** produces very little insulin, she is prone to developing ketoacidosis. When insulin levels are low, HSL of adipose tissue is very active, resulting in increased lipolysis. The fatty acids that are released travel to the liver, where they are converted to the triacylglycerols of VLDL. They also undergo β-oxidation and conversion to ketone bodies. If Dianne does not take exogenous insulin or if her insulin levels decrease abruptly for some physiologic reason, she may develop DKA. In fact, she has had repeated bouts of DKA.

For reasons that are not as well understood, individuals with type 2 diabetes mellitus, such as **Deborah S.**, do not tend to develop ketoacidosis. One possible explanation is that the insulin resistance is tissue specific; the insulin sensitivity of adipocytes may be greater than that of muscle and liver. It has been suggested that the level of insulin required to suppress lipolysis is only 10% that required to enhance glucose use by muscle and adipocyte. Such a tissue-specific sensitivity would lead to less fatty acids being released from adipocytes in type 2 diabetes than in type 1 diabetes, although in both cases, the release of fatty acids would be greater than that of an individual without the disease. If, however, a person with type 2 diabetes has a precipitating event, such as the release of stress hormones, then ketoacidosis is more likely to be found as the stress hormones counteract the effects of insulin on the adipocyte.

## CLINICAL COMMENTS

Diseases discussed in this chapter are summarized in Table 30.4.

**Dianne A.** Diabetes mellitus is a well-accepted risk factor for the development of coronary artery disease; the risk is three to four times higher in the population with diabetes than in the population without diabetes. Although chronically elevated serum levels of chylomicrons and VLDL may contribute to this atherogenic predisposition, the premature vascular disease seen in **Dianne A.** and other patients with type 1 diabetes mellitus, as well as **Deborah S.** and other patients with type 2 diabetes mellitus, is also related to other abnormalities in lipid metabolism. Among these are the increase in glycation (nonenzymatic attachment of glucose molecules to proteins) of LDL apolipoproteins as well as glycation of the proteins of the LDL receptor, which occurs when serum glucose levels are chronically elevated. These glycations interfere with the normal interaction or "fit" of the circulating LDL particles with their specific receptors on cell membranes. As a consequence, the rate of uptake of circulating LDL by the normal target cells is diminished. The LDL particles, therefore, remain in the circulation and eventually bind nonspecifically to "scavenger" receptors located on macrophages adjacent to the endothelial surfaces of blood vessels, one of the early steps in the process of atherogenesis.

**Table 30.4   Diseases Discussed in Chapter 30**

| Disease or Disorder | Environmental or Genetic | Comments |
|---|---|---|
| Diabetic ketoacidosis (type 1 diabetes) | Environmental | Diabetic ketoacidosis occurs due to an elevation of ketone body levels due to reduced levels of insulin in a type 1 diabetic. Diabetic ketoacidosis is not normally seen in type 2 diabetics due to only a partial resistance of adipocytes to circulating insulin. |
| Type 2 diabetes | Both | Reduced ability of tissues to respond to insulin even though insulin is being produced. Different tissues may display a differential sensitivity to insulin, particularly fat cells as compared to muscle cells. |

## REVIEW QUESTIONS-CHAPTER 30

1.  A 20-year-old woman with diabetes mellitus was admitted to the hospital in a semiconscious state with fever, nausea, and vomiting. Her breath smelled of acetone. A urine sample was strongly positive for ketone bodies. Which one of the following statements correctly describes an aspect of this woman's case?

    A.  A blood glucose test would probably show that her blood glucose level was well below 80 mg/dL.
    B.  She should be given a glucose infusion to regain consciousness.
    C.  An insulin injection would decrease her ketone body production.
    D.  Glucagon should be administered to stimulate glycogenolysis and gluconeogenesis in the liver.
    E.  The acetone was produced by decarboxylation of the ketone body β-hydroxybutyrate.

2.  A woman was told by her physician to go on a low-fat diet. She decided to continue to consume the same number of calories by increasing her carbohydrate intake while decreasing her fat intake. Which one of the following blood lipoprotein levels would be decreased as a consequence of her diet?

    A.  Chylomicrons
    B.  VLDL
    C.  IDL
    D.  HDL
    E.  LDL

3.  Assume that an individual has been eating excess calories daily such that they will gain weight. Under which one of the following conditions would the person gain weight most rapidly?

    A.  If all the excess calories were due to carbohydrate
    B.  If all the excess calories were due to triacylglycerol

    C.  If all the excess calories were split 50%/50% between carbohydrate and triacylglycerol
    D.  If all the excess calories were split 25%/75% between carbohydrate and triacylglycerol
    E.  It makes no difference what form the excess calories are in.

4.  A chronic alcoholic has been admitted to the hospital due to a severe hypoglycemic episode brought about by excessive alcohol consumption for the past 5 days. A blood lipid analysis indicates much higher than expected VLDL levels. The elevated VLDL is due to which one of the following underlying causes?

    A.  Elevated NADH levels in the liver
    B.  Alcohol-induced inhibition of lipoprotein lipase
    C.  Alcohol-induced transcription of the apoB-100 gene
    D.  NADH activation of phosphoenolpyruvate carboxykinase
    E.  Acetaldehyde induction of enzymes on the endoplasmic reticulum

5.  Certain patients with abetalipoproteinemia frequently have difficulties in maintaining blood volume; their blood has trouble clotting. This symptom is due to which one of the following?

    A.  Inability to synthesize clotting factors
    B.  Inability to synthesize fatty acids
    C.  Inability to absorb short-chain fatty acids
    D.  Inability to produce chylomicrons
    E.  Inability to produce VLDL

# 31  Protein Digestion and Amino Acid Absorption

## CHAPTER OUTLINE

## KEY POINTS

- Proteases (proteolytic enzymes) break down dietary proteins into peptides and then their constituent amino acids in the stomach and intestine.
- Pepsin initiates protein breakdown in the stomach.
- Upon entering the small intestine, inactive zymogens secreted from the pancreas are activated to continue protein digestion.
- Enzymes produced by the intestinal epithelial cells are also required to fully degrade proteins.
- The amino acids generated by proteolysis in the intestinal lumen are transported into the intestinal epithelial cells, from which they enter the circulation for use by the tissues.
- Transport systems for amino acids are similar to transport systems for monosaccharides; both facilitative and active transport systems exist.
- There are several overlapping transport systems for amino acids in cells.
- Protein degradation (turnover) occurs continuously in all cells.
- Proteins can be degraded by lysosomal enzymes (cathepsins).
- Proteins are also targeted for destruction by being covalently linked to the small protein ubiquitin.
- The ubiquitin-tagged proteins interact with the proteasome, a large complex designed to degrade proteins to small peptides in an adenosine triphosphate–dependent process.
- Amino acids released from proteins during turnover can be used for the synthesis of new proteins, for energy generation, or for gluconeogenesis.

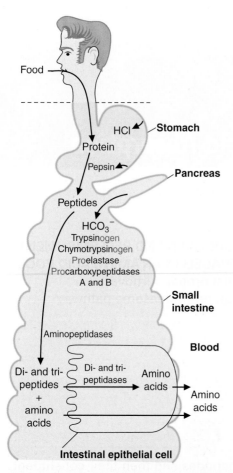

**FIG. 31.1.** Digestion of proteins. The proteolytic enzymes, pepsin, trypsin, chymotrypsin, elastase, and the carboxypeptidases, are produced as zymogens (the "pro-" and "-ogen", in *red*, accompanying the enzyme name) that are activated by cleavage after they enter the gastrointestinal lumen (see Fig. 31.2). Pepsinogen is produced within the stomach and is activated within the stomach (to pepsin) as the pH drops due to HCl secretion.

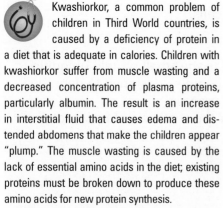

Kwashiorkor, a common problem of children in Third World countries, is caused by a deficiency of protein in a diet that is adequate in calories. Children with kwashiorkor suffer from muscle wasting and a decreased concentration of plasma proteins, particularly albumin. The result is an increase in interstitial fluid that causes edema and distended abdomens that make the children appear "plump." The muscle wasting is caused by the lack of essential amino acids in the diet; existing proteins must be broken down to produce these amino acids for new protein synthesis.

These problems may be compounded by a decreased ability to produce digestive enzymes and new intestinal epithelial cells because of a decreased availability of amino acids for the synthesis of new proteins.

# THE WAITING ROOM

**Susan F.**, a young child with cystic fibrosis (see Chapter 14), has had repeated bouts of bronchitis/bronchiolitis caused by *Pseudomonas aeruginosa*. With each of these infections, her response to aerosolized antibiotics has been good. However, her malabsorption of food continues, resulting in foul-smelling, glistening, bulky stools. Her growth records show a slow decline. She is now in the 24th percentile for height and the 20th percentile for weight. She is often listless and irritable, and she tires easily. When her pediatrician discovered that her levels of the serum proteins albumin and prealbumin were low to low normal (indicating protein malnutrition), Susan was given enteric-coated microspheres of pancreatic enzymes. Almost immediately, the character of Susan's stools became more normal and she began gaining weight. Over the next 6 months, her growth curves showed improvement and she seemed brighter, more active, and less irritable.

For the first few months after a painful episode of renal colic, during which he passed a kidney stone, **David K.** had faithfully maintained a high daily fluid intake and had taken the medication required to increase the pH of his urine. David had been diagnosed with cystinuria, a genetically determined amino acid substitution in the transport protein that normally reabsorbs cystine, arginine, and lysine from the kidney lumen back into the renal tubular cells. Therefore, his urine contained high amounts of these amino acids. Cystine, which is less soluble than the other amino acids, precipitates in the urine to form renal stones (also known as calculi). The measures David was instructed to follow were necessary to increase the solubility of the large amounts of cystine present in his urine and thereby to prevent further formation of kidney stones (calculi). With time, however, he became increasingly complacent about his preventive program. After failing to take his medication for a month, he experienced another severe episode of renal colic with grossly bloody urine. Fortunately, he passed the stone spontaneously, after which he vowed to faithfully comply with therapy.

His mother heard that some dietary amino acids were not absorbed in patients with cystinuria and asked whether any dietary changes would reduce David's chances of developing additional renal stones.

## I. PROTEIN DIGESTION

The digestion of proteins begins in the stomach and is completed in the intestine (Fig. 31.1). The enzymes that digest proteins are produced as inactive precursors (zymogens) that are larger than the active enzymes. The inactive zymogens are secreted from the cells in which they are synthesized and enter the lumen of the digestive tract, where they are cleaved to smaller forms that have proteolytic activity (Fig. 31.2). These active enzymes have different specificities; no single enzyme can completely digest a protein. However, by acting in concert, they can digest dietary proteins to amino acids and small peptides, which are cleaved by peptidases associated with intestinal epithelial cells.

### A. Digestion in the Stomach

Pepsinogen is secreted by the chief cells of the stomach. The gastric parietal cells secrete hydrochloric acid (HCl). The acid in the stomach lumen alters the conformation of pepsinogen so that it can cleave itself, producing the active protease pepsin. Thus, the activation of pepsinogen is autocatalytic.

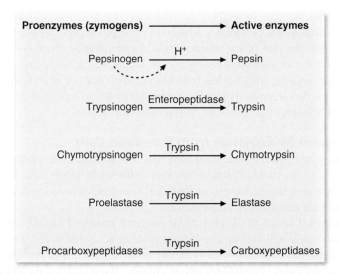

**FIG. 31.2.** Activation of the gastric and pancreatic zymogens. Pepsinogen catalyzes its own cleavage as the pH of the stomach drops. Trypsinogen is cleaved by enteropeptidase in the intestine to form the active protease trypsin. Trypsin then plays a key role by catalyzing the cleavage and activation of the other pancreatic zymogens.

Dietary proteins are denatured by the acid in the stomach. This inactivates the proteins and partially unfolds them such that they are better substrates for proteases. However, at the low pH of the stomach, pepsin is not denatured and acts as an endopeptidase, cleaving peptide bonds at various points within the protein chain. Although pepsin has a fairly broad specificity, it tends to cleave peptide bonds in which the carboxyl group is provided by an aromatic or acidic amino acid. Smaller peptides and some free amino acids are produced.

## B.  Digestion by Enzymes from the Pancreas

As the gastric contents empty into the intestine, they encounter the secretions from the exocrine pancreas. Recall that the exocrine pancreas secretes amylase for starch digestion and lipase and colipase for dietary triacylglycerol digestion. Another pancreatic secretion is bicarbonate, which, in addition to neutralizing the stomach acid, raises the pH such that the pancreatic proteases, which are also present in pancreatic secretions, can be active. As secreted, these pancreatic proteases are in the inactive proenzyme form (zymogens). Because the active forms of these enzymes can digest each other, it is important for their zymogen forms all to be activated within a short span of time. This is accomplished by the cleavage of trypsinogen to the active enzyme trypsin, which then cleaves the other pancreatic zymogens, producing their active forms (see Fig. 31.2).

The zymogen trypsinogen is cleaved to form trypsin by enteropeptidase (a protease) secreted by the brush border cells of the small intestine. Trypsin catalyzes the cleavages that convert chymotrypsinogen to the active enzyme chymotrypsin, proelastase to elastase, and the procarboxypeptidases to the carboxypeptidases. Thus, trypsin plays a central role in digestion because it both cleaves dietary proteins and activates other digestive proteases produced by the pancreas.

Trypsin, chymotrypsin, and elastase are serine proteases (see Chapter 6) that act as endopeptidases. Trypsin is the most specific of these enzymes, cleaving peptide bonds in which the carboxyl (carbonyl) group is provided by lysine or arginine. Chymotrypsin is less specific but favors residues that contain hydrophobic side chains. Elastase cleaves not only elastin (for which it was named) but also other proteins at bonds in which the carboxyl group is contributed by amino acid residues with small side chains (alanine, glycine, and serine). The actions of these pancreatic endopeptidases continue the digestion of dietary proteins begun by pepsin in the stomach.

Elastase is also found in neutrophils, which are white blood cells that engulf and destroy invading bacteria. Neutrophils frequently act in the lung, and elastase is sometimes released into the lung as the neutrophils work. In normal individuals, the released elastase is blocked from destroying lung cells by the action of circulating α1-antitrypsin, a protease inhibitor that is synthesized and secreted by the liver. Certain individuals have a genetic mutation that leads to the production of an inactive α1-antitrypsin protein (α1-antitrypsin deficiency). The lack of this activity leads to the development of emphysema caused by proteolytic destruction of lung cells, which results in a reduction in the expansion and contraction capability of the lungs.

Patients with cystic fibrosis, such as **Susan F.**, have a genetically determined defect in the function of the chloride channels. In the pancreatic secretory ducts, which carry pancreatic enzymes into the lumen of the small intestine, this defect causes inspissation (drying and thickening) of pancreatic exocrine secretions, eventually leading to obstruction of these ducts. One result of this problem is the inability of pancreatic enzymes to enter the intestinal lumen to digest dietary proteins.

The pancreas synthesizes and stores the zymogens in secretory granules. The pancreas also synthesizes a secretory trypsin inhibitor. The need for the inhibitor is to block any trypsin activity that may occur from accidental trypsinogen activation. If the inhibitor were not present, trypsinogen activation would lead to the activation of all of the zymogens in the pancreas, which would lead to the digestion of intracellular pancreatic proteins. Such episodes can lead to pancreatitis.

The smaller peptides formed by the action of trypsin, chymotrypsin, and elastase are attacked by exopeptidases, which are proteases that cleave one amino acid at a time from the end of the chain. Procarboxypeptidases, zymogens produced by the pancreas, are converted by trypsin to the active carboxypeptidases. These exopeptidases remove amino acids from the carboxyl ends of peptide chains. Carboxypeptidase A preferentially releases hydrophobic amino acids, whereas carboxypeptidase B releases basic amino acids (arginine and lysine).

### C. Digestion by Enzymes from Intestinal Cells

Exopeptidases produced by intestinal epithelial cells act within the brush border and also within the cell. Aminopeptidases, located on the brush border, cleave one amino acid at a time from the amino end of peptides. Intracellular peptidases act on small peptides that are absorbed by the cells.

The concerted action of the proteolytic enzymes produced by cells of the stomach, pancreas, and intestine cleave dietary proteins to amino acids. The digestive enzymes digest themselves as well as dietary protein. They also digest the intestinal cells that are regularly sloughed off into the lumen. These cells are replaced by cells that mature from precursor cells in the duodenal crypts. The amount of protein that is digested and absorbed each day from digestive juices and cells released into the intestinal lumen may be equal to or greater than the amount of protein consumed in the diet (50 to 100 g).

## II. ABSORPTION OF AMINO ACIDS

Amino acids are absorbed from the intestinal lumen through secondary active $Na^+$-dependent transport systems and through facilitated diffusion.

### A. Cotransport of Sodium Ions and Amino Acids

Amino acids are absorbed from the lumen of the small intestine principally by semi-specific $Na^+$-dependent transport proteins in the luminal membrane of the intestinal cell brush border, similar to that already seen for carbohydrate transport (Fig. 31.3). The cotransport of $Na^+$ and the amino acid from the outside of the apical membrane to the inside of the cell is driven by the low intracellular $Na^+$ concentration. Low intracellular $Na^+$ results from the pumping of $Na^+$ out of the cell by a $Na^+$, $K^+$-ATPase on the serosal membrane. Thus, the primary transport mechanism is dependent on the creation of a sodium gradient; the secondary transport process involves the coupling of amino acids to the influx of sodium. This mechanism allows the cells to concentrate amino acids from the intestinal lumen. The amino acids are then transported out of the cell into the interstitial fluid principally by facilitated transporters in the serosal membrane (see Fig. 31.3).

At least six different $Na^+$-dependent amino acid carriers are located in the apical brush border membrane of the epithelial cells. These carriers have an overlapping specificity for different amino acids. One carrier preferentially transports neutral amino acids, another transports proline and hydroxyproline, a third preferentially transports acidic amino acids, and a fourth transports basic amino acids (lysine, arginine, the urea cycle intermediate ornithine) and cystine (two cysteine residues linked by a disulfide bond). In addition to these $Na^+$-dependent carriers, some amino acids are transported across the luminal membrane by facilitated transport carriers. Most amino acids are transported by more than one transport system.

As with glucose transport, the $Na^+$-dependent carriers of the apical membrane of the intestinal epithelial cells are also present in the renal epithelium. However, different isozymes are present in the cell membranes of other tissues. Conversely, the facilitated transport carriers in the serosal membrane of the intestinal epithelia are similar to those found in other cell types in the body. During starvation, the intestinal epithelia, like these other cells, take up amino acids from the blood to use as an energy source. Thus, amino acid transport across the serosal membrane is bidirectional.

**Hartnup disease** is a genetically determined and relatively rare autosomal recessive disorder. It is caused by a defect in the transport of neutral amino acids across both intestinal and renal epithelial cells (the amino acid transport system $B^0$ is affected). The signs and symptoms are caused, in part, by a deficiency of essential amino acids (see Clinical Comments). **Cystinuria** (a defect in the amino acid transport system $B^{0+}$) and Hartnup disease involve defects in two different transport proteins. In each case, the defect is present both in intestinal cells, causing malabsorption of the amino acids from the digestive products in the intestinal lumen, and in kidney tubular cells, causing a decreased resorption of these amino acids from the glomerular filtrate and an increased concentration of the amino acids in the urine. Normally, only a few percent of the amino acids that enter the glomerular filtrate are excreted in the urine; most are resorbed. In Hartnup disease (and cystinuria), much larger amounts of the affected amino acids are excreted in the urine, resulting in a hyperaminoaciduria.

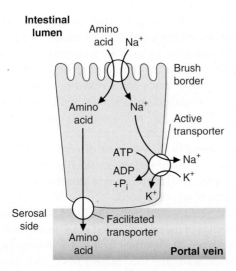

**FIG. 31.3.** Transepithelial amino acid transport. $Na^+$-dependent carriers transport both $Na^+$ and an amino acid into the intestinal epithelial cell from the intestinal lumen. $Na^+$ is pumped out on the serosal side (across the basolateral membrane) in exchange for $K^+$ by the $Na^+,K^+$-ATPase. On the serosal side, the amino acid is carried by a facilitated transporter down its concentration gradient into the blood. This process is an example of secondary active transport. $P_i$, inorganic phosphate.

## B. Transport of Amino Acids into Cells

Amino acids that enter the blood are transported across cell membranes of the various tissues principally by $Na^+$-dependent cotransporters and, to a lesser extent, by facilitated transporters. (A partial listing of such systems is shown in Table A31.1 of the online supplement @.) In this respect, amino acid transport differs from glucose transport, which is $Na^+$-dependent transport in the intestinal and renal epithelium but facilitated transport in other cell types. The $Na^+$ dependence of amino acid transport in liver, muscle, and other tissues allows these cells to concentrate amino acids from the blood. These transport proteins have a different genetic basis, amino acid composition, and somewhat different specificity than those in the luminal membrane of intestinal epithelia. They also differ somewhat between tissues. As with the epithelial cell transporter, there is also some overlap in specificity of the transport proteins, with most amino acids being transported by more than one carrier.

## III. PROTEIN TURNOVER AND REPLENISHMENT OF THE INTRACELLULAR AMINO ACID POOL

The amino acid pool within cells is generated both from dietary amino acids and from the degradation of existing proteins within the cell. All proteins within cells have a half-life ($t_{1/2}$), a time at which 50% of the protein that was synthesized at a particular time will have been degraded. Some proteins are inherently short-lived, with half-lives of 5 to 20 minutes. Other proteins are present for extended periods, with half-lives of many hours or even days. Thus, proteins are continuously being synthesized and degraded in the body, using a variety of enzyme systems to do so (see Table A31.2 of the online supplement @). Examples of proteins that undergo extensive synthesis and degradation are hemoglobin, muscle proteins, digestive enzymes, and the proteins of cells sloughed off from the gastrointestinal tract. Hemoglobin is produced in reticulocytes and reconverted to amino acids by the phagocytic cells that remove mature red blood cells from the circulation on a daily basis. Muscle protein is degraded during periods of fasting, and the amino acids are used for gluconeogenesis. After ingestion of protein in the diet, muscle protein is resynthesized.

**David K.** and other patients with cystinuria have a genetically determined defect in the transport of cystine and the basic amino acids, lysine, arginine, and ornithine, across the brush border membranes of cells in both their small intestine and renal tubules. However, they do not appear to have any symptoms of amino acid deficiency, in part because the amino acids cysteine (which is oxidized in blood and urine to form the disulfide cystine) and arginine can be synthesized in the body (i.e., they are "nonessential" amino acids). Ornithine (an amino acid that is not found in proteins but serves as an intermediate of the urea cycle) can also be synthesized. The most serious problem for these patients is the insolubility of cystine, which can form kidney stones that may lodge in the ureter, causing genitourinary bleeding and severe pain known as renal colic.

Adults cannot increase the amount of muscle or other body proteins by eating an excess amount of protein. If dietary protein is consumed in excess of our needs, it is converted to glycogen and triacylglycerols, which are then stored.

A large amount of protein is recycled daily in the form of digestive enzymes, which are themselves degraded by digestive proteases. In addition, approximately one-fourth of the cells lining the walls of the gastrointestinal tract are lost each day and replaced by newly synthesized cells. As cells leave the gastrointestinal wall, their proteins and other components are digested by enzymes in the lumen of the gut, and the products are absorbed. Additionally, red blood cells have a life span of about 120 days. Every day, $3 \times 10^{11}$ red blood cells dies and are phagocytosed. The hemoglobin in these cells is degraded to amino acids by lysosomal proteases, and their amino acids are reused in the synthesis of new proteins. Only approximately 6% (roughly 10 g) of the protein that enters the digestive tract (including dietary proteins, digestive enzymes, and the proteins in sloughed-off cells) is excreted in the feces each day. The remainder is recycled.

Proteins are also recycled within cells. The differences in amino acid composition of the various proteins of the body, the vast range in turnover times ($t_{1/2}$), and the recycling of amino acids are all important factors that help to determine the requirements for specific amino acids and total protein in the diet. The synthesis of many enzymes is induced in response to physiological demand (such as fasting or feeding). These enzymes are continuously being degraded. Intracellular proteins are also damaged by oxidation and other modifications that limit their function. Mechanisms for intracellular degradation of unnecessary or damaged proteins involve lysosomes and the ubiquitin-proteasome system.

## A. Lysosomal Protein Turnover

Lysosomes participate in the process of autophagy, in which intracellular components are surrounded by membranes that fuse with lysosomes, and endocytosis (see Chapter 8). Autophagy is a complex regulated process in which cytoplasm is sequestered into vesicles and delivered to the lysosomes. Within the lysosomes, the cathepsin family of proteases degrades the ingested proteins to individual amino acids. The recycled amino acids can then leave the lysosome and rejoin the intracellular amino acid pool. The cathespins exhibit optimal activity within the acidic environment of the lysosome. Although the details of how autophagy is induced are still being investigated, starvation of a cell is a trigger to induce this process. This will allow old proteins to be recycled and the newly released amino acids used for new protein synthesis, to enable the cell to survive starvation conditions.

## B. The Ubiquitin-Proteasome Pathway

Ubiquitin is a small protein (76 amino acids) that is highly conserved. Its amino acid sequence in yeast and humans differs by only three residues. Ubiquitin targets intracellular proteins for degradation by covalently binding to the ε-amino group of lysine residues. This is accomplished by a three-enzyme system that adds ubiquitin to proteins targeted for degradation. Oftentimes, the target protein is polyubiquitinylated in which additional ubiquitin molecules are added to previous ubiquitin molecules, forming a long ubiquitin tail on the target protein. After polyubiquitinylation is complete, the targeted protein is released from the three-enzyme complex and is directed to the proteasome via a variety of mechanisms.

A protease complex, known as the proteasome, then degrades the targeted protein into small peptides, releasing intact ubiquitin that can again mark other proteins for degradation (Fig. 31.4). The basic proteasome is a cylindrical 20S protein complex with multiple internal proteolytic sites. Adenosine triphosphate (ATP) hydrolysis is used both to unfold the tagged protein and to push the protein into the core of the cylinder. The complex is regulated by 19S regulatory particles (cap complexes), which bind the ubiquinylated protein (a step that requires ATP) and deliver them to the complex. After the target protein is degraded, the ubiquitin is released intact and recycled. The resulting amino acids join the intracellular pool of free amino acids.

Many proteins that contain regions rich in the amino acids proline (P), glutamate (E), serine (S), and threonine (T) have short half-lives. These regions are known as PEST sequences based on the one-letter abbreviations used for these amino acids. Most of the proteins that contain PEST sequences are hydrolyzed by the ubiquitin-proteasome system.

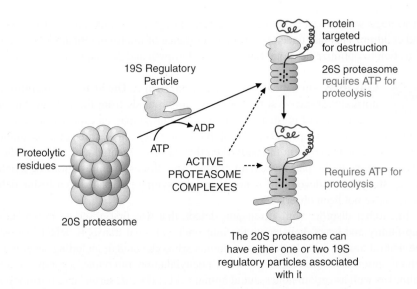

*FIG. 31.4.* The proteasome and regulatory proteins. The regulatory particle regulates the activity of this proteolytic complex by recruiting to the complex the substrates for proteolysis. The ATP requirement is to unfold and denature the proteins targeted for destruction.

## CLINICAL COMMENTS

Diseases discussed in this chapter are summarized in Table 31.1.

**Susan F.** Susan F.'s growth and weight curves were both subnormal until her pediatrician added pancreatic enzyme supplements to her treatment plan. These supplements digest dietary protein, releasing essential and other amino acids from the dietary protein, which are then absorbed by the endothelial cells of Susan's small intestine, through which they are transported into the blood. A discernable improvement in Susan's body weight and growth curves was noted within months of starting this therapy.

Besides the proportions of essential amino acids present in various foods, the quality of a dietary protein is also determined by the rate at which it is digested and, in a more general way, by its capacity to contribute to the growth of the infant. In this regard, the proteins in foods of animal origin are more digestible than are those derived from plants. For example, the digestibility of proteins in eggs is approximately 97%; that for meats, poultry, and fish is 85% to 100%; and that from wheat, soybeans, and other legumes ranges from 75% to 90%.

The official daily dietary "protein requirement" accepted by the United States and Canadian governments is 0.8 g of protein per kilogram of desirable body weight for adults (approximately 56 g for an adult man and 44 g for an adult woman). On

**Table 31.1    Diseases Discussed in Chapter 31**

| Disease or Disorder | Genetic or Environmental | Comments |
|---|---|---|
| Cystic fibrosis | Genetic | Patients with cystic fibrosis often experience a blockage of the pancreatic duct, which necessitates oral ingestion of digestive enzymes for appropriate nutrient degradation and absorption. |
| Cystinuria | Genetic | A mutation in a membrane transport protein ($B^{0+}$) for basic amino acids, including cystine, which is expressed in kidney and intestine. Kidney stones may develop due to this disorder. |
| Kwashiorkor | Environmental | Protein-calorie malnutrition (diet is adequate in calories but lacking in protein), leading to excessive protein degradation in the extremities and edema. |
| Hartnup disease | Genetic | A mutation in a membrane transport protein ($B^0$) for neutral amino acids, including tryptophan, which is expressed in both the kidney and intestine. Some patients may develop pellagralike symptoms due to the lack of tryptophan and inability to synthesize adequate amounts of $NAD(P)^+$. |

an average weight basis, the requirement per kilogram is much greater for infants and children. This fact underscores the importance of improving **Susan F.'s** protein digestion to optimize her potential for normal growth and development.

 **David K.** In patients with cystinuria, such as **David K.**, the inability to normally absorb cystine and basic amino acids from the gut and the increased loss of these amino acids in the urine may be expected to cause a deficiency of these compounds in the blood. However, because three of these amino acids can be synthesized in the body (i.e., they are nonessential amino acids), their concentrations in the plasma remain normal, and clinical manifestations of a deficiency state do not develop. It is not clear why symptoms related to a lysine deficiency have not been observed.

In another disorder with a transport defect, that was first observed in the Hartnup family and bears their name, the intestinal and renal transport defect involves the neutral amino acids (monoamine, monocarboxylic acids), including several essential amino acids (isoleucine, leucine, phenylalanine, threonine, tryptophan, and valine) as well as certain nonessential amino acids (alanine, serine, and tyrosine). A reduction in the availability of these essential amino acids may be expected to cause a variety of clinical disorders. Yet, children with the Hartnup disorder identified by routine newborn urine screening almost always remain clinically normal.

However, some patients with the Hartnup biochemical phenotype eventually develop pellagralike manifestations, which usually include a photosensitivity rash, ataxia, and neuropsychiatric symptoms. Pellagra results from a dietary deficiency of the vitamin niacin or the essential amino acid tryptophan, which are both precursors for the nicotinamide moiety of NAD and NADP. In asymptomatic patients, the transport abnormality may be incomplete and so subtle as to allow no phenotypic expression of Hartnup disease. These patients also may be capable of absorbing some small peptides that contain the neutral amino acids.

The only rational treatment of patients having pellagralike symptoms is the administration of niacin (nicotinic acid) in oral doses up to 300 mg/day. Although the rash, ataxia, and neuropsychiatric manifestations of niacin deficiency may disappear, the hyperaminoaciduria and intestinal transport defect do not respond to this therapy. In addition to niacin, a high-protein diet may benefit some patients.

## REVIEW QUESTIONS-CHAPTER 31

1. An individual with a deficiency in the conversion of trypsinogen to trypsin would be expected to have a more detrimental effect on protein digestion than an individual who was defective in any of the other digestive proteases. This is due to which one of the following?

   A. Trypsin has a greater and wider range of substrates to act on.
   B. Trypsin activates the other zymogens that are secreted by the pancreas.
   C. Trypsin activates pepsinogen, so digestion can begin in the stomach.
   D. Trypsin activates enteropeptidase, which is needed to activate the other pancreatic zymogens.
   E. Trypsin inhibits intestinal motility, so the substrates can be hydrolyzed for longer periods of time.

2. An individual has been shown to have a deficiency in an intestinal epithelial cell amino acid transport system for leucine. However, the individual shows no symptoms of amino acid deficiency. This could be due to which one of the following?

   A. The kidney reabsorbs leucine and sends it to other tissues.
   B. The body synthesizes leucine to compensate for the transport defect.
   C. There are multiple transport systems for leucine.
   D. Isoleucine takes the place of leucine in proteins.
   E. Leucine is not necessary for bulk protein synthesis.

3.  Kwashiorkor can result from which one of the following?

    A.  Consuming a calorie-adequate diet which is deficient in proteins
    B.  Consuming a calorie-deficient diet, which is also deficient in protein
    C.  Consuming a calorie-adequate diet which is deficient in carbohydrates
    D.  Consuming a calorie-adequate diet which is deficient in fatty acids
    E.  Consuming a calorie-deficient diet which is primarily proteins

4.  Children with kwashiorkor usually have a fatty liver. This is due to which one of the following?

    A.  The high fat content of their diet
    B.  The high carbohydrate content of their diet
    C.  The high protein content of their diet
    D.  The lack of substrates for gluconeogenesis in the liver
    E.  The lack of substrates for protein synthesis in the liver
    F.  The lack of substrates for glycogen synthesis in the liver

5.  The Atkins diet promotes meals high in protein and fat but very low in carbohydrates. After 2 weeks on such a diet, the excess amino acids being consumed can be stored within the body as which one of the following?

    A.  As amino acid pools within the muscle
    B.  As plasma proteins synthesized by the liver
    C.  As short, energy-rich peptides stored in the muscle
    D.  As liver glycogen
    E.  As amino acid pools within the liver

# 32 Fate of Amino Acid Nitrogen: Urea Cycle

## CHAPTER OUTLINE

I. **FATE OF AMINO ACID NITROGEN**
  A. Transamination reactions
  B. Removal of amino acid nitrogen as ammonia
  C. Role of glutamate in the metabolism of amino acid nitrogen
  D. Role of alanine and glutamine in transporting amino acid nitrogen to the liver

II. **UREA CYCLE**
  A. Reactions of the urea cycle
    1. Synthesis of carbamoyl phosphate
    2. Production of arginine by the urea cycle
    3. Cleavage of arginine to produce urea
  B. Origin of ornithine
  C. Regulation of the urea cycle
  D. Function of the urea cycle during fasting

III. **DISORDERS OF THE UREA CYCLE**

## KEY POINTS

- Amino acid catabolism generates urea, which is a nontoxic carrier of nitrogen atoms.
- Urea synthesis occurs in the liver. The amino acids alanine and glutamine carry amino acid nitrogen from peripheral tissues to the liver.
- Key enzymes involved in nitrogen disposal are transaminases, glutamate dehydrogenase, and glutaminase.
- The urea cycle consists of four steps and incorporates a nitrogen from ammonia and one from aspartate into urea.
- Disorders of the urea cycle lead to hyperammonemia, a condition toxic to nervous system health and development.

# THE WAITING ROOM

**Percy V.** and a very good friend decided to take a Caribbean cruise, during which they sampled the cuisine of many of the islands on their itinerary. One month after their return to the United States, Percy complained of severe malaise, loss of appetite, nausea, vomiting, and arthralgias (joint pains). He had a low-grade fever and noted a persistent and increasing pain in the area of his liver. His friend noted a yellow discoloration of the whites of Percy's eyes and skin. Percy's urine turned the color of iced tea, and his stool became a light clay color. His doctor found his liver to be enlarged and tender. Liver function tests were ordered.

Serological testing for viral hepatitis types B and C were nonreactive, but tests for antibodies to antigens of the hepatitis A virus (anti-HAV) in the serum were positive for the immunoglobulin M type.

A diagnosis of acute viral hepatitis type A was made, probably contracted from virus-contaminated food Percy had eaten while on his cruise. His physician explained that there was no specific treatment for type A viral hepatitis but recommended symptomatic and supportive care and prevention of transmission to others by the fecal-oral route. Percy took acetaminophen three or four times a day for fever and arthralgias throughout his illness.

## I. FATE OF AMINO ACID NITROGEN

### A. Transamination Reactions

Transamination is the major process for removing nitrogen from amino acids. In most instances, the nitrogen is transferred as an amino group from the original amino acid to α-ketoglutarate, forming glutamate, whereas the original amino acid is converted to its corresponding α-keto acid (Fig. 32.1). For example, the amino acid aspartate can be transaminated to form its corresponding α-keto acid, oxalo-acetate. In the process, the amino group is transferred to α-ketoglutarate, which is converted to its corresponding amino acid, glutamate.

All amino acids except lysine and threonine undergo transamination reactions. The enzymes that catalyze these reactions are known as transaminases or amino-transferases. For most of these reactions, α-ketoglutarate and glutamate serve as one of the α-keto acid–amino acid pairs. Pyridoxal phosphate is the required cofactor for these reactions. Because these reactions are readily reversible, they can be used to remove nitrogen from amino acids or to transfer nitrogen to α-keto acids to form amino acids. Thus, they are involved both in amino acid degradation and in amino acid synthesis.

### B. Removal of Amino Acid Nitrogen as Ammonia

Cells in the body and bacteria in the gut release the nitrogen of certain amino acids as ammonia or ammonium ion ($NH_4^+$) (Fig. 32.2). Because these two forms of nitrogen can be interconverted, the terms are sometimes used interchangeably. $NH_4^+$ releases a proton to form ammonia by a reaction with a pK of 9.3. Therefore, at physiological pH, the equilibrium favors $NH_4^+$ by a factor of approximately 100:1 (see Chapter 2, the Henderson-Hasselbalch equation). However, it is important to note that $NH_3$ is also present in the body because this is the form that can cross cell membranes. For example, $NH_3$ passes into the urine from kidney tubule cells and decreases the acidity of the urine by binding protons, forming $NH_4^+$. Once the $NH_4^+$ is formed, the compound can no longer freely diffuse across membranes.

Glutamate is oxidatively deaminated by a reaction catalyzed by glutamate dehydrogenase that produces $NH_4^+$ and α-ketoglutarate (Fig. 32.3). Either nicotinamide

**A**

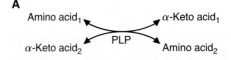

**B**

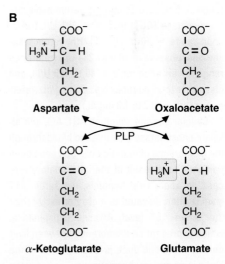

*FIG. 32.1.* Transamination. The amino group from one amino acid is transferred to another. Pairs of amino acids and their corresponding α-keto acids are involved in these reactions. α-Ketoglutarate and glutamate are usually one of the pairs. The reactions, which are readily reversible, use pyridoxal phosphate (PLP) as a cofactor. The enzymes are called transaminases or aminotransferases. **A.** A generalized reaction. **B.** The aspartate transaminase reaction.

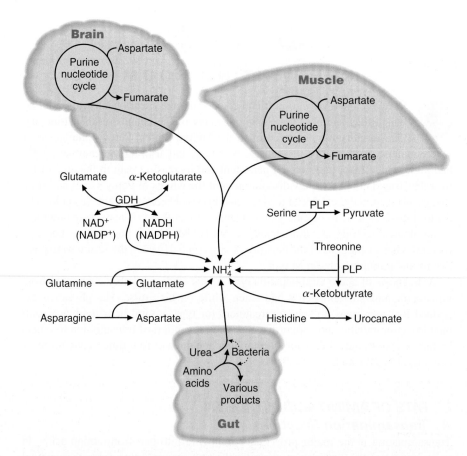

**FIG. 32.2.** Summary of the sources of NH$_4^+$ for the urea cycle. All of the reactions are irreversible except glutamate dehydrogenase (GDH). Only the dehydratase reactions, which produce NH$_4^+$ from serine and threonine, require pyridoxal phosphate as a cofactor. The reactions that are not shown occurring in the muscle or the gut can all occur in the liver, where the NH$_4^+$ generated can be converted to urea. The purine nucleotide cycle of the brain and muscle is further described in Chapter 35. *PLP*, pyridoxal phosphate.

Percy V.'s laboratory studies showed that his serum alanine transaminase (ALT) level was 675 U/L (reference range = 5 to 30 U/L) and his serum aspartate transaminase (AST) level was 601 U/L (reference range = 10 to 30 U/L). His serum alkaline phosphatase level was 284 U/L (reference range for an adult male = 40 to 125 U/L), and his serum total bilirubin was 9.6 mg/dL (reference range = 0.2 to 1.0 mg/dL).

Cellular enzymes such as AST, ALT, and alkaline phosphatase leak into the blood through the membranes of hepatic cells that have been damaged as a result of the inflammatory process. In acute viral hepatitis, the serum ALT level is often elevated to a greater extent than the serum AST level. Alkaline phosphatase, which is present on membranes between liver cells and the bile duct, is also elevated in the blood in acute viral hepatitis.

The rise in serum total bilirubin occurs as a result of the inability of the infected liver to conjugate bilirubin and of a partial or complete occlusion of the hepatic biliary drainage ducts caused by inflammatory swelling within the liver. In fulminant hepatic failure, the serum bilirubin level may exceed 20 mg/dL, a poor prognostic sign.

adenine dinucleotide (NAD$^+$) or oxidized nicotinamide adenine dinucleotide phosphate (NADP$^+$) can serve as the cofactor. This reaction, which occurs in the mitochondria of most cells, is readily reversible; it can incorporate ammonia into glutamate or release ammonia from glutamate. Glutamate can collect nitrogen from other amino acids as a consequence of transmination reactions and then release ammonia through the glutamate dehydrogenase reaction. This process provides one source of the ammonia that enters the urea cycle.

In addition to glutamate, several amino acids release their nitrogen as NH$_4^+$ (see Fig. 32.2). Histidine may be directly deaminated to form NH$_4^+$ and urocanate. The

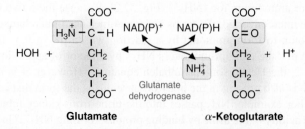

**FIG. 32.3.** Reaction catalyzed by glutamate dehydrogenase. This reaction is readily reversible and can use either NAD$^+$ or NADP$^+$ as a cofactor. The oxygen on α-ketoglutarate is derived from H$_2$O.

deaminations of serine and threonine are dehydration reactions that require pyridoxal phosphate and are catalyzed by serine dehydratase. Serine forms pyruvate, and threonine forms $\alpha$-ketobutyrate. In both cases, $NH_4^+$ is released.

Glutamine and asparagine contain R group amides that may be released as $NH_4^+$ by deamidation. Asparagine is deamidated by asparaginase, yielding aspartate and $NH_4^+$. Glutaminase acts on glutamine, forming glutamate and $NH_4^+$. The glutaminase reaction is particularly important in the kidney, where the $NH_4^+$ produced is excreted directly into the urine, where it forms salts with metabolic acids, facilitating their removal in the urine.

In muscle and brain, but not in liver, the purine nucleotide cycle allows $NH_4^+$ to be released from amino acids (see Fig. 32.2). Nitrogen is collected by glutamate from other amino acids by means of transamination reactions. Glutamate then transfers its amino group to oxaloacetate to form aspartate, which supplies nitrogen to the purine nucleotide cycle (see Chapter 35). The reactions of the cycle release fumarate and $NH_4^+$. The $NH_4^+$ formed can leave the muscle in the form of glutamine.

In summary, $NH_4^+$ that enters the urea cycle is produced in the body by deamination or deamidation of amino acids (see Fig. 32.2). A significant amount of $NH_4^+$ is also produced by bacteria that live in the lumen of the intestinal tract. This $NH_4^+$ enters the hepatic portal vein and travels to the liver.

## C. Role of Glutamate in the Metabolism of Amino Acid Nitrogen

Glutamate plays a pivotal role in the metabolism of amino acids. It is involved in both synthesis and degradation.

Glutamate provides nitrogen for amino acid synthesis (Fig. 32.4). In this process, glutamate obtains its nitrogen either from other amino acids by transamination reactions or from $NH_4^+$ by the glutamate dehydrogenase reaction. Transamination reactions then serve to transfer amino groups from glutamate to $\alpha$-keto acids to produce their corresponding amino acids.

When amino acids are degraded and urea is formed, glutamate collects nitrogen from other amino acids by transamination reactions. Some of this nitrogen is released as ammonia by the glutamate dehydrogenase reaction, but much larger amounts of ammonia are produced from the other sources shown in Figure 32.2. $NH_4^+$ is one of the two forms in which nitrogen enters the urea cycle (Fig. 32.5).

The second form of nitrogen for urea synthesis is provided by aspartate (see Fig. 32.5). Glutamate can be the source of the nitrogen. Glutamate transfers its amino group to oxaloacetate, and aspartate and $\alpha$-ketoglutarate are formed.

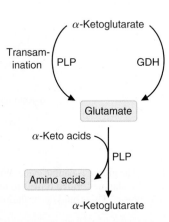

**FIG. 32.4.** Role of glutamate in amino acid synthesis. Glutamate transfers nitrogen by means of transamination reactions to $\alpha$-keto acids to form amino acids. This nitrogen is either obtained by glutamate from transamination of other amino acids or from $NH_4^+$ by means of the glutamate dehydrogenase (GDH) reaction. *PLP*, pyridoxal phosphate, the active form of vitamin $B_6$ (pyridoxine).

 Glutamate dehydrogenase is one of three mammalian enzymes that can fix ammonia into organic molecules. The other two are glutamine synthetase and carbamoyl phosphate synthetase I.

 Vitamin $B_6$ deficiency symptoms include dermatitis; a microcytic, hypochromic anemia; weakness; irritability; and, in some cases, convulsions. Xanthurenic acid (a degradation product of tryptophan) and other compounds appear in the urine because of an inability to metabolize amino acids completely. A decreased ability to synthesize heme from glycine may cause the microcytic anemia (see Chapter 33) and decreased decarboxylation of amino acids to form neurotransmitters (see Chapter 33) may explain the convulsions. Although vitamin $B_6$ is required for a large number of reactions involved in amino acid metabolism, it is also required for the glycogen phosphorylase reaction.

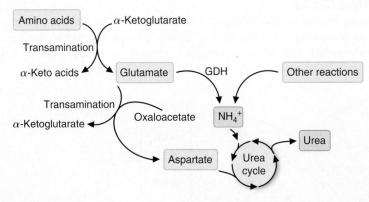

**FIG. 32.5.** Role of glutamate in urea production. Glutamate collects nitrogen from other amino acids by transamination reactions. This nitrogen can be released as $NH_4^+$ by glutamate dehydrogenase (GDH). $NH_4^+$ is also produced by other reactions (see Fig. 32.2). $NH_4^+$ provides one of the nitrogens for urea synthesis. The other nitrogen comes from aspartate and is obtained from glutamate by transamination of oxaloacetate.

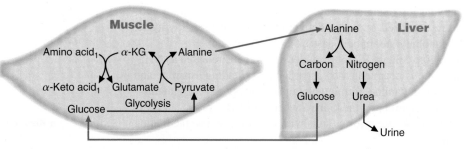

**FIG. 32.6.** The glucose-alanine cycle. Within the muscle, amino acid degradation leads to the transfer of nitrogens to α-ketoglutarate (α-KG) and pyruvate. The alanine formed travels to the liver, where the carbons of alanine are used for gluconeogenesis and the alanine nitrogen is used for urea biosynthesis. This could occur during exercise, when the muscle uses blood-borne glucose.

### D. Role of Alanine and Glutamine in Transporting Amino Acid Nitrogen to the Liver

Protein turnover and amino acid degradation occur in all tissues; however, the urea cycle enzymes are primarily active in the liver. (The intestine expresses low levels of activity of these enzymes.) Thus, a mechanism needs to be in place to transport amino acid nitrogen to the liver. Alanine and glutamine are the major carriers of nitrogen in the blood. Alanine is primarily exported by muscle. Because the muscle is metabolizing glucose through glycolysis, pyruvate is available in the muscle. The pyruvate is transaminated by glutamate to form alanine, which travels to the liver (Fig. 32.6). The glutamate is formed by transamination of an amino acid that is being degraded. Upon arriving at the liver, alanine is transaminated to pyruvate, and the nitrogen is used for urea synthesis. The pyruvate formed is used for gluconeogenesis and the glucose exported to the muscle for use as energy. This cycle of moving carbons and nitrogen between the muscle and liver is known as the glucose-alanine cycle.

Glutamine is synthesized from glutamate by the fixation of ammonia, requiring energy (adenosine triphosphate [ATP]) and the enzyme glutamine synthetase (Fig. 32.7), which is a cytoplasmic enzyme found in all cells. Under conditions of rapid amino acid degradation within a tissue, so that ammonia levels increase, the glutamate that has been formed from transamination reactions accepts another nitrogen molecule to form glutamine. The glutamine travels to the liver, kidney, or intestines where glutaminase (see Fig. 32.7) will remove the amide nitrogen to form glutamate plus ammonia. In the kidney, the release of ammonia, and the formation of $NH_4^+$, serves to form salts with metabolic acids in the urine. In the intestine, the glutamine is used as a fuel. In the liver, the ammonia is used for urea biosynthesis.

> Glutamine synthetase in liver is located in cells surrounding the portal vein. Its major role is to convert any ammonia that has escaped from urea production into glutamine, such that free ammonia does not leave the liver and enter the circulation.

### II. UREA CYCLE

The normal human adult is in nitrogen balance; that is, the amount of nitrogen ingested each day, mainly in the form of dietary protein, is equal to the amount of nitrogen excreted. The major nitrogenous excretory product is urea, which exits

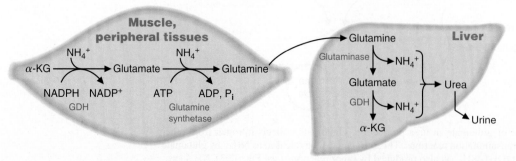

**FIG. 32.7.** Synthesis of glutamine in peripheral tissues and its transport to the liver. Within the liver, glutaminase converts glutamine to glutamate. Note how α-ketoglutarate can accept two molecules of ammonia to form glutamine. *GDH*, glutamate dehydrogenase; α-*KG*, α-ketoglutarate; $P_i$, inorganic phosphate.

from the body in the urine. This innocuous compound, produced mainly in the liver by the urea cycle, serves as the disposal form of ammonia, which is toxic, particularly to the brain and central nervous system. Normally, little ammonia (or $NH_4^+$) is present in the blood. The concentration ranges between 30 and 60 $\mu M$. Ammonia is rapidly removed from the blood and converted to urea by the liver. Nitrogen travels in the blood mainly in amino acids, particularly alanine and glutamine.

## A. Reactions of the Urea Cycle

Nitrogen enters the urea cycle as $NH_4^+$ and aspartate (Fig. 32.8). $NH_4^+$ forms carbamoyl phosphate, which reacts with ornithine to form citrulline. Ornithine is the compound that both initiates and is regenerated by the cycle (similar to oxaloacetate in the tricarboxylic acid [TCA] cycle). Aspartate reacts with citrulline, eventually donating its nitrogen for urea formation. Arginine is formed in two successive steps. Cleavage of arginine by arginase releases urea and regenerates ornithine.

## 1. SYNTHESIS OF CARBAMOYL PHOSPHATE

In the first step of the urea cycle, $NH_4^+$, bicarbonate, and ATP react to form carbamoyl phosphate (see Fig. 32.8). The cleavage of two molecules of ATP is required to form the high-energy phosphate bond of carbamoyl phosphate. Carbamoyl

**Percy V.'s** symptoms and laboratory abnormalities did not slowly subside over the next 6 weeks, as they usually do in uncomplicated viral hepatitis A infections. Instead, his serum total bilirubin, ALT, AST, and alkaline phosphatase levels increased further. His vomiting became intractable, and his friend noted jerking motions of his arms (asterixis), facial grimacing, restlessness, slowed mentation, and slight disorientation. He was admitted to the hospital with a diagnosis of hepatic failure with incipient hepatic encephalopathy (brain dysfunction caused by accumulation of various toxins in the blood), a rare complication of acute type A viral hepatitis alone. The possibility of a superimposed acute hepatic toxicity caused by the use of acetaminophen was considered.

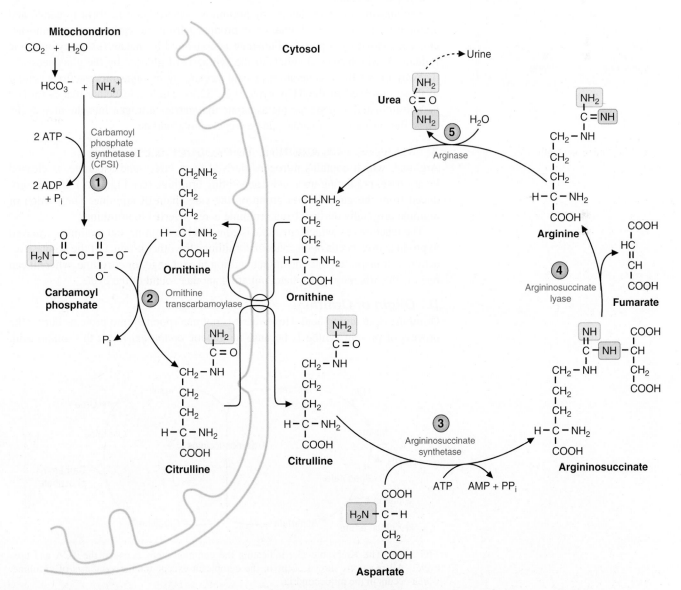

**FIG. 32.8.** Urea cycle. The steps of the cycle are numbered 1 to 5. $P_i$, inorganic phosphate.

When OTC is deficient, the carbamoyl phosphate that normally would enter the urea cycle accumulates and floods the pathway for pyrimidine biosynthesis. Carbamoyl phosphate, produced by a cytoplasmic enzyme (carbamoyl phosphate synthetase II; see Chapter 35), is the precursor for pyrimidine biosynthesis. Under these conditions, excess orotic acid (orotate), an intermediate in pyrimidine biosynthesis, is excreted in the urine. It produces no ill effects but is indicative of a problem in the urea cycle.

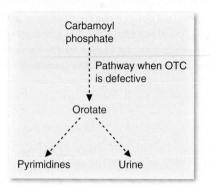

phosphate synthetase I (CPSI), the enzyme that catalyzes this first step of the urea cycle, is found mainly in mitochondria of the liver and intestine. The Roman numeral suggests that another carbamoyl phosphate synthetase exists, and, indeed, carbamoyl phosphate synthetase II (CPSII), located in the cytosol, produces carbamoyl phosphate for pyrimidine biosynthesis using nitrogen from glutamine (see Chapter 35).

## 2. PRODUCTION OF ARGININE BY THE UREA CYCLE

Carbamoyl phosphate reacts with ornithine to form citrulline (see Fig. 32.8). The high-energy phosphate bond of carbamoyl phosphate provides the energy required for this reaction, which occurs in mitochondria and is catalyzed by ornithine transcarbamoylase (OTC). The product citrulline is transported across the mitochondrial membranes in exchange for cytoplasmic ornithine and enters the cytosol. The carrier for this transport reaction catalyzes an electroneutral exchange of the two compounds.

In the cytosol, citrulline reacts with aspartate, the second source of nitrogen for urea synthesis, to produce argininosuccinate (see Fig. 32.8). This reaction, catalyzed by argininosuccinate synthetase, is driven by the hydrolysis of ATP to adenosine monophosphate (AMP) and pyrophosphate. Aspartate is produced by transamination of oxaloacetate.

Argininosuccinate is cleaved by argininosuccinate lyase to form fumarate and arginine (see Fig. 32.8). Fumarate is produced from the carbons of argininosuccinate provided by aspartate. Fumarate is converted to malate (using cytoplasmic fumarase), which is used either for the synthesis of glucose by the gluconeogenic pathway or for the regeneration of oxaloacetate by cytoplasmic reactions similar to those observed in the TCA cycle (Fig. 32.9). The oxaloacetate that is formed is transaminated to generate the aspartate that carries nitrogen into the urea cycle. Thus, the carbons of fumarate can be recycled to aspartate.

## 3. CLEAVAGE OF ARGININE TO PRODUCE UREA

Arginine, which contains nitrogens derived from $NH_4^+$ and aspartate, is cleaved by arginase, producing urea and regenerating ornithine (see Fig. 32.8). Urea is produced from the guanidinium group on the side chain of arginine. The portion of arginine originally derived from ornithine is reconverted to ornithine.

The reactions by which citrulline is converted to arginine and arginine is cleaved to produce urea occur in the cytosol. Ornithine, the other product of the arginase reaction, is transported into the mitochondrion in exchange for citrulline, where it can react with carbamoyl phosphate, initiating another round of the cycle.

### B. Origin of Ornithine

Ornithine is an amino acid. However, it is not incorporated into proteins during the process of protein synthesis because no genetic codon exists for this amino acid.

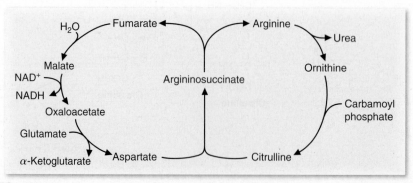

**FIG. 32.9.** The Krebs bicycle, indicating the common steps between the TCA and urea cycles. All reactions shown occur in the cytoplasm except for the synthesis of citrulline, which occurs in the mitochondria.

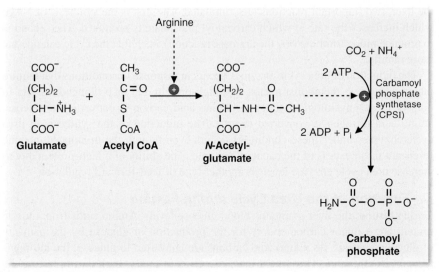

*FIG. 32.10.* Activation of CPSI. Arginine stimulates the synthesis of NAG, which activates CPSI. $P_i$, inorganic phosphate.

Although ornithine is normally regenerated by the urea cycle (as one of the products of the arginase reaction), ornithine also can be synthesized de novo if needed (from glutamate semialdehyde) in an unusual transamination reaction in the intestine.

## C. Regulation of the Urea Cycle

The human liver has a vast capacity to convert amino acid nitrogen to urea, thereby preventing toxic effects from ammonia, which would otherwise accumulate. In general, the urea cycle is regulated by substrate availability; the higher the rate of ammonia production, the higher is the rate of urea formation. Regulation by substrate availability is a general characteristic of disposal pathways, such as the urea cycle, which remove toxic compounds from the body. This is a type of feed-forward regulation, in contrast to the feedback regulation characteristic of pathways that produce functional end products.

Two other types of regulation control the urea cycle: allosteric activation of CPSI by *N*-acetylglutamate (NAG) and induction and repression of the synthesis of urea cycle enzymes. NAG is formed specifically to activate CPSI; it has no other known function in mammals. The synthesis of NAG from acetyl coenzyme A and glutamate is stimulated by arginine (Fig. 32.10). Thus, as arginine levels increase within

 The precise pathogenesis of the central nervous system (CNS) signs and symptoms that accompany liver failure (hepatic encephalopathy) in patients such as **Percy V.** is not completely understood. These changes are, however, attributable in part to toxic materials that are derived from the metabolism of nitrogenous substrates by bacteria in the gut that circulate to the liver in the portal vein. These materials bypass their normal metabolism by the liver cells, however, because the acute inflammatory process of viral hepatitis severely limits the ability of liver cells to degrade these compounds to harmless metabolites. As a result, these toxins are shunted into the hepatic veins unaltered and eventually reach the brain through the systemic circulation ("portal-systemic encephalopathy").

$NH_4^+$ is one of the toxins that results from the degradation of urea or proteins by intestinal bacteria and is not metabolized by the infected liver. The subsequent elevation of ammonia concentrations in the fluid bathing the brain causes depletion of TCA cycle intermediates and ATP in the central nervous system. α-Ketoglutarate, a TCA cycle intermediate, combines with ammonia to form glutamate in a reaction catalyzed by glutamate dehydrogenase. Glutamate subsequently reacts with ammonia to form glutamine. This effectively reduces α-ketoglutarate levels in the mitochondria, thereby reducing the rate at which the TCA cycle can operate.

The absolute level of ammonia and its metabolites, such as glutamine, in the blood or cerebrospinal fluid in patients with hepatic encephalopathy correlates only roughly with the presence or severity of the neurological signs and symptoms. γ-Aminobutyric acid (GABA), an important inhibitory neurotransmitter in the brain, is also produced in the gut lumen and is shunted into the systemic circulation in increased amounts in patients with hepatic failure. In addition, other compounds (such as aromatic amino acids, false neurotransmitters, and certain short-chain fatty acids) bypass liver metabolism and accumulate in the systemic circulation, adversely affecting central nervous system function. Their relative importance in the pathogenesis of hepatic encephalopathy remains to be determined.

In addition to producing urea, the reactions of the urea cycle also serve as the pathway for the biosynthesis of arginine. Therefore, this amino acid is not required in the diet of the adult; however, it is required in the diet for growth.

the liver, two important reactions are stimulated. The first is the synthesis of NAG, which increases the rate at which carbamoyl phosphate is produced. The second is to produce more ornithine (via the arginase reaction), such that the cycle can operate more rapidly.

The induction of urea cycle enzymes occurs in response to conditions that require increased protein metabolism, such as a high-protein diet or prolonged fasting. In both of these physiological states, as amino acid carbon is converted to glucose, amino acid nitrogen is converted to urea. The induction of the synthesis of urea cycle enzymes under these conditions occurs even though the uninduced enzyme levels are far in excess of the capacity required. The ability of a high-protein diet to increase urea cycle enzyme levels is another type of feed-forward regulation.

## D. Function of the Urea Cycle during Fasting

During fasting, the liver maintains blood glucose levels. Amino acids from muscle protein are a major carbon source for the production of glucose by the pathway of gluconeogenesis. As amino acid carbons are converted to glucose, the nitrogens are converted to urea. Thus, the urinary excretion of urea is high during fasting. As fasting progresses, however, the brain begins to use ketone bodies, sparing blood glucose. Less muscle protein is cleaved to provide amino acids for gluconeogenesis, and decreased production of glucose from amino acids is accompanied by decreased production of urea (see Chapter 26).

The major amino acid substrate for gluconeogenesis is alanine, which is synthesized in peripheral tissues to act as a nitrogen carrier (see Fig. 32.6). Glucagon release, which is expected during fasting, stimulates alanine transport into the liver by activating the transcription of transport systems for alanine. Two molecules of alanine are required to generate one molecule of glucose. The nitrogen from the two molecules of alanine is converted to one molecule of urea.

## III. DISORDERS OF THE UREA CYCLE

Disorders of the urea cycle are dangerous because of the accumulation of ammonia in the circulation. Ammonia is toxic to the nervous system, and its concentration in the body must be carefully controlled. Under normal conditions, free ammonia is rapidly fixed into either α-ketoglutarate (by glutamate dehydrogenase, to form glutamate) or glutamate (by glutamine synthetase, to form glutamine). The glutamine can be used by many tissues, including the liver; the glutamate donates nitrogens to pyruvate to form alanine, which travels to the liver. Within the liver, as the nitrogens are removed from their carriers, CPSI fixes the ammonia into carbamoyl phosphate to initiate the urea cycle. However, when a urea cycle enzyme is defective, the cycle is interrupted, which leads to an accumulation of urea cycle intermediates before the block. Because of the block in the urea cycle, glutamine levels increase in the circulation, and because α-ketoglutarate is no longer being regenerated by removal of nitrogen from glutamine, the α-ketoglutarate levels are too low to fix more free ammonia, leading to elevated ammonia levels in the blood. Therefore, defects in any urea cycle enzyme lead to elevated glutamine and ammonia levels in the circulation. However, the extent of the elevation depends on which enzyme is defective. (See the questions at the end of this chapter.)

Ammonia toxicity will lead to brain swelling due, in part, to an osmotic imbalance due to high levels of both ammonia and glutamine in the astrocytes. As ammonia levels increase in the astrocytes, more glutamine is produced (via glutamine synthetase), which only exacerbates the osmotic imbalance. The ammonia levels inhibit glutaminase, leading to glutamine elevation. Additionally, high levels of glutamine alter the permeability of the mitochondrial membrane, leading to an opening of a pore in the mitochondrial membrane (the mitochondrial permeability transition pore), which leads to cell death. Another toxic effect of ammonia is a lowering of glutamate levels (due to the high activity of the glutamine synthetase reaction).

Glutamate is a neurotransmitter, and glutamatergic neurotransmission if impaired causes brain dysfunction, because glutamate is one of the excitatory neurotransmitters and in the absence of glutamate neurotransmission, lethargy and reduced nervous system activity can result.

The most common urea cycle defect is OTC deficiency, which is an X-linked disorder. This disorder occurs with a frequency of between 1 in 20,000 and 1 in 80,000 live births. The reason for the range of values is that there is a late-onset form of OTC deficiency that may be underrepresented in the data used to determine the frequency of the disorder in the population.

The major clinical problem in treating patients with urea cycle defects is reducing the effects of excessive blood ammonia on the nervous system. High ammonia levels can lead to irreversible neuronal damage and mental retardation. So how is hyperammonemia treated?

The key to treating patients with urea cycle defects is to diagnose the disease early and then treat aggressively with compounds that can aid in nitrogen removal from the patient. Low-protein diets are essential to reduce the potential for excessive amino acid degradation. If the enzyme defect in the urea cycle comes after the synthesis of argininosuccinate, massive arginine supplementation has proved beneficial. Once argininosuccinate has been synthesized, the two nitrogen molecules destined for excretion have been incorporated into the substrate; the problem is that ornithine cannot be regenerated. If ornithine could be replenished to allow the cycle to continue, argininosuccinate could be used as the carrier for nitrogen excretion from the body. Thus, ingesting large levels of arginine leads to ornithine production by the arginase reaction, and nitrogen excretion via argininosuccinate in the urine can be enhanced.

Arginine therapy will not work for enzyme defects that exist in steps before the synthesis of argininosuccinate. For these disorders, drugs are used that form conjugates with amino acids. The conjugated amino acids are excreted and the body then has to use its nitrogen to resynthesize the excreted amino acid. The two compounds most frequently used are benzoic acid and phenylbutyrate. (The active component of pheylbutyrate is phenylacetate, its oxidation product. Phenylacetate has a bad odor, which makes it difficult to take orally.) As indicated in Figure 32.11A, benzoic acid, after activation, reacts with glycine to form hippuric acid, which is excreted. As glycine is synthesized from serine, the body now uses nitrogens to synthesize serine, so more glycine can be produced. Phenylacetate (see Fig. 32.11B) forms a conjugate with glutamine, which is excreted. This conjugate removes two nitrogens per molecule and requires the body to resynthesize glutamine from glucose, thereby using another two nitrogen molecules.

Urea cycle defects are excellent candidates for treatment by gene therapy. This is because the defect only has to be repaired in one cell type (in this case, the hepatocyte), which makes it easier to target the vector carrying the replacement gene. Preliminary gene therapy experiments had been carried out on individuals with OTC deficiency (the most common inherited defect in the urea cycle), but the experiments came to a halt when one of the patients died of a severe immunological reaction to the vector used to deliver the gene. This incident has placed gene replacement therapy in the United States "on hold" for the foreseeable future.

## CLINICAL COMMENTS

Diseases discussed in this chapter are summarized in Table 32.1.

**Percy V.** The two most serious complications of acute viral hepatitis found in patients such as **Percy V.** are massive hepatic necrosis leading to fulminant liver failure and the eventual development of chronic hepatitis.

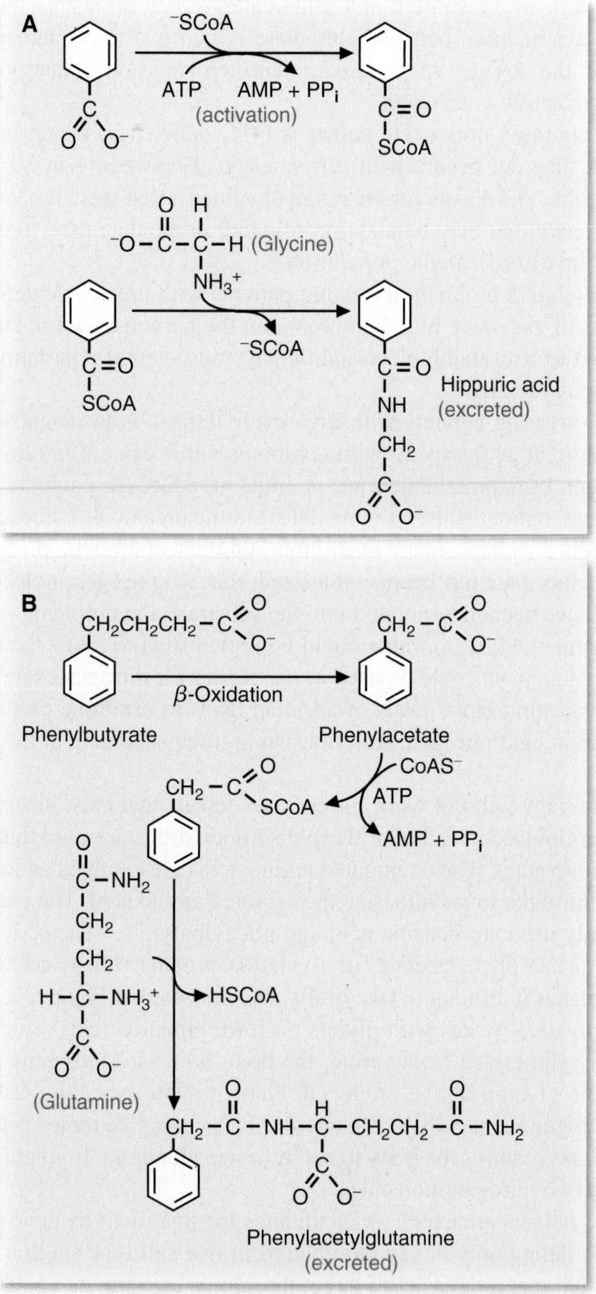

**FIG. 32.11.** The metabolism of benzoic acid (**A**) and phenylbutyrate (**B**), two agents used to reduce nitrogen levels in patients with urea cycle defects.

Both complications are rare in acute viral hepatitis type A, however, suggesting that acetaminophen toxicity may have contributed to Percy's otherwise unexpectedly severe hepatocellular dysfunction and early hepatic encephalopathy.

Fortunately, bed rest, rehydration, parenteral nutrition, and therapy directed at decreasing the production of toxins that result from bacterial degradation of nitrogenous substrates in the gut lumen (e.g., administration of lactulose, which reduces gut ammonia levels by a variety of mechanisms; the use of enemas and certain antibiotics, such as rifaximin, to decrease the intestinal flora; a low-protein diet)

**Table 32.1    Diseases Discussed in Chapter 32**

| Disease or Disorder | Genetic or Environmental | Comments |
|---|---|---|
| Viral hepatitis | Environmental | Infection of the liver by viral hepatitis may lead to liver failure. |
| Pyridoxamine deficiency | Environmental | The lack of vitamin $B_6$ affects many systems, such as heme synthesis, glycogen phosphorylase activity, and neurotransmitter synthesis, leading to possibly dementia, dermatitis, anemia, weakness, and convulsions. |
| Hepatic encephalopathy | Environmental | Liver failure leading to brain dysfunction due to the liver's inability to rid the body of toxins, including ammonia. |
| Ammonia toxicity | Both | Ammonia accumulation interferes with energy production and neurotransmitter synthesis in the brain, altering brain function. |
| Ornithine transcarbamoylase deficiency | Genetic | Most common urea cycle defect, leading to elevated blood ammonia and orotic acid levels and will lead to mental impairment if not treated. |
| CPSI deficiency, argininosuccinate synthetase deficiency, argininosuccinate lyase deficiency, and arginase deficiency | All genetic | Mutations in urea cycle enzymes, leading to various degrees of hyperammonemia and inability to synthesize urea. Can be distinguished by the type of urea cycle intermediates that accumulate in the blood. |

CPSI, carbamoyl phosphate synthetase I.

prevented **Percy V.** from progressing to the later stages of hepatic encephalopathy. As with most patients who survive an episode of fulminant hepatic failure, recovery to his previous state of health occurred over the next 3 months. Percy's liver function studies returned to normal and a follow-up liver biopsy showed no histological abnormalities.

# REVIEW QUESTIONS-CHAPTER 32

*The following case applies to all five questions:*

Deficiency diseases have been described that involve each of the five enzymes of the urea cycle. Clinical manifestations may appear in the neonatal period. Infants with defects in the first four enzymes usually appear normal at birth but after 24 hours progressively develop lethargy, hypothermia, and apnea. They have high blood ammonia levels and the brain becomes swollen. One possible explanation for the swelling is the osmotic effect of the accumulation of glutamine in the brain produced by the reactions of ammonia with α-ketoglutarate and glutamate. Arginase deficiency is not as severe as deficiencies of the other urea cycle enzymes.

Given the following information about five newborn infants (identified as I to V) who appeared normal at birth but developed hyperammonemia after 24 hours, determine which urea cycle enzyme might be defective in each case. All infants had low levels of blood urea nitrogen (BUN). (Normal citrulline levels are 10 to 20 μM.)

| Infant | Urine Orotate | Blood Citrulline | Blood Arginine | Blood Ammonia |
|---|---|---|---|---|
| I | Low | Low | Low | High |
| II | — | High (>1,000 μM) | Low | High |
| III | — | — | High | Moderately high |
| IV | High | Low | Low | High |
| V | — | High (200 μM) | Low | High |

— = Value not determined; low = below normal; high = above normal.

1.  The defect in infant I is in which enzyme?

    A.  Carbamoylphosphate synthetase I (CPSI)
    B.  Ornithine transcarbamoylase
    C.  Argininosuccinate synthetase
    D.  Argininosuccinate lyase
    E.  Arginase

2.   The defect in infant II is in which enzyme?

    A.   Carbamoylphosphate synthetase I (CPSI)
    B.   Ornithine transcarbamoylase
    C.   Argininosuccinate synthetase
    D.   Argininosuccinate lyase
    E.   Arginase

3.   The defect in infant III is in which enzyme?

    A.   Carbamoylphosphate synthetase I (CPSI)
    B.   Ornithine transcarbamoylase
    C.   Argininosuccinate synthetase
    D.   Argininosuccinate lyase
    E.   Arginase

4.   The defect in infant IV is in which enzyme?

    A.   Carbamoylphosphate synthetase I (CPSI)
    B.   Ornithine transcarbamoylase
    C.   Argininosuccinate synthetase
    D.   Argininosuccinate lyase
    E.   Arginase

5.   The defect in infant V is in which enzyme?

    A.   Carbamoylphosphate synthetase I (CPSI)
    B.   Ornithine transcarbamoylase
    C.   Argininosuccinate synthetase
    D.   Argininosuccinate lyase
    E.   Arginase

# 33 Synthesis and Degradation of Amino Acids and Amino Acid–Derived Products

## CHAPTER OUTLINE

## KEY POINTS

- Humans can synthesize only 11 of the 20 amino acids required for protein synthesis; the other 9 are considered to be essential amino acids in the diet.
- Amino acid metabolism uses, to a large extent, the cofactors pyridoxal phosphate, tetrahydrobiopterin ($BH_4$), and tetrahydrofolate ($FH_4$).
  - Pyridoxal phosphate is required primarily for transamination reactions.
  - $BH_4$ is required for ring hydroxylation reactions.
  - $FH_4$ is required for one-carbon metabolism and is discussed further in Chapter 34.
- The nonessential amino acids can be synthesized from glycolytic intermediates (serine, glycine, cysteine, and alanine), TCA cycle intermediates (aspartate, asparagine, glutamate, glutamine, proline, arginine, and ornithine), or from existing amino acids (tyrosine from phenylalanine).

continued

- When amino acids are degraded, the nitrogen is converted to urea, and the carbon skeletons are classified as either glucogenic (a precursor of glucose) or ketogenic (a precursor of ketone bodies).
- Defects in amino acid degradation pathways can lead to disease.
  - Glycine degradation can lead to oxalate production, which may lead to one class of kidney stone formation.
  - Defects in methionine degradation can lead to hyperhomocysteinemia, which has been linked to blood clotting disorders and heart disease.
  - A defect in branched-chain amino acid degradation leads to maple syrup urine disease, which has severe neurological consequences.
  - Defects in phenylalanine and tyrosine degradation lead to phenylketonuria (PKU), alcaptonuria, and albinism.
- Amino acids are also the precursors for the small nitrogen–containing neurotransmitters, such as the catecholamines, serotonin, and histamine.
- Glycine is required for the biosynthesis of heme. Mutations in enzymes involved in heme biosynthesis give rise to a class of diseases known as the porphyrias.

# THE WAITING ROOM

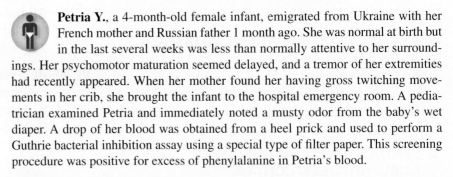

**Petria Y.**, a 4-month-old female infant, emigrated from Ukraine with her French mother and Russian father 1 month ago. She was normal at birth but in the last several weeks was less than normally attentive to her surroundings. Her psychomotor maturation seemed delayed, and a tremor of her extremities had recently appeared. When her mother found her having gross twitching movements in her crib, she brought the infant to the hospital emergency room. A pediatrician examined Petria and immediately noted a musty odor from the baby's wet diaper. A drop of her blood was obtained from a heel prick and used to perform a Guthrie bacterial inhibition assay using a special type of filter paper. This screening procedure was positive for excess of phenylalanine in Petria's blood.

**Horace S.**, a 14-year-old boy, had a sudden grand mal seizure (with jerking movements of the torso and head) in his eighth grade classroom. The school physician noted mild weakness of the muscles of the left side of Horace's face and of his left arm and leg. Horace was hospitalized with a tentative diagnosis of a cerebrovascular accident involving the right cerebral hemisphere, which presumably triggered the seizure.

Horace's past medical history was normal, except for slight intellectual disability requiring placement in a special education group. He also had a downward partial dislocation of the lenses of both eyes for which he had a surgical procedure.

Horace's left-sided neurological deficits cleared within 3 days, but a computerized axial tomogram (CAT) showed changes consistent with a small infarction (a damaged area caused by a temporary or permanent loss of adequate arterial blood flow) in the right cerebral hemisphere. A neurologist noted that Horace had a slight waddling gait, which his mother said began several years earlier and was progressing with time. Further studies confirmed the decreased mineralization (decreased density) of the skeleton (called osteopenia if mild and osteoporosis if more severe) and high methionine and homocysteine but low cystine levels in the blood.

All of this information, plus the increased length of the long bones of Horace's extremities and a slight curvature of his spine (scoliosis), caused his physician to suspect that Horace might have an inborn error of metabolism.

# I.  OVERVIEW OF AMINO ACID METABOLISM

Amino acids, produced by digestion of dietary proteins, are absorbed through intestinal epithelial cells and enter the blood (see Chapter 31). Various cell types take up these amino acids, which enter the cellular pools. They are used for the synthesis of proteins and other nitrogen-containing compounds (such as neurotransmitters, heme, and the purines and pyrimidines), or they are oxidized for energy (Fig. 33.1). They may also be converted to glucose for storage as glycogen or to fatty acids for storage as adipose triacylglycerol. When amino acids are oxidized, they can be classified as either glucogenic (giving rise to a precursor which can synthesize glucose) or ketogenic (giving rise to a precursor which can synthesize ketone bodies but not glucose). There are only two strictly ketogenic amino acids: leucine and lysine. All other amino acids can be used to synthesize glucose.

Eleven of the 20 amino acids used to form proteins are synthesized in the body if an adequate amount is not present in the diet (Table 33.1). Ten of these amino acids can be produced from glucose; the 11th, tyrosine, is synthesized from the essential amino acid phenylalanine. It should be noted that cysteine, 1 of the 10 amino acids produced from glucose, obtains its sulfur atom from the essential amino acid methionine.

Certain amino acids are essential to the human. "Essential" means that the carbon skeleton cannot be synthesized and, therefore, these amino acids are required in the diet (see Table 33.1). Arginine is essential during periods of growth; in adults, it is no longer considered essential.

In this chapter, we will primarily discuss pathways that are associated with disease, although not all disorders of amino acid metabolism will be discussed.

# II.  THE ROLE OF COFACTORS IN AMINO ACID METABOLISM

Amino acid metabolism requires the participation of three important cofactors. Pyridoxal phosphate (PLP) is the quintessential coenzyme of amino acid metabolism (see Chapter 32). It is required for the following types of reactions involving amino acids: transamination, deamination, decarboxylation, β-elimination, racemization, and γ-elimination. Almost all pathways involving amino acid metabolism will require PLP at one step in the pathway.

The coenzyme tetrahydrofolate ($FH_4$), which is derived from the vitamin folate, is required in certain amino acid pathways to either accept or donate a one-carbon group. The carbon can be in various states of oxidation. Chapter 34 describes the reactions of $FH_4$ in much more detail.

The coenzyme tetrahydrobiopterin ($BH_4$) is required for ring hydroxylations. The reactions involve molecular oxygen, and one atom of oxygen is incorporated into the product. The second is found in water. $BH_4$ is important for the synthesis of tyrosine and neurotransmitters (see Section V of this chapter).

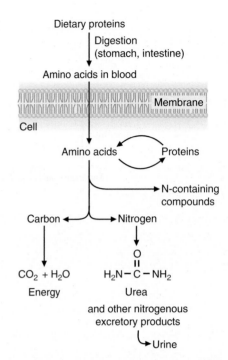

**FIG. 33.1.** Summary of amino acid metabolism. Dietary proteins are digested to amino acids in the stomach and intestine, which are absorbed by the intestinal epithelium, transferred to the circulation, and taken up by cells. Amino acids are used to synthesize proteins and other nitrogen-containing compounds. The carbon skeletons of amino acids are also oxidized for energy, and the nitrogen is converted to urea and other nitrogenous excretory products.

**Table 33.1  Essential and Nonessential Amino Acids**

| Essential in the Diet | Amino Acids Synthesized in the Body[a] | |
| --- | --- | --- |
| | From Glucose | From an Essential Amino Acid |
| Histidine | Alanine | Tyrosine (from phenylalanine) |
| Isoleucine | Arginine | |
| Leucine | Asparagine | |
| Lysine | Aspartate | |
| Methionine | Cysteine[b] | |
| Phenylalanine | Glutamic acid | |
| Threonine | Glutamine | |
| Tryptophan | Glycine | |
| Valine | Proline | |
| Arginine[c] | Serine | |

[a]These amino acids are called "nonessential" or "dispensable," terms that refer to dietary requirements. Of course, within the body, they are necessary. We cannot survive without them.
[b]Although the carbons of cysteine can be derived from glucose, its sulfur is obtained from the essential amino acid methionine.
[c]Arginine is not required by the adult, but is required for growth.

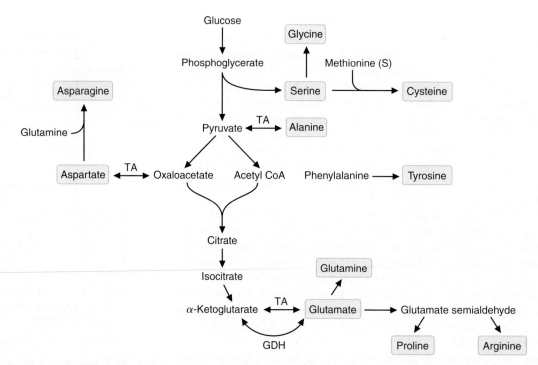

**FIG. 33.2.** Overview of the synthesis of the nonessential amino acids. The carbons of 10 amino acids may be produced from glucose through intermediates of glycolysis or the TCA cycle. The 11th nonessential amino acid, tyrosine, is synthesized by hydroxylation of the essential amino acid phenylalanine. Only the sulfur of cysteine comes from the essential amino acid methionine; its carbons and nitrogen come from serine. Transamination (TA) reactions involve PLP and another amino acid–α-keto acid pair.

## III. BIOSYNTHESIS OF THE NONESSENTIAL AMINO ACIDS

An overview of the biosynthesis of nonessential amino acids is shown in Figure 33.2. Four amino acids are derived from intermediates of glycolysis: serine, glycine, cysteine, and alanine, whereas six amino acids found in proteins are derived from tricarboxylic acid (TCA) cycle intermediates. Tyrosine is synthesized from the essential amino acid phenylalanine.

### A. Serine, Glycine, Cysteine, and Alanine

Serine, which produces glycine and cysteine, is synthesized from 3-phosphoglycerate, and alanine is formed by transamination of pyruvate. Glycine is primarily produced from serine but can also be produced by threonine. The major route of production from serine is by a reversible reaction that involves FH₄ and PLP (Fig. 33.3). The minor pathway for glycine formation involves threonine degradation (in an aldolase-like reaction).

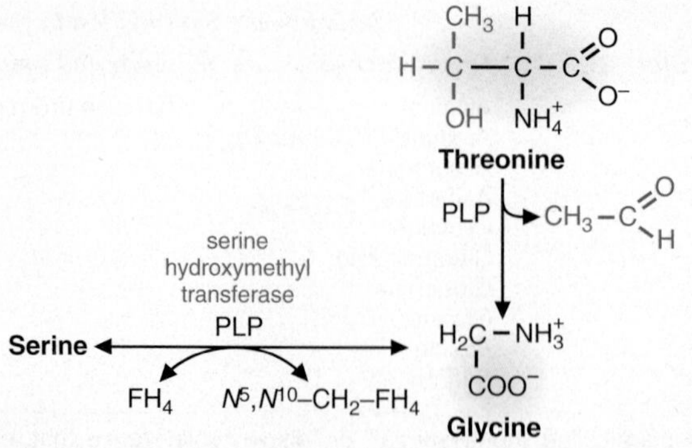

**FIG. 33.3.** Biosynthesis of glycine. Glycine can be synthesized from serine (major route) or threonine. The serine hydroxymethyltransferase reaction requires $FH_4$ and produces $N^5$, $N^{10}$-methylene-$FH_4$ ($N^5$, $N^{10}$-$CH_2$-$FH_4$).

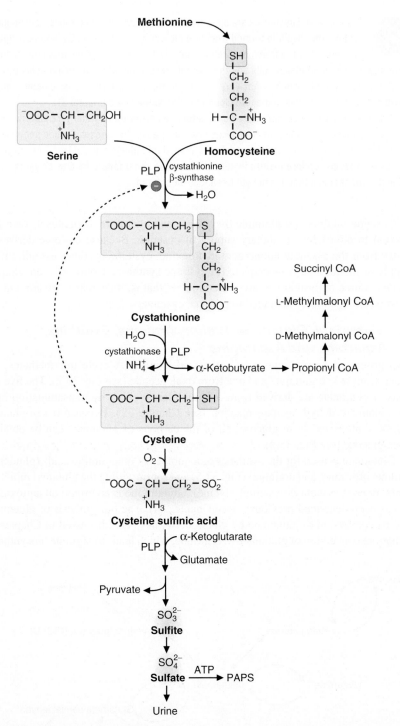

**FIG. 33.4.** Synthesis and degradation of cysteine. Cysteine is synthesized from the carbons and nitrogen of serine and the sulfur of homocysteine (which is derived from methionine). During the degradation of cysteine, the sulfur is converted to sulfate and either excreted in the urine or converted to 3′-phosphoadenosine 5′-phosphosulfate (PAPS; universal sulfate donor), and the carbons are converted to pyruvate. *PLP*, pyridoxal phosphate.

The carbons and nitrogen for cysteine synthesis are provided by serine, and the sulfur is provided by methionine (Fig. 33.4). Serine reacts with homocysteine (which is produced from methionine) to form cystathionine. This reaction is catalyzed by cystathionine β-synthase. Cleavage of cystathionine by cystathionase produces cysteine and α-ketobutyrate, which forms succinyl coenzyme A (CoA) via propionyl CoA. Both cystathionine β-synthase (β-elimination) and cystathionase (γ-elimination) require PLP.

 Cystathioninuria, the presence of cystathionine in the urine, is relatively common in premature infants. As they mature, cystathionase levels rise, and the levels of cystathionine in the urine decrease. In adults, a genetic deficiency of cystathionase causes cystathioninuria. Individuals with a genetically normal cystathionase can also develop cystathioninuria from a dietary deficiency of pyridoxine (vitamin $B_6$) because cystathionase requires the cofactor PLP. No characteristic clinical abnormalities have been observed in individuals with cystathionase deficiency, and it is probably a benign disorder.

Homocysteine is oxidized to a disulfide, homocystine. To indicate that both forms are being considered, the term homocyst(e)ine is used.

### Homocysteine

$$
\begin{array}{c}
COO^- \\
| \\
H_3\overset{+}{N} - CH \\
| \\
CH_2 \\
| \\
CH_2 \\
| \\
\boxed{SH}
\end{array}
\qquad\longleftrightarrow\qquad
\begin{array}{c}
COO^- \\
| \\
H_3\overset{+}{N} - CH \\
| \\
CH_2 \\
| \\
CH_2 \\
| \\
\boxed{S} \\
| \\
\boxed{S} \\
| \\
CH_2 \\
| \\
CH_2 \\
| \\
H - C - \overset{+}{N}H_3 \\
| \\
COO^-
\end{array}
$$

$$
\begin{array}{c}
\boxed{SH} \\
| \\
CH_2 \\
| \\
CH_2 \\
| \\
H - C - \overset{+}{N}H_3 \\
| \\
COO^-
\end{array}
$$

**Homocysteine**          **Homocystine**

Because a colorimetric screening test for urinary homocystine was positive, the doctor ordered several biochemical studies on **Horace S.'s** serum, which included tests for methionine, homocyst(e)ine (both free and protein bound), cystine, vitamin B$_{12}$, and folate. The level of homocystine in a 24-hour urine collection was also measured.

The results were as follows: the serum methionine level was 980 μM (reference range, <30 μM); serum homocyst(e)ine (both free and protein bound) was markedly elevated; cystine was not detected in the serum; the serum B$_{12}$ and folate levels were normal. A 24-hour urine homocystine level was elevated.

Based on these measurements, **Horace S.'s** doctor concluded that he had homocystinuria caused by an enzyme deficiency. What was the rationale for this conclusion?

Cystinuria and cystinosis are disorders involving two different transport proteins for cystine, the disulfide formed from two molecules of cysteine. Cystinuria is caused by a defect in the transport protein that carries cystine, lysine, arginine, and ornithine into intestinal epithelial cells and that permits resorption of these amino acids by renal tubular cells. Cystine, which is not very soluble in the urine, forms renal calculi (stones). **David K.**, a patient with cystinuria, developed cystine stones (see Chapter 31).

Cystinosis is a rare disorder caused by a defective carrier that normally transports cystine across the lysosomal membrane from lysosomal vesicles to the cytosol. Cystine accumulates in the lysosomes in many tissues and forms crystals, leading to a depletion of intracellular cysteine levels. Children with this disorder develop renal failure by 6 to 12 years of age through a mechanism that has not yet been fully elucidated.

Cysteine inhibits cystathionine β-synthase and, therefore, regulates its own production to adjust for the dietary supply of cysteine. Because cysteine derives its sulfur from the essential amino acid methionine, cysteine becomes essential if the supply of methionine is inadequate for cysteine synthesis. Conversely, an adequate dietary source of cysteine "spares" methionine; that is, it decreases the amount that must be endogenously degraded to produce cysteine.

### B. Glutamate, Glutamine, Proline, Arginine, Ornithine, Aspartate, and Asparagine

Two groups of amino acids are synthesized from TCA cycle intermediates; one group from α-ketoglutarate and one from oxaloacetate (see Fig. 33.2). The five carbons of glutamate are derived from α-ketoglutarate either by transamination or by the glutamate dehydrogenase reaction (see Chapter 32). Because α-ketoglutarate can be synthesized from glucose, all of the carbons of glutamate can be obtained from glucose (see Fig. 33.2).

Glutamate is used for the synthesis of a number of other amino acids (glutamine, proline, ornithine, and arginine) (Fig. 33.5) and for providing the glutamyl moiety of glutathione (γ-glutamyl-cysteinyl-glycine). Glutathione is an important antioxidant, as has been described previously (see Chapter 24). The biosynthesis of glutamine, and its conversion to glutamate by glutaminase, has been discussed in Chapter 32, as has the conversion of glutamate to ornithine, which leads to arginine biosynthesis.

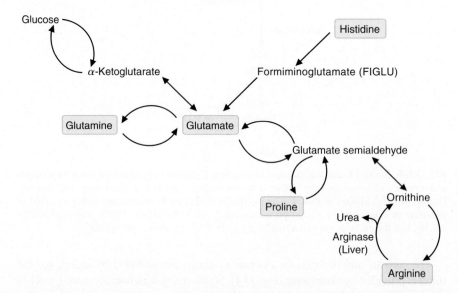

**FIG. 33.5.** Amino acids related through glutamate. These amino acids contain carbons that can be reconverted to glutamate, which can be converted to glucose in the liver. All of these amino acids except histidine can be synthesized from glucose.

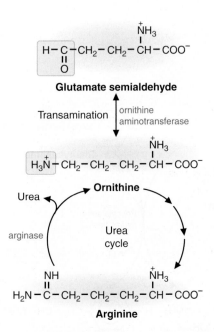

**Glutamate semialdehyde**

Transamination | ornithine aminotransferase

**Ornithine**

Urea

arginase

Urea cycle

**Arginine**

**FIG. 33.6.** Synthesis and degradation of arginine. The carbons of ornithine are derived from glutamate semialdehyde, which is derived from glutamate. Reactions of the urea cycle convert ornithine to arginine. Arginase converts arginine back to ornithine by releasing urea.

 If the blood levels of methionine and homocysteine are very elevated and cystine is low, cystathionine β-synthase could be defective, but a cystathionase deficiency is also a possibility. With a deficiency of either of these enzymes, cysteine could not be synthesized and levels of homocysteine would rise. Homocysteine would be converted to methionine by reactions that require B$_{12}$ and tetrahydrofolate (see Chapter 34). In addition, it would be oxidized to homocystine, which would appear in the urine. The levels of cysteine (measured as its oxidation product cystine) would be low. A measurement of serum cystathionine levels would help to distinguish between a cystathionase or cystathionine β-synthase deficiency.

Arginine is synthesized from glutamate via glutamate semialdehyde, which is transaminated to form ornithine, an intermediate of the urea cycle (see Chapter 32 and Fig. 33.6). This activity (ornithine aminotransferase) appears to be greatest in the epithelial cells of the small intestine (see Chapter 36). The reactions of the urea cycle then produce arginine. However, the quantities of arginine generated by the urea cycle are adequate only for the adult and are insufficient to support growth. Therefore, during periods of growth, arginine becomes an essential amino acid. It is important to realize that if arginine is used for protein synthesis, the levels of ornithine will drop, thereby slowing the urea cycle. This will stimulate the formation of ornithine from glutamate.

Arginine is cleaved by arginase to form urea and ornithine. If ornithine is present in amounts in excess of those required for the urea cycle, it is transaminated to glutamate semialdehyde, which is oxidized to glutamate. The conversion of an aldehyde to a primary amine is a unique form of a transamination reaction and requires PLP.

Aspartate is produced by transamination of oxaloacetate. This reaction is readily reversible, so aspartate can be reconverted to oxaloacetate.

Asparagine is formed from aspartate by a reaction in which glutamine provides the nitrogen for formation of the amide group. Thus, this reaction differs from the synthesis of glutamine from glutamate in which ammonium ion ($NH_4^+$) provides the nitrogen. However, the reaction catalyzed by asparaginase, which hydrolyzes asparagine to $NH_4^+$ and aspartate, is analogous to the reaction catalyzed by glutaminase.

## C.  Tyrosine

Phenylalanine is converted to tyrosine via a ring hydroxylation reaction (Fig. 33.7). The enzyme phenylalanine hydroxylase (PAH) requires molecular oxygen ($O_2$) and BH$_4$. The cofactor BH$_4$ is converted to quininoid dihydrobiopterin by this reaction. BH$_4$ is not synthesized from a vitamin; it can be synthesized in the body from guanosine triphosphate (GTP). However, as is the case with other cofactors, the body contains limited amounts. Therefore, dihydrobiopterin must be converted to BH$_4$ in order for the reaction to continue to produce tyrosine.

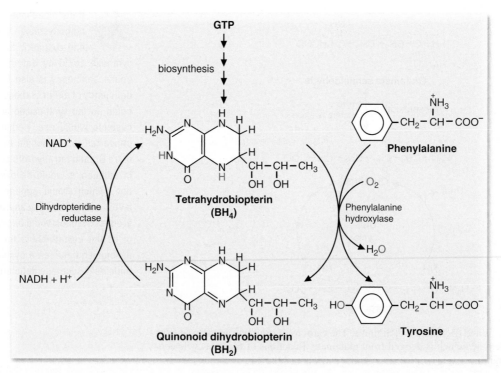

**FIG. 33.7.** Hydroxylation of phenylalanine. PAH is a mixed-function oxidase; that is, molecular $O_2$ donates one atom to water and one to the product, tyrosine. The cofactor, $BH_4$, is oxidized to dihydrobiopterin ($BH_2$) and must be reduced back to $BH_4$ for the PAH to continue forming tyrosine. $BH_4$ is synthesized in the body from GTP. The disease phenylketonuria (PKU) results from deficiencies of PAH (the classic form), dihydropteridine reductase (DHPR), or enzymes in the biosynthetic pathway for $BH_4$.

## IV. AMINO ACID DEGRADATION AND DISEASE

Amino acids, when degraded, give rise to glucogenic or ketogenic carbon skeletons (the nitrogens go to urea). Figure 33.8 shows the ultimate fate of amino acid carbons in degradation. The remainder of this section will focus on selected pathways, which, when interfered with, can lead to disease.

### A. Glycine

Glycine degradation can occur via two routes (Fig. 33.9). One is conversion to carbon dioxide, ammonia, and $N^5,N^{10}$-methylenetetrahydrofolate via glycine cleavage enzyme. This is the only pathway for glycine oxidation that can generate energy. The other is the conversion of glycine to glyoxylate by the enzyme D–amino acid oxidase in a degradative pathway of glycine that is clinically relevant. Once glyoxylate is formed, it can be oxidized to oxalate, which is sparingly soluble and tends to precipitate in kidney tubules, leading to kidney stone formation. Approximately 40% of oxalate formation in the liver comes from glycine metabolism. Dietary oxalate accumulation has been estimated to be a low contributor to excreted oxalate in the urine because of poor absorption of oxalate in the intestine.

Although glyoxalate can be transaminated back to glycine, this is not really considered a biosynthetic route for "new" glycine because the primary route for glyoxylate formation is from glycine oxidation.

### B. Methionine

The methionine degradative pathway is the same as the biosynthesis of cysteine (see Fig. 33.4). Methionine is converted to *S*-adenosylmethionine (SAM), which donates its methyl group to other compounds to form *S*-adenosylhomocysteine (SAH). SAH is then converted to homocysteine (Fig. 33.10). Methionine can be regenerated from homocysteine by a reaction requiring both $FH_4$ and vitamin $B_{12}$ (a topic

Oxalate, produced from glycine or obtained from the diet, forms precipitates with calcium. Kidney stones (renal calculi) are often composed of calcium oxalate. A lack of the transaminase that can convert glyoxylate to glycine (see Fig. 33.9) leads to the disease primary oxaluria type I (PH 1). This disease has a consequence of renal failure attributable to excessive accumulation of oxalate in the kidney.

Homocystinuria is caused by deficiencies in the enzymes cystathionine β-synthase and cystathionase as well as by deficiencies of methyltetrahydrofolate ($CH_3$-$FH_4$) or of methyl-$B_{12}$. The deficiencies of $CH_3$-$FH_4$ or of methyl-$B_{12}$ are caused by either an inadequate dietary intake of folate or $B_{12}$ or by defective enzymes involved in joining methyl groups to tetrahydrofolate ($FH_4$), transferring methyl groups from $FH_4$ to $B_{12}$ or passing them from $B_{12}$ to homocysteine to form methionine (see Chapter 34).

Is **Horace S.'s** homocystinuria caused by any of these problems?

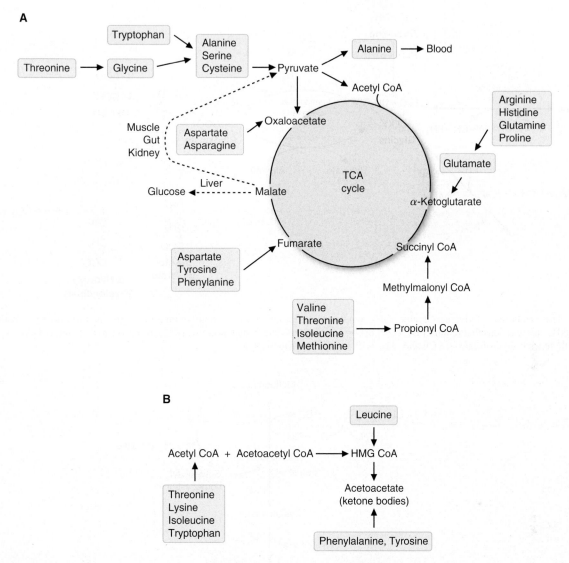

**FIG. 33.8.** Degradation of amino acids. **A.** Amino acids that produce pyruvate or intermediates of the TCA cycle. These amino acids are considered glucogenic because they can produce glucose in the liver. The fumarate group of amino acids produces cytoplasmic fumarate. **B.** Amino acids that produce acetyl CoA or ketone bodies. These amino acids are considered ketogenic.

that is considered in more detail in Chapter 34). Alternatively, by reactions that require PLP, homocysteine can provide the sulfur needed for the synthesis of cysteine (see Fig. 33.4). Carbons of homocysteine are then metabolized to α-ketobutyrate, which undergoes oxidative decarboxylation to propionyl CoA. The propionyl CoA is then converted to succinyl CoA (see Fig. 33.10). Because this is the only degradative route for homocysteine, vitamin B₆ deficiency or congenital cystathionine β-synthase deficiency can result in homocysteinemia, which is associated with cardiovascular disease (see Chapter 34).

## C. Branched-Chain Amino Acids

The branched-chain amino acids (valine, isoleucine, and leucine) are a universal fuel, and the degradation of these amino acids occurs at low levels in the mitochondria of most tissues, but the muscle carries out the highest level of branched-chain amino acid oxidation. The branched-chain amino acids make up almost 25% of the content of the average protein, so their use as fuel is quite significant. The degradative pathway for valine and isoleucine has two major functions, the first being

 **Horace S.'s** methionine levels are elevated, and his B₁₂ and folate levels are normal. Therefore, he does not have a deficiency of dietary folate or vitamin B₁₂ or of the enzymes that transfer methyl groups from tetrahydrofolate to homocysteine to form methionine. In these cases, homocysteine levels are elevated but methionine levels are low.

A biopsy specimen from **Horace S.'s** liver was sent to the hospital's biochemistry research laboratory for enzyme assays. Cystathionine β-synthase activity was reported to be 7% of that found in normal liver.

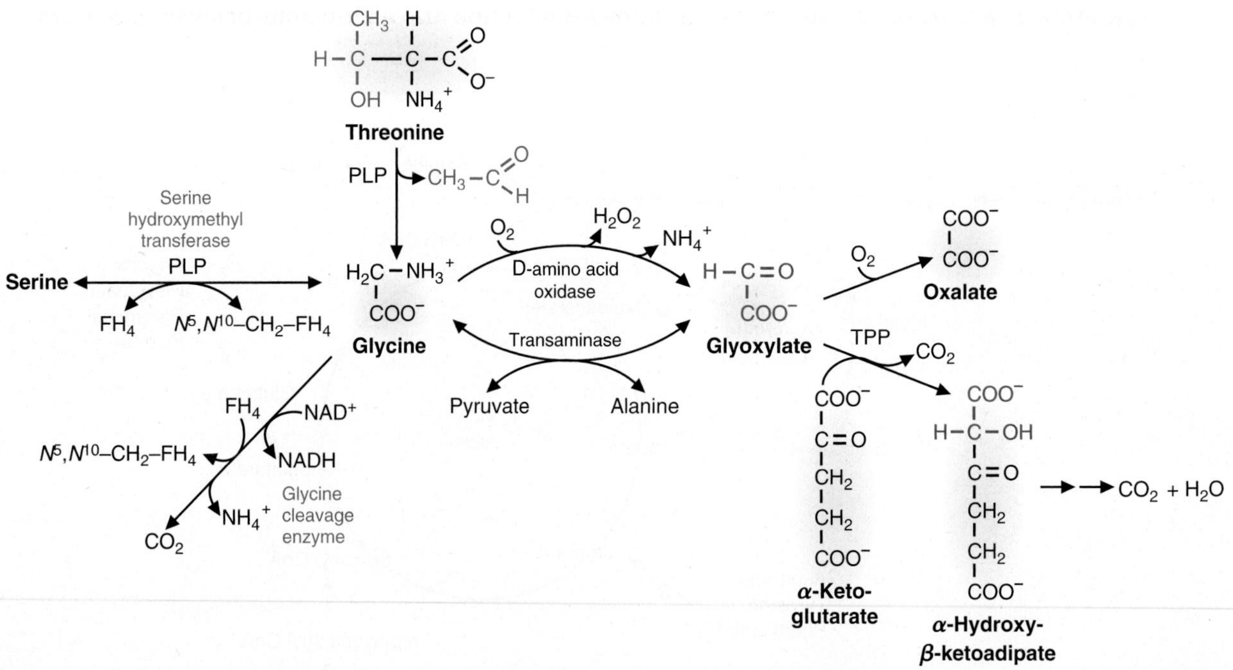

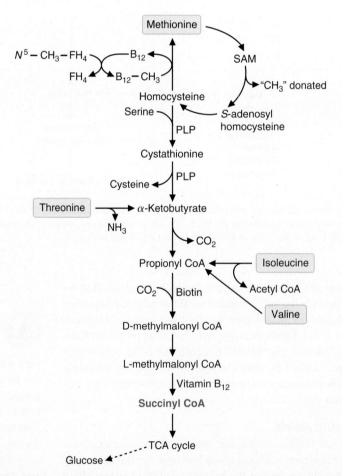

**FIG. 33.9.** The metabolism of glycine. Glycine can be synthesized from serine (major route) or threonine. Glycine forms serine or carbon dioxide ($CO_2$) and $NH_4^+$ by reactions that require $FH_4$. Glycine also forms glyoxylate, which is converted to oxalate or to $CO_2$ and $H_2O$. $N^5,N^{10}$-$CH_2$-$FH_4$, $N^5$, $N^{10}$-methylenetetrahydrofolate (see Chapter 34); *TPP*, thiamine pyrophosphate.

**FIG. 33.10.** Conversion of methionine and other amino acids to succinyl CoA. The amino acids methionine, threonine, isoleucine, and valine, all of which form succinyl CoA via methylmalonyl CoA, are essential in the diet. The carbons of serine are converted to cysteine and do not form succinyl CoA by this pathway. *SAM*, S-adenosylmethionine; *PLP*, pyridoxal phosphate; B12-CH3, methylcobalamin; $N^5$-$CH_3$-$FH_4$, $N^5$-methyl tetrahydrofolate.

energy generation and the second to provide precursors to replenish TCA cycle intermediates (anaplerosis). Both valine and isoleucine contain carbons that form succinyl CoA. The initial step in the degradation of the branched-chain amino acids is a transamination reaction. In the second step of the degradative pathway, the α-keto analogues of these amino acids undergo oxidative decarboxylation by the α-keto acid dehydrogenase complex in a reaction similar in its mechanism and cofactor requirements to pyruvate dehydrogenase and α-ketoglutarate dehydrogenase. As with the first enzyme of the pathway, the highest level of activity for this dehydrogenase is found in muscle tissue. Subsequently, the pathways for degradation of these amino acids follow parallel routes (Fig. 33.11). The steps are analogous to those for β-oxidation of fatty acids so nicotinamide adenine dinucleotide (NADH) and flavin adenine dinucleotide (FAD[2H]) are generated for energy production.

Valine and isoleucine are converted to succinyl CoA (see Fig. 33.10). Isoleucine also forms acetyl CoA. Leucine, the third branched-chain amino acid, does not produce succinyl CoA. It forms acetoacetate and acetyl CoA and is strictly ketogenic. In maple syrup urine disease, the branched-chain α-keto acid dehydrogenase that oxidatively decarboxylates the branched-chain amino acids is defective. As a result, the branched-chain amino acids and their α-keto analogues (produced by transamination) accumulate. They appear in the urine, giving it the odor of maple syrup or burnt sugar. The accumulation of α-keto analogues leads to neurological complications. This condition is difficult to treat by dietary restriction because abnormalities in the metabolism of three essential amino acids contribute to the disease.

Thiamine deficiency will lead to an accumulation of α-keto acids in the blood because of an inability of pyruvate dehydrogenase, α-ketoglutarate dehydrogenase, and branched-chain α-keto acid dehydrogenase to catalyze their reactions. **Al M.** had a thiamine deficiency resulting from his chronic alcoholism. His ketoacidosis resulted partly from the accumulation of these α-keto acids in his blood and partly from the accumulation of ketone bodies used for energy production. Beriberi is the disorder which results from thiamine deficiency.

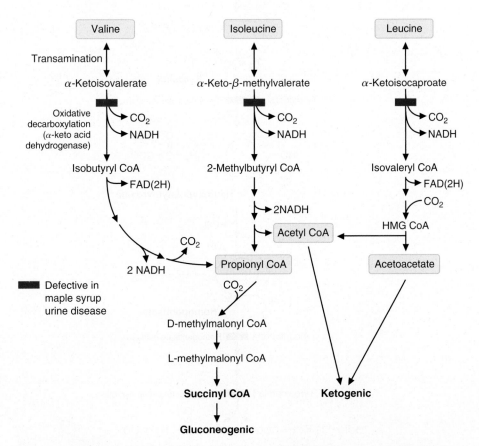

**FIG. 33.11.** Degradation of the branched-chain amino acids. Valine forms propionyl CoA. Isoleucine forms propionyl CoA and acetyl CoA. Leucine forms acetoacetate and acetyl CoA.

### D. Phenylalanine and Tyrosine

The degradation of phenylalanine and tyrosine are the same, as phenylalanine is converted to tyrosine, which then undergoes oxidative degradation (Fig. 33.12). The last step in the pathway produces both fumarate and the ketone body acetoacetate. Deficiencies of different enzymes in the pathway result in phenylketonuria, tyrosinemia, and alcaptonuria.

Alcaptonuria occurs when homogentisate, an intermediate in tyrosine metabolism, cannot be further oxidized because the next enzyme in the pathway, homogentisate oxidase, is defective. Homogentisate accumulates and auto-oxidizes, forming a dark pigment, which discolors the urine and stains the diapers of affected infants. Later in life, the chronic accumulation of this pigment in cartilage may cause arthritic joint pain.

Transient tyrosinemia is frequently observed in newborn infants, especially those that are premature. For the most part, the condition appears to be benign and dietary restriction of protein returns plasma tyrosine levels to normal. The biochemical defect is most likely a low level, attributable to immaturity, of 4-hydroxyphenylpyruvate

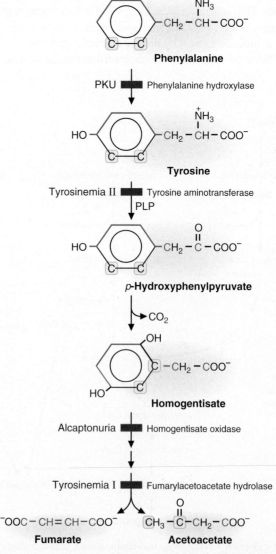

**FIG. 33.12.** Degradation of phenylalanine and tyrosine. The carboxyl carbon forms $CO_2$, and the other carbons form fumarate or acetoacetate as indicated. Deficiencies of enzymes (*dark bars*) result in the indicated diseases. *PKU*, phenylketonuria; *PLP*, pyridoxal phosphate.

dioxygenase. Because this enzyme requires ascorbate, ascorbate supplementation also aids in reducing circulating tyrosine levels.

Other types of tyrosinemia are related to specific enzyme defects (see Fig. 33.12). Tyrosinemia II is caused by a genetic deficiency of tyrosine aminotransferase (TAT) and may lead to lesions of the eye and skin as well as neurological problems. Patients are treated with a low-tyrosine, low-phenylalanine diet.

Tyrosinemia I (also called tyrosinosis) is caused by a genetic deficiency of fumarylacetoacetate hydrolase. The acute form is associated with liver failure, a cabbagelike odor, and death within the first year of life.

A small subset of patients with hyperphenylalaninemia show an appropriate reduction in plasma phenylalanine levels with dietary restriction of this amino acid; however, these patients still develop progressive neurological symptoms and seizures and usually die within the first 2 years of life ("malignant" hyperphenylalaninemia). These infants exhibit normal PAH activity but have a deficiency in dihydropteridine reductase (DHPR), an enzyme required for the regeneration of $BH_4$, a cofactor of PAH (see Fig. 33.7). Less frequently, DHPR activity is normal but a defect in the biosynthesis of $BH_4$ exists. In either case, dietary therapy corrects the hyperphenylalaninemia. However, $BH_4$ is also a cofactor for two other hydroxylations required in the synthesis of neurotransmitters in the brain: the hydroxylation of tryptophan to 5-hydroxytryptophan and of tyrosine to L-dopa (see Section V of this chapter). It has been suggested that the resulting deficit in central nervous system neurotransmitter activity is, at least in part, responsible for the neurological manifestations and eventual death of these patients.

### E.  Tryptophan

When tryptophan is degraded, it is oxidized to produce alanine (from the nonring carbons), formate, and acetyl CoA. Tryptophan is, therefore, both glucogenic and ketogenic. $NAD^+$ and $NADP^+$ can be produced from the ring structure of tryptophan. Therefore, tryptophan "spares" the dietary requirement for niacin. The higher the dietary levels of tryptophan, the lower the levels of niacin required to prevent symptoms of deficiency.

A summary of the amino acid disorders discussed in this chapter is presented in Table 33.2.

### V.  SYNTHESIS AND INACTIVATION OF SMALL NITROGEN-CONTAINING NEUROTRANSMITTERS

Molecules that serve as neurotransmitters fall into two basic structural categories: (a) small nitrogen-containing molecules and (b) neuropeptides. The major small nitrogen-containing molecule neurotransmitters include glutamate, γ-aminobutyric acid (GABA), glycine, acetylcholine, dopamine, norepinephrine, serotonin, and histamine.

If the dietary levels of niacin and tryptophan are insufficient, the condition known as pellagra results. The symptoms of pellagra are dermatitis, diarrhea, dementia, and finally, death. In addition, abnormal metabolism of tryptophan occurs in a vitamin $B_6$ deficiency. Kynurenine intermediates in the tryptophan degradation pathway cannot be cleaved because kynureninase requires PLP derived from vitamin $B_6$. Consequently, these intermediates enter a minor pathway for tryptophan metabolism that produces xanthurenic acid, which is excreted in the urine.

### Table 33.2  Genetic Disorders of Amino Acid Metabolism

| Amino Acid Degradation Pathway | Missing Enzyme | Product that Accumulates | Disease | Symptoms |
|---|---|---|---|---|
| Phenylalanine | Phenylalanine hydroxylase | Phenylalanine | PKU (classical) | Mental retardation |
| | Dihydropteridine reductase | Phenylalanine | PKU (nonclassical) | Mental retardation |
| | Homogentisate oxidase | Homogentisic acid | Alcaptonuria | Black urine, arthritis |
| | Fumarylacetoacetate hydrolase | Fumarylacetoacetate | Tyrosinemia I | Liver failure, early death |
| Tyrosine | Tyrosine aminotransferase | Tyrosine | Tyrosinemia II | Neurological defects |
| Methionine | Cystathionase | Cystathionine | Cystathioninuria | Benign |
| | Cystathionine β-synthase | Homocysteine | Homocysteinemia | Cardiovascular complications and neurological problems |
| Glycine | Glycine transaminase | Glyoxylate | Primary oxaluria type I | Renal failure due to stone formation |
| Branched-chain amino acids (leucine, isoleucine, valine) | Branched-chain α-keto acid dehydrogenase | α-Keto acids of the branched-chain amino acids | Maple syrup urine disease | Mental retardation |

PKU, phenylketonuria.

Additional neurotransmitters that fall into this category include epinephrine, aspartate, and nitric oxide. In general, each neuron synthesizes only those neurotransmitters that it uses for transmission through a neural synapse or to another cell. The neuronal tracts are often identified by their primary neurotransmitter; for example, a dopaminergic tract synthesizes and releases the neurotransmitter dopamine.

### A. General Features of Neurotransmitter Synthesis

A number of features are common to the synthesis, secretion, and metabolism of most small nitrogen-containing neurotransmitters. Most of these neurotransmitters are synthesized from amino acids, intermediates of glycolysis and the TCA cycle, and $O_2$ in the cytoplasm of the presynaptic terminal. The rate of synthesis is generally regulated to correspond to the rate of firing of the neuron as well as the strength of the signal as the membrane is depolarized. Once they are synthesized, the neurotransmitters are transported into storage vesicles by an ATP-requiring pump linked with the proton gradient. Release from the storage vesicle is triggered by the nerve impulse that depolarizes the postsynaptic membrane and causes an influx of calcium ions ($Ca^{2+}$) through voltage-gated calcium channels. The influx of $Ca^{2+}$ promotes fusion of the vesicle with the presynaptic membrane and release of the neurotransmitter into the synaptic cleft (the space between the synapses). The transmission across the synapse is completed by binding of the neurotransmitter to a receptor on the postsynaptic membrane (Fig. 33.13).

In general, the action of the neurotransmitter is terminated through reuptake into the presynaptic terminal, uptake into glial cells, diffusion away from the synapse, or enzymatic inactivation. The enzymatic inactivation may occur in the postsynaptic terminal, the presynaptic terminal, or an adjacent astrocyte microglia cell or in endothelial cells in the brain capillaries.

### B. Dopamine, Norepinephrine, and Epinephrine (the Catecholamines)

#### 1. SYNTHESIS

Dopamine, norepinephrine, and epinephrine are synthesized in a common pathway from the amino acid L-tyrosine. The pathway of catecholamine biosynthesis is shown in Figure 33.14.

Drugs have been developed that block neurotransmitter uptake into storage vesicles. Reserpine, which blocks catecholamine uptake into vesicles, had been used as an antihypertensive and antiepileptic drug for many years, but it was noted that a small percentage of patients on the drug became depressed and even suicidal. Animals treated with reserpine showed signs of lethargy and poor appetite, similar to depression in humans. Thus, a link was forged between monoamine release and depression in humans.

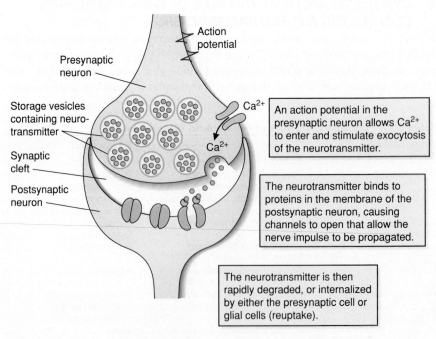

**FIG. 33.13.** Action of neurotransmitters.

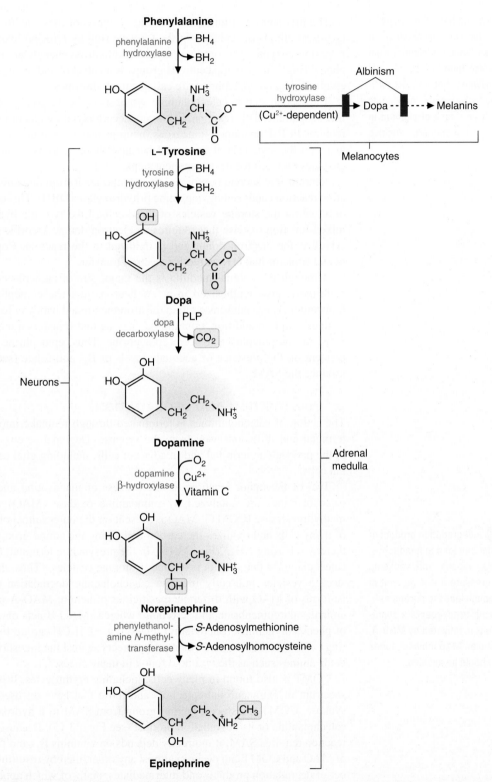

**FIG. 33.14.** The pathways of catecholamine and melanin biosynthesis. The *dark boxes* indicate the enzymes, which, when defective, lead to albinism. *PLP*, pyridoxal phosphate; *BH*4, tetrahydrobiopterin.

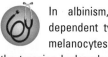

In albinism, either the copper-dependent tyrosine hydroxylase of melanocytes (which is distinct from the tyrosine hydroxylase found in the adrenal medulla) or other enzymes that convert tyrosine to melanins may be defective. Individuals with albinism suffer from a lack of pigment in the skin, hair, and eyes, and they are sensitive to sunlight.

The first and rate-limiting step in the synthesis of these neurotransmitters from tyrosine is the hydroxylation of the tyrosine ring by tyrosine hydroxylase, a $BH_4$-requiring enzyme. The product formed is dihydroxyphenylalanine or DOPA. The phenyl ring with two adjacent OH groups is a catechol and, hence, dopamine, nor-epinephrine, and epinephrine are called **catecholamines**.

The second step in catecholamine synthesis is the decarboxylation of DOPA to form dopamine. This reaction, like many decarboxylation reactions of amino acids, requires PLP. Dopaminergic neurons (neurons using dopamine as a neurotransmitter) stop the synthesis at this point because these neurons do not synthesize the enzymes required for the subsequent steps.

Neurons that secrete norepinephrine synthesize it from dopamine in a hydroxylation reaction catalyzed by dopamine β-hydroxylase (DBH). This enzyme is present only within the storage vesicles of these cells. Like tyrosine hydroxylase, it is a mixed-function oxidase that requires an electron donor. Ascorbic acid (vitamin C) serves as the electron donor and is oxidized in the reaction. Copper ($Cu^{2+}$) is a bound cofactor that is required for electron transfer.

Although the adrenal medulla is the major site of epinephrine synthesis, epinephrine is also synthesized in a few neurons that use epinephrine as a neurotransmitter. These neurons contain the aforementioned pathway for norepinephrine synthesis and, in addition, contain the enzyme that transfers a methyl group from SAM to norepinephrine to form epinephrine. Thus, epinephrine synthesis is dependent on the presence of adequate levels of $B_{12}$ and folate (see Chapter 34) to produce the SAM.

## 2. INACTIVATION AND DEGRADATION

The action of catecholamines is terminated through reuptake into the presynaptic terminal and diffusion away from the synapse. Degradative enzymes are present in the presynaptic terminal and in adjacent cells, including glial cells and endothelial cells.

Two of the major reactions in the process of inactivation and degradation of catecholamines are catalyzed by monoamine oxidase (MAO) and catechol-$O$-methyltransferase (COMT). MAO is present on the outer mitochondrial membrane of many cells and oxidizes the carbon containing the amino group to an aldehyde, thereby releasing $NH_4^+$ (Fig. 33.15). In the presynaptic terminal, MAO inactivates catecholamines that are not protected in storage vesicles. (Thus, drugs that deplete storage vesicles indirectly increase catecholamine degradation.) There are two isoforms of MAO with different specificities of action: MAO-A preferentially deaminates norepinephrine and serotonin, whereas MAO-B acts on a wide spectrum of phenylethylamines (phenylethyl refers to a $-CH_2CH_2$ group linked to a phenyl ring). MAO in the liver and other sites protects against the ingestion of dietary biogenic amines such as the tyramine found in many cheeses.

Tyramine is a degradation product of tyrosine that can lead to headaches, palpitations, nausea and vomiting, and elevated blood pressure if it is present in large quantities. Tyramine leads to norepinephrine release, which binds to its receptors, stimulating them. Tyramine is inactivated by MAO-A, but if a person is taking an MAO inhibitor, foods containing tyramine should be avoided.

COMT is also found in many cells, including erythrocytes. It works on a broad spectrum of extraneuronal catechols and those that have diffused away from the synapse. COMT transfers a methyl group from SAM to a hydroxyl group on the catecholamine or its degradation product (see Fig. 33.15). Because the inactivation reaction requires SAM, it indirectly depends on vitamins $B_{12}$ and folate. The action of MAO and COMT can occur in almost any order, thereby resulting in a large number of degradation products and intermediates, many of which appear in the urine.

## C. Metabolism of Serotonin

The pathway for the synthesis of serotonin from tryptophan is very similar to the pathway for the synthesis of norepinephrine from tyrosine (Fig. 33.16). The first enzyme of the pathway, tryptophan hydroxylase, uses an enzymic mechanism similar to that of tyrosine and PAH and requires $BH_4$ to hydroxylate the ring structure of tryptophan. The second step of the pathway is a decarboxylation reaction catalyzed

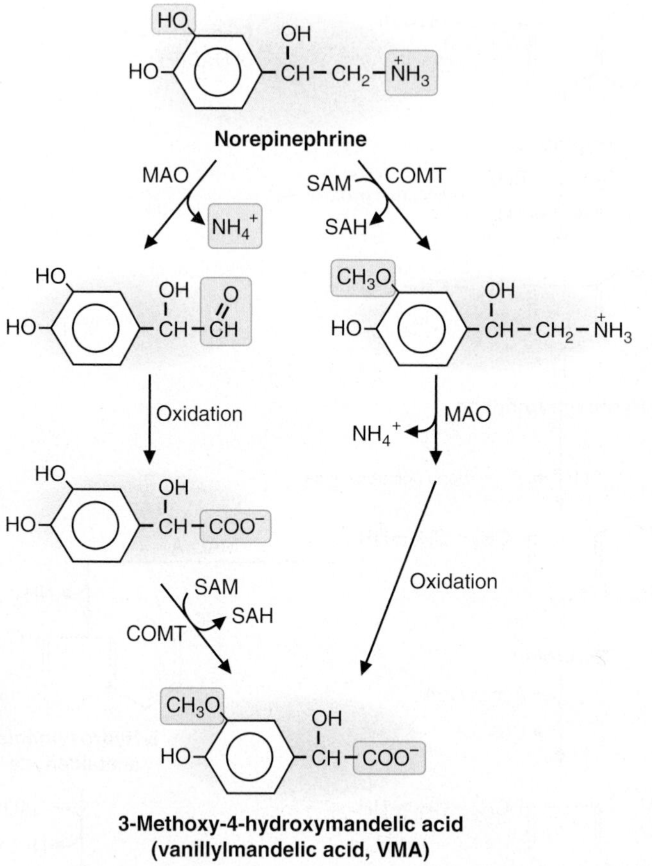

**FIG. 33.15.** Inactivation of catecholamines. Methylation and oxidation may occur in any order. Methylated and oxidized derivatives of norepinephrine and epinephrine are produced, and 3-methoxy-4-hydroxymandelic acid is the final product. These compounds are excreted in the urine. *COMT*, catechol-*O*-methyltransferase; *MAO*, monoamine oxidase; *SAM*, *S*-adenosylmethionine; *SAH*, *S*-adenosylhomocysteine.

by the same enzyme that decarboxylates DOPA. Serotonin, like the catecholamine neurotransmitters, can be inactivated by MAO.

The neurotransmitter melatonin is also synthesized from tryptophan (see Fig. 33.16). Melatonin is produced in the pineal gland in response to the light–dark cycle, its level in the blood rising in a dark environment. It is probably through melatonin that the pineal gland conveys information about light–dark cycles to the body, organizing seasonal and circadian rhythms. Melatonin also may be involved in regulating reproductive functions.

## D. Metabolism of Histamine

Within the brain, histamine is produced both by mast cells and by certain neuronal fibers. Histamine is synthesized from histidine in a single enzymatic step. The enzyme histidine decarboxylase requires PLP, and its mechanism is very similar to that of DOPA decarboxylase (Fig. 33.17).

Like other neurotransmitters, newly synthesized neuronal histamine is stored in the nerve terminal vesicle. Depolarization of nerve terminals activates the exocytotic release of histamine by a voltage-dependent as well as a calcium-dependent mechanism.

The first step in the inactivation of histamine in the brain is methylation (see Fig. 33.17). The enzyme histamine methyltransferase transfers a methyl group from SAM to a ring nitrogen of histamine to form methylhistamine. The second step is

In addition to the catecholamines, serotonin is also inactivated by MAO. The activity of several antipsychotic drugs is based on inhibiting MAO. The first generation of drugs (exemplified by iproniazid, which was originally developed as an antituberculosis drug and was found to induce mood swings in patients) were irreversible inhibitors of both the A and B forms of MAO. Although they did reduce the severity of depression (by maintaining higher levels of serotonin), these drugs suffered from the "cheese" effect. Cheese and other foods that are processed over long periods (such as red wine) contain tyramine, a degradation product of tyrosine (a result of tyrosine decarboxylation). Usually, tyramine is inactivated by MAO-A, but if an individual is taking a MAO inhibitor, tyramine levels will increase. Tyramine induces the release of norepinephrine from storage vesicles, which leads to potentially life-threatening hypertensive episodes. When it was realized that MAO existed in two forms, selective irreversible inhibitors were developed; examples include clorgyline for MAO-A and deprenyl for MAO-B. Deprenyl has been used to treat Parkinson disease (which is caused by a lack of dopamine, which is also inactivated by MAO). Deprenyl, however, is not an antidepressant. Clorgyline is an antidepressant but suffers from the cheese effect. This led to the development of the third generation of MAO inhibitors, which are reversible inhibitors of the enzyme as typified by moclobemide. Moclobemide is a specific, reversible inhibitor of MAO-A and is effective as an antidepressant. More importantly, because of the reversible nature of the drug, the cheese effect is not observed because as tyramine levels increase, they displace the drug from MAO, and the tyramine is safely inactivated.

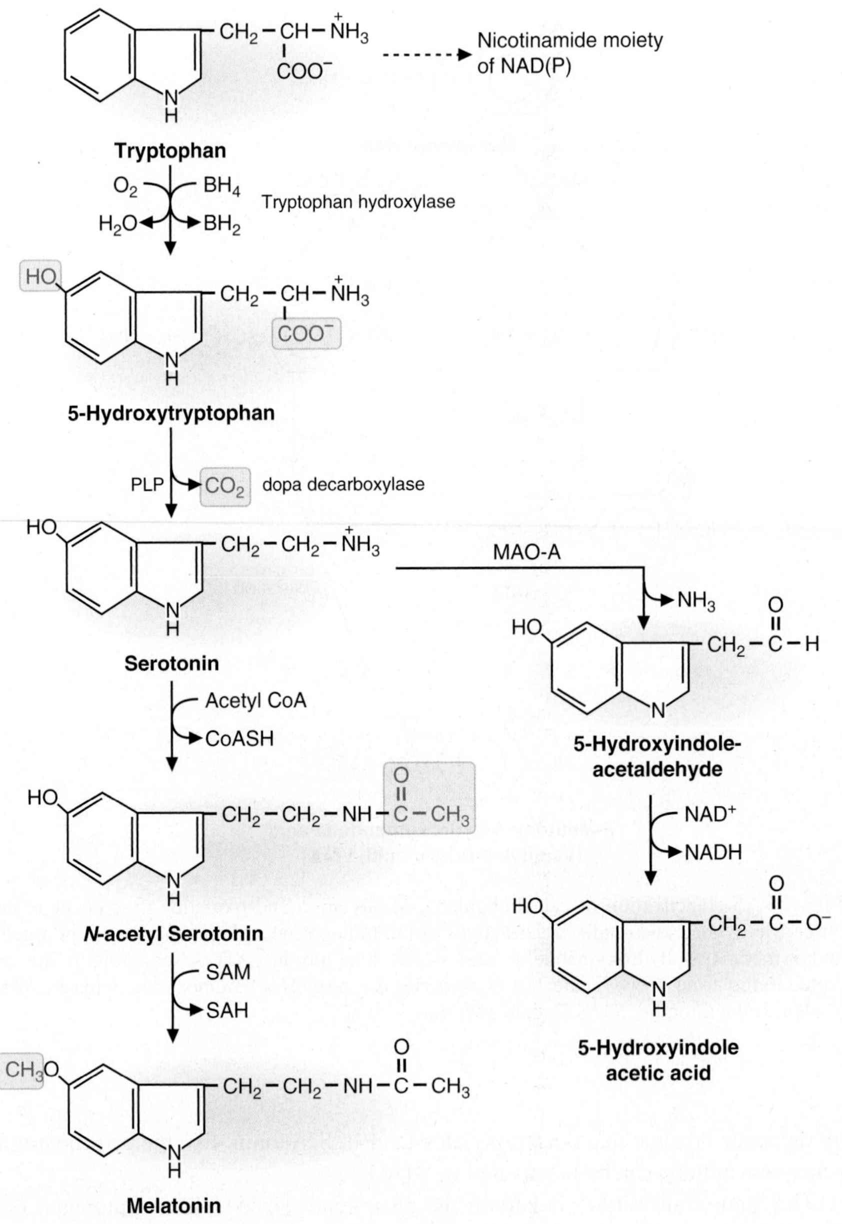

**FIG. 33.16.** Synthesis and inactivation of serotonin.

Histamine elicits several effects on different tissues. Histamine is the major mediator of the allergic response and when released from mast cells (a type of white blood cell found in tissues), it leads to vasodilation and an increase in the permeability of blood vessel walls. This leads to the allergic symptoms of a runny nose and watering eyes. When histamine is released in the lungs, the airways constrict in an attempt to reduce the intake of the allergic material. The ultimate result of this, however, is bronchospasm, which can lead to difficulty in breathing. In the brain, histamine is an excitatory neurotransmitter. Antihistamines block histamine from binding to its receptor. In the tissues, this counteracts histamine's effect on vasodilation and blood vessel wall permeability, but in the brain, the effect is to cause drowsiness. The new generation of "nondrowsy" antihistamines have been modified such that they cannot pass through the blood–brain barrier. Thus, the effects on the peripheral tissues are retained with no effect on central nervous system histamine response.

oxidation by MAO-B followed by an additional oxidation step. In peripheral tissues, histamine undergoes deamination by diamine oxidase followed by oxidation to a carboxylic acid (see Fig. 33.17).

### E. Acetylcholine

#### 1. SYNTHESIS

The synthesis of acetylcholine from acetyl CoA and choline is catalyzed by the enzyme choline acetyltransferase (ChAT) (Fig. 33.18). This synthetic step occurs in the presynaptic terminal. The compound is stored in vesicles and later released through calcium-mediated exocytosis.

Choline is a common component of the diet but also can be synthesized in the human as part of the pathway for the synthesis of phospholipids (see Chapter 28). The only route for choline synthesis is via the sequential addition of three methyl

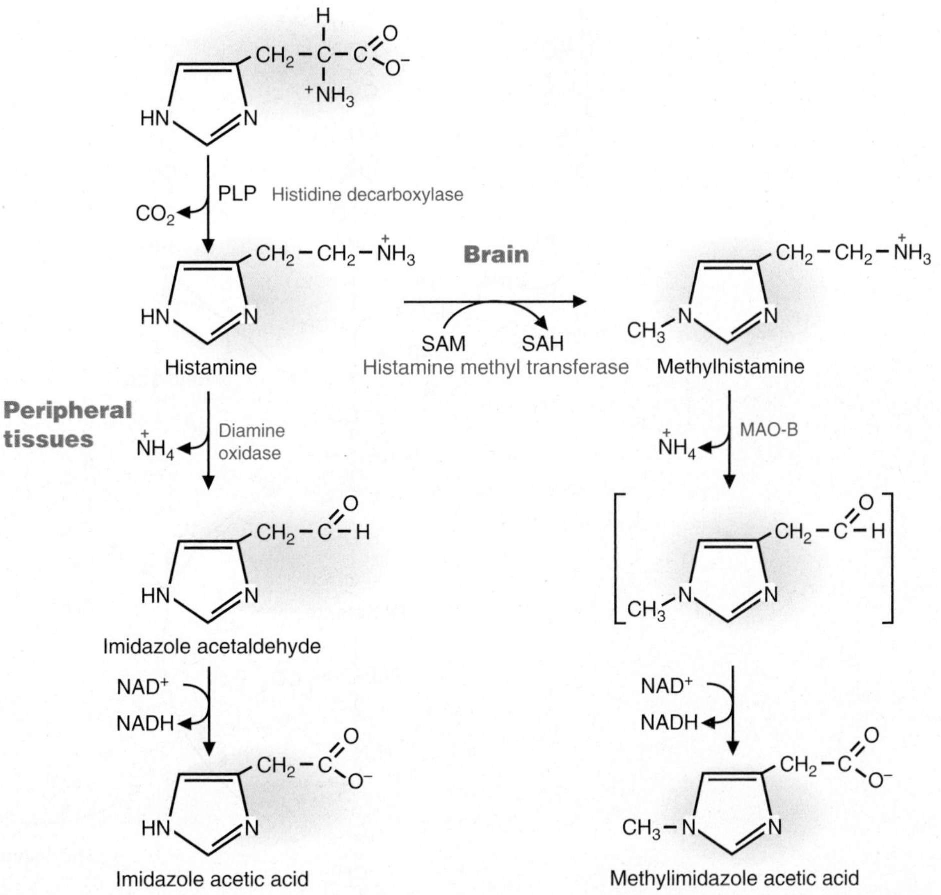

**FIG. 33.17.** Synthesis and inactivation of histamine. Note the different pathways for brain and peripheral tissues. *SAM*, *S*-adenosylmethionine; *SAH*, *S*-adenosylhomocysteine.

groups from SAM to the ethanolamine portion of phosphatidylethanolamine to form phosphatidylcholine. Phosphatidylcholine is subsequently hydrolyzed to release choline or phosphocholine. Conversion of phosphatidylethanolamine to phosphatidylcholine occurs in many tissues, including liver and brain. This conversion is folate and vitamin $B_{12}$ dependent.

## 2. INACTIVATION

Acetylcholine is inactivated by acetylcholinesterase, which is a serine esterase that forms a covalent bond with the acetyl group. The enzyme is inhibited by a wide range of compounds (pharmacological agents and neurotoxins) that form a covalent bond with this reactive serine group. Neurotoxins such as Sarin (the gas used in Japanese subways by a terrorist group) also work through this mechanism. Acetylcholine is the major neurotransmitter at the neuromuscular junctions; inability to inactivate this molecule leads to constant activation of the nerve–muscle synapses, a condition that leads to varying degrees of paralysis.

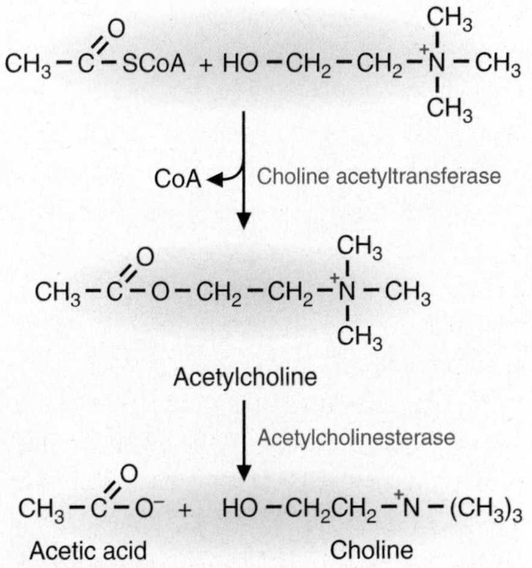

## F. Glutamate and γ-Aminobutyric Acid

### 1. GLUTAMATE

Glutamate functions as an excitatory neurotransmitter within the central nervous system, leading to the depolarization of neurons. Within nerve terminals, glutamate is generally synthesized de novo from glucose rather than taken up from the blood because its plasma concentration is low and it does not readily cross the blood–brain barrier.

**FIG. 33.18.** Acetylcholine synthesis and degradation.

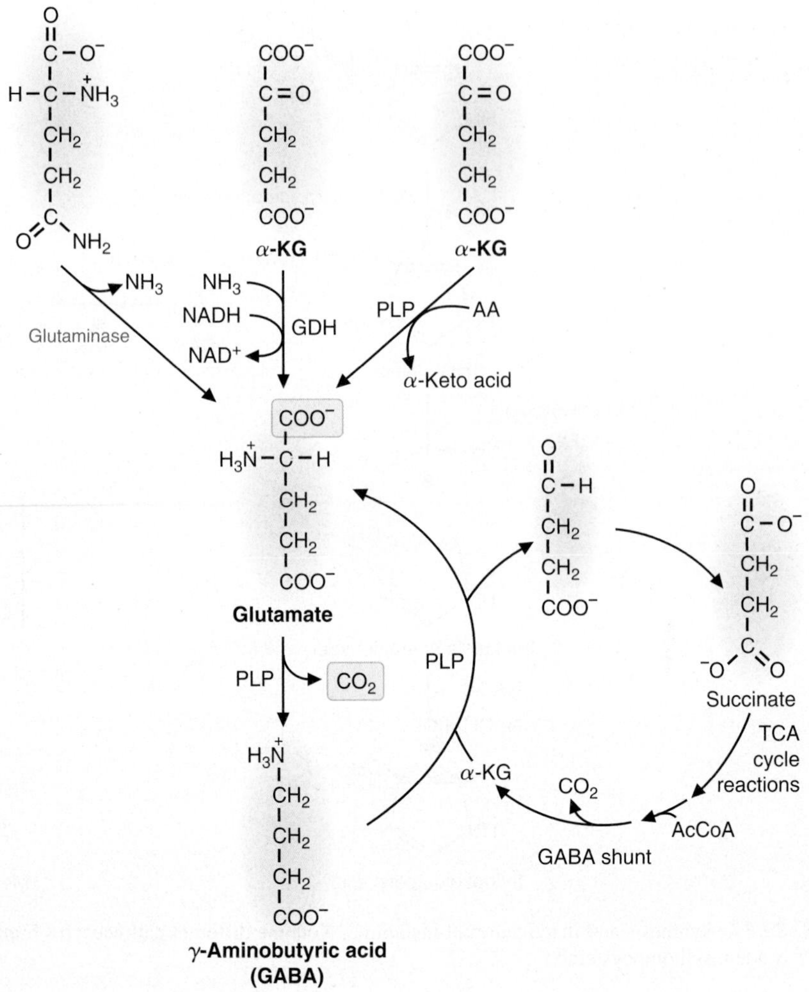

**FIG. 33.19.** Synthesis of glutamate and GABA and the GABA shunt. *GDH*, glutamate dehydrogenase; *PLP*, pyridoxal phosphate; α-*KG*, α-ketoglutarate.

Glutamate is primarily synthesized from the TCA cycle intermediate α-ketoglutarate (Fig. 33.19). This process can occur via either of two routes. The first is via the enzyme glutamate dehydrogenase, which reduces α-ketoglutarate to glutamate, thereby incorporating free ammonia into the carbon backbone. The ammonia pool is provided by amino acid–neurotransmitter degradation or by diffusion of ammonia across the blood–brain barrier. The second route is through transamination reactions in which an amino group is transferred from other amino acids to α-ketoglutarate to form glutamate. Glutamate also can be synthesized from glutamine, using glutaminase. The glutamine is derived from glial cells.

Like other neurotransmitters, glutamate is stored in vesicles, and its release is $Ca^{2+}$ dependent. It is removed from the synaptic cleft by high-affinity uptake systems present in nerve terminals and glial cells.

## 2. γ-AMINOBUTYRIC ACID

GABA (γ-**a**mino**b**utyric **a**cid) is the major inhibitory neurotransmitter in the central nervous system. Its functional significance is far-reaching and altered GABA-ergic function plays a role in many neurological and psychiatric disorders.

GABA is synthesized by the decarboxylation of glutamate (see Fig. 33.19) in a single step catalyzed by the enzyme glutamic acid decarboxylase (GAD). GABA is recycled in the central nervous system by a series of reactions called the **GABA shunt**, which conserves glutamate and GABA (see Fig. 33.19).

# VI. HEME SYNTHESIS AND DEGRADATION

The structure of heme has been presented previously (see Figure 5.12). Heme is the most common porphyrin found in the body. It is complexed with proteins to form hemoglobin, myoglobin, and the cytochromes, including cytochrome P450.

## A. Synthesis of Heme

Heme is synthesized from glycine and succinyl CoA (Fig. 33.20), which condense in the initial reaction to form δ-aminolevulinic acid (δ-ALA) (Fig 33.21). The enzyme that catalyzes this reaction, δ-ALA synthase, requires the participation of PLP, as the reaction is an amino acid decarboxylation reaction (glycine is decarboxylated).

The next reaction of heme synthesis is catalyzed by δ-ALA dehydratase in which two molecules of δ-ALA condense to form the pyrrole, porphobilinogen (Fig. 33.22). Four of these pyrrole rings condense to form a linear chain and then a series of porphyrinogens. The side chains of these porphyrinogens initially contain acetyl (A) and propionyl (P) groups. The acetyl groups are decarboxylated to form methyl groups. Then, the first two propionyl side chains are decarboxylated and oxidized to vinyl groups, forming a protoporphyrinogen. The methylene bridges are subsequently oxidized to form protoporphyrin IX (see Fig. 33.20).

In the final step of the pathway, iron (as $Fe^{2+}$) is incorporated into protoporphyrin IX in a reaction catalyzed by ferrochelatase (also known as heme synthase).

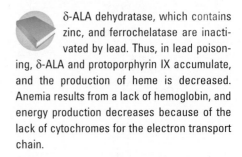

Heme, which is red, is responsible for the color of red blood cells and of muscles that contain a large number of mitochondria. Chlorophyll, the major porphyrin in plants, is similar to heme except that it is coordinated with magnesium rather than iron, and it contains different substituents on the rings, including a long-chain alcohol (phytol). As a result of these structural differences, chlorophyll is green.

δ-ALA dehydratase, which contains zinc, and ferrochelatase are inactivated by lead. Thus, in lead poisoning, δ-ALA and protoporphyrin IX accumulate, and the production of heme is decreased. Anemia results from a lack of hemoglobin, and energy production decreases because of the lack of cytochromes for the electron transport chain.

Porphyrias are a group of rare inherited disorders resulting from deficiencies of enzymes in the pathway for heme biosynthesis (see Fig. 33.20). Intermediates of the pathway accumulate and may have toxic effects on the nervous system that cause neuropsychiatric symptoms. When porphyrinogens accumulate, they may be converted by light to porphyrins, which react with molecular oxygen to form oxygen radicals. These radicals may cause severe damage to the skin. Thus, individuals with excessive production of porphyrins are photosensitive. The scarring and increased growth of facial hair seen in some porphyrias may have contributed to the development of the werewolf legends.

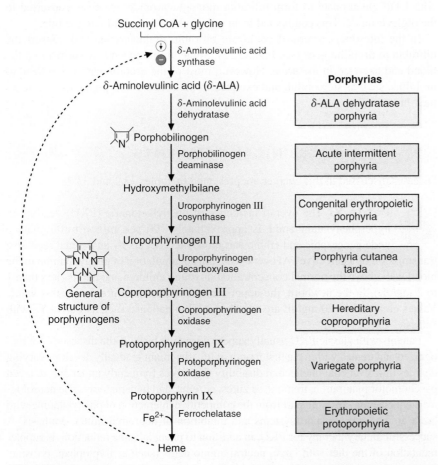

**FIG. 33.20.** Synthesis of heme. To produce one molecule of heme, eight molecules each of glycine and succinyl CoA are required. A series of porphyrinogens are generated in sequence. Finally, iron is added to produce heme. Heme regulates its own production by repressing the synthesis of δ-aminolevulinic acid (δ-ALA) synthase (↓) and by directly inhibiting the activity of this enzyme (−). Deficiencies of enzymes in the pathway result in a series of diseases known as porphyrias (listed on the right, beside the deficient enzyme).

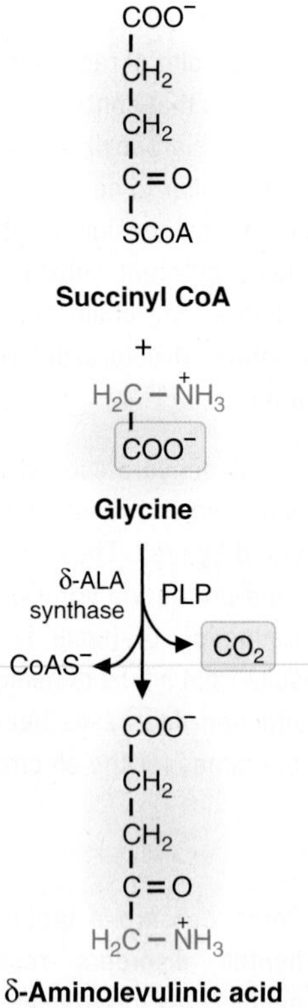

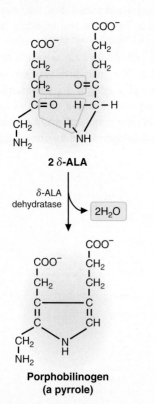

**FIG. 33.21.** Synthesis of δ-ALA. The atoms in *red* in δ-ALA are derived from glycine. *PLP*, pyridoxal phosphate.

**FIG. 33.22.** Two molecules of δ-ALA condense to form porphobilinogen.

## B. Regulation of Heme Synthesis

Heme regulates its own synthesis by mechanisms that affect the first enzyme in the pathway, δ-ALA synthase (see Fig. 33.20). Heme represses the synthesis of this enzyme and also directly inhibits the activity of the enzyme (an allosteric modifier). Thus, heme is synthesized when heme levels fall. As heme levels rise, the rate of heme synthesis decreases.

Heme also regulates the synthesis of hemoglobin by stimulating synthesis of the protein globin. Heme maintains the ribosomal initiation complex for globin synthesis in an active state (see Chapter 13).

## C. Degradation of Heme

Heme is degraded to form bilirubin, which is conjugated with glucuronic acid and excreted in the bile (Fig. 33.23). Although heme from cytochromes and myoglobin also undergoes conversion to bilirubin, the major source of this bile pigment is hemoglobin. After red blood cells reach the end of their life span (approximately 120 days), they are phagocytosed by cells of the reticuloendothelial system. Globin is cleaved to its constituent amino acids, and iron is returned to the body's iron stores. Heme is oxidized and cleaved to produce carbon monoxide and biliverdin. Biliverdin is reduced to bilirubin, which is transported to the liver complexed with serum albumin.

In the liver, bilirubin is converted to a more water-soluble compound by reacting with UDP-glucuronate to form bilirubin monoglucuronide, which is converted to the diglucuronide. This conjugated form of bilirubin is excreted into the bile.

In the intestine, bacteria deconjugate bilirubin diglucuronide and convert the bilirubin to urobilinogens (see Fig. 33.23). Some urobilinogen is absorbed into the blood and excreted in the urine. However, most of the urobilinogen is oxidized to urobilins, such as stercobilin, and excreted in the feces. These pigments give feces their brown color.

### CLINICAL COMMENTS

Diseases discussed in this chapter are presented in Tables 33.2 and 33.3.

**Petria Y.** The overall incidence of phenylketonuria (PKU), leading to hyperphenylalaninemia, is approximately 100 per million births, with a wide geographic and ethnic variation. PKU occurs by autosomal recessive transmission of a defective PAH gene, causing accumulation of phenylalanine in the blood well above the normal concentration in young children and adults (less than 1 to 2 mg/dL). In the newborn, the upper limit of normal is almost twice this value. Values greater than 20 mg/dL are usually found in patients, such as **Petria Y.**, with "classic" PKU.

Patients with classic PKU usually appear normal at birth. If the disease is not recognized and treated within the first month of life, the infant gradually develops varying degrees of irreversible intellectual disability (IQ scores frequently under 50), delayed psychomotor maturation, tremors, seizures, eczema, and hyperactivity. The neurological sequelae may result in part from the competitive interaction of phenylalanine with brain amino acid transport systems and inhibition of neurotransmitter synthesis. A successful dietary therapy for PKU, in addition to phenylalanine reduction, is supplementation of the diet with large, neutral amino acids (such as tryptophan, tyrosine,

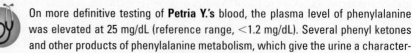

On more definitive testing of **Petria Y.'s** blood, the plasma level of phenylalanine was elevated at 25 mg/dL (reference range, <1.2 mg/dL). Several phenyl ketones and other products of phenylalanine metabolism, which give the urine a characteristic odor, were found in significant quantities in the baby's urine.

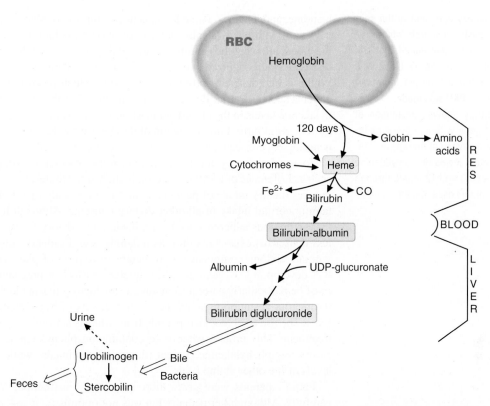

**FIG. 33.23.** Overview of heme degradation. Heme is degraded to bilirubin, carried in the blood by albumin, conjugated to form the diglucuronide in the liver, and excreted in the bile. The iron is returned to the body's iron stores. *RBC*, red blood cells; *RES*, reticuloendothelial system.

**Table 33.3   Diseases Discussed in Chapter 33**

| Disease or Disorder | Environmental or Genetic | Comments |
|---|---|---|
| PKU | Genetic | Classical PKU is due to a defect in phenylalanine hydroxylase, whereas nonclassical PKU is due to a defect in dihydropteridine reductase (or an inability to synthesize tetrahydrobiopterin). Both forms of PKU will lead to intellectual disability if treatment is not initiated at an early age. |
| Alcaptonuria | Genetic | Alcaptonuria is due to a defect in homogentisate oxidase, leading to an accumulation of homogentisic acid. Arthritis may develop later in life. |
| Tyrosinemia | Genetic | Tyrosinemia type 1 is a defect in fumarylacetoacetate hydrolase, leading to liver failure and early death. Tyrosinemia type 2 is a defect in tyrosine aminotransferase, leading to neurological defects. |
| Cystathionuria | Genetic | Defect in cystathionase, leading to an accumulation of cystathionine. No major complications result from this mutation. |
| Homocysteinemia | Genetic | A defect in cystathionine β-synthase leads to accumulation of homocysteine, which can result in cardiologic and neurological complications in the patient. |
| Primary oxaluria type 1 | Genetic | Defect in glycine transaminase leading to oxalate accumulate and renal failure due to stone formation within the kidney. |
| Maple syrup urine disease | Genetic | A defect in the branched-chain α-keto acid dehydrogenase, leading to an accumulation of the α-keto acids of the branched-chain amino acids, resulting in intellectual disability. |
| Cystinosis | Genetic | A defect in the transport protein that carries cystine across lysosomal membranes. Cystine accumulates in lysosomes, interfering with and ultimately destroying their function. |
| Thiamine deficiency | Environmental | A thiamine deficiency leads to accumulation of α-keto acids because the enzymes that catalyze oxidative decarboxylation reactions will not function in the absence of this vitamin. This will interfere with energy production and lead to a ketoacidosis. |
| Porphyrias | Genetic | Inherited defects in almost any step of heme synthesis leading to a series of diseases with different symptoms and outcomes. |
| Iron deficiency | Both | Reduced iron leads to reduced heme synthesis and reduced oxygen delivery to the tissues. |
| Tyramine poisoning | Environmental | Tyramine, a compound found in aged cheeses (for example), is degraded by monoamine oxidase. In the presence of monoamine oxidase inhibitors, tyramine levels can accumulate, triggering the release of high levels of norepinephrine, leading to a hypertensive crisis. |

PKU, phenylketonuria.

A liver biopsy was sent to the special chemistry research laboratory, where it was determined that the level of activity of PAH in Petria's blood was less than 1% of that found in normal infants. A diagnosis of "classic" PKU was made.

Until gene therapy allows substitution of the defective PAH gene with its normal counterpart in vivo, the mainstay of therapy in classic PKU is to maintain levels of phenylalanine in the blood between 3 and 12 mg/dL through dietary restriction of this essential amino acid.

The pathological findings that underlie the clinical features manifested by **Horace S.** are presumed (but not proved) to be the consequence of chronic elevations of homocysteine (and perhaps other compounds, e.g., methionine) in the blood and tissues. The zonular fibers that normally hold the lens of the eye in place become frayed and break, causing dislocation of the lens. The skeleton reveals a loss of bone density (i.e., osteoporosis), which may explain the curvature of the spine. The elongation of the long bones beyond their normal genetically determined length leads to tall stature.

Animal experiments suggest that increased concentrations of homocysteine and methionine in the brain may trap adenosine as *S*-adenosylhomocysteine, diminishing adenosine levels. Because adenosine normally acts as a central nervous system depressant, its deficiency may be associated with a lowering of the seizure threshold as well as a reduction in cognitive function.

histidine, and leucine). These large, neutral amino acids share a transport system (the L-system) with phenylalanine and can overcome the high levels of phenylalanine in the blood, allowing the neurotransmitter precursors to enter the nervous system. If the disease is not recognized in time, the biochemical alterations lead to impaired myelin synthesis and delayed neuronal development, which result in the clinical picture in patients such as Petria. Because of the simplicity of the test for PKU (elevated phenylalanine levels in the blood), all newborns in the United States are required to have a PKU test at birth. Early detection of the disease can lead to early treatment, and the neurological consequences of the disease can be bypassed.

To restrict dietary levels of phenylalanine, special semisynthetic preparations such as Lofenalac or PKUaid are used in the United States. Use of these preparations reduces dietary intake of phenylalanine to 250 mg/day to 500 mg/day while maintaining normal intake of all other dietary nutrients. Although it is generally agreed that scrupulous adherence to this regimen is mandatory for the first decade of life, less consensus exists regarding its indefinite use. Evidence suggests, however, that without lifelong compliance with dietary restriction of phenylalanine, even adults will develop at least neurological sequelae of PKU. A pregnant woman with PKU must be particularly careful to maintain satisfactory plasma levels of phenylalanine throughout gestation to avoid the adverse effects of hyperphenylalaninemia on the fetus. The use of glycomacropeptide from whey is a promising development in PKU treatment. This protein when pure contains no phenylalanine but as isolated has a very low phenylalanine content (due to contaminants) while providing adequate levels of the other amino acids.

Petria's parents were given thorough dietary instruction, which they followed carefully. Although her pediatrician was not optimistic, it was hoped that the damage done to her nervous system before dietary therapy was minimal and that her subsequent psychomotor development would allow her to lead a relatively normal life.

**Horace S.** The most characteristic biochemical features of the disorder that affects **Horace S.**, a cystathionine β-synthase deficiency, are the presence of an accumulation of both homocyst(e)ine and methionine in the blood. Because renal tubular reabsorption of methionine is highly efficient, this amino acid may not appear in the urine. Homocystine, the disulfide of homocysteine, is less efficiently reabsorbed, and amounts in excess of 1 mmol may be excreted in the urine each day.

In the type of homocystinuria in which the patient is deficient in cystathione β-synthase, the elevation in serum methionine levels is presumed to be the result of enhanced rates of conversion of homocysteine to methionine because of increased availability of homocysteine (see Fig. 33.10). In type II and type III homocystinuria, in which there is a deficiency in the synthesis of methyl cobalamin and of $N^5$-methyltetrahydrofolate, respectively (both required for the methylation of homocysteine to form methionine), serum homocysteine levels are elevated but serum methionine levels are low (see Fig. 33.10).

Acute vascular events are common in these patients. Thrombi (blood clots) and emboli (clots that have broken off and traveled to a distant site in the vascular system) have been reported in almost every major artery and vein as well as in smaller vessels. These clots result in infarcts in vital organs such as the liver, the myocardium (heart muscle), the lungs, the kidneys, and many other tissues. Although increased serum levels of homocysteine have been implicated in enhanced platelet aggregation and damage to vascular endothelial cells (leading to clotting and accelerated atherosclerosis), no generally accepted mechanism for these vascular events has yet emerged.

Treatment is directed toward early reduction of the elevated levels of homocysteine and methionine in the blood. In addition to a diet that is low in methionine, very high oral doses of pyridoxine (vitamin B₆) have significantly decreased the plasma levels of homocysteine and methionine in some patients with cystathionine β-synthase deficiency. (Genetically determined "responders" to pyridoxine treatment make up approximately 50% of type I homocystinurics.) PLP serves as a cofactor for cystathionine β-synthase; however, the molecular properties of the defective enzyme that confer the responsiveness to $B_6$ therapy are not known.

The terms *hypermethioninemia*, *homocystinuria* (or *-emia*), and *cystathioninuria* (or *-emia*) designate biochemical abnormalities and are not specific clinical diseases. Each may be caused by more than one specific genetic defect. For example, at least seven distinct genetic alterations can cause increased excretion of homocystine in the urine. A deficiency of cystathionine β-synthase is the most common cause of homocystinuria; more than 600 such proven cases have been studied.

## REVIEW QUESTIONS-CHAPTER 33

1. If an individual has a vitamin $B_6$ deficiency, which one of the following amino acids could still be synthesized and be considered nonessential?

   A. Serine
   B. Alanine
   C. Cysteine
   D. Aspartate
   E. Tyrosine

2. A newborn infant has elevated levels of phenylalanine and phenylpyruvate in her blood. Which one of the following enzymes might be deficient in this baby?

   A. Phenylalanine dehydrogenase
   B. Phenylalanine oxidase
   C. Dihydropteridine reductase
   D. Tyrosine hydroxylase
   E. Tetrahydrofolate synthase

3. An elderly patient is brought to your office by their son. The son is concerned about his father because he does not believe that his father has been eating well. It appears as if the father sometimes forgets to eat and when he does eat, all he consumes is iced tea and romaine lettuce. Upon examination, it is apparent that the patient is malnourished and is often forgetful. Assuming that the patient has some nutritional deficiencies, which one of the following amino acids might also be deficient in this patient?

   A. Phenylalanine
   B. Asparagine
   C. Proline

   D. Serine
   E. Glutamate
   F. Alanine

4. A young couple comes to your office with their 3-month-old daughter who appears to be in excellent health. The parents are concerned because they notice when they change her diaper there are black spots where the urine has been released. Other than that, the patient is on track developmentally and is in perfect health. The disorder this child exhibits is most likely to be caused by a defect in the degradation of which one of the following amino acids?

   A. Methionine
   B. Isoleucine
   C. Cysteine
   D. Arginine
   E. Valine
   F. Phenylalanine

5. The parents of a 10-day-old infant brought their child to your office because the child has become lethargic and refuses to nurse. You also can smell a "burnt sugar" odor from the child's diapers and become suspicious of an inborn error of metabolism. Which of the following tests should be ordered immediately?

   A. Serum tyrosine levels
   B. Serum leucine levels
   C. Serum phenylalanine levels
   D. Serum folate levels
   E. Serum homocysteine levels

# 34 Tetrahydrofolate, Vitamin B$_{12}$, and *S*-Adenosylmethionine

## CHAPTER OUTLINE

**I. TETRAHYDROFOLATE**
A. Structure and forms of tetrahydrofolate
B. The vitamin folate
C. Oxidation and reduction of the one-carbon groups of tetrahydrofolate
D. Sources of one-carbon groups carried by tetrahydrofolate
E. Recipients of one-carbon groups

**II. VITAMIN B$_{12}$**
A. Structure and forms of vitamin B$_{12}$
B. Absorption and transport of vitamin B$_{12}$
C. Functions of vitamin B$_{12}$

**III. *S*-ADENOSYLMETHIONINE**

**IV. RELATIONSHIPS BETWEEN FOLATE, VITAMIN B$_{12}$, AND *S*-ADENOSYLMETHIONINE**
A. The methyl trap hypothesis
B. Hyperhomocysteinemia
C. Neural tube defects

**V. CHOLINE AND ONE-CARBON METABOLISM**

## KEY POINTS

- One-carbon groups at lower oxidation states than carbon dioxide (which is carried by biotin) are transferred by reactions that involve tetrahydrofolate (FH$_4$), vitamin B$_{12}$, and *S*-adenosylmethionine (SAM).
- FH$_4$ is produced from the vitamin folate and obtains one-carbon units from serine, glycine, histidine, formaldehyde, and formic acid.
- The carbon attached to FH$_4$ can be oxidized or reduced, thus producing several different forms of FH$_4$. However, once a carbon has been reduced to the methyl level, it cannot be reoxidized.
- The carbons attached to FH$_4$ are known collectively as the one-carbon pool.
- The carbons carried by folate are used in a limited number of biochemical reactions but are very important in forming deoxythymidine monophosphate (dTMP) and the purine rings.
- Vitamin B$_{12}$ participates in two reactions in the body: conversion of L-methylmalonyl coenzyme A (CoA) to succinyl CoA and conversion of homocysteine to methionine.
- SAM, formed from adenosine triphosphate (ATP) and methionine, transfers the methyl group to precursors forming a variety of methylated compounds.
- Both vitamin B$_{12}$ and methyl-FH$_4$ are required in methionine metabolism; a deficiency of vitamin B$_{12}$ leads to overproduction and trapping of folate in the methyl form, leading to a functional folate deficiency. Such deficiencies can lead to
  - Megaloblastic anemia
  - Neural tube defects in newborn

# THE WAITING ROOM

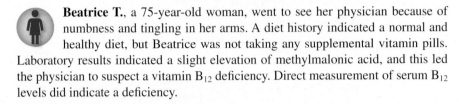**Beatrice T.**, a 75-year-old woman, went to see her physician because of numbness and tingling in her arms. A diet history indicated a normal and healthy diet, but Beatrice was not taking any supplemental vitamin pills. Laboratory results indicated a slight elevation of methylmalonic acid, and this led the physician to suspect a vitamin $B_{12}$ deficiency. Direct measurement of serum $B_{12}$ levels did indicate a deficiency.

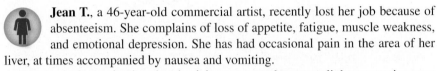**Jean T.**, a 46-year-old commercial artist, recently lost her job because of absenteeism. She complains of loss of appetite, fatigue, muscle weakness, and emotional depression. She has had occasional pain in the area of her liver, at times accompanied by nausea and vomiting.

On physical examination the physician notes tenderness to light percussion over her liver and her abdomen is mildly distended. There is a suggestion of mild jaundice. No obvious neurological or cognitive abnormalities are present.

After detecting a hint of alcohol on Jean's breath, the physician questioned Jean about her drinking. Jean admits that for the last 5 to 6 years she has been drinking gin on a daily basis (approximately 4 to 5 drinks or 68 to 85 g ethanol) and eating infrequently. Laboratory tests showed that her serum ethanol level on the initial office visit was 245 mg/dL (0.245%); values above 150 mg/dL (0.15%) are considered indicative of inebriation.

A battery of liver function studies indicated elevated levels of alanine aminotransferase (ALT) and aspartate aminotransferase (AST) in the blood (indicating liver membrane damage) and a serum total bilirubin of 2.4 mg/mL (reference range, 0.2 to 1.0 mg/mL), indicating reduced liver function. A hematological analysis also indicated that Jean was anemic. Her hemoglobin was 11.0 g/dL (reference range, 12 to 16 g/dL for an adult woman). The erythrocyte (red blood cell) count was 3.6 million cells/mm³ (reference range, 4.0 to 5.2 cells/mm³ for an adult woman). The average volume of her red blood cells (mean corpuscular volume or MCV) was 108 femtoliters (fL; 1 fL = $10^{-12}$ mL) (reference range, 80 to 100 fL), and the hematology laboratory reported a striking variation in the size and shape of the red blood cells in a smear of her peripheral blood. The nuclei of the circulating granulocytic leukocytes had increased nuclear segmentation (polysegmented neutrophils). Because these findings are suggestive of a macrocytic anemia (in which blood cells are larger than normal), measurements of serum folate and vitamin $B_{12}$ (cobalamin) levels were ordered.

## I.  *TETRAHYDROFOLATE*

### A.  *Structure and Forms of Tetrahydrofolate*

Folates exist in many chemical forms. The coenzyme form that functions in accepting one-carbon groups is tetrahydrofolate polyglutamate (Fig. 34.1), generally just referred to as tetrahydrofolate or $FH_4$. It has three major structural components: a bicyclic pteridine ring, paraaminobenzoic acid, and a polyglutamate tail consisting of several glutamate residues joined in amide linkage. The one-carbon group that is accepted by the coenzyme and then transferred to another compound is bound to $N^5$, $N^{10}$, or both.

Sulfa drugs, which are used to treat certain bacterial infections, are analogues of para-aminobenzoic acid. They prevent growth and cell division in bacteria by interfering with the synthesis of folate. Because we cannot synthesize folate, sulfa drugs do not affect human cells in this way.

The Schilling test, now a historical test, involved the patient ingesting radioactive ($Co^{57}$) crystalline vitamin $B_{12}$ after which a 24-hour urine sample was collected. The radioactivity in the urine sample was compared with the input radioactivity, and the difference represents the amount of $B_{12}$ absorbed through the digestive tract. Such tests could distinguish between problems in removing $B_{12}$ from bound dietary proteins or if the deficiency was caused by a lack of intrinsic factor or other proteins involved in transporting $B_{12}$ throughout the body. The Schilling test has been replaced by a competitive-binding luminescence assay, which has recently been criticized for being unreliable, particularly if a patient expresses anti-intrinsic factor antibodies.

Folate deficiencies occur frequently in chronic alcoholics. Several factors are involved: inadequate dietary intake of folate; direct damage to intestinal cells and brush border enzymes, which interferes with absorption of dietary folate; a defect in the enterohepatic circulation, which reduces the absorption of folate; liver damage that causes decreased hepatic production of plasma proteins; and interference with kidney resorption of folate.

Hematopoietic precursor cells, when exposed to too little folate and/or vitamin $B_{12}$, show slowed cell division, but cytoplasmic development occurs at a normal rate. Hence, the megaloblastic cells tend to be large, with an increased ratio of RNA to DNA. Megaloblastic erythroid progenitors are usually destroyed in the bone marrow (although some reach the circulation). Thus, marrow cellularity is often increased but production of red blood cells is decreased, a condition called **ineffective erythropoiesis**.

Jean's serum folic acid level was 3.1 ng/mL (reference range, 6 to 15 ng/mL), and her serum $B_{12}$ level was 154 pg/mL (reference range, 150 to 750 pg/mL). Her serum iron level was normal. It was clear, therefore, that Jean's megaloblastic anemia was caused by a folate deficiency (although her $B_{12}$ levels were in the low range of normal). The management of a pure folate deficiency in an alcoholic patient includes cessation of alcohol intake and a diet that is rich in folate.

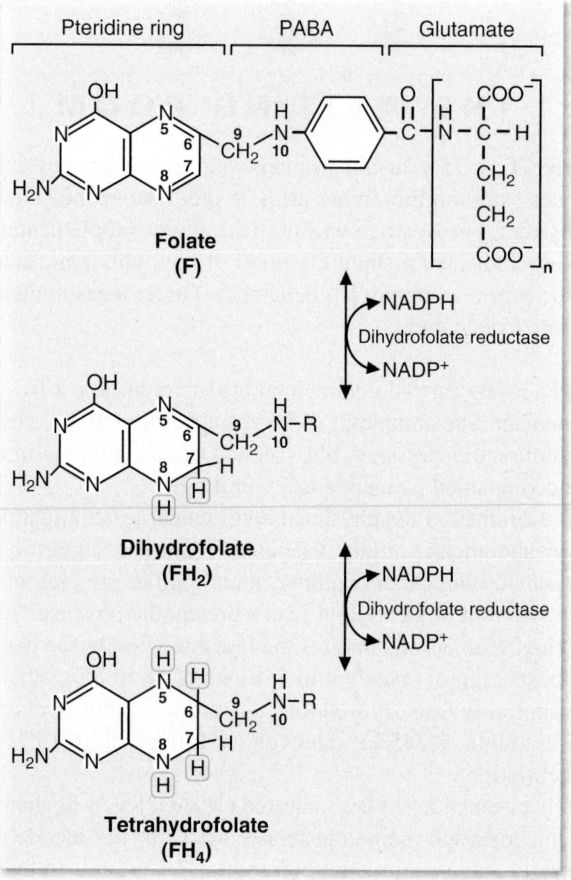

**FIG. 34.1.** Reduction of folate to $FH_4$. The same enzyme, dihydrofolate reductase (DHFR), catalyzes both reactions. Multiple glutamate residues are added within cells (n ~ 5). Plants can synthesize folate but humans cannot. Therefore, folate is a dietary requirement. *R* is the portion of the folate molecule shown to the right of $N^{10}$. The different precursors of $FH_4$ are indicated in the figure. *PABA*, paraaminobenzoic acid.

The current U.S. recommended dietary allowance (RDA) for folate equivalents is approximately 400 μg for adult men and women. In addition to being prevalent in green leafy vegetables, other good sources of this vitamin are liver, yeast, legumes, and some fruits. Protracted cooking of these foods, however, can destroy up to 90% of their folate content. A standard U.S. diet provides 50 to 500 μg absorbable folate each day. Folate deficiency in pregnant women, especially during the month before conception and the month after, increases the risk of neural tube defects, such as spina bifida, in the fetus. To reduce the potential risk of neural tube defects for women capable of becoming pregnant, the recommendation is to take 400 μg of folic acid daily in a multivitamin pill. If the woman has a history of having a child with a neural tube defect, this amount is increased to 4,000 μg/day for the month before and the month after conception. Flour-containing products in the United States are now supplemented with folate to reduce the risk of neural tube defects in newborns.

## B. The Vitamin Folate

Folates are synthesized in bacteria and higher plants and ingested in green leafy vegetables, fruits, and legumes in our diet. The vitamin was named for its presence in green, leafy vegetables (foliage). Most of the dietary folate derived from natural food sources is present in the reduced coenzyme form. However, vitamin supplements and fortified foods contain principally the oxidized form of the pteridine ring.

As dietary folates pass into the proximal third of the small intestine, folate conjugases in the brush border of the lumen cleave off glutamate residues to produce the monoglutamate form of folate, which is then absorbed (see Fig. 34.1, upper structure, when n = 1). Within the intestinal cells, folate is converted principally to $N^5$-methyl-$FH_4$, which enters the portal vein and goes to the liver. Smaller amounts of other forms of folate also follow this route.

The liver, which stores half of the body's folate, takes up much of the folate from the portal circulation; uptake may be through active transport or receptor-mediated endocytosis. Within the liver, $FH_4$ is reconjugated to the polyglutamate form before being used in reactions. A small amount of the folate is partially degraded, and the components enter the urine. A relatively large portion of the folate enters the bile and is subsequently reabsorbed (very similar to the fate of bile salts in the enterohepatic circulation).

$N^5$-Methyl-$FH_4$, the major form of folate in the blood, is loosely bound to plasma proteins, particularly serum albumin.

## C. Oxidation and Reduction of the One-Carbon Groups of Tetrahydrofolate

One-carbon groups transferred by $FH_4$ are attached either to $N^5$ or $N^{10}$ or they form a bridge between $N^5$ and $N^{10}$. The collection of one-carbon groups attached to $FH_4$ is known as the one-carbon pool. While they are attached to $FH_4$, these one-carbon units can be oxidized and reduced (Fig. 34.2). Thus, reactions that require a carbon

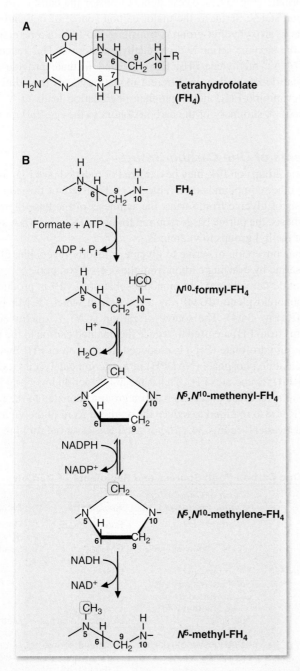

**FIG. 34.2.** One-carbon units attached to $FH_4$. **A.** The active form of $FH_4$. For definition of R, see Figure 34.1. **B.** Interconversions of one-carbon units of $FH_4$. Only the portion of $FH_4$ from $N^5$ to $N^{10}$ is shown, which is indicated by the *green box* in Part **A.** After a formyl group forms a bridge between $N^5$ and $N^{10}$, two reductions can occur. Note that $N^5$-methyl-$FH_4$ cannot be reoxidized. The most oxidized form of $FH_4$ is at the top of the figure, whereas the most reduced form is at the bottom.

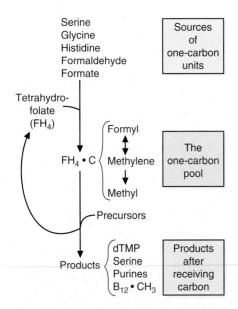

**FIG. 34.3.** Overview of the one-carbon pool. $FH_4 \cdot C$ indicates $FH_4$ containing a one-carbon unit that is at the formyl, methylene, or methyl level of oxidation (see Fig. 34.2). The origin of the carbons is indicated, as are the final products after a one-carbon transfer.

$FH_4$ is required for the synthesis of deoxythymidine monophosphate and the purine bases used to produce the precursors for DNA replication. Therefore, $FH_4$ is required for cell division. Blockage of the synthesis of thymine and the purine bases either by a dietary deficiency of folate or by drugs that interfere with folate metabolism results in a decreased rate of cell division and growth.

in a particular oxidation state may use carbon from the one-carbon pool that was donated in a different oxidation state. The most oxidized form is $N^{10}$-formyl $FH_4$. The most reduced form is $N^5$-methyl-$FH_4$. Once the methyl group is formed, it is *not readily reoxidized back to* $N^5$, $N^{10}$- *methylene-FH$_4$, and thus* $N^5$-*methyl-FH$_4$ tends to accumulate in the cell.*

## D.  Sources of One-Carbon Groups Carried by Tetrahydrofolate

Carbon sources for the one-carbon pool include serine, glycine, formaldehyde, histidine, and formate (Fig. 34.3). These donors transfer the carbons to folate in different oxidation states. Serine is the major carbon source of one-carbon groups in the human. Its hydroxymethyl group is transferred to $FH_4$ in a reversible reaction, catalyzed by the enzyme serine hydroxymethyltransferase. This reaction produces glycine and $N^5,N^{10}$-methylene-$FH_4$. Histidine and formate provide examples of compounds that donate carbon in different oxidation levels (histidine degradation leads to $N^5$-formimino-$FH_4$, and tryptophan degradation leads to $N^{10}$-formyl-$FH_4$ being produced). A summary of the carbon donors to the one-carbon pool is listed in Table 34.1.

## E.  Recipients of One-Carbon Groups

The one-carbon groups on $FH_4$ may be oxidized or reduced (see Fig. 34.2) and then transferred to other compounds (see Table 34.1). Transfers of this sort are involved in the synthesis of glycine from serine, the synthesis of the base thymine required for DNA synthesis, the purine bases required for both DNA and RNA synthesis, and the transfer of methyl groups to vitamin $B_{12}$.

Because the conversion of serine to glycine is readily reversible, glycine can be converted to serine by drawing carbon from the one-carbon pool.

The nucleotide deoxythymidine monophosphate (dTMP) is produced from deoxyuridine monophosphate (dUMP) by a reaction in which dUMP is methylated to form dTMP (Fig. 34.4). The source of carbon is $N^5,N^{10}$-methylene-$FH_4$. Two hydrogen atoms from $FH_4$ are used to reduce the donated carbon to the methyl level. Consequently, dihydrofolate ($FH_2$) is produced. Reduction of $FH_2$ by nicotinamide adenine dinucleotide phosphate (NADPH) in a reaction catalyzed by dihydrofolate reductase (DHFR) regenerates $FH_4$. This is the only reaction involving $FH_4$ in which the folate group is oxidized as the one-carbon group is donated to the recipient. Recall that DHFR is also required to reduce the oxidized form of the vitamin, which is obtained from the diet (see Fig. 34.1). Thus, DHFR is essential for both regenerating

**Table 34.1   One-Carbon Pool: Sources and Recipients of Carbon**

| Source[a] | Form of One-Carbon Donor Produced[b] | Recipient | Final Product |
|---|---|---|---|
| Formate | $N^{10}$-formyl-$FH_4$ | Purine precursor | Purine (C2 and C8) |
| Serine | | dUMP | dTMP |
| Glycine | $N^5,N^{10}$-methylene-$FH_4$ | Glycine | Serine |
| Formaldehyde | | | |
| $N^5,N^{10}$-methylene-$FH_4$ | $N^5$-methyl-$FH_4$ | Vitamin $B_{12}$ | Methylcobalamin |
| Histidine | $N^5$-formimino-$FH_4$ is converted to $N^5$, $N^{10}$-methenyl-$FH_4$ | | |
| Choline | Betaine | Homocysteine | Methionine and dimethylglycine |
| Methionine | *S*-adenosylmethionine (SAM) | Glycine (there are many others; see Fig. 34.7B) | *N*-methylglycine (sarcosine) |

[a]The major source of carbon is serine.
[b]The carbon unit attached to $FH_4$ can be oxidized and reduced (see Fig. 34.2). At the methyl level, reoxidation does not occur.
dUMP, deoxyuridine monophosphate; dTMP, deoxythymidine monophosphate; SAM, *S*-adenosylmethionine.

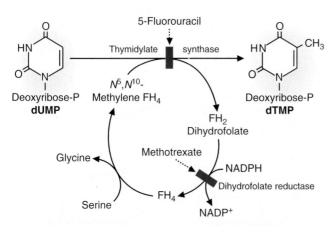

**FIG. 34.4.** Transfer of a one-carbon unit from $N^5$, $N^{10}$-methylene-FH$_4$ to dUMP to form dTMP. FH$_4$ is oxidized to FH$_2$ in this reaction. FH$_2$ is reduced to FH$_4$ by DHFR and FH$_4$ is converted to $N^5$, $N^{10}$-methylene-FH$_4$ using serine as a carbon donor. *Shaded bars* indicate the steps at which the antimetabolites 5-fluorouracil (5-FU) and methotrexate act. 5-FU inhibits thymidylate synthase. Methotrexate inhibits DHFR.

FH$_2$ in the tissues and from the diet. These reactions contribute to the effect of folate deficiency on DNA synthesis because dTMP is only required for the synthesis of DNA.

During the synthesis of the purine bases, carbons 2 and 8 are obtained from the one-carbon pool (see Chapter 35). $N^{10}$-Formyl-FH$_4$ provides both carbons. Folate deficiency would also hinder these reactions, contributing to an inability to replicate DNA because of the lack of precursors.

After the carbon group carried by FH$_4$ is reduced to the methyl level, it is transferred to vitamin B$_{12}$. This is the only reaction through which the methyl group can leave FH$_4$ (recall that the reaction that creates $N^5$-methyl-FH$_4$ is not reversible).

## II.  VITAMIN B₁₂

### A.  Structure and Forms of Vitamin B₁₂

The structure of vitamin B$_{12}$ (also known as cobalamin) is complex (Fig. 34.5). It contains a corrin ring, which is similar to the porphyrin ring found in heme. Its most unusual feature is the presence of cobalt, coordinated with the corrin ring (similar to the iron coordinated with the porphyrin ring). This cobalt can form a bond with a carbon atom. In the body, it reacts with the carbon of a methyl group, forming methylcobalamin, or with the 5′-carbon of 5′-deoxyadenosine, forming 5′-deoxyadenosylcobalamin (note that in this case, the deoxy designation refers to the 5′-carbon, not the 2′-carbon, as is the case in the sugar found in DNA). The form of B$_{12}$ found in vitamin supplements is cyanocobalamin, in which a CN group is linked to the cobalt.

### B.  Absorption and Transport of Vitamin B₁₂

Although vitamin B$_{12}$ is produced by bacteria, it cannot be synthesized by higher plants or animals. The major source of vitamin B$_{12}$ is dietary meat, eggs, dairy products, fish, poultry, and seafood. The animals that serve as the source of these foods obtain B$_{12}$ mainly from the bacteria in their food supply.

Ingested B$_{12}$ can exist in two forms, either free or bound to dietary proteins. If free, the B$_{12}$ binds to proteins known as R-binders (haptocorrins, also known as transcobalamin I), which are secreted by the salivary glands and the gastric mucosa in either the saliva or the stomach. If the ingested B$_{12}$ is bound to proteins, it must be released from the proteins by the action of digestive proteases both in the stomach and small intestine. Once the B$_{12}$ is released from its bound protein, it binds to the haptocorrins. In the small intestine, the pancreatic proteases digest the haptocorrins,

**Jean T.'s** megaloblastic anemia was treated in part with folate supplements (see Clinical Comments). Within 48 hours of the initiation of folate therapy, megaloblastic or "ineffective" erythropoiesis usually subsides, and effective erythropoiesis begins.

Megaloblastic anemia is caused by a decrease in the synthesis of thymine and the purine bases. These deficiencies lead to an inability of hematopoietic (and other) cells to synthesize DNA and, therefore, to divide. Their persistently thwarted attempts at normal DNA replication, DNA repair, and cell division produce abnormally large cells (called megaloblasts) with abundant cytoplasm capable of protein synthesis but with clumping and fragmentation of nuclear chromatin. Some of these large cells, although immature, are released early from the marrow in an attempt to compensate for the anemia. Thus, peripheral blood smears also contain megaloblasts. Many of the large immature cells, however, are destroyed in the marrow and never reach the circulation.

**Q:** Individuals with non-Hodgkin lymphoma receive several drugs to treat the tumor, including methotrexate. The structure of methotrexate is shown below. What compound does methotrexate resemble?

**Methotrexate**

The average daily diet in Western countries contains 5 to 30 μg vitamin B$_{12}$, of which 1 to 5 μg is absorbed into the blood. (The RDA is 2.4 μg/day.) Total body content of this vitamin in an adult is approximately 2 to 5 mg, of which 1 mg is present in the liver. As a result, a dietary deficiency of B$_{12}$ is uncommon and is only observed after a number of years on a diet deficient in this vitamin.

In spite of **Jean T.'s** relatively malnourished state because of her chronic alcoholism, her serum cobalamin level was still within the low to normal range. If her undernourished state had continued, a cobalamin deficiency would eventually have developed.

Methotrexate has the same structure as folate except that it has an amino group on C4 and a methyl group on $N^{10}$. Anticancer drugs such as methotrexate are folate analogues that act by inhibiting dihydrofolate reductase, thereby preventing the conversion of $FH_2$ to $FH_4$ (see Fig. 34.4). Thus, the cellular pools of $FH_4$ are not replenished, and reactions that require $FH_4$ cannot proceed.

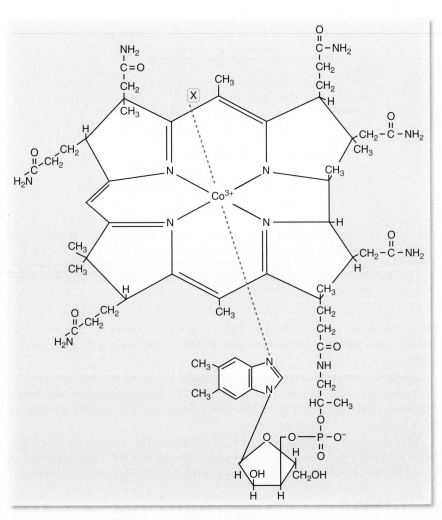

**FIG. 34.5.** Vitamin $B_{12}$. When $X$ is 5′-deoxyadenosine, the vitamin is deoxyadenosylcobalamin; when $X$ is $CH_3$, the product is methylcobalamin; when $X$ is CN, the vitamin is cyanocobalamin (the commercial form found in vitamin tablets).

Pernicious anemia, a deficiency of intrinsic factor, is a relatively common problem that leads to malabsorption of dietary cobalamin. It may result from an inherited defect that leads to a decreased ability of gastric parietal cells to synthesize intrinsic factor, antibodies against parietal cells or intrinsic factor, or from partial resection of the stomach or of the ileum. Production of intrinsic factor often declines with age and may be low in elderly individuals.

How should vitamin $B_{12}$ be administered to a patient with pernicious anemia?

and the released $B_{12}$ then binds to intrinsic factor, a glycoprotein secreted by the parietal cells of the stomach when food enters the stomach. The intrinsic factor–$B_{12}$ complex attaches to specific receptors in the terminal segment of the small intestine known as the ileum, after which the complex is internalized.

The $B_{12}$ within the enterocyte complexes with transcobalamin II before release into the circulation. The transcobalamin II–$B_{12}$ complex delivers $B_{12}$ to the tissues, which contain specific receptors for this complex. The liver takes up approximately 50% of the vitamin $B_{12}$, and the remainder is transported to other tissues. The amount of the vitamin stored in the liver is large enough that 3 to 6 years pass before symptoms of a dietary deficiency occur.

### C. Functions of Vitamin $B_{12}$

Vitamin $B_{12}$ is involved in two reactions in the body: the transfer of a methyl group from $N^5$-methyl-$FH_4$ to homocysteine to form methionine and the rearrangement of L-methylmalonyl CoA to form succinyl CoA (Fig. 34.6).

$FH_4$ receives a one-carbon group from serine or from other sources. This carbon is reduced to the methyl level and transferred to vitamin $B_{12}$, forming methyl-$B_{12}$ (or methylcobalamin). Methylcobalamin transfers the methyl group to homocysteine, which is converted to methionine by the enzyme methionine synthase.

**A**

SH
|
CH₂
|
CH₂
|
H − C − $\overset{+}{N}H_3$
|
COO⁻

**Homocysteine**

B₁₂ • CH₃

Methyl-
cobalamin

B₁₂

CH₃
|
S
|
CH₂
|
CH₂
|
H − C − $\overset{+}{N}H_3$
|
COO⁻

**Methionine**

**B**

H   COO⁻
|   |
H − C − C − H
|   |
H   C ~ SCoA
    ‖
    O

**Methylmalonyl CoA**

B₁₂   Adenosyl
cobalamin

COO⁻
|
H − C − H
|
H − C − H
|
C ~ SCoA
‖
O

**Succinyl CoA**

*FIG. 34.6.* **A,B.** The two reactions involving vitamin B₁₂ in humans.

Methionine can then be activated to *S*-adenosylmethionine (SAM) to transfer the methyl group to other compounds (Fig. 34.7).

Vitamin B₁₂ also participates in the conversion of L-methylmalonyl CoA to succinyl CoA. In this case, the active form of the coenzyme is 5′-deoxyadenosylcobalamin. This reaction is part of the metabolic route for the conversion of carbons from valine, isoleucine, threonine, and the last three carbons of odd-chain fatty acids, all of which form propionyl CoA, to the TCA cycle intermediate succinyl CoA (see Chapter 33).

## III. S-ADENOSYLMETHIONINE

SAM participates in the synthesis of many compounds that contain methyl groups. It is used in reactions that add methyl groups to either oxygen or nitrogen atoms in the acceptor (contrast that to folate derivatives, which can add one-carbon groups to sulfur or to carbon). As examples, SAM is required for the conversion

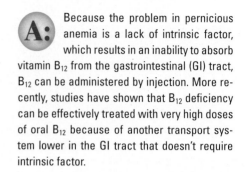

**A:** Because the problem in pernicious anemia is a lack of intrinsic factor, which results in an inability to absorb vitamin B₁₂ from the gastrointestinal (GI) tract, B₁₂ can be administered by injection. More recently, studies have shown that B₁₂ deficiency can be effectively treated with very high doses of oral B₁₂ because of another transport system lower in the GI tract that doesn't require intrinsic factor.

There are two major clinical manifestations of cobalamin (B₁₂) deficiency. One such presentation is hematopoietic (caused by the adverse effects of a B₁₂ deficiency on folate metabolism), and the other is neurological (caused by hypomethylation in the nervous system).

The hemopoietic problems associated with a B₁₂ deficiency are identical to those observed in a folate deficiency and, in fact, result from a folate deficiency secondary to (i.e., caused by) the B₁₂ deficiency (i.e., the methyl trap hypothesis). As the FH₄ pool is exhausted, deficiencies of the FH₄ derivatives needed for purine and dTMP biosynthesis develop, leading to the characteristic megaloblastic anemia.

The classical clinical presentation of the neurological dysfunction associated with a B₁₂ deficiency includes symmetric numbness and tingling of the feet (and less so the hands), diminishing vibratory and position sense, and progression to a spastic gait disturbance. The patient may become somnolent or may become extremely irritable ("megaloblastic madness"). Eventually, blind spots in the central portions of the visual fields develop, accompanied by alterations in gustatory (taste) and olfactory (smell) function. This is believed to be caused by hypomethylation within the nervous system brought about by an inability to recycle homocysteine to methionine and from there to SAM. The latter is the required methyl donor in these reactions. With a B₁₂ deficiency, this pathway is inoperable in the nervous system.

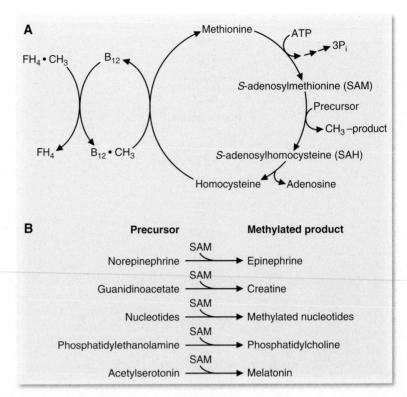

FIG. 34.7. Relationships among $FH_4$, $B_{12}$, and SAM. **A.** Overall scheme. **B.** Some specific reactions that require SAM.

Many health food stores now sell SAMe, a stabilized version of SAM. SAMe has been hypothesized to relieve depression because the synthesis of certain neurotransmitters requires methylation by SAM (see Chapter 33). This has led to the hypothesis that by increasing SAM levels within the nervous system, the biosynthesis of these neurotransmitters will be accelerated. This in turn might alleviate the feelings of depression. There have been reports in the literature indicating that this may occur, but its efficacy as an antidepressant must be confirmed. The major questions that must be addressed include the stability of SAMe in the digestive system and the level of uptake of SAMe by cells of the nervous system.

of phosphatidylethanolamine to phosphatidylcholine, guanidinoacetate to creatine, norepinephrine to epinephrine, acetylserotonin to melatonin, and nucleotides to methylated nucleotides (see Fig. 34.7B). It is also required for the inactivation of catecholamines and serotonin (see Chapter 33). More than 35 reactions in humans require methyl donation from SAM.

SAM is synthesized from methionine and ATP. As with the activation of vitamin $B_{12}$, ATP donates the adenosine. With the transfer of its methyl group, SAM forms $S$-adenosylhomocysteine, which is subsequently hydrolyzed to form homocysteine and adenosine.

Methionine, required for the synthesis of SAM, is obtained from the diet or produced from homocysteine, which accepts a methyl group from vitamin $B_{12}$ (see Fig. 34.7A). Thus, the methyl group of methionine is regenerated. The portion of methionine that is essential in the diet is the homocysteine moiety. If we had an adequate dietary source of homocysteine, methionine would not be required in the diet. However, there is no good dietary source of homocysteine, whereas methionine is plentiful in the diet.

## IV. RELATIONSHIPS BETWEEN FOLATE, VITAMIN $B_{12}$, AND $S$-ADENOSYLMETHIONINE

### A. The Methyl Trap Hypothesis

If one analyzes the flow of carbon in the folate cycle, the equilibrium lies in the direction of the $N^5$-methyl-$FH_4$ form. This appears to be the most stable form of carbon attached to the vitamin. However, in only one reaction can the methyl group be removed from $N^5$-methyl-$FH_4$ and that is the methionine synthase reaction, which requires vitamin $B_{12}$. Thus, if vitamin $B_{12}$ is deficient or if the methionine synthase enzyme is defective, $N^5$-methyl-$FH_4$ will accumulate. Eventually, most folate forms in the body will become "trapped" in the $N^5$-methyl form. A functional folate deficiency results because the carbons cannot be removed from the folate. The appearance of a functional folate deficiency caused by a lack of vitamin B$_{12}$ is known as the "methyl trap" hypothesis, and its clinical implications are discussed in following sections.

## B. Hyperhomocysteinemia

Elevated homocysteine levels have been linked to cardiovascular and neurological disease. Homocysteine levels can accumulate in a number of ways, which are related to both folic acid and vitamin B$_{12}$ metabolism. Homocysteine is derived from SAM, which arises when SAM donates a methyl group (Fig. 34.8). Because SAM is frequently donating methyl groups, there is constant production of *S*-adenosylhomocysteine, which leads to constant production of homocysteine. Recall from Chapter 33 that homocysteine has two biochemical fates. The homocysteine produced can be either remethylated to methionine or condensed with serine to form cystathionine. There are two routes to methionine production. The major one is methylation by $N^5$-methyl-FH$_4$, which requires vitamin B$_{12}$. The liver also expresses a second pathway in which betaine (derived from choline) can donate a methyl group to homocysteine to form methionine (see Section V of this chapter). The conversion of homocysteine to cystathionine requires pyridoxal phosphate. Thus, if an individual is deficient in vitamin B$_{12}$, the conversion of homocysteine to methionine by the major route is inhibited. This directs homocysteine to produce cystathionine, which eventually produces cysteine. As cysteine levels accumulate, the enzyme that makes cystathinonine undergoes feedback inhibition and that pathway is also inhibited (see Fig. 34.8). This, overall, leads to an accumulation of homocysteine, which is released into the blood.

Homocysteine also accumulates in the blood if a mutation is present in the enzyme that converts $N^5,N^{10}$-methylene-FH$_4$ to $N^5$-methyl-FH$_4$. When this occurs, the levels of $N^5$-methyl-FH$_4$ are too low to allow homocysteine to be converted to methionine. The loss of this pathway, coupled with the feedback inhibition by cysteine on cystathionine formation, also leads to elevated homocysteine levels in the blood.

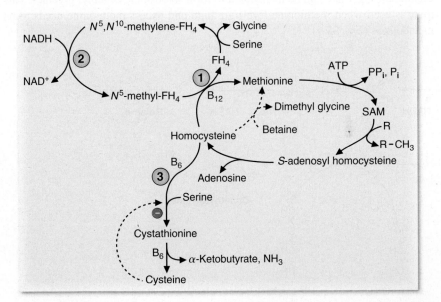

**FIG. 34.8.** Reaction pathways involving homocysteine. Defects in numbered enzymes (*1*, methionine synthase; *2*, $N^5$, $N^{10}$-methylene-FH$_4$ reductase; *3*, cystathionine-β-synthase) lead to elevated homocysteine. Recall that as cysteine accumulates, there is feedback inhibition on cystathionine β-synthase to stop further cysteine production.

A third way in which serum homocysteine levels can be elevated is by a mutated cystathionine β-synthase or a deficiency in vitamin $B_6$, the required cofactor for that enzyme. These defects block the ability of homocysteine to be converted to cysta-thionine, and the homocysteine that does accumulate cannot all be accommodated by conversion to methionine. Thus, an accumulation of homocysteine results.

### C. Neural Tube Defects

Folate deficiency during pregnancy has been associated with an increased risk of neural tube defects in the developing fetus. This risk is significantly reduced if women take folic acid supplements periconceptually. The link between folate defi-ciency and neural tube defects was first observed in women with hyperhomocyste-inemia brought about by a thermolabile variant of $N^5,N^{10}$-methylene-$FH_4$ reductase. This form of the enzyme, which results from a single nucleotide change (C to T) in position 677 of the gene encoding the protein, is less active at body temperature than at lower temperatures. This results in a reduced level of $N^5$-methyl-$FH_4$ being generated and, therefore, an increase in the levels of homocysteine. Along with the elevated homocysteine, the women were also folate deficient. The folate deficiency and the subsequent inhibition of DNA synthesis and reduced SAM levels leads to neural tube defects. The elevated homocysteine is one indication that such a deficit is present. These findings have led to the recommendation that women considering getting pregnant begin taking folate supplements before conception occurs, and for at least 1 month after conception. The Department of Agriculture has, in fact, man-dated that folate be added to flour-containing products in the United States.

### V. CHOLINE AND ONE-CARBON METABOLISM

Other compounds involved in one-carbon metabolism are derived from degradation products of choline. Choline, an essential component of certain phospholipids, is oxidized to form betaine aldehyde, which is further oxidized to betaine (trimethyl-glycine). In the liver, betaine can donate a methyl group to homocysteine to form methionine and dimethyl glycine. This allows the liver to have two routes for homo-cysteine conversion to methionine. This is in contrast to the nervous system, which only expresses the primary $B_{12}$-requiring pathway. Under conditions in which SAM accumulates, glycine can be methylated to form sarcosine (N-methyl glycine). This route is used when methionine levels are high and excess methionine needs to be metabolized (Fig. 34.9).

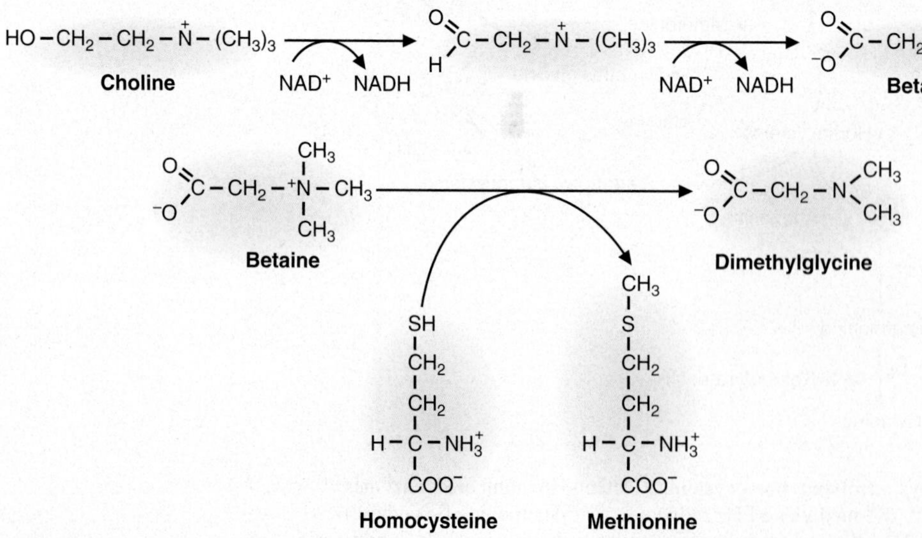

Folate deficiencies lead to decreased methylation of dUMP to form dTMP. This leads to an increase in the in-tracellular dUTP/dTTP ratio. This ratio change causes a significant increase in the incorpora-tion of uracil into DNA. Although much of this uracil can be removed by DNA-repair enzymes, the lack of available dTTP blocks the step of DNA repair that is catalyzed by DNA poly-merase. The result is fragmentation of DNA as well as a blockade of normal DNA replication.

FIG. 34.9. Choline and one-carbon metabolism.

**Table 34.2    Diseases Discussed in Chapter 34**

| Disease or Disorder | Environmental or Genetic | Comments |
|---|---|---|
| Pernicious anemia | Both | Pernicious anemia is due to the lack of intrinsic factor, which leads to a $B_{12}$ deficiency. The $B_{12}$ deficiency indirectly interferes with DNA synthesis. In cells of the erythroid lineage, cell size increases without cell division, leading to megaloblastic anemia. |
| Alcohol-induced megaloblastic anemia | Environmental | Alcohol-induced malnutrition, which can lead to folate and/or $B_{12}$ deficiencies. The folate and/or $B_{12}$ deficiency will lead to the development of megaloblastic anemia. |
| Neural tube defects | Both | A lack of folate derivatives leads to reduced methylation in the nervous system, altering gene expression and increasing the risk of neural tube defects. |

## CLINICAL COMMENTS

Diseases discussed in this chapter are summarized in Table 34.2.

**Jean T.**  **Jean T.** developed a folate deficiency and is on the verge of developing a cobalamin (vitamin $B_{12}$) deficiency as a consequence of prolonged, moderately severe malnutrition related to chronic alcoholism. Before folate therapy is started, the physician must ascertain that the megaloblastic anemia is not caused by a pure $B_{12}$ deficiency or a combined deficiency of folate and $B_{12}$.

If folate is given without cobalamin to a $B_{12}$-deficient patient, the drug only partially corrects the megaloblastic anemia because it will "bypass" the methyl-folate trap and provide adequate $FH_4$ coenzyme for the conversion of dUMP to dTMP and for a resurgence of purine synthesis. As a result, normal DNA synthesis, DNA repair, and cell division occur. However, the neurological syndrome resulting from hypomethylation in nervous tissue may progress unless the physician realizes that $B_{12}$ supplementation is required. In Jean's case, in which the serum $B_{12}$ concentration was borderline low and in which the dietary history supported the possibility of a $B_{12}$ deficiency, a combination of folate and $B_{12}$ supplements is required to avoid this potential therapeutic trap.

**Beatrice T.**  **Beatrice T.** was diagnosed with an inability to absorb dietary $B_{12}$. One of the consequences of aging is a reduced acid production by the gastric mucosa (atrophic gastritis), which limits the ability of pepsin to work on dietary protein. Reduced pepsin efficiency then reduces the amount of bound $B_{12}$ released from dietary protein as a result of which the $B_{12}$ is not available for absorption. Her condition can be treated by taking high-dose vitamin $B_{12}$ supplements orally.

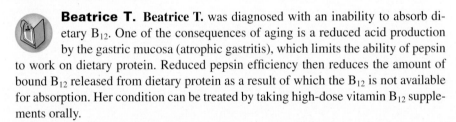

## REVIEW QUESTIONS-CHAPTER 34

1.  Propionic acid accumulation from amino acid degradation would result from a deficiency of which one of the following vitamins?

    A.  Biotin
    B.  Vitamin $B_6$
    C.  Folic acid
    D.  Vitamin C
    E.  Vitamin $B_1$

2.  A patient presents with feelings of lethargy and nausea. During the history, it becomes evident that these feelings are more pronounced after eating a high-protein meal; in fact, the patient is avoiding meals rich in protein so that he can continue to feel well. Laboratory tests taken after the patient eats a high-protein meal indicate elevated levels of methylmalonic acid in the blood and urine. This metabolic defect is most likely caused by a deficiency of which one of the following?

    A.  Thiamine
    B.  Riboflavin
    C.  Vitamin $B_{12}$
    D.  Folic acid
    E.  Vitamin $B_6$

3. A patient presents with feelings of lethargy and nausea. During the history, it becomes evident that these feelings are more pronounced after eating a high-protein meal; in fact, the patient is avoiding meals rich in protein so that he can continue to feel well. Laboratory tests taken after the patient eats a high-protein meal indicate elevated levels of methylmalonic acid in the blood and urine. The ingestion of which one of the following amino acids would be expected to exacerbate the metabolic problem in this patient?

   A. Arginine
   B. Histidine
   C. Leucine
   D. Lysine
   E. Methionine

4. A eukaryotic cell line was developed which contained a thermolabile variant of serine hydroxymethyltransferase. The enzyme had low levels of activity at 37°C but almost normal levels of activity at 32°C. The investigator who developed this line predicted that DNA synthesis would be impaired when the cells were grown at the higher temperature due to a reduction of carbon in the folate pool. However, when the experiment was carried out, normal growth at the higher temperature was observed as long as which one of the following amino acids was also present in the growth media?

   A. Serine
   B. Glycine
   C. Alanine
   D. Aspartate
   E. Glutamate

5. A 65-year-old man visits his primary physician because of tingling in his hands and feet and a sense that he is forgetting things more than usual. A complete blood count (CBC) indicates a mild anemia. The patient states that his diet has not changed, other than eating more red meat than before. This patient can be treated by which one of the following?

   A. Oral administration of vitamin $B_{12}$
   B. Oral administration of folic acid
   C. Oral administration of methionine
   D. Injections of $B_{12}$
   E. Injections of folic acid
   F. Injections of methionine

# 35  Purine and Pyrimidine Metabolism

## CHAPTER OUTLINE

## KEY POINTS

- Purine and pyrimidine nucleotides can both be synthesized from scratch (de novo) or salvaged from existing bases.
- De novo purine synthesis is complex, requiring 11 steps and six molecules of adenosine triphosphate (ATP) for every purine synthesized. Purines are initially synthesized in the ribonucleotide form.
- The precursors for de novo purine synthesis are glycine, ribose 5-phosphate, glutamine, aspartate, carbon dioxide, and $N^{10}$-formyltetrahydrofolate ($FH_4$).
- The initial purine ribonucleotide synthesized is inosine monophosphate (IMP). Adenosine monophosphate (AMP) and guanosine monophosphate (GMP) are each derived from IMP.
- Because de novo purine synthesis requires a large amount of energy, purine nucleotide salvage pathways exist such that free purine bases can be converted to nucleotides.
- Mutations in purine salvage enzymes are associated with severe diseases, such as Lesch-Nyhan syndrome and severe combined immunodeficiency disease (SCID).
- Pyrimidine bases are initially synthesized as the free base and then converted to nucleotides.
- Aspartate and cytoplasmic carbamoyl phosphate are the precursors for pyrimidine ring synthesis.
- The initial pyrimidine nucleotide synthesized is orotate monophosphate, which is converted to uridine monophosphate. The other pyrimidine nucleotides are derived from a uracil-containing intermediate.
- Deoxyribonucleotides are derived by reduction of ribonucleotides, as catalyzed by ribonucleotide reductase. The regulation of ribonucleotide reductase is complex.
- Degradation of purine containing nucleotides results in production of uric acid, which is eliminated in the urine. Elevated uric acid levels in the blood lead to gout.

# THE WAITING ROOM

The initial acute inflammatory process that caused **Lotta T.** to experience a painful attack of gouty arthritis responded quickly to colchicine therapy (see Chapters 3 and 6). Several weeks after the inflammatory signs and symptoms in her right great toe subsided, Lotta was placed on allopurinol (while continuing colchicine), a drug that reduces uric acid synthesis. Her serum uric acid level gradually fell from a pretreatment level of 9.2 mg/dL into the normal range (2.5 to 8.0 mg/dL). She remained free of gouty symptoms when she returned to her physician for a follow-up office visit.

## I. PURINES AND PYRIMIDINES

As has been seen in previous chapters, nucleotides serve numerous functions in different reaction pathways. For example, nucleotides are the activated precursors of DNA and RNA. Nucleotides form the structural moieties of many coenzymes (examples include nicotinamide adenine dinucleotide [NADH], flavin adenine dinucleotide [FAD], and coenzyme A). Nucleotides are critical elements in energy metabolism (adenosine triphosphate [ATP], guanosine triphosphate [GTP]). Nucleotide derivatives are frequently activated intermediates in many biosynthetic pathways. In addition, nucleotides act as second messengers in intracellular signaling (e.g., cyclic adenosine monophosphate [cAMP], cyclic guanosine monophosphate [cGMP]). Finally, nucleotides act as metabolic allosteric regulators. Think about all of the enzymes that have been studied that are regulated by levels of ATP, adenosine diphosphate (ADP), and adenosine monophosphate (AMP).

Dietary uptake of purine and pyrimidine bases is minimal. The diet contains nucleic acids and the exocrine pancreas secretes deoxyribonuclease and ribonuclease, along with the proteolytic and lipolytic enzymes. This enables digested nucleic acids to be converted to nucleotides. The intestinal epithelial cells contain alkaline phosphatase activity, which converts nucleotides to nucleosides. Other enzymes within the epithelial cells tend to metabolize the nucleosides to uric acid (which is released into the circulation) or to salvage them for their own needs. Approximately 5% of ingested nucleotides will make it into the circulation, either as the free base or as a nucleoside. Because of the minimal dietary uptake of these important molecules, de novo synthesis of purines and pyrimidines is required.

## II. PURINE BIOSYNTHESIS

The purine bases are produced de novo by pathways that use amino acids as precursors and produce nucleotides (Fig. 35.1). Most de novo synthesis occurs in the liver, and the nitrogenous bases and nucleosides are then transported to other tissues by red blood cells. The brain also synthesizes significant amounts of nucleotides. Because the de novo pathway requires at least six high-energy bonds per purine produced, a salvage pathway, which is used by many cell types, can convert free bases and nucleosides to nucleotides.

### A. De Novo Synthesis
#### 1. SYNTHESIS OF INOSINE MONOPHOSPHATE

As purines are built on a ribose base, an activated form of ribose is used to initiate the purine biosynthetic pathway. $5'$-Phosphoribosyl-$1'$-pyrophosphate (PRPP) is the activated source of the ribose moiety. It is synthesized from ATP and ribose 5-phosphate (Fig. 35.2), which is produced from glucose through the pentose phosphate pathway (see Chapter 24). The enzyme that catalyzes this reaction, PRPP

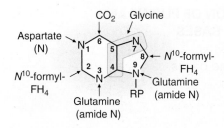

**FIG. 35.1.** Origin of the atoms of the purine base. *FH₄*, tetrahydrofolate; *RP*, ribose 5-phosphate.

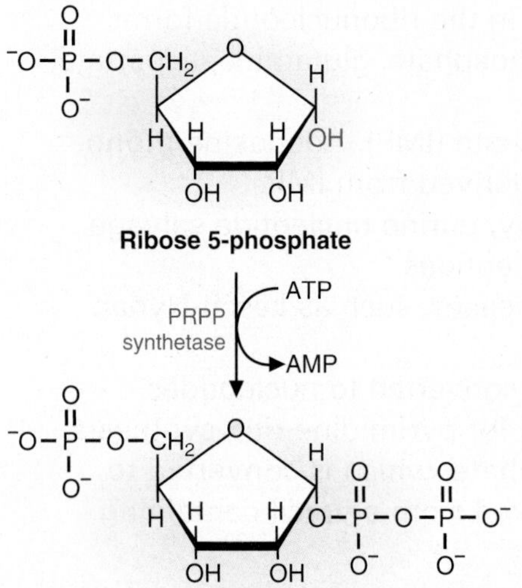

**Ribose 5-phosphate**

PRPP synthetase

ATP
AMP

**5-Phosphoribosyl 1-pyrophosphate (PRPP)**

**FIG. 35.2.** Synthesis of PRPP. Ribose 5-phosphate is produced from glucose by the pentose phosphate pathway.

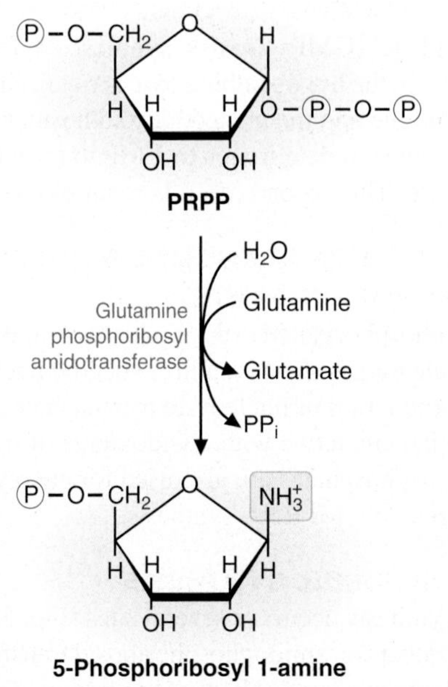

**PRPP**

Glutamine
phosphoribosyl
amidotransferase

$H_2O$

Glutamine

Glutamate

$PP_i$

**5-Phosphoribosyl 1-amine**

**FIG. 35.3.** The first step in purine biosynthesis. The purine base is built on the ribose moiety. The availability of the substrate PRPP is a major determinant of the rate of this reaction.

 Cellular concentrations of PRPP and glutamine are usually below their $K_m$ for glutamine phosphoribosyl amidotransferase. Thus, any situation which leads to an increase in their concentration can lead to an increase in de novo purine biosynthesis.

synthetase, is a regulated enzyme (see Section II.A.5); however, this step is not the committed step of purine biosynthesis. PRPP has many other uses, which are described as the chapter progresses.

In the first committed step of the purine biosynthetic pathway, PRPP reacts with glutamine to form 5′-phosphoribosyl 1′-amine (Fig. 35.3). This reaction, which produces nitrogen 9 of the purine ring, is catalyzed by glutamine phosphoribosyl amidotransferase, a highly regulated enzyme.

In the next step of the pathway, the entire glycine molecule is added to the growing precursor. Glycine provides carbons 4 and 5 and nitrogen 7 of the purine ring (see Fig. 35.1). This step requires energy in the form of ATP.

Subsequently, carbon 8 is provided by $N^{10}$-formyl-FH$_4$, nitrogen 3 by glutamine, carbon 6 by carbon dioxide ($CO_2$), nitrogen 1 by aspartate, and carbon 2 by $N^{10}$-formyl-FH$_4$ (see Fig. 35.1). Note that six high-energy bonds of ATP are required (starting with ribose 5-phosphate) to synthesize the first purine nucleotide, inosine monophosphate (IMP). This nucleotide contains the base hypoxanthine joined by an *N*-glycosidic bond from nitrogen 9 of the purine ring to carbon 1 of the ribose (Fig. 35.4). Hypoxanthine is not found in DNA, but it is the precursor for the other purine bases.

## 2. SYNTHESIS OF ADENOSINE MONOPHOSPHATE

IMP serves as the branch point from which both adenine and guanine nucleotides can be produced. AMP is derived from IMP in two steps (Fig. 35.5). In the first step, aspartate is added to IMP to form adenylosuccinate, a reaction similar to the one catalyzed by argininosuccinate synthetase in the urea cycle. Note how this reaction requires a high-energy bond, donated by GTP. Fumarate is then released from the adenylosuccinate by the enzyme adenylosuccinase to form AMP.

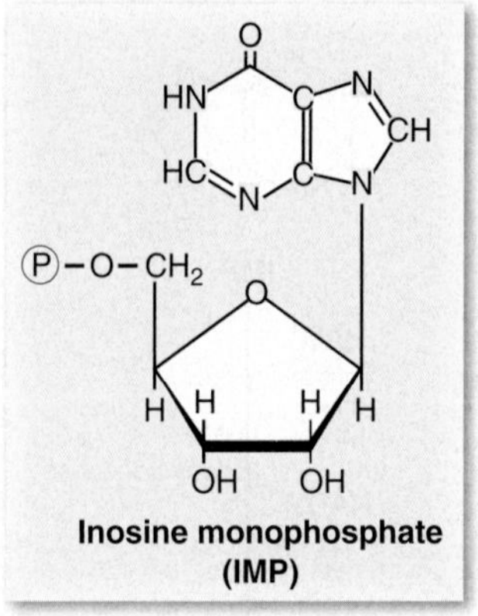

**Inosine monophosphate
(IMP)**

**FIG. 35.4.** Structure of IMP. The base is hypoxanthine.

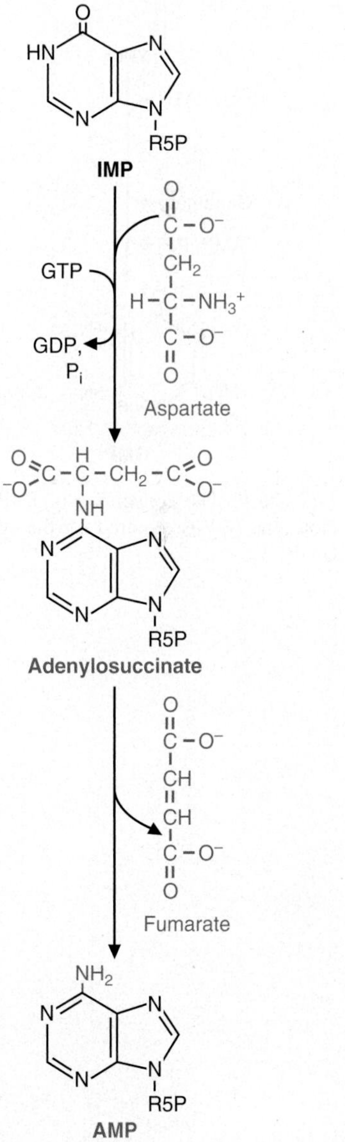

**IMP**

GTP

GDP,
$P_i$

Aspartate

**Adenylosuccinate**

Fumarate

**AMP**

**FIG. 35.5.** The conversion of IMP to AMP. Note that GTP is required for the synthesis of AMP. *R5P*, ribose 5-phosphate.

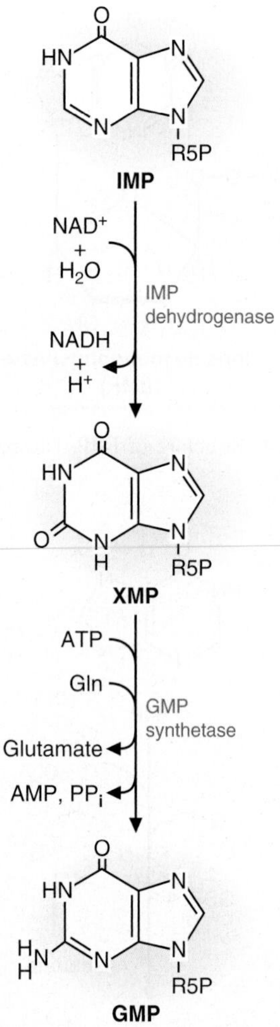

**IMP**

NAD⁺ + H₂O → NADH + H⁺

IMP dehydrogenase

**XMP**

ATP, Gln → Glutamate, AMP, PP_i

GMP synthetase

**GMP**

**FIG. 35.6.** The conversion of IMP to GMP. Note that ATP is required for the synthesis of GMP.

### 3. SYNTHESIS OF GUANOSINE MONOPHOSPHATE

Guanosine monophosphate (GMP) is also synthesized from IMP in two steps (Fig. 35.6). In the first step, the hypoxanthine base is oxidized by IMP dehydrogenase to produce the base xanthine and the nucleotide xanthosine monophosphate (XMP). Glutamine then donates the amide nitrogen to XMP to form GMP in a reaction catalyzed by GMP synthetase. This second reaction requires energy in the form of ATP.

### 4. PHOSPHORYLATION OF ADENOSINE MONOPHOSPHATE AND GUANOSINE MONOPHOSPHATE

AMP and GMP can be phosphorylated to the diphosphate and triphosphate levels. The production of nucleoside diphosphates requires specific nucleoside monophosphate kinases, whereas the production of nucleoside triphosphates requires nucleoside diphosphate kinases, which are active with a wide range of nucleoside diphosphates. The purine nucleoside triphosphates are also used for energy-requiring processes in the cell and also as precursors for RNA synthesis.

### 5. REGULATION OF PURINE SYNTHESIS

Regulation of purine synthesis occurs at several sites (Fig. 35.7). Four key enzymes are regulated: PRPP synthetase, amidophosphoribosyl transferase, adenylosuccinate synthetase, and IMP dehydrogenase. The first two enzymes regulate IMP synthesis; the last two regulate the production of AMP and GMP, respectively.

A primary site of regulation is the synthesis of PRPP. PRPP synthetase is negatively affected by guanosine diphosphate (GDP) and, at a distinct allosteric site, by ADP. Thus, the simultaneous binding of an oxypurine (eg., GDP) and an aminopurine (eg., ADP) can occur with the result being a synergistic inhibition of the enzyme. This enzyme is not the committed step of purine biosynthesis; PRPP is also used in pyrimidine synthesis and both the purine and pyrimidine salvage pathways.

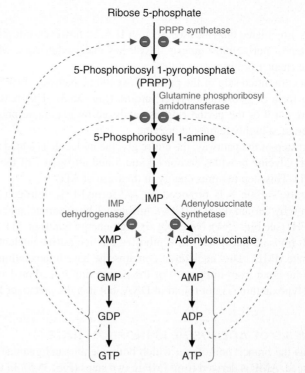

**FIG. 35.7.** The regulation of purine synthesis. PRPP synthetase has two distinct allosteric sites: one for ADP, the other for GDP. Glutamine phosphoribosyl amidotransferase contains adenine nucleotide- and guanine nucleotide–binding sites; the monophosphates are the most important, although the diphosphates and triphosphates will also bind to and inhibit the enzyme. Adenylosuccinate synthetase is inhibited by AMP; IMP dehydrogenase is inhibited by GMP.

The committed step of purine synthesis is the formation of 5′-phosphoribosyl 1′-amine by glutamine phosphoribosyl amidotransferase. This enzyme is strongly inhibited by GMP and AMP (the end products of the purine biosynthetic pathway). The enzyme is also inhibited by the corresponding nucleoside diphosphates and triphosphates, but under cellular conditions, these compounds probably do not play a central role in regulation.

The enzymes that convert IMP to XMP and adenylosuccinate are both regulated. GMP inhibits the activity of IMP dehydrogenase, and AMP inhibits adenylosuccinate synthetase. Note that the synthesis of AMP is dependent on GTP (of which GMP is a precursor), whereas the synthesis of GMP is dependent on ATP (which is made from AMP). This serves as a type of positive regulatory mechanism to balance the pools of these precursors: When the levels of ATP are high, GMP will be made; when the levels of GTP are high, AMP synthesis will take place. GMP and AMP act as negative effectors at these branch points, a classic example of feedback inhibition.

## B.  Purine Salvage Pathways

Most of the de novo synthesis of the bases of nucleotides occurs in the liver, and to some extent in the brain, neutrophils, and other cells of the immune system. Within the liver, nucleotides can be converted to nucleosides or free bases, which can be transported to other tissues via the red blood cell in the circulation. In addition, the small amounts of dietary bases or nucleosides that are absorbed also enter cells in this form. Thus, most cells can salvage these bases to generate nucleotides for RNA and DNA synthesis. For certain cell types, such as the lymphocytes, the salvage of bases is the major form of nucleotide generation.

The overall picture of salvage is shown in Figure 35.8. The pathways allow free bases, nucleosides, and nucleotides to be easily interconverted. The major enzymes required are purine nucleoside phosphorylase, phosphoribosyl transferases, and deaminases.

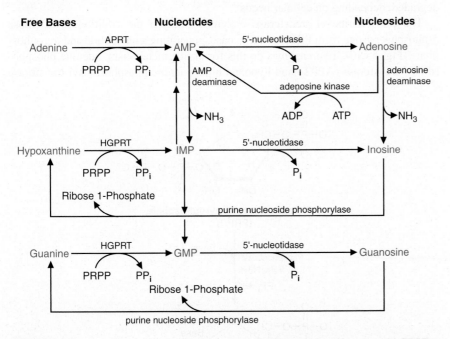

*FIG. 35.8.*   Salvage of bases. The purine bases hypoxanthine and guanine react with PRPP to form the nucleotides IMP and GMP, respectively. The enzyme that catalyzes the reaction is HGPRT. Adenine forms AMP in a reaction catalyzed by APRT. Nucleotides are converted to nucleosides by 5′-nucleotidase. Free bases are generated from nucleosides by purine nucleoside phosphorylase (although adenosine is not a substrate of this enzyme). Deamination of the base adenine occurs with AMP and adenosine deaminase. Of the purines, only adenosine can be phosphorylated directly back to a nucleotide by adenosine kinase.

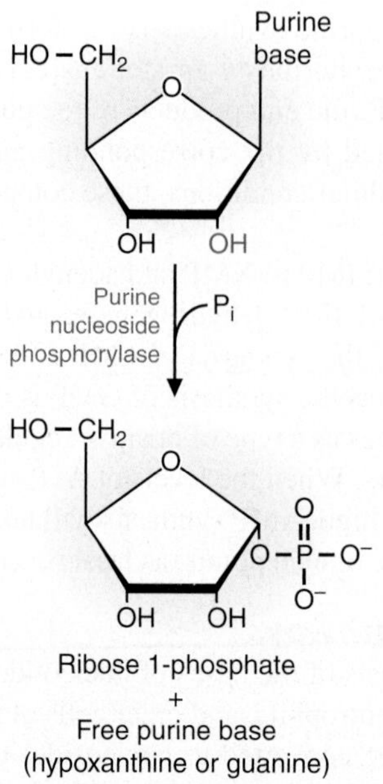

**FIG. 35.9.** The purine nucleoside phosphorylase reaction, converting guanosine or inosine to ribose 1-phosphate plus the free base guanine or hypoxanthine.

A deficiency in purine nucleoside phosphorylase activity leads to an immune disorder in which T-cell immunity is compromised. B-cell immunity, conversely, may be only slightly compromised or even normal. Children lacking this activity have recurrent infections, and more than half display neurological complications. Symptoms of the disorder first appear between 6 months and 4 years of age. It is an extremely rare autosomal recessive disorder.

Purine nucleoside phosphorylase catalyzes a phosphorolysis reaction of the *N*-glycosidic bond that attaches the base to the sugar moiety in the nucleosides guanosine and inosine (Fig. 35.9). Thus, guanosine and inosine are converted to guanine and hypoxanthine, respectively, along with ribose 1-phosphate. The ribose 1-phosphate can be isomerized to ribose 5-phosphate, and the free bases then salvaged or degraded, depending on cellular needs.

The phosphoribosyl transferase enzymes catalyze the addition of a ribose 5-phosphate group from PRPP to a free base, generating a nucleotide and pyrophosphate (Fig. 35.10). Two enzymes do this for purine metabolism: adenine phosphoribosyl transferase (APRT) and hypoxanthine–guanine phosphoribosyl transferase

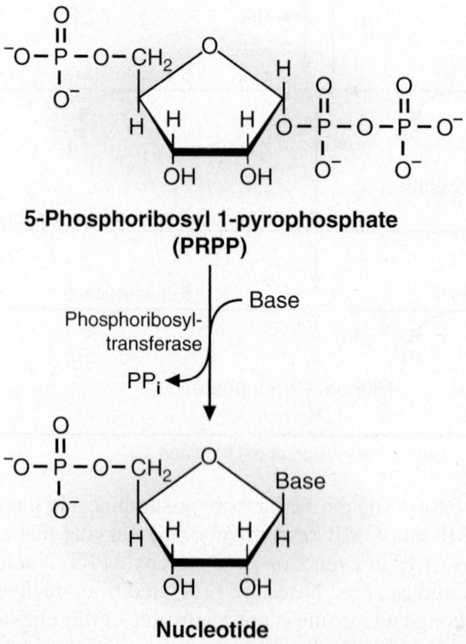

**FIG. 35.10.** The phosphoribosyltransferase reaction. APRT uses the free base adenine; HGPRT can use either hypoxanthine or guanine as a substrate.

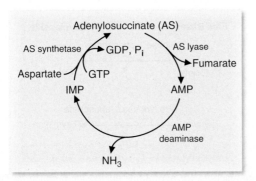

**FIG. 35.11.** The purine nucleotide cycle. Using a combination of biosynthetic and salvage enzymes, the net effect is the conversion of aspartate to fumarate plus ammonia, with the fumarate playing an anaplerotic role in the muscle. *AS*, adenylosuccinate.

(HGPRT). The reactions they catalyze are the same, differing only in their substrate specificity.

Adenosine and AMP can be deaminated by adenosine deaminase and AMP deaminase, respectively, to form inosine and IMP (see Fig. 35.8). Adenosine is also the only nucleoside to be directly phosphorylated to a nucleotide by adenosine kinase. Guanosine and inosine must be converted to free bases by purine nucleoside phosphorylase before they can be converted to nucleotides by HGPRT.

A portion of the salvage pathway that is important in muscle is the purine nucleotide cycle (Fig. 35.11). The net effect of these reactions is the deamination of aspartate to fumarate (as AMP is synthesized from IMP and then deaminated back to IMP by AMP deaminase). Under conditions in which the muscle must generate energy, the fumarate derived from the purine nucleotide cycle is used anaplerotically to replenish tricarboxylic acid (TCA) cycle intermediates and to allow the cycle to operate at a high speed. Deficiencies in enzymes of this cycle lead to muscle fatigue during exercise.

## III. SYNTHESIS OF THE PYRIMIDINE NUCLEOTIDES
### A. De Novo Synthesis

In the synthesis of the pyrimidine nucleotides, the base is synthesized first, and then it is attached to the ribose 5′-phosphate moiety. The origin of the atoms of the ring (aspartate and carbamoyl phosphate, which is derived from $CO_2$ and glutamine) is shown in Figure 35.12. In the initial reaction of the pathway, glutamine combines with bicarbonate and ATP to form carbamoyl phosphate. This reaction is analogous to the first reaction of the urea cycle, except that it uses glutamine as the source of the nitrogen (rather than ammonia) and it occurs in the cytosol (rather than in mitochondria). The reaction is catalyzed by carbamoyl phosphate synthetase II (CPSII), which is the regulated step of the pathway. The analogous reaction in urea synthesis is catalyzed by CPSI.

In the next step of pyrimidine biosynthesis, the entire aspartate molecule adds to carbamoyl phosphate in a reaction catalyzed by aspartate transcarbamoylase. The molecule subsequently closes to produce a ring (catalyzed by dihydroorotase), which is oxidized to form orotic acid (or its anion, orotate) through the actions of dihydroorotate dehydrogenase. The enzyme orotate phosphoribosyl transferase catalyzes the transfer of ribose 5-phosphate from PRPP to orotate, producing orotidine 5′-phosphate, which is decarboxylated by orotidylic acid dehydrogenase to form uridine monophosphate (UMP) (Fig. 35.13). In mammals, the first three enzymes of the pathway (CPSII, aspartate transcarbamoylase, and dihydroorotase) are located on the same polypeptide, designated as CAD. The last two enzymes of the pathway are similarly located on a polypeptide known as UMP synthase (the orotate phosphoribosyl transferase and orotidylic acid dehydrogenase activities).

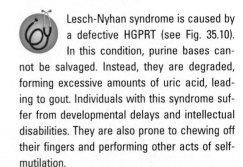

Lesch-Nyhan syndrome is caused by a defective HGPRT (see Fig. 35.10). In this condition, purine bases cannot be salvaged. Instead, they are degraded, forming excessive amounts of uric acid, leading to gout. Individuals with this syndrome suffer from developmental delays and intellectual disabilities. They are also prone to chewing off their fingers and performing other acts of self-mutilation.

A deficiency in adenosine deaminase activity leads to severe combined immunodeficiency disease or SCID. In the severe form of combined immunodeficiency, both T-cells (which provide cell-based immunity) and B-cells (which produce antibodies) are deficient, leaving the individual without a functional immune system. Children born with this disorder do not develop a mature thymus gland and suffer from many opportunistic infections because of their lack of a functional immune system. Death results if the child is not placed in a sterile environment. Administration of polyethylene glycol–modified adenosine deaminase and hematopoietic cell transplantation has been successful in treating the disorder, and the ADA gene was the first to be used in gene therapy in treating the disorder.

In hereditary orotic aciduria, orotic acid is excreted in the urine because the enzymes that convert it to uridine monophosphate, orotate phosphoribosyltransferase and orotidine 5′-phosphate decarboxylase, are defective (see Fig. 35.13). Pyrimidines cannot be synthesized and, therefore, normal growth does not occur. Oral administration of uridine is used to treat this condition. Uridine, which is converted to UMP, bypasses the metabolic block and provides the body with a source of pyrimidines, as both CTP and dTMP can be produced from UMP.

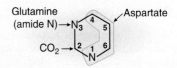

**FIG. 35.12.** The origin of the atoms in the pyrimidine ring.

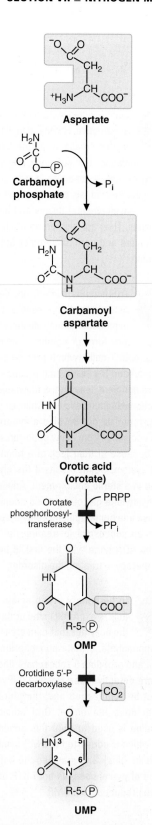

**FIG. 35.13.** Conversion of carbamoyl phosphate and aspartate to UMP. The defective enzymes in hereditary orotic aciduria are indicated by the *dark bars*.

■ Block in hereditary orotic aciduria

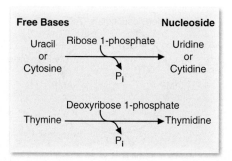

**FIG. 35.14.** Salvage reactions for pyrimidine nucleoside production. Thymine phosphorylase uses deoxyribose 1-phosphate as a substrate, so ribothymidine is rarely formed.

UMP is phosphorylated to uridine triphosphate (UTP). An amino group, derived from the amide of glutamine, is added to carbon 4 to produce cytidine triphosphate (CTP) by the enzyme CTP synthetase (this reaction cannot occur at the nucleotide monophosphate level). UTP and CTP are precursors for the synthesis of RNA. The synthesis of thymidine triphosphate (TTP) will be described in Section IV.

### B. Pyrimidine Salvage Pathways

Pyrimidine bases are normally salvaged by a two-step route. First, a relatively nonspecific pyrimidine nucleoside phosphorylase converts the pyrimidine bases to their respective nucleosides (Fig. 35.14). Notice that the preferred direction for this reaction is the reverse phosphorylase reaction in which phosphate is released and is not being used as a nucleophile to release the pyrimidine base from the nucleoside. The more specific nucleoside kinases then react with the nucleosides, forming nucleotides (Table 35.1). As with purines, further phosphorylation is carried out by increasingly more specific kinases. The nucleoside phosphorylase–nucleoside kinase route for synthesis of pyrimidine nucleoside monophosphates is relatively inefficient for salvage of pyrimidine bases because of the very low concentration of the bases in plasma and tissues.

Pyrimidine phosphorylase can use all of the pyrimidines but has a preference for uracil and is sometimes called **uridine phosphorylase**. The phosphorylase uses cytosine fairly well but has a very, very low affinity for thymine; therefore, a ribonucleoside containing thymine is almost never made in vivo. A second phosphorylase, thymine phosphorylase, has a much higher affinity for thymine and adds a deoxyribose residue (see Fig. 35.14).

### C. Regulation of De Novo Pyrimidine Synthesis

The regulated step of pyrimidine synthesis in humans is CPSII. The enzyme is inhibited by UTP and activated by PRPP. Thus, as pyrimidines decrease in concentration (as indicated by UTP levels), CPSII is activated and pyrimidines are synthesized.

**Table 35.1 Salvage Reactions for Conversion of Pyrimidine Nucleosides to Nucleotides**

| Enzyme | Reaction |
| --- | --- |
| Uridine-cytidine kinase | Uridine + ATP → UMP + ADP |
| | Cytidine + ATP → CMP + ADP |
| Deoxythymidine kinase | Deoxythymidine + ATP → dTMP + ADP |
| Deoxycytidine kinase | Deoxycytidine + ATP → dCMP + ADP |

ATP, adenosine triphosphate; UMP, uridine monophosphate; ADP, adenosine diphosphate; CMP, cytidine monophosphate; dTMP, deoxythymidine monophosphate; dCMP, deoxycytidine monophosphate.

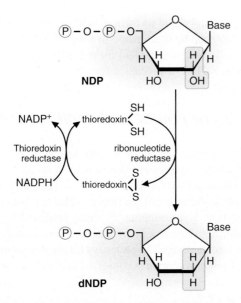

**FIG. 35.15.** Reduction of ribose to deoxyribose. Reduction occurs at the nucleoside diphosphate level. A ribonucleoside diphosphate (NDP) is converted to a deoxyribonucleoside diphosphate (dNDP). Thioredoxin is oxidized to a disulfide, which must be reduced for the reaction to continue producing dNDP.

## IV. THE PRODUCTION OF DEOXYRIBONUCLEOTIDES

For DNA synthesis to occur, the ribose moiety must be reduced to deoxyribose (Fig. 35.15). This reduction occurs at the diphosphate level and is catalyzed by ribonucleotide reductase, which requires the protein thioredoxin. The deoxyribonucleoside diphosphates can be phosphorylated to the triphosphate level and used as precursors for DNA synthesis.

The regulation of ribonucleotide reductase is quite complex. The enzyme contains two allosteric sites, one controlling the activity of the enzyme and the other controlling the substrate specificity of the enzyme. ATP bound to the activity site activates the enzyme; deoxyadenosine triphosphate (dATP) bound to this site inhibits the enzyme. Substrate specificity is more complex. ATP bound to the substrate site activates the reduction of pyrimidines (cytidine diphosphate [CDP] and uridine diphosphate [UDP]) to form deoxycytidine diphosphate (dCDP) and deoxyuridine diphosphate (dUDP). The dUDP is not used for DNA synthesis; rather, it is used to produce deoxythymidine monophosphate (dTMP) (see discussion later). Once dTMP is produced, it is phosphorylated to deoxythymine triphosphate (dTTP), which then binds to the substrate site and induces the reduction of GDP. As deoxyguanosine triphosphate (dGTP) accumulates, it replaces dTTP in the substrate site and allows ADP to be reduced to deoxyadenosine diphosphate (dADP). This leads to the accumulation of dATP, which will inhibit the overall activity of the enzyme. These allosteric changes are summarized in Table 35.2.

 When ornithine transcarbamoylase is deficient (urea cycle disorder), excess carbamoyl phosphate from the mitochondria leaks into the cytoplasm. The elevated levels of cytoplasmic carbamoyl phosphate lead to pyrimidine production, as the regulated step of the pathway, the reaction catalyzed by carbamoyl synthetase II, is being bypassed. Thus, orotic aciduria results.

**Table 35.2   Effectors of Ribonucleotide Reductase Activity**

| Preferred Substrate | Effector Bound to Overall Activity Site | Effector Bound to Substrate Specificity Site |
| --- | --- | --- |
| None | dATP | Any nucleotide |
| CDP | ATP | ATP or dATP |
| UDP | ATP | ATP or dATP |
| GDP | ATP | dTTP |
| ADP | ATP | dGTP |

dATP, deoxyadenosine triphosphate; CDP, cytidine diphosphate; ATP, adenosine triphosphate; UDP, uridine diphosphate; GDP, guanosine diphosphate; dTTP, deoxythymidine triphosphate; ADP, adenosine diphosphate; dGTP, deoxyguanosine triphosphate.

dUDP can be dephosphorylated to form dUMP or, alternatively, deoxycytidine monophosphate (dCMP) can be deaminated to form dUMP. Methylene tetrahydrofolate transfers a methyl group to dUMP to form dTMP (see Fig. 34.4). Phosphorylation reactions produce dTTP, a precursor for DNA synthesis and a regulator of ribonucleotide reductase.

# V. DEGRADATION OF PURINE AND PYRIMIDINE BASES

## A. Purine Bases

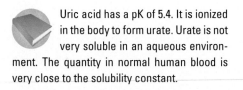

Uric acid has a pK of 5.4. It is ionized in the body to form urate. Urate is not very soluble in an aqueous environment. The quantity in normal human blood is very close to the solubility constant.

The degradation of the purine nucleotides (AMP and GMP) occurs mainly in the liver (Fig. 35.16). Salvage enzymes are used for most of these reactions. AMP is first deaminated to produce IMP (AMP deaminase). Then IMP and GMP are dephosphorylated (5′-nucleotidase), and the ribose is cleaved from the base by purine nucleoside phosphorylase. Hypoxanthine, the base produced by cleavage of IMP, is converted by xanthine oxidase to xanthine, and guanine is deaminated by the enzyme guanase to produce xanthine. The pathways for the degradation of adenine and guanine merge at this point. Xanthine is converted by xanthine oxidase to uric acid,

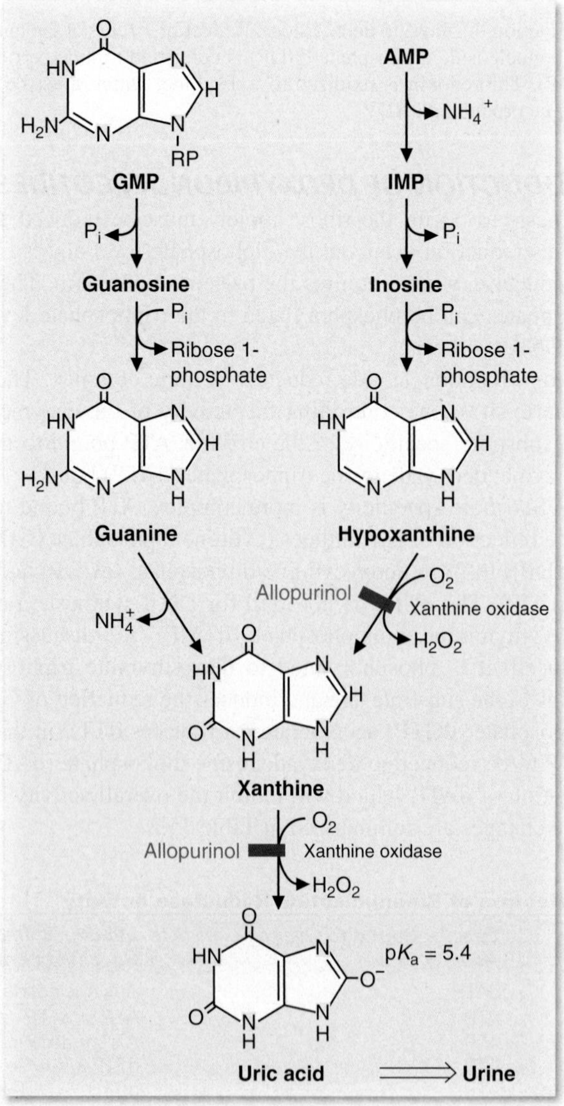

**FIG. 35.16.** Degradation of the purine bases. The reactions inhibited by allopurinol are indicated. A second form of xanthine oxidase exists that uses $NAD^+$ instead of $O_2$ as the electron acceptor.

which is excreted in the urine. Xanthine oxidase is a molybdenum-requiring enzyme that uses molecular oxygen and produces hydrogen peroxide ($H_2O_2$).

Note how little energy is derived from the degradation of the purine ring. Thus, it is to the cell's advantage to recycle and salvage the ring because it costs energy to produce and not much is obtained in return.

## B. Pyrimidine Bases

The pyrimidine nucleotides are dephosphorylated and the nucleosides are cleaved to produce ribose 1-phosphate and the free pyrimidine bases cytosine, uracil, and thymine. Cytosine is deaminated, forming uracil, which is converted to $CO_2$, ammonium ion ($NH_4^+$), and β-alanine. Thymine is converted to $CO_2$, $NH_4^+$, and β-aminoisobutyrate. These products of pyrimidine degradation are excreted in the urine or converted to $CO_2$, $H_2O$, and $NH_4^+$ (which forms urea). They do not cause any problems for the body, in contrast to urate, which is produced from the purines and can precipitate, causing gout. As with the purine degradation pathway, little energy can be generated by pyrimidine degradation.

## CLINICAL COMMENTS

Diseases discussed in this chapter are summarized in Table 35.3.

**Lotta T.** Hyperuricemia in **Lotta T.**'s case arose as a consequence of overproduction of uric acid. Treatment with allopurinol not only inhibits xanthine oxidase, lowering the formation of uric acid with an increase in the excretion of hypoxanthine and xanthine, but also decreases the overall synthesis of purine nucleotides. Hypoxanthine and xanthine produced by purine degradation are salvaged (i.e., converted to nucleotides) by a process that requires the consumption of PRPP. PRPP is a substrate for the glutamine phosphoribosyl amidotransferase reaction that initiates purine biosynthesis. Because the normal cellular levels of PRPP and glutamine are below the $K_m$ of the enzyme, changes in the level of either substrate can accelerate or reduce the rate of the reaction. Therefore, decreased levels of PRPP cause decreased synthesis of purine nucleotides.

 Normally, as cells die, their purine nucleotides are degraded to hypoxanthine and xanthine, which are converted to uric acid by xanthine oxidase (see Fig. 35.16). Allopurinol (a structural analogue of hypoxanthine) is a substrate for xanthine oxidase. It is converted to oxypurinol (also called alloxanthine), which remains tightly bound to the enzyme, preventing further catalytic activity (see Fig. 6.12). Thus, allopurinol is a suicide inhibitor. It reduces the production of uric acid and hence its concentration in the blood and tissues (e.g., the synovial lining of the joints in **Lotta T.**'s great toe). Xanthine and hypoxanthine accumulate, and urate levels decrease. Overall, the amount of purine being degraded is spread over three products rather than appearing in only one. Therefore, none of the compounds exceeds its solubility constant, precipitation does not occur, and the symptoms of gout gradually subside.

 Once nucleotide biosynthesis and salvage was understood at the pathway level, it was quickly realized that one way to inhibit cell proliferation would be to block purine or pyrimidine synthesis. Thus, drugs were developed that would interfere with a cell's ability to generate precursors for DNA synthesis, thereby inhibiting cell growth. This is particularly important for cancer cells, which have lost their normal growth-regulatory properties. Such drugs have been introduced previously with a number of different patients. **Clark T.** (Chapter 9) was treated with 5-fluorouracil, which inhibits thymidylate synthase (dUMP to TMP synthesis). **Mannie W.** (Chapter 13) was treated with hydroxyurea to block ribonucleotide reductase activity, with the goal of inhibiting DNA synthesis in the leukemic cells. Development of these drugs would not have been possible without an understanding of the biochemistry of purine and pyrimidine salvage and synthesis and DNA replication. Such drugs also affect rapidly dividing normal cells, which brings about several side effects of chemotherapeutic regimens.

**Table 35.3 Diseases Discussed in Chapter 35**

| Disease or Disorder | Environmental or Genetic | Comments |
|---|---|---|
| Gout | Both | Painful joints due to the precipation of uric acid in the blood. |
| PNP (purine nucleoside phosphorylase) deficiency | Genetic | A defect in a purine salvage enzyme, leading to a loss of T-cell function, with near-normal B-cell function and a partial immunodeficiency disease. Purine nucleosides will accumulate. |
| Lesch-Nyhan syndrome (lack of hypoxanthine–guanine phosphoribosyl transferase [HGPRT] activity) | Genetic | The loss of HGPRT activity leads to the accumulation of purines and uric acid, with intellectual disabilities and self-mutilation resulting in severe cases. Gout will also occur in these individuals. |
| Hereditary orotic aciduria | Genetic | A defect in uridine monophosphate (UMP) synthase, leading to orotic acid accumulation and growth retardation. |
| Adenosine deaminase deficiency | Genetic | The loss of adenosine deaminase activity leads to severe combined immunodeficiency disease (SCID), with a loss of both T- and B-cell function. Deoxyadenosine (dA) and derivatives of dA accumulate in the blood and blood-borne cells. |
| Cancer | Both | The use of drugs that interfere with DNA replication will destroy rapidly dividing cells at a faster rate than normal cells. |

1. Similarities between carbamoyl phosphate synthetase I and carbamoyl phosphate synthetase II include which **ONE** of the following?

    A. Carbon source
    B. Intracellular location
    C. Nitrogen source
    D. Regulation by *N*-acetyl glutamate
    E. Regulation by UMP

2. Gout can result from a reduction in activity of which one of the following enzymes?

    A. Glutamine phosphoribosyl amidotransferase
    B. Glucose-6-phosphatase
    C. Glucose-6-phosphate dehydrogenase
    D. PRPP synthetase
    E. Purine nucleoside phosphorylase

3. The regulation of ribonucleotide reductase is quite complex. Assuming that an enzyme deficiency leads to highly elevated levels of dGTP, what effect would you predict on the reduction of ribonucleotides to deoxyribonucleotides under these conditions?

    A. Elevated levels of dCDP will be produced.
    B. AMP would begin to be reduced.

    C. Reduced thioredoxin would become rate-limiting, thereby reducing the activity of ribonucleotide reductase.
    D. dGTP would bind to the overall activity site and inhibit the functioning of the enzyme.
    E. The formation of dADP will be favored.

4. Actively exercising muscle utilizes the purine nucleotide cycle to do which one of the following?

    A. Synthesize urea
    B. Synthesize glucose
    C. Synthesize glutamate
    D. Synthesize four-carbon TCA cycle intermediates
    E. Generate NADH for energy

5. DNA synthesis is impaired when individuals have a vitamin $B_{12}$ deficiency. The reason for the reduction in DNA synthesis is which one of the following?

    A. Inability to produce deoxythymidine monophosphate
    B. Inability to make deoxyribonucleotides
    C. Inhibition of PRPP synthetase
    D. Inability to produce orotic acid
    E. Inability to produce 5′-phosphoribosyl 1′-amine

# 36 Intertissue Relationships in the Metabolism of Amino Acids

## CHAPTER OUTLINE

## KEY POINTS

- The body maintains a large free amino acid pool in the blood, even during fasting, allowing tissues continuous access to these building blocks.
- Amino acids are used for gluconeogenesis by the liver, as a fuel source for the gut, and as neurotransmitter precursors in the nervous system. They are also required by all organs for protein synthesis.
- During an overnight fast, and during hypercatabolic states, degradation of labile protein (primarily from skeletal muscle) is the major source of free amino acids.
- The liver is the major site for urea synthesis. Nitrogen from other tissues travel to the liver in the form of glutamine and alanine.
- Branched-chain amino acids (BCAAs) are oxidized primarily in the skeletal muscle.
- Glutamine in the blood serves several roles:
  - The kidney utilizes the ammonium ion carried by glutamine for excretion in the urine to act as a buffer against acidotic conditions.
  - The kidney and the gut utilize glutamine as a fuel source.
  - All tissues use glutamine for protein synthesis.

continued

■ The body can enter a catabolic state characterized by negative nitrogen balance under the following conditions:
  ■ Sepsis (the presence of various pathogenic organisms or their toxins in the blood or tissues)
  ■ Trauma
  ■ Injury
  ■ Burns

■ The negative nitrogen balance results from increased net protein degradation in skeletal muscle brought about by the release of glucocorticoids. The released amino acids are used for protein synthesis and cell division in cells involved in the immune response and wound healing.

## THE WAITING ROOM

**Katherine B.**, a 62-year-old homeless woman, was found by a neighborhood child who heard Katherine's moans coming from an abandoned building. The child's mother called the police, who took Katherine to the hospital emergency room. The patient was semicomatose, incontinent of urine, and her clothes were stained with vomitus. She had a fever of 103°F, was trembling uncontrollably, appeared to be severely dehydrated, and had marked muscle wasting. Her heart rate was very rapid, and her blood pressure was low (85/46 mm Hg). Her abdomen was distended and without bowel sounds. She responded to moderate pressure on her abdomen with moaning and grimacing.

Blood was sent for a broad laboratory profile, and cultures of her urine and blood were taken. Intravenous saline with thiamine and folate, glucose, and parenteral broad-spectrum antibiotics were begun. Radiography performed after her vital signs were stabilized suggested a bowel perforation. These findings were compatible with a diagnosis of a ruptured viscus (e.g., an infected colonic diverticulum that perforated, allowing colonic bacteria to infect the tissues of the peritoneal cavity, causing peritonitis). Further studies confirmed that a diverticulum had ruptured, and appropriate surgery was performed. All of the blood cultures grew out *Escherichia coli*, indicating that Katherine also had a gram-negative infection of her blood (septicemia) that had been seeded by the proliferating organisms in her peritoneal cavity. Intensive fluid and electrolyte therapy and antibiotic coverage were continued. The medical team (surgeons, internists, and nutritionists) began developing a complex therapeutic plan to reverse Katherine's severely catabolic state.

### I. MAINTENANCE OF THE FREE AMINO ACID POOL IN BLOOD

The body maintains a relatively large free amino acid pool in the blood, even in the absence of an intake of dietary protein. The large free amino acid pool ensures the continuous availability of individual amino acids to tissues for the synthesis of proteins, neurotransmitters, and other nitrogen-containing compounds (Fig. 36.1). In a normal, well-fed, healthy individual, approximately 300 to 600 g body protein is degraded per day. At the same time, roughly 100 g of protein is consumed in the diet per day, which adds additional amino acids. From this pool, tissues use amino acids for the continuous synthesis of new proteins (300 to 600 g) to replace those degraded. The continuous turnover of proteins in the body makes the complete complement of amino acids available for the synthesis of new and different proteins, such as antibodies. Protein turnover allows shifts in the quantities of different proteins produced in tissues in response to changes in physiological state and continuously removes modified or damaged proteins. It also provides a complete

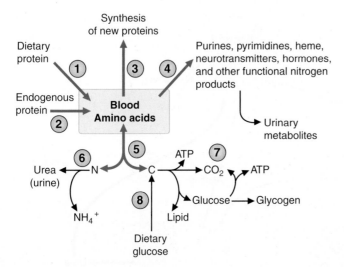

**FIG. 36.1.** Maintenance of the blood amino acid pool. Dietary protein *(1)* and degradation of endogenous protein *(2)* provide a source of essential amino acids (those that cannot be synthesized in the human). *(3)* The synthesis of new protein is the major use of amino acids from the free amino acid pool. *(4)* Compounds synthesized from amino acid precursors are essential for physiological functions. Many of these compounds are degraded to nitrogen-containing urinary metabolites and do not return to the free amino acid pool. *(5)* In tissues, the nitrogen is removed from amino acids by transamination and deamination reactions. *(6)* The nitrogen from amino acid degradation appears in the urine primarily as urea or $NH_4^+$. Ammonia excretion is necessary to maintain the pH of the blood. *(7)* Amino acids are used as fuels either directly or after being converted to glucose by gluconeogenesis. *(8)* Some amino acids can be synthesized in the human provided that glucose and a nitrogen source are available.

pool of specific amino acids that can be used as oxidizable substrates; precursors for gluconeogenesis and for heme, creatine phosphate, purine, pyrimidine, and neurotransmitter synthesis; for ammoniagenesis to maintain blood pH levels; and for numerous other functions.

### A. Interorgan Flux of Amino Acids in the Postabsorptive State

The fasting state provides an example of the interorgan flux of amino acids necessary to maintain the free amino acid pool in the blood and supply tissues with their required amino acids (Fig. 36.2). During an overnight fast, protein synthesis in the liver and other tissues continues but at a diminished rate compared with the postprandial state. Net degradation of labile protein occurs in skeletal muscle (which contains the body's largest protein mass) and other tissues.

### 1. RELEASE OF AMINO ACIDS FROM SKELETAL MUSCLE DURING FASTING

The efflux of amino acids from skeletal muscle supports the essential amino acid pool in the blood (see Fig. 36.2). Skeletal muscle oxidizes the branched-chain amino acids (BCAAs) (valine, leucine, isoleucine) to produce energy and glutamine. The amino groups of the BCAAs and of aspartate and glutamate are transferred out of skeletal muscle in alanine and glutamine. Alanine and glutamine account for approximately 50% of the total α-amino nitrogen released by skeletal muscle.

The release of amino acids from skeletal muscle is stimulated during an overnight fast by the decrease of insulin and increase of glucocorticoid (such as cortisol) levels in the blood. Insulin promotes the uptake of amino acids and the general synthesis of proteins. The fall of blood insulin levels during an overnight fast results in net proteolysis and release of amino acids. As glucocorticoid release from the adrenal cortex increases, an induction of ubiquitin synthesis and increase of ubiquitin-dependent proteolysis also occur.

 The concentration of free amino acids in the blood is not nearly as rigidly controlled as blood glucose levels. The free amino acid pool in the blood is only a small part (0.5%) of the total amino acid pool in whole body protein.

**Q:** What changes in hormone levels and fuel metabolism occur during an overnight fast?

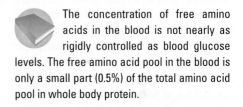 Glucocorticoids, such as cortisol, were named for their ability to raise blood glucose levels. Cortisol will stimulate lipolysis in adipocytes, proteolysis in muscles, and gluconeogenesis in the liver.

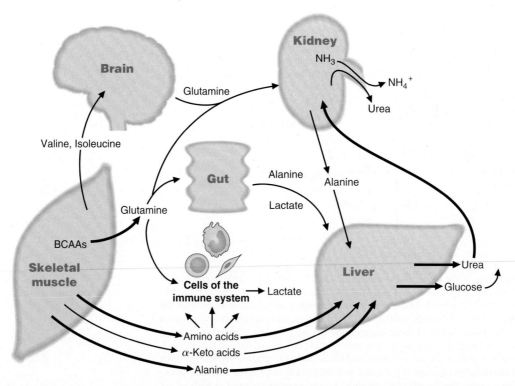

**FIG. 36.2.** Interorgan amino acid exchange after an overnight fast. After an overnight fast (the postabsorptive state), the use of amino acids for protein synthesis, for fuels, and for the synthesis of essential functional compounds continues. The free amino acid pool is supported largely by net degradation of skeletal muscle protein. Glutamine and alanine serve as amino group carriers from skeletal muscle to other tissues. Glutamine brings $NH_4^+$ to the kidney for the excretion of protons and serves as a fuel for the kidney, gut, and cells of the immune system. Alanine transfers amino groups from skeletal muscle, the kidney, and the gut to the liver, where they are converted to urea for excretion. The brain continues to use amino acids for neurotransmitter synthesis.

 The hormonal changes that occur during an overnight fast include a decrease of blood insulin levels and an increase of glucagon relative to levels after a high-carbohydrate meal. Glucocorticoid levels also increase in the blood. These hormones coordinate the changes of fat, carbohydrate, and amino acid metabolism. Fatty acids are released from adipose triacylglycerols and are used as the major fuel by heart, skeletal muscle, liver, and other tissues. The liver converts some of the fatty acids to ketone bodies. Liver glycogen stores are diminished and gluconeogenesis becomes the major support of blood glucose levels for glucose-dependent tissues. The major precursors of gluconeogenesis include amino acids released from skeletal muscle, lactate, and glycerol.

## 2. AMINO ACID METABOLISM IN LIVER DURING FASTING

The major site of alanine uptake is the liver, which disposes of the amino nitrogen by incorporating it into urea (see Fig. 36.2). The liver also extracts free amino acids, α-keto acids, and some glutamine from the blood. Alanine and other amino acids are oxidized and their carbon skeletons converted principally to glucose. Glucagon and glucocorticoids stimulate the uptake of amino acids into liver and increase gluconeogenesis and ureagenesis (Fig. 36.3). Alanine transport into the liver, in particular, is

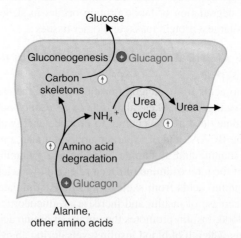

**FIG. 36.3.** Hormonal regulation of hepatic amino acid metabolism in the postabsorptive state. Induction of urea cycle enzymes occurs both during fasting and after a high-protein meal. Because many individuals in the United States normally have a high-protein diet, the levels of urea cycle enzymes may not fluctuate to any great extent. ⊕, glucagon-mediated activation of enzymes or proteins; ⇡, induction of enzyme synthesis mediated by glucagon and glucocorticoids.

enhanced by glucagon. The induction of the synthesis of gluconeogenic enzymes by glucagon and glucocorticoids during the overnight fast correlates with an induction of many of the enzymes of amino acid degradation and an induction of urea cycle enzymes (see Chapter 32). Urea synthesis also increases because of the increased supply of ammonium ions ($NH_4^+$) from amino acid degradation in the liver.

## 3. METABOLISM OF AMINO ACIDS IN OTHER TISSUES DURING FASTING

Glucose, produced by the liver, is used for energy by the brain and other glucose-dependent tissues, such as erythrocytes. The muscle, under conditions of exercise, when the adenosine monophosphate (AMP)-activated protein kinase is active, also oxidizes some of this glucose to pyruvate, which is used for the carbon skeleton of alanine (the glucose–alanine cycle; see Chapter 32).

Glutamine is generated in skeletal muscle from the oxidation of BCAAs and by the lungs and brain for the removal of $NH_4^+$ formed from amino acid catabolism or entering from the blood. The kidney, the gut, and cells with rapid turnover rates such as those of the immune system, are the major sites of glutamine uptake (see Fig. 36.2). Glutamine serves as a fuel for these tissues, as a nitrogen donor for purine synthesis, and as a substrate for ammoniagenesis in the kidney. Much of the unused nitrogen from glutamine is transferred to pyruvate to form alanine in these tissues. Alanine then carries the unused nitrogen back to the liver.

The brain is glucose dependent, but like many cells in the body, can use BCAAs for energy. The BCAAs also provide a source of nitrogen for neurotransmitter synthesis during fasting. Other amino acids released from skeletal muscle protein degradation also serve as precursors of neurotransmitters.

## B. Principles Governing Amino Acid Flux between Tissues

The pattern of interorgan flux of amino acids is strongly affected by conditions that change the supply of fuels (e.g., the overnight fast, a mixed meal, a high-protein meal) and by conditions that increase the demand for amino acids (metabolic acidosis, surgical stress, traumatic injury, burns, wound healing, and sepsis). The flux of amino acid carbon and nitrogen in these different conditions is dictated by several considerations:

1. Ammonia ($NH_3$) is toxic. Consequently, it is transported between tissues as alanine or glutamine. Alanine is the principal carrier of amino acid nitrogen from other tissues back to the liver, where the nitrogen is converted to urea and subsequently excreted into the urine by the kidneys. The amount of urea synthesized is proportional to the amount of amino acid carbon that is being oxidized as a fuel.

   The differences in amino acid metabolism between tissues are dictated by the types and amounts of different enzyme and transport proteins present in each tissue and the ability of each tissue to respond to different regulatory messages (hormones and neural signals).

2. The pool of glutamine in the blood serves several essential metabolic functions (Table 36.1). It provides ammonia for excretion of protons in the urine as $NH_4^+$. It serves as a fuel for the gut, the kidney, and the cells of the immune system. Glutamine is also required by the cells of the immune system and other rapidly dividing cells in which its amide group serves as the source of nitrogen for biosynthetic reactions. In the brain, the formation of glutamine from glutamate and $NH_4^+$ provides a means of removing ammonia and of transporting glutamate between different cell types within the brain. The utilization of the blood glutamine pool is prioritized. During metabolic acidosis, the kidney becomes the predominant site of glutamine uptake, at the expense of glutamine utilization in other tissues. Conversely, during sepsis, in the absence of acidosis, cells involved in the immune response (macrophages, hepatocytes) become the preferential sites of glutamine uptake.

3. The BCAAs (valine, leucine, and isoleucine) form a significant portion of the composition of the average protein and can be converted to tricarboxylic acid

**Katherine B.** was in a severe stage of negative nitrogen balance (see Chapter 1, Section VII.C.2) on admission, which was caused by both her malnourished state and her intra-abdominal infection complicated by sepsis. The physiological response to advanced catabolic status includes a degradation of muscle protein with the release of amino acids into the blood. This release is coupled with an increased uptake of amino acids for acute-phase protein synthesis by the liver (systemic response) and other cells involved in the immune response to general and severe infection.

**Table 36.1   Functions of Glutamine**

Protein synthesis
Ammonia genesis for proton excretion
Nitrogen donor for synthesis of
    Purines
    Pyrimidines
    $NAD^+$
    Amino sugars
    Asparagine
    Other compounds
Glutamate donor for synthesis of
    Glutathione
    γ-Aminobutyric acid (GABA)
    Ornithine
    Arginine
    Proline
    Other compounds

(TCA) cycle intermediates and used as fuels by almost all tissues. Valine and isoleucine are also the major precursors of glutamine. Except for the BCAAs and alanine, aspartate, and glutamate, the catabolism of amino acids occurs principally in the liver.

The ability to convert four-carbon intermediates of the TCA cycle to pyruvate is required for oxidation of both BCAAs and glutamine. This sequence of reactions requires phosphoenolpyruvate (PEP) carboxykinase or decarboxylating malate dehydrogenase (malic enzyme). Most tissues have one, or both, of these enzymes.

4. Amino acids are major gluconeogenic substrates, and most of the energy obtained from their oxidation is derived from oxidation of the glucose formed from their carbon skeletons. A much smaller percentage of amino acid carbon is converted to acetyl coenzyme A (CoA) or to ketone bodies and oxidized. The use of amino acids for glucose synthesis for the brain and other glucose-requiring tissues is subject to the hormonal regulatory mechanisms of glucose homeostasis (see Chapters 21 and 26).

5. The relative rates of protein synthesis and degradation (protein turnover) determine the size of the free amino acid pools available for the synthesis of new proteins and for other essential functions. For example, the synthesis of new proteins to mount an immune response is supported by the net degradation of other proteins in the body.

## II.  UTILIZATION OF AMINO ACIDS IN INDIVIDUAL TISSUES

Because tissues differ in their physiological functions, they have different amino acid requirements and contribute differently to whole body nitrogen metabolism. However, all tissues share a common requirement for essential amino acids for protein synthesis, and protein turnover is an ongoing process in all cells.

### A.  Kidney

One of the primary roles of amino acid nitrogen is to provide ammonia in the kidney for the excretion of protons in the urine. $NH_4^+$ is released from glutamine by glutaminase and from glutamate by glutamate dehydrogenase, resulting in the formation of α-ketoglutarate (Fig. 36.4). α-Ketoglutarate is used as a fuel by the kidney and is oxidized to carbon dioxide ($CO_2$), converted to glucose for use in cells in the renal medulla, or converted to alanine to return ammonia to the liver for urea synthesis.

Glutamine is used as a fuel by the kidney in the normal fed state and, to a greater extent, during fasting and metabolic acidosis. The carbon skeleton forms α-ketoglutarate, which is oxidized to $CO_2$, converted to glucose, or released as the carbon skeleton of serine or alanine (Fig. 36.5). α-Ketoglutarate can be converted to oxaloacetate by TCA cycle reactions, and oxaloacetate is converted to PEP by PEP carboxykinase. PEP can then be converted to pyruvate and subsequently acetyl CoA, alanine, serine, or glucose. The glucose is used principally by the cells of the renal medulla, which have a relatively high dependence on anaerobic glycolysis because of their lower oxygen supply and mitochondrial capacity. The lactate released from anaerobic glycolysis in these cells is taken up and oxidized in the renal cortical cells, which have a higher mitochondrial capacity and a greater blood supply.

### B.  Skeletal Muscle

Skeletal muscle, because of its large mass, is a major site of protein synthesis and degradation in the human. After a high-protein meal, insulin promotes the uptake of certain amino acids and stimulates net protein synthesis. The insulin stimulation of protein synthesis is dependent on an adequate supply of amino acids to undergo protein synthesis. During fasting and other catabolic states, a net degradation of skeletal muscle protein and release of amino acids occur (see Fig. 36.2). The net degradation of protein affects functional proteins, such as myosin, which are sacrificed to meet more urgent demands for amino acids in other tissues. During sepsis, degradation of skeletal muscle protein is stimulated by the glucocorticoid cortisol. The effect of

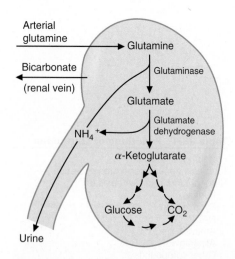

**FIG. 36.4.** Renal glutamine metabolism. Renal tubule cells preferentially oxidize glutamine. During metabolic acidosis, it is the major fuel for the kidney. Conversion of glutamine to α-ketoglutarate generates $NH_4^+$. $NH_4^+$ excretion helps to buffer systemic acidemia.

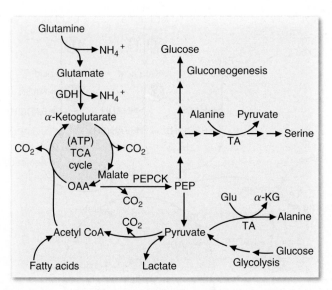

***FIG. 36.5.*** Metabolism of glutamine and other fuels in the kidney. To completely oxidize glutamate carbon to $CO_2$, it must enter the TCA cycle as acetyl CoA. Carbon entering the TCA cycle as α-ketoglutarate (α-KG) exits as oxaloacetate and is converted to PEP by PEP carboxykinase. PEP is converted to pyruvate, which may be oxidized to acetyl CoA. PEP can also be converted to serine, glucose, or alanine. *GDH,* glutamate dehydrogenase; *OAA,* oxaloacetate; *PEPCK,* phosphoenolpyruvate carboxykinase; *TA,* transaminase.

cortisol is exerted through the activation of ubiquitin-dependent proteolysis. During fasting, the decrease of blood insulin levels and the increase of blood cortisol levels increase net protein degradation.

Skeletal muscle is a major site of glutamine synthesis, thereby satisfying the demand for glutamine during the postabsorptive state, during metabolic acidosis, and during septic stress and trauma. The carbon skeleton and nitrogen of glutamine are derived principally from the metabolism of BCAAs. Amino acid degradation in skeletal muscle is also accompanied by the formation of alanine, which transfers amino groups from skeletal muscle to the liver in the glucose–alanine cycle.

## 1. OXIDATION OF BRANCHED-CHAIN AMINO ACIDS IN SKELETAL MUSCLE

The BCAAs play a special role in muscle and most other tissues because they are the major amino acids that can be oxidized in tissues other than the liver. However, all tissues can interconvert amino acids and TCA cycle intermediates through transaminase reactions, that is, alanine ↔ pyruvate, aspartate ↔ oxaloacetate, and α-ketoglutarate ↔ glutamate. The first step of the pathway, transamination of the BCAAs to α-keto acids, occurs principally in brain, heart, kidney, and skeletal muscles. These tissues have a high content of BCAAs transaminase relative to the low levels in liver. The α-keto acids of the BCAAs are then either released into the blood and taken up by liver or oxidized to $CO_2$ or glutamine within the muscle or other tissue (Fig. 36.6). They can be oxidized by all tissues that contain mitochondria.

The oxidative pathways of the BCAAs convert the carbon skeleton to either succinyl CoA or acetyl CoA (see Chapter 33 and Fig. 36.6). The pathways generate nicotinamide adenine dinucleotide (NADH) and flavin adenine dinucleotide (FAD[2H]) for adenosine triphosphate (ATP) synthesis before the conversion of carbon into intermediates of the TCA cycle, thus providing the muscle with energy without loss of carbon as $CO_2$. Leucine is "ketogenic" in that it is converted to acetyl CoA and acetoacetate. Skeletal muscle, adipocytes, and most other tissues are able to use these products and, therefore, oxidize leucine directly to $CO_2$. The portion of isoleucine that is converted to acetyl CoA is also oxidized directly to $CO_2$. For the portion of

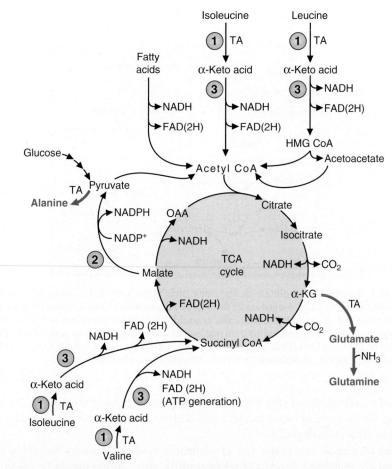

*FIG. 36.6.* Metabolism of the carbon skeletons of BCAAs in skeletal muscle. *(1)* The first step in the metabolism of BCAAs is transamination (TA). *(2)* Carbon from valine and isoleucine enters the TCA cycle as succinyl CoA and is converted to pyruvate by malic enzyme. *(3)* The oxidative pathways generate NADH and FAD(2H) even before the carbon skeleton enters the TCA cycle. The rate-limiting enzyme in the oxidative pathways is the α-keto acid dehydrogenase complex. The carbon skeleton also can be converted to glutamate and alanine, shown in *red*.

valine and isoleucine that enters the TCA cycle as succinyl CoA to be completely oxidized to $CO_2$, it must first be converted to acetyl CoA. To form acetyl CoA, succinyl CoA is oxidized to malate in the TCA cycle, and malate is then converted to pyruvate by malic enzyme (malate + $NADP^+$ → pyruvate + NADPH + $H^+$) (see Fig. 36.6). Pyruvate can then be oxidized to acetyl CoA. Alternatively, pyruvate can form alanine or lactate.

## 2. CONVERSION OF BRANCHED-CHAIN AMINO ACIDS TO GLUTAMINE

The major route of valine and isoleucine catabolism in skeletal muscle is to enter the TCA cycle as succinyl CoA and exit as α-ketoglutarate to provide the carbon skeleton for glutamine formation (see Fig. 36.6). Some of the glutamine and $CO_2$ that is formed from net protein degradation in skeletal muscle may also arise from the carbon skeletons of aspartate and glutamate. These amino acids are transaminated and become part of the pool of four-carbon intermediates of the TCA cycle.

Glutamine nitrogen is derived principally from the BCAAs (Fig. 36.7). The α-amino group arises from transamination reactions that form glutamate from α-ketoglutarate, and the amide nitrogen is formed from the addition of free ammonia to glutamate by glutamine synthetase. Free ammonia in skeletal muscle arises

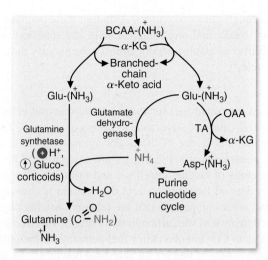

**FIG. 36.7.** Formation of glutamine from the amino groups of BCAAs. The BCAAs are first transaminated with α-ketoglutarate to form glutamate and the branched-chain α-keto acids. The glutamate nitrogen can then follow either of two paths leading to glutamine formation. *α-KG,* α-ketoglutarate; *OAA,* oxaloacetate; *TA,* transamination.

principally from the deamination of glutamate by glutamate dehydrogenase or from the purine nucleotide cycle.

In the purine nucleotide cycle (Fig. 36.8), the deamination of AMP to inosine monophosphate (IMP) releases $NH_4^+$. AMP is resynthesized with amino groups provided from aspartate. The aspartate amino groups can arise from the BCAAs through transamination reactions. The fumarate can be used to replenish TCA cycle intermediates.

## 3. GLUCOSE–ALANINE CYCLE

The nitrogen arising from the oxidation of BCAAs in skeletal muscle can also be transferred back to the liver as alanine in the glucose–alanine cycle (Fig. 36.9). The amino group of the BCAAs is first transferred to α-ketoglutarate to form glutamate and then transferred to pyruvate to form alanine by sequential transamination reactions. The pyruvate arises principally from glucose via the glycolytic pathway. The alanine released from skeletal muscle is taken up principally by the liver, where the amino group is incorporated into urea, and the carbon skeleton can be converted

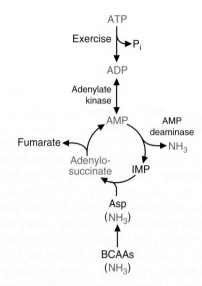

**FIG. 36.8.** Purine nucleotide cycle. In skeletal muscle, the purine nucleotide cycle can convert the amino groups of the BCAAs to $NH_3$, which is incorporated into glutamine. Compare this to Figure 35.11, in which the fumarate generated is used in an anaplerotic role in muscle.

The purine nucleotide cycle is found in skeletal muscle and brain but is absent in the liver and many other tissues. One of its functions in skeletal muscle is to respond to the rapid utilization of ATP during exercise. During exercise, the rapid hydrolysis of ATP increases AMP levels, resulting in an activation of AMP deaminase (see Fig. 36.8). As a consequence, the cellular concentration of IMP increases and ammonia is generated. IMP, like AMP, activates muscle glycogen phosphorylase during exercise (see Chapter 23). The ammonia that is generated may help to buffer the increased lactic acid production occurring in skeletal muscles during strenuous exercise.

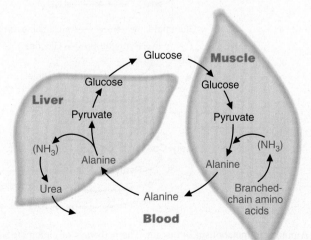

**FIG. 36.9.** Glucose–alanine cycle. The pathway for transfer of the amino groups from BCAAs in skeletal muscle to urea in the liver is shown in *red.*

back to glucose through gluconeogenesis. Although the amount of alanine formed varies with dietary intake and physiological state, the transport of nitrogen from skeletal muscle to liver as alanine occurs almost continuously throughout our daily fasting–feeding cycle.

### C. Gut

Amino acids are an important fuel for the intestinal mucosal cells after a protein-containing meal and in catabolic states such as fasting or surgical trauma (Fig. 36.10). During fasting, glutamine is one of the major amino acids used by the gut. The principal fates of glutamine carbon in the gut are oxidation to $CO_2$ and conversion to the carbon skeletons of lactate, citrulline, and ornithine. The gut also oxidizes BCAAs. Nitrogen derived from amino acid degradation is converted to citrulline, alanine, $NH_4^+$, and other compounds that are released into the blood and taken up by the liver. Although most of the carbon in this alanine is derived from glucose, the oxidation of glucose to $CO_2$ is not a major fuel pathway for the gut. Fatty acids are also not a significant source of fuel for the intestinal mucosal cells, although they do use ketone bodies.

After a protein meal, dietary glutamine is a major fuel for the gut, and the products of glutamine metabolism are similar to those seen in the postabsorptive state. The gut also uses dietary aspartate and glutamate, which enter the TCA cycle. Colonocytes (the cells of the colon) also use short-chain fatty acids, derived from bacterial action in the lumen.

The importance of the gut in whole body nitrogen metabolism arises from the high rate of division and death of intestinal mucosal cells and the need to continuously provide these cells with amino acids to sustain the high rates of protein synthesis required for cellular division. Not only are these cells important for the uptake of nutrients, they maintain a barrier against invading bacteria from the gut lumen and are, therefore, part of our passive defense system. As a result of these important functions, the intestinal mucosal cells are supplied with the amino acids required

Even though the liver is the organ that generates urea, the intestine also contains the enzymes for the urea cycle, including carbamoyl-phosphate synthetase I. However, within the intestine, the maximum velocity ($V_{max}$) for argininosuccinate synthetase and argininosuccinate lyase are very low, suggesting that the primary role of the urea cycle enzymes in the gut is to produce citrulline from the carbons of glutamine (glutamine → glutamate → glutamate semialdehyde → ornithine → citrulline). The citrulline is released in the circulation for use by the liver.

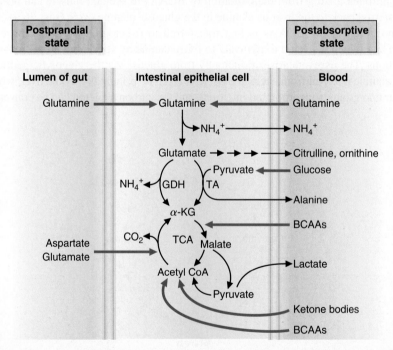

**FIG. 36.10.** Amino acid metabolism in the gut. The pathways of glutamine metabolism in the gut are the same whether it is supplied by the diet (postprandial state) or from the blood (postabsorptive state). Cells of the gut also metabolize aspartate, glutamate, and BCAAs. Glucose is converted principally to the carbon skeleton of alanine. α-*KG*, α-ketoglutarate; *GDH*, glutamate dehydrogenase; *TA*, transaminase.

for protein synthesis and fuel oxidation at the expense of the more expendable skeletal muscle protein. However, glutamine use by the gut is diminished by metabolic acidosis compared with the postabsorptive or postprandial state. During metabolic acidosis, the uptake of glutamine by the kidney is increased and blood glucose levels decrease. As a consequence, the gut takes up less glutamine.

## D.  Liver

The liver is the major site of amino acid metabolism. It is the major site of amino acid catabolism and converts most of the carbon in amino acids to intermediates of the TCA cycle or the glycolytic pathway (which can be converted to glucose or oxidized to $CO_2$) or to acetyl CoA and ketone bodies. The liver is also the major site for urea synthesis. It can take up both glutamine and alanine and convert the nitrogen to urea for disposal (see Chapter 32). Other pathways in the liver give it an unusually high amino acid requirement. The liver synthesizes plasma proteins, such as serum albumin, transferrin, and the proteins of the blood coagulation cascade. It is a major site for the synthesis of nonessential amino acids, the conjugation of xenobiotic compounds with glycine, the synthesis of heme and purine nucleotides, and the synthesis of glutathione.

## E.  Brain and Nervous Tissue

### 1.  AMINO ACID POOL AND NEUROTRANSMITTER SYNTHESIS

A major function of amino acid metabolism in neural tissue is the synthesis of neurotransmitters (see Chapter 33). More than 40 compounds are believed to function as neurotransmitters, and all of these contain nitrogen derived from precursor amino acids. They include amino acids, which are themselves neurotransmitters (e.g., glutamate, glycine), the catecholamines derived from tyrosine (dopamine, norepinephrine, epinephrine), serotonin (derived from tryptophan), γ-aminobutyric acid (GABA, derived from glutamate), acetylcholine (derived from choline and acetyl CoA), and many peptides. The rapid metabolism of neurotransmitters requires the continuous availability of a precursor pool of amino acids for de novo neurotransmitter synthesis.

### 2.  METABOLISM OF GLUTAMINE IN THE BRAIN

The brain is a net glutamine producer owing principally to the presence of glutamine synthetase in astroglial cells, a supporting cell type of the brain. Glutamate and aspartate are synthesized in these cells, using amino groups donated by the BCAAs (principally valine) and TCA cycle intermediates formed from glucose and from the carbon skeletons of BCAAs (Fig. 36.11). The glutamate is converted to glutamine by glutamine synthetase, which incorporates $NH_4^+$ released from deamination of amino acids and deamination of AMP in the purine nucleotide cycle in the brain.

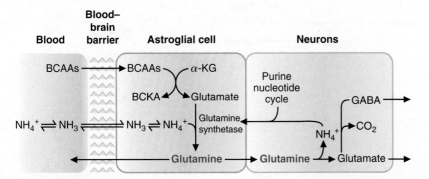

*FIG. 36.11.* Role of glutamine in the brain. Glutamine serves as a nitrogen transporter in the brain for the synthesis of many different neurotransmitters. Different neurons convert glutamine to GABA or to glutamate. Glutamine also transports excess $NH_4^+$ from the brain into the blood. *BCKA*, branched-chain α-keto acids; *α-KG*, α-ketoglutarate.

During hyperammonemia, ammonia ($NH_3$) can diffuse into the brain from the blood. The ammonia is able to inhibit the neural isozyme of glutaminase, thereby decreasing additional ammonia formation in the brain and inhibiting the formation of glutamate and its subsequent metabolism to GABA. This effect of ammonia might contribute to the lethargy associated with the hyperammonemia found in patients with hepatic disease.

This glutamine may efflux from the brain, carrying excess $NH_4^+$ into the blood, or serve as a precursor of glutamate in neuronal cells.

Glutamine synthesized in the astroglial cells is a precursor of glutamate (an excitatory neurotransmitter) and GABA (an inhibitory neurotransmitter) in the neuronal cells (see Fig. 36.11). It is converted to glutamate by a neuronal glutaminase isozyme. In GABA-ergic neurons, glutamate is then decarboxylated to GABA, which is released during excitation of the neuron. GABA is one of the neurotransmitters that is recycled; a transaminase converts it to succinaldehyde, which is then oxidized to succinate. Succinate enters the TCA cycle.

## III. CHANGES IN AMINO ACID METABOLISM WITH DIETARY AND PHYSIOLOGICAL STATE

The rate and pattern of amino acid utilization by different tissues change with dietary and physiological state. Two such states, the postprandial period following a high-protein meal and the hypercatabolic state produced by sepsis or surgical trauma, differ from the postabsorptive state with respect to the availability of amino acids and other fuels and the levels of different hormones in the blood. As a result, the pattern of amino acid use is somewhat different.

### A. High-Protein Meal

After the ingestion of a high-protein meal, the gut and the liver use most of the absorbed amino acids (Fig. 36.12). Glutamate and aspartate are used as fuels by the gut and very little enters the portal vein. The gut may also use some BCAAs. The liver takes up 60% to 70% of the amino acids present in the portal vein. These amino acids, for the most part, are converted to glucose in the gluconeogenic pathway.

After a pure protein meal, the increased levels of dietary amino acids reaching the pancreas stimulate the release of glucagon above fasting levels, thereby increasing amino acid uptake into liver and stimulating gluconeogenesis. Insulin release is also stimulated but not nearly to the levels found after a high-carbohydrate meal. In general, the insulin released after a high-protein meal is sufficiently high that the

**Q:** In what ways does liver metabolism after a high-protein meal resemble liver metabolism in the fasting state?

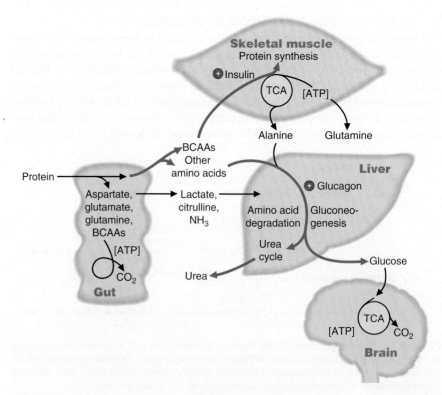

FIG. 36.12. Flux of amino acids after a high-protein meal.

uptake of BCAAs into skeletal muscle and net protein synthesis is stimulated, but gluconeogenesis in the liver is not inhibited. The higher the carbohydrate content of the meal, the higher the insulin/glucagon ratio and the greater the shift of amino acids away from gluconeogenesis into biosynthetic pathways in the liver such as the synthesis of plasma proteins.

Most of the amino acid nitrogen entering the peripheral circulation after a high-protein meal or a mixed meal is present as the BCAAs. Because the liver has low levels of transaminases for these amino acids, it cannot oxidize them to a significant extent, and they enter the systemic circulation. The BCAAs are slowly taken up by skeletal muscle and other tissues. These peripheral nonhepatic tissues use the amino acids derived from the diet principally for net protein synthesis.

## B. Hypercatabolic States

Surgery, trauma, burns, and septic stress are examples of hypercatabolic states characterized by increased fuel use and a negative nitrogen balance. The mobilization of body protein, fat, and carbohydrate stores serves to maintain normal tissue function in the presence of a limited dietary intake as well as to support the energy and amino acid requirements for the immune response and wound healing. The negative nitrogen balance that occurs in these hypercatabolic states results from an accelerated protein turnover and an increased rate of net protein degradation, primarily in skeletal muscle.

The catabolic state of sepsis (acute, generalized, febrile infection) is one of enhanced mobilization of fuels and amino acids to provide the energy and precursors required by cells of the immune system, host defense mechanisms, and wound healing. The amino acids must provide the substrates for new protein synthesis and cell division. Glucose synthesis and release are enhanced to provide fuel for these cells, and the patient may become mildly hyperglycemic.

In these hypercatabolic states, skeletal muscle protein synthesis decreases and protein degradation increases. Oxidation of BCAAs is increased and glutamine production enhanced. Amino acid uptake is diminished. Cortisol is the major hormonal mediator of these responses, although certain cytokines may also have direct effects on skeletal muscle metabolism. As occurs during fasting and metabolic acidosis, increased levels of cortisol stimulate ubiquitin-mediated proteolysis, induce the synthesis of glutamine synthetase, and enhance release of amino acids and glutamine from the muscle cells.

The amino acids released from skeletal muscle during periods of hypercatabolic stress are used in a prioritized manner, with the cellular components of the immune system receiving top priority. For example, the uptake of amino acids by the liver for the synthesis of acute-phase proteins, which are part of the immune system, is greatly increased. Conversely, during the early phase of the acute response, the synthesis of other plasma proteins (e.g., albumin) is decreased. The increased availability of amino acids and the increased cortisol levels also stimulate gluconeogenesis, thereby providing fuel for the glucose-dependent cells of the immune system (e.g., lymphocytes). An increase of urea synthesis accompanies the acceleration of amino acid degradation.

The increased efflux of glutamine from skeletal muscle during sepsis serves several functions. It provides the rapidly dividing cells of the immune system with an energy source. Glutamine is available as a nitrogen donor for purine synthesis, for oxidized nicotinamide adenine dinucleotide ($NAD^+$) synthesis (to convert nicotinic acid to nicotinamide), and for other biosynthetic functions that are essential to growth and division of the cells. Increased production of metabolic acids may accompany stress such as sepsis, so there is an increased use of glutamine by the kidney.

Under the influence of elevated levels of glucocorticoids, epinephrine, and glucagon, fatty acids are mobilized from adipose tissue to provide alternate fuels for other tissues and spare glucose. Under these conditions, fatty acids are the major energy source for skeletal muscle, and glucose uptake is decreased. These changes may lead to a mild hyperglycemia.

High-protein, low-carbohydrate diets are based on the premise that ingesting high-protein, low-carbohydrate meals will keep circulating insulin levels low so that energy storage is not induced, and glucagon release will point the insulin/glucagon ratio to energy mobilization, particularly fatty acid release from the adipocyte and oxidation by the tissues. The lack of energy storage coupled with the loss of fat leads to weight loss.

The degree of the body's hypercatabolic response depends on the severity and duration of the trauma or stress. After an uncomplicated surgical procedure in an otherwise healthy patient, the net negative nitrogen balance may be limited to about 1 week. The mild nitrogen losses are usually reversed by dietary protein supplementation as the patient recovers. With more severe traumatic injury or septic stress, the body may catabolize body protein and adipose tissue lipids for a prolonged period, and the negative nitrogen balance may not be corrected for weeks.

**Katherine B.**'s severe negative nitrogen balance was caused by both her malnourished state and her intra-abdominal infection complicated by sepsis. The systemic and diverse responses the body makes to insults such as an acute febrile illness are termed the acute-phase response. An early event in this response is the stimulation of phagocytic activity. Stimulated macrophages release cytokines, which are regulatory proteins that stimulate the release of cortisol, insulin, and growth hormone. Cytokines also directly mediate the acute-phase response of the liver and skeletal muscle to sepsis.

**A:** Both of these dietary states are characterized by an elevation of glucagon. Glucagon stimulates amino acid transport into the liver; stimulates gluconeogenesis through decreasing levels of fructose 2,6-bisphosphate; and induces the synthesis of enzymes in the urea cycle, the gluconeogenic pathway, and the pathways for degradation of some of the amino acids.

**Table 36.2 Diseases Discussed in Chapter 36**

| Disease or Disorder | Environmental of Genetic | Comments |
| --- | --- | --- |
| Catabolic state | Environmental | The body adapts to a catabolic state by degrading proteins to enhance survival. This change in metabolism is initiated through the stress response, as mediated by cortisol, epinephrine, and norepinephrine, amongst other signaling molecules. |
| Hyperammonemia | Both | Hyperammonemia can result from mutations in urea cycle enzymes or due to a failing liver as caused by a variety of conditions (one of which is alcohol abuse over many years). |

## CLINICAL COMMENTS

Diseases discussed in this chapter are summarized in Table 36.2.

 **Katherine B.** The clinician can determine whether a patient such as **Katherine B.** is mounting an acute-phase response to some insult, however subtle, by determining whether several unique acute-phase proteins are being secreted by the liver. C-reactive protein, so named because of its ability to interact with the C-polysaccharide of pneumococci, and serum amyloid A protein, a precursor of the amyloid fibril found in secondary amyloidosis, are elevated in patients undergoing the acute-phase response as compared with healthy individuals. Other proteins normally found in the blood of healthy individuals are present in increased concentrations in patients undergoing an acute-phase response. These include haptoglobin, certain protease inhibitors, complement components, ceruloplasmin, and fibrinogen. The elevated concentration of these proteins in the blood increases the erythrocyte sedimentation rate (ESR), another laboratory measure of the presence of an acute-phase response.

The weight loss often noted in septic patients is caused primarily by a loss of appetite resulting from the effect of certain cytokines on the medullary appetite center. Other causes include increased energy expenditure from fever and enhanced muscle proteolysis.

## REVIEW QUESTIONS-CHAPTER 36

1. Which one of the profiles indicated below would occur within 2 hours after eating a meal very high in protein and low in carbohydrates?

| | Blood Glucagon Levels | Liver Gluconeogenesis | BCAA Oxidation in Muscle |
| --- | --- | --- | --- |
| A. | ↓ | ↓ | ↑ |
| B. | ↑ | ↓ | ↑ |
| C. | ↓ | ↑ | ↑ |
| D. | ↑ | ↑ | ↑ |
| E. | ↓ | ↓ | ↓ |
| F. | ↑ | ↓ | ↓ |
| G. | ↓ | ↑ | ↓ |
| H. | ↑ | ↑ | ↓ |

2. The gut utilizes glutamine as an energy source, but can also secrete citrulline, synthesized from the carbons of glutamine. Which one of the following compounds is an obligatory intermediate in this conversion (consider only the carbon atoms of glutamine while answering this question)?

A. Glutamate
B. Aspartate
C. Succinyl CoA
D. Serine
E. Fumarate

3. The start of protein degradation in muscle is initiated by which one of the following signals?

    A. Glucagon
    B. Insulin
    C. Cortisol
    D. Epinephrine
    E. Glucose

4. The skeletal muscles convert branched-chain amino acid (BCAA) carbons to glutamine for export to the rest of the body. An obligatory intermediate, which carries carbons originally from the BCAAs, in the conversion of BCAAs to glutamine, is which one of the following?

    A. Pyruvate
    B. Isocitrate

C. Urea
D. Phosphoenolpyruvate
E. Lactate

5. An individual in sepsis would display which one of the following metabolic patterns?

| | Nitrogen Balance | Gluconeogenesis | Fatty Acid Oxidation |
|---|---|---|---|
| A. | Positive | ↑ | ↓ |
| B. | Negative | ↑ | ↑ |
| C. | Positive | ↑ | ↓ |
| D. | Negative | ↑ | ↓ |
| E. | Positive | ↓ | ↑ |
| F. | Negative | ↓ | ↓ |

# Answers to Review Questions

## CHAPTER 1

1. **The answer is D.** Although fuels can be stored as triacylglycerols when food consumption is high, this does not occur during respiration. Respiration is a catabolic pathway (fuels are degraded) as opposed to an anabolic pathway (e.g., synthesis of triacylglycerol). In the process of respiration, oxygen is consumed and fuels are oxidized to $CO_2$ and $H_2O$. The energy from the oxidation reactions is used to generate ATP from ADP and $P_i$. A small amount of energy is also released as heat, but it is a minor amount.

2. **The answer is A.** The resting metabolic rate (RMR) is the calories being expended by a recently awakened resting person who has fasted 12 to 18 hours and is at 20°C. It is equivalent to the energy expenditure of our major organs and resting skeletal muscle. Women generally have a lower RMR per kilogram of body weight because usually more of their body weight is metabolically inactive adipose tissue. Children have a higher RMR per kilogram of body weight because more of their body weight is metabolically active organs such as brain. The RMR increases in a cold environment because more energy is being expended to generate heat. The RMR is not equivalent to our daily energy expenditure, which includes RMR, physical activity, and diet-induced thermogenesis.

3. **The answer is E.** After a high-carbohydrate meal, glucose is the major fuel used for most tissues, including skeletal muscle and adipose tissue. The increase in blood glucose levels stimulates the release of insulin, not glucagon. Insulin stimulates the transport of glucose in skeletal muscle and adipose tissue but not the brain. Liver, not skeletal muscle, converts glucose to fatty acids. Although the red blood cell uses glucose as its only fuel at all times, it generates ATP from conversion of glucose to lactate, not $CO_2$.

4. **The answer is B.** Liver glycogen levels are only sufficient to release glucose for 24 to 30 hours after the initiation of a fast. Once liver glycogen is depleted, the only means the liver has to replenish blood glucose levels is through gluconeogenesis. Muscle glycogenolysis does not provide glucose for the circulation, as the muscle lacks a key enzyme (glucose-6-phosphatase) needed to convert glucose-6-phosphate to free glucose. The muscle, therefore, only uses muscle glycogen when the muscle needs to do work. The muscle also cannot convert amino acid carbon to free glucose due to the lack of the key enzyme referenced earlier. Fatty acid carbons produce acetyl CoA, which cannot be used to synthesize net glucose. Ketone bodies, when metabolized, also produce acetyl CoA, which cannot be used for glucose production.

5. **The answer is E.** Mr. Smith's protein intake of 150 kcal is about 37 g protein (150 kcal at 4 kcal/g = 37 g) below the RDA for protein. His carbohydrate intake of 150 kcal (37 g) is below the glucose requirements of his brain and red blood cells (about 150 g/day). Therefore, he will be breaking down muscle protein to synthesize glucose for the brain and other glucose-dependent tissues and adipose tissue mass to supply fatty acids for muscle and tissues able to oxidize fatty acids. Because he will be breaking down muscle protein to amino acids and converting the nitrogen from both these amino acids and his dietary amino acids to urea, his nitrogen excretion will be greater than his intake and he will be in negative nitrogen balance. It is unlikely that he will develop hypoglycemia while he is able to supply gluconeogenic precursors from muscle protein breakdown.

## CHAPTER 2

1. **The answer is A.** The pH is the negative $\log_{10}$ of the $H^+$ concentration ($[H^+]$). Thus, at pH 7.5, $[H^+]$ is $10^{-7.5}$, and at pH 6.5, it is $10^{-6.5}$. The $[H^+]$ has changed by a factor of $10^{-6.5}/10^{-7.5}$, which is $10^1$ or 10. Any decrease of 1 pH unit is a 10-fold increase of $[H^+]$ or a 10-fold decrease of $[OH^-]$. A shift in the concentration of buffer anions has definitely occurred, but the change in pH reflects the increase in $[H^+]$ in excess of that absorbed by buffers.

2. **The answer is C.** Buffers by definition tend to keep the pH of a solution constant, absorbing protons if an acid is added to the solution and releasing protons if a base is added to the solution. Because they must have the ability to dissociate or reassociate a proton, they work best at the pH at which they are 50% dissociated, the $pK_a$. Buffers cannot be composed of strong acids or strong bases because strong acids and bases are fully dissociated in solution. The higher the buffer concentration, the better the buffer works because the buffer components can absorb or dissociate more protons.

3. **The answer is E.** $NH_3$ is a weak base that associates with a proton to produce $NH_4^+$ ($NH_3 + H^+ \rightarrow NH_4^+$), which has a $pK_a$ of 9.5. Thus, at pH 7.4, most of the ammonia is present as $NH_4^+$. The absorption of $H^+$ will tend to increase, not decrease, the pH of the blood. With the decrease of $H^+$, carbonic acid will dissociate to produce more bicarbonate ($H_2CO_3 \rightarrow HCO_3^- + H^+$), and more $CO_2$ will go toward carbonic acid. Kussmaul breathing, an increased expiration of $CO_2$, occurs during acidosis, the opposite condition.

4. **The answer is B.** Vomiting expels the strong gastric acid HCl. As cells in the stomach secrete more HCl, they draw on $H^+$ in interstitial fluid and blood, thereby tending to increase blood pH and cause alkalosis. The other conditions tend to produce acidosis. Lactic acid is a weak acid secreted into the blood by muscles during exercise. A patient with increased ketone body production can exhibit a fall of blood pH because the ketone bodies acetoacetate and β-hydroxybutyrate are dissociated acids.

As bicarbonate in the intestinal lumen is lost in the watery diarrhea, more bicarbonate is secreted by intestinal cells. As intestinal cells produce bicarbonate, more $H^+$ is also generated ($H_2CO_3 \rightarrow HCO_3^- + H^+$). Although the bicarbonate produced by these cells is released into the intestinal lumen, the protons accumulate in blood, resulting in acidosis. Hypercatabolism, an increased rate of catabolism, generates additional $CO_2$, which produces more acid ($CO_2 + H_2O \rightarrow H_2CO_3 \rightarrow HCO_3^- + H^+$).

5.  **The answer is E.** Blood is buffered principally by the bicarbonate buffering system, by hemoglobin, and by the high concentration of serum proteins, which are able to absorb and release hydrogen ions from multiple amino acid side chains. However, carbonic anhydrase is present principally in the red blood cell and not in serum, which is cell free. Although the phosphate buffering system is present in low concentrations in extracellular fluid, it is principally involved in maintaining intracellular and interstitial fluid pH, which has a low protein content. Normal metabolism produces principally acids: weak acids (e.g., lactic acid), $CO_2$, and strong acids, such as sulfuric acid, but very few bases except for ammonia. The pH is maintained between 7.37 and 7.43; a pH as low as 6.43 is not compatible with life.

## CHAPTER 3

1.  **The answer is B.** Water-soluble compounds are polar (contain an uneven distribution of charge) so that the more positive portion of the molecule hydrogen bonds with the oxygen of water and the more negative portion of the molecule hydrogen bonds with the hydrogens of water. Water-soluble compounds need not contain a full negative or positive charge and generally contain oxygen or nitrogen in addition to carbon and hydrogen. Large C–H portions of a molecule, such as an aromatic ring, are nonpolar and contribute to the water insolubility of a molecule.

2.  **The answer is E.** The compound contains an OH group, which should appear in the name as an "-ol" or a "hydroxy" group. All of the possible answers fit this criterion. The structure also contains a carboxylate group ($COO^-$), which should appear in the name as an "-ate" or "acid." Counting backward from the carboxylate group (carbon 1), the second carbon is $\alpha$, the third is $\beta$, and the fourth carbon, containing the hydroxyl group, is $\gamma$. Thus, the compound is $\gamma$-hydroxybutyrate. Other means of eliminating answers are "meth-" denotes a single carbon, "eth-" denotes two carbons, and the "-ene" in ethylene denotes a double bond, none of which applies to the compound in the question.

3.  **The answer is A.** The term "glycosidic bond" refers to a *covalent* bond formed between the anomeric carbon of one sugar, when it is in a ring form, and a hydroxyl group or nitrogen of another compound. Disaccharides can be linked through their anomeric carbons but not polysaccharides because there would be no anomeric carbon left to form a link with the next sugar in the chain.

4.  **The answer is D.** Triglycerides (triacylglycerols) are composed of a glycerol backbone to which three fatty acids ("tri-") are attached. The carboxylic acid group of each fatty acid forms an ester with one of the three −OH groups on glycerol; thus, the fatty acid is an "acyl" group. Sphingolipids, in contrast, contain one fatty acyl group and one group derived from a fatty acid, attached to a group derived from serine.

5.  **The answer is B.** Sphingolipids contain a ceramide group, which is sphingosine with an attached fatty acid. They do not contain a glycerol moiety. However, different sphingolipids have different substituents on the −$CH_2OH$ group of ceramide. For example, sphingomyelin contains phosphorylcholine and gangliosides contain *N*-acetylneuraminic acid (NANA). No known sphingolipids contain a steroid.

## CHAPTER 4

1.  **The answer is C.** In hydrogen bonds, a hydrogen atom is shared between two electron-rich atoms such as oxygen or nitrogen. Thus, the nitrogen in the peptide bond may share its hydrogen with the oxygen in an aspartate carboxyl group, which will be negatively charged at a pH of 7.4. Leucine is nonpolar and cannot participate in hydrogen bonding, and aspartyl and glutamyl residues are both negatively charged and lack a proton to share. Bonds between two fully charged groups are electrostatic (ionic) bonds, not hydrogen bonds. Sulfhydryl groups do not participate in hydrogen bonding.

2.  **The answer is E.** The peptide backbone contains only carbon and nitrogen atoms covalently linked in a chain (oxygen is not part of the peptide backbone). The amide nitrogen of one amino acid (N) is covalently attached to the $\alpha$-carbon of the same amino acid (C), which is covalently linked to the carboxyl carbon (C) of that amino acid, which forms a peptide bond with the nitrogen of the next amino acid (N). NCCNCCNCC represents a chain of three complete amino acids.

3.  **The answer is A.** The protamine preparation is arginine-rich, and it is the arginine residues which complex with insulin. Arginine is a *basic* amino acid that has a positively charged side chain at neutral pH. It can, therefore, form tight electrostatic bonds with negatively charged *asp* and *glu* side chains in insulin. The $\alpha$-carboxylic acid groups at the *N*-terminals of proteins are bound through peptide bonds to the second amino acid in the protein. The arginine side chain is not hydrophobic, and it cannot form disulfide bonds because it does not contain a sulfhydryl group. Its basic group is a guanidinium group that cannot form peptide bonds.

4.  **The answer is B.** Only serine, threonine, and tyrosine have side chain hydroxyl groups. As a general rule,

serine–threonine protein kinases form one group of proteins kinases and tyrosine protein kinases form another. The side chains of aspartate and glutamate contain carboxylic acid groups. Phenylalanine has a phenyl group as a side chain, and arginine has three methylene groups linked to a guanidinium group. Lysine and arginine are basic amino acids (no hydroxyl groups), and proline does not contain a hydroxyl group.

5. **The answer is D.** Phenylalanine (F) and tyrosine (Y) are both large aromatic amino acids, but tyrosine contains a hydroxyl group that makes it more polar. Phenylalanine is less hydrophilic than tyrosine due to the presence of the hydroxyl group on tyrosine, which is missing in phenylalanine. Neither phenylalanine nor tyrosine is charged. Methionine (M) and leucine (L) are both large nonpolar aliphatic amino acids. The sulfur in methionine is nonpolar.

## CHAPTER 5

1. **The answer is E.** The regular repeating structure of an α-helix is possible because it is formed by hydrogen bonds within the peptide backbone of a single strand. There are no hydrogen bonds between the backbone and amino acid side chains. Thus, α-helices can be formed from a variety of primary structures. However, proline cannot accommodate the bond angles required for an α-helix because the atoms involved in the peptide backbone are part of a ring structure that are severely constrained in the angles they can form. Although glycine may be part of an α-helical structure, a high content of glycine is not required to form an α-helix. Glycine is required, however, for the structure of the fibril-forming collagen molecules in which 33% of the residues are glycine due to steric constraints of the triple helix.

2. **The answer is B.** Globular proteins fold into a sphere-like structure with their hydrophilic residues on the outside to interact with water and their hydrophobic residues on the inside away from water. Secondary structures are formed by hydrogen bonding, not hydrophobic bonding. Disulfide bonds are rare in globular proteins and are not needed to maintain a stable structure. Tertiary structure uses the properties of both amino acid side chains and backbone, whereas secondary structure only uses interactions between backbone atoms.

3. **The answer is C.** When an α-helix is formed, all side chains face the outside of the helix, which in this case is the hydrophobic environment of the lipid membrane. Thus, the side chains should be hydrophobic. Of the amino acids listed, only leucine fits this requirement. Proline interrupts helical structure because the imino bond of its ring structure does not allow the polypeptide backbone to form the angles required for α-helical formation.

4. **The answer is D.** The protein hydrolyzes ATP, which is a characteristic of the actin fold but not of the other

domains listed as potential answers. The substrate receives a phosphate from ATP, and ADP is the other product of the reaction.

5. **The answer is A.** As the pH is increased above the $pK_a$ of positively charged basic groups (usually around 10 to 11), they are converted from $-NH_3^+$ to $-NH_2$, leading to both a loss of ionic interactions and hydrogen bonding. The loss of these interactions will destabilize the tertiary structure of the protein and lead to a loss of structure. The change in pH will not affect the charge on carboxylic acid groups, as the $pK_a$ for those groups is around 4, and at pH 7, they have already lost their protons. Peptide bonds cannot be broken by base; proteases or extensive acid treatment are required to do so.

## CHAPTER 6

1. **The answer is B.** In most reactions, the substrate binds to the enzyme before its reaction with the coenzyme occurs. Thus, the substrate may bind but cannot react with the coenzyme to form the transition state complex. Each coenzyme carries out a single type of reaction, so no other coenzyme can substitute. The three-dimensional geometry of the reaction is so specific that functional groups on amino acid side chains cannot substitute. Free coenzymes are not very reactive because amino acid side chains in the active site are required to activate the coenzyme or the reactants. However, increasing the supply of vitamins to increase the amount of coenzyme bound to the enzyme can sometimes alleviate the condition, particularly if the binding of the vitamin to the enzyme has been altered by the mutation.

2. **The answer is A.** The patient was diagnosed with maturity-onset diabetes of the young (MODY) caused by this mutation. In glucokinase, binding of glucose normally causes a huge conformational change in the actin fold that creates the binding site for ATP. Although proline and leucine are both nonpolar amino acids, proline creates kinks in helices and terminates them. Thus, this change would be expected to disturb the large conformational change required when ATP binds to this site. In general, binding of the first substrate to an enzyme creates conformational changes that increases the binding of the second substrate or brings functional groups into position for further steps in the reaction. Thus, a mutation need not be in the active site to impair the reaction. It would probably take more energy to fold the enzyme into the form required for the transition state complex, and fewer molecules would acquire the necessary energy. In the absence of the conformational change, the active site lacks the functional groups required for an alternate mechanism.

3. **The answer is E.** Enzymes using histidine to abstract a proton from the substrate in acid-base catalysis are active only over a narrow pH range near neutrality because histidine must be able to accept and donate a proton within

this pH range. As the pH falls below 6.5, protons will not readily dissociate from histidine. In contrast, lysine is fully protonated at both pH 6.5 and 5.5. All intestinal hydrolases (proteases, esterases, glycosidases) use acid-base catalysis to add the elements of water across the bonds. Usually, the pH must fall much lower before the hydrogen bonding is disrupted and proteins are denatured and lose their tertiary structure, as the groups involved in stabilizing both secondary and tertiary structure do not gain or lose protons in this pH range.

4. **The answer is C.** Enzymes lower the energy of activation required for the substrate(s) to reach the transition state. This is accomplished through binding of the substrate to the enzyme. Enzymes do not alter the energy levels of either the initial or final states of the reaction nor do they alter the concentration of substrates or products. Enzymes also do not affect diffusion rates and do not control collision frequency between molecules.

5. **The answer is A.** In the conversion of ethanol to acetaldehyde, the ethanol loses electrons (and is oxidized), whereas the $NAD^+$ gains electrons (to form NADH) and is reduced. Neither the active site serine nor zinc atom gains or loses electrons during the course of the reaction. Thiamine pyrophosphate is not a required cofactor for this reaction.

## CHAPTER 7

1. **The answer is B.** The rate of an enzyme-catalyzed reaction is directly proportional to the number of enzyme molecules containing bound substrate. Thus, it is at 50% of its maximal rate when 50% of the enzyme molecules contain bound substrate. The rate of the reaction is also directly proportional to the amount of enzyme present, which is incorporated into the term $V_{max}$ ($V_{max}$ = k [total enzyme]). If the concentration of substrate molecules in the solution is much greater than the number of enzyme molecules, then the enzyme will be at its maximal velocity even though not all substrate molecules are bound.

2. **The answer is A.** The patient's enzyme has a lower $K_m$ than the normal enzyme and therefore requires a lower glucose concentration to reach one-half $V_{max}$. Thus, the mutation may have increased the affinity of the enzyme for glucose, but it has greatly decreased the subsequent steps of the reaction leading to formation of the transition state complex, and thus $V_{max}$ is much slower. The difference in $V_{max}$ is so great that the patient's enzyme is much slower whether you are above or below its $K_m$ for glucose. You can test this by substituting 2 mM glucose and 4 mM glucose into the Michaelis-Menten equation of v = $V_{max}$ S/($K_m$ + S) for the patient's enzyme and for the normal enzyme. The values are 0.0095 and 0.0129 for the patient's enzyme versus 23.2 and 37.2 for the normal enzyme, respectively. At near-saturating glucose concentrations, both enzymes will be near $V_{max}$, which is equal to $k_{cat}$ times the

enzyme concentration. Thus, it will take nearly 500 times as much of the patient's enzyme to achieve the normal rate (93/0.2). The rates of enzyme catalyzed reactions change most as you decrease the substrate concentration below the $K_m$. Thus, the enzyme with the highest $K_m$ will show the largest changes in rate as the substrate concentration is altered.

3. **The answer is E.** Ethanol has a structure very similar to methanol (a structural analogue) and, thus, would be expected to compete with methanol at its substrate binding site. This inhibition is competitive with respect to methanol; therefore, the $V_{max}$ for methanol would not be altered, and ethanol inhibition could be overcome by high concentrations of methanol. It would not be expected that ethanol is a noncompetitive inhibitor when the structures of ethanol and methanol are similar. Because ethanol is an analogue of methanol, it would not be expected to compete for binding with the product of the reaction, formaldehyde.

4. **The answer is D.** Allosteric enzymes generally have more than one subunit, each of which contains a binding site for the substrate. As the substrate binds to one site, it changes the conformation of one or more of the other subunits, leading to cooperativity in substrate binding. Thus, plots of velocity versus substrate concentration are usually S-shaped rather than the rectangular hyperbola of Michaelis-Menten kinetics. Generally, a compound binding in the catalytic site cannot be an activator. Most allosteric inhibitors are reversibly bound at either allosteric sites or the catalytic site because they must be released from the enzyme when the concentration of activator changes. In the absence of effectors, the kinetic curve of allosteric enzymes is sigmoidal due to the cooperative binding explained earlier.

5. **The answer is A.** When monomeric G proteins contain bound GTP, they are in an activated conformation and bind to their target enzymes or proteins. As they hydrolyze this GTP to GDP, they revert back to an inactive conformation. When a guanine nucleotide exchange protein (GEF) binds to the monomeric G protein, it activates the exchange of GTP for bound GDP. GEFs usually do not change the rate of hydrolysis of bound GTP.

## CHAPTER 8

1. **The answer is E.** The transmembrane regions are α-helices with hydrophobic amino acid side chains binding to membrane lipids. The hydrophobic interactions hinder their extraction. Because they are not easily extracted, they are classified as integral proteins. The carboxy and amino terminals of transmembrane proteins extend into the aqueous intra- and extracellular medium and thus need to contain many hydrophilic residues.

2. **The answer is B.** Most of fuel oxidation and ATP generation occurs in the mitochondrion. Although some may also occur in the cytosol, the amount is much smaller in most

cells. The peroxisomes are used primarily for oxidative reactions that generate hydrogen peroxide. The lysosome is the compartment of the cell that degrades unwanted cellular materials. The nucleus contains the genetic material and is the site of RNA synthesis and processing, an energy-requiring process. The Golgi apparatus performs posttranslational modification of proteins and protein sorting.

3. **The answer is E.** Each chemical messenger has a specific protein receptor in a target cell that will generally bind only that messenger, and only that cell responds to the message. Only endocrine messengers reach their target cells through the blood. Many chemical messengers have paracrine actions. Messengers are secreted by only one type of cell. Many messengers bind to extracellular domains of plasma membrane receptors, and do not enter the cells. It is rare for chemical messengers to be metabolized to intracellular second messengers, and this would not be a general characteristic of all chemical messengers.

4. **The answer is A.** Parathyroid hormone is a polypeptide hormone and thus must bind to a plasma membrane receptor instead of an intracellular receptor. Hormones that bind to plasma membrane receptors do not need to enter the cell to transmit their signals. Heptahelical receptors work through heterotrimeric G proteins that have an $\alpha$-subunit, and tyrosine kinase receptors work through monomeric G proteins that have no subunits.

5. **The answer is D.** $G_s\alpha$ normally activates adenylyl cyclase to generate ATP in response to parathyroid hormone. Because the patient has end-organ unresponsiveness, he or she must have a deficiency in the signaling pathway and cAMP would be decreased. Decreased GTPase activity would increase binding to adenylyl cyclase and increase responsiveness. Neither $IP_3$ nor phosphatidylinositol 2,3,5-trisphosphate are involved in signal transduction by the Gs $\alpha$-subunit. A gain-of-function mutation would lead to constant activation of the Gs $\alpha$-subunit, which is not observed.

## CHAPTER 9

1. **The answer is C.** The complementary strand must run in the opposite direction, so the 5′ end must base-pair with the G at the 3′ end of the given strand. Therefore, the 5′ end of the complementary strand must be C. G would then base-pair to C, A to T, and T to A. Recall that the base U is not found in DNA and that this complementary strand must have the opposite polarity of the given strand.

2. **The answer is A.** The RNA strand must be complementary to the DNA strand. An A in DNA pairs with U in RNA, a T in DNA base-pairs with an A in RNA, a G in DNA base-pairs with C in RNA, and C in DNA will base-pair with G in RNA. Thymine (T) is found in DNA but not RNA. Thus, following the above rules, the RNA sequence must begin at the 5′ end with ACGCAAUU.

3. **The answer is D.** The phosphate is in an ester bond to two ribose groups, generating the phosphodiester bond. This is a covalent bond.

4. **The answer is E.** There are 4 possible bases at each position in the molecule, so as a total, there are $4^8$ possibilities (once one strand is defined at a certain position, the base in the complementary strand is known). This comes out to 65,536 possible DNA sequences for a molecule which is only 8 bases long.

5. **The answer is B.** RNA contains a hydroxyl group on the 2′-carbon, which loses its proton in the presence of base and acts as a nucleophile that can break the phosphodiester bond. DNA lacks this hydroxyl group and is stable under basic conditions. Both DNA and RNA form secondary structures, contain negatively charged phosphate groups, contain G-C base pairs, and can be denatured by heat (which disrupts the hydrogen bonds holding complementary bases together).

## CHAPTER 10

1. **The answer is A.** The 3′ to 5′ exonuclease activity is required for proofreading (check the base just inserted, and if it is incorrect, remove it), and reverse transcriptase does not have this activity, whereas polymerase $\delta$ does. Both reverse transcriptase and polymerase $\delta$ synthesize DNA in the 5′ to 3′ directions (all DNA polymerases do this) and both follow standard Watson-Crick base-pairing rules (A with T or U, G with C). Neither polymerase can synthesize DNA in the opposite direction (3′ to 5′) or insert inosine into a growing DNA chain. Thus, the only difference between the two polymerases is the presence or absence of the error-checking exonuclease activity.

2. **The answer is D.** In 50 seconds, each replication origin will have synthesized 100 kilobases of DNA (50 in each direction). Because there are 10 origins, 10 times 100 will yield the 1,000 kilobases needed to replicate the DNA. The first origin would be 50 kilobases from one end, and the remaining 9 origins would each be 100 kilobases apart.

3. **The answer is B.** The role of the primer is to provide a free 3′-OH group for DNA polymerase to add the next nucleotide and form a phosphodiester bond. When DNA repair occurs, one of the remaining bases in the DNA will have a free 3′-OH, which DNA polymerase I will use to begin extension of the DNA. All DNA polymerases require a primer.

4. **The answer is E.** Xeroderma pigmentosum is a set of diseases all related to an inability to repair thymine dimers, leading to an inability to excise UV-damaged DNA. It does not affect bypass polymerases, which can synthesize across the damaged region, sometimes making mutations in their path. The primase gene, or mismatch repair, is not involved in excising thymine dimers. The proofreading ability of DNA polymerases is likewise not specifically involved in the excision of thymine dimers.

5. **The answer is A.** Replication is initiated at an origin of replication and proceeds in both directions from the fork (bidirectional). Replication occurs during the S phase of the cell cycle; the M phase is when the cell divides. DNA replication proceeds in the 5' to 3' direction, which means that the template strand is always copied in a 3' to 5' direction. The daughter molecules each contain one parental strand and one newly synthesized strand (semiconservative replication), and DNA polymerases require a free 3'-hydroxyl group in order to synthesize DNA. A 3'-phosphate group would block replication.

## CHAPTER 11

1. **The answer is E.** The transcript that is produced is copied from the DNA template strand, which must be of the opposite orientation from the transcript. So the 5' end of the template strand should base-pair with the 3' end of the transcript. Thus, CGTACGGAT would base-pair with the transcript and would represent the template strand. Uracil (U) is not found in DNA strands, only RNA.

2. **The answer is B.** Enhancer sequences can be thousands of bases away from the basal promoter and still stimulate transcription of the gene. This is accomplished by looping of the DNA so that the protein binding to the enhancer sequence (transactivators) can also bind to proteins bound to the promoter (coactivators). A promoter proximal element is a DNA sequence near the promoter that can bind transcription factors that aid in recruiting RNA polymerase to the promoter region. The promoter and operator are always adjacent to the gene of interest. Splice donor sites are within a gene, at exon-intron borders, and do not usually regulate gene expression.

3. **The answer is C.** Both prokaryotes and eukaryotes require RNA polymerase binding to an upstream promoter element. Only eukaryotic mRNA is capped and polyadenylated; this does not occur for prokaryotic mRNA. Prokaryotes have no nucleus, thus the 5' end of an mRNA is immediately available for ribosomes binding and initiation of translation; however, this is not true of eukaryotes. Both DNA and RNA synthesis occur in the 5' to 3' direction, never in the opposite direction. The existence of introns in eukaryotic genes means that the mature mRNA is not precisely colinear to the gene from which it is transcribed (although this statement is true for prokaryotic mRNA).

4. **The answer is A.** The nontemplate strand is the message identical strand (with the exception of U for T) and complementary to the template strand. Thus, the sequence of RNA from that stretch of nontemplate strand is AGCUCACUG (identical to the nontemplate or coding strand and complementary to the template strand).

5. **The answer is E.** The promoter-proximal element is a sequence near the promoter that binds transcription factors that enhance RNA polymerase binding to the promoter.

A mutation in that sequence could increase the affinity of the *trans* acting factor such that RNA polymerase was recruited at an enhanced rate, leading to increased RNA synthesis and enhanced expression of the gene. Splice sites are not present upstream of the gene nor does the helix have to be melted upstream of the transcription start site. Because the promoter-proximal element is upstream of the coding sequence, there is no amino acid replacement, and sigma factor is only used for prokaryotic RNA synthesis, and this question concerns eukaryotic RNA synthesis.

## CHAPTER 12

1. **The answer is A.** It is important to note that the question is asking about prokaryotic mechanisms. In prokaryotes, there is no nucleus and translation begins before transcription is terminated (coupled translation–transcription). Thus, before the ribosome can move from one codon to the next (translocation) or the protein synthesis machinery terminates (via termination factors), the initiating tRNA must bind and align with the mRNA to initiate translation.

2. **The answer is C.** Because the extract contains all normal components, the Cys-tRNA charged with alanine will compete with Cys-tRNA charged with cysteine for binding to the cysteine codons. Thus, the protein will have some alanines put in the place of cysteine, leading to a deficiency of cysteine residues.

3. **The answer is E.** There are 64 triplet codes and only 20 amino acids, so some amino acids have more than one codon that codes for them. The other answers do not address this issue.

4. **The answer is B.** Because each codon is three bases long, there are 4 possible bases that can fill each codon position (A, T, C, or G). That means there are $4 \times 4 \times 4$ possible combinations of bases, for a total of 64 codons. There are fewer than 64 aminoacyl-tRNA synthetases due to one tRNA recognizing more than one codon due to wobbling. Not all bases participate in wobbling (I can base-pair with U, and C, A, or U can base-pair with G, but those are the only combinations possible), and only one reading frame is used for each message produced. The rate of protein synthesis is not dependent on the number of codons, but rather, how rapidly the components required to synthesize proteins can be brought to the ribosomes and how much RNA is present to be translated.

5. **The answer is B.** Examination of the sequence indicates that if the reading frame is the first nucleotide and we are looking at the message-identical strand, then the codons will be read as ACA CAC ACA CAC. If you start the reading frame at codon two, the codons will be read as CAC ACA CAC ACA. If you start the reading frame at codon three, the codons will be read as if you started at codon one. Thus, for this stretch of DNA, there are two repeating amino acids corresponding to the codons ACA and CAC. There is no reason

for such a stretch of bases to cause cessation of protein synthesis or alternative splicing if located within an intron.

## CHAPTER 13

1. **The answer is E.** In order to transcribe the *lac* operon, the repressor protein (lac I gene product) must bind allolactose and leave the operator region, and the cAMP-CRP complex must bind to the promoter in order for RNA polymerase to bind. Of the choices offered, only raising cAMP levels can allow transcription of the operon when both lactose and glucose are high. Raising cAMP, even though glucose is present, will allow the cAMP-CRP complex to bind and recruit RNA polymerase. Answers which call for mutations in the repressor will not affect binding of cAMP-CRP. Mutations in the DNA do not allow CRP binding in the absence of cAMP.

2. **The answer is B.** The repressor will bind to the operator and block transcription of all genes in the operon unless prevented by the inducer allolactose. If the repressor has lost its affinity for the inducer, it cannot dissociate from the operator and the genes in the operon will not be expressed. If the repressor has lost its affinity for the operator, then the operon would be constitutively expressed. Because the question states that there is a mutation in the I (repressor) gene, the mutation cannot be in the CAP gene, and mutations in the I gene do not affect *trans*-acting factors from binding to the promoter, although the only other one for the *lac* operon is the CAP.

3. **The answer is D.** The sequence, if read 5′ to 3′, is identical to the complementary sequence read 5′ to 3′. None of the other sequences fits this pattern.

4. **The answer is A.** All DNA binding proteins contain an α-helix which hydrogen bonds to the bases within the major groove in DNA. These proteins do not recognize RNA molecules nor do they form bonds between the peptide backbone and the DNA backbone. Only zinc fingers contain zinc, and dimers are formed by hydrogen bonding—not by disulfide linkages.

5. **The answer is C.** Amino acid side chains within the protein form hydrogen bonds with the nucleotide bases in DNA, which leads to the sequence specificity of protein binding to DNA. It is not base pairing because proteins do not contain nitrogenous bases nor do they contain anticodons or DNA codons. Aminoacyl linkages are found in tRNA, and there is no unwinding of the helix when these proteins initially bind.

## CHAPTER 14

1. **The answer is B.** All DNA fragments are negatively charged and will migrate toward the positive charge in an electric field. The only difference between the fragments is their size, and the smaller fragments will move faster than the larger fragments due to their ability to squeeze through the gel more easily.

2. **The answer is E.** The enzyme recognizes six bases, and the probability that the correct base is in each position is 1 in 4, so the overall probability is $(1/4)^6$ or 1 in 4,096 bases.

3. **The answer is C.** Ethidium bromide is a dye that intercalates between the stacked bases of DNA and can be visualized by UV light. As the gel is run, the smaller fragments migrate farther in the gel, and the DNA migrates toward the positive charge (due to the negative charges on the phosphate backbone). When a huge molecule like human DNA is cut with any endonuclease, many bands will be generated (not just three) and DNA is not denatured before it is run on the gel. When doing a Southern blot, the DNA is denatured after transfer to the filter paper.

4. **The answer is A.** A Northern blot allows one to determine which genes are being transcribed in a tissue at the time of mRNA isolation. The mRNA is run on a gel, transferred to filter paper, and then analyzed with a probe. If albumin is being transcribed, then a probe for albumin should give a positive result in the Northern blot. A genomic library screening will not indicate if a particular gene is being transcribed (although screening a cDNA library will) nor will a Southern blot. Those techniques will only allow one to determine that the gene is present in the genome. A Western blot analyzes protein content, not mRNA content. Analysis of VNTR does not provide information as to whether a gene is transcribed.

5. **The answer is A.** When DNA is run in a gel and transferred to nitrocellulose, and then probed, the blot is a Southern. When RNA is run in a gel, transferred to nitrocellulose, and probed, the blot is a Northern. When protein is run through a gel, transferred to nitrocellulose, and probed, the blot is a Western.

## CHAPTER 15

1. **The answer is C.** The *ras* oncogene has a point mutation in codon 12 (position 35 of the DNA chain) in which T replaces G. This changes the codon from one that specifies glycine to one that specifies valine. Thus, there is a single amino acid change in the protooncogene (a valine for a glycine) that changes *ras* to an oncogene.

2. **The answer is C.** Ras, when it is oncogenic, has lost its GTPase activity and thus remains active for a longer time. Answer A is incorrect because GAP proteins activate the GTPase activity of Ras and this mutation would make Ras less active. cAMP does not interact directly with Ras (thus, B is incorrect), and if Ras could no longer bind GTP, it would not be active (hence, D is also incorrect). Ras is not phosphorylated by the MAP kinase (thus, E is incorrect).

3. **The answer is B.** Retroviral oncogenes were originally obtained from genes on a host's chromosome. All retroviruses do not contain oncogenes (thus, A is incorrect); protooncogenes are found in host cells, not viruses (thus, C is incorrect); the oncogenes that lead to human disease are

very similar to those that are mutated in animals (thus, D is incorrect); and oncogenes are a misexpressed or mutated version of normal cellular genes, not viral genes (thus, E is incorrect).

4. **The answer is D.** When p53 increases in response to DNA damage, it acts as a transcription factor and induces the transcription of p21, which blocks phosphorylation of Rb. Rb then stays bound to transcription factor E2F, and E2F cannot induce the genes required for the $G_1$-to-S transition. p53 does not induce transcription of either cyclin D or cdk4 (thus, A and B are incorrect) nor does p53 bind to E2F (thus, C is incorrect). p53 does not contain kinase activity (thus, E is incorrect).

5. **The answer is B.** Tumor suppressor genes balance cell growth and quiescence. When they are not expressed (via loss-of-function mutations), the balance shifts to cell proliferation and tumorigenesis (thus, A is incorrect). Tumor suppressor genes do not act on viral genes (they help to regulate other cellular genes), so answer C is incorrect. Tumor suppressor genes are not specifically targeted to just one portion of the cell cycle (they regulate genes in every part of the cycle), so answer D is incorrect. A loss of expression of tumor suppressor genes leads to tumor formation, not expression of these genes (thus, answer E is incorrect).

## CHAPTER 16

1. **The answer is A.** Both of the high-energy phosphate bonds in ATP are located between phosphate groups (both the α and β phosphates, and the β and γ phosphates). The phosphate bond between the α-phosphate and ribose (or adenosine) is not a high-energy bond, and there is no phosphate between either the ribose and adenine or the two hydroxyl groups in the ribose ring.

2. **The answer is D.** The change in enthalpy, $\Delta H$, is the total amount of heat that can be released in a reaction. The first law of thermodynamics states that the total energy of a system remains constant and the second law of thermodynamics states the universe tends toward a state of disorder. $\Delta G°'$ is the standard free energy change measured at 25°C and a pH of 7, not at 37°C or pH 7.4. A high-energy bond releases more than about 7 kcal/mole of heat when it is hydrolyzed, not three. The definition of high-energy bond is based on the hydrolysis of one of the high-energy bonds of ATP.

3. **The answer is B.** The concentration of the substrates and products influence the direction of a reaction. Reactions with a positive free energy, at 1 M concentrations of substrate and product, will proceed in the direction of substrate formation, not product formation. The substrate and product concentration do influence the free energy of a reaction, particularly under nonstandard conditions. The standard free energy must be considered (in addition to the substrate and product concentration) in order to determine

the direction of a reaction; it is not just determined by the concentrations of substrates and products. An enzyme's efficiency does not influence the direction of a reaction, only the rate at which the reaction may occur.

4. **The answer is C.** A heart attack results in decreased pumping of blood and thus a decreased oxygen supply to the heart. The lack of oxygen leads to a lack of ATP due to an inability to perform oxidative phosphorylation. The lack of ATP impairs the working of the $Na^+$-$K^+$ ATPase, which pumps sodium out of the cell in exchange for potassium. Therefore, intracellular levels of sodium will increase as $Na^+$ enters the cell through other transport mechanisms. The high intracellular sodium concentration then blocks the functioning of the $Na^+/H^+$ antiporter (which sends protons out of the cell in exchange for sodium. Because intracellular sodium is high, the driving force for this reaction is lost), which leads to increased intracellular $H^+$ or a lower intracellular pH. The intracellular pH also increases because of glycolysis in the absence of oxygen, which produces lactic acid. The loss of the sodium gradient, coupled with the lack of ATP, leads to increased calcium in the cell due to an inability to pump calcium out.

5. **The answer is B.** $NAD^+$ accepts two electrons as hydride ions to form NADH. FAD can accept two single electrons from separate atoms, together with protons, or can accept a pair of electrons. FAD can also accept one electron at a time.

## CHAPTER 17

1. **The answer is E.** Thiamine pyrophosphate is the coenzyme for the α-ketoglutarate dehydrogenase and pyruvate dehydrogenase complexes. With these complexes inactive, pyruvic acid and α-ketoglutaric acid accumulate and dissociate to generate the anion and $H^+$. As α-ketoglutarate is not listed as an answer, the only possible answer is pyruvate. Isocitrate can still be converted to α-ketoglutarate, succinic acid can still be converted to fumarate, and malic acid can still be converted to oxaloacetate under these conditions. Oxaloacetic acid can still condense with acetyl CoA to form citrate under these conditions as well. Because pyruvate is increasing, lactate levels will also be elevated.

2. **The answer is B.** NADH decreases during exercise in order to generate energy for the exercise (if it were increased, it would inhibit the cycle and slow it down), thus the NADH/$NAD^+$ ratio is decreased, and the lack of NADH activates flux through isocitrate dehydrogenase, α-ketoglutarate dehydrogenase, and malate dehydrogenase. Isocitrate dehydrogenase is inhibited by NADH, not activated. Fumarase is not a regulated enzyme of the cycle. The four-carbon intermediates of the cycle are regenerated during each turn of the cycle, so their concentration does not decrease under these conditions. Product inhibition of citrate synthase would slow the cycle and not generate more energy, which does not occur under exercising conditions.

3.  **The answer is D.** ADP is an activator of isocitrate dehydrogenase, which would speed up this reaction and increase the overall flux of metabolites through the cycle. Oxygen is normally present in excess in cells, so having more of it would not speed up the cycle. If the $V_{max}$ of $\alpha$-ketoglutarate dehydrogenase were decreased, flux through the cycle would decrease because this enzyme would not work as rapidly, and, therefore, the rate of carbon dioxide production would decrease. If the $K_m$ of isocitrate dehydrogenase increased, the enzyme would require higher concentrations of isocitrate for the enzyme to reach its normal rate, which would have the effect of decreasing the rate of carbon dioxide production as well. This is also true if the $K_m$ of citrate synthase was also increased; higher concentrations of substrate would be required to reach half-maximal velocity, which would have the effect of slowing down the cycle.

4.  **The answer is A.** The pyruvate dehydrogenase complex is active when it is dephosphorylated. It is inactive when it is phosphorylated by pyruvate dehydrogenase kinase. An increase of NADH would decrease the activity of pyruvate dehydrogenase, both allosterically and by activation of pyruvate dehydrogenase kinase. An increase of acetyl CoA would also decrease the activity of the enzyme in a manner similar to NADH. $Ca^{2+}$ activates the pyruvate dehydrogenase phosphatase, which then dephosphorylates the enzyme, thereby activating it. Thus, calcium works through an indirect mechanism, as calcium itself does not directly activate the pyruvate dehydrogenase complex. An increase in the concentration of ATP would decrease the activity of the pyruvate dehydrogenase complex, again, in an allosteric manner.

5.  **The answer is E.** Oxaloacetate initiates the cycle by condensing with acetyl CoA to produce citrate. Oxaloacetate is then regenerated via the malate dehydrogenase reaction in which malate is converted to oxaloacetate. Thus, oxaloacetate cycles through the reactions, always being regenerated. This is not true for the other members of the TCA cycle.

## CHAPTER 18

1.  **The answer is B.** For a component to be in the oxidized state, it must have donated or never received electrons. Complex II will metabolize succinate to produce fumarate (generating FAD[2H]), but no succinate is available in this experiment. Thus, complex II never sees any electrons and is always in an oxidized state. The substrate malate is oxidized to oxaloacetate, generating NADH, which donates electrons to complex I of the electron transfer chain. These electrons are transferred to coenzyme Q, which donates electrons to complex III, to cytochrome C, and then to complex IV. Cyanide will block the transfer of electrons from complex IV to oxygen, so all previous complexes containing electrons will be backed up and the electrons will be "trapped" in the complexes, making those components reduced.

2.  **The answer is A.** The proton-motive force consists of two components, a $\Delta pH$ and a $\Delta\Psi$ (electrical component). The addition of valinomycin and potassium will destroy the electrical component but not the pH component. Thus, the PMF will decrease but will still be greater than zero.

3.  **The answer is E.** A deficiency of Fe-S centers in the electron transport chain would impair the transfer of electrons down the chain and reduce ATP production by oxidative phosphorylation. The lack of ATP would lead to fatigue, as would the reduced delivery of oxygen to tissues due to reduced hemoglobin levels in the red blood cells. A decreased production of water from the electron transport chain under these conditions would not be of sufficient magnitude to cause the patient to become dehydrated. Iron does not form a chelate with NADH and FAD(2H) nor is it a cofactor for $\alpha$-ketoglutarate dehydrogenase. The establishment of a proton gradient across the mitochondrial inner membrane does not require the cotransport of iron.

4.  **The answer is C.** Because rotenone inhibits the oxidation of NADH, it would completely block the generation of the electrochemical potential gradient in vivo and, therefore, it would block ATP generation. In the presence of rotenone, NADH would accumulate and $NAD^+$ concentrations would decrease. Although the mitochondria might still be able to oxidize compounds like succinate, which transfer electrons to FAD, no succinate would be produced in vivo if the $NAD^+$-dependent dehydrogenases of the TCA cycle were inhibited. Thus, very shortly after rotenone administration, there would not be any substrates available for the electron transfer chain, and NADH dehydrogenase is blocked, so oxidative phosphorylation would be completely inhibited. If glucose supplies were high, anaerobic glycolysis could provide some ATP but not nearly enough to keep the heart pumping.

5.  **The answer is D.** Histones coat nuclear DNA and can protect the DNA from radical damage. Mitochondrial DNA lacks histones, such that when radicals are formed, the DNA can be easily oxidized. Superoxide dismutase reduces radical concentrations, so the fact that it is present in the mitochondria should help to protect the DNA from damage, not enhance it, and glutathione also protects against radical damage, and if the nucleus lacks it, then one would expect higher levels of nuclear DNA damage, not reduced levels. Reactive oxygen species can diffuse across all membranes. Other factors which increase mitochondrial DNA damage relative to nuclear DNA are the proximity of mitochondrial DNA to the membrane, and the fact that most radical species are formed from coenzyme Q, which is found within the mitochondria.

## CHAPTER 19

1.  **The answer is A.** By starting with glyceraldehyde 3-phosphate the energy requiring steps of glycolysis are bypassed. Thus, as glyceraldehyde 3-phosphate is converted to pyruvate, two molecules of ATP will be produced (at the

phosphoglycerate kinase and pyruvate kinase steps) and one molecule of NADH will be produced (at the glyceraldehyde 3-phosphate dehydrogenase step).

2. **The answer is E.** The pathway consumes two ATP at the beginning of the pathway and produces four ATP at the end of the pathway for each molecule of glucose. Therefore, the net energy production is two ATP for each molecule of glucose. Glycolysis synthesizes ATP via substrate-level phosphorylation, not oxidative phosphorylation, and synthesizes two molecules of pyruvate in the process. The pathway is cytosolic and the rate-limiting step is the one catalyzed by PFK-1, not pyruvate kinase.

3. **The answer is B.** Glycolysis and the TCA cycle will be going as fast as possible in order to try to keep up with the increased ATP demand by the muscle. The pyruvate that is being produced from glycolysis accumulates as the TCA cycle is working at maximal capacity and cannot oxidize any more pyruvate to acetyl CoA. Thus, the pyruvate is converted to lactate by lactate dehydrogenase. Because the substrate for this reaction is increasing, the velocity of the reaction is also increasing. NADH is being produced as quickly as possible, in both the cytoplasm and the matrix, so the $NAD^+$:NADH ratio would be low under these conditions. The ratio of ATP:ADP would also be low, as the ATP is being used quickly due to the increased demand. It is the low ATP levels that is actually driving the demand for increased glycolysis and TCA cycle activity. The velocity of the NADH dehydrogenase reaction would increase due to the increased amount of NADH being produced by the TCA cycle, and because of this, $O_2$ consumption would increase due to the increased rate of the electron transport chain.

4. **The answer is D.** Fructose 2,6-bisphosphate allosterically activates PFK-1. Fructose 2,6-bisphosphate is not an intermediate of glycolysis; its role is a regulator of glycolysis. Fructose 2,6-bisphosphate is not an enzyme and does not catalyze a reaction.

5. **The answer is C.** AMP activates the enzyme by shifting the kinetic curve to the left, indicating that a reduced substrate concentration (as compared to the absence of AMP) will lead to 50% maximal velocity. However, the maximal velocity does not change, just the substrate concentration required to reach this activity level.

## CHAPTER 20

1. **The answer is C.** The ETF:CoQ oxidoreductase is required to transfer the electrons from the FAD(2H) of the acyl CoA dehydrogenase to coenzyme Q. When the oxidoreductase is missing, the electrons cannot be transferred and the acyl-CoA dehydrogenase cannot continue to oxidize fatty acids due to having a reduced cofactor instead of an oxidized cofactor. During times of fasting, when fatty acids are the primary energy source, no energy will be forthcoming, gluconeogenesis is shut down, and death may result. The lack of this enzyme does not dramatically affect the other pathways listed as potential answers, as succinate dehydrogenase of the TCA cycle transfers electrons directly to coenzyme Q and does not require the ETF:CoQ oxidoreductase. Electrons carried by the glycerol 3-phosphate shuttle may not be able to be used effectively in the electron transport chain, but this is a minor component of glucose, glycogen, and alcohol oxidation.

2. **The answer is C.** An 18-carbon saturated fatty acid would require eight spirals of fatty acid oxidation, which yields eight NADH, eight FAD(2H), and nine acyl CoA. Because each NADH gives rise to 2.5 ATP, and each FAD(2H) gives rise to 1.5 ATP, the reduced cofactors will give rise to 32 ATP. Each acyl CoA gives rise to 10 ATP, for a total of 90 ATP. This then yields 122 ATP, but we must subtract 2 ATP for the activation step, at which two high-energy bonds are broken. Thus, the net yield is 120 ATPs for each molecule of fatty acid oxidized.

3. **The answer is E.** A lack of carnitine would lead to an inability to transport fatty acyl CoAs into the mitochondria. This would lead to a decrease in fatty acid oxidation, a decrease in ketone body production because fatty acids cannot be oxidized, a decrease in blood glucose levels because gluconeogenesis is impaired due to a lack of energy, and no increase in the levels of very long chain fatty acids because these are initially oxidized in the peroxisomes and do not require carnitine for entry into that organelle. The ω-oxidation system, which creates dicarboxylic acids, is found in the ER, and as the concentration of fatty acyl CoAs increase in tissues, they will be oxidized by this alternative pathway.

4. **The answer is B.** A defect in CPTII activity would lead to the fatty acids being added to carnitine (via CPTI) but not being able to have the carnitine removed. This would lead to a buildup of acylcarnitine levels in the blood. This would also lead to an inability to oxidize fatty acids or synthesize ketone bodies. Because of the lack of energy from fatty acid oxidation for gluconeogenesis, blood glucose levels would be low. The lack of energy would signal adipocytes to release more fatty acids, such that blood fatty acid levels will be increased. The buildup of acylcarnitine in muscle will damage the muscle membranes and release creatine phosphokinase into circulation.

5. **The answer is D.** Because short chain dicarboxylic fatty acids are found in the urine, there is some fatty acid metabolism occurring, but it cannot go to completion, indicating that CPTI, CPTII, and carnitine:acylcarnitine translocase must all be functioning. Even if those enzymes were partially defective, once a fatty acid was transported into the mitochondria, it would be able to be oxidized to completion, and the short chain dicarboxylic acids would not be observed. Because the dicarboxylic acids (products of ω oxidation) are short, it indicates that LCAD is active and MCAD is defective. The lack of energy from fatty acid oxidation resulted in an inability to synthesize sufficient glucose for the circulation, resulting in the lethargy. Eating frequently maintained blood glucose levels such that the brain could function, and the symptoms were alleviated.

## CHAPTER 21

1. **The answer is A.** Once insulin is injected, glucose transport into the peripheral tissues will be enhanced. If the patient does not eat, the normal fasting level of glucose will drop even further due to the injection of insulin, which increases the movement of glucose into muscle and fat cells. The patient becomes hypoglycemic, as a result of which epinephrine is released from the adrenal medulla. This, in turn, leads to the signs and symptoms associated with high levels of epinephrine in the blood. The problems are not due to altered glucagon release; it is the insulin in the absence of additional glucose that causes the problem. Elevated ketone body production does not produce hypoglycemic symptoms nor would they be significantly elevated only a few hours after the insulin shock the patient is experiencing.

2. **The answer is E.** When glucagon binds to its receptor, the enzyme adenylate cyclase is eventually activated (through the action of G proteins), which raises cAMP levels in the cell. The cAMP phosphodiesterase opposes this rise in cAMP and hydrolyzes cAMP to 5'-AMP. If the phosphodiesterase is inhibited by caffeine, cAMP levels would stay elevated for an extended period of time, enhancing the glucagon response. The glucagon response in liver is to export glucose and to inhibit glycolysis. cAMP activates protein kinase A, and the effect of insulin is to reduce cAMP levels.

3. **The answer is B.** Insulin release is dependent on an increase in the [ATP]/[ADP] ratio within the pancreatic β-cell. In MODY, the mutation in glucokinase results in a less active glucokinase at glucose concentrations which normally stimulate insulin release. Thus, higher concentrations of glucose are required to stimulate glycolysis and the TCA cycle to effectively raise the ratio of ATP to ADP. Alterations in cAMP levels are not related to the mechanism of insulin release. Insulin release from the β-cells is due to exocytosis of preformed insulin in secretory vesicles, indicating that gene transcription is not required. The pancreas does not degrade glycogen under conditions of high blood glucose, and lactate is not involved in stimulating insulin release.

4. **The answer is D.** The key to answering this question correctly relates to the absence of detectable C-peptide levels in the blood. An overproduction of insulin by the β-cells can lead to hypoglycemia severe enough to cause loss of consciousness, but because there was no detectable C-peptide in the blood, the loss of consciousness was most likely the result of the administration of exogenous insulin, which lacks the C-peptide. An overdose of glucagon, or epinephrine, would promote glucose release by the liver and not lead to hypoglycemia.

5. **The answer is B.** The high levels of glucagon will antagonize the effects of insulin and will lead to hyperglycemia. Due to the overriding effects of glucagon, blood glucose cannot enter muscle and fat cells, and fat oxidation is stimulated to provide energy for these tissues. This leads to a loss of stored triglyceride, which, in turn, leads to weight loss. Insulin is required to stimulate protein synthesis in muscles, and glucagon signals export of glucose from the liver, which means that the rate of glycolysis is suppressed in hepatic cells under these conditions.

## CHAPTER 22

1. **The answer is C.** The pancreas produces α-amylase that digests starch in the intestinal lumen. If pancreatic α-amylase cannot enter the lumen due to the pancreatitis, the starch would not be digested to a significant extent (the salivary α-amylase begins the process but only for the time period the food is in the mouth, as the acidic conditions of the stomach destroy the salivary activity). The discomfort arises from the bacteria in the intestine digesting the starch and producing acids and gases. Lactose, sucrose, and maltose are all disaccharides that would be cleaved by the intestinal disaccharidases located on the brush border of the intestinal epithelial cells. These enzymes are not derived from the pancreas. These activities might be slightly reduced, as the pancreas would also have difficulty secreting bicarbonate to the intestine, and the low pH of the stomach contents might reduce the activity of these enzymes. However, these enzymes are present in excess and will eventually digest the disaccharides. Dietary fiber cannot be digested by human enzymes.

2. **The answer is A.** Insulin is required to stimulate glucose transport into the muscle and fat cells but not brain, liver, pancreas, or red blood cells. Thus, muscle would be feeling the effects of glucose deprivation and would be unable to replenish its own glycogen supplies due to the inability to extract blood glucose, even though blood glucose levels would be high.

3. **The answer is D.** Flour contains starch, which will lead to glucose production in the intestine. Milk contains lactose, a disaccharide of glucose and galactose, which will be split by lactase in the small intestine. Sucrose is a disaccharide of glucose and fructose, which is split by sucrase in the small intestine. Thus, glucose, galactose, and fructose will all be available in the lumen of the small intestine for transport through the intestinal epithelial cells and into the circulation.

4. **The answer is B.** Salivary and pancreatic α-amylase will partially digest starch to glucose, but maltose and disaccharides will pass through the intestine and exit with the stool due to the limited activity of the brush border enzymes. Because the amylase enzymes are working, there will only be normal levels of starch in the stool. Because not all available glucose is entering the blood, less insulin will be released by the pancreas, which leads to less glucose uptake by the muscles and less glycogen production. Because neither lactose nor sucrose can be digested to a large extent in the intestinal lumen, it would be difficult to have elevated levels of glucose or fructose in the blood.

5. **The answer is D.** Any type of damage to the intestinal epithelial cells results in the loss of membrane-associated enzymes from the brush border membrane, including lactase. Lactase, however, recovers slowly and is not as prevalent as the other brush border enzymes, so in the recovery period from the damage, many individuals become sensitive to lactose. As the other enzymes are in excess, functional deficiencies in their activities are not noted.

## CHAPTER 23

1. **The answer is B.** If, after fasting, the branches were shorter than normal, glycogen phosphorylase must be functional and capable of being activated by glucagon. The branching enzyme (amylo-4,6-transferase) is also normal because branch points are present within the glycogen. Because glycogen is also present, glycogenin is present in order to build the carbohydrate chains. If the debranching activity is abnormal (the amylo-1,6-glucosidase), glycogen phosphorylase would degrade the glycogen to within four residues from branch points, and would then stop. With no debranching activity, the resultant glycogen would contain the normal number of branches, but the branched chains would be shorter than normal.

2. **The answer is E.** The patient has McArdle disease, a glycogen storage disease caused by a deficiency of muscle glycogen phosphorylase. Because she cannot degrade glycogen to produce energy for muscle contraction, she becomes fatigued more readily than a normal person, the glycogen levels in her muscle will be higher than normal due to the inability to degrade them, and her blood lactate levels will be lower due to the lack of glucose for entry into glycolysis. She will, however, draw on the glucose in the circulation for energy, thus her forearm blood glucose levels will be decreased, and because the liver is not affected, blood glucose levels can be maintained by liver glycogenolysis.

3. **The answer is A.** After ingestion of glucose, insulin levels rise, cAMP levels within the liver cell drop, and protein phosphatase I is activated. Glycogen phosphorylase *a* is converted to glycogen phosphorylase *b* by protein phosphatase 1 (so the ratio of form *a* to form b decreases), and glycogen synthase is activated by the phosphatase. Red blood cells continue to use glucose at their normal rate, thus lactate formation will remain the same.

4. **The answer is D.** When glycogen phosphorylase degrades glycogen, glucose-1-phosphate is produced. The glucose-1-phosphate is isomerized to glucose-6-phosphate, and glucose-6-phosphatase removes the phosphate so glucose can be exported from the cell. If glucose-6-phosphatase is defective, glucose would not be exported. The 10% of normal rise in blood glucose is due to the action of the debranching enzyme, which hydrolyzes α (1,6) linkages and releases free glucose. The reason for higher than normal levels of glycogen is the activation of glycogen synthase D

by glucose-6-phosphate, which synthesizes glycogen under conditions in which the synthase should be inactive. A mutation in glycogen phosphorylase would not allow debranching enzyme to work, as the glycogen would never get to branch points of the appropriate size for the debrancher to operate. A defect in glycogen synthase would not result in higher levels of normal glycogen in the muscle. A mutation in protein kinase A would not allow normal glycogen degradation in response to glucagon. A mutation in UDP-glucose pyrophosphorylase would interfere with glycogen synthesis, as UDP-glucose would not be produced, and this is not observed. Such a mutation would not affect glycogen degradation.

5. **The answer is A.** The muscle wants to degrade glycogen when it needs energy, and the best indication that energy stores are low is an elevation in AMP levels. Glucose is an allosteric inhibitor of glycogen phosphorylase in liver, but it has no effect in muscle. Glucose-6-phosphate, ADP, and ATP do not alter muscle glycogen phosphorylase activity.

## CHAPTER 24

1. **The answer is D.** Transketolase requires thiamine pyrophosphate as a cofactor, as does pyruvate dehydrogenase. Alcohol interferes with thiamine absorption in the intestine, thus chronic alcoholics may become thiamine deficient. A thiamine deficiency can lead to beriberi and Wernicke-Korsakoff syndrome due to reduced energy production in the nervous system due to the lack of pyruvate dehydrogenase activity. Niacin (NAD) and riboflavin (FAD) are used in oxidation–reduction reactions, and their absorption is not affected by alcohol consumption. Pantothenic acid is the precursor for Coenzyme A (needed for acyl-group activation), and biotin is required for carboxylation reactions. Alcohol does not affect pantothenic acid or biotin absorption from the intestine. When testing for a thiamine deficiency, the transketolase activity in the red blood cells is assayed both in the presence and absence of exogenous thiamine. If the activity is increased when thiamine is added, the patient has a thiamine deficiency.

2. **The answer is B.** Fructose is converted to fructose 1-phosphate by fructokinase, and aldolase B in the liver splits the fructose-1-P into glyceraldehyde and dihydroxyacetone phosphate. Thus, the major regulated step of glycolysis, PFK-1, is bypassed and PEP is rapidly produced. As the PEP increases, pyruvate kinase produces pyruvate. As the glyceraldehyde-3-phosphate dehydrogenase reaction is proceeding rapidly (remember that fructokinase is a high $V_{max}$ enzyme, so there is a lot of substrate proceeding through the glycolytic pathway), the intracellular [NADH]/[NAD$^+$] ratio is high, and the pyruvate produced is converted to lactate in order to regenerate NAD$^+$. Thus, the pyruvate kinase step is not bypassed. Neither aldolase B nor lactate dehydrogenase is allosterically regulated, and

even though the [ATP]/[ADP] ratio is high in the liver under these conditions, this ratio does not affect lactate formation.

3. **The answer is C.** The oxidizing agent (the drug) is acting on red blood cell membranes and converts the protective, reduced glutathione to oxidized glutathione. Glutathione reductase, the enzyme that converts oxidized glutathione to reduced glutathione, requires NADPH. Because red blood cells contain no mitochondria, their only means of generating NADPH is through the pentose phosphate pathway. If glucose-6-phosphate dehydrogenase is defective, NADPH production in the red cell would be compromised, and the red cells will lyse in the presence of an oxidizing agent. The reaction catalyzed by glucose-6-phosphate dehydrogenase is glucose-6-phosphate to 6-phosphogluconate. Hexokinase, the enzyme which converts glucose to glucose-6-phosphate in the red cells, is not defective in this disorder (the liver enzyme which does this is glucokinase). UDP-glucose pyrophosphorylase (the enzyme which makes UDP-glucose from UTP and glucose-1-phosphate) is needed for galactose metabolism and glycogen synthesis (in order to produce UDP-glucose) but not for glucose metabolism or NADPH production. The lack of phosphohexose isomerase (glucose-6-phosphate to fructose 6-phosphate) or 6-phosphogluconate dehydrogenase (producing ribulose 5-phosphate from 6-phosphogluconate) will not lead to hemolytic anemia, as does glucose-6-phosphate dehydrogenase deficiency.

4. **The answer is A.** Galactose is phosphorylated by galactokinase to form galactose 1-phosphate, which reacts with UDP-glucose in a reaction catalyzed by galactose 1-phosphate uridylyl transferase to form UDP-galactose and glucose-1-phosphate. An epimerase converts UDP-galactose to UDP-glucose. Phosphoglucomutase interconverts glucose-6-phosphate and glucose-1-phosphate. Hexokinase phosphorylates glucose to glucose-6-phosphate. If galactose 1-phosphate levels are low, but galactose and galactitol levels elevated, then the cell has a problem in either transporting galactose into the cell or activating galactose once it enters the cell. A defect in either would result in elevated serum galactose levels, which leads to elevated serum galactitol levels. Because a transport protein is not amongst the list of options, galactokinase is the best choice for an answer. This disorder leads to one of the galactosemia diseases (the other is a defect in the galactose 1-phosphate uridylyl transferase).

5. **The answer is E.** There is an isozyme of aldehyde dehydrogenase that has a dramatically increased $K_m$ (>200-fold), and a 10-fold reduced $V_{max}$. In such individuals, acetaldehyde, the toxic component of alcohol ingestion, accumulates to a large extent due to its slow metabolism, leading to the individual having a very low tolerance for alcohol. Alcohol dehydrogenase converts ethanol to acetaldehyde, as does the microsomal ethanol oxidizing system (MEOS). MEOS is used at high ethanol concentrations. Acetyl CoA carboxylase converts acetyl CoA to malonyl CoA (for fatty acid biosynthesis), and acetyl CoA synthetase converts acetic acid to acetyl CoA.

## CHAPTER 25

1. **The answer is E.** Classical galactosemia is due to a deficiency in the activity of galactose 1-phosphate uridylyltransferase (nonclassical galactosemia is due to a deficiency in the activity of galactokinase). Galactose metabolism requires the phosphorylation of galactose to galactose 1-phosphate, which is then converted to UDP-galactose (which is the step defective in the patient) and then epimerized to UDP-glucose. Although the mother cannot convert galactose to lactose due to the enzyme deficiency, she can make UDP-glucose from glucose-6-phosphate, and once she has made UDP-glucose, she can epimerize it to form UDP-galactose and can synthesize lactose. However, due to her enzyme deficiency, the mother cannot convert galactose 1-phosphate to UDP-galactose, or UDP-glucose, so the dietary galactose cannot be used for glycogen synthesis or glucose production. After ingesting milk, the galactose levels will be elevated in the serum due to the metabolic block in the cells.

2. **The answer is D.** Bilirubin is conjugated with glucuronic acid residues to enhance its solubility. Glucuronic acid is produced from glucose when the glucose is oxidized at position 6; gluconic acid is glucose oxidized at position 1 and is generated by the HMP shunt pathway. Bilirubin is not conjugated with glucose, galactose, or the sugar alcohol galactitol.

3. **The answer is B.** Lactose synthase is composed of two subunits, a galactosyltransferase and α-lactalbumin. In the absence of α-lactalbumin, the galactosyltransferase is active in glycoprotein and glycolipid synthesis but relatively inactive for lactose synthesis. At birth, α-lactalbumin is induced and alters the specificity of the galactosyltransferase such that lactose can now be synthesized. Lactase is the enzyme which digests lactose in the intestine, and a lactosyltransferase enzyme, if such an enzyme did exist, would not be able to synthesize lactose (it would transfer lactose to other substrates).

4. **The answer is A.** Type A blood cells will coexist in individuals with either type A or AB blood. Type O blood cell glycolipids lack the terminal sugar present on type A blood, thus that carbohydrate determinant would be recognized as foreign in a type O individual. Similarly, type B blood cells contain a different terminal sugar on the carbohydrate chain than type A cells, and if type A cells enter a type B individual, an immune reaction would also be generated. Type AB blood has both types of cells present, so the A type carbohydrate would not be recognized as foreign.

5. **The answer is B.** Glycosaminoglycan chains contain negative charges due to the presence of acidic sugars and the sulfated sugars in the molecule. Thus, in their characteristic bottleneck structure, the chains repel each other, yet also

attract positively charged cations and water into the spaces between the chains. The water forms hydrogen bonds with the sugars and a gel-like space is created. This gel acts as a diffusion sieve for materials that either leave or enter this space. Hydroxylation and cross-linking of chains does not occur nor does hydrogen bonding between chains (they are too far apart due to the charge repulsion, but they do form hydrogen bonds with water).

## CHAPTER 26

1. **The answer is A.** Glycerol is converted to glycerol 3-phosphate, which is then oxidized to form dihydroxyacetone phosphate (DHAP). The DHAP is isomerized to glyceraldehyde 3-phosphate (G3P), and the DHAP and G3P condense to form fructose 1,6 bisphosphate, which then follows the gluconeogenic pathway up to glucose. Lactate is converted to pyruvate, which is then carboxylated to form oxaloacetate. The oxaloacetate is decarboxylated to form phosphoenolpyruvate, and then run up through gluconeogenesis to glucose. As glycerol enters the gluconeogenic pathway at the glyceraldehyde 3-phosphate step, and lactate at the PEP step, the only compounds in common between these two starting points are the steps from glyceraldehyde 3-phosphate to glucose. Glucose-6-phosphate satisfies this criterion.

2. **The answer is B.** PEPCK converts oxaloacetate to phosphoenolpyruvate. In combination with pyruvate carboxylase, it is used to bypass the pyruvate kinase reaction. Thus, compounds that enter gluconeogenesis before PEP (such as lactate, alanine, or any TCA cycle intermediate) must use PEPCK to produce PEP. Glycerol enters gluconeogenesis as glyceraldehyde 3-phosphate, bypassing the PEPCK step. Galactose is converted to glucose-1-phosphate, then glucose-6-phosphate, also bypassing the PEPCK step. Even-chain fatty acids can only give rise to acetyl CoA, which cannot be used to synthesize glucose. Odd-chain fatty acids will generate propionyl CoA, which enters the TCA cycle at succinyl CoA, so glucose production from propionyl CoA would also be affected in this patient.

3. **The answer is C.** The hyperglycemia in an untreated diabetic creates an osmotic diuresis, which means that excessive water is lost through urination. This can lead to a contraction of blood volume, leading to low blood pressure and a rapid heartbeat. It also leads to dehydration. The rapid respirations results from an acidosis-induced stimulation of the respiratory center of the brain in order to reduce the amount of acid in the blood. Ketone bodies have accumulated leading to diabetic ketoacidosis (not an alkalosis). Patients with a hypoglycemic coma (which can be caused by an insulin shock) do not exhibit dehydration, low blood pressure, or rapid respirations; in fact, they sweat profusely due to epinephrine release. The lack of a functional pancreas would be a fatal condition, so it cannot be the answer to this question.

4. **The answer is D.** Calcium activates a calmodulin subunit in phosphorylase kinase, which will allow phosphorylase kinase to phosphorylate, and activate, glycogen phosphorylase. Glucose is an allosteric inhibitor of glycogen phosphorylase *a* in liver but has no effect in muscle. Glucose-1-phosphate has no effect on muscle phosphorylase, whereas glucose-6-phosphate is an allosteric inhibitor of muscle glycogen phosphorylase *a*. The levels of magnesium have no effect on muscle glycogen phosphorylase activity. Normally, glucagon or epinephrine would activate the cAMP-dependent protein kinase, but this is not occurring in this individual due to the expression of a mutation that does not allow cAMP to activate PKA.

5. **The answer is B.** The patient is exhibiting some of the symptoms of type II diabetes, a resistance to insulin action. Under these conditions, the muscle and fat cells are not responding to the released insulin, so GLUT 4 transporters are not sent to the cell surface, and glucose levels remain elevated because the peripheral tissues are not taking up glucose at their normal rate. A defective glucokinase in the pancreas would result in insulin being released abnormally, most likely at higher than normal blood glucose levels, and that is not observed. Muscle cells contain hexokinase, not glucokinase. High glucose levels in the liver will stimulate glycogen synthesis, and eventually glycolysis in order to produce acetyl CoA for fat synthesis.

## CHAPTER 27

1. **The answer is E.** Chylomicrons transport dietary lipids, and 80% or more of the chylomicron is triglyceride. All other components within chylomicrons (protein, phospholipid, cholesterol, cholesterol ester) are present at less than 10%.

2. **The answer is A.** HDL transfer apolipoproteins C-II and E to nascent chylomicrons to convert them to mature chylomicrons. Bile salts are required to emulsify dietary lipid, 2-monoacylglycerol is a digestion product of pancreatic lipase, LPL digests triacylglycerol from mature chylomicrons, and the lymphatic system delivers the nascent chylomicrons to the blood stream.

3. **The answer is B.** Both apoB-48 and apoB-100 are derived from the same gene and from the same mRNA (there is no difference in splicing between the two). However, RNA editing introduces a stop codon in the message such that B-48 stops protein synthesis approximately 48% along the message. Thus, proteolytic cleavage is not a correct answer. B-48 is only found in chylomicrons, and B-100 is found in VLDL, IDL, and LDL particles.

4. **The answer is C.** Nascent chylomicrons would be synthesized and can only acquire apoC-II from HDL. The chylomicrons would be degraded in part by lipoprotein lipase, leading to chylomicron remnant formation. However, the chylomicron remnants would remain in circulation due to the lack of apoE, which is necessary for the remnant

to bind to receptors on the liver cell. VLDL particles are not produced immediately after a meal; it is the chylomicrons which transport dietary triglycerides throughout the body. Because the chylomicron remnants still contain a fair amount of triglyceride, serum triglyceride levels would be elevated due to the lack of apoE.

5. **The answer is D.** Obstruction of the pancreatic duct would block pancreatic enzymes from entering the intestinal lumen. Bile salts, however, enter the intestine via the common bile duct, and bile salt metabolism would be normal. Of the pancreatic enzymes which are secreted for lipid digestion, it is pancreatic lipase which is required for triglyceride metabolism. When triglycerides accumulate in the intestine and are excreted with the feces, steatorrhea results.

## CHAPTER 28

1. **The answer is E.** Fatty acids, cleaved from the triacylglycerols of blood lipoproteins by the action of lipoprotein lipase, are taken up by adipose cells and react with coenzyme A to form fatty acyl CoA. Glucose is converted via dihydroxyacetone phosphate to glycerol 3-phosphate, which reacts with fatty acyl CoA to form phosphatidic acid (adipose tissue lacks glycerol kinase so cannot use glycerol directly). After inorganic phosphate is released from phosphatidic acid, the resulting diacylglycerol reacts with another fatty acyl CoA to form a triacylglycerol, which is stored in adipose cells (2-monoacylglycerol is an intermediate of triacylglycerol synthesis only in the intestine). LPL action releases fatty acids from triglycerides and is not involved in triglyceride synthesis, and acetoacetyl CoA is an intermediate in ketone body or cholesterol biosynthesis but not triglyceride synthesis.

2. **The answer is A.** The triacylglycerol is degraded by pancreatic lipase, which releases the fatty acids at positions 1 and 3. The fatty acids released are then transported to the cell surface in a bile salt micelle. The only exception are short-chain fatty acids (shorter than palmitic acid), which can diffuse to the cell surface and enter the intestinal cell in the absence of micelle formation. Chylomicrons are secreted from intestinal epithelial cells, into the lymph, to transport dietary triglyceride to the peripheral tissues. VLDL transports triglyceride from the liver to peripheral tissues. Fatty acids, upon release from adipocytes, bind to albumin for travel through the circulation to tissues that can oxidize fatty acids for energy. LDL, a cholesterol-rich particle, is formed as a degradation product of VLDL.

3. **The answer is B.** Dietary carbohydrate is converted to lipid in the liver and exported via VLDL. Thus, a low-carbohydrate diet would reduce VLDL formation and reduce the hyperlipoproteinemia. Dietary lipid is found in chylomicrons. IDL and LDL are degradation products of VLDL and contain fewer lipids than VLDL. HDL donates apolipoproteins to nascent chylomicrons and nascent VLDL and also participates in reverse cholesterol transport.

4. **The answer is D.** Aspirin leads to the acetylation of COX-1 and COX-2, which inhibits the enzymes. Tylenol contains acetaminophen, which is a competitive inhibitor of both COX-1 and COX-2, but acetaminophen does not covalently attach to the enzymes. Advil contains ibuprofen, which is another competitive inhibitor of the COX enzymes. Vioxx and Celebrex contain inhibitors specific for COX-2, which is the form of cyclooxygenase that is induced during inflammation. Vioxx and Celebrex do not inhibit COX-1 activity and do not work through a covalent modification mechanism.

5. **The answer is C.** When fatty acids are being synthesized, malonyl CoA accumulates, which inhibits carnitine acyltransferase I. This blocks fatty acid entry into the mitochondrion for oxidation. The liver both synthesizes and degrades fatty acids. NADPH blocks the glucose-6-phosphate dehydrogenase reaction but not fatty acid oxidation. Insulin has no effect on the synthesis of the enzymes involved in fatty acid degradation (unlike the effect of insulin on the induction of enzymes involved in fatty acid synthesis). Finally, newly synthesized fatty acids are converted to their CoA derivatives for elongation and desaturation.

## CHAPTER 29

1. **The answer is C.** The presence of chronic hyperglycemia (usually accompanied by high levels of free fatty acids in the blood), as seen in diabetes mellitus, causes diffuse multiorgan toxic effects ("glucose toxicity" and "lipotoxicity") to the extent that it raises the risk for a future atherosclerotic event to a level equal to that posed by a history of the patient having already suffered such an event in the past. Obesity, cigarette smoking, hypertension, and sedentary lifestyle, in the absence of a previous myocardial infarction, do not require the suggested lower limits for circulating cholesterol levels.

2. **The answer is E.** Taurocholic acid has a pK of about 2, glycocholic acid a pK of about 4, palmitic acid a pK of about 4, cholic acid a pK of about 6, and cholesterol a pK of about 12. At pH 3.0, greater than 90% of the taurocholic acid will be ionized, whereas less than 10% of glycocholic acid or palmitic acid will be ionized. Recall that the pK is the pH at which the group in question is 50% ionized.

3. **The answer is A.** Of the blood lipoproteins, LDL contains the highest concentration of cholesterol and lowest concentration of triacylglycerols. Elevation of blood LDL levels (the result of decreased endocytosis of LDL) would result in high blood cholesterol levels and relatively normal triacylglycerol levels. A decreased ability to degrade the triacylglycerols of chylomicrons or to convert VLDL to IDL, as well as an increased ability to produce VLDL, would all result in elevated triacylglycerol levels. Because HDL helps to transfer cholesterol from peripheral cells to the liver, high levels of HDL in the blood are associated with low serum cholesterol levels.

4. **The answer is B.** Phosphorylation of HMG-CoA reductase reduces its activity, thereby reducing endogenous cholesterol synthesis. With reduced endogenous synthesis, there is less VLDL being exported from the liver, and the LDL levels will decrease (also, cells will be upregulating their LDL receptors due to a decrease in endogenous cholesterol synthesis). Altering endogenous cholesterol levels will have no effect on chylomicron production, which is produced from dietary lipids. There is no evidence to suggest that the ingestion of garlic will reduce the frequency of vampire bites.

5. **The answer is D.** As bile salts are lost in the feces, the liver must produce more of them. This leads to upregulation of HMG-CoA reductase and increased cholesterol, which is the precursor of bile acid synthesis. As mevalonate is the product of the HMG-CoA reductase reaction, its levels will also rise. The other potential answers, vitamin K, lecithin, fatty acids, or triglyceride, will not display increased synthesis in the presence of the bile acid binding resin.

## CHAPTER 30

1. **The answer is C.** The acetone on the patient's breath is produced by decarboxylation of acetoacetate, not β-hydroxybutyrate. The ketones in the urine indicate that the woman is in diabetic ketoacidosis. This is caused by low insulin levels, so her blood glucose levels are high because the glucose is not being taken up by the peripheral tissues. An insulin injection would reduce her blood glucose levels and decrease the release of fatty acids from adipose triglycerides. Consequently, ketone body production would decrease. Glucagon, which antagonizes insulin's effects, would just exacerbate the woman's current condition.

2. **The answer is A.** Chylomicrons are blood lipoproteins produced from dietary fat. VLDL are produced mainly from dietary carbohydrate. IDL and LDL are produced from VLDL. HDL does not transport triacylglycerol to the tissues.

3. **The answer is E.** Excess energy is stored as triglyceride; when caloric excess is primarily triglyceride, energy is still required to resynthesize the triglycerides in the intestine, and then again in the adipose tissue. The energy is needed to activate the fatty acids to their CoA derivatives before condensation with glycerol 3-phosphate. When caloric excess is primarily carbohydrate derived, energy must be used to synthesize the fatty acids from glucose; however, that energy is balanced by the energy obtained when glucose is converted to two molecules of acetyl CoA. Thus, the amount of triglyceride that would be stored would be similar regardless of the source of the calories.

4. **The answer is A.** Metabolism of ethanol leads to production of NADH in the liver, which will inhibit fatty acid oxidation in the liver. Because the patient has not eaten for 5 days, the insulin/glucagon ratio is low, hormone-sensitive lipase is activated, and fatty acids are being released by the adipocyte and taken up by the muscle and liver. However,

because the liver NADH levels are high due to ethanol metabolism, the fatty acids received from the adipocyte are repackaged into triacylglycerol (the high NADH promotes the conversion of dihydroxyacetone-phosphate to glycerol 3-phosphate as well) and secreted from the liver in the form of VLDL. Alcohol does not inhibit lipoprotein lipase nor does it induce transcription of the apoB-100 gene. NADH is not an activator of PEP carboxykinase. Acetaldehyde does not induce ER enzymes in general.

5. **The answer is D.** The clotting problems are due to a lack of vitamin K, a lipid-soluble vitamin. Vitamin K is absorbed from the diet in mixed micelles and packaged with chylomicrons for delivery to the other tissues. Because individuals with abetalipoproteinemia lack the microsomal triglyceride transfer protein and cannot effectively produce chylomicrons, vitamin K deficiency can result. Such patients also cannot produce VLDL, but lipid-soluble vitamin distribution does not depend on VLDL particles, only chylomicrons. The disorder does not affect the ability to synthesize fatty acids, clotting factors, or the absorption of short-chain fatty acids (which bypass the mixed micelle step and go directly into the intestinal epithelial cells).

## CHAPTER 31

1. **The answer is B.** Trypsinogen, which is secreted by the intestine, is activated by enteropeptidase, a protein found in the intestine. Once trypsin is formed, it will activate all of the other zymogens secreted by the pancreas. Trypsin does not activate pepsinogen because pepsinogen is found in the stomach and autocatalyzes its own activation when the pH drops due to acid secretion. Trypsin has no effect on intestinal motility and also does not have a much broader base of substrates than any other protease (trypsin cleaves on the carboxy side of the amino acids with basic side chains, lysine and arginine).

2. **The answer is C.** As with many amino acids, leucine can be transported by a number of different amino acid systems. Leucine is an essential amino acid so the body cannot synthesize it. If the intestine cannot absorb leucine, and because leucine is an essential amino acid, then there would be insufficient leucine for the kidneys to reabsorb and send to the tissues of the body. Leucine and isoleucine have different structures and cannot substitute for each other in all positions within a protein. Leucine is an important component of proteins and is required for protein synthesis.

3. **The answer is A.** Kwashiorkor is a disease which results from eating a calorie-sufficient diet which lacks protein. It is not the result of a calorie-deficient diet.

4. **The answer is E.** Due to a lack of protein in the diet, protein synthesis is impaired in the liver (lack of essential amino acids). The liver can still synthesize fatty acids from carbohydrate or fat sources, but VLDL particles cannot be assembled due to a shortage of apoB-100. Thus, the fatty acids remain in the liver, leading to a fatty liver. There are

adequate substrates for glycogen synthesis and gluconeogenesis in this condition.

5. **The answer is D.** Excess amino acids are metabolized and converted to either glycogen or fatty acids for energy storage. They are not stored as amino acid pools in tissues or as short, energy-rich peptides.

## CHAPTER 32

1. **The answer is A.** High blood ammonia, with low orotic acid, citrulline, and arginine suggests an early defect in the urea cycle. If carbamoyl-phosphate were made, but not citrulline (an ornithine transcarbamoylase defect), then orotic acid would be expected to accumulate. If citrulline were made, but not argininosuccinate, then citrulline should accumulate. Because this does not occur, it is most likely that carbamoyl phosphate is not being produced, suggesting a defect in CPSI.

2. **The answer is C.** The high levels of citrulline suggest that citrulline cannot be converted to argininosuccinate in this infant, indicating a block in argininosuccinate synthetase. A CPSI defect would be expected to only exhibit elevated levels of ammonia; an OTC defect elevated levels of orotic acid; an argininosuccinate lyase deficiency elevated levels of argininosuccinate, with mildly elevated levels of citrulline; and an arginase defect would show elevated levels of arginine. The data are only consistent with a defect in argininosuccinate synthetase.

3. **The answer is E.** An arginase deficiency would be expected to result in elevated levels of arginine, and only moderately elevated levels of ammonia. This is due to the location of arginine in the cycle; at this point, two molecules of ammonia have been incorporated into arginine, which reduces the overall ammonia content of the liver. A defect in carbamoyl phosphate synthetase I would be expected to elevate only ammonia levels. A defect in ornithine transcarbamoylase would exhibit elevated orotic acid levels. A defect in argininosuccinate synthetase would display elevated citrulline levels and low arginine levels. A defect in argininosuccinate lyase would display elevated argininosuccinate levels but reduced arginine levels.

4. **The answer is B.** An ornithine transcarbamoylase deficiency results in an inability to convert carbamoyl phosphate to citrulline, resulting in an accumulation of carbamoyl phosphate. The carbamoyl phosphate diffuses from the mitochondria and enters the cytosol, where it bypasses the regulated step of pyrimidine synthesis and leads to the synthesis of orotic acid, which accumulates. Defects in carbamoyl phosphate synthetase I, argininosuccinate synthetase, argininosuccinate lyase, and arginase will not lead to an accumulation of carbamoyl phosphate and will not display elevated orotic acid levels in the patient.

5. **The answer is D.** A defect in argininosuccinate lyase would result in elevated levels of argininosuccinate, and due to product inhibition, a moderate elevation of citrulline. A defect in argininosuccinate synthetase results in markedly elevated levels of citrulline but no argininosuccinate production. Defects in carbamoyl phosphate synthase I or ornithine transcarbamoylase would not lead to citrulline production, and a defect in arginase would result in elevated arginine levels, which is not observed.

## CHAPTER 33

1. **The answer is E.** Tyrosine is derived from phenylalanine, which requires $BH_4$ but not vitamin $B_6$. Vitamin $B_6$ is required in the synthesis of serine (transamination), alanine (another transamination), cysteine (β-elimination, β-addition, γ-elimination), and aspartate (transamination).

2. **The answer is C.** The classical form of PKU, a deficiency of phenylalanine hydroxylase, will result in elevations of phenylalanine and phenylpyruvate. However, this enzyme is not a choice amongst the answers. In the nonclassical variant of PKU, there is a problem in either synthesizing or regenerating $BH_4$. The enzyme which converts $BH_2$ to $BH_4$ is dihydropteridine reductase. Tetrahydrofolate is not involved in phenylalanine metabolism.

3. **The answer is A.** Of the amino acids listed, phenylalanine is the only one which is an essential (in terms of the diet) amino acid. Asparagine, proline, serine, glutamate, and alanine can be synthesized from glucose and a nitrogen source.

4. **The answer is F.** The baby has alcaptonuria, a defect in phenylalanine metabolism which leads to a buildup of homogentisic acid. Homogentisic acid oxidizes in air to form a black compound. Alcaptonuria may lead to arthritis later in life.

5. **The answer is B.** The baby has maple syrup urine disease, a defect in the second step of the oxidation of the branched-chain amino acids. This can be diagnosed by measuring the levels of leucine in the blood. The substrate for the defective enzyme in this disease is the α-keto acids derived from the branched-chain amino acids. These substrates are generated by a transamination reaction. Transaminases usually have an equilibrium constant of 1 so as the α-keto acids accumulate, the transaminases will be inhibited from producing more α-keto acids. This will lead to an accumulation of the nonmodified branched-chain amino acids, which will accumulate in the blood.

## CHAPTER 34

1. **The answer is A.** Propionic acid is derived from an accumulation of propionyl CoA. The normal pathway for the degradation of propionyl CoA is first, a biotin-dependent carboxylation to D-methylmalonyl CoA, racemization to L-methylmalonyl CoA, and then, the $B_{12}$-dependent rearrangement to succinyl CoA. A deficiency of biotin would lead to propionic acid accumulation. A defect in vitamin C

would lead to altered collagen formation. Vitamins $B_6$, $B_1$ (thiamine), $B_2$ (riboflavin), and folate are not required for this pathway.

2. **The answer is C.** The only metabolic route for methylmalonic acid is for it to be converted to succinyl CoA in a reaction that requires vitamin $B_{12}$. This strongly suggests a deficiency in vitamin $B_{12}$, which may be from the diet or may be due to a deficiency in intrinsic factor. A folate deficiency does not result in a functional cobalamin deficiency, whereas a lack of $B_{12}$ can lead to a functional folate deficiency (methyl trap hypothesis). Thiamine ($B_1$), riboflavin ($B_2$), and pyridoxine ($B_6$) are not required for this reaction.

3. **The answer is E.** Methionine is degraded to propionyl CoA, which is converted, by carboxylation to methylmalonyl CoA. The other amino acids, which also produce methylmalonyl CoA, include valine, isoleucine, and threonine. Arginine and histidine degradation lead to glutamate formation, and leucine and lysine are strictly ketogenic and would not produce methylmalonic acid.

4. **The answer is B.** At the nonpermissive temperature, serine is not converted to glycine, such that the cells now require glycine for growth. In addition, the serine to glycine conversion is the major route of adding carbon to $FH_4$, producing $N^5$, $N^{10}$-methylene-$FH_4$ in the reaction. The lack of carbon in the folate pool could then interfere with purine and thymidine synthesis. Supplying glycine to the cells allows protein synthesis to continue, and also will generate $N^5$, $N^{10}$-methylene-$FH_4$ via the glycine cleavage enzyme reaction, thereby replenishing the one-carbon pool and allowing DNA synthesis to proceed. Adding serine to the medium would have no effect, as the serine to glycine reaction is blocked at the nonpermissive temperature. The amino acids alanine, glutamate, and aspartate are all nonessential amino acids whose synthesis is not blocked by the enzyme defect in the cells. None of those amino acids can also donate a carbon to the $FH_4$ pool.

5. **The answer is D.** The patient is experiencing the effects of reduced levels of vitamin $B_{12}$ due to a lack of intrinsic factor. As individuals age, a variety of conditions can give rise to reduced intrinsic factor production by the stomach. Because oral delivery of $B_{12}$ will be impaired if intrinsic factor is lacking, injections of $B_{12}$ are the appropriate treatment for this individual. The patient has a form of pernicious anemia. Folate deficiencies will not give rise to the neurological symptoms (tingling in the hands and feet) observed in this patient. Giving methionine to the patient will not overcome the symptoms brought about by the $B_{12}$ vitamin deficiency.

## CHAPTER 35

1. **The answer is A.** Both carbamoyl phosphate synthetase I and II use carbon dioxide as the carbon source in the production of carbamoyl phosphate. CPSI is located in the mitochondria, whereas CPSII is in the cytoplasm. CPSI can fix ammonia into an organic compound; CPSII requires gluta-

mine as the nitrogen source. $N$-acetyl glutamate activates CPS-I; CSPII is activated by PRPP. UMP inhibits CPSII but has no effect on CPSI.

2. **The answer is B.** A lack of glucose-6-phosphatase activity (von Gierke's disease) leads to an accumulation of glucose-6-phosphate, which will lead to an increase in ribose 5-phosphate levels, and then an increase in PRPP levels. As PRPP levels rise, purine synthesis will be stimulated, leading to excessive levels of purines in the blood. The degradation of the extra purines leads to uric acid production and gout. A loss of either PRPP synthetase activity or glutamine phosphoribosyl amidotransferase activity would lead to reduced purine synthesis and hypouricemia. A lack of glucose-6-phosphate dehydrogenase would hinder ribose 5-phosphate production and, thus, would not lead to excessive purine synthesis. A lack of purine nucleoside phosphorylase would hinder the salvage pathway, leading to an accumulation of nucleosides. Purine nucleoside phosphorylase activity is required to synthesize uric acid, so in the absence of this enzyme, less uric acid would be produced.

3. **The answer is E.** If dGTP were to accumulate in cells, the dGTP would bind to the substrate specificity site of ribonucleotide reductase and direct the synthesis of dADP. This would lead to elevations of dATP levels, which would inhibit the activity of ribonucleotide reductase. The inhibition of ribonucleotide reductase leads to a cessation of cell proliferation, as the supply of deoxyribonucleotides for DNA synthesis become limiting. In order for dCDP to be elevated, ATP would need to bind to the substrate specificity site to direct its synthesis, and ATP is not accumulating. This, then, would not occur under conditions of elevated dGTP levels. Ribonucleotide reductase only reduces nucleotides in the diphosphate form, AMP would not be a substrate for this enzyme. Thioredoxin is always regenerated as the reactions proceed and does not become rate-limiting for the reductase reaction. dGTP does not bind to the activity site of the reductase; only ATP (activator) or dATP (inhibitor) are capable of binding to the activity site.

4. **The answer is D.** The purine nucleotide cycle generates fumarate, which is used in an anaplerotic role to replenish TCA cycle intermediates in order to allow the cycle to continue operating. The purine nucleotide cycle does not directly generate glutamate, urea, glucose, or NADH. Aspartate donates nitrogen to IMP in order to generate adenylosuccinate. Adenylosuccinate loses fumarate and generates AMP. The AMP is deaminated, producing ammonia, to form IMP and completes the cycle.

5. **The answer is A.** Vitamin $B_{12}$ deficiency results in an inability of $N^5$-methyl-$FH_4$ to donate its methyl group to homocysteine in order to form methionine. This leads to an accumulation of $N^5$-methyl-$FH_4$ and the trapping of folic acid in this form. This generates a functional folate deficiency, such that reactions that require different forms of folic acid are inhibited. Under such conditions, de novo purine synthesis is blocked because that pathway requires two carbons from $N^{10}$-formyl-$FH_4$. The synthesis of dTMP

from dUMP is also blocked because that reaction requires $N^5$, $N^{10}$-methylene-FH$_4$. None of the other reactions listed require an FH$_4$ derivative for the reaction to proceed.

## CHAPTER 36

1.  **The answer is D.** High levels of amino acids in the blood stimulate the pancreas to release glucagon, so blood levels of glucagon will be increased. Insulin is also released, but the glucagon/insulin ratio is such that the liver still utilizes the carbons of amino acids to synthesize glucose, so liver gluconeogenesis is still enhanced. However, the insulin levels are high enough to stimulate BCAA uptake into the muscle for oxidation, resulting in increased BCAA oxidation in the muscle.

2.  **The answer is A.** The pathway followed is glutamine to glutamate, to glutamate semialdehyde, to ornithine, and then after condensation with carbamoyl phosphate, to citrulline. Aspartate, succinyl CoA, serine, and fumarate are not a part of this pathway.

3.  **The answer is C.** Cortisol is released during fasting and times of stress and signals muscle cells to initiate ubiquitin-mediated protein degradation. The other hormones listed do not have this effect on muscle protein metabolism. Insulin stimulates protein synthesis; glucagon has no effect on muscle, as muscle lacks glucagon receptors. Epinephrine initiates glycogen degradation, but not protein degradation, and glucose is not a signaling molecule for muscle as it can be for the pancreas.

4.  **The answer is B.** Glutamine is derived from glutamate, which is formed from α-ketoglutarate. Only isoleucine and valine can give rise to glutamine, as leucine is strictly ketogenic. These amino acids give rise to succinyl CoA, which goes around the TCA cycle to form citrate (after condensing with acetyl CoA), which then forms isocitrate (the correct answer), and the isocitrate is converted to α-ketoglutarate. Urea, pyruvate, phosphoenolpyruvate, and lactate are not required intermediates in the conversion of BCAA carbons to glutamine carbons.

5.  **The answer is B.** An individual in sepsis will be catabolic; protein degradation exceeds protein intake, leading to negative nitrogen balance. The liver is synthesizing glucose from amino acid precursors to raise blood glucose levels for the immune cells and the nervous system; thus, gluconeogenesis is active. Fatty acid release and oxidation has also been stimulated to provide an energy source for the liver and skeletal muscle.

# Patient Index

Note: Page numbers followed by *f* denote figures.

# Index

Note: Page numbers followed by *f* denote figures; page numbers followed by *t* denote tables.